handbook of
CLINICAL
DRUG
DATA

handbook of
CLINICAL
DRUG
DATA

SIXTH EDITION

Editors
James E. Knoben, Pharm.D.
Philip O. Anderson, Pharm.D.

Assistant Editors
Larry J. Davis, Pharm.D.
William G. Troutman, Pharm.D.

DRUG INTELLIGENCE PUBLICATIONS, INC., HAMILTON, ILLINOIS 62341

Library of Congress Cataloging in Publication Data

Handbook of clinical drug data.

 Includes bibliographies and index.
 1. Pharmacology — Handbooks, manuals, etc.
 2. Drugs — Handbooks, manuals, etc. I. Knoben, James E.
II. Anderson, Philip O. III. Title. Clinical drug data.
[DNLM: 1. Drugs—handbooks. 2. Pharmacology,
Clinical—handbooks. QV 39 H2358]
RM301.12.H36   1988   615′.1   88-11814
ISBN 0-914768-46-8

First Printing, May 1988
Second Printing, January 1989

PRINTED IN THE UNITED STATES OF AMERICA BY HAMILTON PRESS, INC.

PREFACE TO THE SIXTH EDITION

IN RECENT YEARS, there has been a significant increase in the number of new drugs approved, particularly anti-infective and cardiovascular drugs. This, coupled with important advances in biotechnology, has led to enormous growth in the drug literature. The need for a comprehensive, yet compact, source of authoritative drug information is therefore greater than ever, and the *Handbook of Clinical Drug Data* is designed to meet that need.

The editors and contributors are gratified by the acceptance of previous editions of the *Handbook*. Users will find this new edition familiar in style, yet thoroughly revised and updated with clinically relevant data and extensive documentation (over 3300 cited references). New sections have also been added, including anthropometrics, drug-laboratory test interferences, drug-induced sexual dysfunction and an expanded discussion on enteral nutrition. The high quality of work throughout the book reflects the continued participation of expert contributors, each of whom has written within his or her area of clinical specialization.

The assistance of our editorial colleagues, Larry Davis and Bill Troutman, has been invaluable to the preparation of the Sixth Edition. Bill Ball, whose career has taken him in a new direction, nevertheless continued to provide editorial guidance. The contributors to this edition, many of whom worked on the previous edition, are once again to be congratulated for a superb effort in researching and distilling the current literature; needless to say, the *Handbook* would not be possible without their long hours of painstaking work. Special thanks also go to the following expert medical and pharmacy consultants who reviewed various portions of the manuscript: Steven I. Berk, Pharm.D., Alexander M. Gilderman, Pharm.D., Leslie Hendeles, Pharm.D., J. Edward Jackson, M.D., Orville G. Kolterman, M.D., James R. Lane, Jr., Pharm.D., Richard J. Mangini, Pharm.D., Anthony S. Manoguerra, Pharm.D., Michael T. Reed, Pharm.D., Bruce J. Schrader, Pharm.D., Alfred E. Staubus, Ph.D., Michael Z. Wincor, Pharm.D., Cindy J. Wordell, Pharm.D. and Michael G. Ziegler, M.D. Thanks are also in order to Joanne Goralka, Pharm.D. for her assistance in the preparation of the manuscript and especially to Gloria N. Francke, Pharm.D. and Mary Ann Jaske, B.Sc.Pharm. of Drug Intelligence Publications for their exceptional efforts in readying the manuscript for publication.

JAMES E. KNOBEN
PHILIP O. ANDERSON

NOTICE

THE DRUG INFORMATION presented in this *Handbook* conforms to that found in the medical literature or in the manufacturer's product literature. However, this *Handbook* provides only the more important elements of clinical drug data, and is *not* a complete drug information resource. While great care has been taken to ensure the accuracy of the book's content when it went to press, the editors, contributors and publisher cannot be responsible for the continued accuracy of the information due to ongoing research and new developments in the field. Therefore, the manufacturer's current product information or other standard references should always be consulted for more detailed information, especially before prescribing is undertaken.

The Editors, James E. Knoben, Pharm.D. and Philip O. Anderson, Pharm.D., the Assistant Editors and Contributors have written this book in their private capacities. No official support or endorsement by any Federal Agency, University, Hospital or Pharmaceutical Company is intended or should be inferred.

EDITORS AND CONTRIBUTORS

EDITORS

James E. Knoben, Pharm.D., M.P.H.
Director, Division of Drug Information Resources
Center for Drug Evaluation and Research
Food and Drug Administration
Rockville, Maryland

Philip O. Anderson, Pharm.D.
Director, Drug Information Service
University of California Medical Center
San Diego, California
Associate Clinical Professor of Pharmacy
University of California, San Francisco,
San Diego Program

ASSISTANT EDITORS

Larry Jay Davis, Pharm.D.
Supervisor, Department of Pharmacy
Stanford University Hospital
Stanford Medical Center
Stanford, California
Associate Clinical Professor of Pharmacy
University of California, San Francisco,
San Francisco, California

William G. Troutman, Pharm.D.
Director, New Mexico Poison
and Drug Information Center
Professor of Pharmacy
College of Pharmacy
University of New Mexico
Albuquerque, New Mexico

CONTRIBUTORS

Andrea J. Anderson, Pharm.D.

Director, Drug Information Service
New England Medical Center
Associate Professor, Clinical Pharmacy
College of Pharmacy and Allied Health Professions
Northeastern University
Boston, Massachusetts

William D. Ball, Pharm.D.

Western U.S. District Manager
Schering Laboratories
Laguna Niguel, California

Steven L. Barriere, Pharm.D.

Specialist in Infectious Diseases, Pharmaceutical Services
Adjunct Associate Professor of Medicine and Pharmacology
Departments of Medicine and Pharmacology
University of California Center for the Health Sciences
Los Angeles, California

Jerry L. Bauman, Pharm.D.

Associate Professor of Pharmacy Practice and
  Instructor in Medicine, Section of Cardiology
Colleges of Pharmacy and Medicine, University of Illinois
Chicago, Illinois

Rosemary R. Berardi, Pharm.D.

Clinical Pharmacist, Gastroenterology
Department of Pharmacy, University Hospitals
Associate Professor of Pharmacy
College of Pharmacy, University of Michigan
Ann Arbor, Michigan

Lawrence R. Borgsdorf, Pharm.D.

Clinical Pharmacist, Department of Medicine
Kern Medical Center
Bakersfield, California
Adjunct Associate Professor of Medicine
School of Medicine, University of California, Los Angeles,
Kern Medical Center Program

R. Keith Campbell, B.Pharm., M.B.A.

Director of Externship
Professor of Clinical Pharmacy
College of Pharmacy, Washington State University
Pullman, Washington

Betty J. Dong, Pharm.D.

Clinical Pharmacist, Family Practice and
  Thyroid Clinics
U.C.S.F. and San Francisco General Hospital
Associate Clinical Professor
School of Pharmacy and Department of Family
  and Community Medicine
University of California, San Francisco,
San Francisco, California

Robert T. Dorr, Ph.D.

Research Assistant Professor
Medicine and Pharmacology
The Arizona Cancer Center
University of Arizona
Tucson, Arizona

Michael N. Dudley, Pharm.D.

Division of Infectious Diseases and Department of Pharmacy
Roger Williams General Hospital
Assistant Professor of Pharmacy and
  Adjunct Assistant Professor of Medicine
College of Pharmacy, University of Rhode Island and
  Brown University Program in Medicine
Providence, Rhode Island

Robert C. Eschbach, Pharm.D.

Pharmacy Clinical Services Supervisor
Spohn Hospital
Corpus Christi, Texas

John G. Gambertoglio, Pharm.D.

Adjunct Professor of Pharmacy
School of Pharmacy
University of California, San Francisco,
San Francisco, California

Philip D. Hansten, Pharm.D.

Professor of Clinical Pharmacy
College of Pharmacy
Washington State University
Spokane, Washington

Christine D. Kelley-Buchanan, B.A.

Prevention Coordinator/Teratogen Risk Consultant
Tri-Counties Regional Center for the
  Developmentally Disabled
Santa Barbara, California

H. William Kelly, Pharm.D.

Associate Professor of Pharmacy and Pediatrics
College of Pharmacy and Department of Pediatrics,
  School of Medicine
University of New Mexico
Albuquerque, New Mexico

John M. Kovarik, Pharm.D.

Fellow, The Drug Evaluation Unit
Hennepin County Medical Center
Clinical Instructor, Pharmacy Practice
College of Pharmacy, University of Minnesota
Minneapolis, Minnesota

Gary R. Matzke, Pharm.D.

Co-Director, The Drug Evaluation Unit
Hennepin County Medical Center
Professor, Pharmacy Practice
College of Pharmacy, University of Minnesota
Minneapolis, Minnesota

Thomas J. Mrazik, Pharm.D.

Clinical Pharmacist
Drug Information and Research Division
Department of Pharmacy
Thomas Jefferson University Hospital
Clinical Associate Professor of Pharmacy
Philadelphia College of Pharmacy and Science
Philadelphia, Pennsylvania

Robert E. Pachorek, Pharm.D.

Clinical Pharmacist
Department of Pharmacy
Mercy Hospital and Medical Center
San Diego, California

Lisa C. Rodondi, Pharm.D.

Department of Pharmacy
Veterans Administration Medical Center
Palo Alto, California
Adjunct Professor of Pharmacy
School of Pharmacy, University of the Pacific
Stockton, California

Fred Shatsky, B.S. Pharm.

Pharmacist Specialist, Nutritional Support
University of California Medical Center
San Diego, California
Assistant Clinical Professor of Pharmacy
University of California, San Francisco,
San Diego Program

Lisa L. Stagaman, Pharm.D.

Clinical Assistant Professor
Department of Pharmacology
University of Texas
Health Science Center at San Antonio
San Antonio, Texas

Alfred E. Staubus, Pharm.D., Ph.D.

Director, Clinical Pharmacology/Pharmacokinetic Laboratory
Associate Professor of Pharmaceutics and
  Pharmaceutical Chemistry
College of Pharmacy
The Ohio State University
Columbus, Ohio

Glen L. Stimmel, Pharm.D.

Professor of Clinical Pharmacy, Psychiatry and
  the Behavioral Sciences
Schools of Pharmacy and Medicine
University of Southern California
Los Angeles, California

Dianne E. Tobias, Pharm.D.

Director, Quality Assurance and Education
HealthCare Network
Anaheim, California
Assistant Clinical Professor of Pharmacy
University of California, San Francisco,
Irvine Program

Lai J. Wong, Pharm.D.

Pharmacist Specialist, Inpatient Pharmacy
Kaiser Foundation Hospital
Clinical Instructor of Pharmacy
School of Pharmacy, University of Southern California
Los Angeles, California

Frederick P. Zeller, Pharm.D.

Clinical Pharmacist, Coronary Intensive Care Unit
Assistant Professor of Pharmacy Practice and
  Instructor in Medicine, Section of Cardiology
University of Illinois at Chicago
Chicago, Illinois

CONTENTS

DRUG REVIEWS

1 ABBREVIATIONS, CONVERSION FACTORS AND ANTHROPOMETRICS

THE FOLLOWING medical record and prescription abbreviations are in common usage, but many variations occur by institution or geographic area. When in doubt, always verify the meaning of an abbreviation.

Medical Record Abbreviations

A	Apical; Artery; Assessment (POMR)	**AP**	Antepartum; Anteroposterior; Apical pulse
A2	Aortic second sound		
AAL	Anterior axillary line	**A & P**	Anterior and posterior; Assessment and plans; Auscultation and percussion
Ab	Abort; Abortion; Antibody		
Abd	Abdomen; Abdominal	**Appy**	Appendectomy
ABE	Acute bacterial endocarditis	**APTT**	Activated partial thromboplastin time
ABG	Arterial blood gases	**ARDS**	Adult respiratory distress syndrome
ACLS	Advanced cardiac life support	**ARF**	Acute renal failure; Acute respiratory failure
ACT	Activated clotting time; Allergen challenge test		
		AS	Anal sphincter; Ankylosing spondylitis; Aortic stenosis
ACTH	Adrenocorticotropic hormone		
ADH	Antidiuretic hormone	**ASCVD**	Arteriosclerotic cardiovascular disease
ADL	Activities of daily living	**ASD**	Atrial septal defect
ADM	Admission	**ASHD**	Arteriosclerotic heart disease
ADR	Adverse drug reaction	**ASO**	Arteriosclerosis obliterans
AF	Amniotic fluid; Atrial fibrillation	**AST**	Aspartate aminotransferase (same as SGOT)
AFB	Acid fast bacillus; Aorto-femoral bypass		
Ag	Antigen	**ASVD**	Arteriosclerotic vascular disease
A/G	Albumin/globulin ratio	**ATN**	Acute tubular necrosis
AGL	Acute granulocytic leukemia	**AV**	Arteriovenous; Atrioventricular; Auditory-visual
AGN	Acute glomerular nephritis		
AI	Allergy index; Aortic insufficiency	**A & W**	Alive and well
AIDS	Acquired immune deficiency syndrome	**Ax**	Axillary
AJ	Ankle jerk	**BAC**	Blood alcohol concentration
AK	Above knee	**BaE**	Barium enema
ALL	Acute lymphocytic leukemia	**BBB**	Blood-brain barrier; Bundle branch block
ALS	Advanced life support; Amyotrophic lateral sclerosis		
		BBT	Basal body temperature
ALT	Alanine aminotransferase (same as SGPT)	**BCG**	Bacille Calmette-Guerin
		BCLS	Basic cardiac life support
AMA	Against medical advice	**BCP**	Birth control pill
AML	Acute myelocytic leukemia	**BE**	Bacterial endocarditis; Barium enema
ANA	Antinuclear antibodies	**BF**	Black female
A & O	Alert and oriented	**BJ**	Biceps jerk; Bone and joint
AODM	Adult onset diabetes mellitus	**BK**	Below knee

1

Bl Obs	Bladder observation; Bladder obstruction	**CRP**	C-reactive protein
BLS	Basic life support	**CS**	Cesarean section; Coronary sclerosis
BM	Black male; Bowel movement; Breast milk	**C & S**	Culture and sensitivity
		CS & CC	Culture, sensitivity and colony count
BMR	Basal metabolic rate	**CSF**	Cerebrospinal fluid
BNO	Bladder neck obstruction	**CT**	Circulation time; Clotting time; Coagulation time; Computed tomography
BP	Blood pressure		
BPH	Benign prostatic hypertrophy		
BR	Bathroom; Bedrest	**CUC**	Chronic ulcerative colitis
BRP	Bathroom privileges	**CV**	Cardiovascular; Conjugata vera
BS	Blood sugar; Bowel sounds; Breath sounds	**CVA**	Cerebral vascular accident; Costovertebral angle
BSA	Body surface area	**CVI**	Cerebral vascular insufficiency; Continuous venous infusion
BSO	Bilateral salpingo-oophorectomy		
BTL	Bilateral tubal ligation	**CVP**	Central venous pressure
BUN	Blood urea nitrogen	**Cx**	Cervical; Cervix
BVL	Bilateral vas ligation	**CXR**	Chest x-ray
BW	Birth weight; Body weight	**DC** *or* **D/C**	Discharge; Discontinue
Bx	Biopsy		
C₂	Second cervical vertebra	**D & C**	Dilatation and curettage
CA	Cancer; Carcinoma; Cardiac arrest; Chronologic age	**DD** *or* **DDX**	Differential diagnosis
CAB	Coronary artery bypass	**DDD**	Degenerative disc disease
CAD	Coronary artery disease	**DHL**	Diffuse histiocytic lymphoma
CAPD	Chronic ambulatory peritoneal dialysis	**DHS**	Duration of hospital stay
CAT	Computed axial tomography	**Diff**	Differential blood count
CBC	Complete blood count	**DJD**	Degenerative joint disease
CBF	Cerebral blood flow	**DM**	Diabetes mellitus; Diastolic murmur
CBS	Chronic brain syndrome	**DOA**	Date of admission; Dead on arrival
CC	Chief complaint	**DOE**	Dyspnea on exertion
CCU	Coronary care unit	**DOI**	Date of injury
CF	Cardiac failure; Caucasian female; Complement fixation; Cystic fibrosis	**DPT**	Diphtheria-pertussis-tetanus (immunization, pediatric)
		DRG	Diagnosis-related group(s)
CGL	Chronic granulocytic leukemia	**DSD**	Discharge summary dictated; Dry sterile dressing
CHD	Congenital heart disease; Coronary heart disease		
		DTP	Diphtheria-tetanus-pertussis (immunization, pediatric)
CHF	Congestive heart failure		
CHO	Carbohydrate	**DTR**	Deep tendon reflex
CI	Cardiac index; Color index	**DTs**	Delirium tremens
CIBD	Chronic inflammatory bowel disease	**DU**	Duodenal ulcer
CLL	Chronic lymphocytic leukemia	**DVT**	Deep vein thrombosis
CM	Caucasian male; Contrast media; Culture media	**DW**	Dextrose in water; Distilled water
		D5W	Dextrose 5% in water
CML	Chronic myelocytic leukemia	**Dx**	Diagnosis
CNS	Central nervous system	**EBL**	Estimated blood loss
CO	Cardiac output	**EBV**	Epstein-Barr virus
C/O	Complaint of	**ECF**	Extracellular fluid
COLD	Chronic obstructive lung disease	**ECG**	Electrocardiogram
COPD	Chronic obstructive pulmonary disease	**ECT**	Electroconvulsive therapy; Emission computed tomography; Enhanced computed tomography
C & P	Cystoscopy and pyelogram		
CPAP	Continuous positive airway pressure	**EDV**	End-diastolic volume
CPK	Creatine phosphokinase	**EEG**	Electroencephalogram
CPP	Cerebral perfusion pressure	**EENT**	Eyes, ears, nose, throat
CPPB	Continuous positive pressure breathing	**EF**	Ejection fraction; Extended-field
CPR	Cardiopulmonary resuscitation	**EFA**	Essential fatty acids
CRF	Chronic renal failure; Corticotropin releasing factor	**EFM**	External fetal monitoring
		EGA	Estimated gestational age

EH	Enlarged heart; Essential hypertension	**Hgb**	Hemoglobin
EKG	Electrocardiogram	**HHC**	Home health care
EMG	Electromyogram	**HHD**	Hypertensive heart disease
EMIT	Enzyme multiplied immunoassay technique	**HIV**	Human immunodeficiency virus
		HLA	Human lymphocyte antigen
ENT	Ears, nose and throat	**HO**	House officer
EPIS	Episiotomy	**H/O**	History of
ER	Emergency room; Estrogen receptors	**H & P**	History and physical
ERA	Evoked response audiometry	**HPF**	High power field
ESR	Erythrocyte sedimentation rate	**HPI**	History of present illness
ESRD	End-stage renal disease	**HPLC**	High pressure liquid chromatography
EST	Electroshock therapy	**HPN**	Home parenteral nutrition
ET	Ejection time; Endotracheal; Eustachian tube	**HR**	Heart rate; Hospital record
		HT	Hypertension; Hypodermic tablet
FAS	Fetal alcohol syndrome	**HTN**	Hypertension
FB	Finger breadths; Foreign bodies	**HTVD**	Hypertensive vascular disease
FBS	Fasting blood sugar	**Hx**	History
F Cath	Foley catheter	**I**	Impression (POMR)
FEV₁	Forced expiratory volume in one second	**IA**	Intra-amniotic(ally)
		IASD	Interatrial septal defect
FF	Fat free; Filtration fraction; Force fluids	**IBC**	Iron binding capacity
		IBS	Irritable bowel syndrome
FFA	Free fatty acids	**IBW**	Ideal body weight
FH	Family history; Fetal heart	**ICF**	Intracellular fluid
FHR	Fetal heart rate	**ICG**	Indocyanine green
FHS	Fetal heart sounds	**ICM**	Intercostal margin
FIA	Fluorescence immunoassay	**ICS**	Intercostal space
FRC	Functional residual capacity	**ICU**	Intensive care unit
FSH	Follicle stimulating hormone	**ID**	Infectious disease; Intradermal(ly)
FTA	Fluorescent titer antibody; Fluorescent treponemal antibody	**I & D**	Incision and drainage
		IF	Immunofluorescence; Inspiratory force; Interstitial fluid; Intrinsic factor
FTND	Full-term normal delivery		
FUO	Fever of undetermined origin	**Ig**	Immunoglobulin
FVC	Forced vital capacity	**ILDL**	Intermediate low-density lipoprotein
Fx	Fracture	**IM**	Intramuscular(ly)
GA	Gastric analysis; General anesthesia; General appearance; Gestational age	**IMP**	Impression
		IMV	Intermittent mechanical ventilation
GB	Gallbladder	**I & O**	Intake and output
GC	Geriatric chair; Gonococci	**IOP**	Intraocular pressure
GFR	Glomerular filtration rate	**IP**	Intraperitoneal(ly)
GH	Growth hormone	**IPPB**	Intermittent positive pressure breathing
GI	Gastrointestinal		
GIS	Gastrointestinal series	**IT**	Inhalation therapy; Intrathecal(ly)
G-P-	Gravida-, para-	**IU**	International unit; Intrauterine
G-6-PD	Glucose-6-phosphate dehydrogenase	**IUD**	Intrauterine (contraceptive) device
GTT	Glucose tolerance test	**IUGR**	Intrauterine growth retardation
GU	Genitourinary	**IUP**	Intrauterine pregnancy
Gyn	Gynecology	**IV**	Intravenous(ly)
HA	Headache; Hemolytic anemia; Hyperalimentation	**IVP**	Intravenous push; Intravenous pyelogram
		IVPB	Intravenous piggyback
HAA	Hepatitis-associated antigen	**IVSD**	Intraventricular septal defect
HBAg	Hepatitis B antigen	**JVD**	Jugular-venous distention
HBO	Hyperbaric oxygen	**JVP**	Jugular venous pressure; Jugular venous pulse
HBP	High blood pressure		
HCG	Human chorionic gonadotropin	**KJ**	Knee jerk
HCT	Hematocrit; Histamine challenge test	**KO**	Keep open
HCVD	Hypertensive cardiovascular disease	**KUB**	Kidneys, ureters, bladder
HDL	High-density lipoprotein	**KVO**	Keep vein open
HEENT	Head, eyes, ears, nose, throat		

KW	Keith-Wagener (ophthalmoscopic findings)
L	Left; Liter; Lumbar
L₂	Second lumbar vertebra
LA	Left atrium; Local anesthetic
Lap	Laparotomy
LATS	Long-acting thyroid stimulator
LBBB	Left bundle branch block
LBM	Lean body mass
LCM	Left costal margin
LD	Lethal dose; Liver disease; Loading dose; Longitudinal diameter (of heart)
LDH	Lactic dehydrogenase
LDL	Low-density lipoprotein
LE	Lower extremities; Lupus erythematosus
LFT	Liver function test(s)
LH	Luteinizing hormone
LKS	Liver, kidneys, spleen
LLL	Left lower lobe
LLQ	Left lower quadrant
LMP	Last menstrual period
LOA	Left occipital anterior
LOM	Limitation of motion
LOS	Length of stay
LP	Light perception; Lumbar puncture
LPF	Low power field
LT	Levine tube; Luken's trap
LTC	Long term care
LUL	Left upper lobe
LUQ	Left upper quadrant
LVH	Left ventricular hypertrophy
L & W	Living and well
Lytes	Electrolytes
M	Meter; Molar; Murmur
M₁	Mitral first sound
M/A	Mood and/or affect
MAP	Mean arterial pressure
MBC	Maximum breathing capacity; Minimum bactericidal concentration
MCH	Mean corpuscular hemoglobin
MCHC	Mean corpuscular hemoglobin concentration
MCL	Midclavicular line; Midcostal line
MCV	Mean corpuscular volume
MDV	Multiple dose vial
MF	Myocardial fibrosis
MH	Malignant hyperthermia; Marital history; Menstrual history; Mental health
MI	Mitral insufficiency; Myocardial infarction
MIC	Minimum inhibitory concentration
ML	Midline
MLD	Minimum lethal dose
MMR	Measles, mumps, rubella vaccine
MRI	Magnetic resonance imaging
MS	Mental status; Mitral stenosis; Multiple sclerosis

MSL	Midsternal line
N	Negative; Normal
NAD	No acute distress; No apparent distress
NAS	No added salt
NG	Nasogastric
NGU	Nongonococcal urethritis
NKA	No known allergies
NL	Normal
NMR	Nuclear magnetic resonance
NPN	Nonprotein nitrogen
NPO	Nothing by mouth
NS	Normal saline; Not seen; Not significant
NSAIA	Nonsteroidal anti-inflammatory agent
NSR	Normal sinus rhythm
NSU	Nonspecific urethritis
NSVD	Normal spontaneous vaginal delivery
N & T	Nose and throat
N & V	Nausea and vomiting
NVD	Nausea, vomiting, diarrhea
NYD	Not yet diagnosed
O	Objective data (POMR)
Ob	Obstetrics
OB	Occult blood
OBS	Organic brain syndrome
OC	On call; Oral contraceptive
O/E	On examination
OM	Otitis media
OOB	Out of bed
OPV	Outpatient visit; Oral polio vaccine
OR	Operating room
OT	Occupational therapy; Old tuberculin
P	Plan (POMR); Pulse
PA	Pernicious anemia; Physician's assistant; Posteroanterior; Pulmonary artery
P & A	Percussion and auscultation
PABA	Para-aminobenzoic acid
PAC	Premature atrial contraction
PAT	Paroxysmal atrial tachycardia; Preadmission testing
PC	Porto-caval; Present complaint
PCP	Phencyclidine; Pneumocystis carinii pneumonia; Pulmonary capillary pressure
PCV	Packed cell volume
PE	Physical examination; Pleural effusion; Pulmonary embolism
PEEP	Positive end-expiratory pressure
PEG	Pneumoencephalogram; Polyethylene glycol
PERLA	Pupils equal, reactive to light and accommodation
PET	Positron emission tomography; Pre-eclamptic toxemia
PFT	Pulmonary function test(s)
pHa	Arterial blood pH
PI	Present illness; Pulmonary infarction
PID	Pelvic inflammatory disease

PKU	Phenylketonuria	**RUL**	Right upper lobe
PMH	Past medical history	**RUQ**	Right upper quadrant
PMI	Point of maximal impulse; Point of maximal intensity	**RVH**	Right ventricular hypertrophy
		S	Subjective data (POMR)
PMN	Polymorphonuclear leukocytes	S_1	First heart sound
PM & R	Physical medicine and rehabilitation	S_2	Second heart sound
PMS	Premenstrual syndrome	**SA**	Sinoatrial; Surface area
PND	Paroxysmal nocturnal dyspnea; Post-nasal drip	**SBE**	Subacute bacterial endocarditis
		SBO	Small bowel obstruction
Pnx	Pneumothorax	**SC**	Sickle cell; Subclavian; Subcutaneous(ly)
PO	By mouth		
Polys	Polymorphonuclear leukocytes	**SD**	Senile dementia; Spontaneous delivery; Standard deviation; Surgical drain
POMR	Problem oriented medical record		
POR	Problem oriented record	**SGOT**	Serum glutamic oxaloacetic transaminase
PP	Postpartum; Postprandial		
PPBS	Postprandial blood sugar	**SGPT**	Serum glutamic pyruvic transaminase
PPD	Purified protein derivative	**SH**	Serum hepatitis; Social history
ppm	Parts per million	**SI**	Standard international (units)
PR	Per rectum; Pulse rate	**SIADH**	Syndrome of inappropriate ADH (secretion)
P & R	Pulse and respiration		
PT	Patient; Physical therapy; Prothrombin time	**SIDS**	Sudden infant death syndrome
		SL	Sublingual(ly)
PTA	Plasma thromboplastin antecedent; Prior to admission; Prothrombin activity	**SLE**	Systemic lupus erythematosus
		SMA	Sequential/serial multiple analysis
		SNF	Skilled nursing facility
PTC	Plasma thromboplastin component	**SOAP**	Subjective, objective, assessment and plans (POMR)
PTT	Partial thromboplastin time		
PU	Peptic ulcer	**SOB**	Shortness of breath
PUD	Peptic ulcer disease	**S/P**	Status post
PVC	Premature ventricular contraction	**SQ**	Subcutaneous(ly)
PVT	Paroxysmal ventricular tachycardia	**SR**	Sedimentation rate; Sustained release; Systems review
R	Respiration; Right		
RA	Rheumatoid arthritis; Right atrium	**STD**	Sexually transmitted disease; Skin test dose
RAI	Radioactive iodine		
RBBB	Right bundle branch block	**STS**	Serologic test for syphilis
RBC	Red blood cell; Red blood count	**Sx**	Signs; Symptom(s)
RBF	Renal blood flow	**T**	Temperature
RCM	Radiographic contrast media; Right costal margin	**T & A**	Tonsillectomy and adenoidectomy
		TAb	Therapeutic abortion
RDS	Respiratory distress syndrome	**TAH**	Total abdominal hysterectomy
REM	Rapid eye movement	**TB**	Tuberculin; Tuberculosis
RF	Renal failure; Rheumatic fever; Rheumatoid factor	**TBA**	To be administered; To be admitted
		TBG	Thyroxine-binding globulin
Rh	Rhesus factor	**TBW**	Total body water
RHD	Rheumatic heart disease	**T & C**	Type and crossmatch
RIA	Radioimmunoassay	**Td**	Tetanus and diphtheria toxoids (for adult use)
RK	Radial keratotomy		
RLL	Right lower lobe	**TD**	Tardive dyskinesia; Transverse diameter (of heart); Treatment discontinued
RLQ	Right lower quadrant		
RO	Routine order		
R/O	Rule out	**TEA**	Thromboendarterectomy
ROM	Range of motion	**TET**	Treadmill exercise test
ROS	Review of symptoms; Review of systems	**TIA**	Transient ischemic attack
ROT	Right occipital transverse	**TIBC**	Total iron-binding capacity
RPF	Renal plasma flow	**TKO**	To keep open
RQ	Respiratory quotient	**TL**	Tubal ligation
RR	Recovery room; Respiratory rate	**TLC**	Tender loving care; Thin layer chromatography; Total lymphocyte count
RTA	Renal tubular acidosis		
RTC	Return to clinic		

TM	Trabecular meshwork; Tympanic membrane	**VC**	Vena cava; Vital capacity
		VCT	Venous clotting time
TOPV	Trivalent oral polio vaccine	**VD**	Venereal disease
TP	Thrombophlebitis; Total protein	**VDRL**	Venereal disease research laboratory
TPI	Treponema pallidum immobilization	**VF**	Ventricular fibrillation; Vision field
TPN	Total parenteral nutrition	**VLDL**	Very low-density lipoprotein
TPR	Temperature, pulse, respiration; Total peripheral resistance	**VP**	Venous pressure
		VS	Vital signs
T-set	Tracheotomy set	**VSD**	Ventricular septal defect
TSH	Thyroid-stimulating hormone	**VSS**	Vital signs stable
TURP	Transurethral resection of prostate	**VT**	Ventricular tachycardia
TVC	Triple voiding cystogram	**WB**	Weight bearing; Whole blood
Tx	Therapy; Treatment	**WBC**	White blood cell; White blood count
T & X	Type and crossmatch	**WD**	Well developed
UA	Uric acid; Urinalysis	**WF**	White female
UCG	Urine chorionic gonadotropin	**WM**	White male
UGI	Upper gastrointestinal (series)	**WN**	Well nourished
URI	Upper respiratory infection	**WNL**	Within normal limits
UTI	Urinary tract infection		

Prescription Abbreviations

aa	Of each (ana)	**os**	Left eye (oculus sinister)
ac	Before meals (ante cibum)	**ou**	Each eye (oculus uterque)
ad	Right ear (auris dextra)	**pc**	After meals (post cibum)
ad	Up to (ad)	**po**	By mouth (per os)
ad lib	As desired (ad libitum)	**prn**	As needed (pro re nata)
aq	Water (aqua)	**q**	Each (quaque)
as	Left ear (auris sinistra)	**qd**	Every day (quaque die)*
au	Each ear (auris utro)	**qh** *or*	Every hour (quaque hora)
bid	Twice a day (bis in die)	**qhr**	
c	With (cum)	**qid**	Four times a day (quarter in die)
dos	Dose (dosis)	**qs**	Sufficient quantity (quantum sufficiat)
dtd	Let such doses be given (dentur tales doses)	**qs ad**	Sufficient quantity to make (quantum sufficiat ad)
et	And (et)	**repet**	To be repeated (repetatur)
ft	Make (fiat, fiant)	**s**	Without (sine)
gtt(s)	Drop(s) (gutta)	**ss**	One-half (semis)
h *or* **hr**	Hour (hora)	**Sig**	Mark, write (signa)
hs	At bedtime (hora somni)	**stat**	At once (statim)
M	Mix (misce)	**tid**	Three times a day (ter in die)
mt	Send of such (mitte talis)	**ud** *or*	As directed (ut dictum)
nr	Do not repeat (non repetatur)	**ut dict**	
od	Right eye (oculus dexter)		

For prescription abbreviations not listed, see ''Medical Record Abbreviations.'' For abbreviations related to prescription dosages (volume, weight), see ''Conversion Factors''.

*Use is *not* recommended, due to possibility of being misread as ''qid.''

Conversion Factors

Milliequivalents
Temperature
Weights and Measures

MILLIEQUIVALENTS

An equivalent weight of a substance is that weight which will combine with or replace one gram of hydrogen; a milliequivalent is 1/1000 of an equivalent weight.

Milliequivalents per Liter (mEq/L)

$$mEq/L = \frac{Weight\ of\ salt\ (g) \times Valence\ of\ ion \times 1000}{Molecular\ weight\ of\ salt}$$

$$Weight\ of\ Salt\ (g) = \frac{mEq/L \times Molecular\ weight\ of\ salt}{Valence\ of\ ion \times 1000}$$

Approximate Milliequivalents-Weights of Selected Ions

SALT	MEQ/GRAM SALT	MG SALT/MEQ
Calcium Carbonate [$CaCO_3$]	20.0	50.0
Calcium Chloride [$CaCl_2 \cdot 2H_2O$]	13.6	73.5
Calcium Gluceptate [$Ca(C_7H_{13}O_8)_2$]	4.1	245.2
Calcium Gluconate [$Ca(C_6H_{11}O_7)_2 \cdot H_2O$]	4.5	224.1
Calcium Lactate [$Ca(C_3H_5O_3)_2 \cdot 5H_2O$]	6.5	154.1
Magnesium Gluconate [$Mg(C_6H_{11}O_7)_2 \cdot H_2O$]	4.6	216.3
Magnesium Oxide [MgO]	49.6	20.2
Magnesium Sulfate [$MgSO_4$]	16.6	60.2
Magnesium Sulfate [$MgSO_4 \cdot 7H_2O$]	8.1	123.2
Potassium Acetate [$K(C_2H_3O_2)$]	10.2	98.1
Potassium Chloride [KCl]	13.4	74.6
Potassium Citrate [$K_3(C_6H_5O_7) \cdot H_2O$]	9.2	108.1
Potassium Iodide [KI]	6.0	166.0
Sodium Acetate [$Na(C_2H_3O_2)$]	12.2	82.0
Sodium Acetate [$Na(C_2H_3O_2) \cdot 3H_2O$]	7.3	136.1
Sodium Bicarbonate [$NaHCO_3$]	11.9	84.0
Sodium Chloride [$NaCl$]	17.1	58.4
Sodium Citrate [$Na_3(C_6H_5O_7) \cdot 2H_2O$]	10.2	98.0
Sodium Iodide [NaI]	6.7	149.9
Sodium Lactate [$Na(C_3H_5O_3)$]	8.9	112.1
Zinc Sulfate [$ZnSO_4 \cdot 7H_2O$]	7.0	143.8

Valences and Atomic Weights of Selected Ions

SUBSTANCE	ELECTROLYTE	VALENCE	MOLECULAR WEIGHT
Calcium	Ca^{++}	2	40.1
Chloride	Cl^-	1	35.5
Magnesium	Mg^{++}	2	24.3
Phosphate	$HPO_4^=$ (80%)	1.8	96.0*
pH = 7.4	$H_2PO_4^-$ (20%)		
Potassium	K^+	1	39.1
Sodium	Na^+	1	23.0
Sulfate	$SO_4^=$	2	96.0*

*The molecular weight of phosphorus only is 31, and sulfur only is 32.1.

TEMPERATURE

Fahrenheit to Centigrade: $(°F - 32) \times 5/9 = °C$

Centigrade to Fahrenheit: $(°C \times 9/5) + 32 = °F$

Centigrade to Kelvin: $°C + 273 = °K$

WEIGHTS AND MEASURES

Metric Weight Equivalents

1 kilogram (kg)	= 1,000 grams
1 gram (g)	= 1,000 milligrams
1 milligram (mg)	= 0.001 gram
1 microgram (mcg, μg)	= 0.001 milligram
1 nanogram (ng)	= 0.001 microgram
1 picogram (pg)	= 0.001 nanogram

Metric Volume Equivalents

1 liter (L)	= 1,000 milliliters (ml)
1 deciliter (dl)	= 100 milliliters

Apothecary Weight Equivalents

1 scruple (℈)	= 20 grains (gr)
60 grains	= 1 dram (ℨ)
8 drams	= 1 ounce (ℨ)
1 ounce	= 480 grains
12 ounces	= 1 pound (℔)

Apothecary Volume Equivalents

60 minims (♏)	= 1 fluidram (flℨ)
8 fluidrams	= 1 fluidounce (flℨ)
1 fluidounce	= 480 minims
16 fluidounces	= 1 pint (pt)

Avoirdupois Weight Equivalents

1 ounce (oz) = 437.5 grains
16 ounces = 1 pound (lb)

Weight/Volume Equivalents

1 mg/dl = 10 mcg/ml
1 mg/dl = 1 mg%
1 ppm = 1 mg/L

Conversion Equivalents

1 gram	(g) = 15.43 grains	0.1	mg = 1/600 gr
1 grain	(gr) = 64.8 milligrams	0.12	mg = 1/500 gr
1 ounce	(ʒ) = 31.1 grams	0.15	mg = 1/400 gr
1 ounce	(oz) = 28.35 grams	0.2	mg = 1/300 gr
1 pound	(lb) = 453.6 grams	0.3	mg = 1/200 gr
1 kilogram	(kg) = 2.2 pounds	0.4	mg = 1/150 gr
1 milliliter	(ml) = 16.23 minims	0.5	mg = 1/120 gr
1 minim	(ℳ) = 0.06 milliliter	0.6	mg = 1/100 gr
1 fluidounce	(flʒ) = 29.57 ml	0.8	mg = 1/80 gr
1 pint	(pt) = 473.2 ml	1.0	mg = 1/65 gr

Anthropometrics

CREATININE CLEARANCE FORMULAS

Formulas for Estimating Creatinine Clearance in Patients with Stable Renal Function.

Adults [Age 18 Years and Older][a]

$$Cl_{cr} \text{ (Males)} = \frac{(140 - Age) \times (Weight)}{Cr_s \times 72}$$

$$Cl_{cr} \text{ (Females)} = 0.85 \times \text{Above value}$$

where, Cl_{cr} = creatinine clearance in ml/min
Cr_s = serum creatinine in mg/dl
Age is in years
Weight is in kg.

Children [Age 1 - 18 Years][b]

$$Cl_{cr} = \frac{0.48 \times (Height) \times (BSA)}{Cr_s \times 1.73}$$

where, BSA = body surface area in M^2
Cl_{cr} = creatinine clearance in ml/min
Cr_s = serum creatinine in mg/dl
Height is in cm.

IDEAL BODY WEIGHT

Ideal body weight (IBW) is the weight expected for a nonobese person of a given height. The IBW formulas below, as well as various life insurance tables, can be used to estimate IBW. Another measurement, lean body mass (LBM), is an estimate of the body weight minus the weight of all body fat. Because many drugs are distributed into highly perfused tissues (such as muscle) and not into adipose tissue, LBM probably represents the optimum method upon which to base drug dosage. However, most dosing methods described in the literature utilize IBW as a method in dosing obese patients and, thus, substitution of LBM for IBW in determining a dosage regimen would result in underdosing of the patient.[c]

Adults [Age 18 Years and Older][d]

IBW (Males) = 50 + (2.3 × Height in inches over 5 feet)
IBW (Females) = 45.5 + (2.3 × Height in inches over 5 feet)
where, IBW is in kg.

Children [Age 1 - 18 Years][b]

Children Under 5 Feet Tall:

$$IBW = \frac{(Height^2 \times 1.65)}{1000}$$

where, IBW is in kg
Height is in cm.

Children 5 Feet or Taller:

IBW (Males) = 39 + (2.27 × Height in inches over 5 feet)
IBW (Females) = 42.2 + (2.27 × Height in inches over 5 feet)
where, IBW is in kg.

a. Cockcroft DW, Gault MH. Prediction of creatinine clearance from serum creatinine. Nephron 1976;16:31-41.
b. Traub SL, Johnson CE. Comparison of methods of estimating creatinine clearance in children. Am J Hosp Pharm 1980;37:195-201.
c. Anderson PO, Lane JR. Lean body mass and volume of distribution. Am J Hosp Pharm 1984;41:658. Letter.
d. Devine BJ. Gentamicin therapy. Drug Intell Clin Pharm 1974;8:650-5.

Surface Area Nomograms

Body Surface Area of Adults and Children[a]
Nomogram for Determination of Body Surface Area from Height and Weight
(Adults and Children)

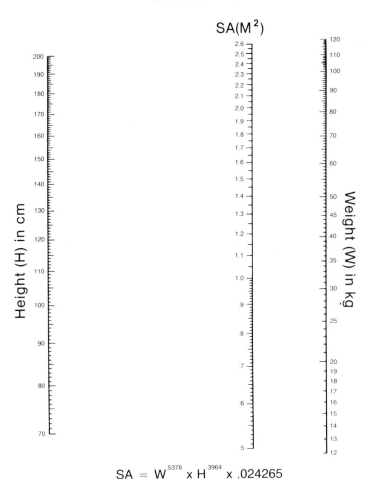

$$SA = W^{5378} \times H^{3964} \times .024265$$

Nomogram representing the relationship between height, weight, and surface area in adults and children. To use the nomogram, a ruler is aligned with the height and weight on the two lateral axes. The point at which the center line is intersected gives the corresponding value for surface area.

a. From Haycock GB, Schwartz GJ, Wisotsky DH. Geometric method for measuring body surface area: a height-weight formula validated in infants, children, and adults. J Pediatr 1978;93:62-6, reproduced with permission.

Body Surface Area of Infants[a]

Nomogram for Determination of Body Surface Area from Height and Weight
(Infants)

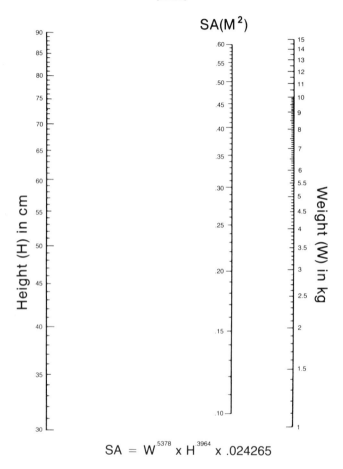

$$SA = W^{5378} \times H^{3964} \times .024265$$

Nomogram representing the relationship between height, weight, and surface area in infants. To use the nomogram, a ruler is aligned with the height and weight on the two lateral axes. The point at which the center line is intersected gives the corresponding value for surface area.

a. From Haycock GB, Schwartz GJ, Wisotsky DH. Geometric method for measuring body surface area: a height-weight formula validated in infants, children, and adults. J Pediatr 1978;93:62-6, reproduced with permission.

2 BIOPHARMACEUTICS AND PHARMACOKINETICS

General Principles, Dosing in Renal Impairment, Dialysis of Drugs

General Principles

BIOPHARMACEUTICS IS THE STUDY of the relationship between physicochemical properties of a drug in a dosage form and the therapeutic response observed after its administration. Pharmacokinetics is concerned with the characterization of the time course of drug absorption, distribution, elimination, the relationship among these processes and the observed therapeutic or adverse effects.

The purpose of this section is to provide a brief review of the more important biopharmaceutical factors that influence drug delivery, the pharmacokinetic concepts used to describe drug disposition in the body and their application to the design of drug dosage regimens. More extensive discussions of these topics are available for less experienced[1-6] as well as advanced practitioners.[7,8]

Familiarity with this information is essential for those individuals involved in clinical practice, but its usefulness must be kept in perspective. The goal of drug therapy is more than just the attainment of desired plasma drug concentrations. It is the successful control or eradication of a disease state through the appropriate selection, proper administration and efficient distribution of drugs. The concepts presented in this section, when used in conjunction with these objectives, will make a useful contribution to rational drug therapy.

Pharmacokinetic Model Systems. The most common method used to describe the pharmacokinetic behavior of a drug in the body is by the use of models depicting the body as a single compartment or series of compartments. These compartments do not usually have any literal anatomic or physiologic reality. However, visualization of the body in this fashion helps explain the observed disposition characteristics of various drugs and allows prediction of drug concentrations in the body as a function of time, dose and route of administration.

The single compartment model with intravenous (IV) bolus administration assumes that a drug is instantaneously available for

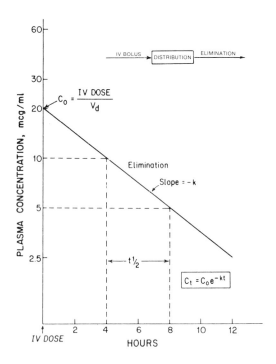

Figure 1. Plasma concentration-time decline after intravenous administration for a drug best characterized by a one-compartment model.

distribution to whatever body fluids and tissues are in equilibrium with the drug's plasma/blood concentration (Figure 1). This model can be most readily applied to drugs that rapidly distribute between plasma and other body fluids and tissues after reaching the systemic circulation. The rate of drug elimination from the body is assumed to follow first-order or linear pharmacokinetics. In other words, the rate of elimination is proportional to the amount (or concentration) of drug present in the body at any given time.

The two-compartment model separates the body into a central compartment, usually with a small volume, and a peripheral compartment with a larger volume (Figure 2). Initial distribution of a drug occurs within the central compartment. The central compartment is assumed to consist of the plasma/blood and other body fluids and tissues which are in rapid equilibrium with the blood. Slower drug distribution occurs between the central and

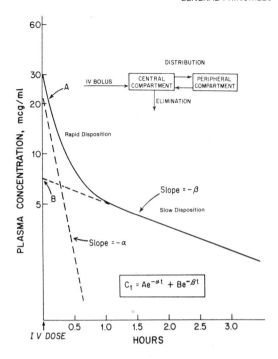

Figure 2. Plasma concentration-time decline after intravenous administration for a drug best characterized by a two-compartment model.

peripheral compartments. The peripheral compartments are those body fluids that slowly equilibrate with the drug in plasma/blood. Both the transfer of drug between compartments and drug elimination from the central compartment are again assumed to obey first-order pharmacokinetics.

Multi-compartment models may be necessary to fully characterize the observed pharmacokinetic behavior of a drug; however, the increased complexity of these models may reduce their clinical usefulness. Simpler models that describe drug disposition in a less complex, but adequate fashion, may prove more useful. For example, while the disposition of gentamicin is more accurately characterized by a two- or three-compartment model,[9,10] the use of a one-compartment model to predict plasma concentrations and individualize dosing regimens for gentamicin has proven successful clinically.[11]

A more mathematical approach to pharmacokinetic modeling is the use of physiologic models to describe drug disposition in the body.[12,13] In such models, physiological parameters are defined such as tissue and organ perfusion, plasma protein binding and the intrinsic capacity of the eliminating organs to remove drug from the body. While possibly being more helpful than compartment modeling in explaining the effects of changes in body hemodynamics on drug disposition, the mathematical complexity of physiological modeling prohibits its use clinically.

Drug Absorption and Bioavailability. Bioavailability can be defined as the rate and the extent (F) to which a drug is absorbed from a particular formulation and reaches the systemic circulation. For routes of administration other than intravenous, the extent of bioavailability of a drug may be less than 100% (F<1) due to incomplete absorption or metabolism that occurs before the drug can reach the systemic circulation. Therefore, it is important to briefly review some of the factors involved in these processes and how they may affect bioavailability.

In order for a drug to be absorbed from the gastrointestinal (GI) tract or an injection site, it must be in solution. This process of dissolution is most often of concern when dealing with compressed oral dosage forms such as tablets and capsules. After administration, these dosage forms must first undergo disintegration before the drug can dissolve sufficiently to be absorbed. Disintegrating agents (eg, starch, methylcellulose) are used in these formulations to promote swelling and break-up into smaller granules which eventually reduce to fine particles. As the size of these particles decreases, the surface area of drug exposed to GI fluids increases, thus enhancing drug dissolution. The water solubility of drugs also plays an important role in dissolution. It is difficult for a drug with a very low water solubility to dissolve and remain in solution long enough to have significant absorption. This problem can often be overcome by administering these drugs as a more soluble salt form instead of the free acid or base.

Disintegration does not ensure dissolution nor does dissolution guarantee absorption. The process of absorption is dependent on many factors including the extent of surface area available for absorption, existence of a drug concentration gradient, adequate blood flow to and from the absorption site and the physicochemical properties of a drug (eg, lipid solubility and degree of ionization).[1,4] The more lipid soluble a drug, the faster it is absorbed. For drugs that are weak acids or bases, an increase in the proportion of unionized drug usually increases their ability to cross lipid membranes. Thus, weakly acidic drugs should be more rapidly absorbed in the stomach due to low pH of gastric fluids. However, the absorption of these compounds is actually much faster and more complete in the more basic environment of the small intestine. This is explained by the greater blood flow to the intestines and the much larger surface area available compared to the stomach. It should be evident that the rate of gastric emptying also influences the rate of drug absorption. The presence of food in the stomach may delay gastric emptying, thereby decreasing the rate of absorption for most drugs.[14] Other conditions that may affect GI drug absorption include malabsorption (due to disease or surgical resection of the intestine), faster GI transit time (due to diarrhea) and chemical reactions in the GI tract such as drug complexation and acid hydrolysis.

When drugs are administered by parenteral or sublingual routes, they directly enter the systemic circulation before significant metabolism can occur. After oral administration, drugs are absorbed from the GI tract, enter the portal circulation and pass through the liver before reaching the systemic circulation. Some drugs (eg, propranolol, nitroglycerin, lidocaine, methyltestosterone) may undergo extensive metabolism either in the wall of the GI tract during absorption or during this initial exposure to the liver immediately after absorption. This "first-pass effect" may considerably reduce the effectiveness of the oral route of administration for these drugs by limiting the amount of unchanged drug reaching the site of action, even if actual absorption of the compound is complete.[7,15]

The extent of bioavailability can be expressed in two ways that have different clinical applications. Absolute bioavailability is measured by comparing the area under the plasma concentration versus time curves (AUC), or the cumulative amount of unchanged drug eventually excreted in the urine after a single oral (or other route of administration) dose and an IV dose of a drug. The extent of bioavailability for the drug product in question can then be calculated by considering the IV dose to be completely available ($F = 1$). If the IV product is a salt of the drug, the F value must be adjusted to reflect the actual amount of drug in the preparation. Absolute bioavailability can also be determined upon multiple dosing by comparison of the AUC or the amount of drug excreted during a dosing interval under steady-state conditions. These estimates of bioavailability may be helpful in determining what dosage adjustment would be required for a patient being switched from IV to the oral route of administration or vice versa.

Relative bioavailability is determined when the intravenous route is not used for comparison either by design or because an IV dosage form is not available. The most common application of this type of bioavailability determination is the comparison of a new oral dosage form of a generic drug to a similar oral product of established efficacy (usually the original product on the market). This type of bioavailability study may also be referred to as a "bioequivalency" study.[16] When evaluating bioequivalency studies, three characteristics of the plasma concentration versus time curve for each of the two products should be examined (Figure 3). Comparison of the *peak concentration* (C_{max}) and time required to achieve this peak (t_{max}) provides an estimate of the rate of absorption of each product. Generally, the faster the rate of absorption, the greater the peak concentration that is attained. At t_{max}, the rate of absorption is equal to the rate of elimination. Absorption continues past t_{max}, but at a rate exceeded by the rate of elimination. Comparison of the *rate of absorption* is important for drugs with a narrow therapeutic index where very rapid absorption may increase the likelihood of toxicity occurring after administration or for drugs that require rapid achievement of a certain peak

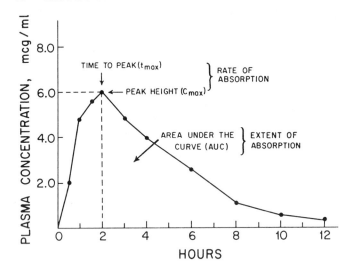

Figure 3. The most important characteristics of the plasma concentration-time curve for determining bioequivalence after oral administration of a drug.

concentration to produce the desired therapeutic effect. Measurement of the AUC provides an estimate of the total amount of drug absorbed for each product. Determination of this *extent of absorption* is usually more important than the rate of absorption when evaluating the bioequivalence of two products. Proper interpretation of study data is essential to ensure the selection of a generic product that is bioequivalent as well as chemically equivalent to an established product. It should be remembered that when bioequivalency studies are conducted in normal healthy volunteers rather than patients, their results may not always be extrapolated to the clinical setting. The reader is referred to other more detailed discussions of the principles of bioavailability testing[7,8,17] and lists of drugs that may experience bioavailability problems.[16,18] It should be noted that not all generic products on the market have FDA approval. Pharmacists should consult the current FDA publication *Approved Drug Products with Therapeutic Equivalence Evaluations* before purchasing a generic product from a different manufacturer.

Drug Distribution. The apparent volume of distribution (V_d) is a proportionality constant that correlates the plasma concentration of a drug at a given time (C) to the total amount of drug in the body at the same time (A) as follows:

$$V_d = \frac{A}{C} \tag{1}$$

This relationship can reasonably predict the dose of a drug required to achieve a desired plasma concentration. The magnitude of V_d for any drug is determined by the extent of tissue and plasma protein binding and the lipid versus water solubility of the drug. Drugs that are more water soluble, extensively bound to plasma proteins or demonstrate little tissue binding may have a V_d as small as the plasma volume (approximately 3 L). A larger V_d (up to several thousand liters) may be observed with drugs (eg, tricyclic antidepressants) that are very lipid soluble or exhibit a large amount of tissue binding. The fact that V_d only represents an *apparent* volume allows for the existence of such large values for many drugs. Even if the value of V_d approximates the volume of an actual body space such as plasma volume, it should not be assumed that distribution of the drug is restricted solely to that space. Great intra- and inter-patient variability in V_d can occur as a result of changes or differences in factors such as age, body weight and surface area, obesity, renal function, metabolic activity, cardiac output and protein binding.

There are several methods for calculating V_d. Due to its simplicity, a common method for estimating V_d in clinical practice is to obtain the difference between the peak concentration (C_{max}) and trough concentration (C_{min}) after multiple administrations of a drug dose (D), such that:[19]

$$V_d = \frac{FD}{C_{max} - C_{min}} \qquad (2)$$

Another method involves extrapolation of the terminal elimination phase of the plasma concentration decline curve back to the y-intercept to obtain the concentration (C_0) that theoretically would have existed if absorption and distribution were instantaneous (Figure 1).[20] Dividing C_0 into the dose administered (D) as in equation (1) would then give V_d. Either method usually provides a usable approximation of V_d for use in dosage calculations, unless absorption is greatly delayed. Other reviews provide more detailed discussions of methods for determining V_d and factors that influence V_d.[21,22]

Protein Binding. The effects of protein binding on drug disposition have been reviewed extensively.[23-27] Acidic drugs are bound largely to albumin while basic drugs are bound primarily to α_1-acid glycoprotein, lipoproteins and also to some degree, albumin. Most often when laboratories report a plasma drug concentration, it is a total concentration (including both bound and unbound drug). The drug bound to proteins is unavailable to the site of action and considered pharmacologically inactive. The unbound (free) drug is considered the active form of the drug, because it has unrestricted access to the site of action. Clinically significant problems with protein binding alterations occur with drugs that have a small V_d, a narrow therapeutic index and are greater than 90% bound to albumin. One of the most common and potentially dangerous problems is partial displacement from albumin binding sites of one highly albumin-bound drug by another. This interaction results in a transient increase in the pharmacologic activity of the displaced drug due to an increase in circulating free drug.[24] With this increase in free drug plasma concentration, more drug is available for distribution, metabolism and elimination, thereby eventually returning the free drug plasma concentration and pharmacologic effect to their previous levels. The free concentration now constitutes an increased percentage (increased free fraction) of the total drug plasma concentration, which is now lower than before displacement. This protein binding interaction is of most importance when a displacing drug is started in a patient already receiving chronic therapy with a highly albumin-bound drug. However, it is also important to note that the displacing agent need not be a drug, but can also be an endogenous compound. Increases in plasma free fatty acids (due to bacterial infection, hyperthyroidism, renal failure, fasting, etc) can cause displacement of highly albumin-bound drugs with similar results.

Conditions that result in decreased albumin concentrations due to altered production or excretion (eg, liver disease, nephrotic syndrome) and/or albumin binding capacity (eg, renal disease) also alter the dose-response curve of drugs that are highly albumin-bound. This occurs because of a decrease in the fraction of total plasma drug concentration bound to albumin, increasing the free fraction. Some drugs (eg, lidocaine, valproic acid) demonstrate concentration-dependent protein binding in their therapeutic plasma level range. As the total plasma concentration of these drugs increases, proportionately less drug is bound to plasma proteins. This results in a curvilinear dose-plasma concentration relationship in which the increase in total plasma drug concentration is less than expected from an increase in dose.

Increased concentrations of α_1-acid glycoprotein (due to acute physiologic stress as in myocardial infarction or surgery) and lipoproteins (due to primary or secondary causes of hyperlipoproteinemia) may increase the protein binding of basic drugs, potentially decreasing their therapeutic effectiveness.[28]

Drug Elimination. The two most important eliminating organs for most drugs are the kidneys and the liver. Prediction of creatinine clearance from serum creatinine provides a reasonable estimation of renal function and some indication of the ability of the kidney to eliminate drugs (see the following section Dosing in Renal Impairment).[29,30] No liver function test consistently provides an accurate indication of the metabolic ability of the liver; therefore, the effect of impaired liver function on the metabolism of different drugs is often difficult or impossible to predict. The effects of renal, hepatic and other disease states on drug pharmacokinetics have been reviewed extensively.[13,26,31-35]

The elimination half-life ($t_{1/2}$) is the time required for the plasma drug concentration to decrease by one-half (Figure 1). The apparent first-order elimination rate constant (k) is a proportionality constant that relates the rate of elimination to A as follows:

$$\frac{dA}{dt} = -kA \tag{3}$$

and represents the fraction of drug removed from plasma per unit time. The relationship between k and $t_{1/2}$ is:

$$k = \frac{\ln 2}{t_{1/2}} \cong \frac{0.693}{t_{1/2}} \tag{4}$$

The decline of the plasma drug concentration during the elimination phase when using logarithms to the base 10 can be described by:

$$\log C_t = \log C_0 - \frac{kt}{2.3} \tag{5a}$$

or using natural logarithms (base e):

$$\ln C_t = \ln C_0 - kt \tag{5b}$$

or

$$C_t = C_0 e^{-kt} \tag{6}$$

where, C_0 = drug concentration at time 0
C_t = drug concentration at time t
e^{-kt} = fraction of dose remaining at time t.

The $t_{1/2}$ and k are often inappropriate expressions of the elimination characteristics of a drug, because they only describe the rate of removal of drug from the plasma and not necessarily from the body. Therefore, the half-life of a drug may reflect the rate of drug distribution between body tissues and plasma as well as elimination from the body. The pharmacokinetic parameter, clearance (Cl), defined as the volume of body fluid (eg, plasma) totally cleared of drug per unit time, is a physiologically more appropriate term than half-life to describe drug elimination from the body.[36] It is a measure of the ability of the eliminating organs (eg, liver, kidneys) to remove drug from the body and is not influenced by drug distribution outside of these organs; this is expressed as:

$$Cl = \frac{\text{Rate of drug removal from body}}{\text{Concentration}} \tag{7}$$

Based on this relationship and equations (1) and (3), Cl can be described in a simple, but clinically useful form:

$$Cl = k V_d \tag{8}$$

for those drugs adequately described by a one-compartment model. It is inappropriate to consider that Cl is dependent on k and V_d simply because of equation (8). Rather, the values for k and $t_{1/2}$ are dependent on Cl and V_d. The V_d or Cl may change independently of one another, resulting in a change in k and $t_{1/2}$. A drug may have a long $t_{1/2}$, because either it has a large V_d or it is slowly removed from the body by the eliminating organs, or both. Clearance can also be calculated experimentally by:

$$Cl = \frac{\text{Dose}}{\text{AUC}} \tag{9}$$

using AUC after a single dose or AUC of a dosing interval (τ) during multiple dosing at steady-state.

Clearance values most often cited in the literature refer to the total body clearance (Cl_t) of a drug. Total body clearance is the sum of all clearance processes in the body and thus, the entire body is considered to be a single drug elimination system. Since the kidneys and liver are the major eliminating organs for most drugs, then:

$$Cl_t = Cl_r + Cl_m \tag{10}$$

where, Cl_r = renal clearance
   Cl_m = metabolic (hepatic) clearance.

Renal drug excretion occurs by a combination of three distinct processes: filtration, active tubular secretion and tubular reabsorption. The plasma drug concentration, degree of plasma protein binding, urine flow rate and pH, and the overall functional state of the kidneys therefore influence renal clearance.

Hepatic clearance is influenced by blood flow to the liver, drug plasma protein binding and the intrinsic metabolic capacity of liver enzymes (intrinsic metabolic clearance, Cl_{int}).[37] Classifying drugs by hepatic extraction ratio (the fraction of drug removed from the blood in a single pass through the liver) helps predict which of these factors will be the primary determinant of Cl_m for a given drug. For drugs with high (greater than 70%) extraction ratios (eg, lidocaine, propranolol), the Cl_m is considered flow-limited and is directly related to changes in hepatic blood flow. Any condition that decreases blood flow to the liver would reduce Cl_m for these drugs. The Cl_m for drugs with low (less than 20%) extraction ratios (eg, theophylline, phenytoin) is capacity-limited and is more dependent on Cl_{int} of the drug than on hepatic blood flow. Alterations in protein binding or changes in the Cl_{int} due to enzyme induction or liver disease may more greatly affect the Cl_m for this latter group of drugs.[26]

The Cl_{int} is considered to be the actual clearance of a drug if the Cl_m were not limited by protein binding or hepatic blood flow.[37] For most drugs, this clearance is an apparent first-order (linear) process; therefore, any change in dose results in a proportional change in plasma drug concentration (ie, doubling the dose doubles the plasma concentration). However, if the drug metabolizing capacity of the hepatic enzymes is limited (saturable), the clearance may follow nonlinear (Michaelis-Menten) pharmacokinetics. In this case, Cl_m would then proceed at a constant or fixed rate regardless of the dose administered. Therefore, larger doses of a drug have lower time-averaged clearances and longer half-lives when compared to smaller doses. This results in a disproportionate increase in plasma drug concentration with increased doses and the decline in these plasma concentrations can no longer be predicted by equation (6). Phenytoin, salicylates and ethanol are drugs that exhibit significant dose-dependent elimination.

Accumulation with Repetitive Drug Administration.
Upon repetitive dosing, the plasma drug concentration gradually

increases until a plateau or steady-state concentration (C_{ss}) is achieved, where the rate of drug administration equals the rate of elimination. The major determinants of the C_{ss} are the maintenance dose of a drug and the patient's clearance. Approximately 95% of the eventual C_{ss} is attained after administration of a fixed drug dose at a given rate for four times the drug's $t_{1/2}$. Equations (11)–(15) are valid only for drugs that obey linear pharmacokinetics and are adequately described by a one-compartment model. Appropriate dosing regimen equations for drugs that exhibit multi-compartment or nonlinear characteristics can be found elsewhere.[7,8]

If a drug is administered by a constant intravenous infusion, then the plasma drug concentration at steady-state is:

$$C_{ss} = \frac{R_o}{kV_d} = \frac{R_o}{Cl} \tag{11}$$

where R_o is the amount of drug infused per unit time. Therefore, the steady-state concentration is directly proportional to the infusion rate for drugs having first-order elimination. Care must be given to increasing the infusion rate or the multiple dosing regimen of nonlinearly eliminated drugs, since the increase in the steady-state plasma concentration will be more than proportional to the increase in the dosing rate.

If the drug is administered intermittently, the average plasma drug concentration at steady-state ($C_{ss\ av}$) is expressed as:

$$C_{ss\ av} = \frac{F\ D}{k\ V_d\ \tau} = \frac{F\ D}{Cl\ \tau} \tag{12}$$

where τ = dosing interval.

With intermittent drug administration, fluctuations in plasma drug concentrations around $C_{ss\ av}$ occur throughout the dosing interval (Figure 4). The maximum ($C_{ss\ max}$) and minimum ($C_{ss\ min}$) concentrations during a dosing interval at steady-state are calculated by:

$$C_{ss\ max} = \frac{F\ D}{V_d\ (1 - e^{-k\tau})} \tag{13}$$

and

$$C_{ss\ min} = \frac{F\ D\ e^{-k\tau}}{V_d\ (1 - e^{-k\tau})} \tag{14}$$

The extent of these fluctuations can therefore be minimized by decreasing each dose and the dosing interval or reducing the rate of absorption. Adaptation of equations (12)-(14) for use after oral administration requires the inclusion of absorption rate constants and increases their complexity.[7,8]

In certain clinical situations, it may be necessary to quickly attain the plasma drug concentrations that will produce the desired

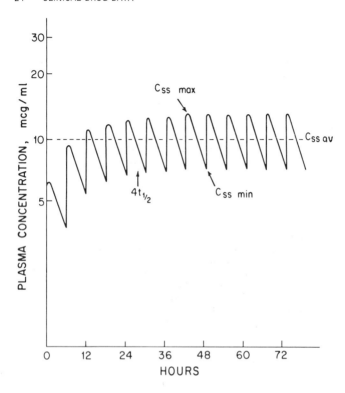

Figure 4. Fluctuations in plasma drug concentrations with intermittent administration of a drug with a $t_{1/2} = 7$ hours.

therapeutic effect. This can be accomplished by the administration of a loading dose (LD):

$$LD = C_{ss} V_d \qquad (15)$$

While administration of this loading dose should produce the
desired concentration, the condition of steady-state is not
achieved because the rate of drug administration does not equal
the rate of drug elimination. Maintenance of this desired plasma
drug concentration requires the selection of an appropriate drug
dose and rate of administration. The importance of the
maintenance dose, rather than the loading dose, in determining
the eventual C_{ss} is readily apparent in Figure 5, where the same
loading and maintenance doses were administered to three patients with markedly different clearances. Several methods that
rapidly predict the maintenance dose required to achieve and sustain a desired steady-state plasma concentration have been pro-

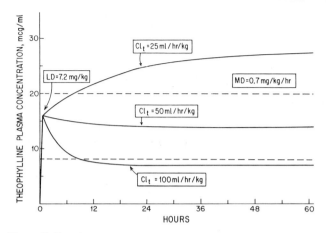

Figure 5. Resultant plasma theophylline concentrations after the administration of a loading dose (LD) = 7.2 mg/kg and a maintenance dose (MD) = 0.7 mg/kg/hr to three patients with differing total body clearances of theophylline.

posed for both continuous infusion[38,39] and intermittent drug administration.[40,41]

Plasma Drug Concentrations. Plasma drug concentrations can improve the ability of the clinician to maximize efficacy and minimize the toxicity of certain drugs by allowing a more precise adjustment of dosing regimens through the calculation of individual patient pharmacokinetic parameters. However, poor correlation between plasma concentrations and therapeutic or toxic effects as well as the restricted availability of accurate assays, limits the clinical application of plasma concentrations for most drugs. Therefore, it is essential that one fully understand the pharmacologic and pharmacokinetic properties of each drug in order to determine whether obtaining plasma concentrations is justified, and if so, how to properly obtain and interpret these concentrations.

Individual drug monographs should be consulted for information that will be helpful in making these decisions. The following section discusses using plasma drug concentrations to determine pharmacokinetic parameters for dosing regimen adjustment in patients with altered drug distribution and/or elimination.

References

1. Gibaldi M. Biopharmaceutics and clinical pharmacokinetics. 3rd ed. Philadelphia: Lea and Febiger, 1984.

2. Benet LZ, Sheiner LB. Design and optimization of dosage regimens: pharmacokinetic data. In: Gilman AG, Goodman LS, Rall TW et al, eds. Goodman and Gilman's The pharmacological basis of therapeutics. 7th ed. New York: Macmillan, 1985:1663-733.

3. Winter ME. Basic clinical pharmacokinetics. San Francisco: Applied Therapeutics, 1980.

4. Rowland M, Tozer TN. Clinical pharmacokinetics: concepts and applications. Philadelphia: Lea and Febiger, 1980.

5. Greenblatt DJ, Koch-Weser J. Clinical pharmacokinetics. N Engl J Med 1975; 294:702-5, 964-70.

6. Atkinson AJ, Kushner W. Clinical pharmacokinetics. Ann Rev Pharmacol Toxicol 1979;19:105-27.

7. Gibaldi M, Perrier D. Pharmacokinetics. 2nd ed. New York: Marcel Dekker, 1982.

8. Wagner JG. Fundamentals of clinical pharmacokinetics. Hamilton, IL: Drug Intelligence Publications, 1975.

9. Schentag JJ, Jusko WJ, Vance JW et al. Gentamicin disposition and tissue accumulation on multiple dosing. J Pharmacokinet Biopharm 1977;5:559-77.

10. Notari RE. Biopharmaceutics and clinical pharmacokinetics: an introduction. 4th ed. New York: Marcel Dekker, 1987:304-10.

11. Sawchuk RJ, Zaske DE. Pharmacokinetics of dosing regimens which utilize multiple intravenous infusions: gentamicin in burn patients. J Pharmacokinet Biopharm 1976;4:183-95.

12. Himmelstein KJ, Lutz RJ. A review of the applications of physiologically based pharmacokinetic modeling. J Pharmacokinet Biopharm 1979;7:127-45.

13. Williams RL, Benet LZ. Drug pharmacokinetics in cardiac and hepatic disease. Ann Rev Pharmacol Toxicol 1980;20:389-413.

14. Toothaker RD, Welling PG. The effect of food on drug bioavailability. Ann Rev Pharmacol Toxicol 1980;20:173-99.

15. Riegelman S, Rowland M. Effect of route of administration on drug disposition. J Pharmacokinet Biopharm 1973;1:419-34.

16. Chodos DJ, DiSanto AR. Basics of bioavailability and description of Upjohn single-dose study design. Kalamazoo, MI: The Upjohn Company, 1974.

17. Deasy PB, Timoney RF, eds. The quality control of medicines. Amsterdam: Elsevier Scientific, 1976.

18. Anon. Holders of approved new drug applications for drugs presenting actual or potential bioequivalence problems. (HEW Publication No. (FDA) 76-3009, June 1976, Revised).

19. Bonora MR, Guaglio R, Terzoni PA. Clinical pharmacokinetics: the pharmacological monitoring of plasmatic levels in therapy. Int J Clin Pharmacol Ther Toxicol 1980;18:73-87.

20. Chiou WL, Huang SM, Huang YC. Mid point back-extrapolation method for the rapid estimation of drugs' volume of distribution and dosage adjustment exhibiting multicompartmental characteristics. Int J Clin Pharmacol Ther Toxicol 1980;18:1-4.

21. Perrier D, Gibaldi M. Relationship between plasma or serum drug concentration and amount of drug in the body at steady state upon multiple dosing. J Pharmacokinet Biopharm 1973;1:17-22.

22. Klotz U. Pathophysiological and disease-induced changes in drug distribution volume: pharmacokinetic implications. Clin Pharmacokinet 1976;1:204-18.

23. Jusko WJ, Gretch M. Plasma and tissue protein binding of drugs in pharmacokinetics. Drug Metab Rev 1976;5:43-140.

24. Koch-Weser J, Sellers EM. Binding of drugs to serum albumin. N Engl J Med 1976;294:311-6, 526-31.

25. Gibaldi M. Drug distribution in renal failure. Am J Med 1977;62:471-4.

26. Blaschke TF. Protein binding and kinetics of drugs in liver diseases. Clin Pharmacokinet 1977;2:32-44.

27. Tillement JP, Lhoste F, Giudicelli JF. Diseases and drug protein binding. Clin Pharmacokinet 1978;3:144-54.

28. Piafsky KM. Disease-induced changes in the plasma binding of basic drugs. Clin Pharmacokinet 1980;5:246-62.

29. Kampmann J, Siersbaek-Nielsen K, Kristensen M et al. Rapid evaluation of creatinine clearance. Acta Med Scand 1974;196:517-20.

30. Cockcroft DW, Gault MH. Prediction of creatinine clearance from serum creatinine. Nephron 1976;16:31-41.

31. Pagliaro LA, Benet LZ. Critical compilation of terminal half-lives, percent excreted unchanged, and changes of half-life in renal and hepatic dysfunction for studies in humans with references. J Pharmacokinet Biopharm 1975;3:333-83.

32. Benowitz NL, Meister W. Pharmacokinetics in patients with cardiac failure. Clin Pharmacokinet 1976;1:389-405.

33. Fabre J, Balant L. Renal failure, drug pharmacokinetics and drug action. Clin Pharmacokinet 1976;1:99-120.

34. du Souich P, McLean AJ, Lalka D et al. Pulmonary disease and drug kinetics. Clin Pharmacokinet 1978;3:257-66.

35. Williams RL, Mamelok RD. Hepatic disease and drug pharmacokinetics. Clin Pharmacokinet 1980;5:528-47.

36. Rowland M, Benet LZ, Graham GG. Clearance concepts in pharmacokinetics. J Pharmacokinet Biopharm 1973;1:123-36.

37. Wilkinson GR, Shand DG. A physiological approach to hepatic drug clearance. Clin Pharmacol Ther 1975;18:377-90.

38. Wagner JG. A safe method for rapidly achieving plasma concentration plateaus. Clin Pharmacol Ther 1974;16:691-700.

39. Zimmerman JJ. Rapid attainment of successively higher steady-state plasma levels using the Wagner two-step infusion method. J Pharm Sci 1978;67:1651-6.

40. Ritschel WA, Erni W. Pharmacokinetic comparison of the one-point method with other methods in predicting steady state drug concentrations in multiple dosing. Int J Clin Pharmacol 1977;15:279-87.

41. Slattery JT, Gibaldi M, Koup JR. Prediction of maintenance dose required to attain a desired drug concentration at steady-state from a single determination of concentration after an initial dose. Clin Pharmacokinet 1980;5:377-85.

Dosing in Renal Impairment

Introduction. Epidemiologic evidence indicates that impaired renal function is a major risk factor in predisposing patients to drug toxicity.[1,2] The primary reason for this relationship is the dependence of many drugs on the kidney for their elimination, with the consequent potential for toxic drug accumulation in the presence of impaired renal function. Careful dosage adjustment can prevent much of this toxicity. Therefore, it is important that practitioners possess a basic understanding of the relationship between drug elimination and renal function, and that they have an ability to make appropriate drug dosage adjustments when managing patients with impaired renal function. This section presents general principles and guidelines which can be applied to drug dosage adjustment in specific patient situations. A general understanding of pharmacokinetic principles is requisite to this discussion—see the preceding section entitled General Principles.

Basic Relationships. The renal clearance (Cl_r) of most drugs closely parallels the glomerular filtration rate (GFR), estimated commonly from creatinine clearance (Cl_{cr}).[3] For drugs eliminated by nonrenal and renal mechanisms, Cl_r should be a product of the ratio of the drug's normal renal clearance to the normal creatinine clearance (R_k), and the creatinine clearance.[4]

$$Cl_r = R_k \times Cl_{cr} \tag{1}$$

The contribution of Cl_r to the total body clearance (Cl_t) of a drug is:

$$Cl_t = Cl_m + R_k \times Cl_{cr} \tag{2}$$

where Cl_m is the nonrenal metabolic clearance of the drug. The effect of a change in renal function, as reflected in a change in Cl_{cr}, on the Cl_t of a drug can be estimated from equation (2). In general, proper dosage adjustment in renal impairment should be to reduce the rate of drug administration in proportion to the decrease in Cl_t from normal. This would maintain the usual average plasma drug level, assuming that bioavailability and Cl_m are unchanged.

These basic concepts have been explored by many investigators in an attempt to develop guidelines for drug dosing in renal impairment. Work in this area has produced three basic approaches: (1) general drug nomograms, (2) drug-specific nomograms and (3) individualized pharmacokinetic analyses. The dosage modification schemes that have been derived from each of these approaches have distinct advantages and disadvantages which must be considered in applying them to specific patients.

General Nomograms. The simplest approach to dosage adjustment in renal impairment utilizes the basic relationship between drug elimination and renal function shown in equation (2). Tozer,[4,5] Dettli[6] and others[7] have used this relationship to develop methods which may be applied to drugs for which there is appropriate basic pharmacokinetic information. If the fraction of the systemically available dose which is excreted unchanged (f_e) for a given drug and the fraction of normal renal function in a given patient are known, modification of the dosage regimen to produce normal plasma levels in renal impairment can be made using the nomogram and equations at the end of the section (Figure 1). The accuracy and usefulness of general nomograms is limited, however, because of the stringent assumptions upon which they are based.[8]

Drug-Specific Nomograms. In recent years, a growing number of drug-specific nomograms have become available. These nomograms are based on studies of the elimination of a particular drug in subjects with varying degrees of renal function. They attempt to describe the relationship between drug elimination in the study population and measures of renal function by means of a mathematical equation or graphical representation. For many drugs, a wide variety of dosage modification schemes have been proposed, and considerable debate exists with regard to their relative merits. Some of the differences can be attributed to methodologic variables and errors in study design and implementation; others are the result of limitations inherent in using nomograms for drug dosing. These factors, which should be considered when evaluating or applying dosing nomograms, are discussed below.

Methodologic Variables and Errors.
1. *Patients of varying age, sex, body build and underlying disease state are commonly used as subjects.* These variables produce wide fluctuations in drug elimination which are not necessarily due to changes in renal function. Also, some measures of renal function (especially Cr_s and BUN) are significantly affected by these nonrenal variables, and many studies using serum creatinine (Cr_s) or BUN do not note or attempt to compensate for this variability. The net result is that the predictive accuracy of these nomograms is greatly reduced.

2. *Some study populations are largely composed of people with essentially normal renal function.* Relationships derived from these populations predict most accurately in patients with near normal renal function. Application of such relationships should not, however, be overextended to patients with severely impaired renal function.

3. *Pharmacokinetic parameters may be determined unscientifically.* Frequently, methods used to determine parameters such as the elimination rate constant (k) or $t_{1/2}$ are not adequately documented (eg, time of obtaining blood samples relative to dosing) or are incorrect and inaccurate (eg, poor assay, improper timing of plasma level determinations, oversimplification of compartmental kinetics).

4. *Statistical evaluations of the significance of the results do not adequately reflect clinical implications.* Despite statistically significant correlation between measured drug concentrations and those predicted by a nomogram, close examination of data (if available) frequently reveals some potentially serious discrepan-

cies between the individual values and those which the nomogram would predict.

Limitations of Nomograms.

1. They are only gross estimates. Even with drugs that are nearly 100% renally eliminated by glomerular filtration (eg, gentamicin, vancomycin), the half-life in individuals with apparently identical renal function can still vary greatly. Also, some subgroups of patients (eg, burn patients) may vary greatly from the relationships found in the nomogram population.[9,29] Even with the most precise pharmacokinetic estimates, the expected relationship between renal function and drug elimination is not always adequate. Therefore, predictability is not good enough to prevent occasional important errors.

2. The errors involved in using nomograms are cumulative. The use of a nomogram for a day or two while waiting for specific plasma drug concentration results is not likely to cause complications, despite some expected errors in prediction. An estimated half-life of 48 hr for a drug which actually has a 60 hr half-life would ultimately result in a 20% overdosage. However, the full expression of this error would not occur for 10-12 days (4-5 half-lives). Errors involving drugs with shorter half-lives would become manifest much sooner.

3. They should not be used in patients with variable renal function. Nomograms based on Cr_s as the measure of renal function are especially susceptible to errors, because Cr_s continues to rise for many days following an acute, drastic decrease in renal function.[10] Frequent plasma drug level determinations are the safest guide to drug dosing in patients with variable renal function.[11]

4. They cannot be used accurately in patients undergoing dialysis. The dialysis of most drugs has not been studied extensively enough to predict the amount of drug which must be given to replace that removed by dialysis. With hemodialysis, the amount of drug removed may vary greatly, depending on the particular dialysis apparatus and techniques used—see the following section entitled Dialysis of Drugs. Consequently, great care should be taken in interpreting published recommendations in this area.

5. Dosage recommendations vary widely for the same drug. Few prospective clinical evaluations of nomograms have been published (see references 12 and 13). However, theoretical interpretations have been conducted which demonstrate clinically important differences between nomogram dosage recommendations for some agents.[8,14,15]

6. In some cases their dosage recommendations may not be suitable. This is most likely to be the case when intermittently dosed drugs with narrow therapeutic indices (eg, gentamicin) are used in patients with severely impaired renal function. Nomograms which recommend dosage reductions by dosing interval extension only may result in dangerously prolonged periods of subtherapeutic plasma concentrations. Nomograms which recommend dosage reductions by individual dose reduction only may result in such minute peak plasma drug levels that optimal therapeutic concentrations may not be reached or maintained long enough.[5, 8, 14]

7. Generally, there has been little or no development of nomograms for use in women or children.

Compiled Dosing Guidelines. Several authors have developed extensive compilations of guidelines for dosing a wide variety of drugs in patients with renal impairment.[16, 17] These recommendations are usually derived from drug-specific nomograms or other general data regarding the elimination of the particular drugs. Usually, the guidelines are presented in tabular form with the specific dosage adjustments classified by broad ranges of renal function. Because of the breadth of these categories, these guidelines may not be as accurate as the nomograms from which they are derived. Also, the data on which these guidelines are based should be examined to determine if they were collected in patients or subjects with physical characteristics similar to those of the patient in question.[8]

Developing Individual Pharmacokinetic Parameters. Specific pharmacokinetic parameters can be determined for individual patients using properly drawn blood samples, accurate and specific assay techniques and general pharmacokinetic principles. These parameters can then be used to calculate dosage adjustments. There are many methods by which this could be accomplished. A relatively simple method is suggested for intermittently administered drugs.

1. Give initial dose(s) as suggested by the best available data.

2. Following any dose, draw one sample at the estimated time of peak plasma concentration (C_{max}).

3. Draw a second sample immediately before the next dose (C_{min}) *(if not at steady-state,* a sample immediately *before* the previous dose must be used as the C_{min} for the calculation of V_d). Note: if C_{min} is less than the lower limits of assay sensitivity, an alternative procedure must be used (see references 18 and 19).

4. Calculate V_d from the equation:

$$V_d = \frac{F\,D}{C_{max} - C_{min}} \qquad (3)$$

where $C_{max} - C_{min}$ equals the change in plasma levels due to the dose administered, D and F, the fraction absorbed (bioavailability). If V_d is being calculated from the first dose, $C_{min} = 0$.

5. Calculate k from the equation:

$$k = \frac{\ln C_{max} - \ln C_{min}}{t} \qquad (4)$$

where t is the time interval between C_{max} and C_{min}.

6. Select the desired maximum and minimum plasma drug concentrations. Select a reasonable dosing interval, τ. For instance, if the desired minimum plasma concentration is one-half of the maximum, then select an interval equal to $t_{1/2}$, as calculated from k. Calculate the new maintenance dose, D, from the following:

$$D = V_d (C_{max} - C_{min}) \qquad (5)$$

Note that these calculations are suitable only for rapidly and completely absorbed parenteral or oral drugs exhibiting first-order kinetics which can be described satisfactorily by a one-compartment model (or a two-compartment model drug having, at most, a small, rapid disposition phase), given rapidly relative to elimination. More complex kinetic models should be used when indicated (see reference 18).

Unified Approach. Based on the foregoing discussion, a unified, stepwise approach to the dosing of drugs in patients with impaired renal function can be synthesized.

STEP I. CONSIDER THE PATIENT

1. To what extent is renal function impaired? Accurately assessing renal function can be very difficult. Potential inaccuracies exist with all measures of renal function. An accurately timed and collected Cl_{cr} is probably the best available assessment of renal function. However, the use of formulas and nomograms can *approximate* Cl_{cr} from Cr_s. Formulas to rapidly estimate the Cl_{cr} are presented in Chapter 1. Formulas and nomograms for estimating creatinine clearance should be applied with careful consideration of their limitations.[8]

2. Is renal function unstable? Cr_s and Cl_{cr} determinations are not reliable indicators during drastic fluctuations in renal function.[10] In this case, plasma drug concentrations should be measured, if possible, to accurately guide dosing.

3. Is the patient to be dialyzed? If so, by what method, for what duration and at what intervals? (See the following section Dialysis of Drugs).

4. Are there any other patient factors which may alter the absorption, distribution, elimination or response to the drug? For example, it is well known that the status of the cardiovascular system and liver may greatly alter the absorption, distribution or elimination of many drugs.[20-22] Also, patients with renal failure may be unusually sensitive to some agents.[23]

STEP II. CONSIDER THE DRUG

1. Are specific and accurate dosing recommendations available? If such recommendations are available and appear to be soundly developed (see *Methodologic Variables and Errors*), they should be used with due regard for their inherent limitations (see *Limitations of Nomograms*).

2. If no such recommendations are available, what are the known relevant pharmacokinetic characteristics of the drug?
    a. To what extent is absorbed drug excreted unchanged in the

urine (f_e)? From these data and the patient's renal function, the nomogram (Figure 1) may be used to calculate an approximate adjustment. However, the points below must also be considered.

b. *What is the therapeutic index of the drug?* Drugs which have a very low toxic potential or wide therapeutic index (eg, penicillin G) may require little or no dosage adjustment despite expected accumulation with impaired renal function. Conversely, drugs possessing a high potential for toxicity or a narrow therapeutic index (eg, gentamicin) must be adjusted carefully if they are largely excreted by the kidneys.

c. *Are any active or toxic metabolites renally eliminated? If so, what are their therapeutic indices?* For most drugs this information is not available. However, for some drugs (eg, procainamide) this is an important consideration.[24]

d. *What is the site of action of the drug? Does impaired renal function change the ability of the drug to reach this site?* As an example, methenamine salts and nitrofurantoin are therapeutically active only in the urinary tract. In the presence of moderate to severe renal impairment they do not achieve therapeutic levels at this site and are ineffective. Also, extrarenal toxicity may occur due to accumulation of such drugs in the body. Dosage adjustments may prevent the latter occurrence, but further decrease urinary tract levels. Consequently, these drugs are contraindicated in moderate to severe renal impairment.

e. *If the patient is to undergo dialysis, to what extent is the drug removed by this procedure?* See previous comments under *Limitations of Nomograms* and the following section Dialysis of Drugs.

f. *Does the elimination of the drug obey first order kinetics? Do absorption, distribution, protein binding and metabolism remain generally constant with changing renal function?* If these questions cannot be answered affirmatively, the Figure 1 dosing nomogram cannot be used with confidence, and other nomograms should be examined to determine if these kinetic parameters have been taken into account. There are many drugs which do not exhibit simple, first-order kinetic behavior and whose distribution and metabolism are altered in patients with renal function impairment (eg, phenytoin).[21,23,25,26] When using such drugs, plasma level determinations are the only safe guide to accurate dosing. Without plasma level determinations, such drugs can only be used with careful monitoring for signs of toxicity or subtherapeutic response.

STEP III. CONSIDER THE ADJUSTMENT

1. *Consider the loading dose.* For most agents, a change in loading dose is unnecessary in the presence of renal impairment. However, for some agents renal impairment may alter the apparent volume of distribution, requiring a change in the loading and maintenance doses.[27] Also, some drugs with normally short

half-lives, which are usually administered without a loading dose, may require a loading dose in the presence of severe renal impairment in order to quickly attain therapeutic levels (eg, carbenicillin, ticarcillin). With these drugs, reduced elimination necessitates the use of smaller maintenance doses to avoid toxic drug accumulation; however, a loading dose equal to the usual therapeutic dose may be advisable to achieve more rapid therapeutic levels.[28]

2. Choose practical, convenient doses and administration schedules. Consider available dosage form sizes (especially with capsules) and usual administration schedules for drugs. Odd doses and schedules may lead to errors in administration and unnecessary inconvenience. Round-off adjustments within reasonable limits (eg, give 60 mg instead of 58 or 62 mg of gentamicin, every 24 hr instead of 23 or 25 hr).

3. Use available nomograms in a flexible way to suit the situation. For intermittently dosed drugs, the choice between decreasing the individual dose or increasing the dosing interval is largely a theoretical one. However, with severely impaired renal function it may be wise to use some combination of these adjustments to achieve the same decrease in administration rate (D / τ) without the potential risks involved in making either adjustment alone.[14] Thus, a nomogram which adjusts a dosage regimen by recommending a decrease in individual dose can be reinterpreted to increase the dosing interval, or to alter the combined administration rate, in order to achieve the same adjustment factor.

4. Measure plasma drug concentrations when indicated. Plasma level determinations are indicated when they are known to be reliable indicators of potential subtherapeutic or toxic effects and when:
   a. Patients have fluctuating renal function.
   b. Patients are to undergo dialysis.
   c. Suitable specific dosage nomograms are being used for extended periods, especially with more toxic agents.
   d. Suitable specific nomograms are not available and a general pharmacokinetic nomogram is being used (eg, Figure 1), especially for drugs having poorly characterized kinetics.
   e. The drug has nonlinear or unpredictable kinetics.

5. Above all, closely monitor the clinical status of the patient with renal impairment. Even the best nomograms and pharmacokinetic calculations occasionally produce serious errors in dosing, due to inherent limitations in predictability and changes in patient status. Careful observation for signs of drug toxicity or suboptimal response is imperative.

Summary. To use drugs safely in patients with impaired renal function, the following approach should be considered:
1. Evaluate the patient carefully, characterizing renal function accurately and noting any other patient factors which may affect absorption, distribution, elimination or efficacy.

2. Choose the best available drug dosing guidelines and use them within their known limitations.
   a. Carefully prepared drug-specific nomograms should be used as initial guides to dosing, if available.
   b. A general nomogram (eg, see Figure 1 and references 5 and 6) should be used if a specific nomogram is not available and the drug in question meets the restrictions imposed on the use of such nomograms.

3. Plasma drug levels should be measured when indicated, to guide dosing.

4. The patient should be closely monitored for any signs of toxicity or subtherapeutic response.

The references for this section follow on page 35.

Figure 1. Estimation of Dosage Regimens in Patients with Renal Function Impairment[a] *

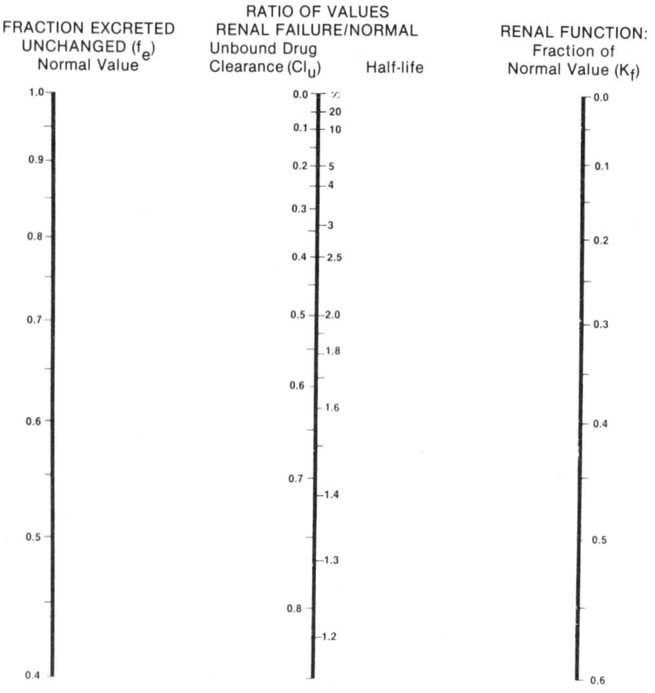

| FRACTION EXCRETED UNCHANGED (f_e) Normal Value | RATIO OF VALUES RENAL FAILURE/NORMAL Unbound Drug Clearance (Cl_u)   Half-life | RENAL FUNCTION: Fraction of Normal Value (K_f) |

a. From Rowland M, Tozer TN. Clinical pharmacokinetics: concepts and applications. Philadelphia: Lea & Febiger, 1980, reproduced with permission. To be used to determine how to change a normal dosage regimen. The normal dosage regimen depends upon age, weight, and condition being treated.
*For Conditions for Use of Nomogram, How to Use Nomogram, and Modification of Dosage Regimen, see page 35.

Conditions for Use of Nomogram (Figure 1)

*NOTE: this nomogram should be used only if the following conditions are met:

1. Metabolites are inactive and nontoxic.
2. Individual variation in metabolism or response are not significant.
3. Altered protein binding, metabolism or distribution do not occur.
4. Cardiac output, hepatic function and all other physiologic factors which might affect absorption or distribution are normal.
5. Renal function is reasonably constant.
6. Pharmacokinetics of the drug are linear.
7. The renal clearance of the drug is proportional to creatinine clearance.

How to use nomogram: *With a ruler, connect the fraction of drug normally excreted unchanged and the patient's kidney function, expressed as a fraction of normal value in a person of the same age. Read off from the center line the clearance of unbound drug (Cl_U) and the half-life relative to their normal values in a patient of the same age.*

Modification of Dosage Regimen

I. Initial dose–no change (see text)
II. Adjustment of rate of administration for maintenance of drug in body.

A. Change in dosing interval, τ, only

$$\tau \text{ (failure)} = \frac{t_{1/2} \text{ (failure)}}{t_{1/2} \text{ (normal)}} \times \tau \text{ (normal)}$$

B. Change in maintenance dose, D, only.

$$D \text{ (failure)} = \frac{Cl_U \text{ (failure)}}{Cl_U \text{ (normal)}} \times D \text{ (normal)}$$

C. Change in rate of administration D / τ

$$(D / \tau) \text{ (failure)} = \frac{Cl_U \text{ (failure)}}{Cl_U \text{ (normal)}} \times [(D / \tau) \text{ (normal)}]$$

References

1. Smith JW, Seidl LG, Cluff LE. Studies on the epidemiology of adverse drug reactions: V. clinical factors affecting susceptibility. Ann Intern Med 1966;65:629-40.

2. Jick H. Adverse drug effects in relation to renal function. Am J Med 1977;62:514-7.

3. Rowland M. Drug administration and regimens. In: Melmon KL, Morrelli HF, eds. Clinical pharmacology: basic principles in therapeutics. New York: Macmillan, 1978:25-70.

4. Tozer TN. Nomogram for modification of dosage regimens in patients with chronic renal function impairment. J Pharmacokinet Biopharm 1974;2:13-28.

5. Rowland M, Tozer TN. Clinical pharmacokinetics: concepts and applications. Philadelphia: Lea & Febiger, 1980.

6. Dettli L. Drug dosage in renal disease. In: Gibaldi M, Prescott L, eds. Handbook of clinical pharmacokinetics. New York: ADIS Health Science Press, 1983: 261-76.

7. Bryan CS, Stone WJ. Antimicrobial dosage in renal failure: a unifying nomogram. Clin Nephrol 1977;7:81-4.

8. Chennavasin P, Brater DC. Nomograms for drug use in renal disease. Clin Pharmacokinet 1981;6:193-214.

9. Sawchuk RJ. Drug absorption and disposition in burn patients. In: Benet LZ, Massoud N, Gambertoglio JG, eds. Pharmacokinetic basis for drug treatment. New York: Raven Press, 1984:333-48.

10. Bjornsson TD. Use of serum creatinine concentrations to determine renal function. In: Gibaldi M, Prescott L, eds. Handbook of clinical pharmacokinetics. New York: ADIS Health Science Press, 1983:277-300.

11. Koch-Weser J. Serum drug concentrations in clinical perspective. Ther Drug Monit 1981;3:3-16.

12. Michelson PA, Miller WA, Warner JF et al. Multiple dose pharmacokinetics of gentamicin in man: evaluation of the Jelliffe nomogram and the adjustment of dosage in patients with renal impairment. In: Benet LZ, ed. The effect of disease states on drug pharmacokinetics. Washington: APhA Academy of Pharmaceutical Sciences, 1976, 207-43.

13. Chow M, Deglin J, Harralson A et al. Prediction of gentamicin serum levels using a 1-compartment open linear pharmacokinetic model. Am J Hosp Pharm 1978;35:1078-81.

14. Schumacher GE. Pharmacokinetic analysis of gentamicin dosage regimens recommended for renal impairment. J Clin Pharmacol 1975;15:656-65.

15. Matzke GR, Kovarik JM, Rybak MJ et al. Evaluation of the vancomycin-clearance: creatinine-clearance relationship for predicting vancomycin dosage. Clin Pharm 1985;4:311-5.

16. Bennett WM, Aronoff GR, Morrison G et al. Drug prescribing in renal failure: dosing guidelines for adults. Am J Kidney Dis 1983;3:155-93.

17. Cheigh JS. Drug administration in renal failure. Am J Med 1977;62:555-63.

18. Wagner, JG. Fundamentals of clinical pharmacokinetics. Hamilton, IL: Drug Intelligence Publications, 1976.

19. Schumacher GE. Choosing optimal sampling times for therapeutic drug monitoring. Clin Pharm 1985;4:84-92.

20. Williams RL, Benet LZ. Drug pharmacokinetics in cardiac and hepatic disease. Annual Rev Pharmacol Toxicol 1980;20:389-413.

21. Tozer TN. Implications of altered plasma protein binding in disease states. In: Benet LZ, Massoud N, Gamber-toglio JG, eds. Pharmacokinetic basis for drug treatment. New York: Raven Press, 1984:173-93.

22. Wilkinson GR, Branch RA. Effects of hepatic disease on clinical pharmacokinetics. In: Benet LZ, Massoud N, Gambertoglio JG, eds. Pharmacokinetic basis for drug treatment. New York: Raven Press, 1984:49-61.

23. Bennett WM. Drug prescribing in renal failure. Drugs 1979;17:111-23.

24. Drayer DE. Pharmacologically active drug metabolites: therapeutic and toxic activities, plasma and urine data in man, accumulation in renal failure. In: Gibaldi M, Prescott L, eds. Handbook of clinical pharmacokinetics. New York: Raven Press, 1983:114-32.

25. Bennett WM, Porter GA, Bagby SP et al. Drugs and renal disease. New York: Churchill Livingstone, 1978.

26. Reidenberg MM, Drayer DE. Drug therapy in renal failure. Annual Rev Pharmacol Toxicol 1980;20:45-54.

27. Gibaldi M. Drug distribution in renal failure. Am J Med 1977;62:471-4.

28. Latos DL, Bryan CS, Stone WJ. Carbenicillin therapy in patients with normal and impaired renal function. Clin Pharmacol Ther 1975;17:692-700.

29. Michael KA, Mohler JL, Blouin RA et al. Failure of creatinine clearance to predict gentamicin half-life in a renal transplant patient with diabetes mellitus. Clin Pharm 1985;4:572-5.

Dialysis of Drugs

OVER THE PAST SEVERAL YEARS, dialysis has become an important therapeutic approach in the treatment of renal failure. It is estimated that approximately 50,000 patients with chronic renal failure are undergoing dialysis. This is primarily in the form of hemodialysis, although an increasing number are now receiving chronic peritoneal dialysis. It has been shown that patients on chronic dialysis receive an average of 8 drugs for a variety of medical indications.[1] Although the purpose of dialysis is to remove unwanted toxic waste products from the body, it also has the effect of removing drugs as well. Thus, it is important to know to what extent drugs administered for therapeutic purposes are removed, as it may affect the patient's therapy. Supplemental doses or a revised dosage regimen may be required under these circumstances.

Dialysis procedures, including hemoperfusion, have also been used in the drug overdose situation as a means of eliminating drug from the body. It is, therefore, important to know how effective these procedures are and whether they offer any substantial advantage over conventional means of treating drug overdoses.

The purpose of this chapter is first, to review various factors involved in assessing the removal of drugs by dialysis and second, to illustrate how the use of pharmacokinetic information can help predict the extent of this removal. This information can be especially useful for drugs whose dialyzability has not been determined. Additionally, the accompanying table lists the effect of hemodialysis, peritoneal dialysis and hemoperfusion on the removal of specific drugs for which information is available.

Methodologic Problems. Several problems are encountered in attempting to assess the removal of drugs by dialysis. The literature is generally anecdotal for many drugs. This is primarily true in the overdose setting in which the effect of dialysis on drug removal is determined by clinical response alone. For example, a comatose patient awakens during or shortly after dialysis and it is assumed that dialysis removed the drug, accounting for the improved clinical status. The amount of drug ingested and/or the amount of drug recovered in the dialysate are often unknown. The type of dialysis system employed is frequently not specified; this is of importance when comparing the system you are using with published data. Also, there is a general lack of patient data, such as weight, hematocrit, renal and liver function. The method used to calculate drug clearance is commonly unspecified. For example, was it determined from the amount of drug recovered in the dialysate or from differences in arterial and venous plasma concentrations across the dialyzer? A more detailed discussion of the proper method for clearance calculations in hemodialysis is described in reference 2.

A common error is misinterpretation of plasma drug concentrations obtained before and after dialysis. A declining plasma level during dialysis is often believed to be the result of the dialysis procedure. However, a declining level could be due to drug elimination by metabolism or renal excretion, and the contribution of dialysis to this decline may be very small. The situation in which drug concentrations are relatively unchanged during dialysis usually means that little or no drug is being removed by dialysis. However, it is possible that the drug is continually being absorbed from the GI tract, as in the delayed and prolonged absorption of drugs observed in overdose cases. Another problem is that of interpreting drug removal rate by dialysis. It has been assumed by some that if 200 mg of a drug were removed in the first hour of dialysis, that five hours of dialysis would remove five times as much (ie, 1000 mg). This is incorrect, because drug removal by dialysis occurs by a first-order process, so that as the amount of drug in the body declines, so does its removal rate. Thus, the total amount removed is less than that calculated from the initial estimates.

For many drugs, there is a lack of correlation between plasma drug concentrations and clinical response. Some drugs have been found to have active or toxic metabolites which correlate well with the toxic effects of the drug. For example, the toxicity of glutethimide is primarily due to an active metabolite, 4-hydroxy-2-ethyl-2-phenylglutarimide. Thus, in attempting to collect information on the dialysis removal of drugs, attention must be given to metabolites as well. A final point relative to the overdose situation is that the pharmacokinetic disposition of a drug may be altered. In making predictions of drug dialyzability, pharmacokinetic data are usually derived from healthy subjects. However, during an overdose, there may be changes in drug metabolism, apparent volume of distribution (V_d) or protein binding. For example, with large amounts of drug in the body, saturation of plasma protein binding may occur, which could alter drug distribution and metabolism. The potential for these changes must be considered.

Pharmacokinetic Factors. There are certain properties of a drug which can be used to make some predictions about drug dialyzability.[3,4] Drugs with a small molecular weight, usually less than 500, cross dialysis membranes readily. Large molecular weight drugs, such as vancomycin (MW 1800) and amphotericin B (MW 960) cross membranes only with difficulty, and thus are not effectively removed by hemodialysis or peritoneal dialysis. However, molecular weight is not a limitation for hemoperfusion techniques where the drug is adsorbed onto a high surface area material.

Drugs with greater water solubility are more easily removed to the aqueous dialysate than more lipid-soluble compounds. In addition, the latter usually have larger volumes of distribution compared to more water-soluble drugs. A large V_d, such as that of digoxin (approximately 500 L), impairs the ability of dialysis to remove a drug from the body. Because the majority of drug is contained in tissue compartments rather than in the blood, it is not accessible for removal. The effect of a large V_d limits the use of hemoperfusion as well.[5] Hemoperfusion may rapidly clear the blood compartment of a drug (evidenced by a dramatic decrease in plasma level); however, once hemoperfusion has ended, plasma drug concentrations can increase as a result of re-equilibration of drug from tissue stores.

Plasma protein binding of a drug also determines how effectively it can be dialyzed. Drugs with a high degree of protein binding, for example propranolol (90–94%) and warfarin (99%), are not significantly removed by dialysis, because the drug-protein complex is too large to cross the dialysis membrane. This is not a limitation of hemoperfusion, because the drug is removed from plasma proteins as the complex passes through the high surface area adsorbent material.[5]

The clearance of a drug by dialysis can be compared to the clearance of the drug by the body. Clearance terms are additive; therefore, the following equation applies:

$$Cl_{TD} = Cl_T + Cl_D$$

where, Cl_{TD} = total body clearance of drug during dialysis
$\quad\quad\; Cl_T$ = total body clearance of drug
$\quad\quad\; Cl_D$ = dialysis clearance of drug.

Thus, if dialysis clearance adds substantially to body clearance, forming a much larger total clearance, then the drug will be eliminated that much faster. For example, if the dialysis clearance of a drug were 50 ml/min and the body clearance were 50 ml/min, then the drug would be eliminated from the body twice as fast during the dialysis period. In order to relate clearance to drug half-life ($t_{1/2}$), the following equations are useful:

$$t_{1/2} = \frac{0.693}{Cl_T} \times V_d \quad\quad \text{(off dialysis)}$$

and

$$t_{1/2} = \frac{0.693}{Cl_T + Cl_D} \times V_d \quad\quad \text{(on dialysis)}$$

Thus, the greater the dialysis clearance adds to the body's clearance, the shorter the drug $t_{1/2}$ will be on dialysis (assuming V_d remains constant). A further extension of this gives the following equation:

$$\text{Fraction Lost During a Dialysis Period} = 1 - e^{-(Cl_T + Cl_D)(\tau/V_d)}$$

where τ is the duration of the dialysis.

This allows calculation of the fraction of drug in the body that is lost during a dialysis period by all routes of elimination (ie, dialysis, metabolism and renal excretion). Thus, it is necessary to acquire from literature sources (keeping in mind the limitations discussed previously) values for V_d, Cl_T and Cl_D. If renal or liver function are diminished, this must be taken into consideration. In addition, changes in V_d in certain disease states (eg, the decreased V_d of digoxin in renal failure) must also be taken into account.

Clearance data are not always available in the literature. Many authors often report only the half-lives of the drugs, on and off dialysis. The following equation may be used to estimate the fraction of drug removed by dialysis alone utilizing half-life data:[7]

$$f = \frac{t_{1/2(off)} - t_{1/2(on)}}{t_{1/2(off)}} \times (1 - e^{[-0.693/t_{1/2(on)}] \times \tau})$$

where, f = fraction of drug removed by dialysis
$t_{1/2(on)}$ = half-life on dialysis
$t_{1/2(off)}$ = half-life off dialysis
τ = duration of dialysis.

The assumptions made when using this equation are as follows:

1. All drug elimination (including dialysis removal) occurs by first-order processes.
2. Dialysis is initiated after the completion of absorption and distribution phases.

The primary limitation of this equation is that inaccurate values of half-lives result in incorrect estimates of drug removal by dialysis. It is important to note the duration of dialysis in relation to the estimate of $t_{1/2(on)}$. For example, if the $t_{1/2(on)}$ were reported as 24 hours, but the dialysis duration was only 4 hours, the half-life value is probably not accurate. On the other hand, if the $t_{1/2(on)}$ were reported as 1 hour during a 4-hour dialysis period, the half-life value might be more reliable.

Two examples illustrate the use of pharmacokinetic data to calculate drug clearance during dialysis. Phenobarbital has a volume of distribution of approximately 50 L, a total body clearance of 5 ml/min and a hemodialysis clearance of 70 ml/min. The half-life off dialysis is 115 hours and would decrease to 8 hours with dialysis. Thus, approximately 50% of the drug would be removed from the body during 8 hours of dialysis. As another example, digoxin has a V_d of about 300 L and a Cl_T of 40 ml/min in an anephric patient. The hemodialysis clearance of digoxin is 20 ml/min. Therefore, the half-life of digoxin in this patient off dialysis is 86 hours, while on dialysis it declines to 58 hours. Although this appears to be a substantial decrease in half-life, it means that the patient would have to be dialyzed 58 hours continuously in order to remove half the digoxin in the body. The fraction of drug lost during a routine hemodialysis period of 4 hours would be only 5%. Thus, a supplemental dose of digoxin following hemodialysis is not warranted.

Use of the Table. The table which follows should be consulted for data on specific drugs. For each drug, a qualitative statement of the range of drug removal by dialysis was derived using pharmacokinetic parameters taken from the literature. The ranges used include: "not dialyzed, 0–5% removed;" "slightly dialyzed, 5–20% removed;" "moderately dialyzed, 20–50% removed;" or "dialyzed, 50–100% removed," each of which describes the extent of removal using the three techniques. Drug removal is intentionally described in a qualitative fashion for a number of reasons. First, much of this information changes quite rapidly (eg, as new dialysis and hemoperfusion techniques are developed). Secondly, a given value for the amount of drug removed or the dialysis clearance determined in one study may be different from that found in another study, due to differences in dialysate or blood flow during dialysis, or the duration of the dialysis. The usual duration of dialysis has changed since earlier studies. Most hemodialysis runs are 4 to 5 hours as compared with 6-hour runs used in the past. Also, data on the amount of drug removed by peritoneal dialysis vary, because estimates of removal were determined from the literature in which both constant dialysis for long periods of time (such as in an overdose situation) or by intermittent dialysis for shorter periods each day were used. Data on hemoperfusion vary depending on such factors as the type of adsorbent material, blood flow through the adsorbent and duration of perfusion. This technique for drug removal is generally recommended and used after conservative management of drug overdose has failed. In addition, the table contains comments for clarification of certain points and selected references are provided for more specific information.

The following abbreviations are used in the table beginning on page 41:

D — Dialyzed (50–100%)	ND — Not Dialyzed (0–5%)
HD — Hemodialysis	PD — Peritoneal Dialysis
MD — Moderately Dialyzed (20–50%)	SD — Slightly Dialyzed (5–20%)

Dialysis of Drugs

DRUG	HEMO-DIALYSIS	PERITONEAL DIALYSIS	HEMO-PERFUSION	COMMENTS	REFERENCES
Acetaminophen	MD	ND	MD	No studies demonstrate HD or hemoperfusion (charcoal) decrease or prevent hepatic or renal toxicity; PD ineffective in removing drug—one case reported.	14-18
Acetazolamide	MD			Data from single case study.	19
Acetohexamide		ND		Active metabolite also not dialyzed.	20
Acyclovir	D			One-half usual dose post-HD.	21,22
Allopurinol				No data available.	
Amantadine	SD	SD			23,24
Amdinocillin	MD-D	SD		One-half to usual dose post-HD.	25,26
Amikacin	D	MD		Dialyzable to the same extent as other aminoglycosides; 50-70% of the loading dose may be given post-dialysis; plasma concentrations should be used as a guide to dosing.	28-30
Amoxicillin	MD			Supplemental post-dialysis dose may be warranted—see reference 32.	31,32
Amphotericin B	ND				33,34
Ampicillin	MD	ND		Supplemental post-dialysis dose may be warranted—see reference 35.	16,35-37
Aspirin	D	D	D	Charcoal may be more effective than resin for hemoperfusion.	38,39
Atenolol	MD				27
Azathioprine	SD-MD				40
Azlocillin	MD			1-2 g dose post-HD.	41 Continued

Dialysis of Drugs

DRUG	HEMO-DIALYSIS	PERITONEAL DIALYSIS	HEMO-PERFUSION	COMMENTS	REFERENCES
Aztreonam	MD	SD		One-half usual dose post-HD.	42,43
Bretylium	MD				49
Captopril	MD				50
Carbamazepine			MD	Insufficient data.	225
Carbenicillin	MD				51-55
Cefaclor	MD			See Cefazolin.	56,57
Cefamandole	MD			See Cefazolin.	58-61
Cefazolin	MD	SD		Maintenance dose after dialysis may be necessary.	62-67
Cefonicid	SD				68
Cefoperazone	SD	ND			69,70
Cefonanide	MD			1-1.5 g post-HD (insufficient data).	71
Cefotaxime	MD	SD		One-half usual dose post-HD.	72-74
Desacetylcefotaxime (active metabolite)	MD	SD			
Cefotetan	SD			Insufficient data.	75
Cefoxitin	MD	SD		One-half usual dose post-HD.	76,77
Cefsulodin	D			One-half usual dose post-HD.	78
Ceftazidime	D	SD		One-half usual dose post-HD.	79-81
Ceftizoxime	MD	SD		One-half usual dose post-HD.	82-84
Ceftriaxone	ND				85
Cefuroxime	MD	SD		Supplemental post-HD dose is warranted.	86,87,226,227

Continued

Dialysis of Drugs

DRUG	HEMO-DIALYSIS	PERITONEAL DIALYSIS	HEMO-PERFUSION	COMMENTS	REFERENCES
Cephalexin	MD	SD		Usual dose post-HD.	88,89
Cephalothin	MD			See Cefazolin.	90
Chloral Hydrate	D			Data are for the trichloroethanol active metabolite.	91,92
Chloramphenicol	SD	ND			93-95
Chlordiazepoxide	ND-SD			Active metabolites.	38,48,96
Chlorpropamide		ND		Single case of PD did not decrease plasma chlorpropamide levels; high protein binding limits its dialyzability.	97
Cimetidine	SD	SD	SD-MD	Supplemental doses after dialysis appear unnecessary; coincide doses around dialysis; PD studied in only 2 patients.	98-107
Ciprofloxacin	SD				229
Clavulanic Acid	D				108
Clindamycin	ND	ND		Insufficient data.	109-111
Clonidine	ND				112,113
Cloxacillin	ND				51
Colchicine	ND			Insufficient data.	114
Cyclosphosphamide	MD				115
Diazepam	ND				48,116
Dicloxacillin	ND				48,117,118
Digitoxin	ND	ND			119
Digoxin	ND	ND	ND		5,120,121

Continued

Dialysis of Drugs

DRUG	HEMO-DIALYSIS	PERITONEAL DIALYSIS	HEMO-PERFUSION	COMMENTS	REFERENCES
Diphenhydramine			ND	Hemoperfusion was not clinically effective in a case report of a diphenhydramine overdose.	50
Disopyramide	ND			Concentration-dependent kinetics.	122
Doxycycline	ND				124
Enalapril	MD				125
Erythromycin	SD			Insufficient data.	126
Ethambutol	SD				2
Ethanol	D				128
Ethchlorvynol	ND-SD	ND	SD-MD	Concentration-dependent kinetics.	5,129-132
Ethosuximide	MD-D			Hemodialysis potentially useful for overdosage.	133
Flecainide	ND			Insufficient data.	134
Flucytosine	D	MD		20 mg/kg post-HD.	33,35
Flurazepam	ND			Insufficient data.	48
Furosemide				Insufficient data.	
Gentamicin	D			See Amikacin.	136-139
Glutethimide	ND-SD	MD	SD-MD	Insufficient information.	140-143
Haloperidol				No data available; probably insignificant removal by dialysis.	48
Heparin	ND	ND			8
Imipenem/ Cilastatin	MD MD			One-half usual dose post-HD.	144 144
Insulin				No data available.	8
Isoniazid	D			Usual dose post-HD.	145,146
					Continued

Dialysis of Drugs

DRUG	HEMO-DIALYSIS	PERITONEAL DIALYSIS	HEMO-PERFUSION	COMMENTS	REFERENCES
Kanamycin	D	MD		See Amikacin.	28-30
Ketoconazole	ND	ND			147
Lidocaine	ND			Active metabolites with unknown dialysis characteristics.	148,149
Lithium	D	D			150,151
Lorazepam	ND-SD			See Diazepam.	48,116,152
Lorcainide	ND-SD			Insufficient data.	153
Mebendazole	ND			Data from only one patient.	157
Meprobamate	MD	SD	SD	Insufficient information; few case reports with PD and hemoperfusion.	125,154-156
Methanol	D	SD-MD			128,158
Methaqualone	SD	SD	SD	Insufficient information.	3,5,159
Methicillin	ND				51
Methotrexate	ND	ND	ND-SD		160-162
Methyldopa	SD	SD		HD reported for 4 patients; PD reported for only 2 patients.	163
Methylprednisolone	SD				164
Metoclopramide	ND				165
Metronidazole	D	SD		Adjust dosing around HD. Active hydroxy metabolite removed by HD to same extent.	166,167
Mexiletene		ND		Insufficient data.	168,169
Mezlocillin	MD	SD		0.5-1 g dose post-HD.	170,171
Miconazole	ND			Insufficient data.	172

Continued

Dialysis of Drugs

DRUG	HEMO-DIALYSIS	PERITONEAL DIALYSIS	HEMO-PERFUSION	COMMENTS	REFERENCES
Minocycline	ND	ND		Insufficient data.	173
Minoxidil				Insufficient data; probably not dialyzable.	174
Moxalactam	D	SD		Give additional dose after HD.	175-177
Nadolol	SD-MD				178
Nafcillin	ND				51,179
Neomycin	D			See Amikacin.	180
Netilmicin	D			See Amikacin.	181
Oxacillin	ND				51
Oxazepam	ND			See Diazepam.	48,116,182
Penicillin G	SD-MD			Insufficient data.	51,183
Pentobarbital	SD	ND-SD	SD-MD		5,44,184,185
Phenobarbital	MD-D	SD-MD	D	Usual dose post-HD.	5,16,184, 186,187
Phenothiazines	ND				188
Phenytoin	ND	ND	SD-MD		189-192
Piperacillin	MD			1 g dose post-HD.	193
Prazosin				Insufficient data; probably insignificantly dialyzed.	194,195
Primidone	MD				196
Procainamide	SD-MD				197-199
N-Acetylprocainamide (active metabolite)	SD-MD				197-199

Continued

Dialysis of Drugs

DRUG	HEMO-DIALYSIS	PERITONEAL DIALYSIS	HEMO-PERFUSION	COMMENTS	REFERENCES
Propoxyphene	ND	ND			200-204
Propranolol	ND				205,206
Quinidine	SD	SD			207,208
Ranitidine	SD			Insufficient data.	209
Reserpine				Insufficient information; probably not dialyzable.	210
Secobarbital	SD	ND-SD	SD-MD		5,184,185
Sulfamethoxazole	SD-MD				48
Teicoplanin		SD			228
Tetracycline	SD				93
Theophylline	MD		D	Efficiently removed by hemoperfusion.	5,211,213
Ticarcillin	D			See Carbenicillin.	51-55
Tobramycin	MD	MD		See Amikacin.	136-139
Tocainide	MD			Insufficient data.	214
Tolbutamide	ND				8
Tricyclic Anti-depressants				Insufficient data; probably not removed by hemoperfusion.	5
Trimethoprim	SD-MD				215
Valproate	ND	ND			216,217
Vancomycin	ND	SD			218-223
Verapamil	ND			Insufficient data.	224

References

1. Anderson RJ, Melikian DM, Gambertoglio JG et al. Prescribing medication in long-term dialysis units. Arch Intern Med 1982;142:1305-8.

2. Lee CS, Marbury TC, Benet LZ. Clearance calculations in hemodialysis: application to blood, plasma, and dialysate measurements for ethambutol. J. Pharmacokinet Biopharm 1980;8:69-81.

3. Takki S, Gambertoglio JG, Honda DH et al. Pharmacokinetic evaluation of hemodialysis in acute drug overdose. J Pharmacokinet Biopharm 1978;6:427-43.

4. Gibson TP, Nelson HA. Drug kinetics and artificial kidneys. Clin Pharmacokinet 1977;2:403-26.

5. Pond S, Rosenberg J, Benowitz NL et al. Pharmacokinetics of haemoperfusion for drug overdose. Clin Pharmacokinet 1979;4:329-54.

6. Gibson TP, Matusik E, Nelson LD et al. Artificial kidneys and clearance calculations. Clin Pharmacol Ther 1976;20:720-6.

7. Gwilt PR, Perrier D. Plasma protein binding and distribution characteristics of drugs as indices of their hemodialyzability. Clin Pharmacol Ther 1978;24:154-61.

8. Bennett WM, Aronoff GR, Morrison G et al. Drug prescribing in renal failure: dosing guidelines for adults. Am J Kidney Dis 1983;3:155-93.

9. Johnson CA, Zimmerman SW, Rogge M. The pharmacokinetics of antibiotics used to treat peritoneal dialysis-associated peritonitis. Am J Kidney Dis 1984;4:3-17.

10. Lee CC, Marbury TC. Drug therapy in patients undergoing haemodialysis: clinical pharmacokinetic considerations. Clin Pharmacokinet 1984;9:42-66.

11. Gibson TP. Problems in designing hemodialysis drug studies. Pharmacotherapy 1985;5:23-9.

12. Rosenberg J, Benowitz NL, Pond S. Pharmacokinetics of drug overdose. Clin Pharmacokinet 1981;6:161-92.

13. Alexander DP, Gambertoglio JG. Drug overdose and pharmacologic considerations in dialysis. In: Cogan MG, Garovoy MR, eds. Introduction to dialysis. New York: Churchill Livingstone, 1985:261-92.

14. Maclean D, Peters TJ, Brown RAG et al. Treatment of acute paracetamol poisoning. Lancet 1968;2:849-52.

15. Watanabe AS. Pharmacokinetic aspects of the dialysis of drugs. Drug Intell Clin Pharm 1977;11:407-16.

16. Winchester JF, Gelfand MC, Knepshield JH et al. Dialysis and hemoperfusion of poisons and drugs — update. Trans Am Soc Artif Intern Organs 1977;23:762-807.

17. Øie S, Lowenthal DT, Briggs WA et al. Effect of hemodialysis on kinetics of acetaminophen elimination by anephric patients. Clin Pharmacol Ther 1975;18:680-6.

18. Rigby RJ, Thomson NM, Parkin GW et al. The treatment of paracetamol overdose with charcoal haemoperfusion and cysteamine. Med J Aust 1978;1:386-99.

19. Vaziri ND, Saiki J, Barton CH et al. Hemodialyzability of acetazolamide. South Med J 1980;73:422-3.

20. Black WD, Acchiardo SR. Acetohexamide hypoglycemia: treatment by peritoneal dialysis. South Med J 1977;70:1240-1.

21. Krasny HC, Liao SHT, de Miranda P et al. Influence of hemodialysis on acyclovir pharmacokinetics in patients with chronic renal failure. Am J Med 1982;73(Suppl):202-4.

22. Laskin OL, Longstreth JA, Whelton A et al. Acyclovir kinetics in end-stage renal disease. Clin Pharmacol Ther 1982;31:594-601.

23. Soung L-S, Ing TS, Daugirdas JT et al. Amantadine hydrochloride pharmacokinetics in hemodialysis patients. Ann Intern Med 1980;93 (part 1):46-9.

24. Ing TS, Mahurkar SD, Dunea G et al. Removal of amantadine hydrochloride by dialysis in patients with renal insufficiency. Can Med Assoc J 1976;115:515.

25. Schapira A. Single-dose kinetics and dosage of mecillinam in renal failure and haemodialysis. Clin Pharmacokinet 1984;9:364-70.

26. Patel IH, Bornemann LD, Brocks VM et al. Pharmacokinetics of intravenous amdinocillin in healthy subjects and patients with renal insufficiency. Antimicrob Agents Chemother 1985;28:46-50.

27. Flouvat B, Decourt S, Aubert P et al. Pharmacokinetics of atenolol in patients with terminal renal failure and influence of haemodialysis. Br J Clin Pharmacol 1980;9:379-85.

28. Madhavan T, Yaremchuk K, Levin N. Effect of renal failure and dialysis on the serum concentration of the aminoglycoside amikacin. Antimicrob Agents Chemother 1976;10:464-6.

29. Sarubbi FA, Hull JH. Amikacin serum concentrations: prediction of levels and dosage guidelines. Ann Intern Med 1978;89:612-8.

30. Regeur L, Colding H, Jensen H et al. Pharmacokinetics of amikacin during hemodialysis and peritoneal dialysis. Antimicrob Agents Chemother 1977;11:214-8.

31. Oe PL, Simonian S, Verhoef J. Pharmacokinetics of the new penicillins. Chemotherapy 1973;19:279-88.

32. Francke EL, Appel GB, Neu HC. Kinetics of intravenous amoxicillin in patients on long-term dialysis. Clin Pharmacol Ther 1979;26:31-5.

33. Block ER, Bennett JE, Livoti LG et al. Flucytosine and amphotericin B: hemodialysis effects on the plasma concentration and clearance. Ann Intern Med 1974;80:613-7.

34. Bindschadler DD, Bennett JE. A pharmacologic guide to the clinical use of amphotericin B. J Infect Dis 1969;120:427-36.

35. Jusko WJ, Lewis GP, Schmitt GW. Ampicillin and hetacillin pharmacokinetics in normal and anephric subjects. Clin Pharmacol Ther 1972;14:90-9.

36. Kunin CM, Finkelberg Z. Oral cephalexin and ampicillin: antimicrobial activity, recovery in urine, and persistence in blood of uremic patients. Ann Intern Med 1970;72:349-56.

37. Ruedy J. The effects of peritoneal dialysis on the physiological disposition of oxacillin, ampicillin and tetracycline in patients with renal disease. Can Med Assoc J 1966;94:257-61.

38. Schreiner GE, Teehan BP. Dialysis of poisons and drugs — annual review. Trans Am Soc Artif Intern Organs 1972;18:563.

39. Kallen RJ, Zaltzman S, Coe FL et al. Hemodialysis in children: technique, kinetic aspects related to varying

body size, and application to salicylate intoxication, acute renal failure and some other disorders. Medicine 1966;45;1-45.

40. Schusziarra V, Ziekursch V, Schlamp R et al. Pharmacokientics of azathioprine under haemodialysis. Int J Clin Pharmacol 1976;14:298-302.

41. Aletta JM, Francke EF, Neu HC. Intravenous azlocillin kinetics in patients on long-term hemodialysis. Clin Pharmacol Ther 1980;27:563-6.

42. Fillastre JP, Leroy A, Baudoin C et al. Pharmacokinetics of aztreonam in patients with chronic renal failure. Clin Pharmacokinet 1985;10:91-100.

43. Gerig JS, Bolton ND, Swabb EA et al. Effect of hemodialysis and peritoneal dialysis on aztreonam pharmacokinetics. Kidney Int 1984;26:308-18.

44. Bloomer HA, Maddock RK. An assessment of diuresis and dialysis for treating acute barbiturate poisoning. In: Matthew H, ed. Acute barbiturate poisoning. Amsterdam: Excerpta Medica, 1971:233-53.

45. Henderson LW, Merrill JP. Treatment of barbiturate intoxication. Ann Intern Med 1966;64:876-91.

46. Frank JT. Barbiturate intoxication. Drug Intell Clin Pharm 1973;7:309-16.

47. Hadden J, Johnson K, Smith S et al. Acute barbiturate intoxication. JAMA 1969;209:893-900.

48. Anderson RJ, Gambertoglio JG, Schrier RW, eds. Clinical use of drugs in renal failure. Springfield, IL: Charles C Thomas, 1976.

49. Josselson J, Narang PK, Adir J et al. Bretylium kinetics in renal insufficiency. Clin Pharmacol Ther 1983;33:144-50.

50. Hirakata H, Onoyama K, Iseki K et al. Captopril (SQ 14225) clearance during hemodialysis treatment. Clin Nephrol 1981;16:321-3.

51. Barza M, Weinstein L. Pharmacokinetics of the penicillins in man. Clin Pharmacokinet 1976;1:297-308.

52. Hoffman TA, Cestero R, Bullock WE. Pharmacodynamics of carbenicillin in hepatic and renal failure. Ann Intern Med 1970;73:173-8.

53. Eastwood JB, Curtis JR. Carbenicillin administration in patients with severe renal failure. Br Med J 1968;1:486-7.

54. Hoffman TA, Cestero R, Bullock WE. Pharmacokinetics of carbenicillin in patients with hepatic and renal failure. J Infect Dis 1970;122 (Suppl):S75-7.

55. Latos DL, Bryan CS, Stone WJ. Carbenicillin therapy in patients with normal and impaired renal function. Clin Pharmacol Ther 1975;17:692-700.

56. Gartenberg G, Meyers BR, Hirschman SZ et al. Pharmacokinetics of cefaclor in patients with stable renal impairment, and patients undergoing haemodialysis. J Antimicrob Chemother 1979;5:465-70.

57. Berman SJ, Boughton WH, Sugihara JG et al. Pharmacokinetics of cefaclor in patients with end stage renal disease and during hemodialysis. Antimicrob Agents Chemother 1978;14:281-3.

58. Gambertoglio JG, Aziz NS, Lin ET et al. Cefamandole kinetics in uremic patients undergoing hemodialysis. Clin Pharmacol Ther 1979;26:592-9.

59. Appel GB, Neu HC, Parry MF et al. Pharmacokinetics of cefamandole in the presence of renal failure and in patients undergoing hemodialysis. Antimicrob Agents Chemother 1976;10:623-5.

60. Campillo JA, Lanao JM, Dominguez-Gil A et al. Pharmacokinetics of cefamandole in patients undergoing hemodialysis. Int J Clin Pharmacol Biopharm 1979;17:416-20.

61. Bliss M, Mayersohn M, Arnold T et al. Disposition kinetics of cefamandole during continuous ambulatory peritoneal dialysis. Antimicrob Agents Chemother 1986;29:649-53.

62. Brogard JM, Pinget M, Brandt C et al. Pharmacokinetics of cefazolin in patients with renal failure; special reference to hemodialysis. J Clin Pharmacol 1977;17:225-30.

63. Craig CP, Rifkin SI. Pharmacokinetics and hemodialyzability of cefazolin in uremic patients. Clin Pharmacol Ther 1976;19:825-9.

64. McCloskey RV, Forland MF, Sweeney MJ et al. Hemodialysis of cefazolin. J Infect Dis 1973;128 (Suppl):S358-60.

65. Linquist JA, Siddiqui JY, Smith IM. Cephalexin in patients with renal disease. N Engl J Med 1970;283:720-3.

66. Kaye D, Wenger N. Agarwal B. Pharmacology of intraperitoneal cefazolin in patients undergoing peritoneal dialysis. Antimicrob Agents Chemother 1978;14:318-21.

67. Levison ME, Levison SP, Ries K et al. Pharmacology of cefazolin in patients with normal and abnormal renal function. J Infect Dis 1973;128 (Suppl):S354-7.

68. Barriere SL, Gambertoglio JG, Alexander DP et al. Pharmacokinetic disposition of cefonicid in patients with renal failure and receiving hemodialysis. Rev Infect Dis 1984;6(Suppl 4):S809-15.

69. Spyker DA, Richmond JD, Scheld WM et al. Pharmacokinetics of multiple-dose cefoperazone in hemodialysis patients. Am J Nephrol 1985;5:355-60.

70. Keller E, Jansen A, Pelz K et al. Intraperitoneal and intravenous cefoperazone kinetics during continuous ambulatory peritoneal dialysis. Clin Pharmacol Ther 1983;35:203-13.

71. Hawkins SS, Alford RH, Stone WJ et al. Ceforanide kinetics in renal insufficiency. Clin Pharmacol Ther 1981;30:468-74.

72. Ings RMJ, Fillastre JP, Godin M et al. The pharmacokinetics of cefotaxime and its metabolites in subjects with normal and impaired renal function. Rev Infect Dis 1982;4(Suppl):S379-91.

73. Aiexander DP, Gambertoglio JG, Barriere SL et al. Cefotaxime in continuous ambulatory peritoneal dialysis. (Submitted for publication 1987).

74. Albin HC, Demotes-Mainard FM, Bouchet JL et al. Pharmacokinetics of intravenous and intraperitoneal cefotaxime in chronic ambulatory peritoneal dialysis. Clin Pharmacol Ther 1985;38:285-9.

75. Ohkawa M, Hirano S, Tokunaga S et al. Pharmacokinetics of cefotetan in normal subjects and patients with impaired renal function. Antimicrob Agents Chemother 1983;23:31-5.

76. Garcia MJ, Dominguez-Gil A, Tabernero JM et al. Pharmacokinetics of cefoxitin in patients undergoing hemodialysis. Int J Clin Pharmacol Biopharm 1979;17:366-70.

77. Greaves WL, Kreeft JH, Ogilvie RI et al. Cefoxitin disposition during peritoneal dialysis. Antimicrob Agents Chemother 1981;19:253-5.

78. Gibson TP, Granneman GR, Kallal JE et al. Cefsulodin kinetics in renal impairment. Clin Pharmacol Ther 1982;31:602-8.

79. Nikolaidis P, Tourkantonis A. Effect of hemodialysis on ceftazidime pharmacokinetics. Clin Nephrol 1985;24:142-6.

80. Leroy A, Leguy F, Borsa F et al. Pharmacokinetics of ceftazidime in normal and uremic subjects. Antimicrob Agents Chemother 1984;25:638-42.

81. Tourkantonis A, Nicolaidis P. Pharmacokinetics of ceftazidime in patients undergoing peritoneal dialysis. J Antimicrob Chemother 1983;12(Suppl A):263-7.

82. Kowalsky SF, Echols RM, Venezia AR et al. Pharmacokinetics of ceftizoxime in subjects with various degrees of renal function. Antimicrob Agents Chemother 1983;24:151-5.

83. Burgess ED, Blair AD. Pharmacokinetics of ceftizoxime in patients undergoing continuous ambulatory peritoneal dialysis. Antimicrob Agents Chemother 1983;24:237-9.

84. Johnson CA, Zimmerman SW, Bayer W et al. Pharmacokinetics of intravenous ceftizoxime in patients on continuous ambulatory peritoneal dialysis. Clin Nephrol 1985;23:120-4.

85. Cohen D, Appel GB, Scully B et al. Pharmacokinetics of ceftriaxone in patients with renal failure and in those undergoing hemodialysis. Antimicrob Agents Chemother 1983;24:529-32.

86. Local FK, Munro AJ, Kerr DNS et al. Pharmacokinetics of intravenous and intraperitoneal cefuroxime in patients undergoing peritoneal dialysis. Clin Nephrol 1981;16:40-3.

87. Chan MK, Browning AK, Poole CJM et al. Cefuroxime pharmacokinetics in continuous and intermittent peritoneal dialysis. Nephron 1985;41:161-5.

88. Bunke CM, Aronoff GR, Brier ME et al. Cefazolin and cephalexin kinetics in continuous ambulatory peritoneal dialysis. Clin Pharmacol Ther 1983;33:66-72.

89. Reisberg BE, Mandelbaum JM, Cephalexin: absorption and excretion as related to renal function and hemodialysis. Infect Immun 1971;3:540-3.

90. Venuto RC, Plaut ME. Cephalothin handling in patients undergoing hemodialysis. Antimicrob Agents Chemother 1970;10:50-2.

91. Stalker NE, Gambertoglio JG, Fukumitsu CJ et al. Acute massive chloral hydrate intoxication treated with hemodialysis: a clinical pharmacokinetic analysis. J Clin Pharmacol 1978;18:136-42.

92. Vaziri ND, Kumar KP, Mirahmadi K et al. Hemodialysis in treatment of acute chloral hydrate poisoning. South Med J 1977;70:377-8.

93. Greenberg PA, Sanford JP. Removal and absorption of antibiotics in patients with renal failure undergoing peritoneal dialysis: tetracycline, chloramphenicol, kanamycin, and colistimethate. Ann Intern Med 1967;66:465-70.

94. Blouin RA, Erwin WG, Dutro MP et al. Chloramphenicol hemodialysis clearance. Ther Drug Monit 1980;2:351-4.

95. Slaughter RL, Cerra FB, Koup JR. Effect of hemodialysis on total body clearance of chloramphenicol. Am J Hosp Pharm 1980;37:1083-6.

96. Cruz IA, Cramer NC, Parrish AE. Hemodialysis in chlordiazepoxide toxicity. JAMA 1967;202:438-40.

97. Graw RG, Clarke PR. Chlorpropamide intoxication-treatment with peritoneal dialysis. Pediatrics 1970;45:106-9.

98. Vaziri ND, Ness RL, Barton CH. Peritoneal dialysis clearance of cimetidine. Am J Gastroenterol 1979;71:572-6.

99. Doherty CC, O'Connor FA, Buchanan KD et al. Cimetidine for duodenal ulceration in patients undergoing haemodialysis. Br Med J 1977;2:1506-8.

100. Jones RH, Lewin MR, Parsons V. Therapeutic effect of cimetidine in patients undergoing haemodialysis. Br Med J 1979;1:650-2.

101. Cutler RE, Blair AD. In: Mackey BB, ed. 12th Annual Contractors' Conference of the Artificial Kidney Program, Bethesda, USA: National Institutes of Health, 1981. (NIH publication no. 81-1979):235. Abstract.

102. Moran DM, Cersosimo RJ, Ziemniak J et al. Effect of hemodialysis on cimetidine pharmacokinetics. 2nd annual American College of Clinical Pharmacy Meeting 1981. Abstract.

103. Bjaeldager PAL, Jensen JB, Larsen N-E et al. Elimination of oral cimetidine in chronic renal failure and during haemodialysis. Br J Clin Pharmacol 1980;9:585-92.

104. Vaziri ND, Ness RL, Barton CH. Hemodialysis clearance of cimetidine. Arch Intern Med 1978;138:1685-6.

105. Personal Communication. Smith, Kline, and French Laboratories, March 27, 1979.

106. Hyneck ML, Murphy JF, Lipshultz DE. Cimetidine clearance during intermittent and chronic peritoneal dialysis. Am J Hosp Pharm 1981;38:1760-2.

107. Pizzella KM, Moore MC, Schultz RW et al. Removal of cimetidine by peritoneal dialysis, hemodialysis, and charcoal hemoperfusion. Ther Drug Monit 1980;2:273-81.

108. Horber FF, Frey FJ, Descoeudres C et al. Differential effect of impaired renal function on the kinetics of clavulanic acid and amoxicillin. Antimicrob Agents Chemother 1986;29:614-9.

109. Eastwood JB, Gower PE. A study of the pharmacokinetics of clindamycin in normal subjects and patients with chronic renal failure. Postgrad Med J 1974;50:710-2.

110. Peddie BA, Dann E, Bailey RR. The effect of impairment of renal function and dialysis on the serum and urine levels of clindamycin. Austral NZ J Med 1975;5:198-202.

111. Malacoff RF, Finkelstein FO, Andriole VT. Effect of peritoneal dialysis on serum levels of tobramycin and clindamycin. Antimicrob Agents Chemother 1975;8:574-80.

112. Hulter HN, Licht JH, Ilmicki LP et al. Clinical efficacy and pharmacokinetics of clonidine in hemodialysis and renal insufficiency. J Lab Clin Med 1979;94:223-31.

113. Lowenthal DT, Affrime MB, Meyer A et al. Pharmacokinetics and pharmacodynamics of clonidine in varying states of renal function. Chest 1983;2(Suppl):386-90.

114. Ellwood MG, Robb GH. Self-poisoning with colchicine. Postgrad Med J 1971;47:129-38.

115. Wang LH, Lee CS, Majeske BL et al. Clearance and recovery calculations in hemodialysis: application to plasma, red blood cell, and dialysate measurements for cyclophosphamide. Clin Pharmacol Ther 1981;29:365-72.

116. Schreiner GE. Dialysis of poisons and drugs — annual review. Trans Am Soc Artif Intern Organs 1970;16:544.

117. Williams TW, Lawson SA, Brook MI et al. Effect of hemodialysis on dicloxacillin concentrations in plasma. Antimicrob Agents Chemother 1967;7:767-9.

118. McCloskey RV, Hayes CP. Plasma levels of dicloxacillin in oliguric patients and the effect of hemodialysis. Antimicrob Agents Chemother 1967;7:770-2.

119. Finkelstein FO, Goffinet JA, Hendler ED et al. Pharmacokinetics of digoxin and digitoxin in patients undergoing hemodialysis. Am J Med 1975;58:525-31.

120. Ackerman GL, Doherty JE, Flanigan WJ. Peritoneal dialysis and hemodialysis of tritiated digoxin. Ann Intern Med 1967;67:718-23.

121. Koup JR, Jusko WJ, Elwood CM et al. Digoxin pharmacokinetics: role of renal failure in dosage regimen design. Clin Pharmacol Ther 1975;18:9-21.

122. Sevka MJ, Matthews SJ, Nightingale CH et al. Disopyramide hemodialysis and kinetics in patients requiring long-term hemodialysis. Clin Pharmacol Ther 1981;29:322-6.

123. Whelton A, von Whittenau MS, Twomey TM et al. Doxycycline pharmacokinetics in the absence of renal function. Kidney Int 1974;5:365-71.

124. Houin G, Brunner F, Nebout T et al. The effects of chronic renal insufficiency on the pharmacokinetics of doxycycline in man. Br J Clin Pharmacol 1983;16:245-52.

125. Lowenthal DT, Irvin JD, Merrill D et al. The effect of renal function on enalapril kinetics. Clin Pharmacol Ther 1985;38:661-6.

126. Vaziri ND, Cesario TC, Valenti J et al. Hemodialysis of erythromycin. Drug Intell Clin Pharm 1980;14:549-51. Letter.

127. Lee CS, Marbury TC, Benet LZ. Clearance calculations in hemodialysis: application to blood, plasma, and dialysate measurements for ethambutol. J Pharmacokinet Biopharm 1980;8:69-81.

128. McCoy HG, Cipolle RJ, Ehlers SM et al. Severe methanol poisoning. Application of a pharmacokinetic model for ethanol therapy and hemodialysis. Am J Med 1979;67:804-7.

129. Tozer TN, Witt LD, Gee L et al. Evaluation of hemodialysis for ethchlorvynol overdose. Am J Hosp Pharm 1974;31:986-9.

130. Hedley-Whyte J, Laasberg LH. Ethchlorvynol poisoning: gas liquid chromatography in management. Anesthesia 1969;30:107-11.

131. Benowitz N, Abolin C, Tozer T et al. Resin hemoperfusion in ethchlorvynol overdose. Clin Pharmacol Ther 1980;27:236-42.

132. Lynn RI, Honig CL, Jatlow PI et al. Resin hemoperfusion for treatment of ethchlorvynol overdose. Ann Intern Med 1979;91:549-53.

133. Marbury TC, Lee C-s C, Perchalski RJ et al. Hemodialysis clearance of ethosuximide in patients with chronic renal disease. Am J Hosp Pharm 1981;38:1757-60.

134. Conard GJ, Ober RE. Metabolism of flecainide. Am J Cardiol 1984;53(Suppl):41B-51B.

135. Cutler RE, Blair AD, Kelly MR. Flucytosine kinetics in subjects with normal and impaired renal function. Clin Pharmacol Ther 1978;24:333-42.

136. Christopher TG, Korn D, Blair AD et al. Gentamicin pharmacokinetics during hemodialysis. Kidney Int 1974;6:38-44.

137. Halpren BA, Axline SG, Coplon NS et al. Clearance of gentamicin during hemodialysis: comparison of four artificial kidneys. J Infect Dis 1976;133:627-36.

138. Jusko WJ, Baliah T, Kim KH et al. Pharmacokinetics of gentamicin during peritoneal dialysis in children. Kidney Int 1976;9:430-8.

139. Danish M, Schultz R, Jusko WJ. Pharmacokinetics of gentamicin and kanamycin during hemodialysis. Antimicrob Agents Chemother 1974;6:841-7.

140. Ozdemir AI, Tannenberg AM. Peritoneal and Hemodialysis for acute glutethimide overdosage. NY State J Med 1972;72:2076-9.

141. Chazan JA, Cohen JJ. Clinical spectrum of glutethimide intoxication: hemodialysis reevaluated. JAMA 1969;208:837-9.

142. King LRH, Decherd JF, Newton JL et al. A clinically efficient and economical lipid dialyzer. JAMA 1970;211:652-3.

143. Maher JF. Determinants of serum half-life of glutethimide in intoxicated patients. J Pharmacol Exp Ther 1970;174:450-5.

144. Gibson TP, Demetriades JL, Bland JA. Imipenem/cilastatin: pharmacokinetic profile in renal insufficiency. Am J Med 1985;78:(Suppl 6A):54-61.

145. Gold CH, Buchanan N, Tringham V et al. Isoniazid pharmacokinetics in patients in chronic renal failure. Clin Nephrol 1976;6:365-9.

146. Cocco AE, Pazourek LJ. Acute isoniazid intoxication — management by peritoneal dialysis. N Engl J Med 1963;269:852-3.

147. Johnson RJ, Blair AD, Ahmad S. Ketoconazole kinetics in chronic peritoneal dialysis. Clin Pharmacol Ther 1985;37:325-9.

148. Collinsworth KA, Strong JM, Atkinson AJ et al. Pharmacokinetics and metabolism of lidocaine in patients with renal failure. Clin Pharmacol Ther 1975;18:59-64.

149. Thomson PD, Melmon KL, Richardson JA et al. Lidocaine pharmacokinetics in advanced heart failure, liver disease, and renal failure in humans. Ann Intern Med 1973;78:499-508.

150. Wilson HP, Donker AJM, Van Der Hem K et al. Peritoneal dialysis for lithium poisoning. Br Med J 1971;2:749-50.

151. Schou M, Amdisen A, Trap-Jensen J. Lithium poisoning. Am J Psychiatry 1968;4:520-6.

152. Morrison G, Chiang ST, Koepke HH et al. Effect of renal impairment and hemodialysis on lorazepam kinetics. Clin Pharmacol Ther 1984;35:646-52.

153. Somani P, Simon V, Gupta RK et al. Lorcainide kinetics and protein binding in patients with end-stage renal disease. Int J Clin Pharmacol Ther Toxicol 1984;22:121-5.

154. Maddock RK, Bloomer HA. Meprobamate overdosage: evaluation of its severity and methods of treatment. JAMA 1967;201:999-1003.

155. Castell DO, Sode J. Meprobamate intoxication treated with peritoneal dialysis. Illinois Med J 1976;131:298-9.

156. Hoy WE, Rivero A, Marin MG et al. Resin hemoperfusion for treatment of a massive meprobamate overdose. Ann Intern Med 1980;93:455-6.

157. Allgayer H, Zahringer J, Bach P et al. Lack of effect of haemodialysis on mebendazole kinetics: studies in a patient with echinococcosis and renal failure. Eur J Clin Pharmacol 1984;27:243-5.

158. Keyvan-Larijarni H, Tannenberg AM. Methanol intoxication: comparison of peritoneal dialysis and hemodialysis treatment. Arch Intern Med 1974;134:293-6.

159. Proudfoot AT, Noble J, Nimmo J et al. Peritoneal dialysis and haemodialysis in methaqualone (Mandrax) poisoning. Scott Med J 1968;13:232-6.

160. Gibson TP, Reich SD, Krumlovsky FA et al. Hemoperfusion for methotrexate removal. Clin Pharmacol Ther 1978;23:351-5.

161. Ahmad S, Shen FH, Bleyer WA. Methotrexate-induced renal failure and ineffectiveness of peritoneal dialysis. Arch Intern Med 1978;138:1146-7.

162. Howell SB, Blair HE, Uren J et al. Hemodialysis and enzymatic cleavage of methotrexate in man. Eur J Cancer 1978;14:787-92.

163. Yeh BK, Dayton PG, Waters WC. Removal of alpha-methyldopa (Aldomet) in man by dialysis. Proc Soc Exp Biol Med 1970;135:840-3.

164. Sherlock JE, Letteri JM. Effect of hemodialysis on methylprednisolone plasma levels. Nephron 1977;18:208-11.

165. Lehmann CR, Heironimus JD, Collins CB et al. Metoclopramide kinetics in patients with impaired renal function and clearance by hemodialysis. Clin Pharmacol Ther 1985;37:284-9.

166. Somogyi A, Kong C, Sabto J et al. Disposition and removal of metronidazole in patients undergoing haemodialysis. Eur J Clin Pharmacol 1983;25:683-7.

167. Guay DR, Meatherall RC, Baxter H et al. Pharmacokinetics of metronidazole in patients undergoing continuous ambulatory peritoneal dialysis. Antimicrob Agents Chemother 1984;25:306-10.

168. Jones TE, Reece PA, Fisher GC. Mexiletine removal by peritoneal dialysis. Eur J Clin Pharmacol 1983;25:839-40. Letter.

169. Wang T, Wuellner D, Woosley RL et al. Pharmacokinetics and nondialyzability of mexiletine in renal failure. Clin Pharmacol Ther 1985;37:649-53.

170. Janicke DM, Mangione A, Schultz RW et al. Mezlocillin disposition in chronic hemodialysis patients. Antimicrob Agents Chemother 1981;20:590-4.

171. Kampf D, Schurig R, Weihermuller K et al. Effects of impaired renal function, hemodialysis, and peritoneal dialysis on the pharmacokinetics of mezlocillin. Antimicrob Agents Chemother 1980;18:81-7.

172. Lewi PJ, Boelaert J, Daneels R et al. Pharmacokinetic profile of intravenous miconazole in man. Comparison of normal subjects and patients with renal insufficiency. Eur J Clin Pharmacol 1976;10:49-54.

173. Carney S, Butcher RA, Dawborn JK et al. Minocycline excretion and distribution in relation to renal function in man. Clin Exp Pharmacol Physiol 1974;1:299-308.

174. Limas CJ, Freis ED. Minoxidil in severe hypertension with renal failure. Am J Cardiol 1973;31:355-61.

175. Jacobson EJ, Zahrowski JJ, Nissenson AR. Moxalactam kinetics in hemodialysis. Clin Pharmacol Ther 1981;30:487-90.

176. Srinivasan S, Neu HC. Pharmacokinetics of moxalactam in patients with renal failure and during hemodialysis. Antimicrob Agents Chemother 1981;20:398-400.

177. Morse G, Janicke D, Cafarell R et al. Moxalactam epimer disposition in patients undergoing continuous ambulatory peritoneal dialysis. Clin Pharmacol Ther 1985;38:150-6.

178. Herrera J, Vukovich RA, Griffith DL. Elimination of nadolol by patients with renal impairment. Br J Clin Pharmacol 1979;7:2275-2315.

179. Rudnick M, Morrison G, Walker B et al. Renal failure, hemodialysis, and nafcillin kinetics. Clin Pharmacol Ther 1976;20:413-23.

180. Krumlovsky FA, Emmerman J, Parker RH et al. Dialysis in treatment of neomycin overdosage. Ann Intern Med 1972;76:443-6.

181. Basile C, Di Maggio A, Curino E et al. Pharmacokinetics of netilmicin in hypertonic hemodiafiltration and standard hemodialysis. Clin Nephrol 1985;24:305-9.

182. Greenblatt DJ, Murray TG, Audet PR et al. Multiple-dose kinetics and dialyzability of oxazepam in renal insufficiency. Nephron 1983;34:234-8.

183. Bryan CS, Stone WJ. ''Comparably massive'' penicillin G therapy in renal failure. Ann Intern Med 1975;82:189-95.

184. Berman LB, Jeghers HJ, Schreiner GE et al. Hemodialysis, an effective therapy for acute barbiturate poisoning. JAMA 1956;161:820-7.

185. Berman LB, Vogelsang P. Removal rates for barbiturates using two types of peritoneal dialysis. N Engl J Med 1964;270:77-80.

186. Kennedy AC, Briggs JD, Young N et al. Successful treatment of three cases of very severe barbiturate poisoning. Lancet 1969;1:995-8.

187. Chow-Tung E, Lau AH, Vidyasagar D et al. Clearance of phenobarbital by peritoneal dialysis in a neonate. Clin Pharm 1982;1:268-71.

188. Avram MM, McGinn JT. Extracorporeal hemodialysis in phenothiazine overdosage. JAMA 1966;197:182-3.

189. Adler DS, Martin E, Gambertoglio JG et al. Hemodialysis of phenytoin in a uremic patient. Clin Pharmacol Ther 1975;18:65-9.

190. Tenckhoff H, Sherrard DJ, Hickman RO et al. Acute diphenylhydantoin intoxication. Am J Dis Child 1968;116:422-5.

191. Martin E, Gambertoglio JG, Adler DS et al. Removal of phenytoin by hemodialysis in uremic patients. JAMA 1977;238:1750-3.

192. Rubinger D, Levy M, Roll D et al. Inefficiency of haemodialysis in acute phenytoin intoxication. Br J Clin Pharmacol 1979;7:405-7.

193. Francke EL, Appel GB, Neu HC. Pharmacokinetics of intravenous piperacillin in patients undergoing chronic hemodialysis. Antimicrob Agents Chemother 1979;16:788-91.

194. Hobbs DC, Twomey TM, Palmer RF. Pharmacokinetics of prazocin in man. J Clin Pharmacol 1978;18:402-6.

195. Curtis JR. Bateman FJA. Use of Prazocin in management of hypertension in patients with chronic renal failure and in renal transplant recipients. Br Med J 1975;4:432-4.

196. Lee CC, Marbury TC, Perchalski RT et al. Pharmacokinetics of primidone elimination by uremic patients. J Clin Pharmacol 1982;22:301-8.

197. Atkinson AJ, Krumlovsky FA, Huang CM et al. Hemodialysis for severe procainamide toxicity: clinical and pharmacokinetic observations. Clin Pharmacol Ther 1976;20:585-92.

198. Gibson TP, Lowenthal DT, Nelson HA et al. Elimination of procainamide in end stage renal failure. Clin Pharmacol Ther 1975;17:321-9.

199. Gibson TP, Atkinson AJ, Matusik E et al. Kinetics of procainamide and N-acetyl procainamide in renal failure. Kidney Int 1977;12:422-9.

200. Gary NE, Maher JF, De Myttenaere MH et al. Acute propoxyphene hydrochloride intoxication. Arch Intern Med 1968;121:453-7.

201. Mauer SM, Paxson CL, von Hartizsch B et al. Hemodialysis in an infant with propoxyphene intoxication. Clin Pharmacol Ther 1974;17:88-92.

202. McCarthy WH, Keenan RL. Propoxyphene hydrochloride poisoning. JAMA 1964;187:164-5.

203. Karliner JS. Propoxyphene hydrochloride poisoning. JAMA 1967;199:152-5.

204. Giacomini KM, Gibson TP, Levy G. Effect of hemodialysis on propoxyphene and norpropoxyphene concentrations in blood of anephric patients. Clin Pharmacol Ther 1980;27:508-14.

205. Lowenthal DT, Briggs WA, Gibson TP et al. Pharmacokinetics of oral propranolol in chronic renal disease. Clin Pharmacol Ther 1974;16:761-9.

206. Bianchetti G, Graziani G, Brancaccio D et al. Pharmacokinetics and effects of propranolol in terminal uraemic patients and in patients undergoing regular dialysis treatment. Clin Pharmacokinet 1976;1:373-84.

207. Woie L. Oyri A. Quinidine intoxication treated with hemodialysis. Acta Med Scand 1974;195:237-9.

208. Ueda CT, Hirschfeld DS, Scheinman MM et al. Disposition kinetics of quinidine. Clin Pharmacol Ther 1975;19:30-6.

209. Garg DC, Baltodano N, Perez GO et al. Pharmacokinetics of ranitidine after intravenous administration in hemodialysis patients. Pharmacology 1985;31:189-93.

210. Zsoter TT, Johnson GE, De Veber GA et al. Excretion and metabolism of reserpine in renal failure. Clin Pharmacol Ther 1973;14:325-30.

211. Russo ME. Management of theophylline intoxication with charcoal-column hemoperfusion. N Engl J Med 1979;300:24-6.

212. Ehlers SM, Zaske DE, Sawchuck RJ. Massive theophylline overdose: rapid elimination by charcoal hemoperfusion. JAMA 1978;240:474-5.

213. Lawyer C, Aitchison J, Sutton J et al. Treatment of theophylline neurotoxicity with resin hemoperfusion. Ann Intern Med 1978;88:516-7.

214. Wiegers U, Hanrath P, Kuck KH et al. Pharmacokinetics of tocainide in patients with renal dysfunction and during haemodialysis. Eur J Clin Pharmacol 1983;24:503-7.

215. Craig WA, Kunin CM. Trimethoprim-Sulfamethoxazole: pharmacodynamic effects of urinary pH and impaired renal function. Ann Intern Med 1973;78:491-7.

216. Marbury TC, Lee CS, Bruni J et al. Hemodialysis of valproic acid in uremic patients. Dial Transplant 1980;9:961-4.

217. Orr JM, Farrell K, Abbott FS et al. The effects of peritoneal dialysis on the single dose and steady state pharmacokinetics of valproic acid in a uremic epileptic child. Eur J Clin Pharmacol 1983;24:387-90.

218. Ayus JC, Eneas JF, Tong TG et al. Peritoneal clearance and total body elimination of vancomycin during chronic intermittent peritoneal dialysis. Clin Nephrol 1979;11:129-32.

219. Alexander MR. A review of vancomycin after 15 years of use. Drug Intell Clin Pharm 1974;8:520-4.

220. Lindholm DD, Murray JS. Persistence of vancomycin in the blood during renal failure and its treatment by hemodialysis. N Engl J Med 1966;274:1047-51.

221. Nielsen HE, Sorensen I, Hansen HE. Peritoneal transport of vancomycin during peritoneal dialysis. Nephron 1979;24:274-7.

222. Moellering RC, Krogstad DJ, Greenblatt DJ. Vancomycin therapy in patients with impaired renal function: a nomogram for dosage. Ann Intern Med 1981;94:343-6.

223. Bunke CM, Aronoff GR, Brier ME et al. Vancomycin kinetics during continuous ambulatory peritoneal dialysis. Clin Pharmacol Ther 1983;34:631-7.

224. Mooy J, Schols M, v.Baak M et al. Pharmacokinetics of verapamil in patients with renal failure. Eur J Clin Pharmacol 1985;28:405-10.

225. de Groot G, van Heijst ANP, Maes RAA. Charcoal hemoperfusion in the treatment of two cases of acute carbamazepine poisoning. Clin Toxicol 1984;22:349-62.

226. Kosmidis J, Stathakis C, Anyfantis A et al. Cefuroxime in renal insufficiency: therapeutic results in various infections and pharmacokinetics including the effects of dialysis. Proc Roy Soc Med 1977;70 (Suppl 9):139-43.

227. Gower PE, Kennedy MRK, Dash CH. The effect of renal failure and dialysis on the pharmacokinetics of cefuroxime. Proc Roy Soc Med 1977;70(Suppl 9):151-6.

228. Traina GL, Gentile MG, Fellin G et al. Pharmacokinetics of teicoplanin in patients on continuous ambulatory peritoneal dialysis. Eur J Clin Pharmacol 1986;31:501-4.

229. Singlas E, Taburet AM, Landru I et al. Pharmacokinetics of ciprofloxacin tablets in renal failure; influence of haemodialysis. Eur J Clin Pharmacol 1987;31:589-93.

3 *DIETARY CONSIDERATIONS*

Potassium and Tyramine Content of Foods and Beverages, Recommended Daily Dietary Allowances, Sodium Content of Selected Drugs

Potassium Content of Selected Foods, Beverages and Salt Substitutes[a,b]

BEVERAGES [8 fl ℥]	MG	MEQ
Apple juice, bottled/canned	296	7.6
Apricot juice, nectar, canned	286	7.3
Grape juice, bottled/canned	334	8.5
Grapefruit juice, canned	378	9.7
Milk, whole, 3.5% fat (high in sodium)	351	9.0
Milk, lowfat, 2% fat (high in sodium)	377	9.6
Milk, skim (high in sodium)	406	10.4
Orange juice, fresh	496	12.7
Orange juice, canned	436	11.2
Pineapple juice, canned	334	8.5
Prune juice, canned	706	18.1
Tangerine juice, canned	443	11.3
Tomato juice, canned (high in sodium)	598	15.3

FRUITS	MG	MEQ
Apricots, raw, 3 medium	313	8.0
Banana, raw, 1 medium	451	11.5
Cantaloupe, raw, 1 cup pieces	494	12.6
Dates, dried, 10	541	13.8
Figs, dried, 10	1332	34.1
Fruit cocktail, canned, 1 cup	230	5.9
Grapefruit, pink, raw, ½ medium	158	4.0
Orange, navel, raw, 1 medium	250	6.4
Peach, raw, 1 medium	171	4.4
Pear, raw, 1 medium	208	5.3
Pineapple, raw, 1 cup pieces	175	4.5
Prunes, dried, 10	626	16.0
Raisins, seedless, ⅔ cup	751	19.2
Strawberries, raw, 1 cup	247	6.3
Watermelon, raw, 1 cup	186	4.8

VEGETABLES	MG	MEQ
Avocado, raw, 1 medium (California)	1097	28.1
Avocado, raw, 1 medium (Florida)	1484	38.0
Beans, green lima, cooked, ½ cup	338	8.6

Continued

VEGETABLES	MG	MEQ
Beans, red kidney, cooked, ½ cup	425	10.9
Broccoli, cooked, ⅔ cup	267	6.8
Brussels sprouts, cooked, 6-8 medium	273	7.0
Carrot, raw, 1 large	341	8.7
Corn, yellow, canned, ½ cup	138	3.5
Mushrooms, raw, 10 small	414	10.6
Potato, baked, 1 medium	503	12.9
Spinach, cooked, ½ cup	291	7.4
Squash, winter, baked, ½ cup	461	11.8
Tomato, raw, 1 medium	366	9.4

SALT SUBSTITUTES	MG	MEQ
Adolph's, 1 g	485	12.4
Co-Salt, 1 g	469	12.0
Diasal, 1 g	442	11.3
Featherweight K, 1 g	465	11.9
Lite-Salt, 1 g (high in sodium)	293	7.4
Morton, 1 g	504	12.9
Neocurtasal, 1 g	470	12.1
NoSalt (Regular), 1 g	500	12.8
NoSalt (Seasoned), 1 g	266	6.8
Nu-Salt, 1 g	434	11.1
Salfree, 1 g	548	14.1

a. Food values adapted from Pennington JAT, Church HN. Bowes and Church's food values of portions commonly used. 14th ed. Philadelphia: JB Lippincott, 1985.
b. Potassium content amounts are approximations. Salt substitute formulations, and hence potassium content, are subject to change by manufacturer. Salt substitute values from: Pearson RE, Fish KH, Potassium content of selected medicines, foods and salt substitutes, Hosp Pharm 1971;6:6-9; Sopko JA, Freeman RM, Salt substitutes as a source of potassium, JAMA 1977;238:608-10; and product information.

Tyramine Content of Foods and Beverages[a,b]

ALCOHOLIC BEVERAGES	ESTIMATED LEVELS[c]
Beer and Ale[d]	Low
Chartreuse[e]	Unknown
Drambuie[e]	Unknown
Sherry[e]	Low
Wine, red[f]	Low
Wine, white[g]	Little or none

CHEESE	ESTIMATED LEVELS[c]
American, processed	Low
Blue	Moderate to high
Boursault	Very high
Brick, natural	Moderate to high
Brie	Moderate to high
Camembert	Very high
Cheddar	Very high
Cottage cheese	Little or none
Cream cheese	Little or none
Emmenthaler	Very high
Gruyere	Moderate to high

Continued

Tyramine Content of Foods and Beverages[a,b]

CHEESE	ESTIMATED LEVELS[c]
Mozzarella	Moderate to high
Parmesan	Moderate to high
Romano	Moderate to high
Roquefort	Moderate to high
Stilton	Very high

FRUITS	ESTIMATED LEVELS[c]
Bananas	Low
Figs, canned, particularly if overripe	Low to moderate

MEAT AND FISH	ESTIMATED LEVELS[c]
Beef liver, unrefrigerated, fermented	Moderate
Caviar	High
Chicken liver, unrefrigerated, fermented	Moderate
Fish, unrefrigerated, fermented	Moderate
Fish, dried	Moderate
Herring, dried salted	Moderate to high
Herring, pickled, if spoiled	Highest levels found
Sausages, fermented:	Very high
Bologna	
Pepperoni	
Salami	
Summer sausage	
Other unrefrigerated, fermented meats	Moderate

VEGETABLES	ESTIMATED LEVELS[c]
Avocado, particularly if overripe	Low to moderate
Broad bean pods	Probably contain dopamine
Fava beans, particularly if overripe	Contain dopamine

OTHER FOODS AND BEVERAGES	ESTIMATED LEVELS[c]
Caffeine, very large amounts	A weak pressor agent
Chocolate, very large amounts	Contains phenylethylamine, a weak pressor agent
Yeast extracts such as Marmite[h]	Very high

a. Anon. Monoamine oxidase inhibitors for depression. Med Lett Drugs Ther 1980;22:58-60, reproduced with permission.

b. For more detailed information, consult McCabe B, Tsuang MT. Dietary considera- tion in MAO inhibitor regimens. J Clin Psychiatry 1982;43:178-81.

c. The tyramine content of most foods is not entirely predictable. These estimates are taken from isolated reports, some based on small samples. The amount of tyramine in food and beverages could vary with different conditions, different samples and dif- ferent manufacturers.

d. Fermentation of beer does not ordinarily involve processes that produce tyramine. However, the amount can vary greatly, and some imported beers have caused reactions in patients taking MAO inhibitors. McCabe and Tsuang (footnote b.) state that beer is among the most important food restrictions and should be avoided.

e. Some patients have had reactions.

f. Fermentation of wine does not ordinarily produce tyramine. However, contamina- tion with other than the usual fermenting organisms and production of appreciable amounts of tyramine has occurred in Chianti and could occur in any red wine.

g. White wine is free of tyramine because it is made without the grape pulp and seeds, which may be the source of amino acids in red wine.

h. But baked goods do not contain appreciable amounts of tyramine.

Recommended Daily Dietary Allowances,[a] Revised 1980[i]

	Age (years)	Weight (kg)	Weight (lb)	Height (cm)	Height (in)	Protein (g)	MINERALS Calcium (mg)	Phosphorus (mg)	Magnesium (mg)	Iron (mg)	Zinc (mg)	Iodine (mcg)
Infants	0.0–0.5	6	13	60	24	kg × 2.2	360	240	50	10	3	40
	0.5–1.0	9	20	71	28	kg × 2.0	540	360	70	15	5	50
Children	1–3	13	29	90	35	23	800	800	150	15	10	70
	4–6	20	44	112	44	30	800	800	200	10	10	90
	7–10	28	62	132	52	34	800	800	250	10	10	120
Males	11–14	45	99	157	62	45	1200	1200	350	18	15	150
	15–18	66	145	176	69	56	1200	1200	400	18	15	150
	19–22	70	154	177	70	56	800	800	350	10	15	150
	23–50	70	154	178	70	56	800	800	350	10	15	150
	51+	70	154	178	70	56	800	800	350	10	15	150
Females	11–14	46	101	157	62	46	1200	1200	300	18	15	150
	15–18	55	120	163	64	46	1200	1200	300	18	15	150
	19–22	55	120	163	64	44	800	800	300	18	15	150
	23–50	55	120	163	64	44	800	800	300	18	15	150
	51+	55	120	163	64	44	800	800	300	10	15	150
Pregnant						+30	+400	+400	+150	h	+5	+25
Lactating						+20	+400	+400	+150	h	+10	+50

Continued

Recommended Daily Dietary Allowances,[a] Revised 1980[i]

	Age (years)	FAT-SOLUBLE VITAMINS			WATER-SOLUBLE VITAMINS						
		Vitamin A (mcg RE)[b]	Vitamin D (mcg)[c]	Vitamin E (mg α-TE)[d]	Vitamin C (mg)	Thiamin (mg)	Riboflavin (mg)	Niacin (mg NE)[e]	Vitamin B-6 (mg)	Folacin[f] (mcg)	Vitamin B-12 (mcg)
Infants	0.0–0.5	420	10	3	35	0.3	0.4	6	0.3	30	0.5[g]
	0.5–1.0	400	10	4	35	0.5	0.6	8	0.6	45	1.5
Children	1–3	400	10	5	45	0.7	0.8	9	0.9	100	2.0
	4–6	500	10	6	45	0.9	1.0	11	1.3	200	2.5
	7–10	700	10	7	45	1.2	1.4	16	1.6	300	3.0
Males	11–14	1000	10	8	50	1.4	1.6	18	1.8	400	3.0
	15–18	1000	10	10	60	1.4	1.7	18	2.0	400	3.0
	19–22	1000	7.5	10	60	1.5	1.7	19	2.2	400	3.0
	23–50	1000	5	10	60	1.4	1.6	18	2.2	400	3.0
	51+	1000	5	10	60	1.2	1.4	16	2.2	400	3.0
Females	11–14	800	10	8	50	1.1	1.3	15	1.8	400	3.0
	15–18	800	10	8	60	1.1	1.3	14	2.0	400	3.0
	19–22	800	7.5	8	60	1.1	1.3	14	2.0	400	3.0
	23–50	800	5	8	60	1.0	1.2	13	2.0	400	3.0
	51+	800	5	8	60	1.0	1.2	13	2.0	400	3.0
Pregnant		+200	+5	+2	+20	+0.4	+0.3	+2	+0.6	+400	+1.0
Lactating		+400	+5	+3	+40	+0.5	+0.5	+5	+0.5	+100	+1.0

Continued

Footnotes to Recommended Daily Dietary Allowances,[a] Revised 1980[i]

a. The allowances are intended to provide for individual variations among most normal persons as they live in the United States under usual environmental stresses. Diets should be based on a variety of common foods in order to provide other nutrients for which human requirements have been less well defined. See text for detailed discussion of allowances and of nutrients not tabulated. See Table 1 (p. 20) for weights and heights by individual year of age. See Table 3 (p. 23) for suggested average energy intakes.

b. Retinol equivalents. 1 retinol equivalent = 1 mcg retinol or 6 mcg β carotene. See text for calculation of vitamin A activity of diets as retinol equivalents.

c. As cholecalciferol. 10 mcg cholecalciferol = 400 IU of vitamin D.

d. α-tocopherol equivalents. 1 mg d-α tocopherol = 1 α-TE. See text for variation in allowances and calculation of vitamin E activity of the diet as α-tocopherol equivalents.

e. 1 NE (niacin equivalent) is equal to 1 mg of niacin or 60 mg of dietary tryptophan.

f. The folacin allowances refer to dietary sources as determined by Lactobacillus casei assay after treatment with enzymes (conjugases) to make polyglutamyl forms of the vitamin available to the test organism.

g. The recommended dietary allowance for vitamin B-12 in infants is based on average concentration of the vitamin in human milk. The allowances after weaning are based on energy intake (as recommended by the American Academy of Pediatrics) and consideration of other factors, such as intestinal absorption; see text.

h. The increased requirement during pregnancy cannot be met by the iron content of habitual American diets nor by the existing iron stores of many women; therefore the use of 30–60 mg of supplemental iron is recommended. Iron needs during lactation are not substantially different from those of nonpregnant women, but continued supplementation of the mother for 2–3 months after parturition is advisable in order to replenish stores depleted by pregnancy.

i. Food and Nutrition Board. Recommended dietary allowances. 9th ed. Washington, D.C.: National Academy of Sciences–National Research Council, 1980, reproduced with permission.

Sodium Content of Selected Drugs[a]

DRUGS (INJECTABLE FORMS UNLESS NOTED OTHERWISE)	MG	MEQ
Aminosalicylate Sodium, 1 g	108	4.7
Ampicillin Sodium, 1 g	67–71	2.9–3.1
Azlocillin Sodium, 1 g	49.8	2.17
Carbenicillin Disodium, 1 g	108[b]	4.7[b]
Cefamandole Nafate, 1 g	77	3.3
Cefazolin Sodium, 1 g	46.0–48.3	2.0–2.1
Cefoperazone Sodium, 1 g	34	1.5
Cefotaxime Sodium, 1 g	50.5	2.2
Cefoxitin Sodium, 1 g	53.8	2.3
Ceftazidime, 1 g	53.8	2.3
Ceftizoxime Sodium, 1 g	60	2.6
Cefuroxime Sodium, 1 g	54.2	2.4
Cephalothin Sodium, 1 g	63	2.8
Cephapirin Sodium, 1 g	54.2	2.36
Chloramphenicol Sodium Succinate, 1 g	52	2.25
Methicillin Sodium, 1 g	60–71	2.6–3.1
Mezlocillin Sodium, 1 g	42.6	1.85
Moxalactam Disodium, 1 g	88.0	3.8
Nafcillin Sodium, 1 g	67	2.9
Oxacillin Sodium, 1 g	64–71	2.8–3.1
Penicillin G Potassium, 1 million units	6.8	0.3
Penicillin G Sodium, 1 million units	46	2.0
Phenytoin Sodium, 1 g	88.0	3.8
Piperacillin Sodium, 1 g	42.5	1.85
Sodium Bicarbonate, 50 ml of 7.5%, 8.4%	1025, 1150	44.6, 50.0
Sodium Polystyrene Sulfonate, 1 g, oral	94-100[c]	4.1-4.3[c]
Ticarcillin Disodium, 1 g	120[b]	5.2[b]
Ticarcillin Disodium and Clavulanate Potassium (Timentin®), 1 g	109	4.75

a. Sodium content amounts are approximations. Product formulations, and hence sodium content, are subject to change by manufacturer.

b. Sodium content per gram of free acid; actual vial content can be as high as 6.5 mEq per gram.

c. Total sodium content; however, only about 33% is liberated in clinical use.

4 DRUG-INDUCED DISCOLORATION OF FECES AND URINE

THE DRUGS AND DRUG CLASSES in the following tables have been associated with the discoloration of feces or urine. Drugs and drug classes are listed generically, with a corresponding proprietary name given in parentheses.

Drugs Which May Discolor Feces

DRUG/DRUG CLASS	COLOR PRODUCED
Antacids, Aluminum Hydroxide Types	Whitish or speckling
Antibiotics, Oral	Greenish gray
Anticoagulants, All	Pink to red or black*
Bismuth Containing Preparations	Greenish black
Charcoal	Black
Clofazimine (Lamprene®)	Red to brownish black
Danthron (Dorbane®, Modane®)	Brownish staining of rectal mucosa
Dithiazanine (Delvex®)	Green to blue
Ferrous Salts	Black
Heparin	Pink to red or black*
Indocyanine Green	Green
Indomethacin (Indocin®)	Green due to biliverdinemia
Nonsteroidal Anti-Inflammatory Agents	Pink to red or black*
Oxyphenbutazone (Oxalid®, Tandearil®)	Pink to red or black*
Phenazopyridine (Pyridium®)	Orange-red
Phenylbutazone (Azolid®, Butazolidin®)	Pink to red or black*
Pyrvinium Pamoate (Povan®)	Red
Rifampin (Rifadin®, Rimactane®)	Red-orange
Salicylates, Especially **Aspirin**	Pink to red or black*
Senna	Yellow

*These colors may indicate intestinal bleeding.

Drugs Which May Discolor Urine

DRUG/DRUG CLASS	COLOR PRODUCED
Acetanilid	Yellow to red
Aloe	Yellow-pink to red-brown in alkaline urine
Aminopyrine	Red
Aminosalicylic Acid (Pamisyl®)	Discoloration; red in hypochlorite solution*
Amitriptyline (Elavil®)	Blue-green
Anisindione (Miradon®)	Orange to red in urine above pH 4
Antipyrine	Yellow to red
Azuresin (Diagnex Blue®)	Blue or green
Cascara	Brown in acid urine; yellow-pink in alkaline urine, black on standing
Chloroquine (Aralen®)	Rust yellow to brown
Chlorzoxazone (Paraflex®)	Orange to purplish red
Clofazimine (Lamprene®)	Red to brownish black
Danthron (Dorbane®, Modane®)	Pink to red or red-brown in alkaline urine
Daunorubicin (Cerubidine®)	Red
Deferoxamine Mesylate (Desferal®)	Reddish
Dimethylsulfoxide (DMSO)	Reddish, due to hemoglobinuria
Diphenadione	Orange to red in urine above pH 4
Doxorubicin (Adriamycin®)	Red
Emodin	Pink to red or red-brown in alkaline urine
Ethoxazene (Serenium®)	Orange to orange-red
Ferrous Salts	Black
Furazolidone (Furoxone®)	Rust yellow to brown
Indigo Carmine	Blue or green
Indomethacin (Indocin®)	Green due to biliverdinemia
Iron Sorbitex (Jectofer®)	Black
Levodopa (Dopar®, Larodopa®)	Dark on standing in hypochlorite solution*
Methocarbamol (Robaxin®)	Dark to brown, black or green on standing
Methyldopa (Aldomet®)	Dark on standing in hypochlorite solution*
Methylene Blue	Blue or green
Metronidazole (Flagyl®)	Dark
Mitoxantrone (Novantrone®)	Dark blue or green
Nitrofurantoin (Furadantin®, Macrodantin®)	Rust yellow to brown
Pamaquine (Plasmochin®)	Rust yellow to brown

Continued

Phenacetin	Dark brown to black on standing
Phenazopyridine (Pyridium®)	Orange to orange-red
Phenindione (Hedulin®)	Orange to red in urine above pH 4
Phenol (Intravenous)	Green
Phenolphthalein	Pink to purplish red in alkaline urine
Phenolsulfonphthalein (PSP)	Pink to red in alkaline urine
Phenothiazines	Pink to red or red-brown
Phensuximide (Milontin®)	Pink to red or red-brown
Phenytoin (Dilantin®)	Pink to red or red-brown
Primaquine	Rust yellow to brown
Quinacrine (Atabrine®)	Deep yellow in acid urine
Quinine	Brown to black
Resorcinol	Dark green
Riboflavin	Yellow fluorescence
Rifampin (Rifadin®, Rimactane®)	Bright red-orange
Santonin	Yellow; pink in alkaline urine
Senna	Yellow-brown in acid urine; pink to red in alkaline urine, brown on standing
Sulfasalazine (Azulfidine®)	Orange-yellow in alkaline urine
Sulfonamides, Antibacterial	Rust yellow to brown
Thiazolsulfone (Promizole®)	Pink or red
Tolonium (Blutene®)	Blue-green
Triamterene (Dyrenium®)	Pale blue fluorescence
Warfarin (Coumadin®)	Orange

*Hypochlorite solution in toilet bowl from prior use of chlorine bleach cleanser.

References

1. Baran RB, Rowles B. Factors affecting coloration of urine and feces. J Am Pharm Assoc 1973;NS13:139-42, 155.

2. Bowling P, Belliveau RR, Butler TJ. Intravenous medications and green urine. JAMA 1981;246:216.

3. Devereaux MW, Mancall EL. Brown urine, bleach, and L-dopa. N Engl J Med 1974;291:1142.

4. Hansten PD. Drug interactions. 4th ed. Philadelphia: Lea & Febiger, 1979:444-8.

5. Lamy PP. Drug interactions: a growing problem. Hosp Formul Manage 1975;10:60-95 passim.

6. McEvoy GK, ed. AHFS drug information 87. Bethesda, MD: American Society of Hospital Pharmacists, 1987.

7. Meyers FH, Jawetz E, Goldfien A. Review of medical pharmacology. 7th ed. Los Altos, CA: Lange Medical Publications, 1980:704-17.

8. Michaels RM, ed. Discolored urine. Physicians' Drug Alert 1981; II(9):71.

9. Muther RS, Bennett WM. Effects of dimethyl sulfoxide on renal function in man. JAMA 1980;244:2081-3.

10. Shirkey HC. Drugs that discolor the urine and feces. In: Shirkey HC, comp. Pediatric therapy. 6th ed. St. Louis: C.V. Mosby, 1980:163-6.

11. Wallach J. Alteration of laboratory test values by drugs. In: Wallach J, comp. Interpretation of diagnostic tests. 4th ed. Boston: Little, Brown & Co., 1986:660-1.

5 *DRUG-INDUCED DISEASES*

Blood Dyscrasias, Hepatotoxicity, Nephrotoxicity, Oculotoxicity, Ototoxicity, Sexual Dysfunction, Skin Disorders

Introduction. The tables in this chapter provide the user with a ready source of information on a selected group of drug-induced diseases. These tables do not include all drugs reported to be the cause of a drug-induced disease, but every effort has been made to include those agents of major significance.

Each table identifies those drugs which are thought to be most frequently implicated in causing the disorder in question and, in most cases, some statement of the clinical significance of the problem is provided. References are listed which will lead the reader to the primary literature discussions and case reports of each particular drug-induced disorder. Since the format of each table is designed to best display the data available on the subject, it is imperative that the user read the introductory statement preceding the table to become aware of any abbreviations, symbols or other signs used to identify the nature and significance of the drug-induced problems discussed.

When several members of a drug class are known to be similarly capable of producing a disorder, the class name (eg, sulfonamides, phenothiazines) is used to conserve space. Occasionally, the available literature reports that a drug is a possible cause of a disorder, but fails to adequately characterize the frequency and severity of the adverse reaction. In these cases, the phrase "scattered reports only" appears in the discussion section of the table.

Drug-Induced Blood Dyscrasias

THE AGENTS IN THE FOLLOWING TABLE have been regularly reported to cause blood dyscrasias in man. Five major types of blood dyscrasias have been selected for inclusion in this table. These do not constitute a complete list of drug-induced hematological problems and the drugs selected are not necessarily the only ones capable of producing these dyscrasias. For a more comprehensive (although aging) list, the reader should consult reference 1. Excluded from the table are the cancer chemotherapeutic agents which are well known for producing dose-related bone marrow suppression. The following abbreviations are used to indicate the specific blood dyscrasia:

AA—Aplastic Anemia	HA—Hemolytic Anemia
AGN—Agranulocytosis, Granulocytopenia or Neutropenia	MA—Megaloblastic Anemia Th—Thrombocytopenia

Drug-Induced Blood Dyscrasias

DRUG	DYSCRASIA	DISCUSSION
Acetaminophen	HA	Scattered reports only; may be an immune reaction.[3,11]
	Th	Scattered reports only; has been reported in overdose; may be an immune reaction.[1,2,5,9,11,12]
Acetazolamide	AA	Scattered reports only.[1,8,13]
	Th	Scattered reports only.[1,7,9]
Alcohol	HA	Most commonly encountered in chronic alcoholism.[1]
	MA	Results from malnutrition, decreased folate absorption and/or utilization; responds rapidly to folate administration.[1,7]
	Th	Transient in many drinkers; persistent thrombocytopenia may accompany advanced alcoholic liver disease.[1]
Allopurinol	AGN	Scattered reports only.[4,14]
Aminopyrine	AGN	Results from an immune reaction and does not appear to be dose-related. The onset is sudden and may be encountered even after long-term therapy. Beware of the presence of this drug or its derivative, **dipyrone**, in foreign products and "herbal" preparations.[1,2,4]
	HA	In G-6-PD deficiency (but not in blacks). May also result from an immune reaction.[1,3]
Amodiaquine	AGN	Prevalence estimated at 1/2,000 among those taking the drug prophylactically.[15]
Amphotericin B	AGN	Scattered reports only.[1,2,16]
	HA	Rare; may be more common in patients with impaired renal function.[1,2]
	Th	Scattered reports only.[1-3,16,17]
Amrinone	Th	18.6% prevalence in one study of oral therapy (oral form not marketed in US);

Continued

Drug-Induced Blood Dyscrasias

DRUG	DYSCRASIA	DISCUSSION
		the prevalence during parenteral therapy is probably less than 5%.[18]
Antidepressants, Heterocyclic	AGN	Idiosyncratic reaction, probably resulting from a direct toxic effect rather than allergy. Most commonly encountered between the 2nd and 8th weeks of therapy.[1,2,4,19,20]
Antipyrine	AGN	Scattered reports only.[4]
	HA	In G-6-PD deficiency (but not in blacks).[1]
Arsenicals, Organic	AA	Occurs both during and after the completion of therapy.[1,8]
	AGN	Occurs both during and after the completion of therapy.[1]
	Th	Scattered reports only.[1,9,21]
Ascorbic Acid	HA	In G-6-PD deficiency with large doses.[1,2,6]
Aspirin	AA	Prevalence is extremely low when the extent of use is considered. Often occurs after long-term high-dose therapy (several kg total dose).[1,2,8,22]
	AGN	Rare; reported patients were usually taking other drugs capable of producing this dyscrasia.[1,2,4]
	HA	In G-6-PD deficiency; usually in conjunction with infection or other complicating factors.[1,2,6]
	Th	May occur in addition to the drug's effects on platelet adhesiveness. Some evidence for an immune reaction.[1,2,5,9,23]
Captopril	AGN	Rare in normal patients, with prevalence estimated at 1/5,000. The prevalence increases significantly in patients with reduced renal function or collagen diseases and reaches 7% in patients with both renal impairment and a collagen disease. Most common during the first 3 weeks of therapy.[2,4,24]
Carbamazepine	AA	20 cases reported from 1964–1986; onset may be delayed until weeks or months after the initiation of therapy.[1,4,25]

Continued

Drug-Induced Blood Dyscrasias

DRUG	DYSCRASIA	DISCUSSION
	AGN	Transient leukopenia is seen in about 10% of patients, usually during the first month of therapy. Persistent leukopenia occurs in 2%.[25]
	Th	Prevalence estimated at 2%.[25,26]
Cephalosporins	AGN	Rare; possibly the result of an immune reaction.[1,2,4,10]
	HA	Positive direct Coombs' tests are common (3–75%, depending on the report) and may persist for up to 2 months after discontinuation of therapy. Hemolysis is rare.[1-3,10]
	Th	Rare; possibly the result of an immune reaction.[1,2,5,9,10]
Chloramphenicol	AA	Prevalence estimated at 1/18,000 to 1/50,000. Most cases develop after discontinuation of therapy and with oral administration, suggesting the development of a toxic metabolite. Aplastic anemia has occurred with parenteral and ophthalmic therapy. Aplastic anemia should not be confused with the dose-related anemia seen with chloramphenicol (NOTE: one case report suggests that a patient's dose-related anemia may have progressed to aplastic anemia, but most sources separate the two dyscrasias).[1,2,8,10,27-29]
	AGN	Rare when compared with the prevalence of aplastic anemia.[1,4]
	HA	In G-6-PD deficiency.[1,6,10]
Chlordiazepoxide	AGN	Scattered reports only.[1,4]
Chloroquine	AGN	Scattered reports only.[1,2]
	HA	Only a few cases have been reported; some association with G-6-PD deficiency is suspected.[1,2,6]
Chlorpropamide	AGN	Scattered reports only.[1,2,4]
	HA	Scattered reports only, with onset usually shortly after the initiation of therapy.[2,30]
	Th	Scattered reports only.[1,2,9]

Continued

Drug-Induced Blood Dyscrasias

DRUG	DYSCRASIA	DISCUSSION
Cimetidine	AA	Scattered reports only, but at least 1 fatality reported.[31,32]
	AGN	Usually occurs in patients with significant systemic disease which may contribute to the dyscrasia.[4,33,34]
Contraceptives, Oral	MA	Results from impaired absorption and/or utilization of folate; of consequence only if patient's folate status is markedly impaired.[1,7]
Dapsone	AGN	Many cases have occurred during combination therapy, so that it is difficult to determine if dapsone alone is the causative agent.[1,2,4]
	HA	In G-6-PD deficiency; may also have other mechanism(s).[1,2,6]
Diazoxide	HA	In G-6-PD deficiency.[6]
Digitoxin	Th	Scattered reports only; evidence of an immune mechanism.[2,5,9,35]
Digoxin	Th	Scattered reports only; evidence of an immune mechanism.[2,9,36]
Dimercaprol	HA	In G-6-PD deficiency.[1,2,6]
Dipyrone		See Aminopyrine.
Diuretics, Thiazide	AA	Scattered reports only.[1,2,8]
	AGN	Scattered reports only.[1,2,4]
	HA	Exact mechanism is unclear; may be an immune reaction.[1,37]
	Th	Mild thrombocytopenia is common, but severe cases are rare. May result from an immune reaction.[1,2,5,9,38]
Flucytosine	AGN	Dose-related; usually requires plasma level of 125 mcg/ml or greater.[2,39]
	Th	Dose-related; usually requires plasma level of 125 mcg/ml or greater.[2,39]
Furosemide	Th	Uncommon, usually mild and asymptomatic.[1,2]
Gold Salts	AA	Not dose-dependent; while this reaction is not common, numerous fatalities have been reported.[1,2,8,40]

Continued

Drug-Induced Blood Dyscrasias

DRUG	DYSCRASIA	DISCUSSION
	AGN	Often brief and self-limiting; usually responds to withdrawal of therapy.[2,41,42]
	Th	Not dose- or duration-dependent; prevalence estimated at 1–3%; onset usually occurs during the loading phase of gold therapy (first 1000 mg), but may be delayed until after the drug has been discontinued. Mechanism is unclear, but probably related to increased peripheral destruction of platelets.[1,2,9,43,44]
Heparin	Th	Mild reduction in platelet count is common, but reduction of 40% or more occurs in 10% or fewer patients. Highest prevalence occurs with beef lung derived products. Intermittent, continuous infusion and "mini-dose" regimens have all been implicated. Onset is rapid, as is recovery after discontinuation of the drug.[1,2,5,45-48]
Hydralazine	Th	Appears to be quite rare, but 3 cases reported in neonates whose mothers were treated with hydralazine near term.[2,49]
Ibuprofen	Th	Scattered reports only with ibuprofen; isolated cases reported with many of the newer nonsteroidal anti-inflammatory agents.[2]
Indomethacin	Th	Mild impairment of platelet function is common, but thrombocytopenia is rare.[1,2]
Interferon	Th	Scattered reports only.[2,50]
Isoniazid	AGN	Scattered reports only; some evidence of an immune reaction.[1,2,4]
	Th	Scattered reports only; some evidence of an immune reaction.[1,2,5,9]
Levamisole	AGN	May be the result of an autoimmune reaction with a prevalence of 4% in some series. The presence of HLA B27 in seropositive rheumatoid arthritis is apparently an important predisposing factor.[2,51,52]
	Th	Scattered reports only.[2,9,53]
Levodopa	HA	Autoimmune reaction; positive direct and indirect Coombs' tests are com-

Continued

Drug-Induced Blood Dyscrasias

DRUG	DYSCRASIA	DISCUSSION
		mon, but hemolysis is rare. **Carbidopa-levodopa** combinations have also produced hemolysis.[1-3]
Mefenamic Acid	HA	Thought to be autoimmune.[1-3]
Mephenytoin	AA	Onset after several months of therapy.[1,2,8]
	AGN	Rare; normalization usually occurs 1-2 weeks after discontinuation of the drug, but some fatalities have been reported.[1,4]
Methicillin		See Penicillins.
Methimazole	AA	Scattered reports only.[2,8]
	AGN	Most cases are encountered in the first 9 weeks of therapy. Prevalence increases with age and may be higher in females. Doses below 30 mg/day seem to have significantly lower risk.[1,2,4,54,55]
Methyldopa	HA	Autoimmune reaction; positive direct Coombs' test occurs in 5-25% of patients, depending on dose; hemolysis occurs in less than 1% and its onset is gradual after 6 months or more of therapy. Recovery is rapid after drug discontinuation.[1-3,56]
	Th	Rare; may be the manifestation of an immune reaction.[1,2,9,57]
Methylene Blue	HA	In G-6-PD deficiency.[1,2,6]
Nalidixic Acid	HA	In G-6-PD deficiency; may also have other mechanisms.[1,2,10]
	Th	Scattered reports only; possibly associated with renal impairment in one series.[58]
Nitrofurantoin	HA	In G-6-PD deficiency; also encountered with enolase deficiency (mechanism unknown).[1,2,6,10]
Oxprenolol	Th	Scattered reports only; also occurs with some of the other beta-blockers.[2,9,59]
Oxyphenbutazone		See Phenylbutazone.
Penicillamine	AA	Develops slowly; results from direct marrow toxicity.[2,8,60,61]

Continued

Drug-Induced Blood Dyscrasias

DRUG	DYSCRASIA	DISCUSSION
	AGN	Most cases occur during the first month of therapy. [1,2,4,61]
	HA	Scattered reports only; may be due to G-6-PD deficiency or fluctuations in copper levels during therapy of Wilson's disease. [2,61,62]
	Th	Prevalence estimated at 10%; some decrease in platelets in 75% of penicillamine-treated patients. May be the result of an immune reaction; most commonly occurs during the first 6 months of therapy. [1,2,61,63]
Penicillins	AA	Prevalence very low when extent of use is considered. [1,2,10]
	AGN	Uncommon with most penicillins, but encountered frequently with **methicillin**; in one report, neutropenia developed in 23 of 68 methicillin-treated patients; resolution occurred within 3 to 7 days after drug withdrawal. [1,2,4,10,64,65]
	HA	Hemolysis rare; positive direct Coombs' test occurs with large IV doses. [1-3,10]
	Th	Prevalence very low when extent of use is considered. [1,2,5,9,10]
Phenacetin	HA	In G-6-PD deficiency; usually requires infection or other complicating factors. Hemolysis may also result from an immune reaction or direct drug toxicity. [1,3,6]
Phenazopyridine	HA	Mechanism unknown; renal insufficiency and overdose may be contributing factors. Often accompanied by methemoglobinemia. [1,2,6,66]
Phenindione	AGN	Usually occurs as part of a hypersensitivity reaction; number of cases is impressive when the limited use of this drug is considered. [1,4]
Phenobarbital	MA	Usually responds to folate administration. [1,7]
Phenothiazines	AGN	Most common during the first 2 months of therapy and in older patients (more than 85% are over 40 yr). Rapid onset and general lack of dose-dependence suggest an idiosyncratic mechanism. [1,2,4,19,67,68]

Continued

Drug-Induced Blood Dyscrasias

DRUG	DYSCRASIA	DISCUSSION
	Th	Scattered reports only.[1,5]
Phenylbutazone	AA	With the more limited use of chloramphenicol, phenylbutazone is the most frequent cause of drug-induced aplastic anemia, with more than 1,000 recorded cases. Most common in the elderly, with onset after weeks to decades of therapy; fatality rate is about 50%.[1,2,8,69,70]
	AGN	Not dose-dependent; onset after days to years of therapy.[1,4]
	Th	Usually occurs during the first 4 weeks of therapy.[1,2,5]
Phenytoin	AA	Fewer than 25 cases reported, but the association with phenytoin is strong.[1,2,8]
	AGN	Scattered reports only; onset after days to years of therapy.[1,4]
	MA	Results from impaired absorption and/or utilization of folate and responds to folate therapy (although folate replacement may lower phenytoin levels). Mild macrocytosis is very common (25% or more); onset is unpredictable, but usually appears after 6 or more months of therapy.[1,2,7]
	Th	Scattered reports only; may be the result of an immune reaction.[1,5,9,71]
Primaquine	HA	In G-6-PD deficiency.[1,2,6]
Primidone	MA	Similar to phenytoin, but prevalence may be lower; onset unpredictable and may be delayed for several years during therapy.[1,2,7]
Procainamide	AGN	Prevalence usually estimated at less than 1%; occurs with both conventional and sustained-release products.[1,2,4,72-74]
Propranolol		See Oxprenolol.
Propylthiouracil	AA	Scattered reports only, but association with propylthiouracil is strong.[2,8]
	AGN	Exact mechanism unclear; may be an immune reaction. Unlike methimazole,

Continued

Drug-Induced Blood Dyscrasias

DRUG	DYSCRASIA	DISCUSSION
		does not appear to be dose-related. Usually occurs during the first few months of therapy with the prevalence increasing with age.[1,2,4,55]
	Th	Scattered reports only.[1,2,9]
Pyrimethamine	AGN	Scattered reports only.[2]
	MA	Results from inhibition of conversion of folic acid to folinic acid.[2]
	Th	Scattered reports only.[2]
Quinacrine	AA	About one-half of the reported cases were preceded by a rash or lichenoid eruption; prevalence estimated at 3/100,000.[1,2,8,75]
	HA	In G-6-PD deficiency; usually requires infection or other complicating factors.[1,8]
Quinidine	AGN	Scattered reports only; an immune mechanism has been described.[2,4,76]
	HA	In G-6-PD deficiency (but not in blacks). An immune mechanism has also been described.[1-3,77]
	Th	Caused by quinidine-specific anti-bodies; little or no cross-reactivity with quinine. Accounts for a significant percentage of drug-induced thrombo-cytopenia.[1,2,5,9,71,78,79]
Quinine	AGN	Scattered reports only.[1,4]
	HA	In G-6-PD deficiency (but not in blacks). An immune mechanism is also suspected.[1-3,80]
	Th	Caused by quinine-specific antibodies; little or no cross-reactivity with quinidine. Reported in people drinking quinine-containing tonic water.[1,2,5,9,81,82]
Ranitidine	AGN	Scattered reports only.[83]
Rifampin	HA	Rare, but a significant number of patients develop positive Coombs' test; onset in hours in some sensitized patients.[1,2]

Continued

Drug-Induced Blood Dyscrasias

DRUG	DYSCRASIA	DISCUSSION
	Th	Peripheral destruction of platelets appears to result from an immune reaction.[1,2,5,9,84,85]
Silver Sulfadiazine		See Sulfonamides.
Sulfasalazine		See Sulfonamides.
Sulfinpyrazone	AGN	Scattered reports only; occurs during prolonged therapy.[2]
Sulfonamides	AA	Historically, an important cause of aplastic anemia, but most cases were reported following use of older sulfonamides; rarely encountered with products currently in use.[1,2,8,10]
	AGN	Occurs mostly with older products; rarely encountered with products currently in use; reported with **silver sulfadiazine.** Onset is usually rapid.[1,2,4,10,69,86]
	HA	In G-6-PD deficiency; also occurs in nondeficient patients. **Sulfasalazine** is the most commonly used oxidative sulfonamide; hemolysis during sulfasalazine therapy may be more common in slow acetylators.[1,2,3,10,87-89]
	Th	Scattered reports only; probably an immune reaction.[2,9,71,90]
Sulfones		See Dapsone.
Tolbutamide	AA	Scattered reports only.[1,2,8]
	Th	Scattered reports only.[1,2]
Triamterene	AA	Reported in patients with hepatic cirrhosis; responds to folate therapy.[91]
	MA	Few cases reported, but it is a potent inhibitor of dihydrofolate reductase; greatest risk in those with low folate levels prior to therapy (eg, alcoholics).[1,2,7]
Trimethoprim	AA	Rare; occurs when used alone and in combination therapy with sulfonamides.[2,10,92]
	AGN	Rare; occurs when used alone and in combination with sulfonamides, with the latter numerically more common.[1,2,4,10,69,93]

Continued

Drug-Induced Blood Dyscrasias

DRUG	DYSCRASIA	DISCUSSION
	MA	Most cases occur after 1–2 weeks of therapy; this drug may have small antifolate action in humans which becomes important only in those with low folate levels prior to therapy (eg, alcoholics).[1,2,7,10]
	Th	Mild thrombocytopenia is common, but severe cases are rare. Most commonly encountered in combination therapy with sulfonamides.[1,2,5,9,10]
Valproic Acid	Th	Exact prevalence and significance are undetermined. Both immune and dose-dependent mechanisms have been suggested.[2,9,94,95]
Vancomycin	AGN	Scattered reports only; may be an immune reaction.[2,96,97]
Vitamin K	HA	In G-6-PD deficiency; usually requires infection or other complicating factors. Hemolysis from high doses contributes to jaundice in neonates; rarely toxic in older children and adults.[1,2,6]

References

1. Swanson M, Cook R. Drugs, chemicals and blood dyscrasias. Hamilton, IL: Drug Intelligence Publications, Inc. 1977.

2. Dukes MNG, ed. Meyler's side effects of drugs. 10th ed. Amsterdam: Elsevier, 1984.

3. Petz LD. Drug-induced immune haemolytic anaemia. Clin Haematol 1980;9:455-82.

4. Young GAR, Vincent PC. Drug-induced agranulocytosis. Clin Haematol 1980;9:483-504.

5. Miescher PA, Graf J. Drug-induced thrombocytopenia. Clin Haematol 1980;9:505-19.

6. Gordon-Smith EC. Drug-induced oxidative haemolysis. Clin Haematol 1980;9:557-86.

7. Scott JM, Weir DG. Drug-induced megaloblastic change. Clin Haematol 1980;9:587-606.

8. Heimpel H, Heit W. Drug-induced aplastic anaemia: clinical aspects. Clin Haematol 1980;9:641-62.

9. Hackett T, Kelton JG, Powers P. Drug-induced platelet destruction. Semin Thromb Hemost 1982;8:116-37.

10. Kucers A, Bennett NMcK. The use of antibiotics. 3rd ed. Philadelphia: JB Lippincott, 1979.

11. Kornberg A, Polliack A. Paracetamol-induced thrombocytopenia and haemolytic anaemia. Lancet 1978;2:1159. Letter.

12. Shoenfeld Y, Shaklai M, Livni E et al. Thrombocytopenia from acetaminophen. N Engl J Med 1980;303:47. Letter.

13. Niven BI, Manoharan A. Acetazolamide-induced anaemia. Med J Aust 1985;142:120. Letter.

14. Hawson GAT, Bain BJ. Allopurinol and agranulocytosis. Med J Aust 1980;1:283-4. Letter.

15. Hatton CSR, Bunch C, Peto TEA et al. Frequency of severe neutropenia associated with amodiaquine prophylaxis against malaria. Lancet 1986;1:411-4.

16. Wilson R, Feldman S. Toxicity of amphotericin B in children with cancer. Am J Dis Child 1979;133:731-4.

17. Chan CSP, Tuazon CU, Lessin LS. Amphotericin-B-induced thrombocytopenia. Ann Intern Med 1982;96:332-3.

18. Ansell J, Tiarks C, McCue J et al. Amrinone-induced thrombocytopenia. Arch Intern Med 1984;144:949-52.

19. Klein DF, Gittelman R, Quitkin F et al. Diagnosis and drug treatment of psychiatric disorders. 2nd ed. Baltimore: Williams and Wilkins, 1980.

20. Albertini RS, Penders TM. Agranulocytosis associated with tricyclics. J Clin Psychiatry 1978;39:483-5.

21. Falconer EH, Epstein NN, Mills ES. Purpura haemorrhagica due to the arsphenamines. Arch Intern Med 1940;66:319-38.

22. Eldar M, Aderka D. Shoenfeld Y et al. Aspirin-induced aplastic anaemia. S Afr Med J 1979;55:318. Letter.

23. Garg SK, Sarker CR. Aspirin-induced thrombocytopenia on an immune basis. Am J Med Sci 1974;267:129-32.

24. Cooper RA. Captopril-associated neutropenia. Who is at risk? Arch Intern Med 1983;143:659-60. Editorial.

25. Hart RG, Easton JD. Carbamazepine and hematological monitoring. Ann Neurol 1982;11:309-12.

26. Bradley JM, Sagraves R, Kimbrough AC. Carbamazepine-induced thrombocytopenia in a young child. Clin Pharm 1985;4:221-3.

27. Plaunt ME, Best WR. Aplastic anemia after parenteral chloramphenicol: warning renewed. N Engl J Med 1982;306:1486. Letter.

28. Fraunfelder FT, Bagby GC, Kelly DJ. Fatal aplastic anemia following topical administration of ophthalmic chloramphenicol. Am J Ophthalmol 1982;93:356-60.

29. Daum RS, Cohen DL, Smith AL. Fatal aplastic anemia following apparent ''dose-related'' chloramphenicol toxicity. J Pediatr 1979;94:403-6.

30. Or R, Merin E, Stupp Y et al. Chlorpropamide-induced hemolytic anemia. Drug Intell Clin Pharm 1984;18:981-2.

31. Chang HK, Morrison SL. Bone-marrow suppression associated with cimetidine. Ann Intern Med 1979;91:580.

32. Tonkonow B, Hoffman R. Aplastic anemia and cimetidine. Arch Intern Med 1980;140:1123-4. Letter.

33. Carloss HW, Tavassoli M, McMillan R. Cimetidine-induced granulocytopenia. Ann Intern Med 1980;93:57-8.

34. Seville P. Cimetidine and agranulocytosis. Med J Aust 1982;1:250. Letter.

35. Young RC, Nachman RL, Horowitz HI. Thrombocytopenia due to digitoxin. Demonstration of antibody and mechanisms of action. Am J Med 1966;41:605-14.

36. Pirovino M, Ohnhaus EE, von Felten A. Digoxin-associated thrombocytopaenia. Eur J Clin Pharmacol 1981;19:205-7.

37. Beck ML, Cline JF, Hardman JT et al. Fatal intravascular immune hemolysis induced by hydrochlorothiazide. Am J Clin Pathol 1984;81:791-4.

38. Okafor KC, Griffin C, Ngole PM. Hydrochlorothiazide-induced thrombocytopenic purpura. Drug Intell Clin Pharm 1986;20:60-1.

39. Kauffman CA, Frame PT. Bone marrow toxicity associated with 5-fluorocytosine therapy. Antimicrob Agents Chemother 1977;11:244-7.

40. Gibson J, McGirr EE, York J et al. Aplastic anemia in association with gold therapy for rheumatoid arthritis. Aust NZ J Med 1983;13:130-4.

41. Gibbons RB. Complications of chrysotherapy: a review of recent studies. Arch Intern Med 1979;139:343-6.

42. Gottlieb NL, Buchoff HS, Vidal AF et al. The course of severe gold-associated granulocytopenia. Clin Res 1982;30:659A. Abstract.

43. Harth M, Hickey JP, Coulter WK et al. Gold-induced thrombocytopenia. J Rheumatol 1978;5:165-72.

44. Coblyn JS, Weinblatt M, Holdsworth D et al. Gold-induced thrombocytopenia. A clinical and immunogenetic study of twenty-three patients. Ann Intern Med 1981;95:178-81.

45. Ayars GH, Tikoff G. Incidence of thrombocytopenia in medical patients on ''mini-dose'' heparin prophylaxis. Am Heart J 1980;99:816. Letter.

46. Bell WR, Royall RM. Heparin-associated thrombocytopenia: a comparison of three heparin preparations. N Engl J Med 1980;303:902-7.

47. King DJ, Kelton JG. Heparin-associated thrombocytopenia. Ann Intern Med 1984;100:535-40.

48. Ramirez-Lassepas M, Cipolle RJ, Rodvold KA et al. Heparin-induced thrombocytopenia in patients with cerebrovascular ischemic disease. Neurology 1984;34:736-40.

49. Widerlov E, Karlman I, Storsater J. Hydralazine-induced neonatal thrombocytopenia. N Engl J Med 1980;303:1235. Letter.

50. McLaughlin P, Talpaz M, Quesada JR et al. Immune thrombocytopenia following alpha-interferon therapy in patients with cancer. JAMA 1985;254:1353-4.

51. Mielants H, Veys EM. A study of the hematological side effects of levamisole in rheumatoid arthritis with recommendations. J Rheumatol 1978;5(Suppl 4):77-83.

52. Drew SI, Carter BM, Nathanson DS et al. Levamisole-associated neutropenia and autoimmune granulocytotoxins. Ann Rheum Dis 1980;39:59-63.

53. El-Ghobarey AF, Capell HA. Levamisole-induced thrombocytopenia. Br Med J 1977;2:555-6.

54. Luther AL, Wade JS, Slaughter JM. Agranulocytosis secondary to methimazole therapy: report of two cases. South Med J 1976;69:1356-7.

55. Cooper DS, Goldminz D, Levin AA et al. Agranulocytosis associated with antithyroid drugs: effects of patient age and drug dose. Ann Intern Med 1983;98:26-9.

56. Kelton JG. Impaired reticuloendothelial function in patients treated with methyldopa. N Engl J Med 1985;313:596-600.

57. Manohitharajah SM, Jenkins WJ, Roberts PD et al. Methyldopa and associated thrombocytopenia. Br Med J 1971;1:494.

58. Meyboom RHB. Thrombocytopenia induced by nalidixic acid. Br Med J 1984;289:962.

59. Dodds WN, Davidson RJL. Thrombocytopenia due to slow-release oxprenolol. Lancet 1978;2:683. Letter.

60. Kay AGL. Myelotoxicity of D-penicillamine. Ann Rheum Dis 1979;38:232-6.

61. Camp V. Hematologic toxicity from penicillamine in rheumatoid arthritis. J Rheumatol 1981;8(Suppl 7):164-5.

62. Lyle WH. D-penicillamine and haemolytic anaemia. Lancet 1976;1:428. Letter.

63. Thomas D, Gallus A, Tampi R et al. A study of d-penicillamine induced thrombocytopenia in rheumatoid arthritis with Cr[51]-labelled autologous platelets. Aust NZ J Med 1981;11:722. Abstract.

64. Corbett GM, Perry DJ, Shaw TRD. Penicillin-induced leukopenia. N Engl J Med 1982;307:1642-3. Letter.

65. Mallouh AA. Methicillin-induced neutropenia. Pediatr Infect Dis 1985;4:262-4.

66. Jeffery WH, Zelicoff AP, Hardy WR. Acquired methemoglobinemia and hemolytic anemia after usual doses of phenazopyridine. Drug Intell Clin Pharm 1982;16:157-9.

67. Hollister LE. Allergic reactions to tranquilizing drugs. Ann Intern Med 1958;49:17-29.

68. Pisciotta AV, Ebbe S, Lennon EJ et al. Agranulocytosis following administration of phenothiazine derivatives. Am J Med 1958;25:210-23.

69. Inman WHW. Study of fatal bone marrow depression with special reference to phenylbutazone and oxyphenbutazone. Br Med J 1977;1:1500-5.

70. Bottiger LE. Phenylbutazone, oxyphenbutazone and aplastic anaemia. Br Med J 1977;2:265. Letter.

71. Cimo PL, Pisciotta AV, Desai RG et al. Detection of drug-dependent antibodies by the ^{51}Cr platelet lysis test: documentation of immune thrombocytopenia induced by diphenylhydantoin, diazepam, and sulfisoxazole. Am J Hematol 1977;2:65-72.

72. Reidy TJ, Upshaw JD. Procainamide-induced agranulocytosis. South Med J 1984;77:1582-4.

73. Kimmel DP, Antignano LV, Barold SS et al. Neutropenia associated with procainamide. NY State J Med 1985;85:197. Letter.

74. Meyers DG, Gonzalez ER, Peters LL et al. Severe neutropenia associated with procainamide: comparison of sustained release and conventional preparations. Am Heart J 1985;109:1393-5.

75. Custer RP. Aplastic anemia in soldiers treated with atabrine (quinacrine). Am J Med Sci 1946;212:211-24.

76. Ascensao JL, Flynn PJ, Slungaard A et al. Quinidine-induced neutropenia: report of a case with drug-dependent inhibition of granulocyte colony generation. Acta Haematol 1984;72:349-54.

77. Geltner D, Chajek T, Rubinger D et al. Quinidine hypersensitivity and liver involvement. A survey of 32 patients. Gastroenterology 1976;70:650-2.

78. Bolton FG, Dameshek W. Thrombocytopenic purpura due to quinidine. I. Clinical studies. Blood 1956;11:527-46.

79. Alperin JB, deGroot WJ, Cimo PL. Quinidine-induced thrombocytopenia with pulmonary hemorrhage. Arch Intern Med 1980;140:266-7.

80. Webb RF, Ramirez AM, Hocken AG et al. Acute intravascular haemolysis due to quinine. NZ Med J 1980;91:14-6.

81. Steinkamp R, Moore CV, Doubek WG. Thrombocytopenic purpura caused by hypersensitivity to quinine. J Lab Clin Med 1955;45:18-29.

82. Murray JA, Abbott I, Anderson DA et al. Bitter lemon purpura. Br Med J 1979;2:1551-2.

83. Shields LI, Files JA, Doll DC et al. Ranitidine and agranulocytosis. Ann Intern Med 1986;104:128. Letter.

84. Blajchman MA, Lowry RC, Pettit JE et al. Rifampicin-induced immune thrombocytopenia. Br Med J 1970;3:24-6.

85. Hadfield JW. Rifampicin-induced thrombocytopenia. Postgrad Med J 1980;56:59-60.

86. Jarrett F, Ellerbe S, Demling R. Acute leukopenia during topical burn therapy with silver sulfadiazine. Am J Surg 1978;135:818-9.

87. Cohen SM, Rosenthal DS, Karp PJ. Ulcerative colitis and erythrocyte G6PD deficiency. Salicylazosulfapyridine-provoked hemolysis. JAMA 1968;205:528-30.

88. Das KM, Eastwood MA, McManus JPA et al. Adverse reactions during salicylazosulfapyridine therapy and the relation with drug metabolism and acetylator phenotype. N Engl J Med 1973;289:491-5.

89. Zinkham WH. Unstable hemoglobins and the selective hemolytic action of sulfonamides. Arch Intern Med 1977;137:1365-6. Editorial.

90. Hamilton HE, Sheets RF. Sulfisoxazole-induced thrombocytopenic purpura. Immunologic mechanism as cause. JAMA 1978;239:2586-7.

91. Buurke EJ. Diuretic drugs. In: Dukes MNG, ed. Side effects of drugs annual 7. Amsterdam: Excerpta Medica, 1983:246-9.

92. Sheehan J. Trimethoprim-associated marrow toxicity. Lancet 1981;2:692. Letter.

93. Principi N, Marchisio P, Biasini A et al. Early and late neutropenia in children treated with cotrimoxazole (trimethoprim-sulfamethoxazole). Acta Paediatr Scand 1984;73:763-7.

94. Morris N, Barr RD, Pai KRM et al. Valproic acid and thrombocytopenia. Can Med Assoc J 1981;125:63-4.

95. Ribera A, Martin-Vega C et al. Autoimmune thrombocytopenia (AT) and valproic acid treatment. Br Med J 1984;288:830.

96. Borland CDR, Farrar WE. Reversible neutropenia from vancomycin. JAMA 1979;242:2392-3. Letter.

97. Mackett RL, Guay DRP. Vancomycin-induced neutropenia. Can Med Assoc J 1985;132:39-40.

Drug-Induced Hepatotoxicity

THE AGENTS IN THE FOLLOWING TABLE have been associated with drug-induced hepatotoxicity in man. Each entry briefly describes the nature and time course of the drug's hepatotoxicity and, when possible, states its prevalence. The table includes only commonly used drugs with a well-established history of hepatotoxicity; the absence of a drug from the table should not be interpreted as meaning that a drug is incapable of producing liver damage. Virtually all drugs have been reported to produce elevations of liver enzymes in serum.

The table begins on page 78.

Drug-Induced Hepatotoxicity

DRUG	NATURE OF HEPATOTOXICITY
Acetaminophen	Hepatic damage may follow overdosage with 140 mg/kg or more. These doses saturate the normal metabolic pathways and produce large quantities of a toxic metabolite. Therapy with **acetylcysteine** to bind the metabolite is indicated when the 4 hr post-ingestion plasma acetaminophen level is over 200 mcg/ml. A nomogram is available to plot the treatment cutoff concentrations for other post-ingestion times. Even without specific therapy, fatalities are uncommon following acetaminophen overdose. Nonfatal cases usually fully recover in a few weeks. Chronic **alcohol** ingestion has long been thought to increase acetaminophen toxicity, but the available evidence is inconclusive. Acute alcohol ingestion is thought by some to have a protective action. Children appear to be at low risk of developing acetaminophen-induced hepatitis. Less destructive, but still detectable, hepatitis has been reported in patients taking therapeutic doses repeatedly for a prolonged time. [1-7]
Alcohol	Fatty infiltration of the liver can be found in 70-100% of alcoholics. Fatty liver is generally without clinical manifestation, but 30% progress to develop alcoholic hepatitis and about 10% develop cirrhosis. Malnutrition may contribute significantly to alcoholic liver disease and alcohol may potentiate the hepatotoxicity of other drugs. [2]
Allopurinol	Hepatitis and hepatic necrosis may accompany other symptoms (especially rash, fever and vasculitis) of allopurinol hypersensitivity. This reaction is uncommon, but serious when it occurs. Renal impairment may be a predisposing factor for allopurinol-induced hepatitis. Cholestasis has also been attributed to allopurinol. [1-3,8,9]
Aminoglutethimide	Laboratory evidence of hepatic dysfunction is common, but clinical evidence is rare. [1,10]
Aminosalicylic Acid	Up to 5% of patients taking aminosalicylic acid may develop a generalized hypersensitivity reaction. 25% of these patients demonstrate evidence of hepatic injury as part of their hypersensitivity reaction. Fatalities have been reported. [1,2,11]
Amiodarone	Mild increases in AST (SGOT) and LDH levels have been encountered in one-half of amiodarone-treated pa- Continued

Drug-Induced Hepatotoxicity

DRUG	NATURE OF HEPATOTOXICITY
	tients. Onset is after 2–4 months of therapy, often returning to normal despite continued therapy. Phospholipidosis, cirrhosis and fatalities have also been reported.[1,3,12-14]
Androgens	See Steroids, C-17-α-Alkyl.
Antidepressants, Heterocyclic	The prevalence of heterocyclic antidepressant-induced hepatic injury has been estimated at about 1% with most of the cases presenting as cholestasis.[1-3]
Asparaginase	Slowly reversible steatosis has been reported in 50–87% of patients taking this drug, apparently as a result of its influence on protein synthesis. Daily doses may be more toxic than weekly doses.[1,2,15,16]
Carbamazepine	Hepatic necrosis, granulomas and cholestasis have all been encountered with this drug. Some cases have shown signs of hypersensitivity. Onset is most often in the first 6 weeks of therapy. Fatalities have been reported.[1-3,17,18]
Chenodiol	Dose-related elevations in plasma levels of hepatic enzymes and a low (0.4–3%) prevalence of "clinically significant" hepatic injury are associated with the use of this drug.[1,3,19]
Chlorpropamide	Most reported hepatotoxic reactions are cholestatic. A 2-month latent period and other evidence point toward an immune mechanism.[1-3]
Cisplatin	Dose-related elevations of hepatic enzymes are commonly encountered.[1]
Contraceptives, Oral	Several hundred cases of jaundice have been reported, with the onset of symptoms usually in the first few months of therapy. Patients who demonstrate jaundice during pregnancy have a greater chance of reacting similarly to oral contraceptives. Withdrawal of the drug is usually followed by prompt resolution of the jaundice. Oral contraceptives are associated with a marked increase in the prevalence of hepatic adenomas and related benign tumors, especially after 5 or more years of use. These tumors may require

Continued

Drug-Induced Hepatotoxicity

DRUG	NATURE OF HEPATOTOXICITY
	resection. The frequency of gall bladder disease is also apparently increased by oral contraceptives. An association between oral contraceptive use and an increase in the prevalence of hepatocellular carcinoma is being debated.[1-3, 20-25]
Cyclosporine	Conjugated hyperbilirubinemia is common (almost 25% in one study) and responds to dosage reduction.[1, 26, 27]
Dantrolene	At least 0.8% of patients develop laboratory evidence of hepatic dysfunction, with symptomatic hepatitis in about 0.4%; the fatality rate among jaundiced patients is about 25%. Predisposing factors seem to include dose (greater than 300 mg/day), sex (females more than males), age (over 30 yr) and duration of therapy (at least 2 months).[1, 2, 28, 29]
Dapsone	Hepatitis may occur as part of the "dapsone syndrome," which is a generalized hypersensitivity reaction including rash, fever and lymphadenopathy. While most dapsone-associated liver injury is hepatocellular, some cases of cholestasis have occurred.[1-3, 30, 31]
Erythromycin	Some literature has described a 2-4% prevalence of jaundice, but a study of over 12,000 patients failed to confirm this number. Laboratory evidence of cholestasis occurs in many patients and some demonstrate laboratory findings consistent with hepatitis; however, these laboratory value changes appear to be benign. The cholestatic reaction is apparently the result of hypersensitivity and appears after 10-14 days of initial therapy or after 1-2 days in patients with a previous history of exposure to the drug. Rapid reversal of symptoms follows withdrawal of the drug. While more than 90% of the reported cases involved the **estolate** salt, hepatotoxicity has occurred with the **ethylsuccinate**, **stearate** and **propionate** salts.[1-3, 32, 33]
Ethionamide	Hepatitis may occur in 3-5% of patients and serum enzyme elevations in 30% or more. Onset of hepatitis usually occurs after several months of therapy.[1-3, 34]
Etretinate	Increased hepatic enzymes occur in up to 25% of patients, but further evidence of hepatocellular damage is Continued

Drug-Induced Hepatotoxicity

DRUG	NATURE OF HEPATOTOXICITY
	rare. Onset occurs most often after several months of therapy.[1,3,35]
Ferrous Salts	Hepatic necrosis may appear within 1–3 days of an acute overdose. The fatality rate is high if the patient is not treated promptly.[2]
Gold Salts	Cholestasis occasionally occurs with normal doses. Onset is most common within the first 5 weeks of therapy. Hepatic necrosis may result from overdose.[1-3,36]
Halothane	Despite extensive publicity, the actual frequency of halothane hepatitis is low, ranging from 1/10,000 to 1/35,000, with reported fatality rates of 14–71%. Susceptibility is greatest in adults, females, obese patients and especially in patients with prior exposure to halothane hepatitis. The mechanism of halothane hepatitis is poorly understood, but the presentation resembles hypersensitivity. Fever precedes jaundice in most patients and the onset of jaundice is usually between 3–14 days after exposure, with the shorter latent periods associated with prior halothane exposure. Mild elevations of hepatic enzymes are common.[1-3,37-39]
Isoniazid	Subclinical hepatitis is common (10–20%); this usually resolves rapidly following withdrawal of the drug and frequently resolves without discontinuation of therapy. Clinical hepatitis is age-related; it seldom occurs in children and increases in prevalence to about 3% in those over 50 yr. The onset of symptoms may occur any time during the first year of therapy, but over one-half of the cases develop during the first 3 months. The fatality rate is about 10% with a poorer prognosis associated with an onset after more than 2 months of therapy. Concomitant administration of rifampin may increase the risk of hepatotoxicity and, while the exact role of acetylator phenotype remains unclear, it appears that slow acetylators (especially those over 35 yr) may be at increased risk.[1-3,40-42]
Ketoconazole	There is a 5–10% prevalence of mild elevation of hepatic enzymes. The risk of potentially serious hepatic injury is about 1/15,000. There have been a few deaths attributed to ketoconazole hepatotoxicity.[1,3,43]

Continued

Drug-Induced Hepatotoxicity

DRUG	NATURE OF HEPATOTOXICITY
Mercaptopurine	Jaundice associated with cholestasis, hepatic necrosis or mixed reactions has been reported in 6–40% of patients. The highest prevalence is associated with doses of 2.5 mg/kg/day or more.[1,2,44]
Methotrexate	Hepatic injury (macrovesicular steatosis, necrosis and bridging fibrosis) is dependent on dose and duration of therapy and may progress to cirrhosis if the drug is not stopped. The prevalence of hepatic injury is 25% or more in some series. Intermittent high doses may pose less of a threat than low daily doses. Hepatic fibrosis is not reflected by standard liver function tests and is best detected by biopsy.[1,2,45–47]
Methyldopa	Mild changes in liver function tests have been reported in up to 35% of patients taking methyldopa, but the prevalence of clinical hepatitis is probably less than 1%. Hepatitis is more common in females and most patients show rapid recovery after withdrawal of the drug. Most cases occur during the first 3 months of therapy. The fatality rate is less than 10% among patients who develop hepatitis. There is evidence to support a hypersensitivity mechanism in some patients.[1–3,48]
Niacin	Hepatic dysfunction (primarily cholestasis) has been reported in as many as 28% of patients on long-term therapy. The prevalence may be highest with sustained-release formulations. Jaundice may be seen in 5% of patients.[1,2,52]
Nitrofurantoin	Hepatic damage from nitrofurantoin is rare. Cholestasis is the major presentation and usually occurs early in therapy. Several later-developing cases of chronic active hepatitis have been reported; almost all are in women after more than 1 yr of therapy.[1–3,53,54]
Papaverine	Numerous reports of hepatocellular injury and elevated liver enzymes in 27–43% of patients suggest a significant hepatotoxic potential.[1,3,55,56]
Penicillamine	Occasional cases of cholestasis have been associated with penicillamine therapy.[1–3,57]
Phenothiazines	Most reports of phenothiazine-induced liver damage involve **chlorpromazine**. The prevalence of hepatic en-

Continued

Drug-Induced Hepatotoxicity

DRUG	NATURE OF HEPATOTOXICITY
	zyme elevation with this drug has been estimated to be as high as 42%, although 10% is probably more realistic. Similarly, cholestatic jaundice has been projected to occur in up to 6% of patients receiving chlorpromazine, but the actual prevalence is closer to 0.1%. The onset of cholestasis frequently follows a prodrome of gastrointestinal or influenza-like symptoms. The mechanism is apparently hypersensitivity and it usually follows a benign course. Despite the dominance of chlorpromazine in the reported cases, other phenothiazines are capable of producing evidence of hepatic impairment. [1-3,58-61]
Phenylbutazone	This drug produces infrequent, but serious, hepatocellular injury often accompanied by cholestasis. Approximately 70% of cases develop during the first 6 weeks of therapy and about one-half show rash, fever or other signs of hypersensitivity. In the reports included in one review, more than 20% of the patients with the reaction died. [1-3,62]
Phenytoin	Rare, but often fatal, hepatocellular necrosis has been associated with phenytoin therapy. It is usually accompanied by other signs of hypersensitivity, frequently as part of a diffuse syndrome of lymphadenopathy, exfoliative dermatitis, high fever and leukocytosis. Onset usually occurs during the first 8 weeks of therapy. [1-3,63,64]
Plicamycin	Dose-related laboratory evidence of hepatotoxicity has been reported in virtually all patients in some studies. Intermittent, rather than continuous, dosing may provide some protection. [1,2,49-51]
Progestins	See Steroids, C-17-α-Alkyl.
Propoxyphene	A small number of cases of propoxyphene-induced cholestasis have been reported; these are thought to be the result of hypersensitivity. [1,2,65,66]
Propylthiouracil	Isolated cases of propylthiouracil-induced hepatocellular damage have been reported. The onset is usually within the first 2 months of therapy. These reactions are probably idiosyncratic, rather than a reflection of intrinsic hepatotoxicity. [1-3,67]

Continued

Drug-Induced Hepatotoxicity

DRUG	NATURE OF HEPATOTOXICITY
Pyrazinamide	Pyrazinamide-induced hepatitis is dependent on dose and duration of therapy. Daily doses appear to present a greater risk than weekly doses.[1-3,68,69]
Quinidine	Hepatic damage is rare and usually accompanied by other signs of hypersensitivity, especially fever. Most reactions occur during the first month of therapy. The pathology is usually a mixture of hepatocellular necrosis and cholestasis; granulomas have also been reported.[1-3,70]
Rifampin	While rifampin may possess hepatotoxic potential, it is difficult to demonstrate, because the drug is rarely used alone. It may hasten the onset or otherwise enhance isoniazid hepatotoxicity when the drugs are used together.[1-3,71,72]
Salicylates	Salicylate-induced hepatitis is uncommon, usually mild, readily reversible and most often associated with high-dose salicylate therapy such as that encountered in the management of rheumatoid arthritis. Hepatotoxicity is most often encountered at plasma salicylate levels above 25 mg/dl and is very rare below 15 mg/dl.[1-3,73,74]
Steroids, C-17-α-Alkyl	Canalicular cholestasis occurs with a minimal amount of hepatic inflammation. The onset of jaundice may or may not be preceded by other clinical signs and usually follows at least several months of therapy. The prevalence appears to be dose-related. Peliosis hepatis has also been associated with these compounds. Examples include **methyltestosterone**, **norethandrolone**, **methandrostenolone**, **fluoxymesterone**, **oxandrolone**, **oxymetholone** and **stanozolol**. C-17-α-ethinyl steroids such as **norethindrone** and **norethynodrel** may produce similar reactions.[1-3,75]
Sulfasalazine	About 20 isolated cases of sulfasalazine-associated hepatic damage have been reported. Hepatic necrosis is apparently part of a generalized hypersensitivity reaction which includes rash, fever, lymphadenopathy and lymphocytosis.[1-3]

Continued

Drug-Induced Hepatotoxicity

DRUG	NATURE OF HEPATOTOXICITY
Sulfonamides, Antibacterial	The sulfonamides currently in use appear to have a lower prevalence of hepatitis than their predecessors, with most reported cases appearing before 1947. Most cases of sulfonamide hepatotoxicity develop during the first 2 weeks of therapy and many are accompanied by other signs of hypersensitivity. The fatality rate may be 10% or more.[1-3,6]
Sulindac	A growing number of isolated cases of cholestatic and mixed hepatocellular-cholestatic liver injury due to sulindac are appearing in the literature. These reactions are most commonly encountered during the first 6 weeks of therapy, but may be delayed. They are almost all associated with signs of generalized hypersensitivity.[1,3]
Tetracyclines	Fatty infiltration of the liver has been encountered in patients receiving large doses of tetracyclines IV, usually in excess of 1.5 g/day. Contributing factors include pregnancy, malnutrition and impaired renal function, but hepatotoxicity has been reported in patients with none of these. Onset is most often during the first 10 days of therapy. The fatality rate is very high. Oral therapy may also produce signs of hepatotoxicity, although far less frequently.[1-3,77-79]
Troleandomycin	30-50% of patients receiving the drug show some laboratory evidence of abnormal liver function and up to 4% develop jaundice. In general, the reaction is similar to that seen with **erythromycin estolate.**[1,2,80,81]
Valproic Acid	Hepatic enzyme elevations have occurred in the majority of patients in some studies. Numerous cases of fatal hepatitis resulting from valproic acid therapy are reported in the literature. Microvesicular steatosis and hepatic necrosis do not appear to be dose-related and are most commonly encountered during the first 6 months of therapy. Serial liver function tests in asymptomatic patients do not predict patients at risk, but are commonly recommended because immediate withdrawal may reverse the condition. Children appear to be at increased risk, especially those with severe epilepsy associated with structural brain damage and mental retardation.[1,3,82-86]
Vitamin A	Hepatomegaly and mild increases in liver enzyme levels are common features of chronic vitamin A toxicity. Perisinusoidal fibrosis and cirrhosis have been reported in cases of chronic intoxication.[1-3]

References

1. Stricker BHCh, Spoelstra P. Drug-induced hepatic injury. Amsterdam: Elsevier, 1985.

2. Zimmerman HJ. Hepatotoxicity: the adverse effects of drugs and other chemicals on the liver. New York: Appleton-Century-Crofts, 1978.

3. Dukes MNG, ed. Meyler's side effects of drugs. 10th ed. Amsterdam: Elsevier, 1984

4. Barker JD, de Carle DJ, Anuras S. Chronic excessive acetaminophen use and liver damage. Ann Intern Med 1977;87:299-301.

5. Rumack BH, Peterson RC, Koch GG et al. Acetaminophen overdose. 662 cases with evaluation of oral acetylcysteine treatment. Arch Intern Med 1981;141:380-5.

6. Prescott LF. Paracetamol overdosage. Pharmacological considerations and clinical management. Drugs 1983;25:290-314.

7. Rumack BH. Acetaminophen overdose in young children. Treatment and effects of alcohol and other additional ingestants in 417 cases. Am J Dis Child 1984;138:428-33.

8. McInnes GT, Lawson DH, Jick H. Acute adverse reactions attributed to allopurinol in hospitalised patients. Ann Rheum Dis 1981;40:245-9.

9. Hande KR, Noone RM, Stone WJ. Severe allopurinol toxicity. Description and guidelines for prevention in patients with renal insufficiency. Am J Med 1984;76:47-56.

10. Nagel GA, Wander H-E, Blossey H-C. Phase II study of aminoglutethimide and medroxyprogesterone acetate in the treatment of patients with advanced breast cancer. Cancer Res 1982;42(Suppl):3442S-4S.

11. Simpson DG, Walker JH. Hypersensitivity of drugs to para-aminosalicylic acid. Am J Med 1960;29:297-306.

12. Heger JJ, Prystowsky EN, Jackman WM et al. Amiodarone. Clinical efficacy and electrophysiology during long-term therapy for recurrent ventricular tachycardia or ventricular fibrillation. N Engl J Med 1981;305:539-45.

13. Simon JB, Manley PN, Brien JF et al. Amiodarone hepatotoxicity simulating alcoholic liver disease. N Engl J Med 1984;311:167-72.

14. Rinder HM, Love JC, Wexler R. Amiodarone hepatotoxicity. N Engl J Med 1986;314:318-9. Letter.

15. Pratt CB, Simone JV, Zee P et al. Comparison of daily versus weekly L-asparaginase for the treatment of childhood acute leukemia. J Pediatr 1970;77:474-83.

16. Pratt CB, Johnson WW. Duration and severity of fatty metamorphosis of the liver following L-asparaginase therapy. Cancer 1971;28:361-4.

17. Zucker P, Daum F, Cohen MI. Fatal carbamazepine hepatitis. J Pediatr 1977;91:667-8.

18. Hopen G, Nesthus I, Laerum OD. Fatal carbamazepine-associated hepatitis. Report of two cases. Acta Med Scand 1981;210:333-5.

19. Schoenfield LJ, Lachin JM, Baum RA et al. Chenodiol (chenodeoxycholic acid) for dissolution of gallstones: the National Cooperative Gallstone Study. A controlled trial of efficacy and safety. Ann Intern Med 1981;95:257-82.

20. Bennion LJ, Ginsberg RL, Garnick MB et al. Effects of oral contraceptives on the gallbladder bile of normal women. N Engl J Med 1976;294:189-92.

21. Edmondson HA, Henderson B, Benton B. Liver-cell adenomas associated with use of oral contraceptives. N Engl J Med 1976;294:470-2.

22. Rooks JB, Ory HW, Ishak KG et al. Epidemiology of hepatocellular adenoma. The role of oral contraceptive use. JAMA 1979;242:644-8.

23. Neuberger J, Forman D, Doll R et al. Oral contraceptives and hepatocellular carcinoma. Br Med J 1986;292:1355-7.

24. Forman D, Vincent TJ, Doll R. Cancer of the liver and the use of oral contraceptives. Br Med J 1986;292:1357-61.

25. Brosens I, Johannisson E, Baulieu E-E et al. Oral contraceptives and hepatocellular carcinoma. Br Med J 1986;292:1667-8. Letter.

26. Klintmalm GBG, Iwatsuki S, Starzl TE. Cyclosporin A hepatotoxicity in 66 renal allograft recipients. Transplantation 1981;32:488-9.

27. Atkinson K, Biggs J, Dodds A et al. Cyclosporine-associated hepatotoxicity after allogeneic marrow transplantation in man: differentiation from other causes of posttransplant liver disease. Transplant Proc 1983;15(Suppl 1):2671-7.

28. Utili R, Boitnott JK, Zimmerman HJ. Dantrolene-associated hepatic injury. Incidence and character. Gastroenterology 1977;72:610-6.

29. Wilkinson SP, Portmann B, Williams R. Hepatitis from dantrolene sodium. Gut 1979;20:33-6.

30. Tomecki KJ, Catalano CJ. Dapsone hypersensitivity. The sulfone syndrome revisited. Arch Dermatol 1981;117:38-9.

31. Kromann NP, Vilhelmsen R, Stahl D. The dapsone syndrome. Arch Dermatol 1982;118:531-2.

32. McCormack WM, George H, Donner A et al. Hepatotoxicity of erythromycin estolate during pregnancy. Antimicrob Agents Chemother 1977;12:630-5.

33. Inman WHW, Rawson NSB. Erythromycin estolate and jaundice. Br Med J 1983;286:1954-5.

34. Conn HO, Binder HJ, Orr HD. Ethionamide-induced hepatitis. A review with a report of an additional case. Am Rev Resp Dis 1964;90:542-52.

35. Glazer SD, Roenigk HH, Yokoo H et al. A study of potential hepatotoxicity of etretinate used in the treatment of psoriasis. J Am Acad Dermatol 1982;6:683-7.

36. Howrie DL, Gartner JC. Gold-induced hepatotoxicity: case report and review of the literature. J Rheumatol 1982;9:727-9.

37. Neuberger J, Williams R. Halothane anaesthesia and liver damage. Br Med J 1984;289:1136-9.

38. Anon. Halothane-associated liver damage. Lancet 1986;1:1251-2. Editorial.

39. Blogg CE. Halothane and the liver: the problem revisited and made obsolete. Br Med J 1986;292:1691-2.

40. Black M, Mitchell JR, Zimmerman HJ et al. Isoniazid-associated hepatitis in 114 patients. Gastroenterology 1975;69:289-302.

41. Mitchell JR, Zimmerman HJ, Ishak KG et al. Isoniazid liver injury: clinical spectrum, pathology, and probable

pathogenesis. Ann Intern Med 1976;84:181-92.

42. Dickinson DS, Bailey WC, Hirschowitz BI et al. Risk factors for isoniazid (INH)-induced liver dysfunction. J Clin Gastroenterol 1981;3:271-9.

43. Lewis JH, Zimmerman HJ, Benson GD et al. Hepatic injury associated with ketoconazole therapy. Analysis of 33 cases. Gastroenterology 1984;86:503-13.

44. Einhorn M, Davidsohn I. Hepatotoxicity of mercaptopurine. JAMA 1964;188:802-6.

45. McIntosh S, Davidson DL, O'Brien RT et al. Methotrexate hepatotoxicity in children with leukemia. J Pediatr 1977;90:1019-21.

46. Zachariae H, Kragballe K, Sogaard H. Methotrexate induced liver cirrhosis. Studies including serial liver biopsies during continued treatment. Br J Dermatol 1980;102:407-12.

47. Roenigk HH, Auerbach R, Maibach HI et al. Methotrexate guidelines—revised. J Am Acad Dermatol 1982;6:145-55.

48. Rodman JS, Deutsch DJ, Gutman SI. Methyldopa hepatitis. A report of six cases and review of the literature. Am J Med 1976;60:941-8.

49. Kennedy BJ. Metabolic and toxic effects of mithramycin during tumor therapy. Am J Med 1970;49:494-503.

50. Kennedy BJ. Mithramycin therapy in advanced testicular neoplasms. Cancer 1970;26:755-66.

51. Green L, Donehower RC. Hepatic toxicity of low doses of mithramycin in hypercalcemia. Cancer Treat Rep 1984;68:1379-81.

52. Parsons WB. Studies of nicotinic acid use in hypercholesteremia. Changes in hepatic function, carbohydrate tolerance, and uric acid metabolism. Arch Intern Med 1961;107:653-67.

53. Hatoff DE, Cohen M, Schweigert BF et al. Nitrofurantoin: another cause of drug-induced chronic active hepatitis? A report of a patient with HLA-B8 antigen. Am J Med 1979;67:117-21.

54. Sharp JR, Ishak KG, Zimmerman HJ. Chronic active hepatitis and severe hepatic necrosis associated with nitrofurantoin. Ann Intern Med 1980;92:14-9.

55. Ronnov-Jessen V, Tjernlund A. Hepatotoxicity due to treatment with papaverine. Report of four cases. N Engl J Med 1969;281:1333-5.

56. Pathy MS, Reynolds AJ. Papaverine and hepatotoxicity. Postgrad Med J 1980;56:488-90.

57. Seibold JR, Lynch CJ, Medsger TA. Cholestasis associated with D-penicillamine therapy: case report and review of the literature. Arthritis Rheum 1981;24:554-6.

58. Zimmerman HJ. Clinical and laboratory manifestations of hepatotoxicity. Ann NY Acad Sci 1963;104:954-87.

59. Bloom JB, Davis N, Wecht CH. Effect on the liver of long-term tranquilizing medication. Am J Psychiatry 1965;121:788-97.

60. Jick H, Walker AM, Porter J. Drug-induced liver disease. J Clin Pharmacol 1981;21:359-64.

61. Jones JK, Van de Carr SW, Zimmerman H et al. Hepatotoxicity associated with phenothiazines. Psychopharmacol Bull 1983;19:24-7.

62. Benjamin SB, Ishak KG, Zimmerman HJ et al. Phenylbutazone liver injury: a clinical-pathologic survey of 23 cases and review of the literature. Hepatology 1981;1:255-63.

63. Haruda F. Phenytoin hypersensitivity: 38 cases. Neurology 1979;29:1480-5.

64. Mullick FG, Ishak KG. Hepatic injury associated with diphenylhydantoin therapy: a clinicopathologic study of 20 cases. Am J Clin Pathol 1980;74:442-52.

65. Lee TH, Rees PJ, Hepatotoxicity of dextropropoxyphene. Br Med J 1977;2:296-7.

66. Ford MJ, Kellett RJ, Busuttil A et al. Dextropropoxyphene and jaundice. Br Med J 1977;2:674.

67. Parker WA. Propylthiouracil-induced hepatotoxicity. Clin Pharm 1982;1:471-4.

68. Hong Kong Chest Service/British Medical Research Council. Controlled trial of four thrice-weekly regimens and a daily regimen all given for 6 months for pulmonary tuberculosis. Lancet 1981;1:171-4.

69. Cohen CD, Sayed AR, Kirsch RE. Hepatic complications of antituberculosis therapy revisited. S Afr Med J 1983;63:960-3.

70. Geltner D, Chajek T, Rubinger D et al. Quinidine hypersensitivity and liver involvement. A survey of 32 patients. Gastroenterology 1976;70:650-2.

71. Pessayre D, Bentata M, Degott C et al. Isoniazid-rifampin fulminant hepatitis. A possible consequence of the enhancement of isioniazid hepatotoxicity by enzyme induction. Gastroenterology 1977;72:284-9.

72. Tsagaropoulou-Stinga H, Mataki-Emmanouilidou T, Karida-Kavalioti S et al. Hepatotoxic reactions in children with severe tuberculosis treated with isoniazid-rifampin. Pediatr Infect Dis 1985;4:270-3.

73. Zimmerman HJ. Effects of aspirin and acetaminophen on the liver. Arch Intern Med 1981;141:333-42.

74. Hamdan JA, Manasra K, Ahmed M. Salicylate-induced hepatitis in rheumatic fever. Am J Dis Child 1985;139:453-5.

75. Haupt HA, Rovere GD. Anabolic steroids: a review of the literature. Am J Sports Med 1984;12:469-84.

76. Dujovne CA, Chan CH, Zimmerman HJ. Sulfonamide hepatic injury. Review of the literature and report of a case due to sulfamethoxazole. N Engl J Med 1967;277:785-8.

77. Dowling HF, Lepper MH. Hepatic reactions to tetracycline. JAMA 1964;188:307-9.

78. Peters RL, Edmondson HA, Mikkelsen WP et al. Tetracycline-induced fatty liver in nonpregnant patients. A report of six cases. Am J Surg 1967;113:622-32.

79. Combes B, Whalley PJ, Adams RH. Tetracycline and the liver. Prog Liver Dis 1972;4:589-96.

80. Ticktin HE, Zimmerman HJ. Hepatic dysfunction and jaundice in patients receiving triacetyloleandomycin. N Engl J Med 1962;267:964-8.

81. Pessayre D, Larrey D, Funck-Brentano C et al. Drug interactions and hepatitis produced by some macrolide antibiotics. J Antimicrob Chemother 1985;16(Suppl A):181-94.

82. Zimmerman HJ, Ishak KG. Valproate-induced hepatic injury: analyses of 23 fatal cases. Hepatology 1982;2:591-7.

83. Zafrani ES, Berthelot P. Sodium valproate in the induction of unusual hepatotoxicity. Hepatology 1982;2:648-9.

84. Green SH. Sodium valproate and routine liver function tests. Arch Dis Child 1984;59:813-4.

85. Isom JB. On the toxicity of valproic acid. Am J Dis Child 1984;138:901-3. Editorial.

86. Jeavons PM. Non-dose-related side effects of valproate. Epilepsia 1984;25(Suppl 1):S50-5.

Drug-Induced Nephrotoxicity

THE AGENTS IN THE FOLLOWING TABLE have been associated with drug-induced nephrotoxicity. Each is accompanied by a brief description of its nephrotoxicity and references which will be of assistance to the reader who wants additional information. In some cases, especially with new drugs, the literature is not definitive in its description of the prevalence of nephrotoxicity or its pathophysiology. Not included in this table are drugs which produce nephrotoxicity as a result of damage to tissues other than the kidney (eg, liver or skeletal muscle).

The table begins on page 89.

Drug-Induced Nephrotoxicity

DRUG	NATURE OF NEPHROTOXICITY
Acetaminophen	Tubular necrosis has been reported, most frequently in association with hepatotoxicity seen in acute overdose. Whether the nephrotoxicity is a direct effect of acetaminophen or the result of the liver damage is the subject of some controversy. It has been reported in cases without evidence of hepatotoxicity and in therapeutic doses. Acetaminophen has also been implicated in some cases of analgesic nephropathy (see Analgesics) and interstitial nephritis.[1,2,6-10]
Acyclovir	Transient rises in serum creatinine and BUN have been encountered in about 10% of acyclovir-treated patients. The significance of these increases is undetermined.[11]
Allopurinol	Tubular necrosis with fibrinoid deposits has been seen in patients experiencing generalized hypersensitivity reactions to allopurinol. A few cases of interstitial nephritis have also been reported.[1,2]
Aminoglycosides	Proximal tubular necrosis is a feature of all members of this class. These drugs accumulate in renal tissues, but there does not appear to be a good correlation between renal tissue concentrations of individual aminoglycosides and their nephrotoxic potential. The reported prevalence of nephrotoxicity varies widely, but has been as high as 20–30% in some series. It has been suggested that patients with higher pretreatment glomerular filtration rates may be more likely to develop nephrotoxicity, because of greater delivery of aminoglycosides in the urine. The relative nephrotoxic potential of aminoglycosides is shown below.

Relative Nephrotoxic Potential

DRUG		DRUG	
Amikacin	+ +	Netilmicin	+ +
Gentamicin	+ +	Sisomicin	+ +
Kanamycin	+ +	Streptomycin	+
Neomycin	+ + +	Tobramycin	+ +

Continued

Drug-Induced Nephrotoxicity

DRUG	NATURE OF NEPHROTOXICITY
	Aminoglycoside-induced acute renal failure is usually nonoliguric, which may delay its recognition. Damage usually occurs at least 5 days after initiation of therapy and may progress after discontinuation of the drug. Recovery of some to all lost renal function may be seen over several weeks after withdrawal. Monitoring of aminoglycoside plasma levels and serial renal function tests may be of value in recognizing nephrotoxicity. Very early evidence of renal damage includes an increased number of casts in the urine and elevated urine levels of β_2-microglobulins.[1,2,4,12-17]
Amphetamines	Renal failure associated with amphetamine use is usually the result of rhabdomyolysis, but it has also been found in patients without evidence of muscle damage or other apparent predisposing factors.[18,19]
Amphotericin B	Some degree of nephrotoxicity is observed in almost all patients treated with amphotericin B. The drug causes a reduction in renal plasma flow as well as glomerular and tubular damage. Distal tubular damage may lead to loss of concentrating ability, renal tubular acidosis and electrolyte disturbances (most commonly hypokalemia, but also hyponatremia and hypomagnesemia). These effects appear to be dose-related and many patients respond favorably to temporary drug discontinuation or a reduction in dose. Sodium repletion may also have a beneficial effect. Some authors suggest that the total dose of amphotericin B should be kept below 4–5 g to minimize nephrotoxicity.[1,2,5,20-22]
Analgesics	Analgesic nephropathy is a syndrome of papillary necrosis and progressive renal medullary impairment seen in persons who have chronically consumed large quantities of oral analgesic products. The syndrome is characterized by proteinuria, reduced renal concentrating ability and the presence of RBCs and WBCs in the urine. Analgesic nephropathy has been historically attributed to **phenacetin**, but the contribution of other analgesics, especially **salicylates**, must be considered. The removal of phenacetin from nonprescription analgesic products in various countries has not been consistently associated with a significant decline in analgesic nephropathy mortality. Historically, this syndrome has been responsible for a significant percentage of chronic renal failure deaths, with a considerable variation in prevalence among nations (high in Australia, low in the US), apparently in response to analgesic abuse patterns. Mild cases are reversible, but severe cases may continue to deteriorate after the withdrawal of analgesics. The prevalence of renal cancer Continued

Drug-Induced Nephrotoxicity

DRUG	NATURE OF NEPHROTOXICITY
	appears higher than normal among chronic analgesic abusers. See also Nonsteroidal Anti-Inflammatory Agents.[1,2,23-26]
Captopril	Proteinuria (over 1 g/day) accompanies membranous glomerulonephritis in 0.3% of patients treated with captopril. The onset of proteinuria may be delayed until as late as the 8th month of therapy. Pre-existing renal disease may predispose patients to proteinuria. The significance of the proteinuria is unknown, because most patients improve despite continued therapy.[1,27]
Cephalosporins	The cephalosporin (and cephamycin) antibiotics are capable of rarely producing interstitial nephritis similar to the penicillins. The nephrotoxicity of the newer cephalosporins appears to be minimal compared to older drugs such as **cephaloridine** and **cephalothin**.[1-3,28]
Cisplatin	Dose-related nephrotoxicity is a major limiting factor in cisplatin therapy and may be encountered in 50-75% of patients. The greatest damage occurs in the first month of therapy and it appears to be more likely when the drug is administered repetitively at close time intervals. Forced hydration and diuretics may reduce renal toxicity. Magnesium and calcium loss are common manifestations of cisplatin-induced nephrotoxicity.[1,2,29-33]
Colistin	See Polymyxins.
Contrast Media	A variety of renal lesions have been associated with the use of radiocontrast media including osmotic nephrosis, medullary necrosis, proximal tubular vacuolation and necrosis, as well as the deposition of oxalate crystals. The most common pattern is acute oliguric renal failure developing within 24 hr after the administration of the contrast agent and lasting 2-4 days. Most patients recover fully, but permanent renal impairment occurs in as many as 30% of those with contrast media-induced nephrotoxicity. Patients with pre-existing renal impairment and diabetics may be at greater risk. Vigorous hydration of the patient and limiting the total dose of iodine in the administered contrast medium to 80 g or less may reduce the risk of nephrotoxicity.[1,2,34-39]

Continued

Drug-Induced Nephrotoxicity

DRUG	NATURE OF NEPHROTOXICITY
Cyclosporine	Increases in serum creatinine and BUN as well as decreased glomerular filtration rates are regularly encountered in cyclosporine-treated patients. Nephrotoxicity associated with long-term cyclosporine therapy has been described as irreversible and potentially progressive. [40,41]
Demeclocycline	This drug is capable of producing nephrogenic diabetes insipidus which is usually, but not always, dose-related. For this reason, it has been used in the management of the syndrome of inappropriate antidiuretic hormone secretion. See also Tetracyclines. [1,2,4,42-44]
Dextrans	Glomerulonephritis resulting from a hypersensitivity reaction has been reported (particularly with high molecular weight dextran), but the most common lesion is osmotic nephrosis and physical plugging of renal tubules with high viscosity urine. Adequate hydration of the patient minimizes this problem. [2,45]
Diuretics, Thiazide	Occasional cases of interstitial nephritis have been reported. These cases may be the result of hypersensitivity reactions. [1,46,47]
Gallium Nitrate	Nephrotoxicity is the most common adverse effect of gallium and increases in BUN and serum creatinine may be seen after only the first dose. At least one death has been associated with gallium-induced nephrotoxicity. [48,49]
Gold Salts	A lesion resembling membranous glomerulonephritis with proteinuria may be encountered in as many as 10% of patients receiving parenteral gold therapy. Microhematuria (3%) and nephrotic syndrome (0.3%) are less common. Occasional cases of acute tubular necrosis and interstitial nephritis have also been reported. Permanent renal impairment is uncommon. There is evidence for both immune and direct toxic mechanisms for gold nephrotoxicity. **Auranofin** appears to be less nephrotoxic than parenteral gold products. [1,2,24,50-53]
Lithium Salts	These drugs can produce a nephrogenic diabetes insipidus which is, at least in part, dose-related. This effect is usually reversible upon withdrawal of the drug, but some prolonged cases have been reported and the drug is thought to irreversibly reduce tubular function in 5-10% of patients on long-term therapy (over 2 yr). Interstitial nephritis and renal fibrosis have also been reported. [1,2,44,54-57] Continued

Drug-Induced Nephrotoxicity

DRUG	NATURE OF NEPHROTOXICITY
Methotrexate	This drug is directly toxic to the kidney when given in large doses, producing acute tubular necrosis. Methotrexate is significantly eliminated through the kidney and its nephrotoxicity compounds itself by causing the plasma level of the drug to rise. Close monitoring of methotrexate plasma levels may help to minimize the risk of nephrotoxicity.[1,2,31,58,59]
Methoxyflurane	Nephrogenic diabetes insipidus has been reported with this drug. Proximal tubular damage and interstitial nephritis are also reported. The nephrotoxicity of methoxyflurane appears to be dose-related and may be due to increased circulating fluoride ion concentrations. Urinary oxylate crystallization has also been reported following methoxyflurane anesthesia.[1,2,60-62]
Mitomycin	Tubular necrosis is encountered most commonly with daily therapy, but has also been reported with the intermittent therapy now recommended. Nephrotoxicity appears to be related to the total dose administered with the risk of renal impairment rising significantly when the total dose exceeds 50 mg/M². Onset may be delayed for many months.[1,31,63]
Nitrosoureas	The nitrosoureas can produce insidious nephrotoxicity in patients on long-term therapy. **Lomustine** and **semustine** seem to have the greatest nephrotoxic potential. Some cases of permanent injury have been reported. See also Streptozocin.[1,31]
Nonsteroidal Anti-Inflammatory Agents	Most of the nonsteroidal anti-inflammatory agents (NSAIA) can reduce creatinine clearance and produce a nonoliguric renal failure, possibly as a result of renal circulatory changes brought about by the inhibition of prostaglandin synthesis. This effect tends to be relatively minor, usually reversible and associated with long-term therapy. It is not possible at this time to accurately categorize the prevalence associated with each NSAIA. Those at greatest risk are patients with chronic renal insufficiency, hepatic cirrhosis and circulatory volume depletion (such as that produced by diuretic use or nephrotic syndrome). More serious renal effects are also occasionally seen, with **indomethacin** being the most commonly reported cause of NSAIA-induced acute renal failure and **fenoprofen** being the NSAIA most commonly associated with interstitial nephritis and nephrotic syndrome. See also Analgesics.[1,2,23,24,64-67] *Continued*

Drug-Induced Nephrotoxicity

DRUG	NATURE OF NEPHROTOXICITY
Penicillamine	Slight to moderate proteinuria occurs in about 15% of patients on long-term therapy with penicillamine. The proteinuria is usually benign and slowly reversible, but nephrotic syndrome is occasionally encountered. The lesions appear to be perimembranous glomerulonephritis resulting from the deposition of antigen-antibody complexes on the renal basement membrane. Cases of glomerular damage without evidence of immune complex involvement have been reported, as have some cases of Goodpasture's syndrome (interstitial pneumonitis and nephritis).[1,2,24]
Penicillins	Interstitial nephritis has been reported with most of the penicillins. **Methicillin** is by far the most frequently implicated penicillin. The reason for its dominance is unknown. Penicillin interstitial nephritis is an immune reaction which is most commonly encountered during a long course of therapy. The reaction is usually accompanied by other signs of hypersensitivity such as fever, rash and eosinophilia. Hematuria may also be encountered. The reduction of renal function may not be oliguric, so urine volume is not a reliable parameter to monitor.[1-3,68]
Pentamidine	Nephrotoxicity is regularly encountered in pentamidine-treated patients (24% in one study). Intramuscular administration and dehydration, such as that due to diarrhea, may be contributing factors.[69]
Plicamycin	High doses (50 mcg/kg) produced renal impairment in 40% of plicamycin-treated patients, including some who died of acute renal failure. Nephrotoxicity is far less likely at the 25–30 mcg/kg (or lower) dosing currently used in most clinical situations.[1,31]
Polymyxins	Adverse reactions involving the kidney occur in about 20% of patients receiving polymyxins. Tubular necrosis is the most commonly described lesion, but interstitial nephritis has also been reported. High doses, long duration of therapy and renal impairment are predisposing factors. Polymyxin-induced renal damage is usually reversible, but some patients continue to deteriorate after drug withdrawal.[1,2,4,70]
Rifampin	There are scattered reports of rifampin-induced acute renal failure resulting from tubulo-interstitial nephritis. This appears to be a hypersensitivity reaction and is most commonly seen in intermittent dosage regimens (even after prolonged drug-free periods), but has also accompanied continuous therapy.[1,2,5,71,72] Continued

Drug-Induced Nephrotoxicity

DRUG	NATURE OF NEPHROTOXICITY
Streptozocin	Nephrotoxicity is the most common dose-limiting side effect. The prevalence increases with prolonged administration until virtually all patients demonstrate renal impairment. The damage is both glomerular and tubular. See also Nitrosoureas.[1,31]
Sulfonamides, Antibacterial	Early sulfonamides were poorly soluble and urinary crystallization was a common problem. Today, the prevalence of crystallization is less than 0.3% with the use of the more soluble sulfonamides and adequate hydration. Interstitial nephritis, glomerulonephritis and tubular necrosis have been reported, although rarely. These reactions are probably allergic in origin.[1,2,5]
Tetracyclines	Fanconi syndrome, characterized by tubular damage with proteinuria, glycosuria, amino-aciduria and electrolyte disturbances, was associated with the use of outdated tetracycline products. This syndrome is no longer likely to occur, because of changes in the manufacturing process. The anti-anabolic effects of tetracyclines can contribute to azotemia in patients with pre-existing renal impairment. See also Demeclocycline.[1,2,4]
Triamterene	About 0.4% of renal calculi contain triamterene, some of which consist almost entirely of triamterene. One report has suggested that one in 1,500 users of the drug will develop triamterene-associated calculi during the course of a year. As a precaution, the drug should probably not be used in patients with a history of renal calculi. Triamterene use may also be associated with the development of interstitial nephritis.[1,2,72,73]
Vancomycin	There were some reports of nephrotoxicity from vancomycin early in its history, but the nephrotoxic potential of the drug currently appears to be slight.[1,4,74,75]

References

1. Dukes MNG, ed. Meyler's side effects of drugs. 10th ed. Amsterdam: Elsevier, 1984.

2. Roxe DM. Toxic nephropathy from diagnostic and therapeutic agents. Review and commentary. Am J Med 1980;69:759-66.

3. Appel GB, Neu HC. The nephrotoxicity of antimicrobial agents (first of three parts). N Engl J Med 1977;296:663-70.

4. Appel GB, Neu HC. The nephrotoxicity of antimicrobial agents (second of three parts). N Engl J Med 1977;296:722-8.

5. Appel GB, Neu HC. The nephrotoxicity of antimicrobial agents (third of three parts). N Engl J Med 1977;296:784-7.

6. Kleinman JG, Breitenfield RV, Roth DA. Acute renal failure associated with acetaminophen ingestion: report of a case and review of the literature. Clin Nephrol 1980;14:201-5.

7. Duggin GG, Mechanisms in the development of analgesic nephropathy. Kidney Int 1980;18:553-61.

8. Jeffery WH, Lafferty WE. Acute renal failure after acetaminophen overdose: report of two cases. Am J Hosp Pharm 1981;38:1355-8.

9. Cobden I, Record CO, Ward MK et al. Paracetamol-induced acute renal failure in the absence of fulminant liver damage. Br Med J 1982;284:21-2.

10. Gabriel R, Caldwell J, Hartley RB. Acute tubular necrosis, caused by therapeutic doses of paracetamol? Clin Nephrol 1982;18:269-71.

11. Keeney RE, Kirk LE, Bridgen D. Acyclovir tolerance in humans. Am J Med 1982;73(Suppl):176-81.

12. Schentag JJ, Gengo FM, Plaut ME et al. Urinary casts as an indicator of renal tubular damage in patients receiving aminoglycosides. Antimicrob Agents Chemother 1979;16:468 74.

13. Schentag JJ, Plaut ME. Patterns of urinary β_2-microglobulin excretion by patients treated with aminoglycosides. Kidney Int 1980;17:654-61.

14. Kaloyanides GJ, Pastoriza-Munoz E. Aminoglycoside nephrotoxicity. Kidney Int 1980;18:571-82.

15. Humes HD, Weinberg JM, Knauss TC. Clinical and pathophysiologic aspects of aminoglycoside nephrotoxicity. Am J Kidney Dis 1982;2:5-29.

16. Moore RD, Smith CR, Lipsky JJ et al. Risk factors for nephrotoxicity in patients treated with aminoglycosides. Ann Intern Med 1984;100:352-7.

17. Kahlmeter G, Dahlager JI. Aminoglycoside toxicity—a review of clinical studies published between 1975 and 1982. J Antimicrob Chemother 1984;13(Suppl A):9-22.

18. Scandling J, Spital A. Amphetamine-associated myoglobinuric renal failure. South Med J 1982;75:237-40.

19. Foley RJ, Kapatkin K, Verani R et al. Amphetamine-induced acute renal failure. South Med J 1984;77:258-9.

20. Maddux MS, Barriere SL. A review of complications of amphotericin-B therapy: recommendations for prevention and management. Drug Intell Clin Pharm 1980;14:177-81.

21. Heidemann HT, Gerkens JF, Spickard WA et al. Amphotericin B nephrotoxicity in humans decreased by salt repletion. Am J Med 1983;75:476-81.

22. Barton CH, Pahl M, Vaziri ND et al. Renal magnesium wasting associated with amphotericin B therapy. Am J Med 1984;77:471-4.

23. Prescott LF. Analgesic nephropathy: a reassessment of the role of phenacetin and other analgesics. Drugs 1982;23:75-149.

24. Sellars L, Wilkinson R. Adverse effects of antirheumatic drugs on the kidney. Adv Drug React Ac Pois Rev 1983;2:51-66.

25. Maher JF. Analgesic nephropathy. Observations, interpretations, and perspective on the low incidence in America. Am J Med 1984;76:345-8.

26. Consensus conference: analgesic-associated kidney disease. JAMA 1984;251:3123-5.

27. Capoten® product information. ER Squibb & Sons, 1986.

28. Barza M. The nephrotoxicity of cephalosporins: an overview. J Infect Dis 1978;137(Suppl):S60-73.

29. Madias NE, Harrington JT. Platinum nephrotoxicity. Am J Med 1978;65:307-14.

30. Blachley JD, Hill JB. Renal and electrolyte disturbances associated with cisplatin. Ann Intern Med 1981;95:628-32.

31. Weiss RB, Poster DS. The renal toxicity of cancer chemotherapeutic agents. Cancer Treat Rev 1982;9:37-56.

32. Meijer S, Mulder NH, Sleijfer DT et al. Influence of combination chemotherapy with cis-diamminedichloroplatinum on renal function: long-term effects. Oncology 1983;40:170-3.

33. Campbell AB, Kalman SM, Jacobs C. Plasma platinum levels: relationship to cisplatin dose and nephrotoxicity. Cancer Treat Rep 1983;67:169-72.

34. Byrd L, Sherman RL. Radiocontrast-induced acute renal failure: a clinical and pathophysiologic review. Medicine 1979;58:270-9.

35. Mudge GH. Nephrotoxicity of urographic radiocontrast drugs. Kidney Int 1980;18:540-52.

36. Lang EK, Foreman J, Schlegel JU et al. The incidence of contrast medium induced acute tubular necrosis following arteriography. Radiology 1981;138:203-6.

37. Cochran ST, Wong WS, Roe DJ. Predicting angiography-induced acute renal function impairment: clinical risk model. Am J Roentgenol 1983;141:1027-33.

38. Martin-Paredero V, Dixon SM, Baker JD et al. Risk of renal failure after major angiography. Arch Surg 1983;118:1417-20.

39. Misson RT, Cutler RE. Radiocontrast-induced renal failure. West J Med 1985;142:657-64.

40. Myers BD, Ross J, Newton L et al. Cyclosporine-associated chronic nephropathy. N Engl J Med 1984;311:699-705.

41. Strom TB, Loertscher R. Cyclosproine-induced nephrotoxicity. Inevitable and intractable? N Engl J Med 1984;311:728-9.

42. Maxon HR III, Rutsky EA. Vasopressin-resistant diabetes insipidus associated with short-term demethylchlortetracycline (Declomycin) therapy. Milit Med 1973;138:500-1.

43. Cherrill DA, Stote RM, Birge JR et al. Demeclocycline treatment in the syndrome of inappropriate antidiuretic hormone secretion. Ann Intern Med 1975;83:654-6.

44. Forrest JN Jr, Cox M, Hong C et al. Superiority of demeclocycline over lithium in the treatment of chronic syndrome of inappropriate secretion of antidiuretic hormone. N Engl J Med 1978;298:173-7.

45. Van Den Berg CJ, Pineda AA. Plasma exchange in the treatment of acute renal failure due to low molecular-weight dextran. Mayo Clin Proc 1980;55:387-9.

46. Magil AB, Ballon HS, Cameron EC et al. Acute interstitial nephritis associated with thiazide diuretics. Clinical and pathologic observations in three cases. Am J Med 1980;69:939-43.

47. Spence JD, Wong DG, Lindsay RM. Effects of triamterene and amiloride on urinary sediment in hypertensive patients taking hydrochlorothiazide. Lancet 1985;2:73-5.

48. Samson MK, Fraile RJ, Baker LH et al. Phase I-II clinical trial of gallium nitrate (NSC-15200). Cancer Clin Trials 1980;3:131-6.

49. Warrell RP Jr, Coonley CJ, Straus DJ et al. Treatment of patients with advanced malignant lymphoma using gallium nitrate administered as a seven-day continuous infusion. Cancer 1983;51:1982-7.

50. Newton P, Swinburn WR, Swinson DR. Proteinuria with gold therapy: when should gold be permanently stopped? Br J Rheumatol 1983;22:11-7.

51. Furst DE. Mechanism of action, pharmacology, clinical efficacy and side effects of auranofin. An orally administered organic gold compound for the treatment of rheumatoid arthritis. Pharmacotherapy 1983;3:284-98.

52. Cramer CR, Hagler HK, Silva FG et al. Chronic interstitial nephritis associated with gold therapy. Arch Pathol Lab Med 1983;107:258-63.

53. Katz WA, Blodgett RC Jr, Pietrusko RG. Proteinuria in gold-treated rheumatoid arthritis. Ann Intern Med 1984;101:176-9.

54. Hwang S, Tuason VB. Long-term maintenance lithium therapy and possible irreversible renal damage. J Clin Psychiatry 1980;41:11-9.

55. Myers JB, Morgan TO, Carney SL et al. Effects of lithium on the kidney. Kidney Int 1980;18:601-8.

56. Perry PJ. Lithium nephrotoxicity. Drug Intell Clin Pharm 1982;16:740-4.

57. Bendz H. Kidney function in lithium-treated patients. A literature survey. Acta Psychiatr Scand 1983;68:303-24.

58. Condit PT, Chanes RE, Joel W. Renal toxicity of methotrexate. Cancer 1969;23:126-31.

59. Stoller RG, Hande KR, Jacobs SA et al. Use of plasma pharmacokinetics to predict and prevent methotrexate toxicity. N Engl J Med 1977;297:630-4.

60. Mazze RI, Shue GL, Jackson SH. Renal dysfunction associated with methoxyflurane anesthesia. A randomized, prospective clinical evaluation. JAMA 1971;216:278-88.

61. Cousins MJ, Mazze RI. Methoxyflurane nephrotoxicity. A study of dose response in man. JAMA 1973;225:1611-6.

62. Desmond JW. Methoxyflurane nephrotoxicity. Can Anaesth Soc J 1974;21:294-307.

63. Valavaara R, Nordman E. Renal complications of mitomycin C therapy with special reference to the total dose. Cancer 1985;55:47-50.

64. Clive DM, Stoff JS. Renal syndromes associated with nonsteroidal antiinflammatory drugs. N Engl J Med 1984;310:563-72.

65. Garella S, Matarese RA. Renal effects of prostaglandins and clinical adverse effects of nonsteroidal antiinflammatory agents. Medicine 1984;63:165-81.

66. Fox DA, Jick H. Nonsteroidal anti-inflammatory drugs and renal disease. JAMA 1984;251:1299-300.

67. Carmichael J, Shankel SW. Effects of nonsteroidal anti-inflammatory drugs on prostaglandins and renal function. Am J Med 1985;78:992-1000.

68. Appel GB. A decade of penicillin related acute insterstitial nephritis—more questions than answers. Clin Nephrol 1980;13:151-4.

69. Stehr-Green JK, Helmick CG. Pentamidine and renal toxicity. N Engl J Med 1985;313:694-5. Letter.

70. Koch-Weser J, Sidel VW, Federman EB et al. Adverse effects of sodium colistimethate. Manifestations and specific reaction rates during 317 courses of therapy. Ann Intern Med 1970;72:857-68.

71. Qunibi WY, Godwin J, Eknoyan G. Toxic nephropathy during continuous rifampin therapy. South Med J 1980;73:791-2.

72. Power DA, Russell G, Smith FW et al. Acute renal failure due to continuous rifampin. Clin Nephrol 1983;20:155-9.

73. Ettinger B, Oldroyd NO, Sorgel F. Triamterene nephrolithiasis. JAMA 1980;244:2443-5.

74. Farber BF, Moellering RC Jr. Retrospective study of the toxicity of preparations of vancomycin from 1974 to 1981. Antimicrob Agents Chemother 1983;23:138-41.

75. Mellor JA, Kingdom J, Cafferkey M et al. Vancomycin toxicity: a prospective study. J Antimicrob Chemother 1985;15:773-80.

Drug-Induced Oculotoxicity

THE AGENTS IN THE FOLLOWING TABLE have been associated with drug-induced oculotoxicity when administered *systemically*. Occasionally, nonspecific blurred vision occurs with almost all drugs; the drugs in this table are those having a definite association with a specific pattern of oculotoxicity. The oculotoxicity of each drug is briefly described and accompanied by references.

The table begins on page 98.

Drug-Induced Oculotoxicity

DRUG	NATURE OF OCULOTOXICITY
Allopurinol	This drug has been found in cataractous lenses taken from patients on long-term therapy (over 2 yr). Allopurinol-treated patients without cataracts did not demonstrate these deposits. Excessive exposure to ultraviolet radiation may contribute to allopurinol-associated cataracts.[4]
Amiodarone	Most patients treated with amiodarone develop corneal microdeposits. These deposits rarely interfere with vision and are apparently dose-related and reversible (disappearing 3–7 months after discontinuation of the drug). Minute lens opacities were observed in 7 of 14 amiodarone-treated patients in one study.[1-3,5,6]
Anticholinergic Agents	Blurring of vision can result from paralysis of accommodation (cycloplegia). These drugs also dilate the pupil (mydriasis) which may produce photophobia and precipitate narrow angle glaucoma. With systemic administration, large doses are usually required to produce mydriasis which is most commonly associated with potent anticholinergics such as **atropine**, **scopolamine** or **benztropine**. Patients under treatment for narrow angle glaucoma should be able to tolerate systemic anticholinergic therapy, but should nevertheless avoid these drugs unless absolutely necessary. Similarly, patients treated with transdermal scopolamine may show ocular signs of systemic anticholinergic action and those with narrow angle glaucoma should avoid this product. Patients with open angle glaucoma, particularly if treated, can receive anticholinergic medications without significant hazard. All of the ocular effects of anticholinergics are dose-related and reversible.[1-3,7-9]
Antidepressants, Heterocyclic	These drugs all possess anticholinergic properties and are capable of precipitating narrow angle glaucoma (see Anticholinergic Agents). The prevalence of blurred vision resulting from cycloplegia ranges from 10–20%, but it is rarely troublesome and is reversible upon drug withdrawal. Gaze paralysis (ophthalmoplegia) has been occasionally encountered with heterocyclic antidepressant overdose. Ophthalmoplegia responds to IV **physostigmine**.[1-3,10,11]
Antihistamine Drugs (H₁-Blockers)	These drugs all possess some degree of anticholinergic activity and are capable of precipitating narrow angle glaucoma and cycloplegia (see Anticholinergic Agents). These effects tend to be minor and are reversible upon drug withdrawal. Antihistamines are thought by some to significantly reduce night vision.[1-3,8,12]

Continued

Drug-Induced Oculotoxicity

DRUG	NATURE OF OCULOTOXICITY
Beta-Adrenergic Blocking Agents	A reduction in tear production can result in a hot, dry and gritty sensation in the eye during beta-blocker therapy. This is rapidly reversible upon drug withdrawal. [1,3,3-16]
Bromocriptine	Myopia appears to be a fairly common complication of long-term bromocriptine therapy. It often goes unappreciated until the patient complains of blurred vision. It may be the result of lens swelling, but this has not been fully determined. Myopia is reversible within 1-2 weeks after drug withdrawal. [1,2,17,18]
Busulfan	Long-term therapy (several years) with busulfan has been associated with the development of posterior subcapsular cataracts. [19-24]
Chloramphenicol	Optic neuritis, papilledema and visual field defects have been occasionally reported in patients receiving chloramphenicol. These effects can occur after weeks or years of therapy, but are most common after several months of chloramphenicol use. Most cases have been reported in children with cystic fibrosis, but the association with this disorder is unclear and it may only reflect the type of patients who receive long-term chloramphenicol therapy. Both permanent visual impairment and recovery after withdrawal have been reported. It has been suggested that large doses of B vitamins may have a beneficial effect, but there is only anecdotal support for this approach. [1-3,25-29]
Chloroquine	The oculotoxicity of chloroquine limits its usefulness. Two general types of ocular changes are associated with chloroquine use: corneal deposits and retinopathy. About 50% of the patients treated with chloroquine demonstrate corneal deposits, less than one-half of whom have visual impairment resulting from these deposits. Opacities present as punctate or whirling patterns and are usually reversible when chloroquine is withdrawn. They may appear after as little as two months of therapy. Early changes in the retina (deposition of pigment in the macula) are usually asymptomatic and reversible. More advanced damage includes hyperpigmentation of the macula surrounded by a depigmented ring and hyperpigmented retina ("bull's eye" retinopathy). Patients complain of reading difficulty, blurred vision, visual field defects and photophobia; some may also report defective color vision and light flashes. The prevalence ranges from 3-45%, depending

Continued

Drug-Induced Oculotoxicity

DRUG	NATURE OF OCULOTOXICITY
	on the report. Chloroquine retinopathy is dose-related with an apparent dosage threshold of 5.1 mg/kg/day. The daily dose seems to be more important than the total dose or duration of therapy for the development of retinopathy. Most authors suggest limiting the daily dose to a maximum of 250 mg. Prognosis is uncertain; the vision of many patients may continue to deteriorate after drug withdrawal.[1-3,35-34]
Clomiphene	Approximately 2–10% of patients taking clomiphene complain of visual disturbances, most commonly blurred vision, which disappear after the drug is withdrawn.[35,36]
Contraceptives, Oral	A variety of retinal vascular disorders have been attributed to oral contraceptives. The association between oral contraceptive use and these vascular changes remains unclear. It has often been stated that some oral contraceptive users cannot tolerate contact lenses, possibly due to ocular edema or dryness. However, a prospective study failed to show any differences in lens tolerance between oral contraceptive users and nonusers.[1,3,37,38]
Corticosteroids	These drugs are capable of producing a variety of ocular disorders, most notably glaucoma and cataracts. Corticosteroid-induced increases in intra-ocular pressure appear to be dose-related and may persist for several months after drug withdrawal. The exact mechanism is unknown, but some have proposed that accumulation of mucopolysaccharides may play a role. Corticosteroid-induced cataracts (usually posterior subcapsular) are found in 10–20% of patients on long-term therapy. Cataract formation has been correlated with total dose (over 10 g prednisone or equivalent) and duration of therapy by some authors, while others have found no correlation. Outcome is variable, ranging from improvement despite continued therapy to loss of sight.[1-3,22,39-43]
Cyclophosphamide	One report showed a 17% prevalence of transient reversible blurred vision during high-dose cyclophosphamide therapy. Recovery took from 1 hr to 14 days.[22-24,44]
Cytarabine	Conjunctivitis, corneal damage and photophobia are common side effects of cytarabine therapy and may be encountered in the majority of patients. Corticosteroid eye drops may have a beneficial effect, but should be used with caution in patients with corneal damage.[1,24,45,46]

Continued

Drug-Induced Oculotoxicity

DRUG	NATURE OF OCULOTOXICITY
Diethylcarbamazine	Iritis and permanent visual field defects have been encountered in diethylcarbamazine-treated patients. An immunologic mechanism may contribute to the development of the visual field defects. [1,47-49]
Digitalis Glycosides	The most unique feature of the ocular effects of these drugs is the frosted or snowy appearance of objects or the appearance of colored halos around them. These effects are most noticeable in bright light. Color vision may be affected so that objects appear yellow (green or other colors have been reported, but far less frequently). With **digoxin**, color changes are usually encountered when the plasma level exceeds 1.5 ng/ml. Digitalis glycosides have also been reported to produce photophobia, blurred vision, scotoma and flickering or light flashes before the eyes. Reversible ocular side effects are seen in as many as 25% of digitalis-intoxicated patients. [1-3,50,51]
Disulfiram	A few cases of retrobulbar neuritis have occurred, manifested by a dramatic decline in visual acuity and impairment of color vision. In most patients, vision returned to normal after the drug was discontinued. [1,2,52]
Doxorubicin	This drug may stimulate excessive lacrimation shortly after administration. [22,23,53]
Ethambutol	Retrobulbar neuritis is the primary ocular complication of ethambutol therapy. Symptoms include blurred vision, scotoma and reduction of the visual field. Color vision defects are also encountered, usually presenting as a reduction in green perception. Retrobulbar neuritis is dose-related, occurring most frequently with doses of 25 mg/kg/day or more. Its onset is usually after 3-6 months of therapy and it is slowly reversible after drug withdrawal. Doses up to 15 mg/kg/day appear relatively free of ocular side effects. [1-3]
Fluorouracil	Reversible excessive lacrimation can be expected in about 50% of patients treated with systemic fluorouracil. Some patients may develop eversion of the eyelid margin (cicatricial ectropion) or potentially irreversible fibrosis of the tear duct (dacryostenosis) with prolonged therapy. [2,54-57]
Gold Salts	These drugs can produce microscopic crystalline deposits in the cornea, most commonly in the superficial

Continued

Drug-Induced Oculotoxicity

DRUG	NATURE OF OCULOTOXICITY
	layers. These deposits are dose-related and are rarely encountered until the total dose of parenteral gold exceeds 1 g. The deposits slowly resolve after withdrawal of gold therapy, do not appear to affect vision and are not a reason to stop gold therapy.[1-3,58,59]
Hydroxychloroquine	This drug can produce the same spectrum of ocular toxicity as chloroquine (see Chloroquine), but the prevalence appears to be lower. The apparent dosage threshold for retinopathy is 7.8 mg/kg/day and most authors suggest limiting the daily dose to a maximum of 400 mg.[1-3,33,34,60]
Indomethacin	A number of ocular effects, including blurred vision, corneal deposits and retinopathies, have been attributed to indomethacin. Recent literature, however, fails to support the earlier reports of these effects, questioning their significance.[1,61,62]
Isoniazid	Optic neuritis is one of the possible neuropathies resulting from isoniazid therapy. It occurs infrequently, most commonly in malnourished or alcoholic patients and often manifests itself as impairment of red-green perception. It responds to **pyridoxine** therapy.[1-3]
Isotretinoin	Blepharoconjunctivitis may be encountered in more than one-half of patients receiving isotretinoin. This painful condition is apparently dose-related.[1,2,63-66]
Methotrexate	The prevalence of ocular irritation associated with methotrexate therapy has been reported to be 14-25%.[22-24,67]
Oxygen	Retrolental fibroplasia is a significant complication of oxygen therapy in neonates, particularly premature or other low birth weight neonates. The risk of retrolental fibroplasia in these patients increases whenever the inspired air oxygen concentration exceeds normal.[1,68-70]
Phenothiazines	Lesions of the lens, cornea and retina are the most important features of phenothiazine-induced oculotoxicity. White to yellow-brown deposits in the lens most frequently occur with long-term, high-dose (over 1 kg)

Continued

Drug-Induced Oculotoxicity

DRUG	NATURE OF OCULOTOXICITY
	chlorpromazine therapy. Similar deposits can also be found in the corneas of chlorpromazine-treated patients. Epithelial keratopathy, possibly resulting from a photosensitivity reaction, can occur after only a few months of high-dose therapy. It is characterized by a diffuse opacification of the corneal epithelium. Lens and corneal deposits usually do not interfere with vision, and all of these effects may be slowly reversible. **Thioridazine** is also capable of producing lens and corneal deposits, but it is most noted for pigmentary retinopathy. As with most phenothiazine-induced ocular effects, pigmentary retinopathy is dose-related. Patients may complain of blurred vision, decreased night vision, brown discoloration of vision and scotoma. Vision may improve if the drug is withdrawn soon enough; however, some cases have continued to deteriorate despite drug withdrawal. Phenothiazines possess mild anticholinergic effects and may precipitate narrow angle glaucoma.[1-3,71]
Psoralens	The combination of psoralens and long-wave ultraviolet light (UVA) radiation is associated with the development of conjunctivitis, photophobia and other signs of ocular irritation. The use of UVA protective lenses greatly reduces the prevalence of this problem. An experimentally demonstrated connection between psoralens plus UVA (PUVA) therapy and cataracts has not been confirmed clinically.[1,2,72]
Quinidine	Amblyopia, scotoma, double or blurred vision, impaired color vision and, very rarely, blindness have been associated with quinidine overdose. Most quinidine-induced ocular changes are reversible.[73]
Quinine	Loss of visual acuity and reduction of the visual field to the point of blindness can be encountered with quinine therapy or overdose. Other reported ocular effects include impaired color vision and night blindness. These effects are usually reversible, but permanent constriction of the visual field and blindness have been reported. The ocular effects of quinine may be the result of changes in the retinal vasculature.[1,2,74,75]
Rifampin	Exudative conjunctivitis, ocular pain and orange staining of tears and contact lenses have been reported with rifampin. These rare effects are rapidly reversible when the drug is withdrawn.[76-78]
Sympathomimetic Agents	These drugs are capable of dilating the pupil and precipitating narrow angle glaucoma. The risk of this reaction is slight unless large doses are administered.[8]

Continued

Drug-Induced Oculotoxicity

DRUG	NATURE OF OCULOTOXICITY
Tamoxifen	Fine, refractile retinal opacities have been reported in some patients taking tamoxifen; some corneal opacities have also been reported. These lesions have been associated with reduced visual acuity.[1,2,22-24,79-81]
Vinca Alkaloids	A variety of ocular disorders have been associated with vinca alkaloid therapy. Most (ptosis, diplopia) are thought to be the result of cranial nerve impairment. **Vincristine** may be more oculotoxic than **vinblastine**.[1,2,22-24,82]

Drug-Induced Ototoxicity

THE AGENTS IN THE FOLLOWING TABLE have been reported to cause ototoxicity in man. Drug-induced ototoxicity can affect hearing (auditory or cochlear function), balance (vestibular function) or both, depending upon the drug. The most common form of ototoxicity is tinnitus, characterized by a ringing or buzzing sound in the ears. Drugs of almost every class have been reported to produce tinnitus, as have placebos. The only drugs represented in this table are those which have demonstrated a clear capability of producing a measurable hearing or vestibular defect.

The table begins on page 108.

Drug-Induced Ototoxicity

DRUG	NATURE OF OTOTOXICITY
Aminoglycosides	Aminoglycosides can cause both cochlear and vestibular toxicity. Cochlear toxicity presents as progressive hearing loss starting with the highest tones and advancing toward lower tones. Thus, significant damage may have been done before the patient is cognizant of it. Vestibular damage presents as dizziness, vertigo or ataxia. Both forms of ototoxicity are usually bilateral and potentially reversible, but permanent damage is common and damage may progress after the discontinuation of aminoglycoside therapy. It is not uncommon for 20–30% of aminoglycoside-treated patients in a series to have measurable hearing loss. Most aminoglycoside-induced ototoxicity is associated with parenteral therapy, but it has followed topical, oral and irrigation use of these drugs, especially **neomycin**. In general, a patient should receive doses by these routes that are no greater than those given by injection. Possible predisposing factors for ototoxicity include reduced renal function, duration of therapy, total dose received, plasma levels exceeding the therapeutic range, previous aminoglycoside use, concurrent use of other ototoxic drugs, dehydration and old age. Serial audiometry may be useful in early detection of ototoxicity. Each aminoglycoside has a slightly different spectrum of ototoxicity. The table below serves as a general guide to the relative ototoxic potential of the aminoglycosides.[1-9]

Relative Ototoxic Potential

DRUG	COCHLEAR	VESTIBULAR
Amikacin	+ +	+
Gentamicin	+	+ +
Kanamycin	+ + +	+
Neomycin	+ + + +	+

Relative Ototoxic Potential

DRUG	COCHLEAR	VESTIBULAR
Netilmicin	+	+ +
Sisomicin	+	+ +
Streptomycin	+	+ + +
Tobramycin	+	+ +

Drug-Induced Ototoxicity

DRUG	NATURE OF OTOTOXICITY
Chlorhexidine	Preoperative disinfection of the ear (before tympanic membrane repair) with a chlorhexidine solution produced deafness in 14 of 97 exposed patients.[1,10]
Chloroquine	Nerve deafness is a rare, but consistent, feature of chloroquine therapy. Its onset is usually delayed and it is usually thought of as irreversible and accompanying long-term therapy. A partially reversible case and a case resulting from only 1 g of chloroquine have been reported.[1,2,11,12]
Cisplatin	Clinically significant hearing loss has been reported in 12.5% of patients receiving cisplatin, with tinnitus and audiographic abnormalities reported in a much larger percentage of patients. Audiographic changes usually appear within 4 days after drug administration and high frequencies are lost first. The effects are dose-related and are probably irreversible. Rapid infusion of a dose is more ototoxic than the same dose administered over a prolonged time. In children treated with cisplatin, the ototoxicity may be inversely related to age. Patients with pre-existing hearing loss appear to be at increased risk.[1,2,13-18]
Diuretics, Loop	Rapid-onset hearing loss is a frequent feature of high-dose, rapid IV administration of **ethacrynic acid** and **furosemide**. Renal failure is usually listed as a predisposing factor, but renal failure patients are the only ones likely to receive large IV doses. Co-administration with **aminoglycoside antibiotics** is often said to result in increased ototoxicity, but a study of their concomitant use failed to find any evidence of increased ototoxicity. The hearing loss is usually transient, but permanent loss has been reported, more often with **ethacrynic acid** than with **furosemide**. Vestibular toxicity and hearing loss after oral therapy have been encountered. **Bumetanide** may produce less ototoxicity than furosemide.[1,2,19-25]
Erythromycin	Hearing loss has occasionally followed high-dose parenteral and oral therapy. It does not seem to be due to any particular salt form. Impaired hepatic or renal function and advanced age may increase the risk of hearing loss. It is usually reversible, but 1 case of irreversible hearing loss has been reported.[1,2,26-28]

Continued

Drug-Induced Ototoxicity

DRUG	NATURE OF OTOTOXICITY
Minocycline	Reversible vestibular toxicity, manifested primarily by dizziness, loss of balance and lightheadedness is a common occurrence in minocycline therapy. This adverse effect was noted in an average of 76% of patients in 6 studies and required 12–52% of affected patients to either discontinue the drug or to stop working. Other studies have encountered lower, but still large, percentages of patients with vestibular toxicity. Females may be more susceptible than males.[1,2,29-32]
Quinidine	Tinnitus and reversible hearing loss are well-known complications of quinidine therapy. Permanent hearing loss has been reported, but is uncommon.[1,2]
Quinine	Tinnitus is common. Permanent hearing impairment has occurred with long-term therapy. Quinine ototoxicity appears to be the result of an idiosyncratic reaction.[1,2]
Salicylates	Tinnitus, high frequency hearing loss and occasional vertigo are common features of salicylate intoxication. Hearing loss appears to be related to plasma salicylate level, although there is significant interpatient variability in the plasma level at which it is first detected. Most patients demonstrating ototoxicity from salicylates are chronically receiving large doses, such as those used in rheumatoid arthritis. Salicylate ototoxicity, even if severe, is usually reversible, but permanent hearing loss has been reported.[1,2,33,34]
Vancomycin	Transient and permanent hearing loss, tinnitus and dizziness have been encountered with vancomycin use. It has been suggested that these effects are associated with high plasma levels of vancomycin; however, this association is unproved. In many of the reported cases, the patient had also been exposed to other ototoxic drugs, especially **aminoglycoside antibiotics.**[1,2,35]

References

1. Dukes MNG, ed. Meyler's side effects of drugs. 10th ed. Amsterdam: Elsevier, 1984.

2. Brummett RE. Drug-induced ototoxicity. Drugs 1980;19:412-28.

3. Kalbian VV. Deafness following oral use of neomycin. South Med J 1972;65:499-501.

4. Dayal VS, Smith EL, McCain WG. Cochlear and vestibular gentamicin toxicity. A clinical study of systemic and topical usage. Arch Otolaryngol 1974;100:338-40.

5. Masur H, Whelton PK, Whelton A. Neomycin toxicity revisited. Arch Surg 1976;111:822-5.

6. Bamford MFM, Jones LF. Deafness and biochemical imbalance after burns treatment with topical antibiotics in young children. Report of 6 cases. Arch Dis Child 1978;53:326-9.

7. Smith CR, Lipsky JJ, Lietman PS. Relationship between aminoglycoside-induced nephrotoxicity and auditory toxicity. Antimicrob Agents Chemother 1979;15:780-2.

8. Kahlmeter G, Dahlager JI. Aminoglycoside toxicity — a review of clinical studies published between 1975 and 1982. J Antimicrob Chemother 1984;13(Suppl A):9-22.

9. Moore RD, Smith CR, Lietman PS. Risk factors for the development of auditory toxicity in patients receiving aminoglycosides. J Infect Dis 1984;149:23-30.

10. Bicknell PG. Sensorineural deafness following myringoplasty operations. J Laryngol Otol 1971;85:957-61.

11. Dwivedi GS, Mehra YN. Ototoxicity of chloroquine phosphate. A case report. J Laryngol Otol 1978;92:701-3.

12. Mukherjee DK. Chloroquine ototoxicity — a reversible phenomenon? J Laryngol Otol 1979;93:809-15.

13. Helson L, Okonkwo E, Anton L et al. cis-Platinum toxicity. Clin Toxicol 1978;13:469-78.

14. Von Hoff DD, Schilsky R, Reichert CM et al. Toxic effects of cis-dichlorodiammineplatinum(II) in man. Cancer Treat Rep 1979;63:1527-31.

15. Aguilar-Markulis NV, Beckley S, Priore R et al. Auditory toxicity effects of long-term cis-dichlorodiammineplatinum II therapy in genitourinary cancer patients. J Surg Oncol 1981;16:111-23.

16. Vermorken JB, Kapteijn TS, Hart AAM et al. Ototoxicity of cis-diamminedichloroplatinum (II): influence of dose, schedule and mode of administration. Eur J Cancer Clin Oncol 1983;19:55-8.

17. McHaney VA, Thibadoux G, Hayes FA et al. Hearing loss in children receiving cisplatin chemotherapy. J Pediatr 1983;102:314-7.

18. Melamed LB, Selim MA, Schuchman D. Cisplatin ototoxicity in gynecologic cancer patients. A preliminary report. Cancer 1985;55:41-3.

19. Schneider WJ, Becker EL. Acute transient hearing loss after ethacrynic acid therapy. Arch Intern Med 1966;117:715-7.

20. Matz GJ. The ototoxic effects of ethacrynic acid in man and animals. Laryngoscope 1976;86:1065-86.

21. Mathog RH. Vestibulotoxicity of ethacrynic acid. Laryngoscope 1977;87:1791-808.

22. Gallagher KL, Jones JK. Furosemide-induced ototoxicity. Ann Intern Med 1979;91:744-5.

23. Tuzel IH. Comparison of adverse reactions to bumetanide and furosemide. J Clin Pharmacol 1981;21:615-9.

24. Rybak LP. Pathophysiology of furosemide ototoxicity. J Otolaryngol 1982;11:127-33.

25. Smith CR, Lietman PS. Effect of furosemide on aminoglycoside-induced nephrotoxicity and auditory toxicity in humans. Antimicrob Agents Chemother 1983;23:133-7.

26. Schwartz JI, Maggini GA. Erythromycin-induced ototoxicity substantiated by rechallenge. Clin Pharm 1982;1:374-6.

27. Schweitzer VG, Olson NR. Ototoxic effect of erythromycin therapy. Arch Otolaryngol 1984;110:258-60.

28. Haydon RC, Thelin JW, Davis WE. Erythromycin ototoxicity: analysis and conclusions based on 22 case reports. Otolaryngol Head Neck Surg 1984;92:678-84.

29. Schofield CBS, Masterton G. Vestibular reactions to minocycline. Morb Mortal Wkly Rep 1976;25:31.

30. Allen JC. Minocycline. Ann Intern Med 1976;85:482-7.

31. Gump DW, Ashikaga T, Fink TJ et al. Side effects of minocycline: different dosage regimens. Antimicrob Agents Chemother 1977;12:642-6.

32. Greco TP, Bonadio M, Lee RV et al. Minocycline toxicity: experience with an altered dosage regimen. Curr Ther Res 1979;25:193-201.

33. Miller RR. Deafness due to plain and long-acting aspirin tablets. J Clin Pharmacol 1978;18:468-71.

34. Jardini L, Findlay R, Burgi E et al. Auditory changes associated with moderate blood salicylate levels. Rheumatol Rehabil 1978;17:233-6.

35. Mellor JA, Kingdom J, Cafferkey M et al. Vancomycin toxicity: a prospective study. J Antimicrob Chemother 1985;15:773-80.

Drug-Induced Sexual Dysfunction

THE AGENTS IN THE FOLLOWING TABLE have been associated with drug-induced sexual dysfunction in humans. The large subjective component of human sexual response makes the evaluation of drug-induced sexual dysfunction difficult. Variations in study design have produced widely divergent reported rates of sexual dysfunction in the "normal" or control populations. Common drug-induced sexual dysfunctions include decreased libido or sexual drive, impotence (failure to achieve or maintain an erection in males), priapism (persistent and often painful erection), delayed ejaculation or failure of ejaculation, retrograde ejaculation (into the urinary bladder), failure to achieve orgasm and decreased vaginal lubrication. Gynecomastia (enlargement of the male breast) is also usually included in discussions of drug-induced sexual dysfunction.

The table begins on page 113.

Drug-Induced Sexual Dysfunction

DRUG	NATURE OF DYSFUNCTION
Alcohol	Low doses result in behavioral disinhibition. As the dose increases, sexual response is impaired, resulting in failure of erection in males and reduced vaginal vasodilation and delayed orgasm in females. Chronic use has been associated with an 8% rate of impotence, one-half of which was irreversible despite abstinence from alcohol. The chronic effects are probably the result of both neurological and endocrine effects; alcohol has been shown to reduce testosterone levels and increase luteinizing hormone levels. The chronic effects are apparently independent of liver disease.[1-4,6-9]
Aminocaproic Acid	May inhibit ejaculation without affecting libido and has produced "dry" ejaculation. Effects are apparently rapidly reversible upon drug withdrawal.[1-3,10]
Amphetamines	Low doses may increase libido and produce a delay in male orgasm while high doses have been associated with failure to achieve an erection in males and loss of orgasm in both sexes.[1,2,11,12]
Anticholinergic Agents	Drugs with anticholinergic properties can theoretically cause impotence. This does not appear to be a common problem with "pure" anticholinergics used alone, but may be a contributor to adverse sexual effects produced by drugs which have anticholinergic actions as a part of their pharmacologic spectrum.[2-4]
Anticonvulsants	Sexual activity in males is thought to be reduced during therapy with anticonvulsants. This may be due to a reduction in the level of free testosterone resulting from hepatic enzyme induction and higher concentrations of sex hormone binding globulins.[2-5,13,14]
Antidepressants, Heterocyclic	Impotence, delayed ejaculation and painful ejaculation have all been reported in males. Females have encountered delayed orgasm. Both increased and, more commonly, decreased libido have been reported. The frequency of these effects varies considerably among the published reports, perhaps reflecting the influence of the underlying depressive illness. See also Trazodone[1-5,15,16]
Beta-Adrenergic Blocking Agents	These drugs have been associated with a variety of sexual problems, most commonly impotence. In a study of 46 patients on **propranolol**, 7 experienced "complete" impotence, 13 noted reduced potency and 2 com-

Continued

Drug-Induced Sexual Dysfunction

DRUG	NATURE OF DYSFUNCTION
	plained of reduced libido. In a larger trial, the frequency of impotence during propranolol therapy was 13.8% and 13.2% after 12 weeks and 2 years, respectively. These figures did not differ significantly from placebo. Most of the published reports implicate propranolol and, while it has been proposed that other more cardioselective β-blockers may have fewer adverse sexual effects, there are scattered reports involving most of the other members of the class. There have been at least 25 patients complaining of sexual dysfunction (18 impotence, 9 decreased libido) while receiving topical ophthalmic treatment with **timolol**. Some of these patients were rechallenged with positive results.[1-5,17-22]
Carbonic Anhydrase Inhibitors	A significant number of patients receiving carbonic anhydrase inhibitors (**acetazolamide, methazolamide**) develop a syndrome of malaise, fatigue, weight loss and depression which often includes loss of libido. These patients appear to be more acidotic than those without the syndrome and some have responded to therapy with sodium bicarbonate. Decreased libido has been encountered in both males and females and usually requires 2 weeks of carbonic anhydrase inhibitor therapy to develop.[1,2,4,5,23,24]
Cimetidine	In a group of 22 male patients being treated with high doses of cimetidine for hypersecretory states, 11 developed gynecomastia and 9 experienced impotence. These effects appear to be dose-related and readily reversible and should not be a significant problem at the doses used for peptic ulcers. Cimetidine has some anti-androgenic properties, possibly the result of hyperprolactinemia, which are thought to be responsible for sexual dysfunction. **Ranitidine** does not have an anti-androgenic action and should be an acceptable alternative.[1-5,25,26]
Clofibrate	In large multicenter trials, impotence has been reported more frequently than with placebo.[1-3,5,22,27,28]
Clonidine	While some reports have indicated no sexual problems with clonidine, others have indicated problems in up to 24% of patients. Impotence is the most frequently mentioned effect, but delayed or retrograde ejaculation, gynecomastia in males and failure of orgasm in females have also been described.[1-5,21,22,29,30]
Cocaine	While cocaine is commonly perceived as a sexual stimulant, its use is associated with difficulty in establishing an erection and delayed ejaculation.[1,2,31-33]

Continued

Drug-Induced Sexual Dysfunction

DRUG	NATURE OF DYSFUNCTION
Digoxin	Digitalis glycosides have some estrogen-like activity and have been associated with decreased libido, increased impotence and gynecomastia in males.[1,2,22,34]
Diuretics, Thiazide	These drugs are commonly included among those alleged to produce adverse sexual effects, but the available data are not conclusive. In one large study, the frequency of impotence was significantly higher with **bendroflumethiazide** than with placebo (23% after 2 years compared with 10% for placebo) and in another, **hydrochlorothiazide** produced significantly more impotence and loss of libido than **propranolol**. Similar effects have been described for **chlorthalidone**.[1-5,19-22]
Estrogens	Estrogens have been used to reduce libido and sexual activity of male sex offenders.[1,2,35]
Fat Emulsion	In one report, 2 of 35 males being treated with intravenous fat emulsion developed priapism. Both were receiving the 20% emulsion. This effect was thought to be the result of vascular thrombosis either from fat embolism or hypercoagulability.[36]
Guanadrel	Poorly characterized "sexual dysfunction" and "ejaculatory disturbances" have been reported in studies evaluating guanadrel. These effects seem to be maximal after 1 to 2 months of therapy.[37,38]
Guanethidine	As many as 54% of males treated with guanethidine have reported failure of ejaculation and as many as 60% have reported failure of ejaculation. Guanethidine does not affect parasympathetic function and would not be expected to produce impotence. Some have suggested that the impotence is secondary to the inhibition of ejaculation. Retrograde ejaculation may occur as a result of the failure of the internal urethral sphincter to close — this action is sympathetically mediated. Patients may describe retrograde ejaculation as "dry" ejaculation. Guanethidine effects are reversible upon withdrawal of the drug and may be alleviated by a reduction in dose.[1-3,21,22,39,40]
Marijuana	Marijuana has been reported to have both positive and negative effects on sexual function. Low doses may have a disinhibiting effect, while large doses have been associated with decreased libido and the inability of males to perform.[1-3,41,42]

Continued

Drug-Induced Sexual Dysfunction

DRUG	NATURE OF DYSFUNCTION
Methyldopa	Impotence, reduced libido and ejaculatory failure have all been described with methyldopa therapy. The frequency of sexual dysfunction has varied from quite low in some reports to greater than 50% in response to direct questioning. These effects are dose-related and reversible. They may be the result of the sympathetic inhibition and mild CNS depression produced by the drug. Gynecomastia in males and painful breast enlargement in females have been occasionally encountered.[1-5,21,22,32,40,43,44]
Monoamine Oxidase Inhibitors	Reported adverse sexual effects of MAOIs are highly variable. Orgasmic failure in both males and females, impotence, ejaculatory delay and spontaneous erections have all been described. The true frequency of these effects cannot be determined from the available data.[1-5,15,45-47]
Narcotics	Chronic narcotic use (especially abuse) is commonly associated with decreased libido, orgasmic failure in both sexes and impotence in men. These effects are dose-related, with the highest frequency of impotence reported in narcotic addicts (80–90% in some series), and are reversible upon drug withdrawal.[1-4,48-52]
Nitrites and Nitrites	These vasodilators have been used (primarily by inhalation) to enhance the perception of orgasm. When used too soon before orgasm, however, they rapidly produce loss of erection. This effect has been used therapeutically to reduce spontaneous erections in males undergoing urological procedures.[1,53,54]
Phenothiazines	These drugs have been implicated in producing a wide variety of adverse sexual effects including impotence and priapism, absent and spontaneous ejaculation, retrograde ejaculation, menstrual irregularities and decreased libido. These effects are the result of the complex actions of the drugs on the patient's hormonal balance and sympathetic and parasympathetic pathways of the CNS. With the exception of priapism, these effects are usually benign and respond to withdrawal of therapy. **Thioridazine** is the most commonly implicated phenothiazine and, in one major study, 60% of thioridazine-treated patients reported sexual dysfunction compared to 25% of patients treated with other antipsychotic drugs. The most frequently reported adverse effects were ejaculatory impairment (including retrograde ejaculation) and impotence. The possible contribution of the underlying disease state cannot be overlooked.[1-5,55,56]

Continued

Drug-Induced Sexual Dysfunction

DRUG	NATURE OF DYSFUNCTION
Phenoxybenzamine	This α-adrenergic blocker is associated with failure of ejaculation, but not interference with orgasm. This effect was present in all 19 patients in one study and was reversed 24-48 hours after drug withdrawal.[1-3,57,58]
Prazosin	Several cases of priapism have been reported following therapeutic use and overdose with prazosin. These reports are scattered and prazosin appears to be relatively free of other sexual side effects.[3,21,59-61]
Progestins	Impotence has been reported in 25-70% of men receiving progestins for prostatic hypertrophy.[1,2,4,62,63]
Reserpine	Reserpine therapy has resulted in failure of ejaculation, impotence and reduced libido. The first may be the result of its sympatholytic effects, while the last two could be explained as the outcome of the drug's depressant properties.[1-3,21,22,40]
Sedative-Hypnotics	In a manner similar to alcohol, low doses may produce some disinhibition, while large doses should reduce sexual performance. The reputation of some sedative-hypnotics, such as **methaqualone**, as aphrodisiacs probably represents a combination of the initial disinhibition and the expectations of the user.[1-4]
Spironolactone	Gynecomastia in males and painful breast enlargement and menstrual irregularities in females are very common with large doses of spironolactone. Less frequently reported effects include impotence, inhibition of vaginal lubrication and loss of libido. The similarity of the drug to estrogens and progestins is thought to play a key role in the genesis of adverse sexual effects. In one study, spironolactone increased the metabolic clearance of testosterone and its rate of peripheral conversion to estradiol. These effects appear to be dose-related.[1-5,21,22,64-66]
Trazodone	There have been at least 12 cases of priapism associated with trazodone therapy, including some which required surgical intervention. See also Antidepressants, Heterocyclic.[67,68]

References

1. Buffum J. Pharmacosexology: the effects of drugs on sexual function. A review. J Psychoactive Drugs 1982;14:5-44.

2. Anon. Drugs that cause sexual dysfunction. Med Lett Drugs Ther 1983;25:73-6.

3. Aldridge SA. Drug-induced sexual dysfunction. Clin Pharm 1982;1:141-7.

4. Beeley L. Drug-induced sexual dysfunction and infertility. Adverse Drug React Acute Pois Rev 1984;3:23-42.

5. Dukes MNG, ed. Meyler's side effects of drugs. 10th ed. Amsterdam: Elsevier, 1984.

6. Lemere F, Smith JW. Alcohol-induced male impotence. Am J Psychiatry 1973;130:212-3.

7. Wilson GT, Lawson DM. Effects of alcohol on sexual arousal in women. J Abnorm Psychol 1976;85:489-97.

8. Gordon GG, Altman K, Southren AL et al. Effect of alcohol (ethanol) administration on sex-hormone metabolism in normal men. N Engl J Med 1976;295:793-7.

9. Dudek FA, Turner DS. Alcoholism and sexual functioning. J Psychoactive Drugs 1982;14:47-54.

10. Evans BE, Aledort LM. Inhibition of ejaculation due to epsilon aminocaproic acid. N Engl J Med 1978;298:166-7. Letter.

11. Greaves G. Sexual disturbances among chronic amphetamine users. J Nerv Ment Dis 1972;155:363-5.

12. Smith DE, Buxton ME, Dammann G. Amphetamine abuse and sexual dysfunction: clinical and research considerations. In: Smith DE, Wesson DR, Buxton ME et al, eds. Amphetamine use, misuse, and abuse: proceedings of The National Amphetamine Conference, 1978. Boston: GK Hall, 1979:228-48.

13. Toone BK, Wheeler M, Fenwick PBC. Sex hormone changes in male epileptics. Clin Endocrinol 1980;12:391-5.

14. Dana-Haeri J, Oxley J, Richens A. Reduction of free testosterone by antiepileptic drugs. Br Med J 1982;284:85-6.

15. Mitchell JE, Popkin MK. Antidepressant drug therapy and sexual dysfunction in men: a review. J Clin Psychopharmacol 1983;3:76-9.

16. Fraser AR. Sexual dysfunction following antidepressant drug therapy. J Clin Psychopharmacol 1984;4:62-3. Letter.

17. Burnett WC, Chahine RA. Sexual dysfunction as a complication of propranolol therapy in men. Cardiovasc Med 1979;4:811-5.

18. Fraunfelder FT, Meyer SM. Sexual dysfunction secondary to topical ophthalmic timolol. JAMA 1985;253:3092-3. Letter.

19. Medical Research Council Working Party on Mild to Moderate Hypertension. Adverse reactions to bendrofluazide and propranolol for the treatment of mild hypertension. Lancet 1981;2:539-42.

20. Veterans Administration Cooperative Study Group on Antihypertensive Agents. Comparison of propranolol and hydrochlorothiazide for the initial treatment of hypertension. II. Results of long-term therapy. JAMA 1982;248:2004-11.

21. Stevenson JG, Umstead GS. Sexual dysfunction due to antihypertensive agents. Drug Intell Clin Pharm 1984;18:113-21.

22. Papadopoulos C. Cardiovascular drugs and sexuality: a cardiologist's review. Arch Intern Med 1980;140:1341-5.

23. Epstein DL, Grant WM. Carbonic anhydrase inhibitor side effects. Serum chemical analysis. Arch Ophthalmol 1977;95:1378-82.

24. Wallace TR, Fraunfelder FT, Petursson GJ et al. Decreased libido—a side effect of carbonic anhydrase inhibitor. Ann Ophthalmol 1979;11:1563-6.

25. Jensen RT, Collen MJ, Pandol SJ et al. Cimetidine-induced impotence and breast changes in patients with gastric hypersecretory states. N Engl J Med 1983;308:883-7.

26. Peden NR, Wormsley KG. Alleged impotence with ranitidine. Lancet 1983;2:798. Letter.

27. The Coronary Drug Project Research Group. Clofibrate and niacin in coronary heart disease. JAMA 1975;231:360-81.

28. Oliver MF, Heady JA, Morris JN et al. A co-operative trial in the primary prevention of ischaemic heart disease using clofibrate. Report from the Committee of Principal Investigators. Br Heart J 1978;40:1069-118.

29. Onesti G, Bock KD, Heimsoth V et al. Clonidine: a new antihypertensive agent. Am J Cardiol 1971;28:74-83.

30. Hogan MJ, Wallin JD, Baer RM. Antihypertensive therapy and male sexual dysfunction. Psychosomatics 1980;21:234-7 passim.

31. Siegel RK. Cocaine: recreational use and intoxication. In Petersen RC, Stillman RC, eds. Cocaine: 1977. Rockville, Maryland: Public Health Service, 1977:119-36 (NIDA Research Monograph #13).

32. Siegel RK. Cocaine and sexual dysfunction: the curse of mama coca. J Psychoactive Drugs 1982;14:71-4.

33. Wesson DR. Cocaine use by masseuses. J Psychoactive Drugs. 1982;14:75-6.

34. Neri A, Aygen M, Zukerman Z et al. Subjective assessment of sexual dysfunction of patients on long-term administration of digoxin. Arch Sex Behav 1980;9:343-7.

35. Bancroft J, Tennent G, Loucas K et al. The control of deviant sexual behaviour by drugs: I. Behavioural changes following oestrogens and anti-androgens. Br J Psychiatry 1974;125:310-5.

36. Klein EA, Montague DK, Steiger E. Priapism associated with the use of intravenous fat emulsion: case reports and postulated pathogenesis. J Urol 1985;133:857-9.

37. Dunn MI, Dunlap JL. Guanadrel. A new antihypertensive drug. JAMA 1981;245:1639-42.

38. Nugent CA, Palmer JD, Ursprung JJ. Guanadrel sulfate compared with methyldopa for mild and moderate hypertension. Pharmacotherapy 1982;2:378-83.

39. Veterans Administration Cooperative Study Group on Antihypertensive Agents. Multiclinic controlled trial of bethanidine and guanethidine in severe hypertension. Circulation 1977;55:519-25.

40. Bulpitt CJ, Dollery CT. Side effects of hypotensive agents evaluated by a self-administered questionnaire. Br Med J 1973;3:485-90.

41. Chopra GS. Man and marijuana. Int J Addict 1969;4:215-47.

42. Halikas J, Weller R, Morse C. Effects of regular marijuana use on sexual performance. J Psychoactive Drugs 1982;14:59-70.

43. Newman RJ, Salerno HR. Sexual dysfunction due to methyldopa. Br Med J 1974;4:106. Letter.

44. Alexander WD, Evans Jl. Side effects of methyldopa. Br Med J 1975;2:501. Letter.

45. Rapp MS. Two cases of ejaculatory impairment related to phenelzine. Am J Psychiatry 1979;136:1200-1.

46. Barton JL. Orgasmic inhibition by phenelzine. Am J Psychiatry 1979;136:1616-7. Letter.

47. Lesko LM, Stotland NL, Segraves RT. Three cases of female anorgasmia associated with MAOIs. Am J Psychiatry 1982;139:1353-4.

48. Cushman P Jr. Sexual behavior in heroin addiction and methadone maintenance. Correlation with plasma luteinizing hormone. NY State J Med 1972;72:1261-5.

49. Parr D. Sexual aspects of drug abuse in narcotic addicts. Br J Addict 1976;71:261-8.

50. Hanbury R, Cohen M, Stimmel B. Adequacy of sexual performance in men maintained on methadone. Am J Drug Alcohol Abuse 1977;4:13-20.

51. Langrod J, Lowinson J, Ruiz P. Methadone treatment and physical complaints: a clinical analysis. Int J Addict 1981;16:947-52.

52. Rosenbaum M. When drugs come into the picture, love flies out the window: women addicts' love relationships. Int J Addict 1981;16:1197-206.

53. Sigell LT, Kapp FT, Fusaro GA et al. Popping and snorting volatile nitrites: a current fad for getting high. Am J Psychiatry 1978;135:1216-8.

54. Welti RS, Brodsky JB. Treatment of intraoperative penile tumescence. J Urol 1980;124:925-6.

55. Kotin J, Wilbert DE, Verburg D et al. Thioridazine and sexual dysfunction. Am J Psychiatry 1976;133:82-5.

56. Mitchell JE, Popkin MK. Antipsychotic drug therapy and sexual dysfunction in men. Am J Psychiatry 1982;139:633-7.

57. Caine M, Perlberg S, Shapiro A. Phenoxybenzamine for benign prostatic obstruction. Review of 200 cases. Urology 1981;17:542-6.

58. Kedia KR, Persky L. Effect of phenoxybenzamine (Dibenzyline) on sexual function in man. Urology 1981;18:620-2.

59. Bhalla AK, Hoffbrand Bl, Phatak PS et al. Prazosin and priapism. Br Med J 1979;2:1039.

60. Ylitalo P, Pasternack A. Priapism—side-effect of prazosin in patients with renal failure. Acta Med Scand 1983;213:319-20.

61. Robbins DN, Crawford ED, Lackner LH. Priapism secondary to prazosin overdose. J Urol 1983;130:975.

62. Meiraz D, Margolin Y, Lev-Ran A et al. Treatment of benign prostatic hyperplasia with hydroxyprogesterone-caproate: placebo-controlled study. Urology 1977;9:144-8.

63. Palanca E, Juco W. Conservative treatment of benign prostatic hypertrophy. Curr Med Res Opin 1977;4:513-20.

64. Spark RF, Melby JC. Aldosteronism in hypertension. The spironolactone response test. Ann Intern Med 1968;68:685-91.

65. Caminos-Torres R, Ma L, Snyder PJ. Gynecomastia and semen abnormalities induced by spironolactone in normal men. J Clin Endocrinol Metab 1977;45:255-60.

66. Rose Ll, Underwood RH, Newmark SR et al. Pathophysiology of spironolactone-induced gynecomastia. Ann Intern Med 1977;87:398-403.

67. Anon. Priapism with trazodone (Desyrel). Med Lett Drugs Ther 1984;26:35.

68. Lansky MR, Selzer J. Priapism associated with trazodone therapy: case report. J Clin Psychiatry 1984;45:232-3.

Drug-Induced Skin Disorders

THE AGENTS IN THE FOLLOWING TABLE have been reported to cause a variety of skin disorders. The difficulty of establishing a correct diagnosis of a skin disorder and the complexity of establishing a causal relationship with drug administration make estimates of the frequency of occurrence of these reactions virtually impossible.

Drugs believed to be among the most common causes of a particular drug-induced skin disorder are designated by "XX" in the table. Only skin disorders resulting from systemic administration of drugs are presented. Stevens-Johnson syndrome, a potentially fatal form of erythema multiforme, is included in the table entries for erythema multiforme. For skin disorders caused by topical administration of drugs, see Cronin E. Contact dermatitis. Edinburgh: Churchill Livingstone, 1980. The following abbreviations are used to indicate specific skin disorders:

> AE —Acneiform Eruptions
> Al —Alopecia

Continued

ED—Exfoliative Dermatitis
EM—Erythema Multiforme
FE —Fixed Eruptions
LE —Lupus Erythematosus-Like Reactions
Ph —Photosensitivity and Phototoxicity Reactions
TN —Toxic Epidermal Necrolysis

Drug-Induced Skin Disorders

DRUG	AE	AI	ED	EM	FE	LE	Ph	TN	REFERENCES
Acetaminophen					X				7
Acetazolamide				X					5
Allopurinol	X		X					X	2,3,5,10
Aminosalicylic Acid			X	X	X				3-5
Amiodarone							X		1,10
Amphetamines		X							6
Androgens	XX	X							2,3
Arsenicals, Organic			X						3-5
Aspirin			X	X	X			X	2-5,10
Barbiturates	X			X	X			XX	1-5,10
Bleomycin		X							11
Boric Acid		X							4,6
Bromides	XX								1-5
Bromocriptine		X							6
Captopril								X	10
Chloramphenicol								X	2,10
Chloroquine					X		X		1,7,9
Cimetidine			X					X	2,10
Clofibrate		X							3,6
Contraceptives, Oral	X	X					X		1,3,6,9
Corticosteroids	XX	X			X		X		1-6,9
Cyclophosphamide		X							4,11
Dacarbazine							X		11
Dactinomycin	X	X	X						3,5,11
Dapsone			X	X	X			X	1,2,4, 5,7,10
Daunorubicin		X							11
Dextran		X							6
Diphenhydramine							X		1-4
Diuretics, Mercurial			X	X	X				2,4,5,7
Diuretics, Thiazide				X			XX		2-5,9

Continued

Drug-Induced Skin Disorders

DRUG	AE	AI	ED	EM	FE	LE	Ph	TN	REFERENCES
Doxorubicin		X							11
Ethosuximide						X			4,8
Fluorouracil		X					X	X	10,11
Furosemide			X	X			X		1-4
Gold Salts			X	X	X		X	X	1-5,10
Griseofulvin			X	X	X		X		1-5,7,9
Heparin		X							1,3-6
Hydralazine					X	XX			1,3-5,7,8
Ibuprofen		X							6
Iodides	XX	X			X				1-7
Isoniazid	X					X			2-5,8
Lithium	X								1-3,5
Methotrexate		X						X	5,10,11
Methyldopa						X			3,8
Nalidixic Acid							X		1-3,5,9
Nitrofurantoin						X		X	1,2,5,8
Oxyphenbutazone			X	X	X			XX	2,4,7,10
Penicillamine						X			1,3,4,8
Penicillins			X	X	X			X	1-5,7,10
Pentamidine								X	2,10
Pentazocine								X	2,10
Phenolphthalein			X	X	XX			X	2-5,7
Phenothiazines				X		X	XX		1-5,8,9
Phenylbutazone			X	X	XX			XX	1-5,7,10
Phenytoin	X		X	X		X		X	2-5,8,10
Procainamide					XX				3,4,8
Propranolol		X							1,3,6
Propylthiouracil		X							1,5,6
Psoralens							XX		2-5,9
Quinacrine		X	X		X				3,5,7
Quinidine			X	X	X	X	X		2,3,5,7-9
Quinine				X	X			X	2,4,5,7,10
Streptomycin					X			X	5,7,10
Sulfonamides			X	X	X	X	XX	XX	1-5,9,10
Sulfonylureas			X	X			XX	X	1-5,9,10
Tetracyclines				X	X	X	XX	X	1-5,8-10
Trimethadione	X	X				X			3,4,6,8

Continued

Drug-Induced Skin Disorders

DRUG	AE	AI	ED	EM	FE	LE	Ph	TN	REFERENCES
Valproic Acid		X							1,3,6
Vinblastine							X		3,11
Vitamin A		X							3-6
Warfarin		X							3-6

References

1. Dukes MNG, ed. Meyler's side effects of drugs. 10th ed. Amsterdam: Elsevier, 1984.

2. Skin disorders. In: Davies DM, ed. Textbook of adverse drug reactions. 2nd ed. Oxford: Oxford University Press, 1981:420-35.

3. Millikan LE. Drug eruptions (dermatitis medicamentosa). In: Moschella SL, Hurley HJ, eds. Dermatology. 2nd ed. Philadelphia: WB Saunders, 1985:425-63.

4. Baker H. Drug reactions. In: Rook A, Wilkinson DS, Ebling FJG, eds. Textbook of Dermatology. 3rd ed. Oxford: Blackwell Scientific Publications, 1979:1111-49.

5. Contact dermatitis; drug eruptions. In: Domonkos AN, Arnold HL Jr, Odom RB. Andrews' diseases of the skin. 7th ed. Philadelphia: WB Saunders, 1982:97-143.

6. Reeves JRT, Maibach HI. Drug- and chemical-induced hair loss. In: Marzulli FN, Maibach HI, eds. Dermatotoxicology. 2nd ed. Washington: Hemisphere Publishing, 1983:501-17.

7. Korkij W, Soltani K. Fixed drug eruption. A brief review. Arch Dermatol 1984;120:520-4.

8. Stratton MA. Drug-induced systemic lupus erythematosus. Clin Pharm 1985;4:657-63.

9. Epstein JH, Wintroub BU. Photosensitivity due to drugs. Drugs 1985;30:42-57.

10. Fabrizio PJ, McCloskey WW, Jeffrey LP. Drugs causing toxic epidermal necrolysis. Drug Intell Clin Pharm 1985;19:733-5.

11. Bronner AK, Hood AF. Cutaneous complications of chemotherapeutic agents. J Am Acad Dermatol 1983;9:645-63.

6 *DRUG INTERACTIONS*

Drug-Drug Interactions, Drug-Laboratory Test Interferences

Drug-Drug Interactions

THE FOLLOWING IS A LIST OF THOSE DRUG INTERACTIONS which are most likely to be important in clinical practice. Minor or poorly documented interactions have been omitted, as have obvious interactions such as drugs with pharmacological actions which are clearly similar (barbiturates-glutethimide) or opposite (isoproterenol-propranolol). For a more comprehensive review, the reader is directed to references 1 and 2 at the end of this section. It is important to remember that the presence of a drug interaction in this list does not imply that the two drugs should not be used together. In the vast majority of cases, the drugs may be used concomitantly as long as appropriate measures are taken.

In preparing this section, collective drug group or drug class names have been used whenever possible; drugs which are a member of one of these groups are not listed individually. The following drug group names are used:

Aminoglycosides
Amphetamines
Anabolic Steroids
Antacids, Oral
Anticholinergic Agents
Anticoagulants, Oral
Antidepressants, Tricyclic
Antidiabetic Agents
Barbiturates
Benzodiazepines
Beta-Adrenergic Blocking Agents
Calcium Channel Blocking
    Agents
Cephalosporins
Contraceptives, Oral
Corticosteroids
Digitalis Glycosides
Diuretics, Potassium-Sparing
Diuretics, Thiazide

Iron Preparations
Methenamine Compounds
Monoamine Oxidase
    Inhibitors
Narcotic Analgesics
Nitrates
Nonsteroidal Anti-
    Inflammatory Agents
Penicillins
Phenothiazines
Polymyxins
Potassium Salts
Salicylates
Skeletal Muscle Relaxants
    (Surgical)
Sulfonamides, Antibacterial
Sympathomimetic Agents
Tetracyclines
Thyroid Hormones

The table begins on page 124.

Drug Interactions

DRUG	INTERACTION AND COMMENTS

Acetaminophen—*Alcohol:* chronic alcohol abuse may increase the likelihood of acetaminophen hepatotoxicity, probably due to increased production of hepatotoxic acetaminophen metabolites; may occur with high therapeutic acetaminophen doses; alcoholics should limit their use of acetaminophen.[3]

Acetazolamide—*Quinidine:* alkalinization of the urine may decrease quinidine elimination, increasing the risk of quinidine toxicity.[1,2]

—See also Methenamine Compounds; Salicylates; Sympathomimetic Agents.

Alcohol—*Chloral Hydrate:* may inhibit each other's metabolism and prolong CNS depression; may also produce vasodilation and hypotension.[1,2]

—*Disulfiram:* ingestion of even small amounts of alcohol may produce the disulfiram reaction, consisting of vasodilation, hypotension, nausea, vomiting, chest pain, weakness and confusion; patients should also be warned about contact with products whose alcohol content may not be obvious (eg, pharmaceuticals, topical preparations).[1]

—*Guanadrel:* response same as Alcohol—Guanethidine.

—*Guanethidine:* alcohol-induced vasodilation may accentuate guanethidine's orthostatic hypotension.[1,2]

—*Methotrexate:* chronic co-administration may increase the risk of methotrexate-induced liver damage; patients receiving methotrexate should minimize their consumption of alcohol.[1,2]

—*Metronidazole:* disulfiram-like reactions have been reported, but are not a consistent problem; although these reactions are not common, patients should be warned about the possibility of their occurrence.[1,2]

—*Nitrates:* the vasodilation produced by both drugs may combine to produce significant hypotension.[1,2]

—*Phenytoin:* chronic use of large quantities of alcohol may stimulate the metabolism of phenytoin; monitor phenytoin levels in alcoholics.[1,2]

—See also Acetaminophen; Anticoagulants, Oral; Antidiabetic Agents; Salicylates.

Allopurinol—*Azathioprine:* allopurinol inhibits the metabolism of **mercaptopurine** (active metabolite of azathioprine) to inactive products, resulting in increased mercaptopurine toxicity; when co-administration cannot be avoided, the azathioprine dose should be reduced.[1,2]

—*Cyclophosphamide:* cyclophosphamide-induced bone marrow suppression may be enhanced by allopurinol administration; mechanism is unknown.[1,2]

—*Mercaptopurine:* See Allopurinol—Azathioprine (note: the interaction described probably does not occur with IV mercaptopurine).

—See also Anticoagulants, Oral.

Amantadine: See Anticholinergic Agents.

Amiloride: See Diuretics, Potassium-Sparing.

Continued

Drug Interactions

DRUG	INTERACTION AND COMMENTS

Aminoglycosides—*Amphotericin B:* possible additive nephrotoxicity; monitor renal function.[1,2]

—*Cephalosporins:* additive nephrotoxicity is a possibility, primarily with **cephalothin**; prolonged therapy merits repeated renal function tests.[1,2]

—*Cisplatin:* possible additive nephrotoxic effect; if combination cannot be avoided, monitor renal function carefully.[4]

—*Digitalis Glycosides:* oral **neomycin** may impair digoxin absorption; monitor digoxin levels if chronic oral neomycin therapy is begun.[1,2]

—*Ethacrynic Acid:* additive ototoxicity has been reported—impaired renal function is an important predisposing factor.[1,2]

—*Methoxyflurane:* additive nephrotoxicity is a possibility; less nephrotoxic antibiotics should be used whenever possible.[1,2]

—*Penicillins:* the absorption of oral **penicillin V** is impaired by as much as 50% by oral **neomycin**; use parenteral penicillin until neomycin therapy is completed; also, **carbenicillin** and other penicillins appear to inactivate aminoglycosides when mixed in vitro, and possibly also in patients with severe renal impairment.[1,2]

—*Skeletal Muscle Relaxants (Surgical):* aminoglycoside antibiotics are capable of producing neuromuscular blockade which can enhance that of the muscle relaxant, prolonging recovery time and sometimes causing respiratory paralysis; avoid co-administration when ventilatory assistance equipment is not available.[1,2]

Aminophylline: See Theophylline.

Aminosalicylic Acid (PAS)—*Probenecid:* renal elimination of PAS may be greatly impaired by probenecid, requiring reduction of PAS dose to avoid toxicity.[1,2]

Amiodarone—*Anticoagulants, Oral:* enhanced anticoagulant response; if combination cannot be avoided, monitor prothrombin time carefully and adjust anticoagulant dose accordingly.[1,2]

—*Digitalis Glycosides:* increased plasma **digoxin** levels; monitor for evidence of increased digoxin effect, using plasma digoxin determinations if possible.[1,2]

—*Quinidine:* possible reduction in quinidine clearance; monitor quinidine response and reduce quinidine dose if needed.[5]

Ammonium Chloride—*Spironolactone:* large doses of ammonium chloride (eg, for acidification of the urine) may result in systemic acidosis in the presence of spironolactone.[1,2]

Amphetamines: See Sympathomimetic Agents.

Amphotericin B—*Cyclosporine:* possible additive nephrotoxic effect; if combination cannot be avoided, monitor renal function carefully.[6]

—See also Aminoglycosides; Corticosteroids; Digitalis Glycosides.

Anabolic Steroids—*Anticoagulants, Oral:* although mechanism is unknown, increase in anticoagulant activity is commonly encountered; monitor prothrombin time carefully.[1,2]

Drug Interactions

DRUG	INTERACTION AND COMMENTS

—*Antidiabetic Agents:* enhanced hypoglycemic effect; antidiabetic agent dosage adjustments may be required.[1,2]

Antacids, Oral—*Digitalis Glycosides:* antacids may reduce the extent of **digoxin** absorption; give digoxin 2 hr before antacids.[1]

—*Diuretics, Thiazide:* large doses of calcium antacids may produce hypercalcemia in presence of thiazides in predisposed patients (eg, high Vitamin D intake, hyperparathyroidism); mechanism is thiazide-induced reduction in urinary calcium excretion.[7]

—*Iron Preparations:* calcium carbonate, sodium bicarbonate and possibly magnesium trisilicate reduce absorption of oral iron, but aluminum/magnesium hydroxides apparently do not; separate doses by 2 hr or more.[1,2,8]

—*Isoniazid:* aluminum-containing antacids may interfere with isoniazid absorption; separate doses by 2 hr or select another antacid.[1,2]

—*Quinidine:* antacid-induced increases in urinary pH can decrease the amount of quinidine excreted by the kidney; watch for evidence of increased quinidine effect.[1,2]

—*Salicylates:* significantly reduced salicylate levels, due to enhanced renal elimination of salicylate; plasma salicylate levels should be monitored in patients requiring long-term salicylate therapy.[9]

—*Sodium Polystyrene Sulfonate:* this resin can bind magnesium and calcium from the antacid in the gut, resulting in systemic alkalosis; rectal use of the resin may avoid this problem.[1,2]

—*Tetracyclines:* antacids containing di- or trivalent ions interfere with the absorption of orally administered tetracyclines; separate doses by 2 hr.[1,2]

Anticholinergic Agents—*Amantadine:* amantadine potentiates the effects of high doses of anticholinergics, especially the CNS activity.[1,2]

Anticoagulants, Oral—*Alcohol:* increases in anticoagulant activity have been noted with large doses of alcohol, but the mechanism has not been clearly defined; 1 or 2 drinks not likely to have any effect.[1,2]

—*Allopurinol:* increase in anticoagulant activity in some patients; monitor prothrombin time.[1,2]

—*Antidiabetic Agents:* **dicumarol** may inhibit sulfonylurea metabolism; **warfarin** appears to be less likely to interact.[1,2]

—*Barbiturates:* decreased anticoagulant effect, mostly due to stimulation of hepatic metabolism of the anticoagulant; monitor prothrombin time carefully if the barbiturate is being used as an anticonvulsant; **benzodiazepines** are more suitable if only sedative or hypnotic effects are desired.[1,2]

—*Carbamazepine:* decreased anticoagulant effect, most likely due to stimulation of hepatic metabolism of anticoagulant; monitor prothrombin time.[1,2]

—*Chloral Hydrate:* chloral hydrate temporarily increases hypoprothrombinemic effect of **warfarin**, due to plasma protein binding displacement; chronic therapy with both drugs unlikely to cause problems.[1,2]

Continued

Drug Interactions

DRUG	INTERACTION AND COMMENTS

—*Chloramphenicol:* marked increase in dicumarol activity is well documented; while less evidence is available for **warfarin**, caution is nevertheless advised.[1,2]

—*Cholestyramine:* decreased absorption of **warfarin**; separate administration by 6 hr; some interaction occurs even if doses are separated, due to enterohepatic circulation of anticoagulant.[1,2]

—*Cimetidine:* enhanced hypoprothrombinemic response to **warfarin** due to inhibition of warfarin metabolism; may necessitate reduction in warfarin dose; **ranitidine** less likely to interact with warfarin.[1,2]

—*Clofibrate:* well documented increase in anticoagulant activity; monitor prothrombin time carefully.[1,2]

—*Colestipol:* response same as Anticoagulants, Oral—Cholestyramine.

—*Danazol:* increased anticoagulant activity; monitor prothrombin time and adjust anticoagulant dose if needed.[1,2]

—*Dextrothyroxine:* well documented increase in anticoagulant effect; monitor prothrombin time.[1,2]

—*Diazoxide:* may displace **coumarin anticoagulants** from plasma protein binding sites; anticoagulant dose may need to be altered if use of diazoxide is planned.[1,2]

—*Disulfiram:* increased anticoagulant acitivity due to inhibition of metabolism; monitor prothrombin time carefully.[1,2]

—*Erythromycin:* increased anticoagulant activity due to inhibition of **warfarin** metabolism; monitor prothrombin time.[10]

—*Ethacrynic Acid:* may displace **coumarin anticoagulants** from plasma protein binding sites; **furosemide** apparently does not have this effect and is the preferred loop diuretic.[1,2]

—*Gemfibrozil:* response same as Anticoagulants, Oral—Clofibrate.

—*Glucagon:* enhanced anticoagulant activity, mechanism unknown; monitor prothrombin time.[1,2]

—*Glutethimide:* decreased anticoagulant effect, probably due to stimulation of hepatic metabolism of anticoagulant; **benzodiazepine** sedative-hypnotics are preferred in patients taking oral anticoagulants.[1,2]

—*Griseofulvin:* decreased anticoagulant effect has been reported; monitor prothrombin time.[1,2]

—*Meclofenamate:* enhanced hypoprothrombinemic response to **warfarin**; avoid concurrent use or monitor prothrombin time carefully.[1,2]

—*Metronidazole:* enhanced hypoprothrombinemic response to **warfarin** due to inhibition of metabolism; monitor prothrombin time.[1,2]

—*Miconazole:* possible increase in anticoagulant activity; monitor prothrombin time and adjust anticoagulant dose as needed.[1,2]

—*Nonsteroidal Anti-Inflammatory Agents (NSAIA):* do not affect hypoprothrombinemic response to oral anticoagulants in most patients; use caution, due to possible GI bleeding and antiplatelet effect of NSAIA.[1,2]

—*Oxyphenbutazone:* response same as Anticoagulants, Oral—Phenylbutazone.

—*Phenylbutazone:* marked increase in anticoagulant effect due to inhibition of metabolism and displacement of anticoagulant from

Continued

Drug Interactions

DRUG	INTERACTION AND COMMENTS

plasma protein binding sites; avoid concurrent use or monitor pro-thrombin time carefully.[1,2]

—*Phenytoin:* **dicumarol** may inhibit phenytoin metabolism, while phenytoin may stimulate dicumarol metabolism; the use of **warfarin** may reduce the significance of this interaction, but, watch for evidence of reduced warfarin effect due to phenytoin-induced enzyme stimulation.[1,2]

—*Quinidine:* may enhance hypoprothrombinemic response to **warfarin** in an occasional patient; monitor prothrombin time.[1,2]

—*Rifampin:* decreases anticoagulant activity by stimulating **warfarin** metabolism; monitor prothrombin time.[1,2]

—*Salicylates:* large doses of salicylates increase anticoagulant effect; monitor prothrombin time; smaller doses may cause problems due to possible GI bleeding and antiplatelet effect.[1,2]

—*Sulfamethoxazole/Trimethoprim:* well documented increase in hypoprothrombinemic response to **warfarin**; does not occur in all patients; probably due to sulfamethoxazole; monitor prothrombin time.[1,2]

—*Sulfinpyrazone:* increased anticoagulant activity, primarily due to inhibition of **warfarin** metabolism; monitor prothrombin time.[1,2]

—*Sulfonamides:* some sulfonamides may enhance hypoprothrombinemic response to oral anticoagulants; monitor prothrombin time.[1,2]

—*Thyroid Hormones:* increased anticoagulant effect, probably due to increased catabolism of clotting factors; monitor prothrombin time carefully.[1,2]

—See also Amiodarone; Anabolic Steroids.

Antidepressants, Tricyclic—*Barbiturates:* may stimulate antidepressant metabolism; watch for evidence of reduced antidepressant effect.[1,2]

—*Bethanidine:* antidepressants inhibit the uptake (and therefore action) of bethanidine by the adrenergic neurons; use another agent (but not guanethidine or clonidine).[1,2]

—*Cimetidine:* inhibition of tricyclic antidepressant metabolism; monitor for excessive tricyclic effect (eg, severe anticholinergic effects) and adjust tricyclic dose as needed; **ranitidine** may be less likely than cimetidine to interact with tricyclics.[1,2]

—*Clonidine:* reduced antihypertensive response to clonidine; use another antihypertensive (but not bethanidine or guanethidine).[1,2]

—*Guanadrel:* response same as Antidepressants, Tricyclic—Guanethidine.

—*Guanethidine:* antidepressants inhibit the uptake (and therefore action) of guanethidine by the adrenergic neurons; effects noted after 2 days of antidepressant therapy; use another antihypertensive agent (but not bethanidine or clonidine).[1,2]

—*Monoamine Oxidase Inhibitors:* symptoms of CNS stimulation with convulsions and death have been reported; combination can be used if large doses are avoided and patient closely monitored.[1,2]

—*Propoxyphene:* possible inhibition of **doxepin** metabolism; monitor for excessive doxepin response and adjust doxepin dose as needed.[1,2]

Continued

Drug Interactions

DRUG	INTERACTION AND COMMENTS

—*Sympathomimetic Agents:* tricyclic antidepressant therapy may increase pressor response to parenteral **epinephrine, norepinephrine, phenylephrine** and possibly other sympathomimetics; effect of oral or nasal sympathomimetics not established, but caution is warranted; monitor blood pressure when sympathomimetics are given to patients receiving tricyclic antidepressants.[1,2]

Antidiabetic Agents—*Alcohol:* alcohol may produce hypoglycemia, especially in fasting patients; moderate increases in blood glucose may occur in nonfasting patients. Alcohol may enhance the risk of lactic acidosis in patients receiving **phenformin**; disulfiram-like reactions have occurred with **sulfonylureas** and patients should be warned of the possibility of their occurrence.[1,2]

—*Beta-Adrenergic Blocking Agents:* prolongation of hypoglycemic episodes; inhibition of tachycardia and tremors as signs of hypoglycemia (sweating is not inhibited); hypertension during hypoglycemia; selective β-blockers (eg, **metoprolol**) less likely to cause problems with antidiabetics than nonselective types (eg, **nadolol, propranolol**).[11a]

—*Chloramphenicol:* prolonged half-lives have been reported for **tolbutamide** and **chlorpropamide**, probably resulting from inhibition of metabolism; reduction of **sulfonylurea** dosage may be necessary if prolonged use of chloramphenicol is planned.[1,2]

—*Cimetidine:* may increase the hypoglycemic effect of **glipizide**. **Tolbutamide** effect may also be increased by cimetidine doses of 1 g/day or more. Reduction of glipizide or tolbutamide dosage may be required.[11b,11c]

—*Clofibrate:* enhanced hypoglycemic effect of **sulfonylureas** may occur; may require adjustment of sulfonylurea dose.[1,2]

—*Corticosteroids:* corticosteroids may increase circulating glucose levels and adjustment of antidiabetic drug dose may be required.[1,2]

—*Diuretics, Thiazide:* thiazides may aggravate diabetes; increased doses of antidiabetic agents may be needed to maintain control; patients stabilized on both drugs are not likely to have problems.[1,2]

—*Methyldopa:* reduced **tolbutamide** metabolism; possible enhanced tolbutamide hypoglycemia; effect on other **sulfonylureas** not known.[12]

—*Monoamine Oxidase Inhibitors:* MAO inhibitors may interfere with the normal adrenergic response to hypoglycemia, prolonging the action of antidiabetic agents; the MAO inhibitors should be avoided in diabetics.[1,2]

—*Phenylbutazone:* prolongs the action of the active metabolite of **acetohexamide** and may enhance the activity of **tolbutamide** by inhibiting its metabolism or displacing it from plasma protein binding sites; **chlorpropamide** may also be enhanced; use alternative to phenylbutazone.[1,2]

—*Rifampin:* stimulates metabolism of **tolbutamide** and possibly other **sulfonylureas**; may require increased sulfonylurea dose.[1,2]

—*Salicylates:* enhanced response to **sulfonylureas** is possible; several possible mechanisms; reduction of antidiabetic agent dosage may be necessary if prolonged high-dose use of salicylates is planned; **chlorpropamide** most likely to be affected.[1,2]

Continued

Drug Interactions

DRUG	INTERACTION AND COMMENTS

—*Sulfonamides, Antibacterial:* several sulfonamides have been reported to increase the activity of **sulfonylureas** by inhibition of metabolism or displacement from plasma protein binding sites; use another antibiotic whenever possible.[1,2]

—*Thyroid Hormones:* may increase antidiabetic drug requirements; mechanism unknown.[1,2]

—See also Anabolic Steroids; Anticoagulants, Oral.

Azathioprine—See Allopurinol.

Barbiturates—*Beta-Adrenergic Blocking Agents:* enhanced metabolism of those β-blockers that are primarily metabolized by the liver (eg, **propranolol, metoprolol, alprenolol**); monitor for reduced β-blocker effect and adjust β-blocker dose as needed.[1,2]

—*Contraceptives, Oral:* barbiturates may stimulate metabolism of contraceptive hormones; menstrual irregularities and unplanned pregnancies may occur; more likely with low-dose oral contraceptives.[1,13]

—*Corticosteroids:* **phenobarbital** has been shown to increase the metabolism of corticosteroids; patients may require increased doses of corticosteroids.[1,2]

—*Griseofulvin:* significant impairment of griseofulvin absorption; numerous small doses of griseofulvin may provide greater absorption than single large doses.[1,2]

—*Phenothiazines:* barbiturates may enhance phenothiazine metabolism; possible decrease in antipsychotic effect.[1,2]

—*Quinidine:* barbiturates may enhance quinidine metabolism; monitor for reduced quinidine effect.[1,2]

—*Tetracyclines:* barbiturates may enhance **doxycycline** metabolism; possible decrease in antimicrobial effect.[1,2]

—*Valproic Acid:* valproic acid inhibits phenobarbital metabolism; reduced phenobarbital dosage may be necessary.[14]

—See also Anticoagulants, Oral; Antidepressants, Tricyclic.

Benzodiazepines—*Cimetidine:* cimetidine may inhibit the elimination of **chlordiazepoxide** and **diazepam**, but not **lorazepam** or **oxazepam**; reduction in diazepam or chlordiazepoxide dose may be necessary.[15,16]

—*Disulfiram:* disulfiram may inhibit the elimination of **chlordiazepoxide** and **diazepam**, but not **lorazepam** or **oxazepam**; reduction in diazepam or chlordiazepoxide dose may be necessary.[17,18]

Beta-Adrenergic Blocking Agents—*Cimetidine:* enhanced **propranolol** effect; may require reduced propranolol dose.[19]

—*Clonidine:* combined use of clonidine and **propranolol** may result in *hyper*tensive reactions, especially if clonidine is rapidly withdrawn.[1,2]

—*Digitalis Glycosides:* β-blockers may worsen congestive heart failure or digitalis-induced bradycardia.[1,2]

—*Nonsteroidal Anti-Inflammatory Agents:* antihypertensive effect of β-blockers may be inhibited; mechanism may be prostaglandin inhibition. **Sulindac** may be less likely to interact.[1,2]

Continued

Drug Interactions

DRUG	INTERACTION AND COMMENTS

—*Prazosin:* enhanced hypotensive reaction to first dose of prazosin; anticipate hypotensive episode and take appropriate precautions (eg, take first prazosin dose at bedtime).[1,2]

—*Rifampin:* enhanced metabolism of those β-blockers that are primarily metabolized by the liver (eg, **propranolol, metoprolol, alprenolol**); monitor for reduced β-blocker effect and adjust β-blocker dose as needed.[1,2]

—*Sympathomimetic Agents:* **epinephrine** may produce hypertensive reactions in patients on **propranolol** (and probably other nonselective blockers such as **nadolol**); may also occur with other sympathomimetics such as **phenylephrine** and **phenylpropanolamine**; avoid such combinations if possible; if used, monitor carefully for hypertensive response.[1,2]

—*Theophylline:* mutual inhibition of effect may occur; β-blockers (especially nonselective) may worsen asthma.[1,2]

—See also Antidiabetic Agents; Barbiturates; Digitalis Glycosides.

Bethanidine: See Antidepressants, Tricyclic.

Bismuth Subsalicylate—*Tetracycline:* bismuth subsalicylate (Pepto-Bismol®) may reduce GI absorption of tetracycline; separate doses by 2 hr, with tetracycline given first.[2]

Calcium Channel Blocking Agents—*Digitalis Glycosides:* increased plasma **digoxin** levels with **verapamil** and to a lesser extent with **diltiazem** (minimal effects with **nifedipine**); monitor for excessive digoxin effect and adjust digoxin dose as needed.[1,2]

Calcium Salts: See Digitalis Glycosides.

Captopril—*Diuretics, Potassium-Sparing:* additive hyperkalemic effect; monitor potassium status carefully.[20]

—*Nonsteroidal Anti-Inflammatory Agents:* **indomethacin** reduces antihypertensive response to captopril (other NSAIA may also interact, but **sulindac** seems less likely to do so); if combination cannot be avoided, monitor blood pressure carefully.[21,22]

Carbamazepine—*Erythromycin:* inhibition of carbamazepine metabolism; monitor for excessive carbamazepine effect and adjust carbamazepine dose as needed.[1,2]

—*Haloperidol:* enhanced haloperidol metabolism; monitor for reduced haloperidol response and increase haloperidol dose if needed.[23]

—*Isoniazid:* inhibition of carbamazepine metabolism; monitor for excessive carbamazepine effect and adjust carbamazepine dose as needed.[1,2]

—*Propoxyphene:* inhibition of carbamazepine metabolism; monitor for excessive carbamazepine effect and adjust carbamazepine dose as needed.[1,2]

—*Theophylline:* enhanced theophylline metabolism; monitor theophylline plasma levels and increase theophylline dose if needed.[24]

—*Troleandomycin:* inhibition of carbamazepine metabolism; monitor

Continued

Drug Interactions

DRUG	INTERACTION AND COMMENTS

for excessive carbamazepine effect and adjust carbamazepine dose as needed.[1,2]

—See also Anticoagulants, Oral; Tetracyclines.

Cephalosporins—*Furosemide:* additive nephrotoxicity is a possibility; large doses of cephalosporins merit repeated renal function tests.[1,2]

—*Polymyxins:* additive nephrotoxicity is a possibility; unavoidable co-administration merits repeated renal function tests.[1,2]

—*Probenecid:* renal elimination of some cephalosporins is reduced.[1,2]

—See also Aminoglycosides.

Chloral Hydrate—*Furosemide:* IV furosemide may produce flushing, sweating and blood pressure variations in patients on chloral hydrate.[1,2]

—See also Alcohol; Anticoagulants, Oral.

Chloramphenicol—*Phenytoin:* concomitant therapy may result in enhanced phenytoin levels through inhibition of phenytoin metabolism; use another antibiotic whenever possible.[1,2]

—See also Anticoagulants, Oral; Antidiabetic Agents.

Chlorthalidone: See Digitalis Glycosides.

Cholestyramine—*Diuretics, Thiazide:* reduced thiazide absorption; administer thiazide at least 2 hr before the cholestyramine and monitor for reduced thiazide response.[1,2]

—*Methotrexate:* reduced methotrexate absorption; separate doses as much as possible and monitor for reduced methotrexate effect.[25]

—See also Anticoagulants, Oral; Digitalis Glycosides; Thyroid Hormones.

Cimetidine—*Lidocaine:* inhibition of lidocaine elimination; monitor for excessive lidocaine effect and adjust lidocaine dose as needed; **ranitidine** less likely to interact with lidocaine.[1,2]

—*Phenytoin:* inhibition of phenytoin metabolism; monitor for increased phenytoin effect and decrease phenytoin dose as needed; **ranitidine** less likely to interact with phenytoin.[26]

—*Procainamide:* inhibition of renal excretion of both procainamide and N-acetylprocainamide; monitor for excessive procainamide effect and adjust procainamide dose as needed; **ranitidine** may also increase procainamide levels, although probably not to the same extent as cimetidine.[1,2]

—*Quinidine:* inhibition of quinidine metabolism; monitor for excessive quinidine response and adjust quinidine dose as needed; **ranitidine** less likely to interact with quinidine.[1,2]

—*Theophylline:* cimetidine may reduce the elimination of theophylline; watch for evidence of theophylline toxicity and monitor theophylline plasma levels; reduced theophylline dosage may be required;[27] **ranitidine** is less likely to interact with theophylline.

—See also Anticoagulants, Oral; Antidepressants, Tricyclic; Antidiabetic Agents; Benzodiazepines.

Continued

Drug Interactions

DRUG	INTERACTION AND COMMENTS

Cisplatin—*Methotrexate:* reduced methotrexate elimination; monitor for increased methotrexate response.[4]

—See also Aminoglycosides.

Clofibrate—*Furosemide:* clofibrate-induced myopathy (eg, muscle pain, stiffness) may be more likely in presence of furosemide; hypoalbuminemia is also a predisposing factor.[1,2]

—See also Anticoagulants, Oral; Antidiabetic Agents.

Clonidine—*Levodopa:* antiparkinson effect of levodopa may be inhibited; avoid combined use or monitor closely for impaired levodopa effect.[1]

—See also Antidepressants, Tricyclic; Beta-Adrenergic Blocking Agents.

Colestipol: Response same as Cholestyramine.

Contraceptives, Oral—*Griseofulvin:* possible inhibition of oral contraceptive efficacy; if combination cannot be avoided, monitor for menstrual irregularities and consider adding another form of contraception during griseofulvin use.[28]

—*Penicillins:* data are inconclusive; **ampicillin** may interfere with enterohepatic circulation of contraceptive hormones; menstrual irregularities and unplanned pregnancies may occur; more likely with low-dose oral contraceptives; use alternative contraception instead of, or in addition to oral contraceptives while on ampicillin.[1,13]

—*Phenytoin:* oral contraceptive metabolism may be increased; menstrual irregularities and unplanned pregnancies may occur; more likely with low-dose oral contraceptives.[13]

—*Rifampin:* rifampin may interfere with the action of oral contraceptives, increasing the risk of unplanned pregnancy; other methods of birth control should be used.[1,13]

—*Tetracyclines:* possibly same effect as penicillins (above), but documentation is poor.

—See also Barbiturates.

Corticosteroids—*Amphotericin B:* enhancement of amphotericin B-induced potassium depletion; monitor serum potassium levels regularly and supplement with potassium salts, if necessary.[1,2]

—*Diuretics, Thiazide:* enhancement of potassium depletion; monitor serum potassium levels regularly and supplement with potassium chloride, if necessary.[1,2]

—*Ethacrynic Acid:* enhancement of potassium depletion; monitor serum potassium levels regularly and supplement with potassium chloride, if necessary.[1,2]

—*Furosemide:* enhancement of potassium depletion; monitor serum potassium levels regularly and supplement with potassium chloride, if necessary.[1,2]

—*Phenytoin:* increase in **dexamethasone** metabolism; other corticosteroids may be similarly affected.[1,2]

—*Rifampin:* increase in corticosteroid metabolism; may require increased corticosteroid dose.[1,2]

Continued

Drug Interactions

DRUG	INTERACTION AND COMMENTS

—*Salicylates:* decreased salicylate levels, possibly due to corticosteroid effects on salicylate elimination; salicylate intoxication possible if patient is on large doses of salicylate and corticosteroid dosage is reduced.[1,2]

—See also Antidiabetic Agents; Barbiturates.

Cyclophosphamide: See Allopurinol.

Cyclosporine—*Erythromycin:* inhibition of cyclosporine metabolism; monitor for increased cyclosporine levels and reduce cyclosporine dose if needed.[29,30]

—*Ketoconazole:* possible inhibition of cyclosporine metabolism; monitor for increased cyclosporine levels and reduce cyclosporine dose if needed.[1,2]

—*Phenytoin:* enhanced cyclosporine metabolism; monitor for reduced cyclosporine response and increase cyclosporine dose if needed.[31]

—*Rifampin:* enhanced cyclosporine metabolism; monitor for reduced cyclosporine response and increase cyclosporine dose if needed.[32]

—*Sulfonamides:* reduced plasma cyclosporine levels and possible enhanced nephrotoxicity; monitor cyclosporine levels and renal function.[33,34]

—See also Amphotericin B.

Dapsone—*Probenecid:* probenecid may reduce the renal elimination of dapsone; reduction of dapsone dosage may be required.[1,2]

Dextrothyroxine: See Anticoagulants, Oral.

Diazoxide: See Anticoagulants, Oral.

Digitalis Glycosides—*Amphotericin B:* amphotericin B-induced potassium loss may contribute to digitalis toxicity; monitor serum potassium levels regularly and supplement with potassium salts, if necessary.[1,2]

—*Calcium Salts:* both have similar myocardial actions; avoid parenteral calcium salts.[1,2]

—*Cholestyramine:* may bind **digitoxin** (and possibly **digoxin**) in the gut; separate doses and monitor for reduced digitalis effect.[1,2]

—*Chlorthalidone:* See Digitalis Glycosides—Diuretics, Thiazide.

—*Colestipol:* response same as Digitalis Glycosides—Cholestyramine.

—*Diuretics, Thiazide:* diuretic-induced potassium loss may contribute to digitalis intoxication; monitor serum potassium levels and supplement with potassium chloride or give a potassium-sparing diuretic, as needed.[1,2]

—*Ethacrynic Acid:* See Digitalis Glycosides—Diuretics, Thiazide.

—*Furosemide:* See Digitalis Glycosides—Diuretics, Thiazide.

—*Kaolin-Pectin:* reduced GI absorption of **digoxin**; give digoxin 2 or more hr before kaolin-pectin.[1,2]

—*Penicillamine:* reduced plasma **digoxin** levels may occur; assess need for increase in digoxin dose.[35]

Continued

Drug Interactions

DRUG	INTERACTION AND COMMENTS

—*Quinidine:* reduced renal clearance and tissue binding of **digoxin** resulting in average twofold increase in plasma digoxin; **digitoxin** may also be affected, probably by different mechanisms; monitor clinically for increased digitalis effect, plasma digoxin levels useful; may necessitate reduction in digitalis dose.[1,36]

—*Rifampin:* enhanced hepatic metabolism of **digitoxin**; monitor for reduced digitoxin effect; **digoxin** probably less likely to interact with rifampin.[1,2]

—*Spironolactone:* reduced elimination of **digitoxin** and **digoxin** reported, but spironolactone metabolites may also produce false increases in plasma levels of digitalis glycosides by some methods; watch especially for clinical evidence of excessive digitalis effect.[1,37]

—*Sulfasalazine:* reduced GI absorption of **digoxin**; spacing doses may not avoid interaction; monitor for reduced digoxin effect.[1,2]

—See also Aminoglycosides; Amiodarone; Antacids, Oral; Calcium Channel Blocking Agents.

Disulfiram—*Isoniazid:* mental changes may result from effects of both drugs on metabolism of adrenergic neurotransmitters; avoid the use of disulfiram in patients who must take isoniazid.[1,2]

—*Metronidazole:* confusion and psychotic episodes have been reported; avoid combination or monitor for psychiatric reactions.[1,2]

—*Phenytoin:* disulfiram inhibits the inactivation of phenytoin by the liver; phenytoin dosage adjustments may be necessary.[1,2]

—See also Alcohol; Anticoagulants, Oral; Benzodiazepines.

Diuretics, Potassium-Sparing: See Captopril; Nonsteroidal Anti-Inflammatory Agents; Potassium Salts.

Diuretics, Thiazide—*Lithium Carbonate:* chronic diuretic use may result in decreased lithium elimination; monitor plasma lithium levels until the patient is stabilized in the therapeutic range.[1,2]

—*Nonsteroidal Anti-Inflammatory Agents (NSAIA):* NSAIA may slightly inhibit the natriuretic and antihypertensive effects of thiazides; dosage changes may be needed in some patients.[38,39]

—See also Antidiabetic Agents; Cholestyramine; Colestipol; Corticosteroids; Digitalis Glycosides.

Dopamine—*Phenytoin:* IV phenytoin has produced hypotension in severely ill patients receiving IV dopamine; monitor blood pressure carefully if combination used.[40]

Erythromycin—*Theophylline:* erythromycin may reduce theophylline elimination in some patients; risk of theophylline toxicity is greatest in patients on relatively large doses of theophylline.[41]

—See also Anticoagulants, Oral; Carbamazepine; Cyclosporine.

Estrogens: See Contraceptives, Oral.

Ethacrynic Acid: See Aminoglycosides; Anticoagulants, Oral; Corticosteroids; Digitalis Glycosides.

Continued

Drug Interactions

DRUG	INTERACTION AND COMMENTS

Famotidine: Response similar to Ranitidine; see Cimetidine.

Furosemide—*Nonsteroidal Anti-Inflammatory Agents (NSAIA):* the hypotensive and natriuretic effects of furosemide may be inhibited by NSAIA; possible need for increased furosemide dosage.[38]
  —See also Cephalosporins; Chloral Hydrate; Clofibrate; Corticosteroids; Digitalis Glycosides.

Gemfibrozil: See Anticoagulants, Oral.

Glucagon: See Anticoagulants, Oral.

Glutethimide: See Anticoagulants, Oral.

Griseofulvin: See Anticoagulants, Oral; Barbiturates; Contraceptives, Oral.

Guanadrel: See Alcohol; Antidepressants, Tricyclic; Phenothiazines; Sympathomimetic Agents.

Guanethidine: See Alcohol; Antidepressants, Tricyclic; Phenothiazines; Sympathomimetic Agents.

Haloperidol—*Lithium:* possible CNS toxicity (eg, lethargy, confusion, extrapyramidal symptoms, fever) in occasional patients on this combination; avoid combination in acute mania if possible; if combination is used, dose carefully and monitor for neurotoxicity.[1,2]
  —*Methyldopa:* combined use may result in dementia (eg, confusion, disorientation); avoid combination or monitor for adverse psychiatric effects.[1,2]
  —See also Carbamazepine.

Heparin: See Salicylates.

Hydralazine—*Nonsteroidal Anti-Inflammatory Agents:* reduced antihypertensive response to hydralazine; monitor blood pressure.[42]

Iron Preparations—*Tetracyclines:* decreased tetracycline absorption, probably due to chelation in the gut; separate doses by at least 2 hr.[1,2]
  —*Vitamin E:* large doses of vitamin E impair the utilization of iron in patients with iron deficiency anemia; avoid vitamin E use in such patients.[1,2]
  —See also Antacids, Oral.

Isoniazid—*Phenytoin:* isoniazid inhibits the hepatic metabolism of phenytoin, increasing the risk of toxicity, particularly in slow acetylators; reduction of phenytoin dose may be required.[1,2]
  —*Rifampin:* metabolism of isoniazid to hepatotoxic metabolites may be enhanced by rifampin; monitor carefully for hepatotoxicity.[1,2]
  —See also Antacids, Oral; Carbamazepine; Disulfiram.

Kaolin-Pectin—*Lincomycin:* marked decrease in absorption of lin-
Continued

Drug Interactions

DRUG	INTERACTION AND COMMENTS

comycin from the GI tract; avoid concurrent use (note that diarrhea may be a sign of impending pseudomembranous colitis).[1,2]

—See also Digitalis Glycosides.

Ketoconazole: See Cyclosporine.

Levodopa—*Papaverine:* antiparkinson effect of levodopa may be inhibited; avoid papaverine in such patients.[1,2]

—*Phenytoin:* antiparkinson effect of levodopa may be inhibited; if phenytoin must be used in a patient on levodopa, monitor for reduced levodopa response; theoretically, increasing levodopa dose might restore antiparkinson response.[1,2]

—*Pyridoxine:* pyridoxine increases levodopa metabolism, significantly decreasing its effectiveness; this interaction is not encountered if a peripheral decarboxylase inhibitor is used in conjunction with levodopa.[1,2]

—See also Clonidine; Monoamine Oxidase Inhibitors; Phenothiazines.

Lidocaine: See Cimetidine.

Lincomycin: See Kaolin-Pectin.

Lithium—*Methyldopa:* patients on lithium may develop signs of lithium intoxication in presence of methyldopa; plasma lithium not elevated; if interaction occurs, select another antihypertensive.[43]

—*Nonsteroidal Anti-Inflammatory Agents (NSAIA):* reduced renal clearance of lithium; monitor for excessive lithium effect and adjust lithium dose as needed; **sulindac** (and possibly **ibuprofen**) may be less likely to increase lithium than other NSAIA.[44-46]

—*Phenytoin:* signs of lithium toxicity may occur with combined use in absence of increased plasma lithium; monitor for clinical evidence of lithium toxicity if combined use cannot be avoided.[47]

—*Sodium Chloride:* excess sodium increases lithium excretion, while sodium deficiency may promote lithium retention and increase the risk of toxicity; patients taking lithium should not be on low salt diets.[1]

—*Theophylline:* enhanced renal lithium clearance; monitor lithium levels and increase lithium dose as needed.[48,49]

—See also Diuretics, Thiazide; Haloperidol.

Meclofenamate: See Anticoagulants, Oral.

Mercaptopurine: See Allopurinol.

Methenamine Compounds—*Acetazolamide:* the alkaline urine resulting from acetazolamide therapy inhibits the conversion of methenamine to its active form, formaldehyde; select an alternative for one of the drugs.[1,2]

—*Sodium Bicarbonate:* the alkaline urine resulting from bicarbonate therapy inhibits the conversion of methenamine to its active form, formaldehyde; select an alternative for one of the drugs.[1,2]

Continued

Drug Interactions

DRUG	INTERACTION AND COMMENTS

Methotrexate—*Nonsteroidal Anti-Inflammatory Agents (NSAIA):* NSAIA such as **ketoprofen, phenylbutazone, indomethacin** (and probably others) may reduce renal methotrexate excretion; avoid combination until risks are better described.[50,51]

—*Para-Aminobenzoic Acid (PABA):* PABA may displace methotrexate from plasma protein binding sites; do not give PABA-containing products during methotrexate therapy.[1,2]

—*Phenylbutazone:* possible increase in methotrexate plasma levels; monitor for methotrexate toxicity.[1,2]

—*Probenecid:* reduced renal excretion of methotrexate; may necessitate decreases in methotrexate dose.[1,2]

—See also Alcohol; Cholestyramine; Cisplatin; Colestipol; Salicylates.

Methoxyflurane: See Aminoglycosides; Tetracyclines.

Methyldopa: See Antidiabetic Agents; Haloperidol; Lithium; Sympathomimetic Agents.

Metronidazole: See Alcohol; Anticoagulants, Oral; Disulfiram.

Mexiletine—*Phenytoin:* enhanced mexiletine metabolism; monitor for reduced mexiletine response and increase mexiletine dose if needed.[52]

—*Rifampin:* enhanced mexiletine metabolism; monitor for reduced mexiletine response and increase mexiletine dose if needed.[53]

Miconazole: See Anticoagulants, Oral.

Monoamine Oxidase (MAO) Inhibitors—*Levodopa:* co-administration may lead to increased levels of dopamine and norepinephrine, and hypertensive reaction may occur; **carbidopa** seems to protect against this interaction.[1,2]

—*Narcotic Analgesics:* use with **meperidine** has produced a variety of reactions, including hypertension, excitement, rigidity and occasionally, hypotension and coma; other narcotics are apparently safer.[1,2]

—*Sympathomimetic Agents:* indirect-acting agents such as **amphetamines, ephedrine, metaraminol, phenylpropanolamine, pseudoephedrine** and possibly **methylphenidate** may produce a hypertensive crisis in patients on MAO inhibitors; of the direct-acting agents, **phenylephrine** may also produce hypertension in patients on MAO inhibitors, while the response to **epinephrine** and **norepinephrine** is minimally affected.[1,2]

—See also Antidepressants, Tricyclic; Antidiabetic Agents.

Narcotic Analgesics—*Rifampin:* may stimulate metabolism of **methadone**; withdrawal symptoms possible in patients on methadone maintenance.[1]

—See also Monoamine Oxidase Inhibitors.

Nitrates: See Alcohol.

Nonsteroidal Anti-Inflammatory Agents (NSAIA)—*Diuretics, Po-*

Continued

Drug Interactions

DRUG	INTERACTION AND COMMENTS

tassium-Sparing: **indomethacin** (and probably other NSAIA) may reduce renal function when combined with **triamterene**; preliminary evidence indicates that **spironolactone** does not produce the same effect.[54]

—See also Anticoagulants, Oral; Beta-Adrenergic Blocking Agents; Captopril; Diuretics, Thiazide; Furosemide; Hydralazine; Lithium; Methotrexate; Sympathomimetic Agents.

Norepinephrine—*Methyldopa:* possible increase in pressor response to norepinephrine; mechanism not established.[1]

Oxyphenbutazone: See Anabolic Steroids; Anticoagulants, Oral.

Papaverine: See Levodopa.

Para-Aminobenzoic Acid: See Methotrexate; Sulfonamides, Antibacterial.

Penicillamine: See Digitalis Glycosides.

Penicillins—*Probenecid:* renal elimination of penicillins is reduced; this may be used to therapeutic advantage when high levels of penicillin are desired.[2]

—*Tetracyclines:* bacteriostatic agents, such as tetracyclines, inhibit bacterial growth, while penicillins require actively growing bacteria to exert their effect; co-administration could nullify the action of the penicillins (may also occur with other bacteriostatic agents); however, clinical problems are probably infrequent in patients receiving adequate doses of both drugs.[1,2]

—See also Aminoglycosides; Contraceptives, Oral.

Phenothiazines—*Guanadrel:* response possibly same as Phenothiazines—Guanethidine.

—*Guanethidine:* phenothiazines may inhibit the uptake of guanethidine (and perhaps **guanadrel**) by the adrenergic neurons, thereby reducing its hypotensive effects; at the same time, phenothiazines possess hypotensive effects of their own, so use of both drugs requires close monitoring of blood pressure.[1,2]

—*Levodopa:* levodopa does not block phenothiazine-induced extrapyramidal symptoms, while phenothiazines may inhibit the antiparkinson activity of levodopa.[1,2]

—See also Barbiturates.

Phenylbutazone—*Phenytoin:* phenylbutazone appears to inhibit phenytoin metabolism; this may necessitate reduction in phenytoin dosage.[1,2]

—See also Anticoagulants, Oral; Antidiabetic Agents; Methotrexate.

Phenylephrine: See Sympathomimetic Agents.

Phenylpropanolamine: See Sympathomimetic Agents.

Phenytoin—*Quinidine:* enhanced quinidine metabolism; monitor for reduced quinidine effect and increase quinidine dose if needed.[1,2]

Continued

Drug Interactions

DRUG	INTERACTION AND COMMENTS

—*Rifampin:* enhanced phenytoin metabolism; monitor for reduced phenytoin levels and increase phenytoin dose if needed.[55,56]

—*Theophylline:* enhanced theophylline metabolism; monitor theophylline plasma levels and increase theophylline dose if needed.[24]

—*Valproic Acid:* valproic acid displaces phenytoin from plasma protein binding sites; total plasma phenytoin levels are reduced; free phenytoin increases only temporarily, so a change in phenytoin dose is usually not necessary.[57,58]

—See also Alcohol; Anticoagulants, Oral; Chloramphenicol; Cimetidine; Contraceptives, Oral; Corticosteroids; Cyclosporine; Disulfiram; Dopamine; Isoniazid; Levodopa; Lithium; Mexiletine; Phenylbutazone; Sulfonamides, Antibacterial; Tetracyclines.

Polymyxins: See Cephalosporins.

Potassium Salts—*Diuretics, Potassium-Sparing:* serious hyperkalemia may result if potassium salts and a potassium-sparing compound such as **amiloride, spironolactone** or **triamterene** are given to the same patient; monitor serum potassium levels very carefully.[1,2]

Prazosin: See Beta-Adrenergic Blocking Agents.

Probenecid: See Aminosalicylic Acid; Cephalosporins; Dapsone; Indomethacin; Methotrexate; Penicillins; Salicylates.

Procainamide: See Cimetidine.

Propoxyphene: See Antidepressants, Tricyclic; Carbamazepine.

Pyridoxine: See Levodopa.

Quinidine—*Rifampin:* rifampin stimulates quinidine metabolism; quinidine dose may need to be increased if combination cannot be avoided.[59]

—*Sodium Bicarbonate:* alkalinization of the urine may decrease quinidine elimination, thereby increasing the risk of quinidine toxicity.[1]

—See also Acetazolamide; Amiodarone; Antacids, Oral; Anticoagulants, Oral; Barbiturates; Cimetidine; Digitalis Glycosides; Phenytoin.

Ranitidine: See Cimetidine.

Rifampin—*Theophylline:* enhanced theophylline metabolism; monitor theophylline plasma levels and increase theophylline dose if needed.[60]

—See also Anticoagulants, Oral; Antidiabetic Agents; Beta-Adrenergic Blocking Agents; Contraceptives, Oral; Corticosteroids; Cyclosporine; Digitalis Glycosides; Isoniazid; Mexiletine; Narcotic Analgesics; Phenytoin; Quinidine.

Salicylates—*Acetazolamide:* acetazolamide may enhance renal salicylate excretion and increase salicylate penetration into the brain; the latter effect may produce CNS salicylate toxicity if patient is on large doses of salicylate.[1,61]

—*Alcohol:* enhanced risk of GI blood loss.[1,2]

—*Heparin:* aspirin effects on platelet adhesiveness might leave the heparin-treated patient more prone to hemorrhage.[1,2]   Continued

Drug Interactions

DRUG	INTERACTION AND COMMENTS

—*Methotrexate:* salicylates displace methotrexate from plasma protein binding sites and also inhibit its renal elimination, thus greatly increasing the risk of methotrexate toxicity; do not give salicylates to patients taking methotrexate; warn patient about the use of OTC products which contain salicylates.[1,2]

—*Probenecid:* salicylates inhibit the uricosuric effects of probenecid, particularly with large doses of salicylate; occasional small doses present no problem.[1,2]

—*Sulfinpyrazone:* salicylates inhibit the uricosuric effects of sulfinpyrazone; occasional small doses present no problem.[1,2]

—See also Antacids, Oral; Anticoagulants, Oral; Antidiabetic Agents; Corticosteroids.

Skeletal Muscle Relaxants (Surgical): See Aminoglycosides.

Sodium Bicarbonate: See Methenamine Compounds; Quinidine; Sympathomimetic Agents; Tetracyclines.

Sodium Chloride: See Lithium.

Sodium Polystyrene Sulfonate: See Antacids, Oral.

Spironolactone: See Ammonium Chloride; Digitalis Glycosides; Potassium Salts.

Sulfamethoxazole/Trimethoprim: See Anticoagulants, Oral.

Sulfinpyrazone: See Anticoagulants, Oral; Salicylates.

Sulfonamides, Antibacterial—*Para-Aminobenzoic Acid (PABA):* PABA antagonizes the antibacterial effects of the sulfonamides which work by competing with PABA in bacteria.[1]

—*Phenytoin:* sulfonamides have been variously reported to inhibit the metabolism of phenytoin and to displace it from plasma protein binding sites; monitor plasma phenytoin levels if more than a few days of sulfonamide therapy are planned.[1,2]

—See also Anticoagulants, Oral; Antidiabetic Agents; Cyclosporine; Digitalis Glycosides.

Sympathomimetic Agents—*Acetazolamide:* alkalinization of the urine decreases elimination of **amphetamines, pseudoephedrine** and possibly other sympathomimetics.[1]

—*Guanadrel:* response possibly same as Sympathomimetic Agents—Guanethidine.

—*Guanethidine:* sympathomimetics with indirect-activity, such as **amphetamines** and **ephedrine**, may inhibit antihypertensive effect of guanethidine (and perhaps **guanadrel**); direct-acting sympathomimetics, such as **norepinephrine** and **phenylephrine** (and perhaps **guanadrel**), may produce an exaggerated response in patients on guanethidine; avoid sympathomimetics, if possible, in patients on guanethidine.[1,2]

—*Nonsteroidal Anti-Inflammatory Agents (NSAIA):* **indomethacin** may predispose to **phenylpropanolamine**-induced hypertension;

Continued

Drug Interactions

DRUG	INTERACTION AND COMMENTS

might also occur with other combinations of NSAIA and sympathomimetics; but clinical evidence is sparse.[62]

—*Methyldopa:* possible increase in pressor response to **norepinephrine**; mechanism not established.[1]

—*Sodium Bicarbonate:* alkalinization of the urine decreases elimination of **amphetamines, pseudoephedrine** and possibly other sympathomimetics.[1]

—See also Antidepressants, Tricyclic; Beta-Adrenergic Blocking Agents; Monoamine Oxidase Inhibitors.

Tetracyclines—*Carbamazepine:* carbamazepine may stimulate **doxycycline** metabolism; possible decrease in antimicrobial effect.[1,2]

—*Methoxyflurane:* additive nephrotoxicity has been reported.[1,2]

—*Phenytoin:* phenytoin may stimulate **doxycycline** metabolism, possibly decreasing antimicrobial effect.[1,2]

—*Zinc Salts:* large doses of zinc salts (eg, 200 mg) may reduce tetracycline absorption; space doses by 2 hr or more and give tetracycline first.[1,2]

—See also Antacids, Oral; Barbiturates; Bismuth Subsalicylate; Contraceptives, Oral; Iron Preparations; Penicillins.

Theophylline—*Troleandomycin:* elevated plasma theophylline levels may occur; mechanism is probably inhibition of theophylline metabolism; monitor theophylline plasma levels; may need to reduce theophylline dose.[1,2]

—*Vaccination, Influenza:* early reports indicated that theophylline elimination may be reduced following influenza vaccination, but this may not occur with purified subviron influenza vaccines; monitor theophylline plasma levels if patient receives whole viron influenza vaccine.[63,64]

—See also Beta-Adrenergic Blocking Agents; Carbamazepine; Cimetidine; Erythromycin; Lithium; Phenytoin; Rifampin.

Thyroid Hormones—*Cholestyramine:* cholestyramine binds both T_3 and T_4 in the gut, preventing their absorption; separate doses by at least 4 hr.[1,2]

—*Colestipol:* response same as Thyroid Hormones—Cholestyramine.

—See also Anticoagulants, Oral; Antidiabetic Agents.

Tolbutamide: See Cimetidine.

Triamterene: See Potassium Salts.

Troleandomycin: See Carbamazepine; Theophylline.

Vaccination, Influenza: See Theophylline.

Valproic Acid: See Barbiturates; Phenytoin.

Vitamin E: See Iron Preparations.

Zinc Salts: See Tetracyclines.

References

1. Hansten PD. Drug interactions. 5th ed. Philadelphia: Lea & Febiger, 1985.

2. Mangini RJ, ed. Drug interaction facts. St. Louis: JB Lippincott, 1986.

3. Hansten PD, Horn JR. Acetaminophen and alcohol—a potentially toxic combination. Drug Interactions Newsl 1986;6:31-4.

4. Hansten PD, Horn JR. Cisplatin drug interactions. Drug Interactions Newsl 1985;5:49-50.

5. Saal AK, Werner JA, Greene HL et al. Effect of amiodarone on serum quinidine and procainamide levels. Am J Cardiol 1984;53:1264-7.

6. Hansten PD, Horn JR. Amphotericin B interaction. Drug Interactions Newsl 1985;5:U-7.

7. Hakim R, Tolls G, Goltzman D et al. Severe hypercalcemia associated with hydrochlorothiazide and calcium carbonate therapy. Can Med Assoc J 1979;121:591-4.

8. O'Neil-Cutting MA, Crosby WH. The effect of antacids on the absorption of simultaneously ingested iron. JAMA 1986;255:1468-70.

9. Hansten PD, Hayton WL. Effect of antacid and ascorbic acid on serum salicylate concentration. J Clin Pharmacol 1980;20:326-31.

10. Hansten PD, Horn JR. Erythromycin and warfarin. Drug Interactions Newsl 1985;5:37-40.

11a. Hansten PD. Beta-blocking agents and antidiabetic drugs. Drug Intell Clin Pharm 1980;14:46-50.

11b. Feely J, Peden N. Enhanced sulfonylurea-induced hypoglycaemia with cimetidine. Br J Clin Pharmacol 1983;15:607P.

11c. Cate EW, Rogers JF, Powell JR. Inhibition of tolbutamide elimination by cimetidine but not ranitidine. J Clin Pharmacol 1986;26:372-7.

12. Gachalyi B, Tornyossy M, Vas A et al. Effect of alphamethyldopa on the half-lives of antipyrine, tolbutamide and D-glucaric acid excretion in man. Int J Clin Pharmacol Ther Toxicol 1980;18:133-5.

13. Hansten PD. Drug interactions that inhibit oral contraceptive efficacy. Drug Interactions Newsl 1981;1:9-11.

14. Patel IH, Levy RH, Cutler RE. Phenobarbital-valproic acid interaction. Clin Pharmacol Ther 1980;27:515-21.

15. Klotz U, Reimann I. Delayed clearance of diazepam due to cimetidine. N Engl J Med 1980;302:1012-4.

16. Patwardhan RV, Yarborough GW, Desmond PV et al. Cimetidine spares the glucuronidation of lorazepam and oxazepam. Gastroenterology 1980;79:912-6.

17. MacLeod SM, Sellers EM, Giles HG et al. Interaction of disulfiram with benzodiazepines. Clin Pharmacol Ther 1978;24:583-9.

18. Sellers EM, Giles HG, Greenblatt DJ et al. Differential effects on benzodiazepine disposition by disulfiram and ethanol. Arzneim Forsch 1980;882-6.

19. Feely J, Wilkinson GR, Wood AJJ. Reduction of liver blood flow and propranolol metabolism by cimetidine. N Engl J Med 1981;304:692-5.

20. Hansten PD, Horn JR. Captopril (Capoten) interactions. Drug Interactions Newsl 1985;5:U-10-1.

21. Fujita T, Yamashita N, Yamashita K. Effect of indomethacin on antihypertensive action of captopril in hypertensive patients. Clin Exp Hyperten 1981;3:939-52.

22. Silberbauer K, Stanek B, Templ H. Acute hypotensive effect of captopril in man modified by prostaglandin synthesis inhibition. Br J Clin Pharmacol 1982;14(Suppl):87S-93S.

23. Hansten PD, Horn JR. Carbamazepine (Tegretol) interactions. Drug Interactions Newsl 1986;6:U-13.

24. Hansten PD, Horn JR. Enzyme inducers and theophylline. Drug Interactions Newsl 1985;5:41-3.

25. Erttmann R, Landbeck G. Effect of oral cholestyramine on the elimination of high-dose methotrexate. J Cancer Res Clin Oncol 1985;110:48-50.

26. Hansten PD, Horn JR. Phenytoin interaction. Drug Interactions Newsl 1985;5:U-1.

27. Jackson JE, Powell JR, Wandell M et al. Cimetidine-theophylline interaction. Pharmacologist 1980;22:231. Abstract.

28. van Dijke CPH, Weber JCP. Interaction between oral contraceptives and griseofulvin. Br Med J 1984;288:1125-6.

29. Freeman DJ, Martell R, Carruthers SG et al. The effect of erythromycin on the pharmacokinetics of cyclosporine. Clin Pharmacol Ther 1986;39:193. Abstract.

30. Kohan DE. Possible interaction between cyclosporine and erythromycin. N Engl J Med 1986;314:448.

31. Hansten PD, Horn JR. Phenytoin interactions. Drug Interactions Newsl 1985;5:U-3.

32. Hansten PD, Horn JR. Rifampin interactions. Drug Interactions Newsl 1985;5:U-8.

33. Ringden O, Myrenfors P, Klintmalm G et al. Nephrotoxicity by co-trimoxazole and cyclosporine in transplanted patients. Lancet 1984;1:1016-7.

34. Jones DK, Hakim M, Wallwork J et al. Serious interaction between cyclosporin A and sulphadimidine. Br Med J 1986;292:728-9.

35. Moezzi B, Fatourechi V, Khozain R et al. The effect of penicillamine on serum digoxin levels. Jpn Heart J 1978;19:366-70.

36. Hansten PD. Quinidine and digoxin. Drug Interactions Newsl 1981;1:13-5.

37. Carruthers SG, Dujovne CA. Cholestyramine and spironolactone and their combination in digitoxin elimination. Clin Pharmacol Ther 1980;27:184-7.

38. Hansten PD, Horn JR. Diuretics and nonsteroidal anti-inflammatory drugs. Drug Interactions Newsl 1986;6:27-9.

39. Watkins J, Abbott EC, Hensby CN et al. Attenuation of hypotensive effect of propranolol and thiazide diuretics by indomethacin. Br Med J 1980;281:702-5.

40. Bivins BA, Rapp RP, Griffen WO et al. Dopamine-phenytoin interaction. Arch Surg 1978;113:245-9.

41. Hansten PD. Erythromycin and theophylline. Drug Interactions Newsl 1981;1:5-6.

42. Cinquegrani MP, Liang C-s. Indomethacin attenuates the hypotensive action of hydralazine. Clin Pharmacol Ther 1986;39:564-70.

43. Hansten PD. Lithium and methyldopa. Drug Interactions Newsl 1981;1:11.

44. Ragheb MA, Powell AL. Failure of sulindac to increase serum lithium levels. J Clin Psychiatry 1986;47:33-4.

45. Frolich JC, Leftwich R, Ragheb M et al. Indomethacin increases plasma lithium. Br Med J 1979;1:1115-6.

46. Furnell MM, Davies J. The effect of sulindac on lithium therapy. Drug Intell Clin Pharm 1985;19:374-6.

47. MacCallum WAG. Interaction of lithium and phenytoin. Br Med J 1980;1:610.

48. Cook BL, Smith RE, Perry PJ et al. Theophylline-lithium interaction. J Clin Psychiatry 1985;46:278-9.

49. Sierles FS, Ossowski MG. Concurrent use of theophylline and lithium in a patient with chronic obstructive lung disease and bipolar disorder. Am J Psychiatry 1982;139:117-8.

50. Thyss A, Kubar J, Milano G et al. Clinical and pharmacokinetic evidence of a life-threatening interaction between methotrexate and ketoprofen. Lancet 1986;1:256-8.

51. Ellison NM, Servi RJ. Acute renal failure and death following sequential intermediate-dose methotrexate and 5-FU. A possible adverse effect due to concomitant indomethacin administration. Cancer Treat Rep 1985;69:342-3.

52. Hansten PD, Horn JR. Mexiletine (Mexitil) interactions. Drug Interactions Newsl 1985;5:U-9.

53. Pentikainen PJ, Koivula IH, Hiltunen HA. Effect of rifampicin treatment on the kinetics of mexiletine. Eur J Clin Pharmacol 1982;23:261-6.

54. Hansten PD, Horn JR. Indomethacin and triamterene. Drug Interactions Newsl 1985;5:43.

55. Kay L, Kampmann JP, Svendsen TL et al. Influence of rifampicin and isoniazid on the kinetics of phenytoin. Br J Clin Pharmacol 1985;20:323-6.

56. Wagner JC, Slama TG. Rifampin-phenytoin drug interaction. Drug Intell Clin Pharm 1984;18:497.

57. Bruni J, Wilder BJ, Willmore LJ et al. Valproic acid and plasma levels of phenytoin. Neurology 1979;29:904-5.

58. Monks A, Richens A. Effect of single doses of sodium valproate on serum phenytoin levels and protein binding in epileptic patients. Clin Pharmacol Ther 1980;27:89-95.

59. Twum-Barima Y, Carruthers SG. Evaluation of rifampin-quinidine interaction. Clin Pharmacol Ther 1980;27:290. Abstract.

60. Hansten PD, Horn JR. Rifampin interactions. Drug Interactions Newsl 1985;5:U-1.

61. Anderson CJ, Kaufman PL, Sturm RJ. Toxicity of combined therapy with carbonic anhydrase inhibitors and aspirin. Am J Ophthalmol 1978;86:516-9.

62. Lee KY, Beilin LJ, Vandongen R. Severe hypertension after ingestion of an appetite suppressant (phenylpropanolamine) with indomethacin. Lancet 1979;1:1110-1.

63. Renton KW, Gray JD, Hall RI. Decreased elimination of theophylline after influenza vaccination. Can Med Assoc J 1980;123:288-90.

64. Hansten PD, Horn JR. Theophylline interactions. Drug Interactions Newsl 1986;6:U-4.

Drug-Laboratory Test Interferences

THE FOLLOWING TABLE LISTS common clinical laboratory tests and drugs which may interfere with those tests. Drugs can affect laboratory test results by causing pharmacologic (or toxic) interference and/or through test interference. Either effect may lead to an inaccurate or missed diagnosis or cause unnecessary changes in treatment. It is therefore essential that practitioners recognize possible drug-laboratory test interferences and make a judgement about the clinical significance of the interference. It is possible that a drug may be causing an interference with a test when:

- results from the same test vary greatly within a short period of time;
- results of different tests which measure the same or related functions vary greatly; or
- test results do not correspond to the clinical picture.

It should be noted that a drug may interfere with one method of laboratory test analysis, but not another. The reader is encouraged to refer to the reference sources listed at the end of this chapter, as well as other comprehensive sources, for further information. The following abbreviations are used in the table:

(B)—Blood   (P)—Pharmacologic/Toxic Effect
(CSF)—Cerebrospinal Fluid   (S)—Serum
(I)—Test Interference   (U)—Urine

The table begins on page 145.

Drug-Laboratory Test Interferences

TEST	DRUGS WHICH MAY ELEVATE RESULTS	CAUSE OF INTERFERENCE	DRUGS WHICH MAY DECREASE RESULTS	CAUSE OF INTERFERENCE
ALKALINE PHOSPHATASE (S)				
	Albumin	I	Clofibrate	P
	Anticonvulsants	P		
	Fluorides	–		
	Hepatotoxic Drugs [See Chapter 5, Drug-Induced Hepatotoxicity]	P		
AMINOTRANSFERASE [ALT (SGPT)/AST (SGOT)] (S)				
	Cholinergic Agents	P		
	Erythromycin	–		
	Hepatotoxic Drugs [See Chapter 5, Drug-Induced Hepatotoxicity]	P		
	IM Injections	P		
	Methyldopa	–		
	Opium Alkaloids	P		
AMMONIA (B)				
	Acetazolamide	P	Kanamycin, Oral	P
	Alcohol	P	Lactulose	P
	Ammonium Chloride	P	Neomycin, Oral	P
	Asparaginase	P	Potassium Salts	P
	Barbiturates	P		
	Diuretics (Loop, Thiazide)	P		
	Hyperalimentation	P		

Continued

Drug-Laboratory Test Interferences

TEST	DRUGS WHICH MAY ELEVATE RESULTS	CAUSE OF INTERFERENCE	DRUGS WHICH MAY DECREASE RESULTS	CAUSE OF INTERFERENCE
AMYLASE (S)				
	Asparaginase	P		
	Chloride Salts	I		
	Cholinergic Agents	P		
	Contraceptives, Oral	P		
	Contrast Media, Iodine-Containing	P		
	Drugs Inducing Acute Pancreatitis	P		
	Alcohol			
	Azathioprine			
	Corticosteroids			
	Diuretics (Loop, Thiazide)			
	Fluorides	I		
	Methyldopa	P		
	Narcotics	P		
BILIRUBIN (S)				
	Ascorbic Acid	I		
	Dextran	I		
	Epinephrine	I		
	Hepatotoxic Drugs	P	Barbiturates	P
	[See Chapter 5, Drug-Induced Hepatotoxicity]		Pindolol	I
	Hemolytic Agents	P		
	[See Chapter 5, Drug-Induced Blood Dyscrasias]			
	Methyldopa	I		
	Rifampin	I		

Continued

Drug-Laboratory Test Interferences

TEST	DRUGS WHICH MAY ELEVATE RESULTS	CAUSE OF INTERFERENCE	DRUGS WHICH MAY DECREASE RESULTS	CAUSE OF INTERFERENCE
CALCIUM (S)				
	Calcium Salts	P	Acetazolamide	P
	Diuretics, Thiazide	P	Anticonvulsants	P
	Hydralazine	–	Asparaginase	–
	Lithium	P	Aspirin	P
	Thyroid Hormones	P	Calcitonin	P
	Vitamin D	P	Cisplatin	P
			Contraceptives, Oral	P
			Corticosteroids	P
			Diphosphonates	P
			Diuretics, Loop	P
			Heparin	–
			Laxatives	P
			Magnesium Salts	P
			Plicamycin	P
			Sulfisoxazole	–
CATECHOLAMINES (U)				
	Acetaminophen	–	Clonidine	P
	Alcohol	P	Contrast Media, Iodine-Containing	–
	Caffeine	P	Disulfiram	P
	Chloral Hydrate	–	Guanethidine	P
	Epinephrine	–	Reserpine	P
	Erythromycin	–	Salicylates	P
	Insulin	P		
	Labetalol	–		
	Levodopa	–		

Continued

Drug-Laboratory Test Interferences

TEST	DRUGS WHICH MAY ELEVATE RESULTS	CAUSE OF INTERFERENCE	DRUGS WHICH MAY DECREASE RESULTS	CAUSE OF INTERFERENCE
	Methenamine	—		
	Methyldopa	—		
	Niacin	—		
	Nitroglycerin	P		
	Tetracyclines	—		
	Triamterene	—		
CHLORIDE (S) [No Major Test Interference]				
	Acetazolamide	P	Aldosterone	P
	Androgens	P	Corticosteroids	P
	Corticosteroids	P	Diuretics (Loop, Thiazide)	P
	Diuretics (Thiazide, Carbonic Anhydrase Inhibitors) (by Alkalosis)	P		
	Estrogens	P		
	Nonsteroidal Anti-Inflammatory Agents	P		
CHOLESTEROL (S)				
	Aspirin	—	Androgens	P
	Beta-Adrenergic Blocking Agents		Captopril	P
	Contraceptives, Oral	P	Chlorpropamide	P
	Corticosteroids	P	Cholestyramine	P
	Diuretics, Thiazide	I,P	Clofibrate	P
	Phenothiazines	P	Colestipol	P
	Sulfonamides	I,P	Haloperidol	P
	Vitamin D	P	Neomycin, Oral	P
		—	Nitrates	—
COLOR (U)				Continued

[See Chapter 4, Drug-Induced Discoloration of Feces and Urine]

Drug-Laboratory Test Interferences

TEST	DRUGS WHICH MAY ELEVATE RESULTS	CAUSE OF INTERFERENCE	DRUGS WHICH MAY DECREASE RESULTS	CAUSE OF INTERFERENCE
COOMBS' [Direct]				
	Positive			
	Ampicillin			
	Captopril			
	Cephalosporins			
	Chlorpropamide			
	Ethosuximide			
	Hydralazine			
	Indomethacin			
	Isoniazid			
	Levodopa			
	Mefenamic Acid			
	Methyldopa			
	Penicillin			
	Quinidine			
	Quinine			
	Rifampin			
CREATINE PHOSPHOKINASE [CPK] (S)				
	Alcohol, Chronic	P		
	Aminocaproic Acid	P		
	Amphotericin B	P		
	Chlorthalidone	P		
	Clofibrate	P		
	IM Injections	P		
CREATININE (S)				
	Cefoxitin (Jaffe Method)	I		

Continued

Drug-Laboratory Test Interferences

TEST	DRUGS WHICH MAY ELEVATE RESULTS	CAUSE OF INTERFERENCE	DRUGS WHICH MAY DECREASE RESULTS	CAUSE OF INTERFERENCE
	Cephalothin	—		
	Cimetidine	P		
	Flucytosine	—		
	Nephrotoxic Drugs [See Chapter 5, Drug-Induced Nephrotoxicity]	P		
GLUCOSE				
	Antidepressants, Tricyclic (B)	P	Acetaminophen (B)	I,P
	Ascorbic Acid (U)	I	Alcohol (B)	P
	Beta-Adrenergic Blocking Agents (B,U) (Nonselective)	P	Anabolic Steroids (B)	P
	Cephalosporins (B,U)	—	Ascorbic Acid (U)	—
	Corticosteroids (B,U)	P	Cephalosporins (U)	—
	Dextrothyroxine (B)	P	Clofibrate (B)	P
	Diazoxide (B)	P	Disopyramide (B)	P
	Diuretics (Loop, Thiazide) (B,U)	P	Gemfibrozil (B)	P
	Epinephrine (B)	P	Levodopa (U) (Clinistix®, Tes-Tape®)	—
	Estrogens (B,U)	P	Monoamine Oxidase Inhibitors (B)	
	Isoniazid (B)	P	Pentamidine (B)	P
	Levodopa (U) (Clinitest®)	—	Phenazopyridine (U) (Clinitest®)	P
	Lithium (B,U)	P	Salicylates (Acute and Chronic Toxicity) (B)	—
	Nalidixic Acid (U)	—		P
	Phenazopyridine (U) (Tes-Tape®)	—		
	Phenothiazines (B,U)	P		
	Phenytoin (B)	P		
	Salicylates (Acute Toxicity) (B)	P		
	Thiabendazole (B)	P		

Continued

Drug-Laboratory Test Interferences

TEST	DRUGS WHICH MAY ELEVATE RESULTS	CAUSE OF INTERFERENCE	DRUGS WHICH MAY DECREASE RESULTS	CAUSE OF INTERFERENCE
IRON (B)				
	Chloramphenicol	P	Cholestyramine	P
	Contraceptives, Oral	P	Colchicine	P
	Estrogens	P	Deferoxamine	I
	Ferrous Salts	I		
	Iron Dextran	I		
	Methyldopa	P		
KETONE (U)				
	Isoniazid	P		
	Levodopa	I		
	Mesna	I		
	Phenazopyridine	I		
	Salicylates	I		
MAGNESIUM				
	Lithium (S)	P	Alcohol (S)	P
	Magnesium Salts (S)	P	Aminoglycosides (S)	P
			Amphotericin B (S)	P
			Calcium Salts (S,U)	I
			Cisplatin (S)	P
			Digitalis (Toxic Levels) (S)	P
			Diuretics	
			(Loop, Thiazide) (S)	P
			(Potassium-Sparing) (U)	P

Continued

Drug-Laboratory Test Interferences

TEST	DRUGS WHICH MAY ELEVATE RESULTS	CAUSE OF INTERFERENCE	DRUGS WHICH MAY DECREASE RESULTS	CAUSE OF INTERFERENCE
PHOSPHORUS, INORGANIC (S) [No Major Test Interference]				
	Vitamin D (Excessive)	P		
			Antacids, Phosphate-Binding (eg, Aluminum, Calcium)	P
			Mannitol	P
POTASSIUM (S) [No Major Test Interference]				
	Angiotensin-Converting Enzyme Inhibitors (Captopril, Enalapril)	P		
			Ammonium Chloride	P
			Amphotericin B	P
			Corticosteroids	P
	Aminocaproic Acid	P		
	Antineoplastic Agents	P		
	Diuretics, Potassium-Sparing	P	Diuretics, Potassium-Wasting	P
	Isoniazid	P	Glucose	P
	Lithium	P	Insulin	P
	Mannitol	P	Laxatives	P
	Nephrotoxic Drugs [See Chapter 5, Drug-Induced Nephrotoxicity]	P	Penicillins, Extended-Spectrum	P
	Succinylcholine	P	Salicylates	P
PROTEIN				
	Aminoglycosides (U)	I	Contraceptives, Oral (S)	P
	Anabolic Steroids (S)	P	Cytarabine (CSF)	I
	Cephalosporins (U)	I,P	Estrogens (S)	P
	Contrast Media, Iodine-Containing (U)	I,P	Hepatotoxic Drugs (S) (Decreased Synthesis) [See Chapter 5, Drug-Induced Hepatotoxicity]	P
	Corticosteroids (S,U)	P		
	Magnesium Sulfate, Large Doses, IV (U)	I		

Continued

Drug-Laboratory Test Interferences

TEST	DRUGS WHICH MAY ELEVATE RESULTS	CAUSE OF INTERFERENCE	DRUGS WHICH MAY DECREASE RESULTS	CAUSE OF INTERFERENCE
	Methicillin (CSF)	—		
	Miconazole (U)	—		
	Nafcillin (U)	I,P		
	Nephrotoxic Drugs (U) [See Chapter 5, Drug-Induced Nephrotoxicity]	P		
	Penicillins (U)	P		
	Phenazopyridine (S,U)	—		
	Phenothiazines (CSF)	—		
	Sulfonamides (CSF,U)	I,P		
	Tolbutamide (U)	—		
	Tolmetin (U)	—		

PROTHROMBIN TIME (S) [Does Not Include Anticoagulants or Drugs Which Potentiate or Antagonize Them]

TEST	DRUGS WHICH MAY ELEVATE RESULTS	CAUSE OF INTERFERENCE	DRUGS WHICH MAY DECREASE RESULTS	CAUSE OF INTERFERENCE
	Asparaginase	P		
	Aspirin	P		
	Azathioprine	P		
	Cefamandole	P		
	Cefoperazone	P		
	Cephalothin	P		
	Chloramphenicol	P		
	Cholestyramine	P		
	Colestipol	P		
	Cyclophosphamide	P		
	Hepatotoxic Drugs [See Chapter 5, Drug-Induced Hepatotoxicity]	P		
			Anabolic Steroids	P
			Contraceptives, Oral	P
			Estrogens	P
			Vitamin K	P

Continued

Drug-Laboratory Test Interferences

TEST	DRUGS WHICH MAY ELEVATE RESULTS	CAUSE OF INTERFERENCE	DRUGS WHICH MAY DECREASE RESULTS	CAUSE OF INTERFERENCE
	Moxalactam	P		
	Propylthiouracil	P		
	Quinidine	P		
	Quinine	P		
	Sulfonamides	P		
	Tetracyclines	P		
SODIUM (S) [No Major Test Interference]				
	Anabolic Steroids	P	Ammonium Chloride	P
	Clonidine	P	Carbamazepine	P
	Contraceptives, Oral	P	Desmopressin Acetate	P
	Corticosteroids	P	Diuretics	P
	Diazoxide	P	Lypressin	P
	Estrogens	P	Sulfonylureas	P
	Guanabenz	P	Vasopressin	P
	Guanadrel	P		
	Guanethidine	P		
	Methyldopa	P		
	Nonsteroidal Anti-Inflammatory Agents	P		
THYROXINE (S)				
	Amiodarone	P	Amiodarone	P
	Contraceptives, Oral	P	Anabolic Steroids	P
	Estrogens	P	Corticosteroids	P
	Heparin	–	Ethionamide	–
	Methadone	P	Heparin	
	Propranolol	P	Lithium	P

Continued

Drug-Laboratory Test Interferences

TEST	DRUGS WHICH MAY ELEVATE RESULTS	CAUSE OF INTERFERENCE	DRUGS WHICH MAY DECREASE RESULTS	CAUSE OF INTERFERENCE
UREA NITROGEN (B)				
	Anabolic Steroids	P	Phenytoin	P
	Chloral Hydrate	—	Salicylates	P
	Nephrotoxic Drugs [See Chapter 5, Drug-Induced Nephrotoxicity]	P	Sulfonylureas	P
URIC ACID (S)				
	Acetazolamide	P	Acetohexamide	P
	Alcohol	P	Allopurinol	P
	Ascorbic Acid	—	Clofibrate	P
	Caffeine	—	Contrast Media, Iodine-Containing	P
	Cisplatin	P	Diflunisal	P
	Diazoxide	P	Glucose Infusions	P
	Diuretics	P	Guaifenesin	P
	Epinephrine	—	Phenothiazines	P
	Ethambutol	P	Phenylbutazone	P
	Levodopa	I,P	Salicylates, Large Doses	P
	Niacin	P	Uricosuric Agents	P
	Pyrazinamide	P		
	Salicylates, Small Doses	P		
	Theophylline	—		

References

1. Dukes MNG, ed. Meyler's side effects of drugs. 10th ed. New York: Elsevier, 1984.

2. Hansten PD. Drug interactions. 4th ed. Philadelphia: Lea and Febiger, 1979.

3. Herrington D, Drusano GL, Smalls U et al. False elevation in serum creatinine levels. JAMA 1984;252:2962. Letter.

4. McEvoy GK, ed. AHFS drug information 87. Bethesda, MD: American Society of Hospital Pharmacists, 1987.

5. Nademanee K, Singh BN, Callahan B et al. Amiodarone, thyroid hormone indexes, and altered thyroid function: long-term serial effects in patients with cardiac arrhythmias. Am J Cardiol 1986;58:981-6.

6. Ryan MP. Diuretics and potassium/magnesium depletion. Directions for treatment. Am J Med 1987;82:38-47.

7. Sher PP. Drug interferences with clinical laboratory tests. Drugs 1982;24:24-63.

8. Souney PF, Mariani G. Effect of various concentrations of flucytosine on the accuracy of serum creatinine determinations. Am J Hosp Pharm 1985;42:621-2.

9. Tryding N, Lindblad C-G, eds. Drug interference and effects in clinical chemistry. 3rd ed. Stockholm: Aρoteksbolaget AB, 1984.

10. Wallach J. Interpretation of diagnostic tests. A synopsis of laboratory medicine. 4th ed. Boston: Little, Brown and Company, 1986.

7 DRUGS AND BREAST FEEDING

WITH THE INCREASING POPULARITY OF BREAST FEEDING, the clinician often must weigh the benefits versus risks of drug therapy in the lactating woman. Unfortunately, reliable information on drug use during lactation is not readily available. Only recently have thorough, pharmacokinetically sound studies in humans been performed and many important drugs have yet to be adequately studied.[1] Recent publications have described the physicochemical and pharmacokinetic factors involved in drug transfer into milk as derived from animal and human data.[2-4] These factors are briefly discussed below.

Physicochemical Factors. Small water-soluble nonelectrolytes pass into milk by simple diffusion through pores in the lipoid membrane separating plasma from milk. Equilibration with plasma is usually rapid and milk levels approximate plasma levels. The lipid soluble, unionized forms of larger molecules pass through the lipoid membrane. Because the pH of milk is generally lower than plasma, milk can act as an "ion trap" for basic compounds. At equilibrium, these compounds attain high levels in milk relative to plasma. Conversely, acidic drugs tend to be inhibited from entering milk. However, there is considerable intra- and interpatient variation in the pH of milk which can dramatically affect the passage of weak acids and bases. Drugs with a pKa in the range of about 6–9 are most susceptible to this variability. The pKa of weak electrolytes is the primary determinant of their equilibrium concentration in milk, with the oil/water partition coefficient being of lesser importance. Protein binding can also be a factor in the passage of drugs into milk. Binding of drugs is much more avid to plasma proteins than to milk proteins and highly protein-bound drugs do not attain high concentrations in milk.

Pharmacokinetic Factors. With drugs having a short half-life, the rate of passage into milk is very important in determining the concentration of drug in milk. Their concentration in plasma falls to low levels before high concentrations are attained in milk. Drugs having a long half-life reach concentrations in milk more closely resembling equilibrium conditions than those with short half-lives.

Milk/Plasma Ratio. The milk/plasma (M/P) ratio is often used as a measure of a drug's passage into milk. However, there are a number of serious limitations of the M/P ratio as a measure of the advisability of breast feeding during drug use. First, there is no standard definition of the M/P ratio. Many authors report the ratio of milk and plasma drug concentrations at the time of the peak plasma level or at random times during a dosing interval, while some report the ratio of the areas under the milk and plasma concentration-time curves. Because concentration-time curves in milk and plasma are usually not parallel, M/P ratios can fluctuate widely during a dosing interval, particularly with drugs having a short half-life.[5]

To assess the potential effects of a drug on the breast-fed infant, an estimate of the total amount of drug ingested by the infant per day is needed. Also, knowledge of the times when drug levels in milk are the highest is useful in determining when breast feeding should be avoided. As currently used, the M/P ratio is essentially useless as a measure of the amount of drug the infant will receive.

Clinical Considerations

When it appears necessary to administer a drug to a breast feeding mother, several factors should be considered.

Maternal Factors. There are often several choices of drugs and routes of administration available to use in a given condition. Other times, drugs are prescribed which have only a slight or transient benefit to the patient. During breast feeding, consideration should be given to the use of alternative drugs, dosing regimens and routes of administration, as well as to the discontinuation of drug therapy, to minimize the risks of infant drug exposure.

Infant Factors. Acute, dose-related toxic effects in infants are rather uncommon; however, drug behavior is often not predictable because of immature excretory mechanisms. This is especially true in neonatal and preterm infants. Another type of dose-related phenomenon may occur in infants receiving low levels of antibiotics in milk. Although insignificant pharmacologically, levels may be sufficient to upset the GI flora and produce candidiasis, diarrhea or thrush. An additional possibility is sensitization of infants to drugs. Any allergenic drug can probably pass into milk in sufficient quantities to sensitize the infant or cause allergic reactions.

Idiosyncratic (nonallergic, non-dose-related) reactions can also be precipitated in susceptible infants. Hemolysis by oxidizing agents in milk has been reported in G-6-PD deficient infants. Neonates, and especially preterm infants, are also susceptible to hemolysis by oxidizing agents. Other apparently non-dose-related reactions such as blood dyscrasias and hepatotoxicity have rarely been reported, but should be considered before prescribing drugs capable of producing these reactions.

The long-term effects of most potent drugs and environmental chemicals on breast-fed infants are unknown. In addition to agents specifically listed in the table, several groups of drugs should be considered potentially hazardous when used continuously throughout lactation. These include anticonvulsants, antituberculars, corticosteroids, hypotensive agents, psychotherapeutic agents and sex hormones.

Use of the Table. In a previous review, data from the primary literature were compiled in a standardized format.[1] In this chapter, previous data and all new reports are summarized in narrative format. For specific numerical data, consult the references listed.

The table begins on page 160.

Drugs Excreted Into Breast Milk

DRUG	NATURE OF EFFECT
ANALGESICS AND ANTIPYRETICS	
Acetaminophen	Peak acetaminophen concentrations occur 1–2 hr after a dose; amounts ingested by infants are small and appear to be harmless.[6-8] One case of rash, apparently due to acetaminophen in milk, was reported in a breast-fed infant.[9]
Aspirin	See Salicylates.
Narcotics	Opiate agonists have been shown to decrease suckling-induced oxytocin release in animals.[10,11] Opioids inhibit the milk-ejection reflex by this mechanism in animals, but there have been no studies in humans to confirm this effect or define its magnitude. Narcotics in analgesic doses are excreted in small amounts which seem insignificant. Those studied have been **butorphanol** 1–2 mg IM and 8 mg PO,[12] **codeine** 60 mg PO,[1,9] **meperidine** 50–100 mg IM,[15,18] **morphine** 16 mg parenterally,[1] **oxycodone** 5–10 mg PO[13] and **propoxyphene** 65 mg PO.[14]

Heroin abuse can result in high enough milk levels to cause addiction or alleviate withdrawal symptoms in infants; however, breast feeding is not reliable enough to be used as a method of preventing withdrawal.[1,2]

Although **methadone** maintenance is not a contraindication to breast feeding,[17-19] it is best to avoid breast feeding 3–4 hr after the dose when peak milk levels occur.[1,19] One death has been reported in a malnourished 5-week-old infant whose mother was on methadone maintenance. Methadone was detected in the infant on autopsy, but it is unclear what part the drug played in the infant's death.[20] |
| **Nonsteroidal Anti-Inflammatory Agents** | Of the nonsteroidal anti-inflammatory agents that have been studied, **Ibuprofen** appears to be the safest to use during breast feeding; amounts in milk are virtually unmeasurable with doses up to |

Continued

Drugs Excreted Into Breast Milk

DRUG	NATURE OF EFFECT
	1.6 g/day.[21,22] **Diclofenac** was not detected in milk after 50 mg IM.[23] **Naproxen, tolmetin** and **suprofen** are probably safe beyond the neonatal period.[24-28] **Diflunisal, piroxicam** and other long-acting agents should be avoided as should **indomethacin, phenylbutazone, mefenamic acid** and the other more toxic agents.[29-32] **Dipyrone,** an analgesic found in many foreign products, caused cyanosis in one breast-fed infant.[33]
Phenacetin	Phenacetin enters milk in small quantities which seem harmless.[7]
Salicylates	**Salicylate** enters milk in low concentrations relative to plasma.[1,7,34-37] At high doses, salicylate has a long half-life in the mother and may accumulate in infants, particularly neonates. There is a report of metabolic acidosis caused by salicylate in a 16-day old breast-fed infant whose mother was taking aspirin 650 mg q 4 hr for arthritis.[38] However, it is unclear whether salicylate in milk was the sole cause. Infant salicylate plasma levels should be monitored during high-dose chronic use, particularly with neonates. Occasional **aspirin** in analgesic doses should pose no hazards to the infant except for the potential antiplatelet effect. Avoiding breast feeding for an hour after a dose should obviate this effect.
ANTICHOLINERGIC AGENTS	Excretion of anticholinergics into milk has not been studied. Theoretical hazards are anti-cholinergic effects such as drying of secretions, temperature elevations and CNS disturbances in the infant. Observe infants carefully if anticholinergics are used. Theoretically, anticholinergics can decrease milk flow by decreasing oxytocin secretion and release,[39] but this has not been documented clinically.
ANTICOAGULANTS	The two most commonly used anticoagulants, **heparin** and **warfarin,** are safe to use during breast feeding.[1,40,41] Heparin does not pass into milk; amounts of warfarin in milk are insignificant with

Continued

Drugs Excreted Into Breast Milk

DRUG	NATURE OF EFFECT
	maternal doses of 10 mg/day or less and cause no problems. Great caution should be used with other anticoagulants, particularly **indandiones.**[1]
ANTICONVULSANTS	Most anticonvulsants can achieve significant plasma levels in breast-fed infants, causing sleepiness or paradoxical hyperexcitability. The long-term effects of such exposure are not well understood, but limited studies have found no serious effects. Mild drowsiness or fussiness during maternal anticonvulsant use is not uncommon. Periodic plasma level monitoring in breast-fed infants may be indicated.
Carbamazepine	Carbamazepine and its major metabolite are excreted in milk and can be detected in nursing infants; infant plasma concentrations are subtherapeutic and no effects have been seen in infants. Carbamazepine can be used cautiously during lactation, but occasional infant plasma level measurements may be indicated.[1,42,43]
Ethosuximide	Breast-fed infants may attain ethosuximide plasma levels near the therapeutic range and some infants may show signs of drowsiness or fussiness.[44-46] Breast feeding should be undertaken with caution and the mother's plasma levels should be kept as low as possible in the therapeutic range. Occasional infant plasma level measurements may be indicated.
Phenobarbital	Phenobarbital has a pKa near the pH of plasma; therefore, slight variations in milk pH cause marked changes in the amount transferred to milk. Although phenobarbital is generally safe, some infants may receive enough to cause drowsiness; enzyme induction may also occur.[1,44] Withdrawal may occur if breast feeding is abruptly terminated.[237]
Phenytoin	Phenytoin is excreted in small amounts; however, occasionally infants may experience idiosyncratic reactions or enzyme induction may occur. One case of cyanosis and methemoglobinemia may have been caused by phenytoin in milk.[1,47]

Continued

Drugs Excreted Into Breast Milk

DRUG	NATURE OF EFFECT
Primidone	Primidone and its metabolites, **phenobarbital** and **PEMA**, have been detected in milk. The drug appears safe during breast feeding, but occasionally drowsiness may occur.[48]
Valproic Acid	Valproic acid passes poorly into milk, but is detectable. Caution should be used until more is known about this drug in infants, particularly with respect to hepatic damage.[48-52]
ANTIHISTAMINE DRUGS	Some antihistamines (eg, **clemastine**) may cause drowsiness in breast-fed infants.[53,54] Single bedtime doses after the last feeding of the day may be adequate for many women and minimize amounts the infant receives. Theoretically, antihistamines might decrease milk flow due to central inhibition of oxytocin release, although this is not well documented clinically.[35] Frequent use of high doses, sustained-release products and/or combinations with a sympathomimetic agent should be avoided, particularly before lactation is well established. See also Anticholinergic Agents and Sympathomimetic Agents.
ANTI-INFECTIVE AGENTS	
Aminoglycosides	Aminoglycosides are very polar and pass poorly and irregularly into milk; milk concentrations do not fluctuate as widely or as rapidly as plasma levels.[1,55-58] Pharmacologic or toxic effects in infants are unlikely, due to the small amounts in milk and poor oral absorption; however, infants should be observed for disruption of the GI flora, such as thrush or diarrhea.
Cephalosporins	Cephalosporins are not excreted in milk in sufficient quantities to treat infections in infants, but do appear in trace amounts which could lead to allergic sensitization or disruption of the GI flora. Breast feeding is not contraindicated with first- and second-generation agents.[59-67] The risk is greatest with the "third generation" cephalosporins which are much more active against gut organisms and caution should be used with these agents.[68-70] Infants should be observed for rashes, thrush or diarrhea with cephalosporins.

Continued

Drugs Excreted Into Breast Milk

DRUG	NATURE OF EFFECT
Penicillins	Penicillins are not excreted in milk in sufficient quantities to treat infections in infants, but do appear in trace amounts which could lead to allergic sensitization or disruption of the GI flora. Breast feeding is not contraindicated, but infants should be observed for rashes, thrush or diarrhea.[1,44,45]
Plasmodicides	Breast feeding should be undertaken cautiously during **chloroquine** or **hydroxychloroquine** treatment, because the importance of the small amounts in milk is unclear.[71-73] Some recommend withholding breast feeding during therapy and for up to 72 hr after the last dose. During weekly prophylaxis with lower doses, the amounts in milk are less than the infant prophylactic dose. The importance of the small amounts of **quinine** in milk is unclear.[74] **Pyrimethamine** may be excreted in sufficient quantities to treat or protect infants less than 6 months of age against malaria, but this is not a reliable method of drug administration.[1,2]
Sulfonamides	Sulfonamides are not absolutely contraindicated, but may increase the risk of kernicterus in neonates and do pass in sufficient quantities to have caused hemolytic anemia in G-6-PD deficient infants. They should be avoided during the first two months of life, in premature infants and in G-6-PD deficient infants. **Sulfamethoxazole**, with or without **trimethoprim**, may be safe to use in older infants.[75] **Sulfisoxazole** is excreted in small amounts and appears to be safe in healthy infants; use caution in stressed or premature infants.[76] **Sulfasalazine's** metabolites, **sulfapyridine** and **5-aminosalicylic acid** are found in milk, but in quantities that seem to pose no hazard in most infants.[77-80] Bloody diarrhea, which occurs rarely in persons taking sulfasalazine, has been reported in a breast-fed infant.[77]
Tetracyclines	Tetracyclines could theoretically cause mottling of teeth if absorbed by the infant. Calcium in milk apparently inhibits absorption, so toxicity is unlikely; nevertheless, other less potentially toxic alternatives are available for most infections.[1]

Continued

Drugs Excreted Into Breast Milk

DRUG	NATURE OF EFFECT
Urinary Germicides	**Methenamine** hippurate and mandelate pass into milk in very small quantities and seem safe to use.[1,81] **Nalidixic acid** has been associated with one case of hemolytic anemia in a breast-fed infant and should not be used if the infant is under 1 month of age.[1] **Nitrofurantoin** is excreted in pharmacologically insignificant amounts, but caution is advised in neonates, premature infants and those with G-6-PD deficiency.[1]
Miscellaneous Anti-Infective Agents	**Acyclovir.** Data in one woman indicate that acyclovir attains rather high levels in milk. Until better studied, acyclovir should probably be avoided during breast feeding.[235]
	Amantadine is contraindicated according to the manufacturer; it reportedly may cause vomiting, urinary retention and skin rashes in infants.[1]
	Chloramphenicol levels are not sufficient to induce "gray baby" syndrome, but may be enough to harm bone marrow. Additionally, a number of adverse reactions in infants, including refusal of the breast, falling asleep during feeding and vomiting after feeding have occurred. Breast feeding is contraindicated during chloramphenicol treatment.[1]
	Clindamycin is excreted in small amounts in milk.[1] It is not known what effects these levels may have on infants' GI flora (eg, induction of pseudomembranous colitis), so it is best avoided, if possible.
	Cycloserine is excreted in small amounts, but no adverse reactions have been reported in infants.[1]
	Erythromycin is excreted in small amounts and may disrupt the GI flora leading to thrush or candidiasis; however, the drug is generally safe, with few hazards to the infant.[1,2]
	Isoniazid is excreted and should be used with caution during lactation. Hepatic damage theoretically might occur.[82]

Continued

Drugs Excreted Into Breast Milk

DRUG	NATURE OF EFFECT
	Lincomycin is excreted, but no adverse effects have been reported.[1] See Clindamycin.
	Metronidazole is detectable in plasma in small amounts in some infants. The dose in milk is too small to cause immediate reactions and no adverse systemic or GI effects have been reported. Because of the theoretical risk of carcinogenicity, it seems prudent to avoid the drug, or if essential to treat trichomoniasis, to give it as a single 2 g dose and use an alternative feeding method for 24–48 hr.[83,84]
	Novobiocin carries the risk of causing hyperbilirubinemia and kernicterus in the infant. Although no infant toxicities have been reported, safer drugs should be used.[1]
	Trimethoprim is excreted and infants absorb about 0.75–1 mg daily; this amount is probably not harmful.[1] See also Sulfonamides.
ANTINEOPLASTIC AND IMMUNOSUPPRESSANT AGENTS	**Breast feeding is generally considered to be contraindicated in women receiving antineoplastic drugs.** Breast feeding during immunosuppression has been performed safely in a limited number of cases.[85,86]
Azathioprine	Three infants have been reported who were safely breast fed during maternal azathioprine use (75–100 mg/day).[85,86] Low levels of **mercaptopurine** were found in milk. Breast feeding should be undertaken with great caution.
Busulfan	Busulfan was taken by one woman in a dose of 4 mg daily for 5 weeks while breast feeding with no adverse effects on her infant's leukocytes or hemoglobin. This study is by no means conclusive, however.[87]
Cisplatin	In one patient, no platinum was detected in milk following an IV infusion.[88] Although any platinum

Continued

Drugs Excreted Into Breast Milk

DRUG	NATURE OF EFFECT
	in the milk would be taken orally by the infant and unlikely to be absorbed, caution should be used.
Cyclophosphamide	Cyclophosphamide is detectable in milk, and two cases of bone marrow depression have been reported in infants of women receiving the drug.[89,90]
Cyclosporine	Milk levels of cyclosporine are lower than plasma levels, but there are no data on the safety of cyclosporine use during breast feeding.[91,92]
Doxorubicin	Doxorubicin and its primary active metabolite, **doxorubicinol**, appear in rather large amounts in milk.[88]
Mercaptopurine	See Azathioprine.
Methotrexate	Methotrexate was measured in milk in one study. The authors concluded that breast feeding presents little hazard if bottle feeding is not possible; however, this study is not conclusive.[1]
CARDIOVASCULAR DRUGS	
Beta-Adrenergic Blocking Agents	The excretion of β-blockers in breast milk varies greatly among the various compounds, based primarily on their plasma protein binding. **Propranolol** has been the best studied and amounts in milk are insignificant. **Labetalol** and **metoprolol** also have relatively low concentrations in milk and appear safe to use beyond the neonatal period. The long-acting, renally excreted β-blockers with low lipid solubility (**acebutolol**, **nadolol** and **atenolol**) should generally be avoided, particularly in neonates, although atenolol has been used safely during breast feeding in a few older infants.[93-105] **Timolol** should also be avoided, even by the ophthalmic route.[93-105] Beta blockade does not lower prolactin levels in hyperprolactinemia.[103]

Continued

Drugs Excreted Into Breast Milk

DRUG	NATURE OF EFFECT
Calcium Channel Blocking Agents	Only **diltiazem** and **verapamil** have been studied; data are insufficient to judge the safety of their use during breast feeding.[106-108] One paper reported rather significant levels in one infant whose mother was taking verapamil. These agents should be used cautiously during breast feeding.
Cardiac Drugs	**Amiodarone** is excreted in amounts that could pose a hazard to the infant and breast feeding should be discontinued if amiodarone therapy is required.[109] **Digoxin** is excreted in milk in levels approaching maternal plasma. This constitutes an insignificant dose for the infant. Breast feeding is safe during digoxin therapy.[110-113] Limited data on **disopyramide** indicate that significant amounts may be excreted in milk; it should be avoided during lactation.[114,115] **Lidocaine** milk levels during continuous IV lidocaine are very low and should pose no hazard to the infant.[116] Levels of **mexiletine** in milk are small and cannot be detected in the plasma of breast-fed infants,[117,118] but adverse effects may occur.[238] **Procainamide** and its active metabolite, **NAPA**, are concentrated in milk with respect to plasma, but absolute amounts are small.[119] It should be used with caution until it has been better studied. **Quinidine** excretion appears to be insignificant, but some authors warn against breast feeding because of potential accumulation and thrombocytopenia. Data are not conclusive, however.[120]
Hypotensive Agents	**Captopril** is found in very small amounts and no adverse effects have occurred in infants.[121] **Clonidine** milk levels are higher than maternal plasma levels and breast-fed infants have plasma levels approaching those of the mother. Although no adverse effects have occurred in breast-fed infants, clonidine should be used with caution during breast feeding.[122] Limited data indicate that low dose, short-term use of **hydralazine**, as for a few days postpartum, is probably safe.[123] It should be used cautiously during long-term therapy and in high doses. **Methyldopa** appears to be excreted in insignificant amounts.[124,125] There is very limited information on **minoxidil** in milk, but amounts appear to be low.[126] It should be used with caution, particularly with larger doses. **Reserpine** may cause nasal stuffiness and increase tracheobronchial secretions. Because safer alternatives are available, reserpine should be avoided.[1]

Continued

Drugs Excreted Into Breast Milk

DRUG	NATURE OF EFFECT
DIURETICS	Low doses of short-acting thiazide-type diuretics should pose no problems during breast feeding.[1,127] Large doses of thiazides or usual doses of loop diuretics or long-acting thiazide-type diuretics (eg, **chlorthalidone, bendroflumethiazide**) can suppress lactation and should be avoided.[1,128,129] Long-acting agents may also accumulate in infants' plasma. **Acetazolamide** appears in milk, but its effects are not known.[130] Theoretically, thrombocytopenia or allergic reactions to sulfonamide diuretics can occur. The amounts of **spironolactone** and its metabolites in milk appear to be insignificant.[131]
GASTROINTESTINAL DRUGS	
Cathartics and Laxatives	Cathartics and laxatives that are nonabsorbable, such as bulk forming, osmotic and stool softening types cause no problems. Some **anthraquinone derivatives**, such as **cascara** and **danthron**, should probably be avoided and others, such as **aloe** and **senna**, may cause problems if high doses are used.[1] **Phenolphthalein** may cause problems in some infants.[1]
Cimetidine	Cimetidine should be used with caution,[1] because unexpectedly large amounts are found in milk and its effects in infants are unknown.[132] Because of its pKa, there may be large intersubject variations in its excretion. Cimetidine can also increase serum prolactin and induce galactorrhea.[133]
Metoclopramide	Metoclopramide has caused increased gas and GI discomfort in breast-fed infants and causes a 15–30% increase in infant plasma prolactin. Avoiding breast feeding for 3–4 hr after the dose should minimize infant exposure. In a dose of 10 mg tid, metoclopramide may increase milk production in mothers who are producing insufficient quantities of milk, although one controlled trial indicated no increase over placebo. Therapy should be limited to 2 weeks for this use. The drug may also cause galactorrhea.[133–140] A related agent, **sulpiride**, also increases prolactin levels and milk yields. It is not detectable in milk.[141,142]

Continued

Drugs Excreted Into Breast Milk

DRUG	NATURE OF EFFECT
Ranitidine	Ranitidine is excreted in rather large amounts in milk and should be used with caution during breast feeding.[143,144]

HORMONES AND SYNTHETIC SUBSTITUTES

Corticosteroids	There are only a few reports of infants being breast-fed during maternal corticosteroid use. Three infants were breast-fed during chronic maternal use of 6–8 mg/day of **methylprednisolone** with apparent safety. The amounts of various corticosteroids excreted in milk have not been well studied. **Prednisone** and **prednisolone** excretion appears to be minimal with doses of 20 mg/day or less. With these two drugs, avoiding feeding for 1–2 hr after the dose minimizes infant intake. With doses over 20 mg/day or a long duration of therapy, it would be prudent to avoid breast feeding during the first 4 hr after a dose. The use of prednisolone rather than prednisone transfers less total drug to milk.[145-147]
Desmopressin	Desmopressin is excreted in very small amounts in milk and is unlikely to be well absorbed orally by the infant.[148]
Oxytocin	Oxytocin, as a nasal spray, brings about milk ejection, thus facilitating lactation and increasing milk volume in mothers of premature infants and adoptive mothers. Use should be limited to a few days, however, because psychological dependence on the spray can develop in the mother, and water intoxication and seizures have occurred in one woman who overused it.[149,150]
Sex Hormones	*Suppression of Lactation* **Estrogens**, **estrogen/progestin** and **estrogen/androgen** combinations were used to suppress lactation; however, even in high doses, these agents are not always effective, because of the numerous factors affecting lactation. The most important factor is cessation of breast feeding, which alone Continued

Drugs Excreted Into Breast Milk

DRUG	NATURE OF EFFECT
	is quite effective. Because of concern with the possibility of thrombophlebitis and other adverse steroid effects, **bromocriptine** is usually used to suppress lactation.[1,151,152]

In the small doses used in **oral contraceptives**, sex steroids seem to have little effect on milk flow in the majority of women. With older, high-estrogen contraceptives, lactation could be suppressed sufficiently to cause discontinuation of breast feeding. When present-day, low-estrogen contraceptives are begun 3 weeks postpartum, when lactation is well established, this effect usually does not occur, but a long-term negative effect on lactation and infant growth may occur.[236] **Progestins** used singly in oral and depot forms for contraception affect milk flow adversely only at high doses (300 mg IM depot **medroxyprogesterone**), but not at lower doses (150 mg IM).[1,153,154]

Milk Composition

Some studies have shown a decrease in protein, fat and minerals in the milk of mothers using older, high-estrogen oral contraceptives. Newer, low-estrogen combination and progestin-only types decrease protein slightly, but levels remain within the normal range in well-nourished women. These changes in the milk of poorly nourished women (eg, in developing countries) may be of greater importance.[154] Large (600 mg) IM doses of depot **medroxyprogesterone** acetate (DMPA) used as a contraceptive significantly reduce the nutrient quality of milk, while the usual dose of 150 mg increases protein content.[1,153,155]

Excretion into Milk

Rarely, cases of contraceptives possibly causing breast enlargement in infants and proliferation of the vaginal epithelium in female infants have been attributed to combination oral contraceptives; however, a cause-and-effect relationship has not been firmly established.[1,156,157] Assays of estrogens and progestins in milk show that both are found in low levels.[158-163] Although amounts received by infants are small and are readily metabolized,[164] there is concern over the long-term effects of steroids, especially estrogens, in breast-fed infants. Follow-up of infants breast-fed during maternal use of DMPA, although not conclusive, has shown no adverse effects on growth and development. If hormonal contraception is essential, low-dose oral progestin or IM DMPA are the preferred methods.[155,165,166]

Continued

Drugs Excreted Into Breast Milk

DRUG	NATURE OF EFFECT
Thyroid and Antithyroid Agents	**Antithyroid.** In the past, it was felt that any antithyroid therapy was a contraindication to breast feeding. While use of ^{131}I remains a contraindication,[1] recent studies on the **thionamides** now in use indicate that **propylthiouracil** may be excreted in small enough amounts to be used during lactation.[167,169] This cannot necessarily be said for **methimazole**, however.[167,170] Careful monitoring of the infant is mandatory because of the limited knowledge of the safety of propylthiouracil.
	Thyroid. Milk levels of thyroid hormones have not been measured after exogenous administration. Although somewhat controversial, it appears that **thyroxine** (T_4) passes into milk poorly, while **liothyronine** (T_3) may pass in more physiologically significant amounts. The amounts of thyroid hormones in milk are apparently not sufficient to interfere with the diagnosis of hypothyroidism. Because of the conversion of T_4 to T_3 in the body, administration of T_4 to the mother may increase milk T_3 levels. Replacement doses of thyroid hormone to a breast-feeding mother would not be expected to result in excessive thyroid administration to the infant. However, observe the infant carefully if supraphysiologic doses are administered to the mother.[171–179]
PSYCHOTHERAPEUTIC AGENTS	
Antidepressants, Heterocyclic	Most heterocyclic antidepressants have not been well studied during lactation and there is no consensus on their use during lactation.[180–186] Respiratory depression has been reported in one breast-fed infant whose mother was taking **doxepin** 25 mg tid,[187] while maternal doses of **imipramine** (up to 150 mg/day) or **amitriptyline** (up to 150 mg/day) have not caused effects in infants. Single 50 mg doses of **trazodone** produce very low levels in milk, but effects on infants have not been studied.[188] Close monitoring and caution is warranted with all of these drugs during breast feeding.
Tranquilizers	**Butyrophenones. Haloperidol** has been studied in only 2 patients; small quantities have been found which did not affect the infants, but long-term effects are unknown.[189,190]

Continued

Drugs Excreted Into Breast Milk

DRUG	NATURE OF EFFECT
	Phenothiazines pass into milk somewhat unpredictably, but usually in insignificant amounts.[1,181,191,192] Drowsiness with the more sedating agents, such as **chlorpromazine**, has occurred.[192] Other effects, such as extrapyramidal symptoms, seem possible, but have not been reported. Follow-up ranging from 15 months to 6 yr indicates no long-term effects on infant development.[193-195]
Lithium	Lithium in milk can adversely affect the infant when lithium elimination in infants is impaired, as in dehydration or in neonates and premature infants (who may already have lithium in plasma acquired transplacentally).[196-199] The long-term effects of lithium in infants are not known, and some authors consider lithium therapy a contraindication to breast feeding.[181,199] Lithium should be used cautiously during lactation, and breast feeding discontinued if the infant appears restless or looks ill. A plasma lithium level in the infant can help rule out lithium toxicity.
SEDATIVES AND HYPNOTICS	Most sedative-hypnotics pass into breast milk in measurable and potentially significant amounts. Sedative-hypnotic intake should be minimized during lactation; and, agents with unique toxicities in the infant (eg, **bromides, diazepam**) should be avoided.
Barbiturates	Barbiturates can stimulate metabolism of endogenous compounds in the infant if small amounts pass into milk. "Short-acting" agents appear to be preferable to "long-acting" agents, because smaller amounts are excreted in milk. High single doses may have more potential for causing infant drowsiness than do multiple small doses.[1] See also Anticonvulsants.
Benzodiazepines	Benzodiazepines pass into milk in small amounts, but can accumulate in infants, especially neonates, because of their immature excretory mechanisms. Drugs with long-acting metabolites, such as **diazepam**, are particularly troublesome and have caused adverse effects in infants. It is not possible to avoid peak metabolite milk levels, because they occur up to 1-2 days after the dose. Benzodiazepines should be avoided during breast feeding, particularly in neonates.[1,200-203] After a single dose, milk should be discarded for 8 hr after the dose. Continued

Drugs Excreted Into Breast Milk

DRUG	NATURE OF EFFECT
Bromides	Bromides have caused drowsiness and rash and should be avoided during breast feeding.[1]
Chloral Hydrate	Chloral hydrate and its metabolite, **trichloroethanol** reached 50–100% of maternal blood levels in most of 50 women given 1.3 g rectally. Drug and metabolites were detectable for up to 24 hr; the maximum dose that an infant could have received approximates a sedative dose. In another study, drowsiness was noted in 1 infant the morning after a bedtime hypnotic dose of a chloral hydrate derivative in the mother.[1]
Ether	Ether milk levels are about equal to blood levels for 8–10 hr.[1]
Glutethimide	Glutethimide has been detected in minute amounts 8–12 hr after a dose.[1]
Halothane	Halothane milk levels equal or surpass levels in maternally inhaled air.[204]
Meprobamate	Meprobamate concentrations peak in milk at 4 hr, 2 hr after peak plasma levels.[1]
Phenobarbital	See Anticonvulsants.
MISCELLANEOUS AGENTS	
Baclofen	Baclofen appears in milk in small amounts and it should be used with caution.[205]
Dihydrotachysterol	Dihydrotachysterol is considered contraindicated during breast feeding by some authors, because of renal calcifications that occurred in animal studies.[1]
Ergot Alkaloids	**Bromocriptine** inhibits lactation by suppressing prolactin release;[1,34] and rebound galactorrhea has been reported following withdrawal of high-dose bromocriptine.[206] Related agents, **lisuride** and **metergoline**, also inhibit lactation.[207,208]

Continued

Drugs Excreted Into Breast Milk

DRUG	NATURE OF EFFECT
	While **ergonovine** has been reported to lower prolactin levels slightly, **methylergonovine** does not, nor is it found in milk in significant quantities.[1,209] It appears that short-term, low-dose regimens of these two agents postpartum pose no hazard to the infant nor do they affect milk flow.
	Older crude ergot preparations were found to produce toxic effects in infants, but they are no longer used.[1] The use and excretion of **ergotamine** during lactation has not been studied and its long-term use in migraine probably should be avoided during lactation until it has been studied.
Gold	Gold is excreted in milk and can be detected in the blood and urine of nursing infants. The exact amounts of gold that infants receive has not been well quantified, but sufficient amounts may be ingested to cause adverse effects.[210-213] Gold therapy appears to be a reason for withholding breast feeding.
Iodides	Iodides are probably contraindicated during breast feeding, because of possible thyroid suppression and rashes.[1] **Iopanoic acid** contains free iodide which can be detected in milk. Although no adverse effects have been reported in infants, breast feeding should probably be withheld for 24–36 hr after a dose.[1]
Magnesium	IV magnesium therapy increases milk magnesium levels only slightly and causes no effects in the infant. Oral absorption of magnesium is poor in the infant and maternal magnesium therapy is not a contraindication to breast feeding.[214]
Pentoxifylline	The amounts of pentoxifylline in milk appear to be small, but caution should be used until further experience is gained.[215]
Pyridostigmine	Pyridostigmine has been used safely during breast feeding in 2 patients.[216] It should be used cautiously, especially in infants with impaired renal function.

Continued

Drugs Excreted Into Breast Milk

DRUG	NATURE OF EFFECT
Sympathomimetic Agents	In one case report of a mother taking **amphetamine** 20 mg/day therapeutically, milk levels were found to be less than plasma levels and no adverse effects on the infant were noted.[217] However, there is likely to be substantial intersubject variation in excretion, and levels during high dose use and abuse of amphetamines have not been studied. It is likely that some infants would experience agitation and fussiness. One anecdotal case exists of infant irritability, crying and disturbed sleep during maternal intake of a long-acting preparation containing **pseudoephedrine** and **dexbrompheniramine.**[54] In general, sympathomimetics are safe, but infants should be carefully observed with maternal use of high doses and long-acting products. Theoretically, sympathomimetics can decrease milk flow by central inhibition of secretion and release of oxytocin and by peripheral vasoconstriction which limits the access of oxytocin to myoepithelial cells in the breast.[39] Although this effect is not well documented, the use of sympathomimetic nasal sprays is recommended over oral decongestants in order to minimize systemic effects. **Terbutaline** use for asthmatic symptoms caused no problems in breast-fed infants.[218]
Theophylline	Theophylline has been reported to cause irritability and fretful sleep in one infant.[1] Sustained-release products and continuous infusion should tend to maximize the dose received by infants, but amounts in infant plasma should remain below the therapeutic range in most cases.[1,219] There is no need to avoid theophylline products, but infant plasma levels may be measured if side effects occur.
Tolbutamide	Tolbutamide is excreted in very small amounts which should cause no harm.[1]
Vaccines	Much contradictory literature on **poliovirus** has been published about the possibility that antibodies in milk could prevent active immunization in infants. It has been recommended that breast feeding be withheld for 2–6 hr before and after immunization; however, if infants are immunized after 6 weeks of age, breast feeding has a negligible effect on antibody titers.[1] **Rubella** is transferred into milk and results in an immune response in about one-half of infants.[220,221] However,

Continued

Drugs Excreted Into Breast Milk

DRUG	NATURE OF EFFECT
	this appears to be of little consequence and breast feeding is allowable following maternal vaccination.

DRUGS FOR NONMEDICAL USE

Alcohol

Alcohol equilibrates rapidly between blood and milk; milk levels are about 90–95% of simultaneous blood levels. Low to moderate maternal intake appears to produce no effects in the infant; however, prolonged intake of large amounts, as in the alcoholic, may be detrimental. One case of drunkenness has been reported in an 8-day-old infant whose mother drank 750 ml of port wine in a 24-hr period.[1] A case report of pseudo-Cushing's syndrome has been reported in an infant whose mother drank "at least 50 12-ounce cans of beer weekly plus generous amounts of more concentrated alcoholic beverages."[222] Doses of alcohol higher than 1 g/kg may inhibit the milk ejection reflex and doses higher than 2 g/kg probably completely block suckling-induced oxytocin release.[1] Alcohol should be used in moderation during lactation. Recent studies indicate that an unknown substance in beer increases plasma prolactin. This effect also occurs with nonalcoholic beer.[223,224]

Caffeine

Caffeine is excreted in relatively small amounts; most infants are not affected at usual levels of maternal intake.[225-228] However, one infant reportedly developed jitteriness with very high maternal intake (4–5 cups of coffee and 2–3 480 ml bottles of cola daily).[229]

Cocaine

There has been one report in the literature of the measurement of cocaine in milk, and the effects of the drug on a breast-fed infant.[239] The chemical nature of cocaine is such that it would be expected to appear in milk in amounts that might affect the infant, particularly with high doses. Breast feeding is not recommended in the chronic cocaine abuser and occasional use is discouraged during breast feeding.

Continued

Drugs Excreted Into Breast Milk

DRUG	NATURE OF EFFECT
Marijuana	Marijuana has not been well studied, but THC can reach rather high levels in milk, particularly with heavy use.[230] Although adverse effects in infants have not been reported, breast feeding should probably be avoided in heavy users and during therapeutic **dronabinol** use. Breast feeding should probably be withheld for several hours after occasional marijuana use. Caution should also be used to avoid exposing the infant to marijuana smoke.
Phencyclidine	Phencyclidine is concentrated in milk and remains detectable for weeks after heavy use.[231,232] Breast feeding should be avoided after phencyclidine use, but a sufficient duration of abstinence is undefined.
Tobacco	Nicotine is excreted in breast milk in measurable amounts which are not sufficient to harm the infant.[233,234] However, other toxins from tobacco have not been studied and additional nicotine and toxins in tobacco smoke may be inhaled by the infant.

References

1. Anderson PO. Drugs and breast feeding: a review. Drug Intell Clin Pharm 1977;11:208-23. Revised and reprinted in Knoben JE, Anderson PO, Watanabe AS, eds. Handbook of clinical drug data. 4th ed. Hamilton, IL: Drug Intelligence Publications, 1978:89-118.

2. Anderson PO. Drugs and breast feeding. Semin Perinatol 1979;3:271-8.

3. Wilson JT, Brown RD, Cherek DR et al. Drug excretion in human milk: principles, pharmacokinetics and projected consequences. Clin Pharmacokinet 1980;5:1-65. Revised and reprinted as Wilson JT, ed. Drugs in breast milk. New York: ADIS Press, 1981.

4. Rasmussen F. Excretion of drugs by milk. In: Brodie BB, Gillette JR, eds. Concepts in biochemical pharmacology, part 1. New York: Springer-Verlag, 1971:390-402.

5. Wilson JT, Brown D, Hinson JL et al. Pharmacokinetic pitfalls in the estimation of the breast milk/plasma ratio for drugs. Ann Rev Pharmacol Toxicol 1985;25:667-89.

6. Berlin CM, Yaffe SJ, Ragni M. Disposition of acetaminophen in milk, saliva and plasma of lactating women. Pediatr Pharmacol 1980;1:135-41.

7. Findlay JWA, DeAngelis RL, Kearney MF et al. Analgesic drugs in breast milk and plasma. Clin Pharmacol Ther 1981;29:625-33.

8. Bitzen P-O, Gustafsson B, Jostell KG et al. Excretion of paracetamol in human breast milk. Eur J Clin Pharmacol 1981;20:123-5.

9. Matheson I, Lunde PKM, Notarianni L. Infant rash caused by paracetamol in breast milk? Pediatrics 1985:76:651-2. Letter.

10. Clarke G, Wright DM. A comparison of analgesia and suppression of oxytocin release by opiates. Br J Pharmacol 1984;83:799-806.

11. Wright DM. Evidence for a spinal site at which opioids may act to inhibit the milk-ejection reflex. J Endocrinol 1985;106:401-7.

12. Pittman KA, Smyth RD, Losada M et al. Human perinatal distribution of butorphanol. Am J Obstet Gynecol 1980;138:797-800.

13. Marx CM, Pucino F, Carlson JD et al. Oxycodone excretion in human milk in the puerperium. Drug Intell Clin Pharm 1986;20:474. Abstract.

14. Kunka RL, Venkataramanan R, Stern RM et al. Excretion of propoxyphene and norpropoxyphene in breast milk. Clin Pharmacol Ther 1984;35:675-80.

15. Peiker G, Muller B, Inh W et al. Ausscheidung von pethidin durch die muttermilch. Zentralb Gynaekol 1980;102:537-41. Abstract.

16. Freeborn SF, Calvert RT, Black P et al. Saliva and blood pethidine concentrations in the mother and the newborn baby. Br J Obstet Gynaecol 1980;87:966-9.

17. Kreek MJ, Schecter A, Gutjahr CL et al. Analyses of methadone and other drugs in maternal and neonatal body fluids: use in evaluation of symptoms in a neonate of mother maintained on methadone. Am J Drug Alcohol Abuse 1974;1:409-19.

18. Shaffer H. Methadone and pregnancy: perspectives and prescriptions. J Psychedelic Drugs 1979;11:191-202.

19. Anon. Methadone in breast milk. Med Lett Drugs Ther 1979;21:52.

20. Smialek JE, Monforte JR, Aronow R et al. Methadone deaths in children: a continuing problem. JAMA 1977;238:2516-7.

21. Weibert RT, Townsend RJ, Kaiser DG et al. Lack of ibuprofen secretion into human milk. Clin Pharm 1982;1:457-8.

22. Townsend RJ, Benedetti TJ, Erickson SH et al. Excretion of ibuprofen into breast milk. Am J Obstet Gynecol 1984;149:184-6.

23. Fowler PD. Voltarol: diclofenac sodium. Clin Rheum Dis 1979;5:427-64.

24. Jamali F, Stevens DRS. Naproxen excretion in breast milk and its uptake by the infant. Drug Intell Clin Pharm 1983;17:910-1. Letter.

25. Sagraves R, Waller ES, Goehrs HR. Tolmetin in breast milk. Drug Intell Clin Pharm 1985;19:55-6. Letter.

26. Chaikin P, Chasin M, Kennedy B et al. Suprofen concentrations in human breast milk. J Clin Pharmacol 1983;23:385-90.

27. Steelman SL, Breault GO, Tocco D et al. Pharmacokinetics of MK-647, a novel salicylate. Clin Pharmacol Ther 1975;17:245. Abstract.

28. Ostensen M. Piroxicam in human milk. Eur J Clin Pharmacol 1983;25:829-30.

29. Strobel E, Herrmann B. Zur frage des uberganges von oxyphenbutazon in den fetalen kreislauf und die muttermilch. Arzneim Forsch 1962;12:302-5.

30. Leuxner E, Pulver R. Verabreichung von irgapyrin bei schwangeren und wochnerinnen. Schweigeisch Med Mchschr 1956;98:84-7.

31. Gensichen E, Klingmuller V. Verlauf der konzentrationen von phenylbutazon und isopyrin in serum, nabelschnurserum und frauenmilch. N-S Arch Exp Path Pharmakol 1963;246:52.

32. Eeg-Olofsson O, Elwin C-E, Steen B. Convulsions in a breast-fed infant after maternal indomethacin. Lancet 1978;2:215.

33. Rizzoni G, Furlanut M. Cyanotic crises in a breast-fed infant from mother taking dipyrone. Human Toxicol 1984;3:505-7.

34. Erickson SH, Oppenheim GL. Aspirin in breast milk. J Fam Pract 1979;8:189-90.

35. Levy G. Salicylate pharmacokinetics in the human neonate. In: Morselli PL, Sarattini S, Sereni F, eds. Basic and therapeutic aspects of perinatal pharmacology. New York: Raven Press, 1975:319-30.

36. Levy G. Clinical pharmacokinetics of aspirin. J Pediatr 1978;62(Suppl):867-72.

37. Putter J. Quantitative analysis of the main metabolites of acetylsalicylic acid. Z Geburtsh Perinatol 1974;178:135-8.

38. Clark JH, Wilson WG. A 16-day-old breast-fed infant with metabolic acidosis caused by salicylate. Clin Pediatr 1981;20:53-4.

39. Tucker HA. Endocrinology of lactation. Semin Perinatol 1979;3:199-223.

40. Orme ML'E, Lewis PJ, de Swiet M et al. May mothers given warfarin breast-feed their infants? Br Med J 1977;1:1564-5.

41. McKenna R, Cole ER, Vasan U. Is warfarin sodium contraindicated in the lactating mother? J Pediatr 1983;103:325-7.

42. Pynnonen S, Kanto J, Sillanpaa M et al. Carbamazepine: placental transport, tissue concentrations in foetus and newborn and level in milk. Acta Pharmacol Toxicol 1977;41:244-53.

43. Niebyl JR, Blake DA, Freeman JM et al. Carbamazepine levels in pregnancy and lactation. Obstet Gynecol 1979;53:139-40.

44. Kaneko S, Sato T, Suzuki K. The levels of anticonvulsants in breast milk. Br J Clin Pharmacol 1979;7:624-6.

45. Kuhnz W, Koch S, Jakob S et al. Ethosuximide in epileptic women during pregnancy and lactation period. Br J Clin Pharmacol 1984;18:671-7.

46. Koup JR, Rose JQ, Cohen ME. Ethosuximide pharmacokinetics in a pregnant patient and her newborn. Epilepsia 1978;19:535-9.

47. Rane A, Garle M, Borga O et al. Plasma disappearance of transplacentally transferred diphenylhydantoin in the newborn studied by mass fragmentography. Clin Pharmacol Ther 1974;15:39-45.

48. Espir MLE, Benton P, Will E et al. Sodium valproate (Epilim)—some clinical and pharmacological aspects. In: Legg NJ, ed. The treatment of epilepsy. Tunbridge Wells, England: MCS Consultants, 1976:145-51.

49. Nau H, Rating D, Hauser I et al. Placental transfer and pharmacokinetics of primidone and its metabolites phenobarbital, PEMA and hydroxyphenobarbital in neonates and infants of epileptic mothers. Eur J Clin Pharmacol 1980;18:31-42.

50. Alexander FW. Sodium valproate and pregnancy. Arch Dis Child 1979;54:240. Letter.

51. Dickinson RG, Harland RC, Lynn RK et al. Transmission of valproic acid (Depakene) across the placenta: half-life of the drug in mother and baby. J Pediatr 1979;94:832-5.

52. von Unruh GE, Froescher W, Hoffmann F et al. Valproic acid in breast milk: how much is really there? Ther Drug Monit 1984;6:272-6.

53. Kok THHG, Taitz LS, Bennett MJ et al. Drowsiness due to clemastine transmitted in breast milk. Lancet 1982;1:914-5.

54. Mortimer Jr. EA. Drug toxicity from breast milk? Pediatrics 1977;60:780-1. Letter.

55. Takase Z, Shirafuji H, Uchida M. Fundamental studies and clinical trials with sisomycin in obstetrics and gynecology. Chemotherapy (Tokyo) 1978;26:298-302.

56. Takase Z, Shirafuji H, Uchida M et al. Laboratory and clinical studies on tobramycin in the field of obstetrics and gynecology. Chemotherapy (Tokyo) 1975;23:1402-7.

57. Uwaydah M, Bibi S, Salman S. Therapeutic efficacy of tobramycin—a clinical and laboratory evaluation. J Antimicrob Chemother 1975;1:429-37.

58. Fujimori H, Imai S. Studies on dihydrostreptomycin administered to the pregnant and transferred to their fetuses. J Japanese Obstet Gynecol Soc 1957;4:133-49.

59. Yoshioka H, Cho K, Takimoto M et al. Transfer of cefazolin into human milk. J Pediatr 1979;94:151-2.

60. Kobyletzki D, Sas D, Dingeldein E et al. Pharmacokinetic investigations of cefazedone in gynecology and obstetrics. Arzneim Forsch 1979;29:1763-8.

61. Santo GH, Huch A. Ubergang von cefoxitin in muttermilch. Infection 1979;7(Suppl):S90-1.

62. Geddes AM, Schnurr LP, Ball AP et al. Cefoxitin: a hospital study. Br Med J 1977;1:1126-8.

63. Matsuda S, Tanno M, Kashiwagura T et al. Basic and clinical studies on cefotiam (SCE-963) in the field of obstetrics and gynecology. Chemotherapy (Tokyo) 1979;27(S-3):655-60.

64. Mischler TW, Corson SL, Larranaga A et al. Cephradine and epicillin in body fluids of lactating and pregnant women. J Reprod Med 1978;21:130-6.

65. Kafetzis DA, Siafas CA, Georgakopoulos PA et al. Passage of cephalosporins and amoxicillin into the breast milk. Acta Paediatr Scand 1981;70:285-8.

66. Dresse A, Lambotte R, Dubois R et al. Transmammary passage of cefoxitin: additional results. J Clin Pharmacol 1983;23:438-40.

67. Lou MA, Wu YH, Jacob LS et al. Penetration of cefonicid into human breast milk and various body fluids and tissues. Rev Infect Dis 1984;6(Suppl 4):S816-20.

68. Kafetzis DA, Lazarides CV, Siafas CA et al. Transfer of cefotaxime in human milk and from mother to foetus. J Antimicrob Chemother 1980;6(Suppl A):135-41.

69. Blanco JD, Jorgensen JH, Castaneda YS et al. Ceftazidime levels in human breast milk. Antimicrob Agents Chemother 1983;23:479-80.

70. Miller RD, Keegan KA, Thrupp LD et al. Human breast milk concentration of moxalactam. Am J Obstet Gynecol 1984;148:348-9.

71. Deturmeny E, Vaila A, Durand A et al. Le passage de la chloroquine dans le lait, sur 1 cas. Therapie 1984;39:438-40. Letter.

72. Katz M. Treatment of protozoan infections: malaria. Pediatr Infect Dis 1983;2:475-80.

73. Nation RL, Hackett LP, Dusci LJ et al. Excretion of hydroxychloroquine in human milk. Br J Clin Pharmacol 1984;17:368-9. Letter.

74. White NJ. Clinical pharmacokinetics of antimalarial drugs. Clin Pharmacokinet 1985;10:187-215.

75. Miller RD, Salter AJ. The passage of trimethoprim/sulfamethoxazole into breast milk and its significance. In: Progress in chemotherapy, Vol. 1, Antibacterial chemotherapy. Athens. 1974:687-91.

76. Kauffman RE, O'Brien C, Gilford P. Sulfisoxazole secretion into human milk. J Pediatr 1980;97:839-41.

77. Branski D, Kerem E, Gross-Kieselstein E et al. Bloody diarrhea — a possible complication of sulfasalazine transferred through human breast milk. J Pediatr Gastroenterol 1986;5:316-7.

78. Jarnerot G, Into-Malmberg M-B. Sulfasalazine treatment during breast feeding. Scand J Gastroenterol 1979;147:869-71.

79. Azad Kahn AK, Truelove SC. Placental and mammary transfer of sulfasalazine. Br Med J 1979;2:1553.

80. Berlin CM Jr, Yaffe SJ. Disposition of salicylazosulfapyridine (Azulfidine) and metabolites in human breast milk. Develop Pharmacol Ther 1980;1:31-9.

81. Allgen LG, Holmberg G, Persson B et al. Biological fate of methenamine in man. Acta Obstet Gynecol Scand 1979;58:287-93.

82. Berlin CM, Lee C. Isoniazid and acetylisoniazid disposition in human milk, saliva and plasma. Fed Proc 1979;38(3) (part 1):426. Abstract.

83. Moore B, Collier J. Drugs and breast feeding. Br Med J 1979;2:211. Letter.

84. Erickson SH, Oppenheim GL, Smith GH. Metronidazole in breast milk. Obstet Gynecol 1981;57:48-50.

85. Coulam CB, Moyer TP, Jiang N-S et al. Breast feeding after renal transplantation. Transplant Proc 1982;13:605-9.

86. Grekas DM, Vasilou SS, Lazarides AN. Immunosuppressive therapy and breast-feeding after renal transplantation. Nephron 1984;37:68. Letter.

87. Bounameaux Y, Durenne JM. Un cas de luecemie chez une femme allaitante: effects du traitment par le busulfan sur le nourisson. Ann Soc Belge Med Trop 1964;44:381-4.

88. Egan PC, Costanza ME, Dodion P et al. Doxorubicin and cisplatin excretion into human milk. Cancer Treat Rep 1985;69:1387-9.

89. Amato D, Niblett JS. Neutropenia from cyclophosphamide in breast milk. Med J Aust 1977;1:383-4.

90. Durodola JI. Administration of cyclophosphamide during late pregnancy and early lactation: a case report. J Natl Med Assoc 1979;71:165-6.

91. Flechner SM, Katz AR, Rogers AJ et al. The presence of cyclosporine in body tissues and fluids during pregnancy. Am J Kidney Dis 1985;5:60-3.

92. Lewis GJ, Lamont CAR, Lee HA et al. Successful pregnancy in a renal transplant recipient taking cyclosporine A. Br Med J 1983;286:603. Letter.

93. Devlin RG, Duchin KL, Fleiss PM. Nadolol in human serum and breast milk. Br J Clin Pharmacol 1981;12:393-6.

94. Liedholm H, Melander A, Bitzen P-O et al. Accumulation of atenolol and metoprolol in human breast milk. Eur J Clin Pharmacol 1981;20:229-31.

95. Thorley KJ, McAinsh J. Levels of the beta blockers atenolol and propranolol in the breast milk of women treated for hypertension in pregnancy. Biopharm Drug Disp 1983;4:299-301.

96. Tillement JP, Albengres E, Lemaire M. Le lait, compartiment de diffusion d'un mediciment. Therapie 1982;37:357-62.

97. Michael CA. Use of labetalol in the treatment of severe hypertension during pregnancy. Br J Clin Pharmacol 1979;8(Suppl):211S-5S.

98. Lunell NO, Kulas J, Rane A. Transfer of labetalol into amniotic fluid and breast milk in lactating women. Eur J Clin Pharmacol 1985;28:597-9.

99. Lustgarten JS, Podos SM. Topical timolol and the nursing mother. Arch Ophthalmol 1983;101:1381-2.

100. White WB, Andreoli JW, Wong S et al. Atenolol in human plasma and breast milk. Obstet Gynecol 1984;63(Suppl):42S-4S.

101. Kulas J, Lunell N-O, Rosig U et al. Atenolol and metoprolol. A comparison of their excretion into human breast milk. Acta Obstet Gynecol Scand 1984;118(Suppl):65-9.

102. Boutroy MJ, Bianchetti G, Dubruc C et al. To nurse when receiving acebutolol: is it dangerous for the neonate? Eur J Clin Pharmacol 1986;30:737-9.

103. Board JA, Fierro RJ, Wasserman HJ et al. Effects of α- and β- adrenergic blocking agents on serum prolactin levels in women with hyperprolactinemia and galactorrhea. Am J Obstet Gynecol 1977;127:285-7.

104. Sandstrom B, Regardh C-G. Metoprolol excretion into breast milk. Br J Clin Pharmacol 1980;9:518-9.

105. Bauer JH, Pape B, Zajicek J et al. Propranolol in human plasma and breast milk. Am J Cardiol 1979;43:860-2.

106. Andersen HJ. Excretion of verapamil in human milk. Eur J Clin Pharmacol 1983;25:279-80. Letter.

107. Inoue H, Unno N, Ou M-C et al. Level of verapamil in human milk. Eur J Clin Pharmacol 1984;26:657-8. Letter.

108. Okada M, Inoue H, Nakamura Y et al. Excretion of diltiazem in human milk. N Engl J Med 1985;312:992-3. Letter.

109. McKenna WJ, Harris L. Rowland E et al. Amiodarone therapy during pregnancy. Am J Cardiol 1983;51:1231-3.

110. Levy M, Granit L, Laufer N. Excretion of drugs in milk. N Engl J Med 1977;297:789. Letter.

111. Loughnan PM. Digoxin excretion in human breast milk. J Pediatr 1978;92:1019-20.

112. Chan V, Tse TF, Wong V. Transfer of digoxin across the placenta and into breast milk. Br J Obstet Gynaecol 1978;85:605-9.

113. Finley JP, Waxman MB, Wong PY et al. Digoxin excretion in human milk. J Pediatr 1979;94:339-40.

114. Barnett DB, Hudson SA, McBurney A. Disopyramide and its N-monodesalkyl metabolite in breast milk. Br J Clin Pharmacol 1982;14:310-2.

115. MacKintosh D, Buchanan N. Excretion of disopyramide in human breast milk. Br J Clin Pharmacol 1985;19:856-7. Letter.

116. Zeisler JA, Gaarder TD, DeMesquita SA. Lidocaine excretion in breast milk. Drug Intell Clin Pharm 1986;20:691-3.

117. Lewis AM, Johnston A, Patel L et al. Mexiletine in human blood and breast milk. Postgrad Med J 1981;57:546-7.

118. Timmis AD, Jackson G, Holt DW. Mexiletine for control of ventricular dysrhythmias in pregnancy. Lancet 1980;2:647-8. Letter.

119. Pittard III WB, Glazier H. Procainamide excretion in human milk. J Pediatr 1983;102:631-3.

120. Hill LM, Malkasin GD. The use of quinidine sulfate throughout pregnancy. Obstet Gynecol 1979;54:366-8.

121. Devlin RG, Fleiss PM. Captopril in human blood and breast milk. J Clin Pharmacol 1981;21:110-3.

122. Hartikainen-Sorri A-L, Heikkinen JE, Koivisto M. Pharmacokinetics of clonidine during pregnancy and nurs-

ing. Obstet Gynecol 1987;69:598-600.

123. Liedholm H, Wahlin-Boll E, Hanson A et al. Transplacental passage and breast milk concentration of hydralazine. Eur J Clin Pharmacol 1982;21:417-9.

124. Jones HMR, Cummings AJ. A study of the transfer of α-methyldopa to the human foetus and newborn infant. Br J Clin Pharmacol 1978;6:432-4.

125. White WB, Andreoli JW, Cohn RD. Alpha-methyldopa disposition in mothers with hypertension and in their breast-fed infants. Clin Pharmacol Ther 1985;37:387-90.

126. Valdivieso A, Valdes G, Spiro TE et al. Minoxidil in breast milk. Ann Intern Med 1985;102:135. Letter.

127. Miller ME, Cohn RD, Burghart PH. Hydrochlorothiazide disposition in a mother and her breast-fed infant. J Pediatr 1982;101:789-91.

128. Cominos DC, Van Der Walt A, Van Rooyen AJL. Suppression of postpartum lactation with furosemide. S Afr Med J 1976;50:251-2.

129. Mulley BA, Parr GD, Pau WK et al. Placental transfer of chlorthalidone and its elimination in maternal milk. Eur J Clin Pharmacol 1978;13:129-31.

130. Soderman P, Hartvig P, Fagerlund C. Acetazolamide excretion into human breast milk. Br J Clin Pharmacol 1984;17:599-600. Letter.

131. Phelps DL, Karim A. Spironolactone: relationship between concentration of dethioacetylated metabolite in human serum and milk. J Pharm Sci 1977;66:1203.

132. Somogi A, Gugler R. Cimetidine excretion into breast milk. Br J Clin Pharmacol 1979;7:627-9.

133. Bateson MC, Browning MCK, Maconnachie A. Galactorrhoea with cimetidine. Lancet 1977;1:247-8.

134. Kauppila A, Kivinen S, Ylikorkala O. Metoclopramide increases prolactin release and milk secretion in puerperium without stimulating the secretion of thyrotropin and thyroid hormones. J Clin Endocrinol Metab 1981;52:436-9.

135. Kauppila A, Arvela P, Koivisto M et al. Metoclopramide and breast feeding: transfer into milk and the newborn. Eur J Clin Pharmacol 1983;25:819-23.

136. Gupta AP, Gupta PK. Metoclopramide as a lactagogue. Clin Pediatr 1985;24:269-72.

137. Lewis PJ, Devenish C, Kahn C. Controlled trial of metoclopramide in the initiation of breast feeding. Br J Clin Pharmacol 1980;9:217-9.

138. Guzman V, Toscano G, Canales ES et al. Improvement of defective lactation by using oral metoclopramide. Acta Obstet Gynecol Scand 1979;58:53-5.

139. Kauppila A, Kivinen S, Ylikorkala O. A dose response relation between improved lactation and metoclopramide. Lancet 1981;1:1175-7.

140. Finnis WA, Bird CE, Wilson DL. Metoclopramide hydrochloride and galactorrhea. Can Med Assoc J 1976;115:845. Letter.

141. Badraoui MHH, Hefnawi F, Hegab M et al. The effect of a nonhormonal drug used as a contraceptive method and lactation stimulant after delivery. Fertil Steril 1978;30:742.

142. Aono T, Shioji T, Aki T et al. Augmentation of puerperal lactation by oral administration of sulpiride. J Clin Endocrinol Metab 1979;48:478-82.

143. Riley AJ, Crowley P, Harrison C. In: Misiewicz JJ, Wormsley KG, eds. The clinical use of ranitidine. Oxford. Medicine Publishing Foundation. 1981;5:77-86.

144. Kearns GL, McConnell Jr RF, Trang JM et al. Appearance of ranitidine in breast milk following multiple dosing. Clin Pharm 1985;4:322-4.

145. Ost L, Wettrell G, Bjorkhem I et al. Prednisolone excretion in human milk. J Pediatr 1985;106:1008-11.

146. Berlin CM, Kaiser DG, Demers L. Excretion of prednisone and prednisolone in human milk. Pharmacologist 1979;21:264. Abstract.

147. Sagraves R, Kaiser D, Sharpe GL. Prednisone and prednisolone concentrations in the milk of a lactating mother. Drug Intell Clin Pharm 1981;15:484. Abstract.

148. Burrow GN, Wassenaar W, Robertson GL et al. DDAVP treatment of diabetes insipidus during pregnancy and the post-partum period. Acta Endocrinol 1981;97:23-5.

149. Ruis H, Rolland R, Doesburg W et al. Oxytocin enhances onset of lactation among mothers delivering prematurely. Br Med J 1981;283:340-2.

150. Seifer DB, Sandberg EC, Ueland K et al. Water intoxication and hyponatremic encephalopathy from the use of an oxytocin nasal spray. J Reprod Med 1985;30:225-8.

151. Rosa FW. Resolving the ''public health dilemma'' of steroid contraception and its effects on lactation. Am J Public Health 1976;66:791-2..

152. Harrison RG. Suppression of lactation. Semin Perinatol 1979;3:287-97.

153. Toddywalla VS, Joshi L, Virkar K. Effect of contraceptive steroids on human lactation. Am J Obstet Gynecol 1977;127:245-9.

154. Lonnerdal B, Forsum E, Hambraeus L. Effect of oral contraceptives on composition and volume of breast milk. Am J Clin Nutr 1980;33:816-24.

155. IPPF International Medical Advisory Panel. Injectable contraception. IPPF Med Bull 1980;14(6):1-3.

156. Nilsson S, Nygren K-G, Johansson EDB. Ethinyl estradiol in human milk and plasma after oral administration. Contraception 1978;17:131-9.

157. Madhavapeddi R, Ramachandran P. Side effects of oral contraceptive use in lactating women—enlargement of breast in a breast-fed child. Contraception 1985;32:437-43.

158. Saxena BN, Shrimanker K, Grudzinskas JG. Levels of contraceptive steroids in breast milk and plasma of lactating women. Contraception 1977;16:605-13.

159. Nilsson S, Nygren K-G, Johansson EDB. Megestrol acetate concentrations in plasma and milk during administration of an oral contraceptive containing 4 mg megestrol acetate to nursing women. Contraception 1977;16:615-24.

160. Thomas MJ, Danutra V, Read GF et al. The detection and measurement of d-norgestrel in human milk using sephadex LH 20 chromatography and radioimmunoassay. Steroids 1977;30:349-61.

161. Nilsson S, Nygren K-G, Johansson EDB. Transfer of estradiol to human milk. Am J Obstet Gynecol 1978;132:653-7.

162. Toddywalla VS, Mehta S, Virkar KD et al. Release of 19-nor-testosterone type of contraceptive steroids through different drug delivery systems into the serum and breast milk of lactating women. Contraception 1980;21:217-23.

163. Stoppelli I, Rainer E, Humpel M. Transfer of cyproterone to the milk of lactating women. Contraception 1980;22:485-93.

164. Nilsson S, Nygren K-G, Johansson EDB. d-Norgestrel concentrations in maternal plasma, milk and child plasma during administration of oral contraceptives to nursing women. Am J Obstet Gynecol 1977;129:178-84.

165. Nilsson S, Nygren K-G. Transfer of contraceptive steroids to human milk. Res Reprod 1979;11(1):1-2.

166. Kincl FA. Debate on the use of hormonal contraceptives during lactation. Res Reprod 1980;12(2):1.

167. Low LCK, Lang J, Alexander WD. Excretion of carbimazole and propylthiouracil in breast milk. Lancet 1979;2:1011.

168. Kampmann JP, Hansen JM, Johansen K et al. Propylthiouracil in human milk: revision of a dogma. Lancet 1980;1:736-8. Letter.

169. Lamberg B-A, Ikonen E, Osterlund K et al. Antithyroid treatment of maternal hyperthyroidism during lactation. Clin Endocrinol 1984;21:81-7.

170. Cooper DS. Antithyroid drugs: to breast-feed or not to breast-feed. Am J Obstet Gynecol 1987;157:234-5.

171. Letarte J, Guyda H, Dussault JH et al. Lack of protective effect of breast-feeding in congenital hypothyroidism: report of 12 cases. Pediatrics 1980;65:703-5.

172. Mallol J, Obregon MJ, de Escobar GM. Analytical artifacts in radioimmunoassay of L-thyroxine in human milk. Clin Chem 1982;28:1277-82.

173. Sato T, Suzuki Y. Presence of triiodothyronine, no detectable thyroxine and reverse triiodothyronine in human milk. Endocrinol Jpn 1979;26:507-13.

174. Oberkotter LV, Tenore A. Separation and radioimmunoassay of T3 and T4 in human breast milk. Hormone Res 1983;17:11-8.

175. Sack J, Amado O, Lunenfeld B. Thyroxine concentration in human milk. J Clin Endocrinol Metab 1977;45:171-3.

176. Bode HH, Vanjonack WJ, Crawford JD. Mitigation of cretinism by breast-feeding. Pediatrics 1978;62:13-6.

177. Varma SK, Collins M, Row A et al. Thyroxine, tri-iodothyronine and reverse tri-iodothyronine concentrations in human milk. J Pediatr 1978;93:803-6.

178. Strbak V, Macho R, Kovak R et al. Thyroxine (by competitive protein binding analysis) in human and cow milk and in infant formulas. Endocrinol Exp 1976;10:167-74.

179. Abbassi V, Steinour TA. Successful diagnosis of congenital hypothyroidism in four breast-fed infants. J Pediatr 1980;97:259-61.

180. Lloyd AH. Practical considerations in the use of maprotiline (Ludiomil) in general practice. J Int Med Res 1977;5(Suppl 4):122-38.

181. Ananth J. Side effects in the neonate from psychotropic agents excreted through breast-feeding. Am J Psychiatry 1978;135:801-5.

182. Gelenberg AJ. Amoxapine, a new antidepressant, appears in milk. J Nerv Ment Dis 1979;167:635-6.

183. Rees JA, Glass RC, Sporne GA. Serum and breast milk concentration of dothiepin. Practitioner 1976;217:686.

184. Sovner R, Orsulak PJ. Excretion of imipramine and desipramine in human breast milk. Am J Psychiatry 1979;136:451-2.

185. Erickson SJ, Smith GH, Heidrich F. Tricyclics and breast feeding. Am J Psychiatry 1979;136:1483.

186. Bader TF, Newman K. Amitriptyline in human breast milk and the nursing infant's serum. Am J Psychiatry 1980;137:855-6.

187. Matheson I, Pande H, Alertsen AR. Respiratory depression caused by N-desmethyldoxepin in breast milk. Lancet 1985;2:1124. Letter.

188. Verbeeck RK, Ross SG, McKenna EA. Excretion of trazodone in breast milk. Br J Clin Pharmacol 1986;22:367-70.

189. Stewart RB, Karas B, Springer PK. Haloperidol excretion in human milk. Am J Psychiatry 1980;137:849-50.

190. Whalley LJ, Blain PG, Prime JK. Haloperidol secreted in breast milk. Br Med J 1981;282:1746-7.

191. Citterio C. Riconoscimento e dosaggio di derivati fenotiazinici nella secrezione lattea. Neuropsichiatria 1964;20:141-6.

192. Wiles DH, Orr MW, Kolakowska T. Chlorpromazine levels in plasma and milk of nursing mothers. Br J Clin Pharmacol 1978;5:272-3.

193. Kris EB, Carmichael DM. Chlorpromazine maintenance therapy during pregnancy and confinement. Psychiatric Quarterly 1957;31:690-5.

194. Kris EB. Children born to mothers maintained on pharmacotherapy during pregnancy and postpartum. Rec Adv Biol Psychiatr 1962;4:180-7.

195. Ayd FJ Jr. Children born of mothers treated with chlorpromazine during pregnancy. Clin Med 1964;71:1758-63.

196. Skausig OB, Schou M. Diegivning under litiumbehandling. Ugeskr Laeg 1977;139:400-1.

197. Schou M, Weinstein MR. Problems of lithium maintenance treatment during pregnancy, delivery and lactation. Agressologie 1980;21(special issue A):7-9.

198. Rane A, Tomson G, Bjarke B. Effects of maternal lithium therapy in a newborn infant. J Pediatr 1978;93:296-7.

199. Tunnessen WW, Hertz CG. Toxic effects of lithium in newborn infants: a commentary. J Pediatr 1972;81:804-7.

200. Wesson DR, Camber S, Harkey M et al. Diazepam and desmethyldiazepam in breast milk. J Psychoac Drugs 1985;17:55-6.

201. Rey E, Giraux P, d'Athis P et al. Pharmacokinetics of the placental transfer and distribution of clorazepate and its metabolite nordiazepam in the fetoplacental unit and in the neonate. Eur J Clin Pharmacol 1979;15:181-5.

202. Kanto J, Aaltonen L, Kangas L et al. Placental transfer and breast milk levels of flunitrazepam. Curr Ther Res 1979;26:539-46.

203. Pacifici GM, Placidi GF. Rapid and sensitive electron-capture gas chromatographic method for the determination of pinazepam and its metabolites in human plasma, urine and milk. J Chromatogr 1977;135:133-9.

204. Cote CJ, Kenepp NB, Reed SB et al. Trace concentrations of halothane in human breast milk. Br J Anaesth 1976;48:541-3.

205. Eriksson G, Swahn C-G. Concentrations of baclofen in serum and breast milk from a lactating woman. Scand J Clin Lab Invest 1981;41:185-7.

206. Pentland B, Sawers JSA. Galactorrhoea after withdrawal of bromocriptine. Br Med J 1980;281:716.

207. De Cecco L, Venturini PL, Ragni N et al. Effect of lisuride on inhibition of lactation and serum prolactin. Br J Obstet Gynaecol 1979;86:905-8.

208. Delitala G, Masala A, Alagna S et al. Metergoline in the inhibition of puerperal lactation. Br Med J 1977;1:744-6.

209. Erkkola R, Kanto J, Allonen H et al. Excretion of methylergometrine (methylergonovine) into the human breast milk. Int J Clin Pharmacol 1978;16:579-80.

210. Blau SP. Metabolism of gold during lactation. Arthritis Rheum 1973;16:777-8. Letter.

211. Gottlieb NL. Suggested errata. Arthritis Rheum 1974;17:1057. Letter.

212. Bell RAF, Dale IM. Gold secretion on maternal milk. Arthritis Rheum 1976;19:1374. Letter.

213. Ostensen M, Husby G. Antirheumatic drug treatment during pregnancy and lactation. Scand J Rheumatol 1985;14:1-7.

214. Cruikshank DP, Varner MW, Pitkin RM. Breast milk magnesium and calcium concentrations following magnesium sulfate treatment. Am J Obstet Gynecol 1982;143:685-8.

215. Witter FR, Smith RV. The excretion of pentoxifylline and its metabolites into human breast milk. Am J Obstet Gynecol 1985;151:1094-7.

216. Hardell L-I, Lindstrom B, Lonnerholm G et al. Pyridostigmine in human breast milk. Br J Clin Pharmacol 1982;14:565-7. Letter.

217. Steiner E, Villen T, Hallberg M et al. Amphetamine secretion in breast milk. Eur J Clin Pharmacol 1984;27:123-4.

218. Lindberg C, Boreus LO, de Chateau P et al. Transfer of terbutaline into breast milk. Eur J Resp Dis 1984;65(Suppl 134):87-91.

219. Stec GP, Greenberger P, Ruo TI et al. Kinetics of theophylline transfer into breast milk. Clin Pharmacol Ther 1980;28:404-8.

220. Buimovici-Klein E, Hite RL, Byrne T et al. Isolation of rubella virus in milk after postpartum immunization. J Pediatr 1977;91:939-41.

221. Losonsky GA, Fishaut JM, Strussenberg J et al. Effect of immunization against rubella on lactation products (2 parts). J Infect Dis 1982;145:654-66.

222. Binkiewicz A, Robinson MJ, Senior B. Pseudo-Cushing syndrome caused by alcohol in breast milk. J Pediatr 1978;93:965-7.

223. De Rosa G, Corsello SM, Ruffilli MP et al. Prolactin secretion after beer. Lancet 1981;2:934. Letter.

224. Carlson HE, Wasser HL, Reidelberger RD. Beer-induced prolactin secretion: a clinical and laboratory study of the role of salsolinol. J Clin Endocrinol Metab 1985;60:673-7.

225. Tyrala EE, Dodson WE. Caffeine secretion into breast milk. Arch Dis Child 1979;54:787-800.

226. Hill R, Craig JP, Chaney MD et al. Utilization of over-the-counter drugs during pregnancy. Clin Obstet Gynecol 1977;20:381-4.

227. Brazier J-L, Renaud H, Ribon B et al. Plasma xanthine levels in low birthweight infants treated or not treated with theophylline. Arch Dis Child 1979;54:194-9.

228. Sagraves R, Bradley JM, Delgado MJM et al. Pharmacokinetics of caffeine in human breast milk after a single oral dose of caffeine. Drug Intell Clin Pharm 1984;18:507. Abstract.

229. Rivera-Calimlin L. Drugs in breast milk. Drug Ther (Dec) 1977:59-63.

230. Perez-Reyes M, Wall ME. Presence of delta-9 tetrahydrocannabinol in human milk. N Engl J Med 1982;307:819-20. Letter.

231. Kaufman KR, Petrucha RA, Pitts Jr FN et al. PCP in amniotic fluid and breast milk: case report. J Clin Psychiatry 1983;44:269-70.

232. Nicholas JM, Lipshitz J, Schreiber EC et al. Phencyclidine: its transfer across the placenta as well as into breast milk. Am J Obstet Gynecol 1982;143:143-6.

233. Luck W, Nau H. Nicotine and cotinine concentrations in serum and milk of nursing smokers. Br J Clin Pharmacol 1984;18:9-15.

234. Schwartz-Bickenbach D, Schulte-Hobein B, Abt S et al. Smoking and passive smoking during pregnancy and early infancy: effects on birth weight, lactation period, and cotinine concentrations in mother's milk and infant's urine. Toxicol Lett 1987;35:73-81.

235. Lau RJ, Emery MG, Galinsky RE. Unexpected accumulation of acyclovir in breast milk with estimation of infant exposure. Obstet Gynecol 1987;69:468-71.

236. Diaz S, Peralta D, Juez G et al. Fertility regulation in nursing women. Contraception 1983;27:1-38.

237. Knott C, Reynolds F, Clayden G. Infantile spasms on weaning from breast milk containing anticonvulsants. Lancet 1987;2:272-3. Letter.

238. Lownes HE, Ives TJ. Mexiletine use in pregnancy and lactation. Am J Obstet Gynecol 1987;157:446-7.

239. Chasnoff W, Lewis DE, Squires L. Cocaine intoxication in a breast-fed infant. Pediatrics 1987;80:836-8.

8 DRUGS AND PREGNANCY

IN THE UNITED STATES, FETAL MALFORMATIONS occur in approximately 4% of pregnancies. This includes major and minor malformations from any cause, be it drug, infection, genetics or pollutants. Drug use during pregnancy may be associated with risk to the developing fetus as well as to the pregnant woman. Several factors influence pregnancy outcome after fetal exposure to drugs.[1] The genetic makeup of both the fetus and the mother influence the extent to which an agent may affect the developing fetus. For example, the rates of absorption, metabolism and elimination of an agent by the mother, its rate of placental transfer or the way it interacts with cells and tissues of the embryo are all genetically determined factors. Thus, human teratogenicity cannot be predicted based only on animal data or extrapolated from one pregnancy to another.

The timing of fetal exposure is an important factor. Major malformations are usually the result of first trimester exposure during critical periods of organogenesis. Exposures during the second and third trimester may result in alterations or damage in fine structure and function. Intrauterine growth retardation (IUGR) is, perhaps, the most reliable indicator that a teratogen was present during the second and third trimester of fetal development. Several organs and systems (eg, the kidney, CNS, liver and endocrine) continue to develop after birth. Therefore, exposure to agents later in pregnancy carries some risk and may result in more debilitating alterations in development such as mental retardation. Figure 1 depicts the stages of human structural development in relation to teratogenic potential.[2]

Accumulating evidence suggests that most chemicals in the maternal blood stream cross the placenta. Each drug has a threshold dose above which fetal defects can occur and below which no effects are discernible. Therefore, placental transfer of an agent does not necessarily imply teratogenicity. Whether or not an agent reaches a "threshold concentration" in the fetus depends on maternal factors (eg, rate of absorption and metabolism) as well as on the chemical nature of the agent (eg, ionic charge, protein binding, lipophilicity, molecular size, mechanism of placental transfer, affinity for specific receptors).

Teratogenic substances rarely cause a single defect. Most often, a spectrum of defects occurs which corresponds with the systems undergoing major development at the time of exposure. The fetal alcohol syndrome and fetal hydantoin syndrome are examples of this principle.

Figure 1. Human Development with Particular Reference to Potential Teratogenic Drug Insults.[a]

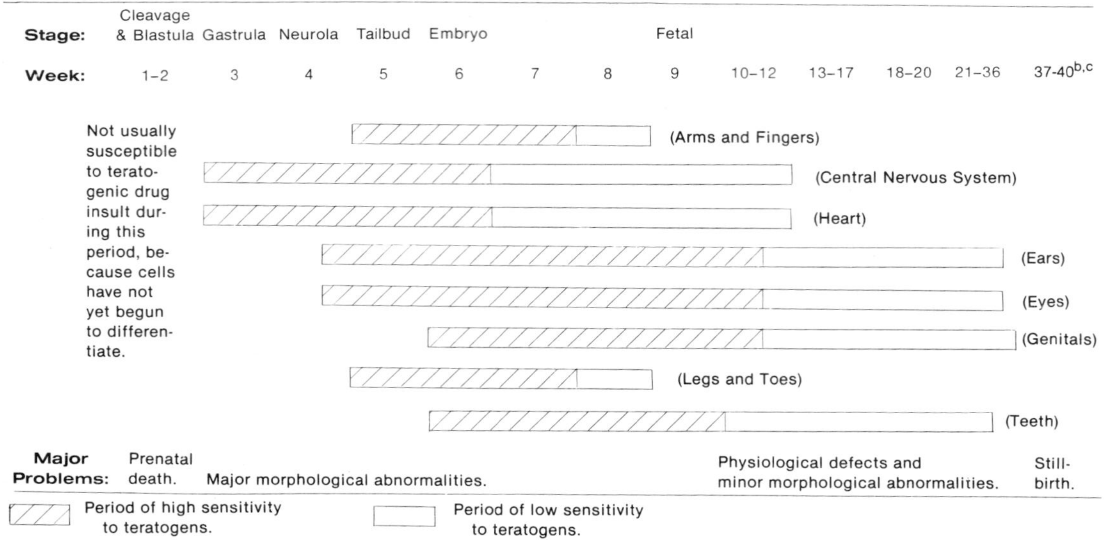

| Stage: | Cleavage & Blastula | Gastrula | Neurola | Tailbud | Embryo | | | | Fetal | | | | | |

Stage: Cleavage & Blastula — Gastrula — Neurola — Tailbud — Embryo — Fetal

Week: 1–2 3 4 5 6 7 8 9 10–12 13–17 18–20 21–36 37–40[b,c]

Not usually susceptible to teratogenic drug insult during this period, because cells have not yet begun to differentiate.

(Arms and Fingers)

(Central Nervous System)

(Heart)

(Ears)

(Eyes)

(Genitals)

(Legs and Toes)

(Teeth)

Major Problems: Prenatal death.   Major morphological abnormalities.   Physiological defects and minor morphological abnormalities.   Stillbirth.

⬛ Period of high sensitivity to teratogens.

☐ Period of low sensitivity to teratogens.

a. From reference 2, reproduced with permission.
b. Average time from fertilization to parturition is 38 weeks.
c. Drugs administered during this period may cause neonatal depression at birth (or other effects directly related to the pharmacological effect of the administered drug).

There are few controlled prospective trials of drug use in pregnancy. Most of the information available comes from case reports or retrospective studies. Cause-and-effect relationships between drugs and teratogenicity are difficult to establish retrospectively, because of the numerous variables associated with each report. These include maternal dose of drug, time of ingestion in relation to date of conception, duration of therapy, concomitant exposures to other potential teratogens and questionable study design or methodology.

Administration of drugs near term poses another threat to the fetus. Before birth, the fetus relies on maternal systems for drug elimination. After birth, the infant must rely on its own metabolic capabilities, which have not yet fully developed. Drugs given near term or during birth, especially those with long half-lives, may have an even more prolonged action in the neonate. Drugs which cause maternal addiction are also known to cause fetal addiction. Neonatal withdrawal symptoms may occur when mothers have been addicted to drugs during pregnancy or when they have taken addicting drugs near term, even though the mothers themselves are not addicted.

Maternal physiology changes as pregnancy progresses and may have an effect on drug disposition and clearance. Maternal blood volume increases by about 20–30% throughout pregnancy and then falls during the last few weeks. The volume of distribution for many drugs increases as the fetal compartment enlarges, causing changes in maternal plasma drug levels. Drugs with narrow therapeutic ranges require careful monitoring during pregnancy, possibly necessitating dosage increases. As maternal plasma volume returns to normal, doses of many drugs require reduction.

The following table presents those drugs for which a known, theoretical or highly suspected increased risk to either the fetus or the mother exists. For a more thorough discussion of the principles of teratology, the reader should consult reference 1.

The following abbreviation is used in the table: IUGR—intrauterine growth retardation.

Drugs and Pregnancy

DRUG	NATURE OF EFFECT
ANALGESICS AND ANTIPYRETICS	
Acetaminophen	Acetaminophen use in pregnancy, although not systematically evaluated, does not appear to be associated with congenital malformations. Acetaminophen is the analgesic-antipyretic of choice for use near term, because it does not affect platelet function or peripheral prostaglandin synthesis.[3]
Aspirin	Maternal aspirin ingestion is associated with a decrease in factor XII, an increase in prothrombin time, platelet dysfunction and bleeding in the neonate. Neonatal clotting may be affected by as little as 650 mg taken two weeks before delivery. An increased length of gestation, which may be due to aspirin's antiprostaglandin effect, and an increased rate of perinatal mortality has been suggested in long-term salicylate users.[3]
Indomethacin	Indomethacin, and other prostaglandin inhibitors, used for the prevention of premature delivery and for the control of uterine activity at term have been associated with persistent fetal circulation (patent ductus arteriosus). This effect is presumably due to its antiprostaglandin activity.[3,4]
Narcotics	Narcotic analgesic use during pregnancy is not associated with any major or minor fetal malformations. Maternal narcotic abuse during pregnancy may lead to maternal and fetal addiction. Withdrawal symptoms, including irritability, tremulousness, high-pitched crying, weak sucking and seizures may occur in neonates born to narcotic-addicted women and nonaddicted women using narcotics near term. Neonatal respiratory depression may occur when narcotic analgesics are given during labor.[5,6] Obstetrical use of **butorphanol** has been compared to **meperidine**. No differences were observed between drugs relative to neonatal neurobehavior or frequency of depressant effects on the newborn.[7a] However, butorphanol frequently causes sinusoidal fetal heart rate pattern.[7b] **Methadone** use during pregnancy is not associated with any structural defects.

Continued

Drugs and Pregnancy

DRUG	NATURE OF EFFECT
	However, IUGR occurs in approximately 35% of infants born to methadone addicts.[6,8,9] 70-90% of infants born to narcotic-addicted mothers exhibit neonatal withdrawal symptoms (see Heroin).[9,10] Prolonged thrombocytosis has been observed in children born to women taking methadone alone or with other addictive drugs.[11] Anecdotal case reports of **pentazocine** use alone or with **triplelennamine** ("T's and Blues") throughout pregnancy have described normal infants who demonstrate withdrawal symptoms similar to those reported in offspring of heroin and methadone addicts.[12] IUGR and prematurity have also been observed.[13] Neonatal respiratory depression may occur when pentazocine is used during delivery.[14] Maternal **propoxyphene** use may also lead to neonatal withdrawal symptoms.[15]
Nonsteroidal Anti-Inflammatory Agents	Systematic evaluation of commonly used drugs in this class have not been conducted in humans. Extrapolating from observations with **indomethacin** and **salicylates**, concern exists for premature closure of the ductus arteriosus, persistent pulmonary hypertension of the newborn and possibly prolonged gestation and labor when used at or near term.[3,4]
ANTICOAGULANTS **Heparin**	The greatest risks with heparin use during pregnancy are increased fetal morbidity and mortality due to spontaneous abortion and prematurity.[16] The frequency of stillbirths and prematurity was as high as 15-33% in two retrospective reviews.[16,17] Maternal thrombocytopenia and hemorrhage may also occur. Heparin has not been associated with an increased risk for structural or functional defects or with IUGR.[16,17]
Warfarin	Warfarin and related anticoagulants may produce the "fetal warfarin syndrome" or "warfarin embryopathy" when ingested during pregnancy. The critical period of risk appears to be between 6-9 weeks of gestation. Features of the syndrome include nasal hypoplasia, neonatal respiratory

Continued

Drugs and Pregnancy

DRUG	NATURE OF EFFECT
	distress secondary to upper airway obstruction, stippled epiphyses, IUGR and varying degrees of hypoplasia of the extremities. Eye abnormalities, including blindness, have also been reported. About one-third of exposed cases resulted in adverse pregnancy outcomes. One-half of these were spontaneous abortions or stillbirths and the other half exhibited some type of congenital abnormality.[16,18] CNS defects occur in about 3% of those exposed and appear to occur independently of the "fetal warfarin syndrome". Dorsal midline dysplasia, Dandy-Walker malformation, midline cerebellar atrophy and ventral midline dysplasia have been reported in many cases. Mental retardation, growth failure, deafness, seizures and spasticity also occur. Critical periods of risk for CNS effects appear to be during the second and third trimesters. Warfarin also increases the risk for fetal as well as maternal hemorrhage, especially when used near term.[18]
ANTICONVULSANTS **Carbamazepine**	A paucity of data on carbamazepine use during pregnancy precludes any conclusions regarding its teratogenicity. A characteristic pattern of malformation has not emerged and the majority of offspring are normal. A reduction in head circumference was observed in a small number of infants; a single case of cranial nerve agenesis and a few cases of unrelated minor abnormalities have been noted after prenatal exposure to carbamazepine alone or in combination with other anticonvulsants. Cause and effect cannot be established.[19]
Phenobarbital	Abnormalities have been reported with phenobarbital used alone and in combination, but causality has not been convincingly established. Malformations similar to those seen with **phenytoin** have been reported when phenobarbital was used alone or in combination with **primidone.** These include craniofacial anomalies (ie, short noses with low nasal bridges, hypertelorism, low-set ears, wide mouth, prominent lips and a cleft soft palate) and digital hypoplasia.[20,21] These effects may be more likely when maternal plasma levels exceed usual therapeutic levels.[22] Anecdotal reports of tumors in 10 children prenatally exposed to phenytoin and a barbiturate have caused concern

Continued

Drugs and Pregnancy

DRUG	NATURE OF EFFECT

Phenytoin — that in utero exposure may potentiate cancer.[23] Barbiturate derivatives can cause a decrease in vitamin K-dependent clotting factors leading to hemorrhagic diatheses in the newborn.[24] Decreased folic acid levels have been reported; some suggest folic acid supplementation may decrease the risk of abnormal offspring.[25] Neonatal withdrawal has been associated with phenobarbital use during pregnancy.

The risk of developing the full-blown fetal hydantoin syndrome (FHS) is about 11% when phenytoin is taken throughout pregnancy. The risk of a less serious effect on prenatal development is 30%. Plasma anticonvulsant levels were higher in mothers with malformed infants than in mothers with normal infants.[22] The principal features of the FHS are craniofacial anomalies (ie, bowed upper lip, ocular hypertelorism, broad nasal bridge, short nose, microcephaly, cleft lip and/or palate), digital hypoplasia with small or absent nails, cardiac defects, pre- and postnatal growth deficiency. Umbilical and inguinal hernias and hypospadias have also been reported.[26,27] Anecdotal reports of tumors in 10 children prenatally exposed to phenytoin and a barbiturate have caused concern that in utero exposure may potentiate cancer.[23] Phenytoin can cause a decrease in vitamin K-dependent clotting factors leading to hemorrhagic diatheses in the newborn.[24] Decreased folic acid levels have been reported; some suggest folic acid supplementation may decrease the risk of abnormal offspring.[25]

Primidone — The teratogenicity of primidone is difficult to assess, because there are few reported cases in the literature and, in most of these, primidone was taken in conjunction with other anticonvulsants, primarily **phenytoin**. Anecdotal reports and one small prospective study have reported abnormalities in offspring of women taking primidone alone. Although no specific pattern has been established, reported malformations include craniofacial alterations (ie, short nose, bowed upper lip, broad nasal bridge, ocular hypertelorism), cardiac defects, pre- and postnatal growth retardation, digital hypoplasia with small or flat nails, inguinal hernias and hypospadias.[20,26,28] Some developmental delay has also been reported. These effects may be more likely when maternal

Continued

Drugs and Pregnancy

DRUG	NATURE OF EFFECT
	plasma levels exceed usual therapeutic levels.[22] Phenobarbital is one metabolite of primidone, and barbiturate derivatives are known to cause a decrease in vitamin K-dependent clotting factors leading to hemorrhagic diatheses of the newborn.[24] Decreased folic acid levels have been reported; some suggest folic acid supplementation may decrease the risk of abnormal offspring.[25] Neonatal withdrawal has been associated with primidone use during pregnancy.
Trimethadione	Use of trimethadione or **paramethadione** during pregnancy has resulted in children with significant anomalies. Abnormalities include varying features of the following: mental deficiency, speech disorders, IUGR, mild midfacial hypoplasia, short upturned nose with broad and low nasal bridge, prominent forehead with V-shaped eyebrows, epicanthal folds, cleft lip and palate, ventricular septal defects, ambiguous genitalia, hypospadias and clitoral hypertrophy. The frequency of spontaneous abortion may also be increased.[27,29]
Valproic Acid	While data are not conclusive that valproic acid is a teratogen, consistency in reported defects raises concern regarding its safety. Spina bifida (following exposure during the first 28 days of gestation), external ear anomalies, congenital heart defects, hypospadias and craniofacial anomalies (ie, epicanthal folds, flat nasal bridge, small mouths with downturned angles and thin upper vermillion borders) have all been reported. Low birth weight and small head circumference have also been reported in offspring of women taking valproic acid alone or in combination with another anticonvulsant.[30-32]
ANTIHISTAMINE DRUGS	Despite reports implicating both **meclizine** and **Bendectin®** (**doxylamine** and **pyridoxine**) as teratogens, large scale studies have shown no association between either of these agents (or the previous formulation of Bendectin® which also included **dicyclomine**) and fetal malformation.[29] **Brompheniramine** or **chlorpheniramine** use during pregnancy has not been associated with an in-

Continued

Drugs and Pregnancy

DRUG	NATURE OF EFFECT
	creased risk of fetal malformations.[29,33,34] **Diphenhydramine** has been suggested by a retrospective study to be a cause of cleft lip and/or palate in the neonate. No other data have confirmed these observations.[29,34]
ANTI-INFECTIVE AGENTS	
Chloramphenicol	Because of its known toxicity (ie, the "gray baby" syndrome) in neonates, there is concern about the use of chloramphenicol during pregnancy. Even though no toxic effects have been reported, chloramphenicol should be used cautiously in the third trimester.[35]
Chloroquine	Chloroquine, when given in doses appropriate for malaria prophylaxis, has not been associated with adverse fetal effects. Larger anti-inflammatory doses, however, have resulted in spontaneous abortion and fetal retinal and vestibular damage.[36]
Dapsone	Extensive, but uncontrolled experience and two surveys on dapsone use in pregnancy have not shown dapsone use to increase the risk of fetal abnormalities.[37]
Erythromycin	Erythromycin estolate can cause hepatotoxicity in pregnant patients. About 10% of 161 women treated with the estolate in the second trimester had abnormally elevated AST (SGOT) levels, which normalized when therapy was discontinued.[29] There is no evidence that erythromycin is harmful to the fetus.[29,35]
Ethambutol	Ethambutol does not appear to cause malformations when used during pregnancy. A 2.1% malformation rate occurred in 655 reported exposures. Although this is below the expected frequency in the normal population and no pattern of malformation was revealed, several anomalies involved the CNS. Exposures were confounded by concomitant isoniazid therapy.[29,38]
Isoniazid	Of the 1480 reported isoniazid exposures during pregnancy, only 1% demonstrated any malforma- Continued

Drugs and Pregnancy

DRUG	NATURE OF EFFECT
	tions. A pattern of malformation was not revealed, but several abnormalities involved the CNS.[29,38] Exposures were confounded by concomitant ethambutol therapy.[38]
Metronidazole	Data from five prospective studies in 1344 women who took metronidazole during pregnancy do not show any increased risk for adverse pregnancy outcome in terms of birth weight, prematurity, perinatal loss, Apgar scores or malformations, and no pattern of specific defects was identified. Time of exposure information was available for 1231 of these exposures. There were 135 first trimester, 540 second trimester and 598 third trimester exposures. No malformation correlated with the time of exposure.[39,40]
Nitrofurantoin	No fetal abnormalities or neonatal hemolytic anemia have been observed with nitrofurantoin use during pregnancy. The drug can produce hemolysis in G-6-PD deficiency.[41]
Primaquine	There are no reports of primaquine teratogenicity. Primaquine may induce hemolysis in G-6-PD deficiency.[29,38]
Pyrimethamine	The recognition that methotrexate, a mammalian folate antagonist, is teratogenic has raised concern over the teratogenicity of all folate antagonists. To date, there is no evidence that pyrimethamine is teratogenic in humans. Folic acid supplementation may be warranted during treatment with pyrimethamine during pregnancy.[29,38]
Quinine	Quinine has been used as a "folk-remedy" for inducing abortion, despite its poor efficacy. When abortion attempts fail, quinine produces a statistically greater number of maternal deaths and fetal anomalies compared with successful therapeutically induced abortion. Fetal anomalies include blindness, optic nerve hypoplasia, deafness and hearing impairment.[29,42]
Rifampin	Rifampin use during pregnancy has not been associated with fetal malformations. Although, in

Continued

Drugs and Pregnancy

DRUG	NATURE OF EFFECT
	most reports rifampin was taken in combination with either isoniazid or ethambutol. Neonatal hypoprothrombinemia has been reported and raises some concern about the use of this drug in pregnancy, especially near term. If rifampin is given during pregnancy, maternal oral prophylactic **vitamin K** 20 mg/day for 2 weeks prior to delivery is recommended.[29,38] Infants should receive 0.5–1.0 mg vitamin K IM or SC immediately after delivery and repeated if necessary 6–8 hr later.[29]
Streptomycin	Streptomycin and **dihydrostreptomycin** have been reported to cause congenital hearing loss ranging from minor high frequency loss to total deafness, when given to pregnant women for the treatment of tuberculosis. Incidence is low, especially with careful dosage calculation and limited duration of therapy.[29,38] Insufficient data are available on the use of other aminoglycosides during pregnancy, but they may pose the same risks.[29,38]
Sulfonamides	Animal data demonstrating an increased rate of cleft palate and bony abnormalities have not been supported by human data. There are occasional reports of abnormalities, but no distinct malformation pattern has emerged. Evidence associating sulfonamide use near term with neonatal kernicterus is lacking, despite the theory that sulfas may displace bilirubin from albumin binding sites.[43-45] **Sulfasalazine** has been associated with IUGR.[46] However, one large survey found the prevalence of IUGR, prematurity, pregnancy loss and developmental defects to be lower in women taking sulfasalazine than in the general population.[46]
Tetracyclines	Tetracycline, and perhaps other tetracyclines, can cause permanent staining of the deciduous teeth when taken after the 20th week of pregnancy. The risk of discoloration increases with dose, duration of therapy and advancing pregnancy; one-third to one-half of third trimester exposures may be affected. Tetracycline is also incorporated into calcifying bone, the clinical significance of which is not established. As bone is resorbed, the tetracycline is released.[47,48]
Trimethoprim	Because trimethoprim is a folate antagonist, caution is advised for its use in pregnancy (see Methotrexate, Pyrimethamine). However, there are data which suggest a lack of teratogenicity.[29]

Continued

Drugs and Pregnancy

DRUG	NATURE OF EFFECT
ANTINEOPLASTIC AGENTS	Antineoplastic agents have both teratogenic and mutagenic potential; reports of infertility and congenital defects do exist. Nevertheless, several studies indicate that fertility is preserved, with normal pregnancy outcome, among both women and men treated for cancer prior to conception. While aggressive treatment of malignancy is necessary on occasion, avoidance or minimum use of these drugs during the first trimester is recommended. First trimester use of the folate antagonists, **aminopterin** and **methotrexate**, is known to cause spontaneous abortions and congenital abnormalities, primarily cranial dysplasia. However, normal pregnancy outcome has been reported after use in the second and third trimesters. **Busulfan** use has been associated with IUGR and multiple malformations, although no specific pattern is evident. **Chlorambucil** use during the first and second trimesters may cause spontaneous abortion and urogenital malformation. **Cyclophosphamide** use during the first trimester has resulted in fetal malformations, particularly of the toes. No malformations have been reported with second and third trimester use. **Fluorouracil** use during pregnancy is limited, but has been reported to cause malformations consistent with inhibition of cell division and cell growth. **Procarbazine** use in pregnancy is limited, but has been associated with several fetal abnormalities, all occurring with first trimester exposure. **Thioguanine** has had reported abnormalities associated with its use in both the first and second trimesters.[49,50]
CARDIOVASCULAR DRUGS	
Diazoxide	Diazoxide, when administered by rapid IV bolus, has been associated with excessive maternal hypotension and fetal distress. Slow IV infusion or mini-bolus administration may prevent this occurrence. Other reported effects include neonatal hyperglycemia when exposure preceded delivery, and alopecia, hypertrichosis languinosa and decreased bone age after exposure in the last 19–70 days of gestation. Other investigators report no problems after long-term oral administration of diazoxide.[51,52]

Continued

Drugs and Pregnancy

DRUG	NATURE OF EFFECT
Digoxin	Digoxin is not known to be a teratogen. It may be given to the pregnant woman to treat fetal CHF. Maternal digitalis toxicity has been associated with fetal toxicity and miscarriage in one case and neonatal EKG changes with subsequent death in another. Maternal levels should be monitored closely, because as pregnancy progresses plasma levels decrease due to an increase in the volume of distribution.[53]
Disopyramide	Disopyramide use during pregnancy has been associated with the initiation of uterine contractions which subsided when the drug was discontinued.[53]
Hydralazine	Hydralazine use in pregnancy may cause reduced uteroplacental blood flow, fetal heart rate changes after acute administration and neonatal hypothermia and thrombocytopenia.[52]
Labetalol	Labetalol given IV to control severe hypertension has caused neonatal bradycardia. Although not statistically significant, labetalol was shown to increase uteroplacental perfusion and decrease uterine vascular resistance.[52]
Methyldopa	Methyldopa use during pregnancy has been more extensively studied than any other antihypertensive agent. Available data suggest no evidence of teratogenicity. Transient reduction in neonatal blood pressure has been noted after maternal methyldopa ingestion. There is a questionable association of IUGR after maternal treatment with methyldopa. One study suggested IUGR was due to chronic hypertension rather than methyldopa.[51,52]
Propranolol	Propranolol use in pregnancy has been associated with IUGR, prolonged labor and neonatal respiratory depression, bradycardia and hypoglycemia. These effects may be dose-related. Maternal disease and concomitant drug therapy make cause-and-effect difficult to establish.[51]
Reserpine	Reserpine, when given to mothers within 24 hr of delivery, produces edema of the nasal mucosa

Continued

Drugs and Pregnancy

DRUG	NATURE OF EFFECT
	in the neonate. This effect is especially significant, because the newborn infant is an obligate nose breather. Lethargy, hypothermia and bradycardia have also been reported in infants whose mothers received antenatal reserpine.[29,51,54]
DIURETICS	Diuretics should be used with great caution during pregnancy. Prophylactic use of diuretics does not appear to reduce the frequency of pre-eclampsia. Diuretics can cause a decrease in maternal intravascular volume and consequently diminish uteroplacental perfusion, thus compromising fetal oxygenation. This effect is most rapid and severe with **loop diuretics**. **Furosemide** increases fetal urine production. IV administration to the pregnant mother has enabled ultrasonic imaging of the fetal bladder. **Thiazide** use in pregnancy may produce neonatal hypoglycemia, hyponatremia, hypokalemia and thrombocytopenia.[51,52,55]
GASTROINTESTINAL DRUGS	
H$_2$-Antagonists	No reports link **cimetidine** or **ranitidine** to adverse pregnancy outcome. Manufacturer data on cimetidine use in 50 pregnant women reveal no increased risk to the developing fetus, although time of exposure was not noted. The use of H$_2$-antagonists as pre-anesthetic agents to prevent aspiration of acidic gastric contents, leading to Mendelson's syndrome, has no reported adverse effects on the course of delivery or in the neonate.[43,56]
HORMONES AND SYNTHETIC SUBSTITUTES	
Clomiphene	Most investigations fail to detect an increase in congenital anomalies in clomiphene-induced conceptions and no recognizable pattern of malformation has been detected.[57] Some evidence suggests an increase in spontaneous abortions associated with clomiphene use; abnormal karyotypes

Continued

Drugs and Pregnancy

DRUG	NATURE OF EFFECT
	have been detected in the abortuses of women receiving ovulation-inducing drugs.[58] One study reports a risk of trisomy 21 (Down's syndrome) similar to that observed in women over age 35 in clomiphene-induced pregnancies.[59]
Corticosteroids	Corticosteroids, while teratogenic in animals, have not been demonstrated to be teratogenic in humans. Large prospective investigations, together with cases of pregnant women with inflammatory bowel disease, asthma or rheumatoid arthritis, do not show an increase in spontaneous abortions or congenital defects in infants prenatally exposed to corticosteroids. Neonates born to women taking steroids chronically should be monitored for adrenal insufficiency.[43,60] Maternal **betamethasone** therapy has been used to prevent respiratory distress in infants born between 28–34 weeks of gestation with no apparent adverse effects.[61]
Danazol	Danazol exposure from the 8th to 12th week postconception is associated with virilization of the female fetus, with clitoromegaly and fusion of labialscrotal folds. Exposure beyond the 12th week of gestation is expected to produce only clitoral hypertrophy. Differentiation of external genitalia occurs 10–12 weeks postconception. The extent of the defect is correlated with the time of exposure. Internal genitalia are reportedly unaffected. The male fetus does not appear to be adversely affected, although genital development may be advanced for gestational age.[62,63]
Diethylstilbestrol (DES)	Daughters of DES-exposed mothers have an increased frequency of adenosis; clear cell adenocarcinoma (0.14–1.4/1000 exposed); and structural defects of the cervix (22–58% of exposed), vagina (22–58% of exposed), uterus (67% of exposed), and fallopian tubes; and reproductive complications. Adverse reproductive effects include infertility, spontaneous abortion (18–47%), ectopic pregnancy (2.6–6.5%), premature deliveries (10–30%) and perinatal deaths.[84] Data on DES-exposed males are suggestive of an increased risk for infertility, various urogenital abnormalities and testicular cancer.[65,66]
Sulfonylureas	Maternal diabetes is known to increase the rate of malformations and perinatal mortality.

Continued

Drugs and Pregnancy

DRUG	NATURE OF EFFECT
	Sulfonylureas may cause prolonged hypoglycemia/hyperinsulinism in the newborn. Pregnant diabetics should be treated with insulin.[29]
Synthetic Progestins	Progestin use (**norethindrone, norethynodrel, ethisterone, medroxyprogesterone**) during pregnancy may cause malformation of external genitalia (clitoral hypertrophy in the female and hypospadias in the male). This is most likely to occur during the period of external genitalia development (8–12 weeks postconception). The suggested linkage of progestin use during pregnancy to the VACTERL syndrome (an acronym for a spectrum of anomalies: vertebral, anal, cardiac, tracheal, esophageal, renal, limb), cardiac defects or limb abnormalities is unfounded.[29,63,66]
Thyroid and Antithyroid Agents	**Propylthiouracil** and **methimazole** were associated with neonatal goiter in early reports, possibly due to the use of iodine in addition to unnecessarily high doses of antithyroid medication. Current practice dictates careful monitoring of the pregnant patient and treatment with the minimum effective drug dose. Such conservative management does not completely eliminate the risk of congenital goiter. Transient neonatal hypothyroidism and neonatal thyrotoxicosis may occur. Monitor infants for thyrotoxicosis, because it may be masked by the antithyroid agent. Hypothyroidism may be prevented by withdrawing the drug, if the mother has remained euthyroid, four to six weeks before delivery. Case reports of four infants with ulcer-like midline scalp defects have been associated with maternal **methimazole** use. Mothers with significant hyperthyroidism, not receiving treatment, have an increased risk of maternal and neonatal complications, including toxemia, small-for-gestational-age babies and perinatal morbidity.[66,67] Excessive **iodine** use during pregnancy is associated with congenital goiter and hypothyroidism. Goiters vary in size, but may be large enough to cause tracheal compression and interfere with delivery. Severe maternal iodine deficiency produces hypothyroidism and cretinism.[66,67]

Maternal exposure to high doses of ^{131}I prior to conception has not been associated with an in- |

Continued

Drugs and Pregnancy

DRUG	NATURE OF EFFECT
	crease in malformations or cytogenic abnormalities. No adverse effects have been reported after inadvertent exposure to ^{131}I prior to 10 weeks gestation. After 10 weeks gestation, the fetal thyroid actively concentrates iodine; any radioactive iodine ingested by the mother will cross the placenta and destroy fetal thyroid tissue.[67,68]
PSYCHOTHERAPEUTIC AGENTS	
Antidepressants, Heterocyclic	Maternal use of **tricyclic antidepressants (clomipramine, desipramine, imipramine)** during pregnancy has produced neonatal withdrawal, characterized by breathlessness, cyanosis, tachypnea, irritability and feeding difficulties. In one case, maternal **nortriptyline** was associated with antenatal urinary retention.[69]
Lithium	Lithium use during the first trimester of pregnancy, particularly from the 3rd to 8th weeks of gestation, is associated with an increased risk of cardiovascular abnormalities, including Ebstein's anomaly. Symptoms of lithium toxicity, including lethargy, hypotonia, poor sucking reflex, respiratory distress, cyanosis, arrhythmias and hypothermia have been reported in newborns of women on chronic lithium therapy. Newborn blood levels were 0.6–1 mEq/L. Monitor maternal levels frequently during pregnancy, because lithium metabolism varies as pregnancy progresses.[70,71]
Phenothiazines	The majority of data do not implicate phenothiazines as teratogens. However, a re-analysis of early data questions the initial negative findings and suggests an increased risk of malformations in association with first trimester phenothiazine use, specifically the 6th to 10th weeks of gestation. Phenothiazine use near term has resulted in some cases of extrapyramidal effects in the neonate, including hypertonicity with tremors and hyperreflexia; effects have persisted up to nine months.[8,72]

Continued

Drugs and Pregnancy

DRUG	NATURE OF EFFECT
SEDATIVES AND HYPNOTICS	High doses of any sedative-hypnotic close to or during delivery may result in neonatal CNS and respiratory depression.
Barbiturates	Barbiturate addiction during pregnancy can cause neonatal withdrawal. Symptoms include tremors, irritability, restlessness, high-pitched increased crying, increased tone, hyperphagia and overreaction to stimuli, which may persist up to 6 months. See also Phenobarbital and Primidone.[66,73]
Chlordiazepoxide	In nearly 42,000 infants exposed to chlordiazepoxide in utero, with the exception of one study, there has not been an association with increased risk to the developing fetus. In one prospective investigation involving 172 women, an increase in fetal death and nonspecific abnormalities was noted in association with maternal ingestion of chlordiazepoxide in the first 42 days of pregnancy. Withdrawal symptoms and neonatal depression have been observed with the use of this drug near term or during delivery.[68,69,74]
Diazepam	Early studies implied that diazepam increased the risk of cleft lip with or without cleft palate by two- to fourfold in infants exposed in the first trimester. This association did not establish a causal relationship. Recent data do not support an association between diazepam and oral cleft-ing.[75,76] However, there is a case report describing an acentric craniofacial cleft in a child whose mother took 580 mg as a single dose about 43 days after her last menstrual period.[77] Neonatal withdrawal symptoms, including tremors, irritability, hypertonicity and sucking difficulties have been reported. Pronounced muscular hypotonia (floppy baby syndrome) has also been described.[75,76]
Inhalation Anesthetics	Inhalation anesthetic use during labor is associated with CNS and respiratory depression in the neonate. In addition, a two- to fourfold increase in the rate of spontaneous abortion in pregnant women chronically exposed to inhalation anesthetics (eg, operating room and dental personnel) has been suggested, although poor study design makes conclusions suspect.[78,79] Continued

Drugs and Pregnancy

DRUG	NATURE OF EFFECT
Meprobamate	In one study, meprobamate ingestion during the first 42 days of pregnancy resulted in eight children with abnormalities (12.1% of exposed), five of whom had cardiovascular malformations.[74] Other large-scale investigations have not confirmed these findings.[29]
SYMPATHOMIMETIC AGENTS	The treatment of hypotension during pregnancy with sympathomimetic agents is complicated by the fact that the uterine vasculature is supplied solely with α-adrenergic receptors and is maximally dilated under basal conditions. Pure α-adrenergic agents significantly constrict uterine vessels and decrease blood flow, thereby compromising the fetus. β-adrenergic agents cause peripheral vasodilation and tend to shunt blood away from the uterus and also may cause fetal compromise. Volume expanding agents seem to be the most prudent treatment for sudden hypotension in the pregnant patient. Use of sympathomimetics for treatment of nasal congestion may be associated with an increase in fetal activity and fetal tachycardia. Sympathomimetics should be avoided in patients with hypertension or toxemia or situations in which there is poor fetal reserve.[29,80]
Amphetamines	Data on the effect of prenatal amphetamines, both prescribed and abused, are conflicting; however, no consistent pattern of abnormalities has emerged. A large prospective evaluation of amphetamines prescribed during pregnancy found no increase in severe congenital malformations, but did report three cases of oral clefts. Another prospective study evaluating infants of amphetamine-addicted women failed to demonstrate an increase in birth defects, but did note an increase in premature births, respiratory distress and jitteriness. The use of other drugs and alcohol may have confounded these findings.[82,83]
VACCINES	See Chapter 10, Immunization, page 238, and reference 81 for information regarding vaccination during pregnancy.

Continued

Drugs and Pregnancy

DRUG	NATURE OF EFFECT
MISCELLANEOUS AGENTS	
Etretinate	Etretinate is a known teratogen in humans. Fetal abnormalities include facial dysmorphia, syndactylies, absence of terminal phalanges, neural tube closure defects, malformations of hip, ankle and forearm, low set ears, high palate, decreased cranial volume and alterations of the skull and cervical vertebrae.[84] Etretinate has been detected in the serum of some patients up to three years after discontinuing therapy. The significance of this, relative to the risk of teratogenicity, is unknown. An effective form of contraception must be used for at least one month before etretinate therapy, during therapy and following discontinuation of therapy for an indefinite period of time.[84,85]
Gold Salts	While shown to be teratogenic in animals, gold salts have not been demonstrated to be harmful to the human fetus. Several anecdotal reports have described normal children born to women using gold salts during pregnancy. Definitive conclusions await further study.[86]
Isotretinoin	Isotretinoin use during pregnancy is associated with the following malformations: CNS (hydrocephalus, microcephaly, optic nerve hypoplasia and posterior fossa cyst); cardiac (conotruncal anomalies or brachial arch mesenchymal tissue defects); ear (microtia or anotia); and thymus (extopia, hypoplasia or aplasia).[87] Other reported malformations include cleft palate, microphthalmia, micrognathia and facial dysmorphia. One case of limb reduction defects of all four limbs has been reported; exposure time correlated with the observed defect.[88] The risk for spontaneous abortion is also increased.[89]
Local Anesthetics	Local anesthetics have been associated with fetal and neonatal depression following maternal use during labor, especially in infants who develop fetal heart rate changes. Fetal bradycardia may occur after as many as 5–70% of paracervical blocks.[89,90]
Oxytocin	Oxytocin given for induction of labor may cause tetanic uterine contractions causing decreased

Continued

Drugs and Pregnancy

DRUG	NATURE OF EFFECT
	uterine blood flow and fetal distress. The use of **ergonovine** or **ergotamine** before delivery carries the same risk. Oxytocin may cause neonatal hypoglycemia.[91]
Penicillamine	Penicillamine in the treatment of 89 pregnant women (46 treated throughout gestation) for rheumatoid arthritis, cystinuria or Wilson's disease resulted in three offspring born with connective tissue defects. Two of the infants had additional defects and died. Penicillamine use during pregnancy should be reserved for treatment of cystinuria and Wilson's disease. Doses should be kept as low as possible.[43,92,93]
Theophylline	No adverse fetal effects from long-term theophylline use during pregnancy are known. Theophylline toxicity was reported in three newborns whose mothers received theophylline or aminophylline in late pregnancy and during labor. Symptoms included jitteriness, vomiting, tachycardia and irritability, all of which resolved in all cases.[29,66]
Tretinoin	Although tretinoin is a vitamin A analogue, no reports of teratogenicity associated with its use have been located. Data demonstrate that topical application of 1 g of a 0.1% tretinoin preparation daily, assuming a maximum penetration of 33%, would result in absorption of approximately 12 IU/kg/day. Most prenatal vitamins contain 5000 IU of vitamin A and result in absorption of about 80 IU/kg/day.[94]
Vaginal Spermicides	Vaginal spermicide use has been associated with major congenital anomalies in one large retrospective analysis. The association, however, has not been substantiated. No one syndrome of malformation was identified; actual use of spermicide by the mother was not verified and the prevalence of major anomalies was only 2.2% in the study group, a rate well within that expected for major malformations in the United States.[95,96] Other studies substantiate the lack of association.[119,120]

Continued

Drugs and Pregnancy

DRUG	NATURE OF EFFECT
Vitamins	Vitamin toxicity has been reported with the use of excessive doses of fat-soluble vitamins during pregnancy.

Vitamin A toxicity is teratogenic in experimental animals, producing defects in almost all organ systems. Such research and the discovery of the teratogenicity of **isotretinoin** and **etretinate** (vitamin A analogues) has raised concern about the effects of excess vitamin A on the human fetus. Human data consist of only a few anecdotal reports. Of five reported cases, four describe abnormalities which involve the urogenital system. Definitive conclusions await further study.[97-99]

Vitamin D excess has been associated with an idiopathic hypercalcemic syndrome including cardiovascular malformation, abnormal bone mineralization, elfin facies, mental retardation, hypercalcemia and nephrocalcinosis. Definitive conclusions await further investigation.[100-102] |
| **DRUGS FOR NONMEDICAL USE** | |
| **Alcohol** | Alcohol consumption during pregnancy should be avoided, because the dose which may produce adverse effects has not been established. A twofold increase in spontaneous abortion was noted among women who drank 1–2 drinks daily for the first two months of pregnancy; the rate was higher in those who drank more than two drinks daily. Moderate drinking (1–2 fluid ounces of absolute alcohol per day) is associated with an increase in some of the features of the fetal alcohol syndrome (FAS). Chronic heavy alcohol consumption is associated with the full-blown FAS in 10–50% of children exposed in utero. Features of FAS include IUGR, microcephaly, postnatal growth deficiency, developmental delay, mental retardation and craniofacial anomalies (ie, microphthalmia and/or short palpebral fissures, poorly developed philtrum, thin upper vermilion border and maxillary hypoplasia). Joint, limb, cardiac and renal defects along with eustachian tube dysfunction are also reported. Neonatal withdrawal symptoms similar to those in adults also occur.[103-105] |

Continued

Drugs and Pregnancy

DRUG	NATURE OF EFFECT
Caffeine	Caffeine is not suspected of causing fetal malformations. A very small reduction in birth weight has been observed when caffeine consumption during pregnancy exceeded 300 mg daily; cigarette smoking may have contributed to these findings. There is conflicting evidence about whether 400-600 mg of caffeine daily increases the risk of miscarriage, stillbirth or prematurity.[66,106]
Cocaine	There is no strong evidence to suggest that intrauterine cocaine exposure causes fetal malformation. However, there may be an association between maternal cocaine use and spontaneous labor and abruptio placentae as well as an increase in spontaneous abortion.[107,108] A case of perinatal cerebral infarction associated with maternal cocaine use has been reported. The mother used cocaine intranasally during her first 5 weeks of pregnancy and then discontinued until the 3 days just prior to delivery, during which time she used 5 grams of cocaine intranasally. The infant's initial exam was within normal limits except for mild decreased muscle tone of the right upper extremity and tachycardia as high as 180 beats per minute. He later had several episodes of apnea and cyanosis and suffered multiple focal seizures. A CT scan at 24 hours of life showed a cerebral hemorrhage. At 3 months of age the infant's head circumference had fallen from the 50th percentile at birth to the 5th percentile.[109]
Heroin	Reports of withdrawal-like symptoms similar to those which occur in adults exist. Neonates exhibit jitteriness, abnormal sleep patterns, poor feeding and irritability.[110] Heroin addiction during pregnancy, although not associated with structural defects, does cause an increase in fetal distress, stillbirths, prematurity and neonatal morbidity and mortality. Over 80% of exposed infants may exhibit asphyxia neonatorum, intracranial hemorrhage, hyaline membrane disease, IUGR, hypoglycemia, septicemia and hyperbilirubinemia. 70-90% of infants born to narcotic-addicted mothers exhibit neonatal withdrawal symptoms including irritability, tremulousness, high-pitched crying, weak sucking and seizures.[111,112]

Continued

Drugs and Pregnancy

DRUG	NATURE OF EFFECT
Marijuana	Marijuana use during pregnancy has not been associated with any specific pattern of malformation. There are unsubstantiated reports of prematurity, increased precipitate labor, meconium passage, IUGR, features compatible with the fetal alcohol syndrome and short-term neurological abnormalities. Exposures were confounded by other drug use (alcohol, nicotine and other nonmedical drugs).[113,114]
Phencyclidine	Chronic phencyclidine use during pregnancy, especially near term, may produce neonatal withdrawal symptoms of lethargy contrasted with coarse flappy tremors after stimulation. The narcotic withdrawal symptoms of voracious sucking, sweating and fine tremors are absent. Lack of data does not allow for generalizations regarding its teratogenicity.[115,116]
Tobacco	Smoking during pregnancy is associated with increased rates of IUGR, prematurity, spontaneous abortion, neonatal and postnatal deaths and placenta previa. Such conditions occur particularly in women who are regular smokers of more than 10 cigarettes daily. Tobacco chewing during pregnancy is also associated with a greatly increased rate of stillbirth, IUGR and prematurity.[86,117,118]

References

1. Wilson JG, Fraser FC, eds. Handbook of teratology. Vol I. General principles and etiology. New York: Plenum Press, 1977.

2. Pagliaro LA, Hays DP. Teratogenesis. In: Pagliaro LA, Pagliaro AM, eds. Problems in pediatric drug therapy 2nd ed. Hamilton, IL: Drug Intelligence Publications, 1987:58.

3. Rudolph AM. Effects of aspirin and acetaminophen in pregnancy and in the newborn. Arch Intern Med 1981;141:358-63.

4. Levin DL, Mills LJ, Weinberg AG. Hemodynamic, pulmonary vascular, and myocardial abnormalities secondary to pharmacologic constriction of the fetal ductus arteriosus: a possible mechanism for persistent pulmonary hypertension and transient tricuspid insufficiency in the newborn infant. Circulation 1979;60:360-4.

5. Mangurten HH, Benawra R. Neonatal codeine withdrawal in infants of nonaddicted mothers. Pediatrics 1980;65:159-60.

6. Ostrea CM, Chavez CJ, Strauss ME. A study of factors that influence the severity of neonatal narcotic withdrawal. J Pediatr 1976;88:642-5.

7a. Maduska AL, Hajghassemali M. A double-blind comparison of butorphanol and meperidine in labour: maternal pain relief and effect on the newborn. Can Anaesth Soc J 1978;25:398-404.

7b. Hatjis CG, Meis PJ. Sinusoidal fetal heart rate pattern associated with butorphanol administration. Obstet Gynecol 1986;67:377-80.

8. Finnegan LP. Management of pregnant drug-dependent women. Ann NY Acad Sci 1978;311:135-46.

9. Newman RG, Bashkow S, Calko D. Results of 313 consecutive live births of infants delivered to patients in the New York City methadone maintenance treatment program. Am J Obstet Gynecol 1975;121:233-7.

10. Blinick G, Jerez E, Wallach RC. Methadone maintenance, pregnancy, and progeny. JAMA 1973;225:477-9.

11. Burstein Y, Rausen AR, Peterson CM. Duration of thrombocytosis in infants of polydrug (including methadone) users. J Pediatr 1982;100:506. Letter.

12. Kopelman AE. Fetal addiction to pentazocine. Pediatrics 1975;55:888-9.

13. Wapner RJ, Fitzsimmons J, Ross RD et al. A quantitative evaluation of fetal growth failure in a drug-abusing population. National Institute on Drug Abuse Research Monographs 1981;34:131-2.

14. Refstad SO, Lindbaek E. Ventilatory depression of the newborn of women receiving pethidine or pentazocine. Br J Anaesth 1980;52:265-70.

15. Golden NL, King KC, Sokol RJ. Propoxyphene and acetaminophen: possible effects on the fetus. Clin Pediatr 1982;21:752-4.

16. Hall JG, Pauli RM, Wilson KM. Maternal and fetal sequelae of anticoagulation during pregnancy. Am J Med 1980;68:122-40.

17. Nageotte MP, Freeman RK, Garite TJ et al. Anticoagulation in pregnancy. Am J Obstet Gynecol 1981;141:472-3. Letter.

18. Whitfield MF. Chondrodysplasia punctata after warfarin in early pregnancy. Case report and summary of the literature. Arch Dis Child 1980;55:139-42.

19. Butler CD. Carbamazepine, seizure disorders, and pregnancy. JAMA 1983;250:3164. Letter.

20. Seip M. Growth retardation, dysmorphic facies and minor malformations following massive exposure to phenobarbitone in utero. Acta Paediatr Scand 1976;65:617-21.

21. Berkowitz FE. Fetal malformation due to phenobarbitone: a case report. S Afr Med J 1979;55:100-1.

22. Dansky L, Andermann E, Andermann F et al. Maternal epilepsy and congenital malformations: correlation with maternal plasma anticonvulsant levels during pregnancy. In: Janz D et al, eds. Epilepsy, pregnancy, and the child. New York: Raven Press, 1982:251-8.

23. Lipson A, Bale P. Ependymoblastoma associated with prenatal exposure to diphenylhydantoin and methylphenobarbitone. Cancer 1985;55:1859-62.

24. Srinivasan G, Seeler RA, Tiruvury A et al. Maternal anticonvulsant therapy and hemorrhagic disease of the newborn. Obstet Gynecol 1982;59:250-2.

25. Biale Y, Lewenthal H. Effect of folic acid supplementation on congenital malformations due to anticonvulsive drugs. Eur J Obstet Gynecol Reprod Biol 1984;18:211-6.

26. Hanson JW, Myrianthopoulos NC, Sedgwick-Harvey MA et al. Risks to the offspring of women treated with hydantoin anticonvulsants, with emphasis on the fetal hydantoin syndrome. J Pediatr 1976;89:662-8.

27. Smith DW. Recognizable patterns of human malformation. 3rd ed. Philadelphia: WB Saunders, 1982.

28. Rating D, Nau H, Jager-Roman E et al. Teratogenic and pharmacokinetic studies of primidone during pregnancy and in the offspring of epileptic women. Acta Paediatr Scand 1982;71:301-11.

29. Briggs GG, Freeman RK, Yaffe SJ. Drugs in pregnancy and lactation. 2nd ed. Baltimore: Williams & Wilkins, 1986.

30. Clay SA, McVie R, Chen H. Possible teratogenic effect of valproic acid. J Pediatr 1981;99:828. Letter.

31. Garden AS, Benzie RJ, Hutton EM et al. Valproic acid therapy and neural tube defects. Can Med Assoc J 1985;132:933-6.

32. Tein I, MacGregor DL. Possible valproate teratogenicity. Arch Neurol 1985;42:291-3.

33. Nelson MM, Forfar JO. Associations between drugs administered during pregnancy and congenital abnormalities of the fetus. Br Med J 1971;1:523-7.

34. Saxen I. Cleft palate and maternal diphenhydramine intake. Lancet 1974;1:407-8. Letter.

35. Landers DV, Green JR, Sweet RL. Antibiotic use during pregnancy and the postpartum period. Clin Obstet Gynecol 1983;26:391-406.

36. Wolfe MS, Cordero JF. Safety of chloroquine in chemosuppression of malaria during pregnancy. Br Med J 1985;290:1466-7.

37. Anon. Dapsone package insert. Princeton, NJ: Jacobus Pharmaceutical, 1985. In: Barnhart ER, ed. Physicians' desk reference. Oradell, NJ: Medical Economics, 1986:951-2.

38. Snider DE, Layde PM, Johnson MW et al. Treatment of tuberculosis during pregnancy Am Rev Respir Dis 1980;122:65-79.

39. Peterson WF, Stauch JE, Ryder CD. Metronidazole in pregnancy. Am J Obstet Gynecol 1966;94:343-9.

40. Morgan I. Metronidazole treatment in pregnancy. Int J Gynaecol Obstet 1978;15:501-2.

41. Powell RD, DeGowin RL, Alving AS. Nitrofurantoin-induced hemolysis. J Lab Clin Med 1963;62:1002-3. Abstract.

42. Dannenberg AL, Dorfman SF, Johnson J. Use of quinine for self-induced abortion. S Med J 1983;76:846-9.

43. Lewis JH, Weingold AB, and the Committee on FDA-related Matters, American College of Gastroenterology. The use of gastrointestinal drugs during pregnancy and lactation. Am J Gastroenterol 1985;80:912-23.

44. Baiocco PJ, Korelitz BI. The influence of inflammatory bowel disease and its treatment on pregnancy and fetal outcome. J Clin Gastroenterol 1984;6:211-6.

45. Jarnerot G, Into-Malmberg MB, Esbjorner E. Placental transfer of sulphasalazine and sulphapyridine and some of its metabolites. Scand J Gastroenterol 1981;16:693-7.

46. Mogadam M, Dobbins WO, Korelitz BI et al. Pregnancy in inflammatory bowel disease: effect of sulfasalazine and corticosteroids on fetal outcome. Gastroenterology 1981;80:72-6.

47. Davis JS, Kaufman RH. Tetracycline toxicity. A clinicopathologic study with special reference to liver damage and its relationship to pregnancy. Am J Obstet Gynecol 1966;95:523-9.

48. Genot MT, Golan HP, Porter PJ et al. Effect of administration of tetracycline in pregnancy on the primary dentition of the offspring. J Oral Med 1970;25:75-9.

49. Gililland J, Weinstein L. The effects of cancer chemotherapeutic agents on the developing fetus. Obstet Gynecol Surv 1983;38:6-13.

50. Blatt J, Mulvihill JJ, Ziegler JL et al. Pregnancy outcome following cancer chemotherapy. Am J Med 1980;69:828-32.

51. Wilson AL, Matzke GR. The treatment of hypertension in pregnancy. Drug Intell Clin Pharm 1981;15:21-6.

52. Naden RP, Redman CWG. Antihypertensive drugs in pregnancy. Clin Perinatol 1985;12:521-38.

53. Rotmensch HH, Elkayam U, Frishman W. Antiarrhythmic drug therapy during pregnancy. Ann Intern Med 1983;98:487-97.

54. Mabie WC, Pernoll ML, Biswas MK. Chronic hypertension in pregnancy. Obstet Gynecol 1986;67:197-205.

55. Sibai BM, Grossman RA, Grossman HG. Effects of diuretics on plasma volume in pregnancies with long-term hypertension. Am J Obstet Gynecol 1984;150:831-5.

56. Qvist N, Storm K, Holmskov A. Cimetidine as pre-anesthetic agent for cesarean section: perinatal effects on the infant, the placental transfer of cimetidine and its elimination in the infants. J Perinat Med 1985;13:179-83.

57. Kurachi K, Aono T, Minagawa J et al. Congenital malformations of newborn infants after clomiphene-induced ovulation. Fertil Steril 1983;40:187-9.

58. Boue JG, Boue A. Increased frequency of chromosomal anomalies in abortions after induced ovulation. Lancet 1973;1:679-80. Letter.

59. Oakley GP, Flynt JW. Increased prevalence of Down's syndrome (Mongolism) among the offspring of women treated with ovulation-inducing agents. Teratology 1972;5:264. Abstract.

60. Bongiovanni AM, McPadden AJ. Steroids during pregnancy and possible fetal consequences. Fertil Steril 1960;11:181-6.

61. MacArthur BA, Howie RN, Dezoete JA et al. Cognitive and psychosocial development of 4-year-old children whose mothers were treated antenatally with betamethasone. Pediatrics 1981;68:638-43.

62. Saenger P. Abnormal sex differentiation. J Pediatr 1984;104:1-17.

63. Schardein JL. Congenital abnormalities and hormones during pregnancy: a critical review. Teratology 1980;22:251-70.

64. Herbst AL. Diethylstilbestrol and other sex hormones during pregnancy. Obstet Gynecol 1981;58:35S-40S.

65. Leary FJ, Resseguie LJ, Kurland LT et al. Males exposed in utero to diethylstilbestrol. JAMA 1984;252:2984-9.

66. Hill RM, Stern L. Drugs in pregnancy: effects on the fetus and newborn. Drugs 1979;17:182-97.

67. Mestman JH. Thyroid disease in pregnancy. Clin Perinatol 1985;12:651-67.

68. Einhorn J, Hulten M, Lindsten J et al. Clinical and cytogenetic investigation in children of parents treated with radioiodine. Acta Radiol 1972;11:193-208.

69. Calabrese JR, Gulledge AD. Psychotropics during pregnancy and lactation: a review. Psychosomatics 1985;26:413-29.

70. Park JM, Sridaromont S, Ledbetter EO et al. Ebstein's anomaly of the tricuspid valve associated with prenatal exposure to lithium carbonate. Am J Dis Child 1980;134:703-4.

71. Rane A, Tomson G, Bjarke B. Effects of maternal lithium therapy in a newborn infant. J Pediatr 1978;93:296-7.

72. Edlund MJ, Craig TJ. Antipsychotic drug use and birth defects: an epidemiologic reassessment. Comprehen Psychiatry 1984;25:32-7.

73. Desmond MM, Schwanecke RP, Wilson GS et al. Maternal barbiturate utilization and neonatal withdrawal symptomatology. J Pediatr 1972;80:190-7.

74. Milkovich L, van den Berg BJ. Effects of prenatal meprobamate and chlordiazepoxide hydrochloride on human embryonic and fetal development. N Engl J Med 1974;291:1268-71.

75. Rosenberg L, Mitchell AA, Parsells JL et al. Lack of relation of oral clefts to diazepam use during pregnancy. N Engl J Med 1983;309:1282-5.

76. Shiono PH, Mills JL. Oral clefts and diazepam use during pregnancy. N Engl J Med 1984;311:919-20. Letter.

77. Rivas F, Hernandez A, Cantu JM. Acentric craniofacial cleft in a newborn female prenatally exposed to a high dose of diazepam. Teratology 1984;30:179-80.

78. Tannenbaum TN, Goldberg RJ. Exposure to anesthetic gases and reproductive outcome. A review of the epidemiologic literature. J Occupational Med 1985;27:659-68.

79. Vessey MP, Nunn JF. Occupational hazards of anaesthesia. Br Med J 1980;281:696-8.

80. Shirkey HC, Ericson AJ. Adverse reactions to drugs — their relation to growth and development. In: Shirkey HC, ed. Pediatric therapy. 6th ed. St. Louis: CV Mosby, 1980;110-51.

81. Blanco JD, Gibbs RS. Immunizations in pregnancy. Clin Obstet Gynecol 1982;25:611-7.

82. Milkovich L, van den Berg BJ. Effects of antenatal exposure to anorectic drugs. Am J Obstet Gynecol

1977;129:637-42.

83. Larsson G. The amphetamine addicted mother and her child. Acta Paediatr Scand 1980;278(Suppl):8-24.

84. Stamatos MN. The most important step forward in years (etretinate). Nutley, NJ: Roche Laboratories, 1986. Promotional letter.

85. Anon. Etretinate approved. FDA Drug Bull 1986;16(2):16-7.

86. Cohen DL, Orzel J, Taylor A. Infants of mothers receiving gold therapy. Arthritis Rheum 1981;24:104-5. Letter.

87. Lammer EJ, Chen DT, Hoar RM et al. Retinoic acid embryopathy. N Engl J Med 1985;313:837-41.

88. McBride WG. Limb reduction deformities in child exposed to isotretinoin in utero on gestation days 26-40 only. Lancet 1985;1:1276. Letter.

89. Stern RS, Rosa F, Baum C. Isotretinoin and pregnancy. J Am Acad Dermatol 1984;10:851-4.

90. Shnider SM. Choice of anesthesia for labor and delivery. Obstet Gynecol 1981;58:24S-34S.

91. Singhi S,Chookang E, Hall JStE et al. Iatrogenic neonatal and maternal hyponatraemia following oxytocin and aqueous glucose infusion during labour. Br J Obstet Gynaecol 1985;92:356-63.

92. Scheinberg IH, Sternlieb I. Pregnancy in penicillamine-treated patients with Wilson's disease. N Engl J Med 1975;293:1300-2.

93. Linares A, Zarranz JJ, Rodriguez-Alarcon J et al. Reversible cutis laxa due to maternal d-penicillamine treatment. Lancet 1979;2:43. Letter.

94. Zbinden G. Investigations on the toxicity of tretinoin administered systemically to animals. Acta Dermatovener (Stockholm) 1975;Suppl 74:36-40.

95. Shapiro S, Slone D, Heinonen OP et al. Birth defects and vaginal spermicides. JAMA 1982;247:2381-4.

96. Jick H, Walker AM, Rothman KJ et al. Vaginal spermicides and congenital disorders. JAMA 1981;245:1329-32.

97. Bernhardt IB, Dorsey DJ. Hypervitaminosis A and congenital renal anomalies in a human infant. Obstet Gynecol 1974;43:750-5.

98. Parkinson CE, Tan JCY. Vitamin A concentration in amniotic fluid and maternal serum related to neural-tube defects. Br J Obstet Gynaecol 1982;89:935-9.

99. Geelen JAG. Hypervitaminosis A induced teratogenesis. Crit Rev Toxicol 1979;6:351-75.

100. Friedman WF. Vitamin D and the supravalvular aortic stenosis syndrome. Adv Teratol 1968;3:85-96.

101. Martin NDT, Snodgrass GJAI, Makin HLJ et al. Increased plasma 1,25-dihydroxyvitamin D in infants with hypercalcemia and elfin facies. N Engl J Med 1985;313:889-9. Letter.

102. Chesney RW, DeLuca HF, Gertner JM et al. Increased plasma 1,25-dihydroxyvitamin D in infants with hypercalcemia and elfin facies. N Engl J Med 1985;313:889-90. Letter.

103. Kline J, Stein Z, Shrout P et al. Drinking during pregnancy and spontaneous abortion. Lancet 1980;2:176-80.

104. Harlap S, Shiono PH. Alcohol, smoking, and incidence of spontaneous abortions in the first and second trimester. Lancet 1980;2:173-6.

105. Streissguth AP, Clarren SK, Jones KL. Natural history of the fetal alcohol syndrome: a 10-year follow-up of eleven patients. Lancet 1985;2:85-91.

106. Watkinson B, Fried PA. Maternal caffeine use before, during and after pregnancy and effects upon offspring. Neurobehav Toxicol Teratol 1985;7:9-17.

107. Acker D, Sachs BP, Tracey KJ et al. Abruptio placentae associated with cocaine use. Am J Obstet Gynecol 1983;146:220-1.

108. Chasnoff IJ, Burns WJ, Schnoll SH et al. Cocaine use in pregnancy. N Engl J Med 1985;313:666-9.

109. Chasnoff IJ, Bussey ME, Savich R et al. Perinatal cerebral infarction and maternal cocaine use. J Pediatr 1986;108:456-9.

110. Personal Communication. Xlina Bean, MD. Neonatalogy. Associate Professor, Pediatrics; Associate Director, Special Care Nursery, King-Drew Medical Center, Los Angeles, CA.

111. Finnegan LP. The effects of narcotics and alcohol on pregnancy and the newborn. Ann NY Acad Sci 1981;362:136-57.

112. Vargas GC, Pildes RS, Vidyasagar D et al. Effect of maternal heroin addiction on 67 liveborn neonates. Clin Pediatr 1975;14:751-7.

113. Fried PA. Marijuana use by pregnant women: neurobehavioral effects in neonates. Drug Alcohol Depend 1980;6:415-24.

114. O'Connell CM, Fried PA. An investigation of prenatal cannabis exposure and minor physical anomalies in a low risk population. Neurobehav Toxicol Teratol 1984;6:345-50.

115. Chasnoff IJ, Burns WJ, Hatcher RP et al. Phencyclidine: effects on the fetus and neonate. Dev Pharmacol Ther 1983;6:404-8.

116. Strauss AA, Modanlou HD, Bosu SK. Neonatal manifestations of maternal phencyclidine (PCP) abuse. Pediatrics 1981;68:550-2.

117. Cole H. Studying reproductive risks, smoking. JAMA 1986;255:22-3.

118. Papoz L, Eschwege E, Pequignot G et al. Maternal smoking and birth weight in relation to dietary habits. Am J Obstet Gynecol 1982;142:870-6.

119. Louik C, Mitchell AA, Werler MM et al. Maternal exposure to spermicides in relation to certain birth defects. N Engl J Med 1987;317:474-8.

120. Warburton D, Neugut RH, Lustenberger A et al. Lack of association between spermicide use and trisomy. N Engl J Med 1987;317:478-82.

9 *GERIATRIC DRUG USE*

GERIATRIC DRUG THERAPY HAS BECOME AN IMPORTANT SPECIALTY area, due to several factors. Among these are the increasing numbers of elderly, particularly those over 80 years; the elderly use more medications than other age groups; the elderly make significant medication errors; and the prevalence of adverse drug reactions is greatest in the elderly.[1-3] It is important, therefore, that health professionals recognize that the elderly can react to drugs differently than other adults and, therefore, may require closer monitoring and/or modification of their drug regimens.

Researchers have begun to examine why the elderly may react differently to drugs. Alterations in the physiological and pharmacological characteristics described below have been suggested as explanations for specific drug responses in the elderly. See references 4–14 for a more detailed discussion.

Absorption. With aging, there is a decrease in gastric secretions, acidity, peristalsis, the number of microvilli, splanchnic blood flow and gastric emptying,[15,16] all of which suggest altered absorption of orally administered drugs in elderly patients. However, a number of studies indicate that the quantity or extent of absorbed drug is *not* affected by age, probably because most drug absorption is passive and primarily dependent on concentration gradients.[4,6] Because of an age-related decrease in intestinal perfusion, it has been hypothesized that the rate of oral drug absorption might be slowed.[11] From a limited number of studies of a few drugs, this hypothesis does not appear to be true. Pathological conditions, meals and concurrent drug therapy are probably more important factors affecting drug absorption than age alone.

Distribution. Body weight generally decreases and body composition changes with age; these factors can alter the volume of distribution (V_d) of drugs in the elderly. Total body water and lean body mass decrease, while body fat increases in proportion to total body weight. The percent of body weight contributed by fat changes from 18% and 33% in young men and women, respectively, to 36% and 45% in their elderly counterparts.[17] Therefore, elderly patients are particularly susceptible to overdosage from drugs which should be dosed on ideal body weight (IBW). Theoretically, highly lipid soluble drugs may have an increased V_d and a prolonged effect. Conversely, highly water soluble drugs may have a decreased V_d, and at least transiently increased plasma levels and effect.[8]

Although cardiac output does not appear to decrease with age,[18] some chronic diseases affecting the elderly do contribute to a decrease in cardiac output and regional blood flow. There is some evidence that blood is preferentially shunted to the brain, heart and muscles and away from the liver and kidneys.[8] These changes could explain the slowed elimination of some drugs and the heightened sensitivity to others.

Protein Binding. The proportion of albumin among total plasma proteins decreases with age and with some chronic diseases.[19] Serum albumin can be significantly decreased despite a normal total serum protein value. One study showed a drop in serum albumin from 3.97 g/dl in those less than 40 years to 3.58 g/dl in those older than 80 years.[20] This phenomenon could alter the percentage of free drug available for pharmacological effect and elimination, and may be more pronounced in seriously or chronically ill elderly where albumin levels are more depressed. An exception are those drugs which are bound to α_1-acid glycoprotein (eg, propranolol); this protein appears to be increased in the elderly and therefore binding may increase.[14] The net effect on clearance varies depending on whether metabolism or elimination is also altered. There is also some evidence that the elderly may have a greater potential for protein displacement drug interactions.[21]

Metabolism. Liver size and hepatic blood flow decrease with age. It has been estimated that hepatic blood flow decreases 40% from age 25 to 65 years.[12] Metabolism of drugs with high hepatic extraction ratios depends to a large part on liver blood flow,[22] and several of these drugs show decreased clearances in the elderly. Age appears to affect oxidation by microsomal enzyme systems more than genetically determined acetylation and other oxidative metabolic processes.[23] Several studies show a large intersubject variation in metabolic rate which is unexplained by age. Continued study into the role of aging in hepatic drug metabolism is needed before more definitive explanations can be made.

Renal. The effect of aging on the renal disposition of drugs is probably the most completely understood and important aspect of geriatric drug therapy. Glomerular filtration and tubular secretion both decrease significantly with age and renal blood flow decreases about 1% per year.[14,24] Creatinine clearance decreases approximately 35% between ages 20 and 90 in patients without evidence of renal disease.[24] In addition, volume depletion, congestive heart failure and renal disease can decrease organ function further. Because creatinine production also decreases with age, serum creatinine may be normal despite a significant decrease in renal function. It is therefore recommended that creatinine clearance be measured or estimated using a method which incorporates age and weight[25,26] when adjusting doses of renally excreted drugs in the elderly. Plasma levels of potentially toxic, renally excreted drugs should be closely monitored even if the drug has not been specifically studied in the elderly.

Pharmacodynamic Factors. Heightened drug effects which have not been explained by altered pharmacokinetic variables have been hypothesized to be caused by changed tissue sensitivity, altered homeostasis or complications of chronic diseases seen in the elderly.[7] More research is needed, especially in quantitatively comparing the changes seen in the elderly with younger adult populations.

Other. Although cigarette smoking has been shown to induce metabolism of some drugs in young patients, this phenomenon may not be as pronounced in the elderly.[4] Some heretofore unexplained interpatient variations of pharmacokinetic data may be explained by smoking history; unfortunately, many published studies do not indicate smoking history.

Nutritional intake can be diminished in the elderly and can lead to nutritional and vitamin deficiencies.[27,28] The nutritional status of the elderly may be important in their handling of some drugs.[29]

Use of the Table. The table which follows provides pharmacologic and pharmacokinetic data for drugs which have been studied in the elderly. Some conflicts in data may be due to health status of the elderly; status is not always stated, methods of classification vary, and degree of ambulation may differ. When a dosage change is recommended due to decreased renal function, consult specific drug literature or general references such as reference number 30.

The following abbreviations are used in the table:

> (E) —Elderly; ages vary for different studies, but uniformly older than 50 years.
>
> (Y) —Young; uniformly younger than 50 years, usually in the 20–30 year range.
>
> Cl —Total body clearance.
>
> Cl_{cr} —Creatinine clearance.
>
> Cr_s —Serum creatinine.
>
> IBW —Ideal body weight.
>
> $t_{1/2}$ —Half-life.
>
> V_d —Apparent volume of distribution.

The table begins on page 215.

Geriatric Drug Use

DRUG	CLINICAL FINDINGS AND MANAGEMENT	DRUG-SPECIFIC DATA
ALCOHOL	Increased blood levels in (E) correlated with decreased V_d; rate of elimination is no different in (Y) vs (E).[31] The (E) should be especially cautioned not to ingest alcohol with other sedative-hypnotics.	Peak alcohol level after infusion: 155 mg/dl (Y) vs 176 mg/dl (E)[31] V_d: 35 L (Y) vs 32 L (E).[31]
ANALGESICS AND ANTIPYRETICS		
Acetaminophen	There are large interpatient variations; alteration of dose is not necessary. No data on comparative toxicity.	No difference in extent or rate of PO absorption or V_d in (Y) vs (E).[32] $t_{1/2}$: 1.8 hr (Y) vs 2.2 hr (E).[32,33] Cl: 0.34 L/hr/kg (Y) vs 0.25 L/hr/kg (E).[32]
Aspirin	Single-dose studies indicate no dosage alteration needed for analgesia; more study is needed in chronic anti-inflammatory doses. Monitor carefully for dose-related toxicities and gastrointestinal ulceration; plasma levels may be helpful in (E) with hearing impairment.	No difference in extent or rate of PO absorption (Y) vs (E).[34-36] $t_{1/2}$: 2.4 hr (Y) vs 3.7 hr (E).[35] V_d: 3.8 L (Y) vs 5.5 L (E).[35] Tinnitus is not a reliable symptom of toxicity in patients with hearing loss.[37]

Continued

Geriatric Drug Use

DRUG	CLINICAL FINDINGS AND MANAGEMENT	DRUG-SPECIFIC DATA
Meperidine and Morphine	The (E) may have increased sensitivity to narcotic analgesics and require lower doses to achieve pain relief.[4,38] The (E) may have increased potential for side effects such as respiratory depression, because of decreased protein binding and initially higher plasma levels.[39,40] Monitor for respiratory depression, especially with IV doses in (E) with lung disease.	Morphine: $t_{1/2}$: 3 hr (Y) vs 4.5 hr (E). V_d: 3.2 L/kg (Y) vs 4.7 L/kg (E). Cl: 0.88 L/hr/kg (Y) vs 0.74 L/hr/kg (E).
Nonsteroidal Anti-Inflammatory Agents	Acute renal failure associated with nonsteroidal agents is more frequent in (E), especially with concomitant gout and atherosclerotic vascular disease.[43] Unbound **naproxen** in (E) found to be twice that of (Y); may explain increased side effects seen in (E).[42] Risk of gastrointestinal hemorrhage may be greater in (E) when agents with extended duration of action are used (eg, **piroxicam**), although increased plasma levels seen in (E) do not appear to correlate with prevalence of adverse effects.[44,45]	
Phenylbutazone	Sodium retention and ulcerogenic potential are especially undesirable in (E); avoid if at all possible or use with caution in (E).	No difference in extent or rate of PO absorption or V_d (Y) vs (E).[32] $t_{1/2}$: somewhat increased in (E),[32] possibly due to decreased serum albumin and drug binding.[19]

Continued

Geriatric Drug Use

DRUG	CLINICAL FINDINGS AND MANAGEMENT	DRUG-SPECIFIC DATA
ANTICHOLINERGICS	The (E) appear to be more sensitive,[4] and many other drugs (E) take have anticholinergic properties. Monitor for confusion, nightmares, urinary hesitancy and retention, and constipation which can lead to fecal impaction.	
ANTICOAGULANTS		
Heparin	Age does not increase risk of minor bleeding, but evidence is inconclusive with respect to risk of major bleeding. Females of all ages were found to have a higher risk of bleeding than males of all ages.[46] Limit anticoagulant treatment in (E) to conditions in which anticoagulants have demonstrated clinical benefit. Dose conservatively; monitor frequently for evidence of bleeding.	
Warfarin	Two studies[47,48] found an increased frequency of bleeding with age, while one study[49] showed no correlation. Difference is probably the result of how bleeding was categorized. The (E) and especially (E) women are probably at higher risk of bleeding while on anticoagulants. (E) have a higher risk of major trauma (eg, hip fracture) and physiological changes in subcutaneous tissues and joint spaces, which may allow bleeding to expand unchecked. The dose of warfarin to achieve the same degree of anticoagulation was found	No difference in V_d, Cl, $t_{1/2}$; degree or affinity of protein binding in (Y) vs (E). Increased sensitivity may be due to dietary deficiency and/or altered kinetics of vitamin K in (E).[50]

Continued

Geriatric Drug Use

DRUG	CLINICAL FINDINGS AND MANAGEMENT	DRUG-SPECIFIC DATA
	to be 40% lower in (E), indicating increased sensitivity,[51,52] although one study failed to show increased sensitivity.[53]	
ANTICONVULSANTS		
Phenytoin	Increased Cl in (E) is correlated with decreased serum albumin and phenytoin binding.[54] Overdosage and underdosage are possible in (E) due to increased free phenytoin. Monitor free phenytoin levels, if possible. One recommendation is to initiate therapy with 200 mg/day[55] and monitor carefully for dose-related toxicities and seizure activity, especially in patients with low serum albumin. Time to reach steady-state after dosage adjustment may be longer in (E).[56]	Cl: 0.026 L/hr/kg (Y) vs 0.042 L/hr/kg (E).[54] Total phenytoin plasma levels increase with age.[57]
ANTI-INFECTIVE AGENTS		
Aminoglycosides	Although one study showed no change in pharmacokinetic parameters using **gentamicin** in (Y) vs (E) with Cl_{cr} greater than 80 ml/min,[58] there was much interpatient variation, and the potential exists for accumulation and overdosage because (E) have decreased lean body mass and likelihood of decreased renal clearance of drug. Dose conservatively based on IBW after determining estimated or actual Cl_{cr}. Monitor and adjust regimen using plasma aminoglycoside levels. Consider audiometry	**Kanamycin:** $t_{1/2}$: 1.78 hr (Y) vs 4.7 hr (E) despite comparable Cr_s.[59]

Continued

Geriatric Drug Use

DRUG	CLINICAL FINDINGS AND MANAGEMENT	DRUG-SPECIFIC DATA
	and vestibular function monitoring, especially in (E) with severe renal or hearing impairment.	
Amoxicillin and Ampicillin	Both drugs have high therapeutic indices; therefore, dosage reduction is considered only in moderate to severe renal impairment.	Amoxicillin: $t_{1/2}$: 1 hr (Y) vs 2.7 hr (E).[60]
		Ampicillin: No difference in extent or rate of PO absorption or V_d.[61]
		$t_{1/2}$: 1.68 hr (Y) vs 6.7 hr (E).[61]
		Cl: 0.18 L/hr/kg (Y) vs 0.08 L/hr/kg (E).[61]
Isoniazid	No need to alter dosage regimen unless (E) can be identified as a "slow acetylator". Increased risk of hepatitis with age, especially in age group 50–64 yr.[62] Routine prophylaxis with isoniazid for recent PPD converters older than 35 yr is not recommended unless additional risk factors for TB are present.[64]	$t_{1/2}$: no difference in (Y) vs (E) although both groups had fast and slow acetylators.[23,63]
Penicillin G	Because of its high therapeutic index, dosage reduction is considered only in moderate to severe renal impairment.	No difference in rate of absorption of **procaine penicillin G** from IM injection site in (Y) vs (E).[65]
Sulfamethizole	Dosage reduction is necessary in moderate to severe renal impairment; consider alternate drug. Maintain adequate fluid intake.	No difference in extent or rate of PO absorption or V_d in (Y) vs (E).

Continued

Geriatric Drug Use

DRUG	CLINICAL FINDINGS AND MANAGEMENT	DRUG-SPECIFIC DATA
		Renal clearance: 8.7 L/hr/1.73 M^2 (Y) vs 3.6 L/hr/1.73 M^2 (E).[32]
Sulfamethoxazole-Trimethoprim	Minor differences between (Y) and (E) pharmacokinetic parameters. No need to alter dose unless there is significant renal impairment.[66]	
Tetracyclines	Dosage alteration is probably not necessary; consider **doxycycline** or non-tetracycline in severe renal impairment.	No difference in extent or rate of PO tetracycline absorption in (E) with achlorhydria.
		Rate of elimination slower in (E) probably due to decreased renal clearance.[67]
CARDIAC DRUGS		
Digoxin	There is a higher prevalence of side effects in (E), probably due to improper dosing and electrolyte imbalance in most cases. (E) with ischemic disease may have increased sensitivity to arrhythmogenic effects of digoxin. Avoid loading method of digitalization in CHF when possible; try to digitalize with maintenance dosing and treat CHF acutely with diuretics. Dose conservatively using IBW and estimated or measured Cl$_{cr}$ (see Digoxin monograph). Maintain adequate serum potassium. Monitor usual parameters for toxicity, especially CNS symptoms such as listlessness, agitation and pseudo-	No difference in extent of PO absorption, although rate of absorption is somewhat slower in (E).
		$t_{1/2}$: 36.8 hr (range 24–53 hr) (Y) vs 70 hr (range 24–129 hr) (E). Note large interpatient variation despite normal Cr$_s$ in all patients.[70]
		V$_d$: No difference in (Y) vs (E).[70]

Continued

Geriatric Drug Use

DRUG	CLINICAL FINDINGS AND MANAGEMENT	DRUG-SPECIFIC DATA
	hallucinations.[4] Periodically review the need for continued therapy, because some evidence suggests digoxin withdrawal may not result in cardiac decompensation in certain (E).[68,69]	Cl: 6.37 L/hr (Y) vs 2.24 L/hr (E).[70]
Diltiazem	Absorption is similar in (Y) vs (E), but Cl is significantly decreased in (E); suggest initiating with lower dose.[72] Diltiazem may have a slower onset of action in (E).[73]	Cl: 4.98 L/hr/1.73 M^2 (Y) vs 3.18 L/hr/1.73 M^2 (E).[71] $t_{1/2}$: 6.6 hr (Y) vs 10.9 hr (E).[72]
Disopyramide	(E) show increased V_d, prolonged $t_{1/2}$ and decreased Cl when compared to (Y). Smoking increases Cl significantly in (E) over nonsmoking (E). Lower initial dose by 30% in nonsmoking (E).[74]	
Lidocaine	The (E) have an increased prevalence of certain side effects, probably related to underlying cardiac disease.[4] Cl is significantly decreased in patients with CHF or liver disease. A nomogram has been developed for dosing of these patients.[78] One study showed no difference in pharmacokinetic parameters in (Y) vs (E) females without cardiac or hepatic disease, while significant differences existed among males;[77] an older study showed general differences between (Y) and (E) subjects.[75] (E) males without chronic disease may need the equivalent loading dose (but a 35% lower infusion rate) as (Y) males.[77] Because of wide interpatient variation in data, plasma levels are suggested.	$t_{1/2}$: 1.66 hr (Y) males vs 2.7 hr (E) males.[77] V_d: No difference (Y) vs (E).[77] Cl: 0.77 L/hr/kg (Y) males vs 1.19 L/hr/kg (E) males.[77] Cl: 42 L/hr (all healthy) vs 26.58 L/hr (CHF) and 25.14 L/hr (liver disease).[76]

Continued

Geriatric Drug Use

DRUG	CLINICAL FINDINGS AND MANAGEMENT	DRUG-SPECIFIC DATA
Propranolol	Serious side effects such as complete heart block, pulmonary edema and profound bradycardia are more common in (E).[78] CNS symptoms of disorientation, visual hallucinations and psychosis have been reported in (E).[79-81] Higher plasma levels in (E) are thought to be the result of decreased hepatic extraction and metabolism.[82] The (E) seem to have a decreased sensitivity to the drug which may be related to reduced β-adrenoreceptor responsiveness or decreased binding.[84,85] The (E) appear to be less sensitive to propranolol-induced bradycardia during exercise;[4] therefore, be wary of using this as an end-point in dosing. Smoking and presence of hyperthyroidism appear to increase rate of metabolism in (Y) and (E).[86,88,89]	Single IV dose: $t_{1/2}$: 152 min (Y) vs 254 min (E).[82] V_d: No difference (Y) vs (E).[82,83] Cl: 0.79 L/hr/kg (Y) vs 0.47 L/hr/kg (E).[82] Multiple PO dosing: (E) plasma levels 3.1 times higher than (Y);[82] no difference found in plasma levels and quantity absorbed in extremely healthy (E).[87]
Quinidine	The (E) may be predisposed to toxicity because of prolonged elimination; optimal dosing may require less frequent administration in (E) or lower dose.[90,91] Plasma levels may be helpful in establishing optimal dosing regimen.	$t_{1/2}$: 7.3 hr (Y) vs 9.7 hr (E). V_d and % bound: no difference in (Y) vs (E). Cl: 0.24 L/hr/kg (Y) vs 0.16 L/hr/kg (E).[90]
DIURETICS	The (E) respond to IV **furosemide** more slowly than (Y), but total 24-hr diuresis is greater in (E); IV dosing in (E) may need to be higher for initial diuretic effect.[92] Although pharmacokinetic changes lead to higher plasma levels of furosemide in (E), one study showed	Fasting blood sugar increases an average 9.6 mg/dl after 2 yr of diuretic therapy in (E), which correlates with the degree of hypokalemia.[96] Continued

Geriatric Drug Use

DRUG	CLINICAL FINDINGS AND MANAGEMENT	DRUG-SPECIFIC DATA
	there was no increase in effect because of decreased GFR in (E).[93] The (E) have a high prevalence of hypokalemia and other side effects.[94,95] Maintain adequate serum potassium and hydration. Monitor for symptoms of glucose intolerance and postural hypotension. Periodically re-evaluate the need for continued therapy.	Diuretics can be withdrawn in certain (E) without deleterious effect.[97]
HORMONES AND SYNTHETIC SUBSTITUTES		
Insulin	Dose and monitor insulin therapy as in (Y).	No altered kinetics in (E).[4]
Sulfonylureas	The (E) have a higher prevalence of hypoglycemia precipitated by sulfonylureas than (Y).[98] Evidence of longer $t_{1/2}$ and increased V_d occurs with **gliclazide**.[99] Use long-acting agents such as **chlorpropamide** and **glyburide** with caution; hypoglycemia may be pronounced and prolonged in (E).	Unbound **tolbutamide** is 25% higher in (E), because of lower serum albumin.[100]
HYPOTENSIVE AGENTS	Although some caution is needed, and controversy exists, treatment of systolic and diastolic hypertension in (E) appears to be indicated, because the risk of cardiovascular morbidity and mortality in general is reduced with treatment.[7,101] Prevalence of postural hypotension[102] and CNS side effects[103] are higher in (E) taking antihypertensive medications.	

Continued

Geriatric Drug Use

DRUG	CLINICAL FINDINGS AND MANAGEMENT	DRUG-SPECIFIC DATA
Labetalol	Bioavailability increases significantly with age; initiate with smaller doses. [104]	

PSYCHOTHERAPEUTIC AGENTS

DRUG	CLINICAL FINDINGS AND MANAGEMENT	DRUG-SPECIFIC DATA
Antidepressants, Heterocyclic	The agent should be chosen based on side effect profile, since (E) are more sensitive to the side effects of sedation, postural hypotension, anticholinergic (especially urinary retention) and cardiac toxicities of this class. [112-114] Newer agents, especially **trazodone**, may offer benefit because of less anticholinergic effect, however potential for cardiac toxicity exists and development of priapism, although rare, may be irreversible. [114] Wait longer to assess therapeutic effect and adjust dosage in (E), because of prolonged $t_{1/2}$. **Dexamethasone suppression test** results may be altered in (E). [105] Monitor for excessive anticholinergic effects such as urinary hesitancy and retention and constipation. Maintain adequate hydration.	**Imipramine:** $t_{1/2}$: 19 hr (Y) vs 34 hr (E). [111] **Desipramine:** $t_{1/2}$: 23 hr (Y) vs 75 hr (E). [111]
Lithium	The (E) may have a higher prevalence of side effects, especially neurological, and may be more susceptible to volume depletion leading to lithium toxicity; [105] up to 50% lowering of initial dose has been recommended in (E) with further dosage adjustment based on plasma levels. [106] Monitor (E) carefully, especially if on concurrent diuretic therapy.	$t_{1/2}$: 24 hr (Y) vs 36 hr (E). [107] Cl: 1.69 L/hr (Y) vs 0.82 L/hr (E). [108]

Continued

Continued

Geriatric Drug Use

DRUG	CLINICAL FINDINGS AND MANAGEMENT	DRUG-SPECIFIC DATA
Phenothiazines	The (E) can be more sensitive to sedative, anti-cholinergic, cardiac, extrapyramidal and autonomic side effects,[105,109] and (E) women have a higher prevalence of drug-induced tardive dyskinesia than other groups.[110] Use these agents only with an established diagnosis and then start with small dose and increase slowly. Consider using a short-acting benzodiazepine if sedation is the objective.	Frequency of choreiform side effects is 6 times higher in (E).[109]
SEDATIVES AND HYPNOTICS		
Barbiturates	The (E) have shown both prolonged CNS depression and a paradoxical CNS stimulation which can present as restlessness, agitation and psychosis.[4] Avoid using as sedatives in (E). A short-acting benzodiazepine is recommended, if a sedative-hypnotic is indicated.	
Benzodiazepines	Benzodiazepines may accumulate to produce excessive sedation, decreased sexual desire, reduced energy level and aggravation of depression in (E).[115,116] Effects may persist after discontinuation; shorter-acting agents which are eliminated by glucuronidation, such as **oxazepam** and **lorazepam**, may be preferred in the (E).[117,118] (See also individual agents below).	
Chloral Hydrate	Chloral hydrate may be useful, because it causes little effect on normal sleep cycles; however, it can displace protein-bound drugs often used by (E).[114]	

Geriatric Drug Use

DRUG	CLINICAL FINDINGS AND MANAGEMENT	DRUG-SPECIFIC DATA
Chlordiazepoxide	Frequency of drowsiness higher in (E), especially non-smokers.[120,121] Use small initial dose and monitor for signs of accumulation. (See also Benzodiazepines).	$t_{1/2}$: 10 hr (Y) vs 18 hr (E). V_d: 0.4 L/kg (Y) vs 0.5 L/kg (E). Cl: 0.036 L/hr/kg (Y) vs 0.018 L/hr/kg (E). No difference in plasma protein binding.[122]
Diazepam	Frequency of drowsiness is higher in (E).[120,123] May take longer to achieve steady-state levels and effect in (E), especially (E) females, because of increased V_d. Altered pharmacokinetics are especially seen in (E) males.[124-126] No difference in PO or IM absorption in (Y) vs (E).[119] (See also Benzodiazepines).	$t_{1/2}$: 20 hr (Y) vs 90 hr (E). $t_{1/2}$: 31.9 hr (Y) males vs 100.7 hr (E) males.[119] $t_{1/2}$: 44.2 hr (Y) females vs 99.2 hr (E) females.[119] V_d: 1.2 L/kg (Y) males vs 1.7 L/kg (E) males, 1.7 L/kg (Y) females vs 3.0 L/kg (E) females.[127]
Flurazepam	Increased prevalence of dose-related residual drowsiness in (E).[128] Start with 15 mg as initial dose in (E). (See also Benzodiazepines).	**Desalkylflurazepam:** $t_{1/2}$: 74 hr (Y) males vs 160 hr (E) males.[129] $t_{1/2}$: 90 hr (Y) females vs 120 hr (E) females.[129]
Lorazepam	Accumulation and side effects in (E) are less likely than with long-acting benzodiazepines. (See also Benzodiazepines).	$t_{1/2}$: 14.3 hr (Y) vs 15.9 hr (E). V_d: 1.1 L/kg (Y) vs 1 L/kg (E).

Continued

Geriatric Drug Use

DRUG	CLINICAL FINDINGS AND MANAGEMENT	DRUG-SPECIFIC DATA
		Cl: 0.059 L/hr/kg (Y) vs 0.047 L/hr/kg (E).[130]
Nitrazepam	Healthy (E) demonstrated poorer psychomotor performance than (Y), despite unchanged pharmacokinetics.[131] Hospitalized (E) with various diseases had prolonged $t_{1/2}$.[132] Start (E) with lower initial dose than (Y). (See also Benzodiazepines).	$t_{1/2}$: 24.2 hr (Y) vs 39.6 hr (E). V_d: 2.4 L/kg (Y) vs 4.8 L/kg (E).[132]
Oxazepam	Accumulation and side effects are less likely than with long-acting benzodiazepines; oxazepam may be agent of choice, especially in (E) with liver disease.[8,119] (See also Benzodiazepines).	$t_{1/2}$: 5.1 hr (Y) vs 5.6 hr (E). V_d: 0.6 L/kg (Y) vs 0.8 L/kg (E). Cl: 6.78 L/hr (Y) vs 8.16 L/hr (E).[133] Cl: not significantly different in (Y) vs (E).[134]
MISCELLANEOUS AGENTS		
Acetazolamide	An increased frequency of side effects may occur in (E), possibly due to increased binding of drug to RBCs and decreased Cl.[135]	
Cimetidine	Severe confusion has been reported in (E).[136] Determine or estimate Cl$_{cr}$ and reduce dose appropriately.[137] Observe for change in sensorium in (E).	Cl decreased in (E).[137]

Continued

Geriatric Drug Use

DRUG	CLINICAL FINDINGS AND MANAGEMENT	DRUG-SPECIFIC DATA
Iron	There appears to be no age-related difference in iron absorption. Red cell uptake of iron appears to be diminished in (E) because of decreased erythropoiesis. This may explain "resistant" iron deficiency anemia in (E).	No difference between (Y) and (E) in mucosal iron uptake, mucosal transfer or retention. Utilization of retained iron: 91% (Y) vs 66% (E).[139]
Levodopa	Postural hypotension may be more common in females over 70 yr[140] and patients over 70 yr with a history of myocardial infarction.[141] Paradoxical behavioral reactions have been described which include depression, paranoid ideations, disorientation or increased alertness and improvement in depression.[142]	Possible increased absorption in (E).[143]
Ranitidine	The half-life of ranitidine is prolonged in (E).[138] Observe for change in sensorium in (E).	
Theophylline	The (E) appear to have a somewhat increased frequency of side effects, especially arrhythmias, if underlying cardiovascular disease is present; but, it is not known if (E) are inherently more sensitive to other effects.[4] Significant decrease in Cl of unbound theophylline in (E) suggests decreased plasma protein binding in (E).[144] Cigarette smoking appears to increase Cl of theophylline and decrease frequency of side effects,[145,146] although this effect is less pronounced in (E). Presence of CHF or liver disease decreases Cl and requires lowering of dose.[147,148]	No difference in extent or rate of PO absorption or V_d between (Y) and (E). $t_{1/2}$: 5.9 hr (Y) smokers vs 7.6 hr (Y) nonsmokers; 5.9 hr (E) smokers vs 8 hr (E) nonsmokers. Cl: 55% higher in (Y) smokers than (Y) nonsmokers; 40% higher in (E) smokers than (E) nonsmokers.[146]

Continued

Geriatric Drug Use

DRUG	CLINICAL FINDINGS AND MANAGEMENT	DRUG-SPECIFIC DATA
VITAMINS	The possibility of vitamin deficiencies should be explored in (E) and therapy monitored for efficacy.	Vitamin B_6, B_{12}, niacin, folate and thiamine deficiencies were documented in 39% of (E) patients despite oral vitamin supplementation; deficiencies were corrected with intramuscular vitamin administration.[149] (E) absorbed riboflavin, vitamin B_6 and pantothenate from yeast (natural source) as well as (Y), but did not absorb natural folates as well as (Y); synthetic folates were an absorbable source for (E).[150]

References

1. Haynes SG, Feinleib M. eds. Second conference on the epidemiology of aging. Bethesda, MD: National Institutes of Health 1980. (NIH publication no. 80-969).

2. Vestal RE. Drugs and the elderly. National Institute on Aging Science Writer Seminar Series. Bethesda, MD: National Institutes of Health, 1979. (NIH publication no. 79-1449).

3. Schwartz D, Wang M, Zeitz L et al. Medication errors made by elderly, chronically ill patients. Am J Public Health 1962;52:2018-29.

4. Vestal RE. Drug use in the elderly: a review of problems and special considerations. Drugs 1978;16:358-82.

5. Vestal RE, Dawson GW. Pharmacology and aging. In: Finch CE, Schneider EL, eds. Handbook of the biology of aging. New York: Van Nostrand Reinhold, 1983:744-819.

6. Crooks J, O'Malley K, Stevenson IH. Pharmacokinetics in the elderly. Clin Pharmacokinet 1976;1:280-96.

7. O'Malley K, Judge TG, Crooks J. Geriatric clinical pharmacology and therapeutics. In: Avery GS, ed. Drug treatment. New York: ADIS Press, 1980:158-81.

8. Schumacher GE. Using pharmacokinetics in drug therapy VII: pharmacokinetic factors influencing drug therapy in the aged. Am J Hosp Pharm 1980;37:559-62.

9. Vestal RE. Drug treatment in the elderly. Boston: ADIS Health Science Press, 1984.

10. Vestal RE. Clinical pharmacology. In: Andres R, Bierman EL, Hazzard WR, eds. Principles of geriatric medicine. New York: McGraw Hill, 1985:424-43.

11. Greenblatt DJ, Sellers EM, Shader RI. Drug disposition in old age. N Engl J Med 1982;306:1081-8.

12. Ho PC, Triggs EJ. Drug therapy in the elderly. Aust NZ J Med 1984;14:179-90.

13. Massoud N. Pharmacokinetic considerations in geriatric patients. In: Benet LZ, Massoud N, Gambertoglio JG, eds. Pharmacokinetic basis for drug treatment. New York: Raven Press, 1984:283-310.

14. Mayersohn M. Special pharmacokinetic considerations in the elderly. In: Evans WE, Schentag JJ, Jusko WJ, eds. Applied pharmacokinetics: principles of therapeutic drug monitoring. 2nd ed. Spokane, WA: Applied Therapeutics, 1986;229-93.

15. Geokas MC, Haverback BJ. The aging gastrointestinal tract. Am J Surg 1969;117:881-92.

16. Bender AD. Effect of age on intestinal absorption: implications for drug absorption in the elderly. J Am Geriatr Soc 1968;16:1331-9.

17. Novak LP. Aging, total body potassium, fat-free mass, and cell mass in males and females between ages 18 and 85 years. J Gerontol 1972;27:438-43.

18. Rodeheffer RJ, Gerstenblith G, Becker LC et al. Exercise cardiac output is maintained with advancing age in healthy human subjects: cardiac dilatation and increased stroke volume compensate for a diminished heart rate. Circulation 1984;69:208-13.

19. Cammarata RJ, Rodnan GP, Fennell RH. Serum anti-gamma-globulin and antinuclear factors in the aged. JAMA 1967;199:455-8.

20. Greenblatt DJ. Reduced serum albumin concentration in the elderly: a report from the Boston collaborative drug surveillance program. J Am Geriatr Soc 1979;27:20-2.

21. Wallace S, Whiting B, Runcie J. Factors affecting drug binding in plasma of elderly patients. Br J Clin Pharmacol 1976;3:327-30.

22. Mooney H, Roberts R, Cooksley WGE et al. Alterations in the liver with ageing. Clin Gastroenterol 1985;14:757-71.

23. Farah F, Taylor W, Rawlins MD et al. Hepatic drug acetylation and oxidation: effects of aging in man. Br Med J 1977;2:155-6.

24. Rowe JW, Andres R, Tobin JD et al. The effect of age on creatinine clearance in men: a cross-sectional and longitudinal study. J Gerontol 1976;31:155-63.

25. Siersbaek-Nielsen K, Hansen JM, Kampmann J et al. Rapid evaluation of creatinine clearance. Lancet 1971;1:1133-4.

26. Cockcroft DW, Gault MH. Prediction of creatinine clearance from serum creatinine. Nephron 1976;16:31-41.

27. Todhunter EN, Darby WJ. Guidelines for maintaining adequate nutrition in old age. Geriatrics 1978;33:49-56.

28. Krehl WA. The influence of nutritional environment on aging. Geriatrics 1974;29:65-76.

29. Smithard DJ, Langman MJS. Drug metabolism in the elderly. Br Med J 1977;3:520-1.

30. Bennett WM, Muther RS, Parker RA et al. Drug therapy in renal failure: dosing guidelines for adults. Ann Intern Med 1980;93:62-89, 286-325.

31. Vestal RE, McGuire EA, Tobin JD et al. Aging and ethanol metabolism. Clin Pharmacol Ther 1977;21:343-54.

32. Triggs EJ, Nation RL, Long A et al. Pharmacokinetics in the elderly. Eur J Clin Pharmacol 1975;8:55-62.

33. Briant RH, Dorrington RE, Cleal J et al. The rate of acetaminophen metabolism in the elderly and the young. J Am Geriatr Soc 1976;24:359-61.

34. Salem SAM, Stevenson IH. Absorption kinetics of aspirin and quinine in elderly subjects. Br J Clin Pharmacol 1977;4:397P.

35. Cuny G, Royer RJ, Mur JM et al. Pharmacokinetics of salicylates in elderly. Gerontology 1979;25:49-55.

36. Castleden CM, Volans CN, Raymond K. The effects of ageing on drug absorption from the gut. Age Ageing 1977;6:138-43.

37. Mongan E, Kelly P, Nies K et al. Tinnitus as an indication of therapeutic serum salicylate levels. JAMA 1973;226:142-5.

38. Bellville JW, Forrest WH, Miller E et al. Influence of age on pain relief from analgesics. A study of postoperative patients. JAMA 1971;217:1835-41.

39. Mather LE, Tucker GT, Pflug AE et al. Meperidine kinetics in man. Clin Pharmacol Ther 1975;17:21-30.

40. Berkowitz BA, Ngai SH, Yang JC et al. The disposition of morphine in surgical patients. Clin Pharmacol Ther 1975;17:629-35.

41. Stanski DR, Greenblatt DJ. Lowenstein E. Kinetics of intravenous and intramuscular morphine. Clin Pharmacol Ther 1978;24:52-9.

42. Upton RA, Williams RL, Kelly J et al. Naproxen pharmacokinetics in the elderly. Br J Clin Pharmacol

1984;18:207-14.

43. Dunn MJ. Nonsteroidal antiinflammatory drugs and renal function. Ann Rev Med 1984;35:411-28.

44. Hobbs DC. Piroxicam pharmacokinetics: recent clinical results relating kinetics and plasma levels to age, sex, and adverse effects. Am J Med 1986;81(Suppl 5B):22-8.

45. Rugstad HE. The Norway Study: plasma concentrations, efficacy, and adverse events. Am J Med 1986;81(Suppl 5B):11-4.

46. Walker AM, Jick H. Predictors of bleeding during heparin therapy. JAMA 1980;244:1209-12.

47. Coon WW, Willis PW. Hemorrhagic complications of anticoagulant therapy. Arch Intern Med 1974;133:386-92.

48. Husted S, Andreasen F. Problems encountered in long-term treatment with anticoagulants. Acta Med Scand 1976;200:379-84.

49. Fortar JC. A 7-year analysis of haemorrhage in patients on long-term anticoagulant treatment. Br Heart J 1979;42:128-32.

50. Shepherd AMM, Hewick DS, Moreland TA et al. Age as a determinant of sensitivity to warfarin. Br J Clin Pharmacol 1977;4:315-20.

51. O'Malley K, Stevenson IH, Ward CA et al. Determinants of anticoagulant control in patients receiving warfarin. Br J Clin Pharmacol 1977;4:309-14.

52. Husted S, Andreasen F. The influence of age on the response to anticoagulants. Br J Clin Pharmacol 1977;4:559-65.

53. Jones BR, Baran A, Reidenberg MM. Evaluating patients' warfarin requirements. J Am Geriatr Soc 1980;28:10-12.

54. Hayes MJ, Langman MJS, Short AH. Changes in drug metabolism with increasing age: 2. phenytoin clearance and protein binding. Br J Clin Pharmacol 1975;2:73-9.

55. Bauer LA, Blouin RA. Age and phenytoin kinetics in adult epileptics. Clin Pharmacol Ther 1982;31:301-4.

56. Lambie DC, Caird FL. Phenytoin dosage in the elderly. Age Ageing 1977;6:133-7.

57. Houghton GW, Richens A, Leighton M. Effect of age, height, weight and sex on serum phenytoin concentration in epileptic patients. Br J Clin Pharmacol 1975;2:251-6.

58. Bauer LA, Blouin RA. Gentamicin pharmacokinetics: effect of aging in patients with normal renal function. J Am Geriatr Soc 1982;30:309-11.

59. Kristensen M, Hansen JM, Kampmann J et al. Drug elimination and renal function. J Clin Pharmacol 1974;14:307-8.

60. Ball P, Barford T, Gilbert J et al. Prolonged serum elimination half-life of amoxycillin in the elderly. J Antimicrob Chemother 1978;4:385-6.

61. Triggs EJ, Johnson JM, Learoyd B. Absorption and disposition of ampicillin in the elderly. Eur J Clin Pharmacol 1980;18:195-8.

62. Kopanoff DE, Snider DE, Caras GJ. Isoniazid-related hepatitis. Am Rev Respir Dis 1978;117:991-1001.

63. Gobert C, Houin G, Abengres E et al. Pharmacokinetics of isoniazid in the elderly. Br J Clin Pharmacol 1980;10:167-8.

64. American Thoracic Society. Preventive therapy of tuberculous infection. Am Rev Respir Dis 1974;110:371-4.

65. Leikola E, Vartia KO. On penicillin levels in young and geriatric subjects. J Gerontol 1957;12:48-52.

66. Varoquaux O, Lajoie D, Gobert C et al. Pharmacokinetics of the trimethoprim-sulphamethoxazole combination in the elderly. Br J Clin Pharmacol 1985;20:575-81.

67. Kramer PA, Chapron DJ, Benson J et al. Tetracycline absorption in elderly patients with achlorhydria. Clin Pharmacol Ther 1978;23:467-72.

68. Whiting B, Wandless I, Sumner DJ et al. Computer-assisted review of digoxin therapy in the elderly. Br Heart J 1978;40:8-13.

69. Dall JLC. Maintenance digoxin in elderly patients. Br Med J 1970;2:705-6.

70. Cusack B, Kelly J, O'Malley K et al. Digoxin in the elderly: pharmacokinetic consequences of old age. Clin Pharmacol Ther 1979;25:772-6.

71. Ewy GA, Kapadia GG, Yao L et al. Digoxin metabolism in the elderly. Circulation 1969;39:449-53.

72. Chaffman M, Brogden RN. Diltiazem: a review of its pharmacological properties and therapeutic efficacy. Drugs 1985;29:387-454.

73. Hermann P, Morselli PL. Pharmacokinetics of diltiazem and other calcium entry blockers. Acta Pharmacol Toxicol 1985;57(Suppl II):10-20.

74. Bonde J, Pedersen LE, Bodtker S et al. The influence of age and smoking on the elimination of disopyramide. Br J Clin Pharmacol 1985;20:453-8.

75. Nation RL, Triggs EJ, Selig M. Lignocaine kinetics in cardiac patients and aged subjects. Br J Clin Pharmacol 1977;4:439-48.

76. Thomson PD, Melmon KL, Richardson JA et al. Lidocaine pharmacokinetics in advanced heart failure, liver disease, and renal failure in humans. Ann Intern Med 1973;78:499-508.

77. Abernethy DR, Greenblatt DJ. Impairment of lidocaine clearance in elderly male subjects. J Cardiovasc Pharmacol 1983;5:1093-6.

78. Greenblatt DJ, Koch-Weser J. Adverse reactions to propranolol in hospitalized medical patients: a report from the Boston collaborative drug surveillance program. Am Heart J 1973;86:478-84.

79. Whitlock FA, Bonfield AR. Propranolol psychosis. Med J Aust 1980;1:184-5.

80. Kurland ML. Organic brain syndrome with propranolol. N Engl J Med 1979;300:366.

81. Fleminger R. Visual hallucinations and illusions with propranolol. Br Med J 1978;1:1182.

82. Castleden CM, George CF. The effect of ageing on the hepatic clearance of propranolol. Br J Clin Pharmacol 1979;7:49-54.

83. Vestal RE, Wood AJJ, Shand DG. Reduced beta-adrenoreceptor sensitivity in the elderly. Clin Res 1978;26:488A.

84. Feldman RD, Limbird LE, Nadeau J et al. Alterations in leukocyte β-receptor affinity with aging. A potential explanation for altered β-adrenergic sensitivity in the elderly. N Engl J Med 1984;310:815-9.

85. Vestal RE, Wood AJJ, Shand DG. Reduced β-adrenoceptor sensitivity in the elderly. Clin Pharmacol Ther 1979;26:181-6.

86. Vestal RE, Wood AJJ, Branch RA et al. Effects of age and cigarette smoking on propranolol disposition. Clin Pharmacol Ther 1979;26:8-11.

87. Schneider RE, Bishop H, Yates RA et al. Effect of age on plasma propranolol levels. Br J Clin Pharmacol 1980;10:169-70.

88. Wood AJJ, Vestal RE, Branch RA et al. Age related effects of smoking on elimination of propranolol, antipyrine and indocyanine green. Clin Res 1978;26:14A.

89. Feely J, Crooks J, Stevenson IH. The influence of age, smoking and hyperthyroidism on plasma propranolol steady state concentration. Br J Clin Pharmacol 1981;12:73-8.

90. Ochs HR, Greenblatt DJ, Woo E et al. Reduced quinidine clearance in elderly persons. Am J Cardiol 1978;42:481-5.

91. Drayer DE, Hughes M, Lorenzo B et al. Prevalence of high (3S)-3-hydroxyquinidine/quinidine ratios in serum, and clearance of quinidine in cardiac patients with age. Clin Pharmacol Ther 1980;27:72-5.

92. Andreasen F, Hansen U, Husted SE et al. The influence of age on renal and extrarenal effects of frusemide. Br J Clin Pharmacol 1984;18:65-74.

93. Kerremans ALM, Tan Y, van Baars H et al. Furosemide kinetics and dynamics in aged patients. Clin Pharmacol Ther 1983;34:181-9.

94. Hamdy RC, Tovey J, Perera N. Hypokalaemia and diuretics. Br Med J 1980;1:1187.

95. Williamson J, Chopin JM. Adverse reactions to prescribed drugs in the elderly: a multicentre investigation. Age Ageing 1980;9:73-80.

96. Amery A, Berthaux P, Bulpitt C et al. Glucose intolerance during diuretic therapy. Lancet 1978;1:681-3.

97. Burr ML, King S, Davies HEF et al. The effects of discontinuing long-term diuretic therapy in the elderly. Age Ageing 1977;6:38-45.

98. Seltzer HS. Drug-induced hypoglycemia. Diabetes 1972;21:955-66.

99. Holmes B, Heel RC, Brogden RN et al. Gliclazide: a preliminary review of its pharmacodynamic properties and therapeutic efficacy in diabetes mellitus. Drugs 1984;27:301-27.

100. Miller AK, Adir J, Vestal RE. Tolbutamide binding to plasma proteins of young and old human subjects. J Pharm Sci 1978;67:1192-3.

101. Dyer AR, Stamler J, Shekelle RB et al. Hypertension in the elderly. Med Clin N Am 1977;61:513-29.

102. Caird FI, Andrews GR, Kennedy RD. Effect of posture on blood pressure in the elderly. Br Heart J 1973;35:527-30.

103. Hale WE, Stewart RB, Marks RG. Central nervous system symptoms of elderly subjects using antihypertensive drugs. J Am Geriatr Soc 1984;32:5-10.

104. McNeill JJ, Louis WJ. Clinical pharmacokinetics of labetalol. Clin Pharmacokinet 1984;9:157-67.

105. Thompson TL, Moran MG, Nies AS. Psychotropic drug use in the elderly (second of two parts). N Engl J Med 1983;308:194-9.

106. Hewick DS, Newbury P, Hopwood S et al. Age as a factor affecting lithium therapy. Br J Clin Pharmacol 1977;4:201-5.

107. Schou M. Lithium in psychiatric therapy and prophylaxis. J Psychiatr Res 1968;6:67-95.

108. Chapron DJ, Cameron IR, White LB et al. Observations on lithium disposition in the elderly. J Am Geriatr Soc 1982;30:651-5.

109. Shillcutt SD, Easterday JL, Anderson RJ. Geriatric therapeutics: safe and effective use of antipsychotic agents. Hosp Formul 1986;21:462-77.

110. Simpson GM, Pi EH, Sramek JJ. Management of tardive dyskinesia: current update. Drugs 1982;23:381-93.

111. Nies A, Robinson DS, Friedman MJ et al. Relationship between age and tricyclic antidepressant plasma levels. Am J Psychiatry 1977;134:790-3.

112. Norman TR, Burrows GD, Scoggins BA et al. Pharmacokinetics and plasma levels of antidepressants in the elderly. Med J Aust 1979;1:273-4.

113. Goff DC, Jenike MA. Treatment-resistant depression in the elderly. J Am Geriatr Soc 1986;34:63-70.

114. Coccaro EF, Siever LJ. Second generation antidepressants: a comparative review. J Clin Pharmacol 1985;25:241-60.

115. Thompson TL, Moran MG, Nies AS. Psychotropic drug use in the elderly (first of two parts). N Engl J Med 1983;308:134-8.

116. Finlayson RE, Martin LM. Recognition and management of depression in the elderly. Mayo Clin Proc 1982;57:115-20.

117. Salzman C, Shader RI, Greenblatt DJ et al. Long v short half-life benzodiazepines in the elderly. Arch Gen Psychiatry 1983;40:293-7.

118. Kraus JW, Desmond PV, Marshall JP et al. Effects of aging and liver disease on disposition of lorazepam. Clin Pharmacol Ther 1978;24:411-9.

119. Divoll M, Greenblatt DJ, Ochs HR et al. Absolute bioavailability of oral and intramuscular diazepam: effects of age and sex. Anesth Analg 1983;62:1-8.

120. Boston Collaborative Drug Surveillance Program. Clinical depression of the central nervous system due to diazepam and chlordiazepoxide in relation to cigarette smoking and age. N Engl J Med 1973;288:277-80.

121. Roberts RK, Wilkinson GR, Branch RA et al. Effect of age and parenchymal liver disease on the disposition and elimination of chlordiazepoxide (Librium). Gastroenterology 1978;75:479-85.

122. Shader RI, Greenblatt DJ, Harmatz JS et al. Absorption and disposition of chlordiazepoxide in young and elderly male volunteers. J Clin Pharmacol 1977;17:709-18.

123. Reidenberg MM, Levy M, Warner H et al. Relationship between diazepam dose, plasma level, age and central nervous system depression. Clin Pharmacol Ther 1978;23:371-4.

124. Ochs HR, Greenblatt DJ, Divoll M et al. Diazepam kinetics in relation to age and sex. Pharmacology 1981;23:24-30.

125. Klotz U, Muller-Seydlitz P. Altered elimination of desmethyldiazepam in the elderly. Br J Clin Pharmacol

1979;7:119-20. Letter.

126. Macklon AF, Barton M, James O et al. The effect of age on the pharmacokinetics of diazepam. Clin Sci 1980;59:479-83.

127. Greenblatt DJ, Allen MD, Locniskar A et al. Age, sex, and diazepam kinetics. Clin Pharmacol Ther 1979;25:227. Abstract.

128. Greenblatt DJ, Allen MD, Shader RI. Toxicity of high-dose flurazepam in the elderly. Clin Pharmacol Ther 1977;21:355-61.

129. Greenblatt DJ, Divoll M,, Harmatz JS et al. Kinetics and clinical effects of flurazepam in young and elderly noninsomniacs. Clin Pharmacol Ther 1981;30:475-86.

130. Greenblatt DJ, Allen MD, Locniskar A et al. Lorazepam kinetics in the elderly. Clin Pharmacol Ther 1979;25:227. Abstract.

131. Castleden CM, George CF, Marcer D et al. Increased sensitivity to nitrazepam in old age. Br Med J 1977;1:10-2.

132. Iisalo E, Kangas L, Ruikka I. Pharmacokinetics of nitrazepam in young volunteers and aged patients. Br J Clin Pharmacol 1977;4:646P-7P.

133. Shull HJ, Wilkinson GR, Johnson R et al. Normal disposition of oxazepam in acute viral hepatitis and cirrhosis. Ann Intern Med 1976;84:420-5.

134. Greenblatt DJ, Divoll M, Harmatz JS et al. Oxazepam kinetics: effects of age and sex. J Pharmacol Exp Ther 1980;215:86-91.

135. Chapron DJ, Sweeney KR, Feig PU et al. Influence of advanced age on the disposition of acetazolamide. Br J Clin Pharmacol 1985;19:363-71.

136. McMillan M, Ambis D, Siegel J. Cimetidine and mental confusion. N Engl J Med 1978;298:284-5.

137. Redolfi A, Borgogelli E, Lodola E. Blood level of cimetidine in relation to age. Eur J Clin Pharmacol 1979;15:257-61.

138. Zeldis JB, Friedman LS, Isselbacher KJ. Ranitidine: a new H_2-receptor antagonist. N Engl J Med 1983;309:1368-73.

139. Marx JJM. Normal iron absorption and decreased red cell iron uptake in the aged. Blood 1979;53:204-11.

140. Grad B, Wener J, Rosenberg G et al. Effects of levodopa therapy in patients with parkinson's disease: statistical evidence for reduced tolerance to levodopa in the elderly. J Am Geriatr Soc 1974;22:489-94.

141. Wener J, Rosenberg G, Grad B et al. Cardiovascular effects of levodopa in aged versus younger patients with parkinson's disease. J Am Geriatr Soc 1976;24:185-8.

142. Riklan M. An L-dopa paradox: bipolar behavioral alterations. J Am Geriatr Soc 1972;20:572-5.

143. Evans MA, Triggs EJ, Broe GA et al. Systemic availability of orally administered L-dopa in the elderly parkinsonian patient. Eur J Clin Pharmacol 1980;17:215-21.

144. Antal EJ, Kramer PA, Mercik SA et al. Theophylline pharmacokinetics in advanced age. Br J Clin Pharmacol 1981;12:637-45.

145. Pfeifer HJ, Greenblatt DJ. Clinical toxicity of theophylline in relation to cigarette smoking. Chest 1978;73:455-9.

146. Cusack B, Kelly JG, Lavan J et al. Theophylline kinetics in relation to age: the importance of smoking. Br J Clin Pharmacol 1980;10:109-14.

147. Anon. IV dosage guidelines for theophylline products. FDA Drug Bull 1980;10:4-6.

148. Murphy J, Ward E. Letter to the editor. N Engl J Med 1980;303:760-1.

149. Baker H, Frank O, Jaslow SP. Oral versus intramuscular vitamin supplementation for hypovitaminosis in the elderly. J Am Geriatr Soc 1980;28:42-5.

150. Baker H, Jaslow SP, Frank O. Severe impairment of dietary folate utilization in the elderly. J Am Geriatr Soc 1980;26:218-21.

10 IMMUNIZATION

General Recommendations on Immunization*

Introduction. Recommendations for immunization of infants, children and adults are based on facts about immunobiologics and scientific knowledge about the principles of active and passive immunization and on judgments by public health officials and specialists in clinical and preventive medicine. Benefits and risks are associated with the use of all products—no vaccine is completely safe or completely effective. The benefits range from partial to complete protection from the consequences of disease, and the risks range from common, trivial and inconvenient side effects to rare, severe and life-threatening conditions. Thus, recommendations on immunization practices balance scientific evidence of benefits, costs and risks to achieve optimal levels of protection against infectious or communicable diseases.

These recommendations of the Advisory Committee on Immunization Practices (ACIP) describe this balance and attempt to minimize the risk by providing specific advice regarding dose and spacing of immunobiologics and by delineating situations warranting precautions or contraindicating their use. These recommendations may apply only in the United States, as epidemiological circumstances and vaccines may differ in other countries.

Spacing of Immunobiologics.

A. Multiple doses of same antigen: Some products require more than one dose for full protection. In addition, it is necessary to give periodic reinforcement (booster) doses of some preparations to maintain protection. In recommending the ages and/or intervals for multiple doses, the ACIP takes into account current risks from disease and the objective of inducing satisfactory protection. Intervals between doses that are longer than those recommended do not lead to a reduction in final antibody levels. Therefore, it is unnecessary to re-start an interrupted series of an immunobiologic or to add extra doses. By contrast, giving doses of a vaccine or toxoid at less than recommended intervals may lessen the antibody response; doses given at less

---

*Excerpted from Advisory Committee on Immunization Practices, Centers for Disease Control. General recommendations on immunization. Morb Mortal Wkly Rep 1983;32:1-8, 13-7. Consult that report and the references at the end of this chapter for more complete information.

than recommended intervals should not be counted as part of a primary series.

B. Different antigens: Experimental evidence and extensive clinical experience have strengthened the scientific basis for giving certain vaccines at the same time. Most of the widely used antigens can safely and effectively be given simultaneously. This knowledge is particularly helpful in circumstances that include imminent exposure to several infectious diseases, preparation for foreign travel or uncertainty that the patient will return for further doses of vaccine.

In general, inactivated vaccines can be administered simultaneously at separate sites. It should be noted, however, that when vaccines commonly associated with local or systemic side effects (such as cholera, typhoid and plague vaccines) are given simultaneously, the side effects theoretically might be accentuated. When practical, these vaccines should be given on separate occasions.

Field observations indicate that simultaneous administration (on the same day) of the most widely used live-virus vaccines has not resulted in impaired antibody response or increased rates of adverse reactions. Observation of children indicates that antibody responses to trivalent oral polio vaccine (OPV) given simultaneously with licensed combination measles-mumps-rubella (MMR) vaccine are comparable to those obtained when the same vaccines are given at separate visits. It is reasonable to expect equivalent immunologic responses when other licensed combination or live, attenuated-virus vaccines or their component antigens are given simultaneously with OPV. While data are lacking on potential interference with antibody responses to measles, mumps, rubella, and/or trivalent oral polio vaccines administered at different times within one month of one another, there are theoretical concerns and data showing that the immune response to a live virus vaccine might be impaired if the vaccine is administered within the month following another live virus vaccine. When feasible, live virus vaccines not administered on the same day should be given at least one month apart.

No data indicate that simultaneous administration of individual measles, mumps or rubella antigens at different sites yields different results from administration of the combined vaccines in a single site. Sufficient data are now available to recommend the simultaneous administration of diphtheria and tetanus toxoids and pertussis vaccine (DTP), OPV and MMR vaccine to all children 15 months of age or older who are eligible to receive these vaccines (Table 1)—the protective response is satisfactory and evidence suggests there is no increased risk of adverse reactions (see reference 16). Simultaneous administration of all these antigens is also recommended when individuals require multiple antigens and there is doubt that the recipient will return to receive further doses of vaccine; children 15 months of age or older who have received fewer than the recommended number of DTP and OPV doses fall into this category (Table 2). Simultaneous administration of pneumococcal polysaccharide vaccine and whole-virus influenza vaccine gives satisfactory antibody response without increasing the occurrence of adverse reactions. Simultaneous administration of the pneumococcal vaccine and split-virus influenza vaccine may also be expected to yield satisfactory results. However, it should be kept in mind that influenza vaccine should be administered annually to the target population, whereas, under current recommendations, pneumococcal polysaccharide vaccine should only be administered in a single dose.

An inactivated vaccine and a live, attenuated-virus vaccine can be administered simultaneously at separate sites, with the precautions that apply to the individual vaccines. Some data suggest that the simultaneous administration of cholera and yellow fever vaccines may interfere with the immune response to each other. Decreased levels of antibodies have been observed when the vaccines are administered within three weeks of each other, compared with administration of the vaccines at longer intervals. However, there is no evidence that protection to either of these diseases diminishes when these vaccines are administered simultaneously. Therefore, the ACIP believes that yellow fever and cholera vaccines can be administered simultaneously, if necessary.

C. Immune globulin: Immune globulin [IG, formerly called Immune Serum Globulin (ISG)] and various specific immune globulins contain antibodies common to the population from which the pooled plasma used in their preparation was obtained. These antibodies may interfere with the effectiveness of live, attenuated vaccines administered shortly after IG or specific IG has been given.

In general, such interference is of little practical importance with inactivated products. They can, therefore, be given anytime after IG use. With live, attenuated vaccines, passively acquired antibody may interfere with replication of vaccine virus and thus with the antibody response of the patient. Parenterally administered live vaccines (eg, MMR or other combinations) should, therefore, not be given for at least six weeks, but preferably three months, after the administration of IG. Preliminary data indicate that IG does not interfere with the immune response either to OPV or yellow fever vaccine.

If IG administration becomes necessary after a live vaccine has been given, interference may occur. In general, vaccine virus replication and stimulation of immunity will occur within 7–10 days. Thus, if the interval between vaccine and IG is less than 14 days, vaccine should be repeated about three months after IG was given, unless serologic testing indicates that antibodies have been produced; if the interval was longer, vaccine need not be readministered. If administration of IG becomes necessary because of imminent exposure to disease, live virus vaccines may be administered simultaneously with IG, with the recognition that vaccine-induced immunity may be compromised. The vaccine should be administered in a site remote from that chosen for IG inoculation. Vaccination should be repeated about three months later, unless serologic testing indicates antibodies have been produced.

Hypersensitivity to Vaccine Components. Vaccine antigens produced in systems or with substrates containing allergenic substances (eg, antigens derived from growing microorganisms in embryonated chicken eggs) may cause hypersensitivity reactions. These reactions may include anaphylaxis when the final vaccine contains a substantial amount of the allergen. Yellow fever vaccine is such an antigen. Vaccines with such characteristics should not be given to persons with known hypersensitivity to components of the substrates. Contrary to this generalization, influenza vaccine antigens (whole or split), although prepared from viruses grown in embryonated eggs, are highly purified during preparation and have only very rarely been reported to be associated with hypersensitivity reactions.

Live virus vaccines prepared by growing viruses in cell cultures are essentially devoid of potentially allergenic substances related to host tissue. On very rare occasions, hypersensitivity reactions to measles vaccine have been reported in persons with anaphylactic hypersensitivity to eggs. Measles vaccine, however, can be given safely to egg-allergic individuals provided the allergies are not manifested by anaphylactic symptoms. Since mumps vaccine is grown in similar cell cultures, the same precautions apply.

Screening persons by history of ability to eat eggs without adverse effects is a reasonable way to identify those possibly at risk from receiving measles, mumps and influenza vaccine. Individuals with anaphylactic hypersensitivity to eggs (hives, swelling of the mouth and throat, difficulty breathing, hypotension or shock)* should not be given these vaccines.

Rubella vaccine is grown in human diploid cell culture and can be safely given, regardless of a history of allergy to eggs or egg proteins.

Bacterial vaccines, such as cholera, DTP, plague and typhoid, are frequently associated with local or systemic adverse effects; these common reactions do not appear to be allergic.

Some vaccines contain preservatives (eg, thimerosal, a mercurial) or trace amounts of antibiotics (eg, neomycin) to which patients may be hypersensitive. Those administering vaccines should carefully review the information provided with the package insert before deciding whether the rare patients with known hypersensitivity to such preservatives or antibiotics should be given the vaccine(s). No currently recommended vaccine contains penicillin or its derivatives.

Some vaccines (eg, MMR vaccine or its individual component vaccines) contain trace amounts of neomycin. This amount is less than would usually be used for the skin test to determine hypersensitivity. Persons who have experienced anaphylactic reactions to neomycin should not receive these vaccines. Most often, neomycin allergy is a contact dermatitis, a manifestation of a delayed-type (cell-mediated) immune response rather than anaphylaxis. In such individuals, the adverse reaction, if any, to neomycin in the vaccines would be an erythematous, pruritic

---

Any of these signs or symptoms constitutes a systemic anaphylactic response.

papule at 48–96 hours. A history of delayed-type reactions to neomycin is not a contraindication to receiving these vaccines.

Altered Immunocompetence. Virus replication after administration of live, attenuated-virus vaccines may be enhanced in persons with immune deficiency diseases, and in those with suppressed capability for immune response, as occurs with leukemia, lymphoma, generalized malignancy, or therapy with corticosteroids, alkylating agents, antimetabolites or radiation. Patients with such conditions should not be given live, attenuated-virus vaccines. Because of the possibility of familial immunodeficiency, live, attenuated-virus vaccines should not be given to a member of a household in which there is a family history of congenital or hereditary immunodeficiency until the immune competence of the potential recipient is known. OPV should not be given to a member of a household in which there is a family history of immunodeficiency or immunosuppression, regardless whether acquired or hereditary, until the immune status of the recipient and the other family members is known. Individuals residing in the household of an immunocompromised individual should not receive OPV, because vaccine viruses are excreted by the recipient of the vaccine and may be communicable to other persons.

Severe Febrile Illnesses. Minor illnesses, such as mild upper-respiratory infections, should not postpone vaccine administration. However, immunization of persons with severe febrile illnesses should generally be deferred until they have recovered. This precaution is to avoid superimposing adverse effects from the vaccine on the underlying illness or mistakenly identifying a manifestation of the underlying illness as a result of the vaccine. In persons whose compliance with medical care cannot be assured, it is particularly important to take every opportunity to provide appropriate vaccinations.

Vaccination During Pregnancy. On the grounds of a theoretical risk to the developing fetus, live, attenuated-virus vaccines are not generally given to pregnant women or to those likely to become pregnant within three months after receiving vaccine(s). With some of these vaccines—particularly rubella, measles, and mumps—pregnancy is a contraindication. Both yellow fever vaccine and OPV can be given to pregnant women at substantial risk of exposure to natural infection. When vaccine is to be given during pregnancy, waiting until the second or third trimester to minimize any concern over teratogenicity is a reasonable precaution. If a pregnant woman receives a live, attenuated-virus vaccine, there is not necessarily any real risk to the fetus. In particular, although there are theoretical risks in giving rubella vaccine during pregnancy, data on previously and currently available rubella vaccines indicate that the risk, if any, of teratogenicity from live rubella vaccine is quite small. There has been no evidence of congenital rubella syndrome in infants born to susceptible mothers who received rubella vaccine during pregnancy.

Since persons given measles, mumps or rubella vaccine viruses do not transmit them, these vaccines may be administered with safety to children of pregnant women. Although live polio virus is shed by children recently immunized with OPV (particularly following the first dose), this vaccine can also be administered to children of pregnant women. Polio immunization of children should not be delayed because of pregnancy in close adult contacts. Experience to date has not revealed any risks of poliovaccine virus to the fetus.

There is no convincing evidence of risk to the fetus from immunization of pregnant women using inactivated virus vaccines, bacterial vaccines, or toxoids. Tetanus and diphtheria toxoid (Td) should be given to inadequately immunized pregnant women, because it affords protection against neonatal tetanus. There is no risk to the fetus from passive immunization of pregnant women with IG. For further information regarding immunization of pregnant women, refer to the American College of Obstetricians and Gynecologists (ACOG) Technical Bulletin Number 14, May 1982 and reference 16.

Dosage. The recommended doses of immunobiologics are derived from theoretical considerations, experimental trials and clinical experience. Administration of dose volumes smaller than those recommended, such as split doses or intradermal administration (unless specifically recommended), may result in inadequate protection. Exceeding the recommended dose volumes might be hazardous, because of excessive local or systemic concentrations of antigens.

Some practitioners use divided doses of vaccine [particularly diphtheria and tetanus toxoids and pertussis vaccine (DTP)] to reduce reaction rates. There has not been adequate study of the efficacy of such practices by serologic confirmation or clinical efficacy or of the effects on the subsequent frequency and severity of adverse reactions. The ACIP does not recommend dividing doses of any vaccine.

Age At Which Immunobiologics Are Administered. Several factors influence recommendations concerning the age at which vaccine is administered. (Tables 1–3). These include: age-specific risks of disease, age-specific risks of complications, ability of individuals of a given age to respond to the vaccine(s) and potential interference with the immune response by passively transferred maternal antibody. In general, vaccines are recommended for the youngest age group at risk with an acceptable level of antibody response following vaccine administration. For example, while infants as young as six months of age may be at risk for measles, most are protected by maternal antibody, which may inhibit successful active immunization at this age. In the United States, measles vaccine is routinely administered at 15 months of age, by which time maternal antibody is no longer detectable.

In certain measles epidemics, public health officials may recommend measles vaccine for infants as young as six months of age. Although a smaller proportion of those given vaccine before the first birthday develop antibody to measles, compared with older infants, the higher risk of disease during an epidemic may justify earlier immunization. Such infants should be reimmunized at the recommended age for measles vaccination to achieve protection.

Table 1. New Recommended Schedule for Active Immunization of Normal Infants and Children*

RECOMMENDED AGE[a]	VACCINE(S)[b]	COMMENTS
2 months	DTP-1,[c] OPV-1[d]	Can be given earlier in areas of high endemicity or during epidemics.
4 months	DTP-2, OPV-2	6-week to 2-month interval desired between OPV doses to avoid interference.
6 months	DTP 3, (OPV)	An additional dose of OPV at this time is optional for use in areas with a high risk of polio exposure.
15 months[e]	MMR,[f] DTP-4, OPV-3	Completion of primary series of DTP and OPV (see footnote e).
18 months	Haemophilus b Conjugate Vaccine	See footnote i.
4–6 years[g]	DTP-5, OPV-4	Preferably at or before school entry.
14–16 years	Td[h]	Repeat every 10 years throughout life.

*Advisory Committee on Immunization Practices, Centers for Disease Control. New recommended schedule for active immunization of normal infants and children. Morb Mortal Wkly Rep 1986;35:577-9. See reference 2 and individual ACIP recommendations (references 3–15, 17, 18) for details.

a. These recommended ages should not be construed as absolute (ie, 2 months can be 6–10 weeks, etc.).

b. For all products used, consult manufacturer's package enclosure for instructions for storage, handling, and administration. Immunobiologics prepared by different manufacturers may vary, and those of the same manufacturer may change from time to time. The package insert should be followed for a specific product.

c. DTP–Diphtheria and Tetanus Toxoids with Pertussis Vaccine Adsorbed.

d. OPV–Poliovirus Vaccine Live Oral; contains poliovirus strains Types 1, 2, and 3.

e. Provided at least 6 months have elapsed since DTP-3 or, if fewer than three DTPs have been received, at least 6 weeks since last previous dose of DTP or OPV. MMR vaccine should not be delayed just to allow simultaneous administration with DTP and OPV. Administering MMR at 15 months and DTP-4 and OPV-3 at 18 months continues to be an acceptable alternative.

f. MMR-Measles, Mumps, and Rubella Virus Vaccine, Live.

g. Up to the seventh birthday.

h. Td-Tetanus and Diphtheria Toxoids Adsorbed (for adult use)—contains the same dose of tetanus toxoid as DTP or DT and a reduced dose of diphtheria toxoid.

i. Haemophilus b Conjugate Vaccine (Diphtheria Toxoid-Conjugate) was licensed in December 1987 for the prevention of infections due to *Haemophilus influenzae* type b.

Because of its significantly greater immunogenicity as compared with Haemophilus b polysaccharide vaccines or "plain" capsular polysaccharide vaccines (referred to as HbPV), the Advisory Committee on Immunization Practices (ACIP), Centers for Disease Control, has issued the following recommendations (excerpted from ACIP, Centers for Disease Control. Update: prevention of *Haemophilus influenzae* type b disease. Morb Mortal Wkly Rep 1988;37:13-6. NOTE: the entire ACIP statement should be reviewed prior to utilizing this vaccine): (1) The ACIP recommends that all children receive conjugate vaccine at 18 months of age. Although the efficacy of conjugate vaccine in children 18 months of age or older has not been determined in field trials, the ACIP recommends use of conjugate vaccine in all children vaccinated against Haemophilus b disease. (2) Until further information is available, revaccination is not recommended for children receiving conjugate vaccine at 18 months of age or older. (3) Vaccination of children more than 24 months of age who have not yet received Haemophilus b vaccine should be based on risk of disease. Children considered at high risk for Haemophilus b disease, including those attending day-care centers, those with anatomic or functional asplenia, and those with malignancies associated with immunosuppression, should receive the vaccine. Although risk of disease decreases with increasing age, physicians may wish to vaccinate previously healthy children between 2 and 5 years of age to prevent disease that can occur in this group. (4) Because many children who received polysaccharide vaccine between the ages of 18 and 23 months may have had a less than adequate response to the vaccine, they should be revaccinated with a single dose of conjugate vaccine. Revaccination should take place a minimum of 2 months after the initial dose of polysaccharide vaccine. (5) There is no need to routinely revaccinate children who received polysaccharide vaccine at 24 months of age or older. (6) Children who had invasive Haemophilus b disease when they were less than 24 months of age should still receive vaccine according to the above recommendations, since most children less than 24 months of age fail to develop adequate immunity following natural infection. (7) Although increases in serum diphtheria anti-toxin levels can follow administration of conjugate vaccine, this vaccine should not be considered an immunizing agent against diphtheria. (8) Vaccination with either polysaccharide vaccine or conjugate vaccine probably does not inhibit asymptomatic carriage of Haemophilus b organisms. Therefore, chemoprophylaxis of household or day-care contacts of children with Haemophilus b disease should be directed at vaccinated as well as unvaccinated contacts. (9) Conjugate vaccine and DTP may be given simultaneously at different sites. Data are lacking on concomitant administration of conjugate vaccine and measles-mumps-rubella (MMR) or oral polio (OPV) vaccines. However, if the recipient is unlikely to return for further vaccination, simultaneous administration of all vaccines appropriate to the recipient's age and previous vaccination status is recommended (including DTP, OPV, MMR, and conjugate vaccine).

Table 2. Recommended Immunization Schedule for Infants and Children Under 7 Years of Age Not Immunized at the Recommended Time in Early Infancy*

RECOMMENDED TIME	VACCINE(S)	COMMENTS
First visit[a]	DTP-1,[b] OPV-1,[c] (If child is ≥ 15 months of age, MMR[d])	DTP, OPV and MMR can be administered simultaneously to children ≥ 15 months of age.
Unspecified	Haemophilus b Conjugate Vaccine	For children 2–5 years of age. See footnote g.
2 months after first DTP, OPV	DTP-2, OPV-2	
2 months after second DTP	DTP-3	An additional dose of OPV at this time is optional for use in areas with a high risk of polio exposure.
6–12 months after third DTP	DTP-4, OPV-3	

Continued

Table 2. Recommended Immunization Schedule for Infants and Children Under 7 Years of Age Not Immunized at the Recommended Time in Early Infancy*

RECOMMENDED TIME	VACCINE(S)	COMMENTS
Preschool[e] (4–6 years)	DTP-5, OPV-4	Preferably at or before school entry.
14–16 years	Td[f]	Repeat every 10 years throughout life.

*Advisory Committee on Immunization Practices, Centers for Disease Control. General recommendations on immunization. Morb Mortal Wkly Rep 1983;32:1-17 passim. See reference 2 and individual ACIP recommendations (references 3-15, 17, 18) for details.

a. If initiated in the first year of life, give DTP-1, 2, and 3, OPV-1 and 2 according to this schedule and give MMR when the child becomes 15 months old.

b. DTP–Diphtheria and tetanus toxoids with pertussis vaccine. DTP may be used up to the seventh birthday.

c. OPV–Oral, attenuated poliovirus vaccine contains poliovirus types 1, 2, and 3.

d. MMR–Live measles, mumps, and rubella viruses in a combined vaccine (see text for discussion of single vaccines versus combination).

e. The preschool dose is not necessary if the fourth dose of DTP and third dose of OPV are administered after the fourth birthday.

f. Td–Adult tetanus toxoid and diphtheria toxoid in combination, which contains the same dose of tetanus toxoid as DTP or DT and a reduced dose of diphtheria toxoid.

g. See Table 1., footnote i.

Table 3. Recommended Immunization Schedule for Persons 7 Years of Age or Older Not Immunized at the Recommended Time in Early Life*

RECOMMENDED TIME	VACCINE(S)	COMMENTS
First visit	Td-1,[a] OPV-1,[b] and MMR[c]	OPV not routinely administered to those with altered immune status or those ≥ 18 years of age. See footnote b.
2 months after first Td, OPV	Td-2, OPV-2	
6–12 months after second Td, OPV	Td-3, OPV-3	OPV-3 may be given as soon as 6 weeks after OPV-2.
10 years after Td-3	Td	Repeat every 10 years throughout life.

*Advisory Committee on Immunization Practices, Centers for Disease Control. General recommendations on immunization. Morb Mortal Wkly Rep 1983;32:1-17 passim. See reference 2 and individual ACIP recommendations (references 3-15, 17, 18) for details.

a. Td–Tetanus and diphtheria toxoids (adult type) are used after the seventh birthday. The DTP doses given to children under 7 years who remain incompletely immunized at age 7 years or older should be counted as prior exposure to tetanus and diphtheria toxoids (eg, a child who previously received 2 doses of DTP, only needs 1 dose of Td to complete a primary series).

b. OPV–Oral, attenuated poliovirus vaccine contains poliovirus types 1, 2, and 3. When polio vaccine is to be given to individuals with altered immune status or those 18 years or older, enhanced-potency inactivated poliovirus vaccine (IPV) is preferred. See ACIP statement on polio vaccine immunization schedule for enhanced-potency IPV, reference 18.

c. MMR–Live measles, mumps, and rubella viruses in a combined vaccine. Persons born before 1957 can generally be considered immune to measles and mumps and need not be immunized. Rubella vaccine may be given to persons of any age, particularly to women of childbearing age. MMR may be used since administration of vaccine to persons already immune is not deleterious. (See text for discussion of single vaccines versus combination.)

For detailed vaccination information, consult the following references:

References

1. ACIP,* Centers for Disease Control. General recommendations on immunization. Morb Mortal Wkly Rep 1983;32:1-8, 13-7.

2. American Academy of Pediatrics. Report of the committee on infectious diseases (the Red Book). 20th ed. Elk Grove Village, IL: AAP, 1986.

3. ACIP,* Centers for Disease Control. Rubella vaccine. Morb Mortal Wkly Rep 1978;27:451-4, 459.

4. ACIP,* Centers for Disease Control. BCG vaccines. Morb Mortal Wkly Rep 1979;28:241-4.

5. ACIP,* Centers for Disease Control. Poliomyelitis prevention. Morb Mortal Wkly Rep 1982;31:22-6, 31-4. See also reference 18.

6. ACIP,* Centers for Disease Control. Measles prevention. Morb Mortal Wkly Rep 1987;36:409-18, 423-5.

7. ACIP,* Centers for Disease Control. Mumps vaccine. Morb Mortal Wkly Rep 1982;31:617-20, 625.

8. ACIP,* Centers for Disease Control. Supplementary statement of contraindications to receipt of pertussis vaccine. Morb Mortal Wkly Rep 1984;33:169-71.

9. ACIP,* Centers for Disease Control. Rubella prevention. Morb Mortal Wkly Rep 1984;33:301-10, 315-8.

10. ACIP,* Centers for Disease Control. Polysaccharide vaccine for prevention of Haemophilus influenzae type b disease. Morb Mortal Wkly Rep 1985;34:201-5.

11. ACIP,* Centers for Disease Control. Diphtheria, tetanus, and pertussis: guidelines for vaccine prophylaxis and other preventive measures. Morb Mortal Wkly Rep 1985;34:405-14, 419-26.

12. ACIP,* Centers for Disease Control. Update: Haemophilus influenzae b polysaccharide vaccine. Morb Mortal Wkly Rep 1986;35:144-5. See also reference 17.

13. ACIP,* Centers for Disease Control. Update: prevention of Haemophilus influenzae type b disease. Morb Mortal Wkly Rep 1986;35:170-4, 179-80. See also reference 17.

14. ACIP,* Centers for Disease Control. Prevention and control of influenza. Morb Mortal Wkly Rep 1987;36:373-80, 385-7.

15. ACIP,* Centers for Disease Control. New recommended schedule for active immunization of normal infants and children. Morb Mortal Wkly Rep 1986;35:577-9.

16. Blanco JD, Gibbs RS. Immunizations in pregnancy. Clin Obstet Gynecol 1982;25:611-7.

17. ACIP,* Centers for Disease Control. Update: prevention of Haemophilus influenzae type b disease. Morb Mortal Wkly Rep 1986;35:373-6.

18. ACIP,* Centers for Disease Control. Poliomyelitis prevention: enhanced-potency inactivated poliomyelitis vaccine—supplementary statement. Morb Mortal Wkly Rep 1987;36:795-8.

For detailed information on adult immunization, consult the following references:

1. ACIP,* Centers for Disease Control. Adult immunization: recommendations of the immunization practices advisory committee. Morb Mortal Wkly Rep Supplement 1984;33(1S).

2. American College of Physicians. Guide for adult immunization. 1st ed. Philadelphia: ACP, 1985.

3. Anon. Routine immunization for adults. Med Lett Drugs Ther 1985;27:98-100.

*Advisory Committee on Immunization Practices.

11 *MEDICAL EMERGENCIES*

Outline of Drug Therapy

THE THERAPEUTIC APPROACHES, DRUGS AND ADULT DOSES given below have been compiled from somewhat divergent and conflicting sources of information. In addition, some recommendations have been made based upon the authors' experience, and suggestions from specialists and researchers in the field. As a result, the therapeutic concepts and dosages contained herein may differ from those advocated by specific practitioners and institutions.

Anaphylaxis

AN ANAPHYLACTIC REACTION is an *urgent* medical problem which can prove fatal. Although the onset of symptoms can vary from minutes to hours, most reactions occur within 5-30 minutes following ingestion or parenteral administration of an antigen. Symptoms may progress from extreme apprehension and cutaneous reactions to more severe systemic manifestations, such as severe respiratory distress and/or profound shock. Reactions include the following: conjunctivitis; gastrointestinal edema (nausea, vomiting, diarrhea); cutaneous reactions (urticaria, pruritus, angioedema); rhinitis, laryngeal edema, and bronchospasm (coughing, wheezing, dyspnea, cyanosis); vascular collapse, cardiac arrhythmias and cardiac arrest.

Definitive Therapy (see also Adjunctive Therapy.) *Adult doses only are given in this section.*

1a. Treatment of anaphylaxis is always initiated with *immediate* **Epinephrine HCl (aqueous), SC or IM, 0.3-0.5 mg** (0.3-0.5 ml of 1:1000), may repeat q 5-20 minutes.

or, for nonresponding or severe reactions
Epinephrine HCl, IV slow push, 0.2-0.5 mg (0.2-0.5 ml of 1:1000 diluted to 10 ml with saline, or 2-5 ml of 1:10,000), may repeat q 5-20 minutes.

1b. Patient should be in recumbent position with legs elevated, patent airway established and oxygen given; if applicable, a tourniquet should be placed proximal to the antigen injection site (remove temporarily q 10-15 minutes), and give

Epinephrine HCl, infiltrate 0.1-0.3 mg (0.1-0.3 ml of 1:1000) at injection site.

2. *Bronchospasm* (without shock) not responding to epinephrine therapy may require
   Aminophylline, IV slow infusion, 250-500 mg (10-20 ml of 25 mg/ml solution in 500 ml fluid, infusion rate not to exceed 50 mg/minute); may begin continuous infusion if necessary—see theophylline monograph in Drug Reviews Section.

3a. *Hypotension* not responding to epinephrine may be overcome by the use of fluids (see 3b.) and vasopressor agents; for example, **Dopamine HCl, IV slow infusion,** adjust rate to response (400 mg in 500 ml NS or D5W = 800 mcg/ml).

   or
   Norepinephrine Bitartrate, IV infusion, adjust rate to maintain a systolic blood pressure of about 90-100 mm Hg (2 ml of 0.2% solution in 500 ml D5W = 4 mcg base/ml).

3b. *Hypovolemia* may be the underlying cause of hypotension, and this requires rapid expansion of the intravascular fluid volume with **saline, plasma, albumin, hetastarch or whole blood** until the central venous pressure is 15 cm H_2O (constant CVP monitoring is required).

Adjunctive Therapy. *Adult doses only are given in this section.*

1. To prevent further cutaneous reactions, give **Diphenhydramine HCl, PO, IM or slow IV, 25-50 mg,** may repeat q 6 hours.

2. To prevent prolonged antigen-antibody reactions, give **Hydrocortisone Phosphate/Succinate, IV, 100 mg,** may repeat q 6 hours (may administer after the initial epinephrine injection). *This is controversial, however.*

3. To treat cardiac arrest, see the following section on cardiac arrest.

References

1. Austen KF. Systemic anaphylaxis in the human being. N Engl J Med 1974;291:661-4.
2. Kelly JF, Patterson R. The treatment of anaphylaxis. Ration Drug Ther 1973;7(11):1-5.
3. Kelly JF, Patterson R. Anaphylaxis—course, mechanisms and treatment. JAMA 1974;227:1431-6.
4. Lockey RF, Bukantz SC. Allergic emergencies. Med Clin North Am 1974;58:147-56.
5. MacFarlane MD, McCarron MM. Anaphylactic shock and anaphylactoid reaction—analysis of 62 cases. Drug Intell Clin Pharm 1973;7:394-407.
6. Parker CW. Drug allergy. N Engl J Med 1975;292:511-4, 732-6, 957-60.
7. Plaut M, Lichtenstein LM. Treatment of immediate hypersensitivity reactions to drugs. Ration Drug Ther 1974;8(7):1-6.

Cardiac Arrest

A CARDIAC ARREST IS A MEDICAL EMERGENCY requiring a systematic approach. Early recognition (unconsciousness, apnea, no pulse) must be followed by prompt, effective application of Basic Cardiac Life Support (BCLS) techniques to sustain the patient until Advanced Cardiac Life Support (ACLS) capabilities are available. With ACLS capabilities, a definitive treatment plan can then be attempted.

Thus, management of cardiac arrest is a four-step approach:
- **Diagnosis**
- **Emergency Treatment (BCLS)**
- **Definitive Therapy (ACLS)**
- **Postresuscitation Care**

Diagnosis

Verify that respiration and perfusion have ceased:

1. Loss of consciousness.

2. Loss of functional ventilation (apnea).

3. Loss of functional perfusion (no pulse).

Emergency Treatment (BCLS)

The findings listed above are sufficient to justify the immediate application of BCLS techniques listed below. The goal of BCLS is to rapidly and effectively reperfuse the CNS with oxygenated blood. It is well recognized that either delays in initiating BCLS or providing ineffective BCLS can result in irreversible hypoxic brain damage in an otherwise "successful" resuscitation.

1. Summon help and resuscitation equipment.

2. If witnessed arrest:
   a. Defibrillate with 200 joules of direct current shock if a defibrillator is immediately available, *or*
   b. Deliver sharp precordial blow.

3. If no response to above, or if an unwitnessed arrest, start artificial ventilation:
   a. Establish an adequate airway.
   b. Ventilate by mouth-to-mouth, mouth-to-nose, mouth-to-tube or bag-valve-mask techniques.
   c. The first few ventilations should be rapid (hyperventilation), then decrease rate to approximately 12 per minute.

4. Begin artificial perfusion via external chest compressions:
   a. Position patient supine on firm surface.
   b. Ensure proper placement of hands on sternum.
   c. Depress sternum at rate of 80 cycles per minute (50% of cycle should be compression).

Definitive Therapy (ACLS). *Adult doses only are given in this section.*

Initiate attempts by trained personnel to maintain a patent airway, establish an intravenous route for administration of fluids and drugs, establish an electrocardiographic diagnosis, and apply specific treatments to correct a recognized electrical and/or mechanical abnormality.

Definitive therapy can be divided into **General Therapy** —

modalities to be considered in all cases of cardiac arrest before a specific electrical abnormality has been identified; and **Specific Therapy** — modalities designed for specific electrocardiographic or mechanical abnormalities.

General Therapy

Management of Acidosis. Severe acidosis can develop within 5 minutes after cardiac arrest and will continue unless BCLS is provided. Acidosis is due primarily to a respiratory component (hypoventilation) and, to a lesser extent, a metabolic component (lactic acidosis), which occurs later.

1. *Respiratory acidosis:*
   a. Etiology: Accumulation of CO_2 secondary to hypoventilation.
   b. Treatment: Adequate ventilation; *no* role for sodium bicarbonate.

2. *Metabolic acidosis:*
   a. Etiology: Slow accumulation of lactic acid secondary to anaerobic metabolism within hypoperfused (hypoxic) tissues.
   b. Treatment: Adequate perfusion of oxygenated blood will delay development of significant lactic acidosis. Thus, early administration of sodium bicarbonate (buffer) is not indicated unless pre-existing acidosis or hyperkalemia is documented. Inappropriate bicarbonate can produce devastating complications including: shift of oxyhemoglobin saturation curve to the left (decreasing release of oxygen); hyperosmolarity; hypernatremia; paradoxical intracellular acidosis (due to production of carbon dioxide which diffuses readily into cells); exacerbation of central venous acidosis; and, possible inactivation of simultaneously administered catecholamines.

Therefore:
Do *not* administer sodium bicarbonate until after specific therapy (eg, intubation; antidysrhythmics) has been employed.

Thereafter:
If *ABGs not available,* then empiric administration of **Sodium Bicarbonate, IV slow push, 1 mEq/kg initially,** then not more than **0.5 mEq/kg** q 10 minutes [50 ml of 7.5% solution = 44.6 mEq (0.9 mEq/ml); 50 ml of 8.4% solution = 50 mEq (1 mEq/ml)].

If *ABGs available,* then sodium bicarbonate doses can be calculated from the base deficit:

$$NaHCO_3 \text{ Dose in mEq} =$$
Base Deficit in mEq/L $\times$ 0.2 $\times$ Body Weight in kg

Epinephrine—Empiric Use. Epinephrine is often given empirically at the start of definitive therapy, even before an EKG diagnosis has been made. The basis for this empiric use is epinephrine's α-adrenergic receptor agonist activity, which increases systemic vascular resistance, enhancing perfusion of the myocardium and CNS during CPR. Thus, the following may be appropriate:

Epinephrine HCl, IV slow push, 0.5-1 mg (5-10 ml of 1:10,000 solution, or 0.5-1 ml of 1:1000 diluted to 10 ml with saline).

If IV access has not been established or has been lost, *then:*
Epinephrine HCl, via endotracheal tube, 0.5-1 mg (5-10 ml of 1:10,000 solution), followed by 3-4 rapid ventilations to disperse drug.

Specific Therapy

In order to simplify the pharmacologic management of cardiopulmonary arrest, disturbances of cardiac activity associated with cardiac arrest may be grouped into three major categories each of which can be approached in a logical manner: ventricular tachydysrhythmias, asystole and electromechanical dissociation.

Ventricular Tachydysrhythmias. Considered in this category, and treated in the same way, are ventricular fibrillation, ventricular flutter and ventricular tachycardia when associated with ineffective cardiac output.

1. *Electrical defibrillation, 200 joules delivered.*

2. Epinephrine HCl, IV slow push, 0.5-1 mg (5-10 ml of 1:10,000 solution) is commonly stated to be an effective adjunct for successful defibrillation, especially when ventricular fibrillation is monitored as "fine" fibrillatory waves. There are no scientific data to support this concept; thus, epinephrine is not recommended as an aid to defibrillation specifically, but rather as an aid to myocardial perfusion (see Epinephrine-Empiric Use).

3. In intractable ventricular tachydysrhythmias or when there is repeated .reversion to tachydysrhythmias following electrical defibrillation, an irritable focus in the myocardium may be the source of persistent tachydysrhythmias and an antidysrhythmic drug is indicated. (If digitalis toxicity is suspected, see item 7).
   Lidocaine HCl, IV slow push, 50-100 mg (1 mg/kg) (2.5-5 ml of 2% or 5-10 ml of 1% solution), may repeat q 3-5 minutes to total of 300 mg.

   If IV access has not been established or has been lost, *then*:
   Lidocaine HCl via endotracheal tube, 150-300 mg (3 mg/kg) (7.5-15 ml of 2% solution), followed by 3-4 rapid ventilations to disperse drug.

   If response to loading dose occurs, *then maintenance*:
   Lidocaine HCl, IV infusion, 1-4 mg/minute (20-50 mcg/kg/minute) (10 ml of 20% in 500 ml D5W = 4 mg/ml).

4. If lidocaine fails to maintain electrical stability, then:
   Bretylium Tosylate, IV rapid push, 500 mg (5 mg/kg) (50 mg/ml, 10 ml vial), may repeat with 10 mg/kg q 15 minutes to total of 30 mg/kg. Note that bretylium frequently has a slow onset of action (>10 minutes). While waiting for this effect, one could ad-

minister procainamide HCl (see item 5) in an attempt to gain control of the dysrhythmia rapidly. The important point to recognize is that once primary therapy fails, second-line agents are not predictably effective. Should procainamide fail to suppress tachydysrhythmias, the slower acting bretylium will already have been administered. Should procainamide be effective, then subsequent doses of bretylium will not be necessary.

If response to loading dose occurs, *then maintenance:* **Bretylium Tosylate, IV infusion, 1–4 mg/minute.**

5. If lidocaine- and bretylium-resistant dysrhythmias persist, or if one elects to administer procainamide concurrently with bretylium, *then:*
Procainamide HCl, IV slow push, 500 mg (5 ml of 100 mg/ml vial, or 1 ml of 500 mg/ml vial), may repeat in 5 minutes to total of 1 g.

Note that this rate is greater than the commonly reported 25–50 mg/minute; however, this is a life-threatening dysrhythmia and delays in drug administration may prove ineffective.

If response to loading dose occurs, *then maintenance:* **Procainamide HCl, IV Infusion, 2–6 mg/minute** (30–80 mcg/kg/minute).

6. If lidocaine-, bretylium- and procainamide-resistant dysrhythmias persist, *then:*
Propranolol HCl, IV slow push, 1 mg over 1 minute (1 mg/ml ampule), may repeat q 5 minutes to total of 0.1 mg/kg.

7. If all of above fail or if digitalis toxicity is suspected, *consider:*
Magnesium Sulfate, IV slow push, 1 g (8 mEq) over 1 minute (2 ml of 50% solution), may repeat after 5 minutes if no response.

Bradydysrhythmias. Considered in this category, and treated in the same way, are asystole, complete heart block, slow ventricular focus, sinus bradycardia and agonal rhythm. In dealing with any of these dysrhythmias (except asystole), transvenous pacing is probably the best long-term approach, but is generally not readily available. Thus, drugs are used to enhance or initiate cardiac activity, at least until transvenous equipment is available.

It is important to note that true asystole, unless the result of excessive vagal tone (bradyasystole event), is frequently associated with irreversible cardiac damage.

1. Treatment of bradydysrhythmias should be initiated with:
Atropine Sulfate, IV push, 0.5–1 mg (5–10 ml of 0.1 mg/ml solution), may repeat with 0.5–1 mg q 5 minutes to total of 4 mg.

If IV access has not been established or has been lost, *then:* **Atropine sulfate, via endotracheal tube, 1 mg** (10 ml of 0.1 mg/ml solution), followed by 3–4 rapid ventilations to disperse drug.

2. For bradydysrhythmias failing to respond to atropine, *then:*
Epinephrine HCl, IV push, 0.5–1 mg (5–10 ml of 1:10,000), may repeat after 5 minutes.

3. For bradydysrhythmias failing to respond to the above, some experts have recommended isoproterenol. However, the use of isoproterenol, although supported by AHA-ACLS guidelines, may be inappropriate, because β-adrenergic agonist mediated vasodilation may actually lower perfusion pressures during CPR. Thus, the use of isoproterenol cannot be justified. However, as a "last resort," the following standard dose may be used:

Isoproterenol HCl, IV push, 0.02–0.04 mg (1–2 ml of 1:50,000 solution which is 1 ml of 1:5000 diluted with 9 ml of NS), may repeat q 3–5 minutes. If isoproterenol is effective, *then maintenance:*
Isoproterenol HCl, IV infusion, beginning with 1–2 mcg/minute, titrated to response (5 ml of 1:5000 in 250 ml D5W = 4 mcg/ml).

Electromechanical Dissociation. Considered in this category are ineffective cardiac output (hypotension) in face of EKG evidence of electrical myocardial activity, hypotension secondary to inadequate peripheral vasoconstriction, volume depletion or cardiac tamponade.

1. Rapidly assess volume status—if depleted, fluid challenge with crystalloid (NS or lactated Ringer's injection).

2. If volume is adequate and no evidence of tamponade, then consider cardiac sympathomimetics for vasoconstricting and inotropic/chronotropic effects. Begin with:
Dopamine HCl, IV infusion, 5 mcg/kg/minute initially, increasing prn to maximum of 20 mcg/kg/minute, adjusting rate to keep systolic blood pressure between 90–100 mm Hg (400 mg in 500 ml D5W = 800 mcg/ml).

3. If dopamine fails, *then:*
Norepinephrine Bitartrate, IV infusion, 8 mcg/minute initially, adjusting, as needed, to keep systolic blood pressure between 90–100 mm Hg [8 ml of 0.1% solution (1 mg/ml) in 500 ml D5W = 16 mcg/ml].

4. If norepinephrine fails, *then add:*
Calcium Chloride, IV slow push, 0.5–1 g
(5–10 ml of 10% solution = 6.8–13.6 mEq), *or:*
Calcium Gluconate, IV slow push, 1–2 g
(10–20 ml of 10% solution = 4.7–9.4 mEq), *or:*
Calcium Gluceptate, IV slow push, 1.1–2.2 g
(5–10 ml = 4.5–9 mEq).
Note that calcium administration in the therapy of electromechanical dissociation has not been shown to be effective and, in fact, may be harmful. Therefore, its use should be confined to situations in which acceptable therapy has failed or in situations in which calcium therapy is antidotal (ie, hyperkalemia, hypocalcemia, calcium channel blocker toxicity).

Postresuscitation Care
Patients who have been successfully resuscitated are at great risk

of experiencing subsequent events. Thus, if the patient is not already in an intensive care setting with constant monitoring, readily available resuscitation equipment and skilled nursing staff, transport the patient to such an area as soon as possible. The cause of the initial episode must be sought and corrected if possible.

Special Considerations/Precautions

Systemic circulation times are grossly prolonged during external chest compression. Remember to allow *at least* 2 minutes between the time of peripheral injection of pharmacologic agents and anticipated response.

Endotracheal administration of epinephrine, lidocaine and atropine can be utilized in situations in which IV access has not been established or has been lost.

Intracardiac injections of drugs play no role in modern management of cardiopulmonary arrest. Drugs do not work within the chambers of the heart, but rather at the cellular level after delivery via the coronary circulation. Stopping BCLS to attempt intracardiac injections only serves to interrupt vital CNS perfusion.

Be aware of the possible physical incompatibilities of sodium bicarbonate and catecholamines. In addition, sodium bicarbonate and calcium-containing solutions may form a precipitate if infused at the same time in the same IV line.

References

1. Anon. Standards and guidelines for cardiopulmonary resuscitation (CPR) and emergency cardiac care (ECC). JAMA 1986;255:2905-84.

2. Bishop RL, Weisfeldt ML. Sodium bicarbonate administration during cardiac arrest. JAMA 1976;235:506-9.

3. Goldberg AH. Cardiopulmonary arrest. N Engl J Med 1974;290:381-5.

4. Greenblatt DJ, Gross PL, Bolognini V. Pharmacotherapy of cardiopulmonary arrest. Am J Hosp Pharm 1978;33:579-83.

5. Mattar JA, Weil MH, Shubin H et al. Cardiac arrest in the critically ill. II. Hyperosmolal states following cardiac arrest. Am J Med 1974;56:162-8.

6. Otto CW, Eisenberg MS, Bircher NG, eds. Wolf Creek III conference on cardiopulmonary resuscitation. Crit Care Med 1985;13:881-951.

7. Raehl CL. Endotracheal drug therapy in cardiopulmonary resuscitation. Clin Pharm 1986;5:572-9.

Poisoning

General Information. Management of the poisoned patient involves procedures designed to prevent the absorption, minimize the toxicity and hasten elimination of the suspected contaminant. The prompt employment of appropriate emergency management procedures can often prevent unnecessary morbidity and mortality.

A regional poison information center is a practitioner's best source of definitive treatment information and should be consulted in all poisonings, regardless of the apparent simplicity of the case. Contact the regional poison information center in your area to learn of their staffing, resources and capabilities before a need for their services arises. Well-qualified regional centers are certified by the American Association of Poison Control Centers.

In all cases, every attempt should be made to accurately identify the contaminant, estimate the quantity involved and determine the time which has expired since the exposure. These data plus patient-specific parameters such as age, weight, sex and underlying medical conditions or drug use will assist you and the regional poison information center in designing an appropriate therapeutic plan for the patient.

The techniques described below are intended for the initial management of the poisoned patient using materials which should be readily available.

Topical Exposures

1. Irrigate affected areas with a copious amount of water; use soap only if a stubborn, oily substance is the contaminant. Skin should be gently washed, not scrubbed, and special attention should be paid to the hair, skin folds, umbilicus and other areas where the contaminant might be trapped.

2. If the patient's clothes have been contaminated, remove them during the irrigation and either destroy them or clean them before the patient is allowed to wear them again. Clothing can interfere with the irrigation process and can serve as a reservoir of toxic material.

3. Do not attempt to "neutralize" the contaminant with another chemical (eg, acids and alkalis). Attempts at neutralization waste valuable time, are of no benefit and may be harmful.

4. Do not cover the affected area with emollients. These may trap unremoved contaminant against the skin. Severely damaged skin may be temporarily covered with a light, dry dressing.

5. Protect yourself from contamination. Gloves, aprons or a change of clothes may be necessary.

6. After the irrigation is complete, contact a regional poison information center for definitive treatment information.

Eye Exposure

1. *Immediately* irrigate the eye; damage can occur within seconds. The stream of water from the tap or a pitcher should strike the patient on the forehead, temple or bridge of the nose and then flow into the eye.

2. The eyelids should be open with frequent blinking during the irrigation.

3. The irrigation should continue for at least 15 minutes (by the clock) to ensure adequate removal of the contaminant and normalization of the conjunctival pH. Body temperature water or saline may be substituted for tap water as the irrigation proceeds, but only if they can be obtained without interrupting the irrigation.

4. After the irrigation is complete, contact a regional poison information center for definitive treatment information.

Inhalation Exposures
1. Remove the patient from the contaminated area, regardless of its apparent safety. Carbon monoxide, a common inhaled toxin, cannot be detected by sight, smell or taste.

2. Institute artificial respiration, if necessary, and provide supplementary hydrated oxygen if available and needed.

3. Protect yourself from contamination at all times.

4. Contact a regional poison information center for definitive treatment information.

Ingestions
1. Remove any remaining contaminant from inside and around the mouth of the patient.

2. Give a small amount of water to clear the mouth and esophagus.

3. Contact a regional poison information center for definitive treatment information.

4. In many cases, it will not be necessary to take further steps. The following information can be utilized if additional care is recommended by the regional poison center.

Induction of Emesis
a. Do not induce emesis if the patient has evidence of CNS depression, seizures, loss of gag reflex or if the patient has ingested a caustic substance.
b. Induce emesis only with syrup of ipecac. Salt water, mustard water, other "home remedies" or gagging have no place in the management of the poisoned patient. These techniques are only marginally effective and can be dangerous.
c. The usual initial dose of **syrup of ipecac is 30 ml in persons over 5 years of age, 15 ml in children 1–5 years old** and **10 ml in children between 6 months and one year of age.**
d. Give the patient additional water to drink: 4 to 8 fluidounces in children, 8 to 16 fluidounces in adults. Activated charcoal should not be given until after ipecac-induced emesis has occurred.
e. Emesis usually occurs within 15–20 minutes. If 30 minutes have passed without emesis, it may be necessary to give an additional dose of syrup of ipecac and more water.
f. When emesis occurs, the risk of aspiration is minimized if the patient's head is lower than his hips. With a small child, this can be accomplished by having the child lie face down across the lap of an adult.
g. Have the patient vomit into a bowl or other container so that the vomitus can be inspected for the presence of the contaminant.

Gastric Lavage
a. An alternative to syrup of ipecac for stomach emptying is

gastric lavage. Lavage has the advantage of being useful in patients with CNS depression.

b. If the patient's gag reflex is weak or absent, the airway should be protected by the use of a cuffed endotracheal tube.

c. The largest possible orogastric tube should be used (26–28 F for children and 34–42 F for adults). The larger the tube diameter, the more efficient the lavage. The tube may be introduced through either the mouth or nose with the aid of a water-soluble lubricant.

d. Gastric lavage may be done with water, but a solution like 0.45% NaCl may be used to minimize the risk of dilutional hyponatremia, especially in children. Aliquots of fluid up to 100 ml in children and 200 ml in adults are introduced through the tube and then removed by gravity or suction-assisted drainage. The lavage should be continued for several cycles after the returning fluid is clear.

Note: Neither ipecac-induced emesis nor gastric lavage should be presumed to provide complete gastric emptying. Comparative studies have shown only limited success with these techniques, with gastric lavage through a large bore tube usually being somewhat superior. There is considerable interpatient variability in response to emesis and lavage.

Activated Charcoal

a. Activated charcoal is a nonspecific adsorbent which is used to bind unabsorbed poison within the GI tract. It is administered orally or by gastric tube in doses which range from 30–120 g. There is some evidence to support the use of activated charcoal as an alternative to ipecac-induced emesis or gastric lavage as an initial approach to the poisoned patient, rather than using it as an adjunct to these therapies. Repeated oral doses of activated charcoal (eg, q 4 hours) have been used to enhance the elimination of some drugs, most notably phenobarbital and theophylline.

b. Activated charcoal must be dispersed in a liquid like water or 35% sorbitol before administration. Gentle encouragement may be needed to make children swallow the charcoal. Having the child take the liquid through a drinking straw from an opaque container is sometimes helpful.

c. Activated charcoal may be followed by the administration of a cathartic.

d. Alert the patient that charcoal will cause the stools to turn black.

Cathartics

a. Cathartics may hasten elimination of unabsorbed drug and charcoal-adsorbed drug. The role of cathartics in the management of poisoning is currently being questioned, because there is little evidence to suggest that they reduce morbidity or mortality. Overuse of cathartics may result in significant losses of body water, sodium, potassium and bicarbonate.

b. The most commonly used cathartics and their doses are:

- **Magnesium sulfate (Epsom salt)** or **sodium sulfate (Glauber's salt), 15–20 g in adults; 250 mg/kg in children** given as 20% solutions. Solutions of these salts taste bad and some patients may reject them.

- **Citrate of magnesia, 4 ml/kg, up to 300 ml.** Although better tasting than the sulfate salts, the major limitation of this agent is the volume of fluid consumed.

- **Sorbitol (20–35% solution), 1 g/kg.** The palatability of this solution makes it easy to administer but, nevertheless, it can produce the same fluid and electrolyte losses associated with other cathartics.

References

1. McGuigan MA. Treatment of poisoning. Clin Symp 1984;36(5):1-32.
2. Haddad LM. A general approach to the emergency management of poisoning. In: Haddad LM, Winchester JF, eds. Clinical management of poisoning and drug overdose. Philadelphia: WB Saunders, 1983;4-18.
3. Tandberg D, Troutman WG. Gastric lavage in the poisoned patient. In: Roberts JR, Hedges JR, eds. Clinical procedures in emergency medicine. Philadelphia: WB Saunders, 1985;762-80.
4. Tandberg D, Diven BG, McLeod JW. Ipecac-induced emesis versus gastric lavage: a controlled study in normal adults. Am J Emerg Med 1986;4:205-9.
5. Auerbach PS, Osterloh J, Braun O et al. Efficacy of gastric emptying: gastric lavage versus emesis induced with ipecac. Ann Emerg Med 1986;15:692-8.
6. Wheeler-Usher DH, Wanke LA, Bayer MJ. Gastric emptying: risk versus benefit in the treatment of acute poisoning. Med Toxicol 1986;1:142-53.
7. Neuvonen PJ, Vartiainen M, Tokola O. Comparison of activated charcoal and ipecac syrup in prevention of drug absorption. Eur J Clin Pharmacol 1983;24:557-62.
8. Kulig K, Bar-Or D, Cantrill SV et al. Management of acutely poisoned patients without gastric emptying. Ann Emerg Med 1985;14:562-7.
9. Pond SM. Role of repeated oral doses of activated charcoal in clinical toxicology. Med Toxicol 1986;1:3-11.
10. Riegel JM, Becker CE. Use of cathartics in toxic ingestions. Ann Emerg Med 1981;10:254-8.
11. Sketris IS, Mowry JB, Czajka PA et al. Saline catharsis: effect on aspirin bioavailability in combination with activated charcoal. J Clin Pharmacol 1982;22:59-64.
12. Krenzelok EP, Keller R, Stewart RD. Gastrointestinal transit times of cathartics combined with charcoal. Ann Emerg Med 1985;14:1152-5.
13. Shannon M, Fish SS, Lovejoy FH. Cathartics and laxatives. Do they still have a place in management of the poisoned patient? Med Toxicol 1986;1:247-52.

Status Epilepticus

STATUS EPILEPTICUS IS DEFINED AS SEIZURES of sufficient duration or frequency to produce an enduring epileptic condition. Thus, status epilepticus is a serious neurological emergency which requires immediate recognition and prompt treatment to reduce morbidity and mortality.

Although status epilepticus can be subdivided into two major categories, convulsive and nonconvulsive status, the approach below deals only with generalized convulsive status. This type of status occurs most commonly, is most serious in terms of morbidity and mortality, and presents the greatest possibility for therapeutic error.

There is limited agreement on the most appropriate treatment regimen for convulsive status epilepticus, because there are no controlled studies from which objective data can be obtained. These guidelines present an approach which, if followed, will result in adequate control for most patients while minimizing drug toxicity.

The emergency treatment of generalized convulsive status epilepticus centers on four major approaches:

- **Protection From Physical Harm**
- **Airway Maintenance**
- **Drug Therapy**
- **Identification and Treatment of Precipitating Factors**

Protection from Physical Harm

1. If patient is on the ground or floor, move potentially harmful objects.

2. If patient is on a bed and side rails are available, they should be raised and padded.

3. A padded tongue blade or similar device can be inserted carefully between the teeth to decrease trauma to tongue, teeth and lips. Never force a tongue blade; insert during interictal period only.

Airway Maintenance

1. Position patient properly to decrease aspiration.

2. Insert soft plastic airway during interictal period.

3. Suction secretions.

4. Intubate if necessary (nasotracheal; orotracheal if interictal).

Drug Therapy. *Adult doses only are given in this section.*
If a rapidly identifiable and treatable cause for seizure activity can be found (see the section, Identification and Treatment of Specific Precipitating Factors, page 257), general pharmacologic management of the seizure may be unnecessary. However, when such an etiology cannot be identified, drug therapy should be considered.

The principal goal of pharmacologic treatment of convulsive status is to quickly control the seizure state by administering a rapid-acting anticonvulsant. This is followed by the administration of an adequate loading dose of a long-acting anticonvulsant to initiate maintenance therapy.

1. For initial control, administer the following rapid-acting anticonvulsant:
   Diazepam, IV slow push (5 mg/minute), 5–10 mg initially (1–2 ml of 5 mg/ml solution), may repeat, if necessary, at 5 minute intervals to a total of 30 mg. If diazepam is effective, consider initiating long-term control with a second agent (phenytoin or phenobarbital).
   Lorazepam, IV slow push (2 mg/minute), 2–4 mg initially (1–2 ml of 2 mg/ml solution) may be an effective (although unapproved) alternative to diazepam.

2. If initial control is not successful with diazepam, *then add:*
Phenytoin Sodium, IV slow push (50 mg/minute), 18 mg/kg (using 50 mg/ml solution). If seizure control is established, then begin maintenance therapy with phenytoin.

3. If seizure control is not established by completion of infusion, *then add:*
Phenobarbital Sodium, IV slow push (100 mg/minute), 5 mg/kg (using 130 mg/ml solution). If seizure control is established with phenobarbital, then begin maintenance therapy with phenobarbital. If seizure control is not established within 20 minutes of completing infusion, may repeat dose.

For patients who continue to have seizures despite full therapeutic doses of the above drugs, the following alternatives can be attempted:

1. **Paraldehyde, IM, 0.1-0.15 ml/kg,** may repeat in 2 hours.

2. **Lidocaine HCl, IV slow push (50 mg/minute), 2-3 mg/kg** (using 20 mg/ml solution). This agent is not approved for status epilepticus, but has demonstrated effectiveness in refractory cases.

3. **Neuromuscular Blocking Agents.** These agents suppress neuromuscular evidence of seizure activity, but do not prevent or attenuate continued cerebral seizure activity; they should only be used with continuous EEG monitoring.

   For example:
   Pancuronium Bromide, IV push, 0.06-0.1 mg/kg, for initial induction of paralysis, *then maintenance:*
   Pancuronium Bromide, IV push, 0.01 mg/kg at 25-60 minute intervals prn.

   or

   Pancuronium Bromide, IV continuous infusion, 0.03-0.06 mg/kg/hr (50 ml of 1 mg/ml solution in 50 ml D5W or NS = 0.5 mg/ml).

4. **General Anesthesia.** Very little information is available as to proper agent, monitoring or duration.

Identification and Treatment of Specific Precipitating Factors

Generalized convulsive status epilepticus occurs primarily in patients with a known seizure disorder and a specific, identifiable precipitating factor. Although most cases of generalized seizures can be temporarily controlled with drugs, it is important to simultaneously attempt to determine the presence of a treatable precipitating factor.

The following list of precipitating factors, although not complete, should be considered.

1. Anticonvulsant drug withdrawal.

2. Drug withdrawal states (sedatives, rarely alcohol).

3. Metabolic abnormalities (eg, hypoxia, hypoglycemia, hyponatremia).

4. Febrile state.

5. Drug toxicity (eg, isoniazid, theophylline, heterocyclic antidepressants).

6. Recent CNS diagnostic procedures.

7. New CNS lesions (eg, infarction, tumor, encephalitis, meningitis).

Special Considerations/Precautions

Only patients who present with active seizure activity should be treated vigorously. The aggressive use of diazepam or phenobarbital in a patient who has stopped convulsing sedates the patient and interferes with the subsequent work-up.

Generalized seizures in pediatric patients present special problems, not only with respect to recognition of precipitating factors, but also with treatment. Practitioners who deal with pediatric seizure patients should refer to specific reviews of these special problems.

References

1. Browne TR. Drug therapy reviews: drug therapy of status epilepticus. Am J Hosp Pharm 1978;35:915-22.
2. Celesia GG. Modern concepts of status epilepticus. JAMA 1976;235:1571-4.
3. Cranford RE, Leppik IE, Patrick B et al. Intravenous phenytoin in acute treatment of seizures. Neurology 1979;29:1474-9.
4. Delagado-Escueta AV, Wasterlain C, Treiman DM et al. Management of status epilepticus. N Engl J Med 1982;306:1337-40.
5. Leppik IE, Derivan AT, Homan RW et al. Double-blind study of lorazepam and diazepam in status epilepticus. JAMA 1983;249:1452-4.
6. Nicol CF. Status epilepticus. JAMA 1975;234:419-20.
7. Tharp BR. Recent progress in epilepsy—diagnostic procedures and treatment. Calif Med 1973;119:19-48.
8. Wilder BJ, Ramsay RE, Willmore LJ et al. Efficacy of intravenous phenytoin in the treatment of status epilepticus: kinetics of central nervous system penetration. Ann Neurol 1977;1:511-8.

The following is a cross-reference index of the generic and proprietary drug names used throughout the Medical Emergencies chapter.

Generic-Proprietary Name Index

Dopamine HCl—Intropin®, Various
Epinephrine HCl—Adrenalin®, Various
Hetastarch—Hespan®
Hydrocortisone Phosphate/Succinate—
    Hydrocortone®/Solu-Cortef®
Isoproterenol HCl—Isuprel®, Various
Lidocaine HCl—Xylocaine®, Various
Lorazepam—Ativan®, Various
Norepinephrine Bitartrate—Levophed®, Various
Paraldehyde—Various
Pancuronium Bromide—Pavulon®
Phenobarbital Sodium—Various
Phenytoin Sodium—Dilantin®, Various
Procainamide HCl—Pronestyl®, Various
Propranolol HCl—Inderal®, Various
Sodium Bicarbonate—Various
Syrup of Ipecac—Various

12 *NUTRITIONAL SUPPORT*

NUTRITIONAL STATUS IS A MAJOR DETERMINANT of patients' morbidity and mortality. Morbidity increases with malnutrition as manifested by depressed cell-mediated immunity and impaired wound healing.[1,2] Conditions that indicate a possible need for nutritional support include inadequate oral nutrition for longer than 7 days, recent body weight loss greater than 10%, an illness lasting more than 3 weeks, recent major surgery, a lymphocyte count of less than 1500/cu mm, serum albumin less than 3.5 g/dl and impaired cellular immunity demonstrated by anergy with skin testing.

The term "nutritional support" can be applied to any nutritional regimen that is provided for conditions that preclude the use of regular foods. There are two broad categories of nutritional support, enteral and parenteral, determined by their route of administration. Enteral nutrition applies to regimens provided via any portion of the gastrointestinal (GI) tract. Parenteral nutrition, although implying all routes other than the GI tract, refers only to regimens provided by the intravenous route of administration.

Whenever possible, maintenance rather than repletion should be the primary objective of nutritional support. Early provision of nutritional requirements without exceeding energy balance will promote synthesis of lean body mass rather than adipose tissue.[3]

Nutritional Assessment

NUTRITIONAL ASSESSMENT OF THE PATIENT can aid in diagnosing malnutrition and determining its degree of severity, so that a proper nutritional support regimen can be formulated. The patient's physical and dietary history should be obtained to establish baseline data. Clinical parameters for assessing the patient's nutritional status can be most effectively evaluated through the use of an assessment form (Table 1). Because a patient's nutritional status is best reflected by body protein,[4] nutritional assessment should focus on the protein compartments. Protein compartments are classified into two types: somatic (muscle protein) and visceral (all other protein).

Somatic Protein Assessment Parameters
Percent Ideal Body Weight. The simplest initial measurement of a patient's nutritional status is body weight expressed as a percentage of ideal body weight (see Chapter 1, section on Anthropometrics).

Table 1. Nutritional Assessment

NAME: AGE: HT (cm):		DEPLETION		
DATE: SEX: WT (kg):	STANDARD	Mild	Moderate	Severe
1. **FAT STORES** $\dfrac{\text{TSF}}{\text{Standard TSF}} \times 100 =$	100%	90%	90–60%	< 60%
2. **SOMATIC PROTEIN** (Marasmus) Triceps Skinfold (TSF) mm =	M 12.5 F 16.5	11.3 14.9	11.3–7.5 14.9–9.9	< 7.5 < 9.9
% Ideal Body Weight $\dfrac{\text{ABW}}{\text{IBW}} \times 100 =$	100%	90%	90–60%	< 60%
Mid-Upper Arm Circumference (MUAC) cm =	M 29.3 F 28.5	26.4 25.7	26.4–17.6 25.7–17.1	< 17.6 < 17.1
Mid-Upper Arm Muscle Circumference MUAC (cm)–[0.314 × TSF (mm)] =	M 25.3 F 23.2	22.8 21.0	22.8–15.2 21.0–13.9	< 15.2 < 13.9
Urinary Creatinine mg/24 hours =				
Creatinine/Height Index $\dfrac{Cr_u}{ICr_u \text{ for height}} \times 100 =$	100%	90%	90–60%	< 60%
3. **VISCERAL PROTEIN** (Kwashiorkor) Serum Albumin g/dl =	3.5–5.0	3.5–3	3–2.5	< 2.5
Serum Prealbumin mg/dl	>20	20–15	15–10	<10
Serum Transferrin mg	200–400	200–180	180–160	< 160
Total Lymphocyte/cu mm $\dfrac{\text{WBC/cu mm} \times \text{\% Lymphocytes}}{100}$	1800–3000	1800–1500	1500–900	< 900
4. **CELLULAR IMMUNITY** mm Candida albicans Mumps PPD Tetanus Toxoid Trichophyton	>5			

Abbreviations:

ABW	—	Actual body weight
IBW	—	Ideal body weight
ICr_u	—	Ideal urinary creatinine
MUAC	—	Mid-upper arm circumference
TSF	—	Triceps skin fold
Cr_u	—	Urinary creatinine

$$\text{Percent Ideal Body Weight} = \frac{\text{Actual Body Weight}}{\text{Ideal Body Weight}} \times 100$$

Creatinine/Height Index. Creatinine/height index (CHI), when accurately obtained, is a more sensitive indicator of somatic protein and nutritional status than is percent ideal body weight.[5] Creatinine, a product of muscle metabolism, is normally excreted in urine at a constant rate proportional to the amount of skeletal muscle and lean body mass catabolized. CHI is calculated from a 24-hour urinary creatinine measurement and the ideal urinary creatinine value found in Table 2, using the following formula:

$$CHI = \frac{\text{Actual Urinary Creatinine}}{\text{Ideal Urinary Creatinine for Height}} \times 100$$

It is important that the urine sample be an aliquot drawn from a 24-hour collection of urine rather than a random sample.

Table 2. Ideal Urinary Creatinine[a]

MALES[b]		FEMALES[c]	
Height (cm)	Ideal Creatinine (mg/24 hr)	Height (cm)	Ideal Creatinine (mg/24 hr)
157.5	1288	147.3	830
160.0	1325	149.9	851
162.6	1359	152.4	875
165.1	1386	154.9	900
167.6	1426	157.5	925
170.2	1467	160.0	949
172.7	1513	162.6	977
175.3	1555	165.1	1006
177.8	1596	167.6	1044
180.3	1642	170.2	1076
182.9	1691	172.7	1109
185.4	1739	175.3	1141
188.0	1785	177.8	1174
190.5	1831	180.3	1206
193.0	1891	182.9	1240

a. From Blackburn GL, Bistrian BR, Maini BS et al. Nutritional and metabolic assessment of the hospitalized patient. JPEN 1977;1:11-22, reproduced with permission.
b. Creatinine coefficient (men) = 23 mg/kg of ideal body weight.
c. Creatinine coefficient (women) = 18 mg/kg of ideal body weight.

There are certain limitations in using CHI as an indicator of malnutrition. Patients sometimes excrete amounts of creatinine and nitrogen that vary with different diets or conditions of illness or stress. Administration of corticosteroids, androgens or nitrofuran derivatives is reported to increase urinary levels of creatinine, whereas thiazides are reported to decrease levels.[6]

Anthropometric Measurements. Anthropometric measurements should be taken on the mid-upper portion of the nondominant arm by trained personnel. Detailed procedures and methods of measurement are available.[7,8] Triceps skin fold (TSF) measurement with calipers is compared to the standards in Table 1 to give a reasonable estimate of subcutaneous fat reserves.[4] Both TSF and mid-upper arm circumference (MUAC), obtained with a metric tape measure, can be used to derive the mid-upper arm muscle circumference (MUAMC) by the formula:[4]

$$MUAMC = MUAC \text{ (cm)} - [0.314 \times TSF \text{ (mm)}]$$

Visceral Protein Assessment Parameters

The status of visceral protein reflects the patient's ability to respond to stress by means such as immunocompetence and wound healing. Visceral protein status can be determined by measurements of serum albumin, serum thyroxine-binding prealbumin (now referred to as transthyretin or prealbumin), serum transferrin and total lymphocytes. Serum albumin and transferrin levels usually decrease after trauma or surgical procedures; however, consistently low levels for a period of at least 1 week may indicate a degree of malnutrition.[8] Serum albumin is unreliable as an assessment parameter in patients with hepatic or renal disease, severe burns or following intravenous administration of albumin.[9] Albumin levels are also known to be elevated as a result of dehydration, shock, hemoconcentration or anabolic hormones. Decreased levels can result from malabsorption, nephrosis, hepatic insufficiency, neoplastic disease, leukemia, overhydration or severe burns.

Prealbumin and transferrin are visceral proteins with a more rapid turnover than albumin. They are regarded as effective assessment parameters with half-lives of two days and seven days, respectively. Laboratory values must be interpreted carefully. Prealbumin serum levels are reported to decline postoperatively.[10] Transferrin levels are known to be elevated in patients who are iron deficient, pregnant, or those who are taking estrogens or oral contraceptives. Serum prealbumin and transferrin values indicative of varying degrees of depletion are given in Table 1.

Cell Mediated Immunity. Skin test data have been the most widely used parameters for assessment of the effect of nutritional depletion on cellular immunity.[11] Skin test antigens are injected intradermally and the response is measured after 24–48 hours. A diameter of induration greater than 5 mm to any one of the antigens listed below (Table 3) indicates an immune response. A lack of response to all of the antigens indicates anergy and possibly malnutrition. Other possible causes of anergy include shock, infection, trauma, burns, therapeutic immunosuppression and old age. The response to skin test antigens that may indicate nutritional depletion are designated in Table 1.

Table 3. Skin Testing for Anergy[8,12]

ANTIGEN	DILUTION	INJECT
Candida albicans	1:100	0.1 ml (1 PNU)
Mumps	Undiluted	0.1 ml
PPD	5 t.u.	0.1 ml
Tetanus Toxoid	1:5	0.1 ml
Trichophyton	1:500	0.1 ml

Periodic Reassessment

AN INITIAL ASSESSMENT can be made prior to beginning a nutritional support regimen. Periodic reassessment of the patient, using some or all of the previously mentioned parameters can provide a means of objectively evaluating the efficacy of the nutritional support. Additional parameters to consider during this stage of assessment are nitrogen balance and body weight.

Nitrogen Balance

Nitrogen balance determinations will indicate the extent to which exogenous protein is being utilized and can serve as a method for evaluating the efficacy of nutritional support selected for the patient. Because nitrogen balance data are subject to errors of collection and other variables, it should be used only as a relative index of daily change and not an absolute measure of depletion or improvement. Nitrogen balance is calculated for a 24-hour period using the following formula:[8]

Nitrogen Balance = Total Nitrogen In − Total Nitrogen Out

Estimation of nitrogen balance by measuring urinary urea nitrogen is a reasonable alternative and is summarized as follows:

$$\text{Nitrogen Balance} = \frac{\text{Protein Intake (g)}}{6.25} - [\text{Urinary Urea Nitrogen (g)} + 4]$$

Urinary urea nitrogen (UUN) is usually reported as a mg/dl value; therefore, to derive the amount in grams for use in the above formula, the value must be multiplied by the total 24-hour volume of urine output. The urine sample sent to the laboratory must be a 24-hour volume or an aliquot drawn from an accurate 24-hour urine collection. The factor "4" is added as an empirical number to account for nonurinary nitrogen, such as that excreted in feces, sweat and other normal losses. Excessive nitrogen losses that cannot be measured, such as nitrogen lost in exudates from severe burns or in dialysate fluids, render nitrogen balance data less reliable.

Positive nitrogen balance can indicate a retention of nitrogen both as newly synthesized body protein tissue and as nitrogen retained in body fluids. Because only synthesized protein is of therapeutic interest, elevations in BUN should be subtracted from total nitrogen balance. This calculation is summarized:

$$\text{Corrected Nitrogen Balance} = \text{Nitrogen Balance} - \text{BUN Increment (g)}$$

To derive the BUN increment above baseline in grams, the total body water volume of the patient must be considered. If the actual volume cannot be established for the patient, body water can be assumed to be 55% of total body weight (0.55 L/kg).[13] A BUN of 10 mg/dl above baseline in a 70 kg patient represents a BUN increment of 3.85 g (70 kg × 0.55 L/kg × 100 mg/L = 3.85 g).

Body Weight

The weight difference between tissue and body water is indistinguishable unless water balance can be measured. Body weight gain alone is therefore not a reliable maintenance assessment parameter. It is known, however, that weight gain in excess of 250 g/day is undesirable because patients cannot synthesize tissue at a greater rate.[14] Despite its shortcomings as a monitoring parameter, body weight should nevertheless be measured throughout the support regimen at the same time each day as an index of progress. Intake and output should be considered in the interpretation of body weight changes.

Nutrient Requirements

THE NUTRIENTS REQUIRED for enteral or parenteral nutrition are virtually the same. Either mode of nutritional support must consist of the basic components of a normal diet: water, carbohydrate, fat, protein, electrolytes, vitamins and trace elements.

Caloric Requirements

Depending upon the nutritional status and clinical condition of the patient, daily caloric requirements can be calculated as a multiple of the patient's basal energy expenditure (BEE). BEE is the amount of energy required to maintain basic metabolic functions in the resting state and can be derived from the Harris-Benedict formulas:[16]

BEE (Men): 66 + (13.7 × wt in kg) + (5 × ht in cm)
— (6.8 × age in yr)
BEE (Women): 665 + (9.6 × wt in kg) + (1.7 × ht in cm)
— (4.7 × age in yr)

Trauma increases energy and protein requirements, and the nutritional support regimen should be adjusted accordingly.[15] Based on the amount of urinary urea nitrogen excreted per 24 hours, the severity of catabolism in stress conditions can be determined. Caloric requirements can then be estimated as a multiple of BEE as follows:[16]

Table 4. Caloric Requirements During Catabolism

24-HOUR UUN	DEGREE OF NET CATABOLISM	CALORIC REQUIREMENTS
0–5 g	1° (normal)	1.0 × BEE
5–10 g	2° (mild)	1.5 × BEE
10–15 g	3° (moderate)	1.75 × BEE
> 15 g	4° (severe)	2.0 × BEE

Sepsis increases oxygen consumption, and presumably energy consumption, about 7% with each degree F of fever.[17] Alternative methods of estimating caloric requirements are also available.[18]

In estimating the calories to be provided by each calorigenic substrate, yields may be considered as: dextrose, 3.4 kcal/g; fat, 9 kcal/g; and protein, 4 kcal/g. Protein, however, should not be relied upon in meeting total energy requirements, because protein should be utilized for the preservation or synthesis of lean body mass.

Protein Requirements

The normal adult protein requirement is suggested to be about 0.6–0.8 g/kg/day.[19] This requirement may be doubled in severely ill or traumatized patients. For optimal synthesis of protein, concurrent provision of nonprotein calories must be sufficient. The optimal ratio of nonprotein calories to nitrogen for efficient nitrogen retention and nitrogen balance has been reported to be anywhere from 150:1 to 450:1.[20] This ratio is presumably not constant, but varies with the metabolic state of the patient.

Enteral Nutrition

FOR BOTH PHYSIOLOGIC AND ECONOMIC REASONS, the enteral route should be used whenever possible. The intravenous route should be reserved for patients who cannot be adequately nourished by the enteral route or whose GI tract is dysfunctional or in need of rest.

Before enteral nutrition can be provided, adequacy of the GI tract must be established. This may be confirmed by bowel sounds and the passage of flatus and stool.

Formulas for enteral nutrition are available for supplemental oral feeding or forced enteral feeding through various types of tubes. When the oral route is not feasible, transnasal passage of a feeding tube into the stomach (nasogastric) or intestine (nasoduodenal or nasojejunal) is generally the feeding route employed. Feeding ostomies, most commonly the gastrostomy, jejunostomy, or combination gastrostomy-jejunostomy, are generally indicated when insertion through the nares is not feasible or when long-term feeding is anticipated.

Formula Selection. The abundance of products available for enteral nutrition may present confusion in the selecting of a formula for a patient. It is not within the scope of this chapter to fully describe criteria for formula selection or provide a complete compendium of formulas. Some enteral formulas that are suitable for a variety of patients are presented in Table 5. Because patients with abnormal intestinal function are usually lactose intolerant, only lactose-free products are included. Disease-specific formulas, such as those with high content of branched chain amino acids for liver disease or essential amino acids for renal disease, are not included because of inadequate evidence of their superiority.

Administration. Either of two types of feeding schedules may be employed, *continuous* or *intermittent*.

Continuous drip infusion is the preferred method of administration, particularly for patients who have not eaten for a long time. Large 24-hour volumes may be given by infusion without challenging the GI tract, thereby allowing readaptation of the starved gut. Although gravity may be used, an infusion pump is recommended. For most patients, it is recommended that the first day's feeding be infused at a rate of 50 ml/hr using a lactose-free, nutrient intact formula of 1 kcal/ml. Many protocols recommend diluting the initial formula to one-half strength; however, this practice has recently been questioned.[21] On the second day, a full strength for-

Table 5. Representative Enteral Formulas

PRODUCT	CALORIES (per ml)	PROTEIN (g/L)	FAT (g/L)	CARBOHYDRATE (g/L)	NONPROTEIN CALORIES (cal/g Nitrogen)	SODIUM (mEq/L)	POTASSIUM (mEq/L)	CALCIUM (mg/L)	PHOSPHORUS (mg/L)	OSMOLARITY (mOsm/L)
Isocal®	1.0	34	44	133	192	23	34	630	530	300
Trauma Cal®	1.5	83	68	143	113	52	36	750	750	550
Ensure Plus®	1.5	55	53	200	170	50	57	625	625	600
Isocal HCN®	2.0	75	102	200	167	35	43	1000	667	740
Precision LR®	1.0	25	0.7	224	263	27	22	556	556	525
Criticare HN®	1.0	36	3	210	174	26	34	530	530	650
Vivonex TEN®	1.0	38	2.8	206	164	20	20	500	500	630

mula is used, maintaining the rate of 50 ml/hr. Thereafter, daily incremental rate increases of 25 ml/hr are attempted until the desired rate (usually 100–125 ml/hr) is achieved. To minimize the risk of aspiration, the tube must be properly placed and the patient's head and shoulders, if not upright, must be kept at a 30- to 45-degree angle.

Once a patient has been stabilized on maintenance therapy, *intermittent* infusions may be used, allowing the patient to rest from the feedings at selected hours. A volume of 250–400 ml may be administered five to eight times per day. This method is preferred for ambulatory patients, because it permits more freedom of movement than does continuous feeding.

Formulas should be given at room temperature and should be kept no longer than 12 hours after the time of preparation to avoid bacterial growth. The delivery system, including bag and tubing, should be changed every 24 hours.

Complications. Mechanical and GI complications known to occur with tube feedings are summarized in Table 6. Metabolic complications that are known to occur with enteral nutrition can similarly occur with parenteral nutrition and are included in Table 13 on page 277.

Table 6. Tube Feeding Complications and Management

COMPLICATION	PREVENTION OR MANAGEMENT
Mechanical	
Clogged Tube	Flush with water, replace tube if necessary.
Nasal, Pharyngeal, Esophageal Irritation	Use small lumen flexible tube. Provide daily care of nose and mouth.
Aspiration	Ensure proper tube placement and verify location. Maintain patient at 30°–45° position during and for 1 hr after feeding. Monitor for gastric reflux and abdominal distention. Stop infusion if vomiting occurs. Check residual volumes prior to and q 2–4 hr during infusion.
Dislocated Tube	Verify tube location and mark tube at insertion site.
Gastrointestinal	
Diarrhea and Cramps	Reduce flow rate, dilute formula or consider alternative formula. If persistent, add antidiarrheal agent.
Vomiting or Bloating	Check stool output and formula residual in gut q 2–4 hr. If necessary, stop or reduce flow.
Constipation	Consider different formula or laxative.

To prevent metabolic complications, monitoring of the patient as suggested in Table 14 on page 279 is recommended.

Parenteral Nutrition

THE PARENTERAL OR INTRAVENOUS (IV) ROUTE of nutrition should be reserved for patients who cannot be adequately maintained by the GI tract or who are in need of bowel rest. The IV route is used to supplement enteral administration or for total parenteral nutrition (TPN).

Intravenous Administration Routes

Parenteral nutrition may be administered by either of two routes of access: peripheral veins or larger central veins. The peripheral route is indicated for those patients who require only short-term supplementation or supplementation in addition to enteral support, or for those in whom the risks of central venous administration are too great. Peripheral veins are predisposed to thrombophlebitis, particularly when the osmolarity of the solution exceeds 600 mOsm/L. Therefore, it is recommended that formulas for peripheral administration not exceed final concentrations of 5% dextrose and 2.75% amino acids (AA) plus electrolyte and vitamin additives. Addition of small amounts of hydrocortisone (5 mg/L) and heparin (1000 units/L) to dextrose and AA solutions has been reported to prevent thrombophlebitis;[25] however, this should not be considered a routine practice. Concurrent administration of IV fat emulsion, which is a concentrated, isoosmotic calorie source, is vital, because it increases the caloric content of a peripheral regimen.

The complete nutritional needs of the malnourished or hypermetabolic patient are difficult to provide via peripheral vein for long periods of time. The concentrated, hyperosmolar solutions required by such patients for TPN *must* be administered into a large central vein, such as the superior vena cava where rapid dilution occurs. Such infusion requires surgical implantation of a catheter and subsequent monitoring. For such techniques and procedures the reader is referred elsewhere.[22-24,31]

Parenteral Nutrients

Each of the following nutrient substrate groups are required in formulas for effective TPN.

Water. The average healthy adult can tolerate a fluid infusion volume of about 5 L/day. The patient who is fluid restricted might be limited to an intake of 2 L/day or less. This may be the deciding factor in selecting a hypertonic concentrated solution for infusion through a large central vein rather than a more dilute solution for peripheral administration.

Carbohydrate. Presently the only carbohydrate substrate recommended for TPN is dextrose. The concentration of dextrose should be determined by the osmotic limitation of the administration route and the nonprotein caloric requirement of the patient. The concentrations of available dextrose solutions with their corresponding caloric concentrations and osmolarities are as follows:

Table 7. IV Dextrose Solutions

CONCENTRATION	kcal/L	mOsm/L
5%	170	252
10%	340	505
20%	680	1010
40%	1360	2020
50%	1700	2520
60%	2040	3030
70%	2380	3530

When not precluded by osmotic or metabolic limitations, about 2/3 of the caloric goal should be provided by dextrose calories.[18] On a calorie for calorie basis, carbohydrate is more efficient than fat in sparing body protein during hypocaloric feedings; however, the inclusion of both dextrose and fat is recommended in TPN regimens.

Fat. Fat is valued as a parenteral substrate for three major reasons: (1) it is a concentrated source of calories in an isotonic medium which makes it useful for peripheral administration; (2) it is a source of essential fatty acids (EFA) required for prevention or treatment of EFA deficiency, which may develop during extensive parenteral nutrition with dextrose;[26] and (3) it is a useful substitute for carbohydrate when dextrose calories must be limited due to glucose intolerance or excessive respiratory load. Metabolism of fat results in an increase in heat production, a decrease in respiratory quotient (RQ) and an increase in oxygen consumption. The RQ of fat is 0.7 versus 1 for carbohydrate.[27] Having a lower RQ, fat produces less CO_2 for a given number of calories, thereby minimizing the respiratory effort required to eliminate CO_2.

Fat is available as emulsions of 10 or 20% soybean oil or 10 or 20% soybean-safflower oil mixtures. Clinical studies have not shown any major advantages of one formulation over the other. The major differences in these products are their fatty acid contents which are summarized as follows:

Table 8. IV Fat Emulsions

FATTY ACID	SOYBEAN OIL	SOYBEAN OIL/ SAFFLOWER OIL
Linoleic Acid	54%	65.8%
Linolenic Acid	8%	4.2%
Oleic Acid	26%	17.7%
Palmitic Acid	9%	8.8%
Stearic Acid	2.5%	3.4%

The caloric density of 10% fat emulsions is 1.1 kcal/ml of which 1 kcal is supplied by lipid and 0.1 kcal by glycerol (carbohydrate); the 20% emulsion has a caloric density of 2 kcal/ml, of which 0.1 kcal/ml is glycerol. The average particle size (0.5 microns) is the same in both concentrations, and both are nearly iso-osmotic: 10% = 280 mOsm/L; 20% = 330 mOsm/L. Although the manufacturers recommend not to exceed 60% of total calories as fat, some researchers advocate the use of fat as 80% of daily nonprotein calories when peripheral IV regimens are used.[28] For further information on dosage, administration and precautions of fat emulsion, the product literature should be consulted.

Protein. Various brands and concentrations of AA solutions are available as sources of protein for parenteral use. The profile of amino acids differs in each, and therefore their nitrogen contents are not equivalent. A comparison of popular brands and concentrations are summarized in Table 9. It is generally recommended that 5–5.5% AA be used in regimens for maintenance or repletion of slightly catabolic patients. Furthermore, the lower osmolarity of these concentrations when mixed with an equal volume of a low concentration of dextrose (eg, 10%), makes them more suitable for peripheral administration than the more concentrated AA solutions. The higher concentrations of AA are more suited for maintenance or repletion of patients who are in greater need of protein.

Special Amino Acid Formulas

Protein Sparing. It has been demonstrated that a low concentration of amino acids infused with or without concurrent nonprotein calories conserves endogenous nitrogen more efficiently than the

Table 9. Amino Acid Solutions Comparison Chart

AA SOLUTION AND CONCENTRATION	TOTAL ESSENTIAL AA (g/dl)	TOTAL N (g/dl)	ELECTROLYTES (mEq/L)						PO$_4$ (mM)	OSMOLARITY (mOsm/L)
			Na$^+$	K$^+$	Mg^{++}	Cl$^-$	Ac$^-$			
For General Purpose										
Aminosyn® 3.5%	1.6	0.55	7	-	-	-	46		-	357
Aminosyn® 5%	2.35	0.79	-	5.4	-	-	86		-	500
Travasol® 5.5%	2.15	0.92	-	-	-	22	48		-	575
(with Electrolytes)------	------	------	70	60	10	70	102		30	850
Aminosyn® 7%	3.3	1.1	-	5.4	-	-	105		-	700
(with Electrolytes)------	------	------	70	66	10	96	124		30	1013
Veinamine® 8%	2.8	1.33	40	30	6	50	50		-	950
Aminosyn® 8.5%	4.0	1.34	-	5.4	-	35	90		-	850
(with Electrolytes)------	------	------	70	66	10	98	142		30	1160
Travasol® 8.5%	3.3	1.42	-	-	-	34	73		-	890
(with Electrolytes)------	------	------	70	60	10	70	141		30	1160
FreAmine® III 8.5%	3.9	1.3	10	-	-	<3	72		10	810
Novamine® 8.5%	3.8	1.35	-	-	-	-	88		-	785 Continued

Table 9. Amino Acid Solutions Comparison Chart

AA SOLUTION AND CONCENTRATION	TOTAL ESSENTIAL AA (g/dl)	TOTAL N (g/dl)	Na+	K+	Mg++	Cl-	Ac-	PO4 (mM)	OSMOLARITY (mOsm/L)
Aminosyn® 10%	4.7	1.57	–	5.4	–	–	148	–	1000
FreAmine® III 10%	4.6	1.53	10	–	–	<2	88	10	950
Travasol® 10%	4.1	1.65	–	–	–	40	87	–	1000
Novamine® 11.4%	5.1	1.8	–	–	–	–	114	–	1049
For Protein Sparing ProcalAmine® 3% [a]	1.4	0.46	35	24	5	41	47	3.5	735
FreAmine® III 3% with Electrolytes	1.4	0.46	35	24	5	40	44	3.5	405
Aminosyn® 3.5% M	1.6	0.55	40	18.4	3	40	68	–	460
3.5% Travasol® M with Electrolyte 45	1.4	0.6	25	15	5	25	54	8	450
For Renal Failure Aminosyn® RF 5.2%	4.6	0.8	–	5.4	–	–	105	–	475
NephrAmine® 5.4%	5.4	0.65	5	–	–	<3	44	–	435

Continued

Table 9. Amino Acid Solutions Comparison Chart

AA SOLUTION AND CONCENTRATION	TOTAL ESSENTIAL AA (g/dl)	TOTAL N (g/dl)	ELECTROLYTES (mEq/L)						OSMOLARITY (mOsm/L)
			Na$^+$	K$^+$	Mg^{++}	Cl$^-$	Ac$^-$	PO$_4$ (mM)	
RenAmin® 6.5%	4.3	1.0	–	–	–	31	60	–	600
For Trauma									
4% BranchAmin® b	4^c	0.44	–	–	–	–	–	–	316
FreAmine® HBC 6.9% b	4.3	0.97	10	–	–	<3	57	–	620
For Liver Disease									
HepatAmine® 8% b	4.2	1.2	10	–	–	<3	62	10	785
For Pediatrics									
TrophAmine® 6%	3.6	0.93	5	–	–	3	56	–	525
Aminosyn® PF 7%	3.5	1.07	3.4	–	–	–	33	–	586

a. Contains glycerol as a nonprotein calorie source.

b. Branched-chain amino acid enriched products. Each of these products has distinct indications for use and should not be interchanged.

c. Contains only the branched-chain amino acids. Other essential amino acids are not included.

traditional 5% dextrose infusion alone.[29] For a limited infusion of no more than 1 week's duration in patients who are not severely catabolic, low concentration AA formulas merit consideration. Low concentration AA formulas are available with or without electrolytes and with or without a nonprotein calorie source (see Table 9).

Renal Failure. The objective of parenteral nutrition in patients with renal failure is to provide sufficient amino acids and calories for protein synthesis without exceeding the renal capacity for excretion of fluid and metabolic wastes. Three formulas which contain primarily essential amino acids have been developed for this purpose are commercially available (see Table 9). There are many special considerations in the nutritional support of renal patients and the reader is referred elsewhere for guidelines.[22,30]

Hepatic Failure. Treatment of patients in hepatic failure in whom muscle breakdown contributes to hepatic encephalopathy may require a special AA formula with relatively greater amounts of branched chain amino acids (BCAA—leucine, isoleucine and valine) and smaller amounts of the aromatic amino acids (phenylalanine, tyrosine, tryptophan and methionine).[31] One formula is currently available specifically for therapeutic and nutritional support of patients with liver disease (see Table 9).

Stress and Trauma. The hypermetabolism that occurs in response to stress and trauma presents difficulty in providing nutritional support. BCAA, in addition to their useful effect in metabolic support of the patient with liver disease, are reported to be useful for the patient with stress and trauma.[32,33] Two products are available (see Table 9). FreAmine® HBC is a solution of nonessential and essential AA enriched with 45% BCAA. 4% BranchAmin® is a solution of only BCAA intended for use as a supplement to be admixed with a complete amino acid and a caloric source.

Pediatrics. It is beyond the scope of this chapter to describe procedures for nutritional support of the pediatric patient except in this brief mention of parenteral amino acid products. Currently, two cystalline AA solutions are marketed for infants (see Table 9) based on the essentiality of certain AA in these patients.[34] As compared to adult AA formulations, these products contain taurine, glutamic and aspartic acids, increased amounts of tyrosine and histidine, and lower amounts of phenylalanine, methionine and glycine. Although cysteine is also assumed to be essential for infants, adequate amounts cannot be included in AA formulas, because of limited solubility. A cysteine solution (50 mg/ml) is available separately for admixture to the formula prior to administration.

Electrolytes. Formulas are available with standard electrolyte compositions which may be suitable for most patients, after the addition of certain additives. Electrolyte provision, however, should be based on close monitoring of patients' laboratory values. Average daily requirements are summarized in Table 10.

Table 10. Electrolytes and Requirements

ELECTROLYTES	AVERAGE DAILY[22,30] TPN REQUIREMENT	DOSAGE FORMS	COMMENTS
Cations Sodium	60–150 mEq	Sodium chloride concentrate (4 mEq/ml) Sodium acetate (2 mEq/ml) Sodium phosphate (4 mEq Na$^+$/ml)	Requirements during parenteral nutrition should not differ from normal fluid therapy requirements unless there is excessive sodium loss. Lactate and bicarbonate salts of sodium should not be used.
Potassium	40–240 mEq	Potassium chloride (2 mEq/ml) Potassium acetate (2 mEq/ml) Potassium phosphate (4.4 mEq K$^+$/ml)	Requirements are related to glucose metabolism and therefore increase with higher concentrations of dextrose infused.
Magnesium	10–45 mEq	Magnesium sulfate (4 mEq/ml)	Requirements increase with anabolism; however, with less variation than does potassium.
Calcium	5–30 mEq	Calcium gluconate 10% (4.5 mEq/10 ml) Calcium chloride 10% (13 mEq/10 ml)	Calcium requirements increase only slightly during parenteral nutrition. Calcium may be combined in solution with phosphate, but should be well diluted before mixing. Concentration should be kept under 5 mEq of calcium and 40 mmol of phosphate in each liter.
Anions Phosphate	10 mmol/1000 kcal	Potassium phosphate (3 mmol P/ml—Abbott) Sodium phosphate (3 mmol P/ml—Abbott) (other concentrations may vary according to manufacturer)	Requirements increase with anabolism. Safe empirical dosing guidelines should be developed, taking into account the amount of sodium or potassium in solution as well as the amount of phosphate.

Acetate and Chloride: The amounts of acetate and chloride contained in each amino acid solution varies (see Table 9). To avoid acid/base disturbances, keep the ratio of sodium to chloride in the formula close to 1:1.[30] This guideline should not replace the monitoring of serum electrolytes to determine electrolyte requirements.

Vitamins. Vitamin requirements for parenteral nutrition have been suggested in a report by an advisory group to the American Medical Association (AMA).[35] Multiple vitamins are now available in adult and pediatric formulations for once daily IV administration (see Table 11). The usual daily dosage of the adult formulation is 10 ml to provide the amounts of vitamins specified in Table 11. The pediatric formula daily dosage for infants who weigh less than 1 kg is 30% of the contents of the vial. For infants weighing 1 to 3 kg, the daily dose is 65% of the vial contents. For infants and children weighing 3 kg or more up to 11 years of age, the daily dose is the contents of one vial. Vitamin K is included in the pediatric product only. Phytonadione 2–4 mg may be given to adults weekly by IM or SC administration.[35] See the Phytonadione drug monograph.

Table 11. IV Multivitamins

	AMOUNT PER DOSE	
TYPICAL FORMULA	ADULT	PEDIATRIC
Ascorbic Acid (C)	100 mg	80 mg
Vitamin A	3300 IU	2300 IU
Vitamin D	200 IU	400 IU
Vitamin E	10 IU	7 IU
Thiamine (B_1)	3 mg	1.2 mg
Riboflavin (B_2)	3.6 mg	1.4 mg
Niacinamide (B_3)	40 mg	17 mg
Pantothenic Acid (B_5)	15 mg	5 mg
Pyridoxine (B_6)	4 mg	1 mg
Biotin	60 mcg	20 mcg
Folic Acid	400 mcg	140 mcg
Cyanocobalamin (B_{12})	5 mcg	1 mcg
Phytonadione (K)	0	200 mcg

Trace Elements. Solutions of *individual* trace elements are available in several concentrations from various manufacturers. Solutions of multiple trace elements are also commercially available in products containing 2, 3, 4, 5, 6 or 7 elements and in concentrations suitable for adult or pediatric use. Guidelines for the use of trace elements in parenteral nutrition have been reported in an AMA statement[36] and the recommended daily dosages appear in Table 12. Although the need for selenium, molybdenum and iodine in long-term TPN has been described, there is no official definition of requirements for these elements.[37-39]

Iron. Iron deficiency can occur in patients deprived of iron during long-term TPN. Although other parenteral sources of iron have been tested, the only commercially available iron product for intravenous use at this time is iron dextran.[40] At least one study has concluded that iron dextran can be safely added to TPN solutions,[41] but dosing recommendations by this route have not been established. Methods of IV and IM administration are given in the Iron Dextran drug monograph.

Insulin. Insulin may be added to parenteral formulas to control hyperglycemia and glycosuria, if necessary. Human insulin is the least immunogenic and is therefore the insulin of choice. Guidelines for dosage are empirical and 10–50 units of regular insulin may be added to each liter of solution. Standardized admixture procedures should be used to minimize variations of insulin activity due to adsorption loss. Other alternatives to control hyperglycemia and glycosuria should be investigated before insulin is employed.[22]

Table 12. Suggested Daily IV Dosage of Trace Elements[a]

TRACE ELEMENT	PEDIATRIC PATIENTS, mcg/kg[b]	STABLE ADULT	ADULT IN ACUTE CATABOLIC STATE[c]	STABLE ADULT WITH INTESTINAL LOSSES[c]
Zinc	300[d] 100[e]	2.5–4.0 mg	Additional 2.0 mg	Add 12.2 mg/L small-bowel fluid lost; 17.1 mg/kg of stool or ileostomy output.[f]
Copper	20	0.5–1.5 mg	—	—
Chromium	0.14–0.2	10–15 mcg	—	20 mcg[g]
Manganese	2–10	0.15–0.8 mg	—	—

a. From American Medical Association Department of Foods and Nutrition. Guidelines for essential trace element preparations for parenteral use: a statement by an expert panel. JAMA 1979;241:2051-4, reproduced with permission.

b. Limited data are available for infants weighing less than 1,500 g. Their requirements may be more than the recommendations because of their low body reserves and increased requirements for growth.

c. Frequent monitoring of plasma levels in these patients is essential to provide proper dosage.

d. Premature infants (weight less than 1,500 g) up to 3 kg of body weight. Thereafter, the recommendations for full-term infants apply.

e. Full-term infants and children up to 5 years old. Thereafter, the recommendations for adults apply, up to a maximum dosage of 4 mg/day.

f. Values derived by mathematical fitting of balance data from a 71-patient-week study in 24 patients.

g. Mean from balance study.

Monitoring the Patient

METABOLIC COMPLICATIONS known to occur with enteral or parenteral nutrition are summarized in Table 13. Most of these can be avoided by proper precautions and close monitoring of the patient. Laboratory parameters for patient monitoring are summarized in Table 14. More complete discussions are found in references 22–24 and 30.

Table 13. Nutritional Support: Metabolic Complications and Management

COMPLICATION	FREQUENT CAUSES	MANAGEMENT
Hyponatremia	Excessive GI or urinary sodium losses. Water intoxication.	Increase sodium in formula based on patient's

Continued

Table 13. Nutritional Support:
Metabolic Complications and Management

COMPLICATION	FREQUENT CAUSES	MANAGEMENT
	Inadequate sodium intake.	requirements. Limit free water intake to treat water intoxication.
Hypokalemia	Excessive GI or urinary potassium losses. Deficit of potassium in formula. Large glucose infusion.	Increase potassium in formula based on patient's requirements.
Hypomagnesemia	Excessive GI or urinary losses. Insufficient magnesium in formula.	Increase magnesium in formula. In an emergency, IV magnesium sulfate may be given.
Hypophosphatemia	Usually due to inadequate inorganic phosphate in formula (concentrated glucose infusion may precipitate syndrome).	Increase phosphate in formula based on patient's requirements.
Hypoglycemia	Usually due to abrupt interruption of formula infusion.	Immediately begin dextrose infusion and monitor blood glucose and potassium.
Hyperglycemia	Deficit of potassium or phosphorus. Insufficient insulin for relatively high glucose infusion. Sepsis. Corticosteroid use.	Increase potassium or phosphate in formulas based on patient's requirements. Give insulin. Reduce rate of glucose infusion. Check for signs of sepsis.
Elevated BUN— Azotemia	Dehydration. Calorie:nitrogen imbalance. Renal dysfunction.	Correct dehydration. Give insulin if hyperglycemia present. Increase nonprotein calories to achieve higher calorie:nitrogen ratio.
Hyperammonemia	Hepatic dysfunction. Excess free ammonia. Excess glycine. Insufficient arginine.	Slow infusion rate. Change amino acid formula to specific infant formula. Discontinue infusion.

Continued

Table 13. Nutritional Support:
Metabolic Complications and Management

COMPLICATION	FREQUENT CAUSES	MANAGEMENT
Metabolic Acidosis	Excessive GI or urinary losses of base. Inadequate amount of base-producing substance in formula to neutralize acid products of amino acid degradation.	Increase acetate in formula.
Osmotic Diuresis	Failure to recognize initial hyperglycemia and increased glucose in urine.	Reduce infusion rate. Give insulin to correct hyperglycemia. Give 5% dextrose and hypertonic saline (¼ to ½ strength) rather than TPN solution to correct dehydration. Continue to monitor blood glucose, sodium, and potassium.
Essential Fatty Acid Deficiency	Insufficient provision of fat during TPN.	Provision of fat.

Table 14. Routine Patient Monitoring Parameters

PARAMETER	FREQUENCY[a]
Urinary glucose and specific gravity.	Every voided specimen until stable, then daily.
Vital signs, weight, intake & output.	Daily.
Serum glucose, electrolytes, creatinine and BUN.	Daily until stable, then twice weekly.
Magnesium, calcium and phosphorus.	Daily until stable, then once weekly.
CBC, hemoglobin, WBC, platelets and prothrombin time.	Baseline, then weekly.
Serum protein and liver function tests.	Baseline, then weekly.
Serum cholesterol and triglycerides.	Baseline, then weekly.
Blood ammonia.	Baseline, then weekly in renal and hepatic patients.

a. Frequency should be increased in critically ill patients.

References

1. Irvin TT. Effects of malnutrition and hyperalimentation on wound healing. Surg Gynecol Obstet 1978;146:33-7.

2. Bistrian BR, Blackburn GL, Scrimshaw NS et al. Cellular immunity in semistarved states in hospitalized adults. Am J Clin Nutr 1975;28:1148-55.

3. Elwyn DH. Nutritional requirements of adult surgical patients. Crit Care Med 1980;8:9-19.

4. Bistrian BR, Blackburn GL, Hallowell E et al. Protein status of general surgical patients. JAMA 1974;230:858-60.

5. Bistrian BR, Blackburn GL, Sherman M et al. Therapeutic index of nutritional depletion in hospitalized patients. Surg Gynecol Obstet 1975;141:512-6.

6. Martin EW, ed. Hazards of medication. Philadelphia: JB Lippincott, 1971:200.

7. Butterworth CE, Blackburn GL. Hospital malnutrition and how to assess the nutritional status of a patient. Nutrition Today 1975;10:8-18.

8. Blackburn GL, Bistrian BR, Maini BS et al. Nutritional and metabolic assessment of the hospitalized patient. JPEN 1977;1:11-22.

9. Vanlandingham S, Spiekerman AM, Newmark SR. Prealbumin: a parameter of visceral protein levels during albumin infusion. JPEN 1982;6:230-1.

10. Surks MI, Oppenheimer JH. Postoperative changes in the concentration of thyroxine-binding prealbumin and serum free thyroxine. J Clin Endocrinol 1964;24:794-802.

11. Miller CL. Immunological assays as measurements of nutritional status: a review. JPEN 1978;2:554-63.

12. Borut TC, Ank BJ, Gard SE et al. Tetanus toxoid skin test in children: correlation with in vitro lymphocyte stimulation and monocyte chemotaxis. J Pediatr 1980;97:567-73.

13. Kinney JM, Moore FD. Surgical metabolism in metabolism of body fluids. In: Zimmerman LM, Levine R, eds. Physiologic principles of surgery. 2nd ed. Philadelphia: WB Saunders, 1964:136-60.

14. Kinney JM, Long CL, Gump FE et al. Tissue composition of weight loss in surgical patients. Ann Surg 1968;168:459-74.

15. Bistrian BR. A simple technique to estimate severity of stress. Surg Gynecol Obstet 1979;148:675-8.

16. Rutten P, Blackburn GL, Flatt JP et al. Determination of optimal hyperalimentation infusion rate. J Surg Res 1975;18:477-83.

17. Kinney JM. Energy requirements for parenteral nutrition. In: Fischer JE, ed. Total parenteral nutrition. Boston: Little, Brown, 1976:135-70.

18. Wilmore DW. The metabolic management of the critically ill. New York: Plenum, 1977.

19. Munro HN. Nutritional requirements in health. Crit Care Med 1979;8:2-8.

20. Chen W-J, Ohashi E, Kasai M. Amino acid metabolism in parenteral nutrition: with special reference to the calorie:nitrogen ratio and the blood urea nitrogen level. Metabolism 1974;23:1117-23.

21. Rees RGP, Keohane PP, Grimble GK et al. Elemental diet administered nasogastrically without starter regimens to patients with inflammatory bowel disease. JPEN 1986;10:258-62.

22. Grant JP. Handbook of total parenteral nutrition. Philadelphia: WB Saunders, 1980.

23. Goldfarb IW, Yates AP. Total parenteral nutrition: concepts and methods. Pittsburgh: Synapse, 1978.

24. Anon. Insights into parenteral nutrition. Deerfield, IL: Travenol Laboratories, 1977.

25. Isaacs JW, Millikan WJ, Stackhouse J et al. Parenteral nutrition of adults with a 900 milliosmolar solution via peripheral veins. Am J Clin Nutr 1977;30:552-9.

26. Kellenberger TA, Johnson TA, Zaske DE. Essential fatty acid deficiency: a consequence of fat-free total parenteral nutrition. Am J Hosp Pharm 1979;36:230-4.

27. Askanazi J, Rosenbaum SH, Hyman AI et al. Respiratory changes induced by the large glucose loads of total parenteral nutrition. JAMA 1980;243:1444-7.

28. Jeejeebhoy KN, Anderson GH, Sanderson I et al. Total parenteral nutrition: nutrient needs and technical tips (part 1). Mod Med Can 1974;29(9).

29. Blackburn GL, Flatt JP, Clowes GHA et al. Peripheral intravenous feeding with isotonic amino acid solutions. Am J Surg 1973;125:447-54.

30. Deitel M, ed. Nutrition in clinical surgery. 2nd ed. Baltimore: Williams & Wilkins, 1985.

31. Freund H, Dienstag J, Lehrich J et al. Infusion of branched-chain enriched amino acid solution in patients with hepatic encephalopathy. Ann Surg 1982;196:209-20.

32. Freund H, Hoover HC, Atamian S et al. Infusion of the branched chain amino acids in postoperative patients: anticatabolic properties. Ann Surg 1979;190:18-23.

33. Cerra FB, Upson D, Angelico R et al. Branched chains support postoperative protein synthesis. Surgery 1982;92:192-9.

34. Zenk KE. Crystalline amino acid solutions for infants. Infusion 1985;9:104-8.

35. American Medical Association Department of Foods and Nutrition. Multivitamin preparations for parenteral use: a statement by the nutrition advisory group. JPEN 1979;3:258-62.

36. American Medical Association Department of Foods and Nutrition. Guidelines for essential trace element preparations for parenteral use: a statement by an expert panel. JAMA 1979;241:2051-4.

37. Van Rij AM, McKenzie JM, Thomson DC et al. Selenium supplementation in total parenteral nutrition. JPEN 1981;5:120-4.

38. Abumrad NN, Schneider AJ, Steel D et al. Amino acid intolerance during prolonged total parenteral nutrition reversed by molybdate therapy. Am J Clin Nutr 1981;34:2551-9.

39. Ruhlman ES, Schneider PJ. Iodine requirements in TPN patients. Infusion 1985;9:19-21.

40. Sayers MH, Johnson DK, Schumann LA et al. Supplementation of total parenteral nutrition solutions with ferrous citrate. JPEN 1983;7:117-20.

41. Peters ML, Maher M, Brennan MF. Minimal IV iron requirements in TPN. JPEN 1980;4:601. Abstract.

13 *DRUG REVIEWS*

Introduction

THE DRUG REVIEWS SECTION PROVIDES INFORMATION on over 600 drugs having widespread usage and/or therapeutic importance. In general, combination products are not listed. Information on drugs is presented in three formats: monographs, mini-monographs and comparison charts. The monograph format (described below) is utilized for drugs of major importance and prototype agents. The mini-monograph is used for investigational and recently marketed drugs for which only limited information is available, drugs for which a prototype monograph appears and for drugs of lesser importance within a drug class. Comparison charts are used to present information on members of the same chemical class (eg, thiazide diuretics) or different drugs within the same therapeutic class (eg, diuretics). Comparison charts are also used to contrast specific properties of related agents (eg, antiplatelet effects, electrophysiologic properties) and to present information on nontherapeutic agents (eg, blood glucose testing methods).

Monographs and charts are categorized and grouped according to the American Hospital Formulary Service (AHFS) Pharmacologic-Therapeutic Classification System.[a] All drugs are arranged alphabetically by generic name within each category. Comparison charts are located immediately following the monographs to which they relate. References for each major AHFS category (eg, 8:00, 92:00) are found immediately following the last monograph of that category. The user will find that the easiest method to gain access to information on a particular drug is to use the index at the end of the book. The index also directs the user to other pertinent information on the drug elsewhere in the book.

a. Permission to use the pharmacologic-therapeutic classification system of the *American Hospital Formulary Service* has been granted by the American Society of Hospital Pharmacists. These data are a part of the *AHFS Drug Information;* the Society is not responsible for the accuracy of transpositions, or additions, or excerpts from the original context. Copyright © 1959-1988, American Society of Hospital Pharmacists, Inc. All rights reserved.

Monograph Format

The following is a description of the monograph format. The absence of any heading for a given drug indicates that such information was either unavailable at the time of writing or that the information available was not considered to be applicable to the drug or clinical situation.

Common brand names are given directly across from the generic name. This is for identification purposes only and is not meant to imply that the brand name products listed are superior to other brand name or generic products. "Various" indicates the availability of numerous brand and/or generic products.

Pharmacology.   A description of the chemistry, major mechanism(s) of action and human pharmacology of the drug.

Administration and Adult Dose.   Route of administration and usual adult dosage ranges are given for the most common uses of the drug. Doses correspond to those given in the manufacturer's product information or in standard reference sources unless specifically referenced otherwise.

Dosage Individualization.   Any known dosing alterations that are needed in various disease states and patient subgroups are presented. Changes in pharmacokinetic parameters occurring in these disease states are presented in **Pharmacokinetics** rather than under this heading.

Pediatric Dose.   Route of administration and dosage ranges are given for the most common uses of the drug. Dosages correspond to those given in the product information or in standard reference sources unless specifically referenced otherwise. When a dosage based on body surface area is given, the body surface area nomogram found in Anthropometrics, Chapter 1, may be utilized.

Dosage Forms.   The most commonly used dosage forms and available strengths are listed. Combination products are generally not listed. See the abbreviations list on page 284 for dosage form abbreviations.

Patient Instructions.   Key information that should be given to the patient when prescribing or dispensing the drug is presented in order to optimize efficacious, safe and compliant use. When instructions pertain to an entire drug category, the reader is referred to **Class Instructions** which appear at the beginning of the drug category.

Pharmacokinetics.   *Onset and Duration.*   The onset, peak and duration of the pharmacologic and/or therapeutic effect are listed when appropriate.

Plasma Levels.   The therapeutic and/or toxic plasma levels are given when a correlation has been made between these concentrations and the effects of the drug.

Fate.   The fate of the drug in the body is traced. Absorption, bioavailability, distribution, metabolism and excretion are discussed and alterations in disease states are mentioned. The pharmacokinetic data given in this section may be affected by variables in the study design and among patients.

$t_{1/2}$.   The range and/or average distribution (α phase) and elimination (β phase) half-life of the drug, obtained from the best sources available are listed. Many studies only measure half-lives in a small number of normal subjects and often these do not apply to diseased patients. Changes in half-life due to the disease state or age group of the patient are given when these are known.

Adverse Reactions.   This section is intended to be a brief list limited to reactions that are important due to their frequency or seriousness. Some indication of the frequency of the reaction and its relationship to dosage is made.

Contraindications.   Absolute contraindications are given as they are found in the manufacturer's product information. In general, a person should not be given a drug to which he is allergic or hypersensitive. Therefore, "hypersensitivity" is not listed as a contraindication in each monograph, but should be understood to be a contraindication unless otherwise specified.

Precautions.   Cautions against the use of a drug in various groups of patients and/or disease states are listed, together with any cross-sensitivities with other drugs. Unusual drug interactions which are not included in Drug Interactions (Chapter 6) are listed here. The words "pregnancy" or "lactation" appearing alone means that insufficient data have been accumulated to ensure drug safety in these conditions; also refer to the Chapters on Drugs and Pregnancy and Drugs and Breast Feeding.

Parameters to Monitor.   The clinical signs and laboratory tests that should be monitored in order to ensure safe and efficacious therapy are listed. The frequency with which such signs should be monitored may also be given; however, in most cases, the optimal frequency has not been determined and is dependent upon the condition of the patient and other variables.

Notes.   Under this heading, miscellaneous information is presented that relates to the physicochemical properties, handling, relative cost, distinguishing characteristics, therapeutic usefulness and relative efficacy of the drug. Occasionally, information on similar drugs is also provided.

Abbreviations

The following are the abbreviations used in the drug monographs:

ANA antinuclear antibody
AV atrioventricular
Cap capsule
CBC complete blood count
Chew chewable
CHF congestive heart failure
Cl clearance
Cl$_{cr}$ creatinine clearance
CNS central nervous system
Crm cream
Cr$_s$ serum creatinine concentration
CVP central venous pressure
D5W dextrose 5% in water
Drp drops
EC enteric coated
EKG electrocardiogram
Elxr elixir
GFR glomerular filtration rate
GI gastrointestinal
Gran granules
Hyp hypodermic
IM intramuscular(ly)
Inhal inhalation
Inj injection
IP intraperitoneal(ly)
IU international units
IV Intravenous(ly)
Lot lotion
mM millimolar
mol mole(s)

NS normal saline
Oint ointment
Ophth ophthalmic
PO oral(ly)
PR rectal(ly)
PT prothrombin time
PTT partial thromboplastin time
PVC premature ventricular contraction
Pwdr powder
RBC red blood cell
SC subcutaneous(ly)
SD standard deviation
SL sublingual(ly)
SLE systemic lupus erythematosus
Soln solution
SR sustained-release
Supp suppository
Susp suspension
Tab tablet
Top topical(ly)
Vag vaginal(ly)
V$_c$ apparent volume of distribution in the central compartment
V$_d$ apparent volume of distribution
V$_{dss}$ apparent steady-state volume of distribution
WBC white blood cell

Limitations

It should be noted that the information in the Drug Reviews section is not exhaustive; rather an attempt has been made to provide the most important aspects relating to each drug's use. For medicolegal purposes, the reader should always be familiar with the manufacturer's product information or other comprehensive drug information sources, especially before prescribing.

4:00 ANTIHISTAMINE DRUGS

General References: 1–3

Class Instructions. These drugs may cause drowsiness and dry mouth or, on occasion, dizziness (with the exceptions of astemizole and terfenadine). Until the extent of drowsiness is known, caution should be used when driving, operating machinery or performing other tasks requiring mental alertness. Avoid excessive concurrent use of alcohol and other drugs which cause drowsiness.

Astemizole (Investigational - Janssen)   Hismanal®

Astemizole is a long-acting antihistamine that is pharmacologically similar to terfenadine. With doses of 10 mg/day, an improvement in nasal symptoms occurs in 5 days; histamine-induced wheal and flare suppression lasts for 20–32 days after single doses of 10–40 mg. Food decreases oral bioavailability by about 60%. The drug is about 97% plasma protein bound and is extensively and rapidly metabolized; the plasma half-life was about 20 hr in one patient after a single 300 mg dose, while it was 18–20 days for the drug and metabolites after chronic administration of 10 mg/day. Like terfenadine, the frequency of CNS side effects is about equal to placebo; appetite stimulation and weight gain have been reported during the first 8–14 weeks of therapy, but they did not progress with continued therapy. The usual oral dose in adults is 30 mg/day for up to a week as a loading dose, then 10 mg/day. In children under 6 yr of age, a dose of 0.2 mg/kg/day has been used, while in children 6–12 yr old, one-half the adult dose has been used.[4-10]

Chlorpheniramine Maleate   Chlor-Trimeton®, Various

Pharmacology. A competitive antagonist of histamine at the H_1-histamine receptor. It also has anticholinergic and transient sedative effects when used intermittently.

Administration and Adult Dose. PO for acute allergic reactions 12 mg in 1–2 divided doses. **PO for seasonal allergic rhinitis** (effectiveness is maximized if given continuously just prior to the pollen season) 4 mg hs (2 mg in children) initially, increasing gradually over 10 days as tolerated to 24 mg/day (12 mg/day in children) in 1–2 divided doses until the end of season.[11] **IV as adjunctive treatment in anaphylaxis, or IM or IV for allergic reactions to blood or plasma** 10–20 mg, to maximum of 40 mg/day.

Pediatric Dose. PO 0.35 mg/kg/day. **PO for seasonal allergic rhinitis** (2–6 yr) 1 mg tid up to 6 mg/day; (6–12 yr) 1–2 mg tid up to 12 mg/day titrated as above. SR not recommended.

Dosage Forms. SR Cap 8, 12 mg (see Notes); **Syrup** 2 mg/5 ml; **Chew Tab** 2 mg; **Tab** 4 mg; **SR Tab** 8, 12 mg (see Notes); **Inj** 10 mg/ml (IM, IV, SC); 100 mg/ml (IM, SC only).

Patient Instructions. This drug effectively suppresses seasonal allergic rhinitis only when taken continuously. See also Class Instructions.

Pharmacokinetics. *Onset and Duration.* Onset 0.5–1 hr; duration of suppression of wheal and flare response (IgE mediated) to skin tests with allergenic extract 2 days.[12]

    Plasma Levels. (Children) 2.3–12.1 ng/ml suppresses allergic rhinitis symptoms; (children) 4.1–10 ng/ml suppresses histamine-induced wheal and flare.[13]

    Fate. About 34% oral bioavailability;[14] V_d (adults) 3.4–7.5 L/kg, (children) 4.3–7 L/kg.[8,13] 72% plasma protein bound.[15] Cl (adults) 0.06–0.2 L/hr/kg,[8] (children) 0.32–0.43 L/hr/kg.[8,13] Rapidly and extensively metabolized to mono- and didesmethylchlorpheniramine and unidentified metabolites which are excreted in urine; a small amount of drug is excreted unchanged in urine.[15]

$t_{1/2}$. (Adults) 14–30 hr;[8,16] (children) 9.6–13 hr;[8,13] (chronic renal failure) 280–330 hr.[8]

Adverse Reactions. Drowsiness, dry mouth, dizziness and irritability occur frequently with intermittent therapy; however, most patients develop tolerance to these side effects during continuous therapy, particularly if dose is increased slowly.

Contraindications. Lactation; premature and newborn infants.

Precautions. Use with caution in the elderly (60 yr and older). May cause paradoxical CNS stimulation in children. OTC labeling states to avoid in patients with asthma, glaucoma or symptomatic prostatic hypertrophy, except under physician supervision.

Parameters to Monitor. In seasonal allergic rhinitis, observe for sneezing, rhinorrhea, itchy nose and conjunctivitis.

Notes. Not effective for nasal stuffiness. Inexpensive generic formulations are available, but bioavailability has not been documented for many products. SR formulations offer no advantage over syrup or plain, uncoated tablets, because the drug is eliminated slowly.[1]

Cyproheptadine Hydrochloride   Periactin®, Various

Pharmacology. See Chlorpheniramine. Also has antiserotonin activity.[17]

Administration and Adult Dose. PO 4–20 mg/day, usually 4 mg tid-qid, to maximum of 0.5 mg/kg/day.

Pediatric Dose. PO 0.25 mg/kg/day, usually. (Under 2 yr) dosage information not available; (2–6 yr) 2 mg bid-tid, to maximum of 12 mg/day; (7–14 yr) 4 mg bid-tid, to maximum of 16 mg/day.

Dosage Forms. Syrup 2 mg/5 ml; Tab 4 mg.

Patient Instructions. See Class Instructions.

Pharmacokinetics. *Fate.* Well absorbed after oral administration; about 70% excreted in urine, primarily as a quaternary ammonium glucuronide conjugate; the remainder is excreted in feces.[18] Unchanged drug is not detectable in urine.

Adverse Reactions. See Chlorpheniramine.

Contraindications. Premature and newborn infants; lactation. Manufacturer states contraindicated in asthma; however, this was not supported in a controlled study, except during prolonged acute asthma symptoms (ie, status asthmaticus).[1,19] Avoid in patients with narrow angle glaucoma, symptomatic prostatic hypertrophy, pyloroduodenal or bladder neck obstruction, stenosing peptic ulcer or those on MAO inhibitors.

Precautions. Use with caution in the elderly (60 yr and older). May cause paradoxical CNS stimulation in children.

Notes. May have potential as an inhibitor of ACTH release in patients with Cushing's disease due to its antiserotonin activity;[20] long-term use of cyproheptadine and **human growth hormone** enhances growth of children with hypopituitarism.[20] Effective for appetite stimulation[21] and cold urticaria.[22] Relatively ineffective as an antipruritic.[23-25] **Loratadine** is a nonsedating antihistamine structurally related to cyproheptadine and azatadine with a half-life of about 14 hr.[26]

Diphenhydramine Hydrochloride   Benadryl®, Various

Pharmacology. See Chlorpheniramine.

Administration and Adult Dose. PO as an antihistamine 25–50 mg tid-qid. **PO for motion sickness** 50 mg 30 min before exposure, and ac and hs; **PO as an antitussive** (syrup only) 25 mg q 4 hr, to maximum of 150 mg/day; **PO as a nighttime sleep aid** 50 mg hs. **Deep IM or IV as an antihistamine, for adjunctive treatment of anaphylaxis or for parkinsonism including extrapyramidal reactions** 10–50 mg/dose, to maximum of 400 mg/day.

Dosage Individualization. Increase dosing interval by 1½–2 times in moderate to severe renal impairment.[27]

Pediatric Dose. PO as an antihistamine (over 9 kg) 5 mg/kg/day, usually 12.5–25 mg tid-qid, to maximum of 300 mg/day. **PO as an antitussive** (syrup only) (6–12 yr) 12.5 mg q 4 hr, to maximum of 75 mg/day; **deep IM or IV** 5 mg/kg/day, in 4 divided doses, to maximum of 300 mg/day.

Dosage Forms. Cap 25, 50 mg; **Elxr** 12.5 mg/5 ml; **Syrup** 12.5, 13.3 mg/5 ml; **Tab** 25, 50 mg; **Inj** 10, 50 mg/ml.

Patient Instructions. See Class Instructions.

Pharmacokinetics. *Onset and Duration.* Onset 15 min after single oral dose; duration of wheal and flare suppression lasts up to 1.9 days.[12]
   Plasma Levels. Frequency of sedation is increased over 50 ng/ml.[28]
   Fate. As a result of first-pass metabolism, oral bioavailability ranges from 40–70%.[8,29] A single 50 mg oral dose in adults usually produces plasma concentrations between 25–50 ng/ml.[28] V_d is 3.3–4.5 L/kg,[8,29] larger in Orientals[30] and in cirrhosis.[31] 85% plasma protein bound, lower in Orientals[30] and in cirrhotic patients.[31] Metabolized to N-dealkylated and acidic metabolites.[29,32] Cl is 0.4–0.7 L/hr/kg,[29] higher in Orientals.[30] Less than 4% excreted unchanged in urine.[33]
   $t_{1/2}$. 3–10 hr in young and elderly subjects;[28,33,34] 15 hr in cirrhosis.[31] However, wheal and flare reaction is suppressed for about 2 days.[12] Thus, duration of effect does not appear related to plasma levels and qid dosing appears unnecessary.

Adverse Reactions. See Chlorpheniramine.

Contraindications. See Chlorpheniramine.

Precautions. See Chlorpheniramine. OTC labeling also advises patients with emphysema, chronic pulmonary disease or breathing difficulties to avoid the drug unless supervised by physician.

Notes. Because of its low degree of efficacy for pruritus and relatively weak suppression of IgE-mediated skin tests, diphenhydramine is not the antihistamine of choice. **Dimenhydrinate** (Dramamine®), used for motion sickness, is the 8-chlorotheophyllinate salt of diphenhydramine; by weight, 100 mg dimenhydrinate is about equal to 50 mg diphenhydramine.

Hydroxyzine Hydrochloride   Atarax®, Various
Hydroxyzine Pamoate   Vistaril®, Various

Pharmacology. A competitive antagonist of histamine at the H_1-histamine receptor. Also has antiemetic and sedative effects, thought to be a result of CNS subcortical suppression. Claims of long-term antianxiety properties have not been substantiated by well-designed studies.

Administration and Adult Dose. PO for pruritus 25 mg tid-qid. **PO for seasonal allergic rhinitis** (effectiveness is maximized if given continuously just prior to the pollen season) 25 mg (10 mg for children) initially q hs until no sedation in morning, then increase dose q 2–3 days, to maximum of 150 mg/day (25–75 mg/day for children) in 1–2 divided doses and maintain until end of season. Reduce dose by one-third or more if sedation persists. Dosage may be increased, if tolerated, for symptoms during peak of pollen season.[35] **IM for sedation pre- and post-general anesthesia** 50–100 mg. **IM for nausea and vomiting, and pre- and postoperative adjunctive medication** 25–100 mg. Preferred IM injection site is upper outer quadrant of gluteus maximus or midlateral thigh. **Not for SC or intra-arterial use.** While labeled "not for IV use" it has been given IV (diluted to at least 50 ml in normal saline) over 4 min, but care *must* be taken to avoid intra-arterial injection.[36]

Pediatric Dose. **PO for pruritus** (under 6 yr) 50 mg/day in 2–3 divided doses; (over 6 yr) 50–100 mg/day in divided doses. **PO for seasonal allergic rhinitis** titrate as above. **IM for pre- and postoperative sedation** 0.7 mg/kg.[37] **IM for nausea and vomiting and pre- and postoperative adjunctive medication** 1.1 mg/kg.

Dosage Forms. **Cap** (as pamoate equivalent of HCl salt) 25, 50, 100 mg; **Susp** (as pamoate equivalent of HCl salt) 25 mg/5 ml; **Syrup** (as HCl) 10 mg/5 ml; **Tab** (as HCl) 10, 25, 50, 100 mg; **Inj** (as HCl) 25, 50 mg/ml (IM only).

Patient Instructions. See Chlorpheniramine.

Pharmacokinetics. *Onset and Duration.* Onset 15–30 min after oral administration. Duration of suppression of wheal and flare response to allergenic extract skin tests is 4 days.[12,23]

  Plasma Levels. (Children) 5.6–41.8 ng/ml significantly suppresses pruritus.[37]

  Fate. Peak plasma level of 72.5 ng/ml occurs 2.1 hr after a 0.7 mg/kg dose (mean dose 39 mg).[38] V_d (healthy adults) is 19.5 L/kg,[38] (children) 18.5 L/kg.[37] Cl (healthy adults) is 0.6 L/hr/kg,[38] (children) 1.9 L/hr/kg.[37]

  $t_{1/2}$. (Healthy adults) 20 hr;[38] (children) 7.1 hr, increasing with age;[38] however, pharmacologic effect is longer than plasma half-life.

Adverse Reactions. Transient drowsiness occurs frequently and dry mouth occasionally when taken intermittently. Most patients develop tolerance to these effects when the drug is taken continuously, particularly if the dose is slowly increased over 7–10 days. IM injection may be painful and has caused sterile abscess. Hemolysis has been associated with IV administration and tissue necrosis with SC or intra-arterial administration.

Contraindications. Early pregnancy; SC or intra-arterial use of injectable solution.

Precautions. Potentiation of other CNS depressants; may require a dosage reduction. Use with caution in the elderly.

Parameters to Monitor. See Chlorpheniramine.

Notes. Suppresses wheal and flare response to the greatest degree and for the longest duration of all antihistamines,[12,23] including the newer nonsedating antihistamines.[4]

Terfenadine   Seldane®

Pharmacology. A nonsedating competitive histamine H_1-receptor antagonist which lacks anticholinergic activity.

Administration and Adult Dose. **PO for seasonal allergic rhinitis** 60 mg bid.

Pediatric Dose. PO for seasonal allergic rhinitis (3–5 yr) 15 mg bid; (6–12 yr) 30–60 mg bid.[39]

Dosage Forms. Tab 60 mg.

Patient Instructions. See Chlorpheniramine.

Pharmacokinetics. *Onset and Duration.* Duration of suppression of histamine-induced wheal and flare response is 12 hr.[40]

Fate. Peak plasma level of 1.5 ng/ml occurs 1–2 hr after a 60 mg oral dose.[39] Rapidly and extensively (99.5%) metabolized to 2 main metabolic products, an active carboxylic acid analogue (metabolite I) and α, α-diphenyl-4-piperidinylmethanol (metabolite II).[41] About 40% of dose is eliminated in urine and about 60% in feces in 12 days after a 60 mg oral dose.[41,42] 11–13% of a dose is eliminated in urine as metabolite I after 24 hr.[41]

$t_{1/2}$. α phase 3.6 hr; β phase 16.1–22.7 hr.[43]

Adverse Reactions. Frequency of sedation is comparable to placebo and about 50% less frequent than with chlorpheniramine or other antihistamines. Little or no anticholinergic side effects reported.[39]

Parameters to Monitor. See Chlorpheniramine.

Notes. Other nonsedating antihistamines under investigation include **acrivastine** (Burroughs Wellcome), **cetirizine** (Pfizer) and **temelastine** (SKF).

Triprolidine Hydrochloride   Actidil®, Various

Pharmacology. See Chlorpheniramine.

Administration and Adult Dose. PO 2.5 mg q 4–6 hr, to maximum of 10 mg/day.

Pediatric Dose. PO (4 months–2 yr) 0.3 mg tid-qid; (2–5 yr) 0.6 mg tid-qid; (6–12 yr) 1.25 mg q 4–6 hr, to a maximum of 4 doses/day.

Dosage Forms. Syrup 1.25 mg/5 ml; Tab 2.5 mg; Syrup 1.25 mg with pseudoephedrine HCl 30 mg/5 ml (Actifed®, various); Tab, Cap 2.5 mg with pseudoephedrine HCl 60 mg (Actifed®, various).

Patient Instructions. See Class Instructions.

Pharmacokinetics. *Onset and Duration.* Histamine-induced wheal and flare response is suppressed approximately 50% after 5 mg, about 90% after 10 mg.[44]

Fate. Peak plasma level of 15.4 ng/ml occurs 2 hr after a 0.04 mg/kg oral dose (average dose 2.7 mg).[45] Cl is 0.62 L/hr/kg.[8] 1.3% excreted unchanged in urine in 24 hr.[45]

$t_{1/2}$. (Healthy adults) 2.1–5 hr.[45]

Adverse Reactions. See Chlorpheniramine.

Precautions. See Chlorpheniramine.

Parameters to Monitor. See Chlorpheniramine.

Antihistamine Drugs Comparison Chart[a]

DRUG	DOSAGE FORMS	ADULT DOSE	PEDIATRIC DOSE	SIDE EFFECTS[b] SEDATION	SIDE EFFECTS[b] ANTI-CHOLINERGIC
ALKYLAMINES **Brompheniramine Maleate** Dimetane® Various	Elxr 2 mg/5 ml Tab 4 mg SR Tab 8, 12 mg Inj 10, 100 mg/ml.	PO 4 mg q 4–6 hr, to maximum of 24 mg/day; SC, IM or IV (slowly) 5–20 mg q 12 hr, to maximum of 40 mg/day.	PO (2–6 yr) 1 mg q 4–6 hr, to maximum of 6 mg/day; (6–12 yr) 2 mg q 4–6 hr, to maximum of 12 mg/day; IM, SC or IV 0.5 mg/kg/day in 3–4 divided doses.	+ +	+ + +
Chlorpheniramine Maleate Chlor-Trimeton® Various	SR Cap 8, 12 mg Syrup 2 mg/5 ml Chew Tab 2 mg Tab 4 mg SR Tab 8, 12 mg Inj 10, 100 mg/ml.	PO (acute allergic reactions) 12 mg/day in 1–2 divided doses; PO (seasonal allergic rhinitis) 24 mg/day in 1–2 divided doses; IV (acute allergic reactions) 10–40 mg/day.	PO 0.35 mg/kg/day; PO (seasonal allergic rhinitis) (2–6 yr) 1 mg tid up to 6 mg/day; (6–12 yr) 1–2 mg tid up to 12 mg/day; SR not recommended.	+ +	+ + +
Dexchlorpheniramine Maleate Polaramine® Various	Syrup 2 mg/5 ml Tab 2 mg SR Tab 4, 6 mg.	PO 2 mg q 4–6 hr, to maximum of 12 mg/day.	PO (2–5 yr) 0.5 mg q 4–6 hr, to maximum of 3 mg/day; SR not recommended. PO (6–11 yr) 1 mg q	+ +	+ + +

Continued

Antihistamine Drugs Comparison Chart[a]

DRUG	DOSAGE FORMS	ADULT DOSE	PEDIATRIC DOSE	SIDE EFFECTS[b] SEDATION	SIDE EFFECTS[b] ANTI-CHOLINERGIC
Triprolidine HCl Actidil® Various	Syrup 1.25 mg/5 ml Tab 2.5 mg.	PO 2.5 mg q 4–6 hr, to maximum of 10 mg/day.	PO (4 months–2 yr) 0.3 mg tid-qid; (2–5 yr) 0.6 mg tid-qid; (6–12 yr) 1.25 mg q 4–6 hr, to maximum of 4 doses/day.	+ +	+ + +
ETHANOLAMINES **Carbinoxamine Maleate** Clistin®	Tab 4 mg.	PO 4–8 mg tid-qid.	PO 0.2–0.4 mg/kg/day; (1–3 yr) 2 mg tid-qid; (3–6 yr) 2–4 mg tid-qid; (over 6 yr) 4–6 mg tid-qid.	+ + +	+ + + +
Clemastine Fumarate Tavist® Tavist-1®	Syrup 0.67 mg (equivalent to 0.5 mg clemastine) /5 ml Tab 1.34, 2.68 mg (equivalent to 1 and 2 mg clemastine, respectively).	PO 1.34 mg bid-2.68 mg tid, to maximum of 8.04 mg/day.	PO (6–12 yr) 0.67–1.34 mg tid, to maximum of 4.02 mg/day.	+ + +	+ + + +

Continued

Antihistamine Drugs Comparison Chart[a]

DRUG	DOSAGE FORMS	ADULT DOSE	PEDIATRIC DOSE	SIDE EFFECTS[b]	
				SEDATION	ANTI-CHOLINERGIC
Diphenhydramine HCl Benadryl® Various	Cap 25, 50 mg Elxr 12.5 mg/5 ml Syrup 12.5, 13.3 mg/5 ml Tab 25, 50 mg Inj 10, 50 mg/ml.	PO (antihistamine) 25–50 mg tid-qid; PO (motion sickness) 50 mg 30 min before exposure, ac and hs; PO (antitussive) 25 mg q 4 hr to maximum of 150 mg/day; PO (nighttime sleep aid) 50 mg hs; IM, IV 10–50 mg, to maximum of 400 mg/day.	PO (over 9 kg) 5 mg/kg/ day, usually 12.5–25 mg tid-qid, to maxi- mum of 300 mg/day; PO (antitussive) (6–12 yr) 12.5 mg q 4 hr, to maximum of 75 mg/day.	+ + + +	+ + + +
ETHYLENEDIAMINES					
Pyrilamine Maleate Various	Tab 25 mg.	PO (allergy) 25–50 mg tid; (sleep aid) 50–100 mg hs.	Safety and efficacy not established under 12 yr.	+ +	+
Tripelennamine HCl PBZ® Various	Elxr 37.5 mg (citrate salt equivalent to 25 mg HCl) /5 ml Tab 25, 50 mg SR Tab 100 mg.	PO 25–50 mg q 4–6 hr, to maximum of 600 mg/day.	PO 5 mg/kg/day in 4–6 divided doses, to maximum of 300 mg/day; SR not recommended.	+ + +	+

Continued

Antihistamine Drugs Comparison Chart[a]

DRUG	DOSAGE FORMS	ADULT DOSE	PEDIATRIC DOSE	SIDE EFFECTS[b]	
				SEDATION	ANTI-CHOLINERGIC
PHENOTHIAZINES					
Methdilazine HCl Tacaryl®	Syrup 4 mg/5 ml Chew Tab 4 mg (equivalent to 3.6 mg methdilazine) Tab 8 mg.	PO 8 mg bid-qid.	PO (over 3 yr) 4 mg bid-qid.	+ +	+ + + +
Promethazine HCl Phenergan® Various	Syrup 6.25, 25 mg/5 ml Tab 12.5, 25, 50 mg Inj 25, 50 mg/ml Supp 12.5, 25, 50 mg.	PO (allergy) 25 mg hs or 12.5 mg ac and hs; (nausea and vomiting) 25 mg initial dose, then 12.5–25 mg q 4–6 hr prn; (adjunctive preoperative use) 50 mg; (adjunctive postoperative use) 25–50 mg/dose; IM, IV or PR (allergy) 25 mg, may repeat in 2 hr; (nausea and vomiting) 12.5–25 mg q 4 hr prn; (adjunctive pre- and postoperative use) 25–50 mg/dose.	PO (allergy) 25 mg hs or 6.25–12.5 mg tid; (nausea and vomiting) 0.25–0.5 mg/kg q 4–6 hr prn; (adjunctive preoperative use) 1.1 mg/kg/ dose; (adjunctive postoperative use) 12.5–25 mg/dose; IM, IV or PR (under 12 yr) (adjunctive preoperative use) 1 mg/kg/dose, maximum dose not to exceed one-half of adult dose.	+ + + +	+ + + +

Continued

Antihistamine Drugs Comparison Chart[a]

DRUG	DOSAGE FORMS	ADULT DOSE	PEDIATRIC DOSE	SIDE EFFECTS[b]	
				SEDATION	ANTI-CHOLINERGIC
Trimeprazine Tartrate Temaril®	SR Cap 5 mg Syrup 2.5 mg/5 ml Tab 2.5 mg.	PO 2.5 mg qid; SR 5 mg q 12 hr.	PO (6 months–3 yr) 1.25 mg hs or tid prn; (over 3 yr) 2.5 mg hs or tid prn; SR not recommended under 6 yr; SR (over 6 yr) 5 mg/day.	+ + +	+ + + +
PIPERAZINES **Hydroxyzine HCl** Atarax® Various **Hydroxyzine Pamoate** Vistaril® Various	Cap (as pamoate equivalent of HCl salt) 25, 50, 100 mg Susp (as pamoate equivalent of HCl salt) 25 mg/5 ml Syrup (as HCl) 10 mg/5 ml Tab (as HCl) 10, 25, 50, 100 mg Inj (as HCl) 25, 50 mg/ml.	PO (pruritus) 25 mg tid-qid; (seasonal allergic rhinitis) titrate up to 150 mg/day in 1–2 divided doses; IM 25–100 mg.	PO (pruritus) (under 6 yr) 50 mg/day in 2–3 divided doses; (over 6 yr) 50–100 mg/day in divided doses; (seasonal allergic rhinitis) 25–75 mg/day in 1–2 divided doses; IM (perioperative sedation) 0.7 mg/kg/dose; (nausea, vomiting, perioperative adjunctive medication) 1.1 mg/kg.	+ + +	+ +

Continued

Antihistamine Drugs Comparison Chart[a]

DRUG	DOSAGE FORMS	ADULT DOSE	PEDIATRIC DOSE	SIDE EFFECTS[b] SEDATION	ANTI-CHOLINERGIC
PIPERIDINES					
Azatadine Maleate Optimine®	Tab 1 mg.	PO 1-2 mg bid.	Safety and efficacy not established under 12 yr.	+ + +	+ + +
Cyproheptadine HCl Periactin® Various	Syrup 2 mg/5 ml Tab 4 mg.	PO 4-20 mg/day, usually 4 mg tid-qid, to maximum of 0.5 mg/kg/day.	PO (2-6 yr) 2 mg bid-tid, to max of 12 mg/day; (7-14 yr) 4 mg bid-tid, to max of 16 mg/day.	+ +	+ + +
Loratadine Claritin®	Tab 10 mg.	PO 10 mg/day.	Safety and efficacy not established under 12 yr.	+	+
MISCELLANEOUS					
Terfenadine Seldane®	Tab 60 mg.	PO 60 mg bid.	PO (3-5 yr) 15 mg bid; (6-12 yr) 30-60 mg bid.	+	+
Astemizole Hismanal® (Investigational-Janssen)	—	PO 10 mg/day; For severe symptoms, 30 mg/day up to 1 week, then 10 mg/day.	PO (under 6 yr) 0.2 mg/kg/day; (6-12 yr) 5 mg/day. Safety and efficacy not established.	+	+

a. From references 46-48. b. Tolerance usually occurs during chronic therapy.

References, 4:00 Antihistamine Drugs

1. Hendeles L, Weinberger M, Wong L. Medical management of noninfectious rhinitis. Am J Hosp Pharm 1980;37:1496-504.

2. Simons FER, Simons KJ. H_1 receptor antagonists: clinical pharmacology and use in allergic disease. Pediatr Clin North Am 1983;30:899-914.

3. Drouin MA. H_1-antihistamines: perspective on the use of the conventional and new agents. Ann Allergy 1985;55:747-52.

4. Gendreau-Reid L, Simons KJ, Simons FER. Comparison of the suppressive effect of astemizole, terfenadine, and hydroxyzine on histamine-induced wheals and flares in humans. J Allergy Clin Immunol 1986;77:335-40.

5. Wihl J-A, Petersen BN, Petersen LN et al. Effect of the nonsedative H_1-receptor antagonist astemizole in perennial allergic and nonallergic rhinitis. J Allergy Clin Immunol 1985;75:720-7.

6. Richards DM, Brogden RN, Heel RC et al. Astemizole: a review of its pharmacodynamic properties and therapeutic efficacy. Drugs 1984;28:38-61.

7. Howarth PH, Emanuel MB, Holgate ST. Astemizole, a potent histamine H_1-receptor antagonist: effect in allergic rhinoconjunctivitis, on antigen and histamine induced skin weal responses and relationship to serum levels. Br J Clin Pharmacol 1984;18:1-8.

8. Paton DM, Webster DR. Clinical pharmacokinetics of H_1-receptor antagonists (the antihistamines). Clin Pharmacokinet 1985;10:477-97.

9. Chapman PH, Rawlins MD. A randomized single-blind study of astemizole and chlorpheniramine in normal volunteers. Br J Clin Pharmacol 1982;13:593P.

10. Heykants J. The pharmacokinetics and metabolism of astemizole in man. In: Astemizole: a new, non-sedative, long-acting H_1-antagonist. Medicine Publishing Foundation Symposium Series 11. Oxford: Medicine Publishing Foundation 1984:25-34.

11. Wong L, Hendeles L, Weinberger M. Pharmacologic prophylaxis of allergic rhinitis: relative efficacy of hydroxyzine and chlorpheniramine. J Allergy Clin Immunol 1981;67:223-8.

12. Cook TJ, MacQueen DM, Wittig HJ et al. Degree and duration of skin test suppression and side effects with antihistamines. J Allergy Clin Immunol 1973;51:71-7.

13. Simons FER, Luciuk GH, Simons KJ. Pharmacokinetics of chlorpheniramine in children. J Allergy Clin Immunol 1982;69:376-81.

14. Huang SM, Athanikar NK, Sridhar K et al. Pharmacokinetics of chlorpheniramine after intravenous and oral administration in normal adults. Eur J Clin Pharmacol 1982;22:359-65.

15. Peets EA, Jackson M, Symchowicz S. Metabolism of chlorpheniramine maleate in man. J Pharmacol Exp Ther 1972;180:464-74.

16. Chiou WL, Athanikar NK, Huang S-M. Long half-life of chlorpheniramine. N Engl J Med 1979;300:501. Letter.

17. Krieger DT, Amorosa L, Linick F. Cyproheptadine-induced remission of Cushing's disease. N Engl J Med 1975;293:893-6.

18. Hintze KL, Wold JS, Fischer LJ. Disposition of cyproheptadine in rats, mice, and humans and identification of a stable epoxide metabolite. Drug Metab Dispos 1975;3:1-9.

19. Karlin JM. The use of antihistamines in asthma. Ann Allergy 1972;30:342-7.

20. Kenien AG, Zeidner DL, Pang SJ et al. The effect of cyproheptadine and human growth hormone on adrenocortical function in children with hypopituitarism. J Pediatr 1978;92:491-4.

21. Anon. Cyproheptadine as an appetite stimulant. Drug Ther Bull 1970;8:71-2.

22. Wanderer AA, St. Pierre J-P, Ellis EF. Primary acquired cold urticaria. Arch Dermatol 1977;113:1375-7.

23. Rhoades RB, Leifer KN, Cohan R et al. Suppression of histamine-induced pruritus by three antihistaminic drugs. J Allergy Clin Immunol 1975;55:180-5.

24. Baraf CS. Treatment of pruritus in allergic dermatoses: an evaluation of the relative efficacy of cyproheptadine and hydroxyzine. Curr Ther Res 1976;19:32-8.

25. Klein GL, Galant SP. A comparison of the antipruritic efficacy of hydroxyzine and cyproheptadine in children with atopic dermatitis. Ann Allergy 1980;44:142-5.

26. Radwanski E, Moritzen V, Parks A et al. Multiple dose pharmacokinetics of loratadine. J Clin Pharmacol 1986;26:557. Abstract.

27. Bennett WM, Aronoff GR, Morrison G et al. Drug prescribing in renal failure: dosing guidelines for adults. Am J Kidney Dis 1983;3:155-93.

28. Carruthers SG, Shoeman DW, Hignite CE et al. Correlation between plasma diphenhydramine level and sedative and antihistamine effects. Clin Pharmacol Ther 1978;23:375-82.

29. Blyden GT, Greenblatt DJ, Scavone JM et al. Pharmacokinetics of diphenhydramine and a demethylated metabolite following intravenous and oral administration. J Clin Pharmacol 1986;26:529-33.

30. Spector R, Choudhury AK, Chiang C-K et al. Diphenhydramine in Orientals and Caucasians. Clin Pharmacol Ther 1980;28:229-34.

31. Meredith CG, Christian CD, Johnson RF et al. Diphenhydramine disposition in chronic liver disease. Clin Pharmacol Ther 1984;35:474-9.

32. Glazko AJ, Dill WA, Young RM et al. Metabolic disposition of diphenhydramine. Clin Pharmacol Ther 1974;16:1066-76.

33. Albert KS, Hallmark MR, Sakmar E et al. Pharmacokinetics of diphenhydramine in man. J Pharmacokinet Biopharm 1975;3:159-70.

34. Berlinger WG, Goldberg MJ, Spector R et al. Diphenhydramine: kinetics and psychomotor effects in elderly women. Clin Pharmacol Ther 1982;32:387-91.

35. Schaaf L, Hendeles L, Weinberger M. Suppression of seasonal allergic rhinitis symptoms with daily hydroxyzine. J Allergy Clin Immunol 1979;63:129-33.

36. Anon. Drug Consult: hydroxyzine intravenous use. Drugdex D7-E7, edition expiring 11/30/86.

37. Simons FER, Simons KJ, Becker AB et al. Pharmacokinetics and antipruritic effects of hydroxyzine in children with atopic dermatitis. J Pediatr 1984;104:123-7.

38. Simons FER, Simons KJ, Frith EM. The pharmacokinetics and antihistaminic of the H_1 receptor antagonist hydroxyzine. J Allergy Clin Immunol 1984;73:69-75.

39. Sorkin EM, Heel RC. Terfenadine: a review of its pharmacodynamic properties and therapeutic efficacy. Drugs 1985;29:34-56.

40. Huther KJ, Renftle G, Barraud N et al. Inhibitory activity of terfenadine on histamine-induced skin wheals in man. Eur J Clin Pharmacol 1977;12:195-9.

41. Garteiz DA, Hook RH, Walker BJ et al. Pharmacokinetics and biotransformation studies of terfenadine in man. Arzneimittelforsch 1982;32:1185-90.

42. Okerholm RA, Weiner DL, Hook RH et al. Bioavailability of terfenadine in man. Biopharm Drug Disp 1981;2:185-90.

43. Woodward JK, Munro NL. Terfenadine, the first non-sedating antihistamine. Arzneimittelforsch 1982;32:1154-6.

44. Fowle ASE, Hughes DTD, Knight GJ. The evaluation of histamine antagonists in man. Eur J Clin Pharmacol 1971;3:215-20.

45. Simons KJ, Singh M, Gillespie CA et al. An investigation of the H_1-receptor antagonist triprolidine: pharmacokinetics and antihistaminic effects. J Allergy Clin Immunol 1986;77:326-30.

46. Kastrup EK, ed. Facts and comparisons. St. Louis. JB Lippincott. 1987.

47. Levander S, Hagermark O, Stahle M. Peripheral antihistamine and central sedative effects of three H_1-receptor antagonists. Eur J Clin Pharmacol 1985;28:523-9.

48. Schuller DE, Turkewitz D. Adverse effects of antihistamines. Postgrad Med 1986;79:75-86.

8:00 ANTI-INFECTIVE AGENTS

For **Antimicrobial Drugs of Choice,** see the Table on the following pages.

8:00 ANTI-INFECTIVE AGENTS

Antimicrobial Drugs of Choice*†

INFECTING ORGANISM	DRUG OF FIRST CHOICE	ALTERNATIVE DRUGS
GRAM-POSITIVE COCCI		
Staphylococcus aureus or epidermidis		
Non-penicillinase-producing	Penicillin G or V.[1]	A cephalosporin;[2,3] vancomycin; imipenem; clindamycin; ciprofloxacin.[4]
Penicillinase-producing	A penicillinase-resistant penicillin.[5]	A cephalosporin;[2,3] vancomycin; amoxicillin-clavulanic acid; ticarcillin-clavulanic acid; ampicillin-sulbactam; imipenem; clindamycin; ciprofloxacin.[4]
Methicillin-resistant[6]	Vancomycin, with or without rifampin[7] and/or gentamicin.	Trimethoprim-sulfamethoxazole;[7] ciprofloxacin.[4]
Streptococcus pyogenes (Group A) and Groups C and G	Penicillin G or V.[1]	An erythromycin;[8] a cephalosporin;[2,3] vancomycin.
Streptococcus, Group B	Penicillin G or ampicillin.	A cephalosporin;[2,3] vancomycin;[7] an erythromycin.
Streptococcus, viridans group[9]	Penicillin G with or without gentamicin.[7]	A cephalosporin;[2,3] vancomycin.
Streptococcus bovis[9]	Penicillin G.	A cephalosporin;[2,3] vancomycin.
Streptococcus, enterococcus group[9] Endocarditis[9] or other severe infection	Penicillin G or ampicillin with gentamicin.[7]	Vancomycin with gentamicin.[7]

Continued

Antimicrobial Drugs of Choice*†

INFECTING ORGANISM	DRUG OF FIRST CHOICE	ALTERNATIVE DRUGS
Uncomplicated urinary tract infection[10]	Ampicillin or amoxicillin.	Norfloxacin;[4] ciprofloxacin;[4] nitrofurantoin.
Streptococcus, anaerobic or Peptostreptococcus	Penicillin G.	Clindamycin; a cephalosporin;[2,3] vancomycin.[7]
*Streptococcus pneumoniae[11] (pneumococcus)	Penicillin G or V.[1]	An erythromycin;[8] a cephalosporin;[2,3] chloramphenicol;[12] vancomycin.[7]
GRAM-NEGATIVE COCCI Branhamella (Neisseria) catarrhalis	Amoxicillin-clavulanic acid.	Trimethoprim-sulfamethoxazole;[7] an erythromycin;[7] a tetracycline;[7,13] cefuroxime;[2,7] cefotaxime;[2,7] ceftizoxime;[2,7] ceftriaxone;[2,7] cefuroxime axetil.[2]
*Neisseria gonorrhoeae[14] (gonococcus)	Ceftriaxone.[2]	Penicillin G; amoxicillin with probenecid; spectinomycin; cefoxitin;[2] trimethoprim-sulfamethoxazole;[7] chloramphenicol;[12] ciprofloxacin.[4,7]
Neisseria meningitidis[15] (meningococcus)	Penicillin G.	Chloramphenicol;[12] cefuroxime;[2] cefotaxime;[2] ceftizoxime;[2,7] ceftriaxone;[2] trimethoprim-sulfamethoxazole;[7] a sulfonamide.[16]
GRAM-POSITIVE BACILLI Bacillus anthracis (anthrax)	Penicillin G.	An erythromycin;[7] a tetracycline.[13]
Clostridium perfringens[17]	Penicillin G.	Chloramphenicol;[12] metronidazole; clindamycin; a tetracycline.[13]

Antimicrobial Drugs of Choice*†

INFECTING ORGANISM	DRUG OF FIRST CHOICE	ALTERNATIVE DRUGS
Clostridium tetani[18]	Penicillin G.	A tetracycline.[13]
Clostridium difficile[19]	Vancomycin.	Metronidazole; bacitracin.[7]
Corynebacterium diphtheriae[20]	An erythromycin.	Penicillin G.
Corynebacterium, JK group	Vancomycin.[7]	
Listeria monocytogenes	Ampicillin[7] with or without gentamicin.[7]	Trimethoprim-sulfamethoxazole;[7] an erythromycin.
ENTERIC GRAM-NEGATIVE BACILLI		
Bacteroides Oropharyngeal strains	Penicillin G.[7,21]	Clindamycin; cefoxitin;[2] metronidazole; chloramphenicol;[12] cefotetan.[2,7]
Gastrointestinal strains[22]	Clindamycin or metronidazole.	Cefoxitin;[2] chloramphenicol;[12] mezlocillin, ticarcillin, or piperacillin; imipenem; ticarcillin-clavulanic acid;[7] ampicillin-sulbactam; cefotetan.[2]
Campylobacter jejuni	An erythromycin[7] or ciprofloxacin.[4]	A tetracycline;[13] gentamicin;[7] chloramphenicol.[12]
Enterobacter	Cefotaxime,[2,23] ceftizoxime,[2,23] or ceftriaxone.[2,23]	Gentamicin, tobramycin, or amikacin; imipenem;[23] carbenicillin,[24] ticarcillin,[24] mezlocillin,[24] piperacillin,[24] or azlocillin;[7,24] aztreonam; ceftazidime;[2,23] trimethoprim-

Continued

Antimicrobial Drugs of Choice*†

INFECTING ORGANISM	DRUG OF FIRST CHOICE	ALTERNATIVE DRUGS
*Escherichia coli;[26]	Ampicillin[27] with or without gentamicin, tobramycin, or amikacin.	sulfamethoxazole; ciprofloxacin;[4] norfloxacin.[4,25] chloramphenicol.[12] A cephalosporin;[2,3,23] carbenicillin,[24] ticarcillin,[24] mezlocillin,[24] piperacillin,[24] or azlocillin;[24] gentamicin, tobramycin, or amikacin; amoxicillin-clavulanic acid;[23] ticarcillin-clavulanic acid;[24] ampicillin-sulbactam;[23] trimethoprim-sulfamethoxazole; imipenem.[23] aztreonam; a tetracycline;[13] ciprofloxacin;[4] norfloxacin.[4,25] chloramphenicol.[12]
*Klebsiella pneumoniae[26]	A cephalosporin.[2,3,23]	Gentamicin, tobramycin, or amikacin; amoxicillin-clavulanic acid;[23] ticarcillin-clavulanic acid;[24] ampicillin-sulbactam;[23] trimethoprim-sulfamethoxazole; imipenem;[23] ciprofloxacin;[4] aztreonam; a tetracycline;[13] chloramphenicol;[4,25] norfloxacin;[4,25] chloramphenicol[24] or piperacillin.[24]
*Proteus mirabilis[26]	Ampicillin.[28]	A cephalosporin;[2,3,23] carbenicillin,[24] ticarcillin,[24] mezlocillin,[24] piperacillin,[24] or azlocillin;[24] gentamicin, tobramycin, or amikacin; trimethoprim-sulfamethoxazole; imipenem;[23] aztreonam; ciprofloxacin;[4] norfloxacin;[4,25] chloramphenicol.[12]

Continued

Antimicrobial Drugs of Choice*†

INFECTING ORGANISM	DRUG OF FIRST CHOICE	ALTERNATIVE DRUGS
Proteus, indole-positive (including Providencia rettgeri, Morganella morganii, and Proteus vulgaris)	Cefotaxime,[2,7,23] ceftizoxime,[2,23] or ceftriaxone.[2,23]	Gentamicin, tobramycin, or amikacin; carbenicillin,[24] ticarcillin,[24] mezlocillin,[24] piperacillin,[24] or azlocillin;[7,24] amoxicillin-clavulanic acid;[7,23] ticarcillin-clavulanic acid;[7,24] ampicillin-sulbactam;[7,23] imipenem;[7,23] aztreonam;[7] ceftazidime;[2,23] trimethoprim-sulfamethoxazole; a tetracycline;[7,13] ciprofloxacin;[4] norfloxacin;[4,25] chloramphenicol.[12]
Providencia stuartii	Cefotaxime,[2,7,23] ceftizoxime,[2,7,23] or ceftriaxone.[2,7,23]	Imipenem;[7,23] ticarcillin-clavulanic acid;[7,24] gentamicin,[7] tobramycin, or amikacin; carbenicillin,[7,24] ticarcillin,[7,24] mezlocillin,[7,24] piperacillin,[7,24] or azlocillin;[7,24] aztreonam;[7] ceftazidime;[2,7,23] trimethoprim-sulfamethoxazole;[7] ciprofloxacin;[4] norfloxacin;[4,7,25] chloramphenicol.[12]
Salmonella typhi[29]	Chloramphenicol.[12]	Ampicillin; amoxicillin;[7] trimethoprim-sulfamethoxazole;[7] ciprofloxacin.[4,7]
other Salmonella[30]	Ampicillin or amoxicillin.[7]	Trimethoprim-sulfamethoxazole;[7] ciprofloxacin;[4,7] chloramphenicol;[12] cefotaxime[2,7] or ceftriaxone.[2,7]
Serratia	Cefotaxime,[2,31] ceftizoxime,[2,31] or ceftriaxone.[2,31]	Gentamicin or amikacin; imipenem;[31] aztreonam; ceftazidime;[2,31] trimethoprim-

Continued

Antimicrobial Drugs of Choice*†

INFECTING ORGANISM	DRUG OF FIRST CHOICE	ALTERNATIVE DRUGS
		sulfamethoxazole;[7] carbenicillin,[7,32] ticarcillin,[7,32] mezlocillin,[7,32] piperacillin,[32] or azlocillin;[7,32] ciprofloxacin;[4] norfloxacin.[4,7,25]
Shigella	Trimethoprim-sulfamethoxazole.	Ciprofloxacin;[4] ampicillin; nalidixic acid.[7]
Yersinia enterocolitica	Trimethoprim-sulfamethoxazole.[7]	Ciprofloxacin;[4,7] gentamicin,[7] tobramycin,[7] or amikacin;[7] a tetracycline;[7,13] cefotaxime[2,7] or ceftizoxime.[2,7]
OTHER GRAM-NEGATIVE BACILLI *Acinetobacter* (Mima, Herellea)	Imipenem.[23]	Tobramycin,[7] gentamicin,[7] or amikacin; carbenicillin,[7,24] ticarcillin,[7,24] mezlocillin,[7,24] piperacillin,[24] or azlocillin;[7,24] trimethoprim-sulfamethoxazole;[7] minocycline,[13] doxycycline.[13]
Aeromonas hydrophila	Trimethoprim-sulfamethoxazole.[7]	Gentamicin[7] or tobramycin;[7] imipenem;[7] a tetracycline.[7,13]
Bordetella pertussis (whooping cough)	An erythromycin.	Trimethoprim-sulfamethoxazole;[7] ampicillin.[7]
Brucella (brucellosis)	A tetracycline[13] with streptomycin.	Chloramphenicol[12] with or without streptomycin; trimethoprim-sulfamethoxazole;[7] rifampin[7] with a tetracycline.[13]
Calymmatobacterium granulomatis (granuloma inguinale)	A tetracycline.[13]	Streptomycin.

Continued

Antimicrobial Drugs of Choice*†

INFECTING ORGANISM	DRUG OF FIRST CHOICE	ALTERNATIVE DRUGS
Eikenella corrodens	Ampicillin.[7]	An erythromycin;[7] a tetracycline;[7,13] amoxicillin-clavulanic acid;[7] ampicillin-sulbactam.[7]
Francisella tularensis (tularemia)	Streptomycin or gentamicin.[7]	A tetracycline;[13] chloramphenicol.[12]
Fusobacterium	Penicillin G.	Metronidazole; clindamycin; chloramphenicol.[12]
Gardnerella (Haemophilus) *vaginalis*[33]	Metronidazole.[7]	Ampicillin.[7]
Haemophilus ducreyi (chancroid)	Ceftriaxone[2,7] or an erythromycin.[7]	Trimethoprim-sulfamethoxazole.[7]
Haemophilus influenzae Meningitis, epiglottitis, arthritis, and other serious infections	Cefotaxime[2] or ceftriaxone.[2]	Cefuroxime;[2] ampicillin plus chloramphenicol initially.[34]
Other infections	Ampicillin or amoxicillin.	Trimethoprim-sulfamethoxazole; cefuroxime;[2] a sulfonamide with or without an erythromycin; amoxicillin-clavulanic acid; cefuroxime axetil;[2] cefaclor;[2] cefotaxime;[2] ceftizoxime;[2] ceftriaxone;[2,7] a tetracycline.[13]
Legionella micdadei (L. pittsburgensis)	An erythromycin[7] with or without rifampin.[7,35]	Trimethoprim-sulfamethoxazole.[7]
Legionella pneumophila	An erythromycin with or without rifampin.[7,35]	Trimethoprim-sulfamethoxazole.[7]

Continued

Antimicrobial Drugs of Choice*†

INFECTING ORGANISM	DRUG OF FIRST CHOICE	ALTERNATIVE DRUGS
Leptotrichia buccalis	Penicillin G.[7]	A tetracycline;[7,13] clindamycin.[7]
Pasteurella multocida	Penicillin G.[7]	A tetracycline;[7,13] a cephalosporin;[2] amoxicillin-clavulanic acid;[7] ampicillin-sulbactam.[7]
Pseudomonas aeruginosa Urinary tract infection	Carbenicillin or ticarcillin.	Piperacillin, mezlocillin, or azlocillin; ceftazidime;[2] imipenem; aztreonam; gentamicin; tobramycin; amikacin; norfloxacin;[4] ciprofloxacin.[4]
Other infections	Carbenicillin, ticarcillin, mezlocillin, piperacillin, or azlocillin plus tobramycin, gentamicin, or amikacin.[36]	Tobramycin, gentamicin, or amikacin with ceftazidime,[2] imipenem, or aztreonam; ciprofloxacin.[4]
Pseudomonas mallei (glanders)	Streptomycin[7] with a tetracycline.[7,13]	Streptomycin[7] with chloramphenicol.[12]
Pseudomonas maltophilia (Xanthomonas maltophilia)	Trimethoprim-sulfamethoxazole.[7]	Minocycline;[7,13] ceftazidime;[2] ciprofloxacin.[4,7]
Pseudomonas pseudomallei (melioidosis)	Trimethoprim-sulfamethoxazole.[7]	A tetracycline[7,13] with or without chloramphenicol;[12,37] chloramphenicol[12] plus kanamycin,[7] gentamicin,[7] or tobramycin;[7] a sulfonamide.

Continued

Antimicrobial Drugs of Choice*†

INFECTING ORGANISM	DRUG OF FIRST CHOICE	ALTERNATIVE DRUGS
Pseudomonas cepacia	Trimethoprim-sulfamethoxazole.[7]	Chloramphenicol;[12] ceftazidime;[2] imipenem.[7]
Spirillum minus (rat bite fever)	Penicillin G.	A tetracycline;[7,13] streptomycin.[7]
Streptobacillus moniliformis (rat bite fever; Haverhill fever)	Penicillin G.	A tetracycline;[7,13] streptomycin.[7]
Vibrio cholerae (cholera)[38]	A tetracycline.[13]	Trimethoprim-sulfamethoxazole.[7]
Vibrio vulnificus	A tetracycline.[7,13]	Penicillin G.[7]
Yersinia pestis (plague)	Streptomycin.	A tetracycline;[13] chloramphenicol;[12] gentamicin.[7]
ACID FAST BACILLI *Mycobacterium tuberculosis*[39]	Isoniazid with rifampin.[40]	Ethambutol; streptomycin;[12] pyrazinamide; aminosalicylic acid (PAS); cycloserine;[12] ethionamide;[12] kanamycin;[7,12] capreomycin.[12]
Mycobacterium kansasii[39]	Isoniazid[7] with rifampin[7] with or without ethambutol.[7]	Streptomycin;[7,12] ethionamide;[7,12] cycloserine.[7,12]
Mycobacterium avium-intracellulare-scrofulaceum complex[39]	Isoniazid,[7] rifampin,[7] ethambutol,[7] and streptomycin.[7,12]	Clofazimine; capreomycin;[7,12] ethionamide;[7,12] cycloserine;[7,12] rifabutine (ansamycin);[41] imipenem;[7] amikacin.[7]
Mycobacterium fortuitum complex[39]	Amikacin[7,12] and doxycycline.[7]	Cefoxitin; rifampin;[7] an erythromycin;[7] a sulfonamide.

Continued

Antimicrobial Drugs of Choice*†

INFECTING ORGANISM	DRUG OF FIRST CHOICE	ALTERNATIVE DRUGS
Mycobacterium marinum (balnei)[42]	Minocycline.	Trimethoprim-sulfamethoxazole;[7] rifampin;[7] cycloserine.[7,12]
Mycobacterium leprae (leprosy)	Dapsone[12] with rifampin[7] with or without clofazimine.	Acedapsone;[12,41] ethionamide;[7,12] protionamide.[41]
ACTINOMYCETES		
Actinomyces israelii (actinomycosis)	Penicillin G.	A tetracycline.[13]
Nocardia	Trisulfapyrimidines.	Trimethoprim-sulfamethoxazole;[7] amikacin;[7] minocycline;[7] trisulfapyrimidines with minocycline, ampicillin,[7] or erythromycin;[7] cycloserine.[7,12]
CHLAMYDIAE		
Chlamydia psittaci (psittacosis; ornithosis)	A tetracycline.[13]	Chloramphenicol.[12]
Chlamydia trachomatis (trachoma)	A tetracycline[13] (topical plus oral).	A sulfonamide (topical plus oral).
(inclusion conjunctivitis)	An erythromycin (oral or IV).	A sulfonamide.
(pneumonia)	An erythromycin.	A sulfonamide.[7]
(urethritis or pelvic inflammatory disease)	A tetracycline[13] or an erythromycin.	Sulfisoxazole.[7]

Continued

Antimicrobial Drugs of Choice*†

INFECTING ORGANISM	DRUG OF FIRST CHOICE	ALTERNATIVE DRUGS
(lymphogranuloma venereum)	A tetracycline[13] or an erythromycin.[7]	
MYCOPLASMA *Mycoplasma pneumoniae*	An erythromycin or a tetracycline.[13]	
Ureaplasma urealyticum	An erythromycin.	A tetracycline.[7,13]
RICKETTSIA Rocky Mountain spotted fever, endemic typhus (murine), tick bite fever, trench fever, typhus, scrub typhus, Q fever	A tetracycline.[13]	Chloramphenicol.[12]
SPIROCHETES *Borrelia burgdorferi*[43] (Lyme disease)	A tetracycline.[7,13]	Penicillin G[7] or V;[7] ceftriaxone;[2,7] an erythromycin.[7]
Borrelia recurrentis (relapsing fever)	A tetracycline.[13]	Penicillin G.[7]
Leptospira	Penicillin G.[7]	A tetracycline.[7,13]
Treponema pallidum	Penicillin G.[1]	A tetracycline;[13] an erythromycin.
Treponema pertenue (yaws)	Penicillin G.[7]	A tetracycline.[13]

Continued

Antimicrobial Drugs of Choice*†

INFECTING ORGANISM	DRUG OF FIRST CHOICE	ALTERNATIVE DRUGS
VIRUSES		
Cytomegalovirus	Ganciclovir.[41]	
Herpes simplex (keratitis)	Trifluridine (topical).	Vidarabine (topical); idoxuridine (topical).
(genital)	Acyclovir.	
(encephalitis)	Acyclovir.[7]	Vidarabine.
(neonatal)	Acyclovir.[7]	Vidarabine.
(disseminated, adult)	Acyclovir.[7]	Vidarabine.[7]
Human immunodeficiency virus	Zidovudine (azidothymidine).	
Influenza A	Amantadine.	
Respiratory syncytial virus	Ribavirin.	
Varicella-zoster	Acyclovir.[7]	Vidarabine.

*Resistance may be a problem; susceptibility tests should be performed.
†From Med Lett Drugs Ther 1988;30:33-40, 43-4 and 1986;28:33-40. Reproduced with permission.
NOTE: This 1988 revision of the chart "Antimicrobial Drugs of Choice" was included, beginning with the Second Printing, Sixth Edition, of the Handbook of Clinical Drug Data.

1. Penicillin V is preferred for oral treatment of infections caused by nonpenicillinase-producing staphylococci and other gram-positive cocci. For initial therapy of severe infections, penicillin G, administered parenterally, is first choice. For somewhat longer action in less severe infections due to Group A streptococci, pneumococci, or Treponema pallidum, procaine penicillin G, an intramuscular formulation, is given once or twice daily. Benzathine penicillin G, a slowly absorbed intramuscular preparation, is usually given in a single monthly injection for prophylaxis of rheumatic fever, once for treatment of Group A streptococcal pharyngitis, and once or more for treatment of syphilis.
Continued

2. The cephalosporins have been used as alternatives to penicillins in patients allergic to penicillins, but such patients may also have allergic reactions to cephalosporins.

3. For parenteral treatment of staphylococcal or nonenterococcal streptococcal infections, a "first-generation" cephalosporin such as cephalothin, cephapirin, cephradine or cefazolin can be used; for staphylococcal endocarditis, some Medical Letter consultants prefer cephalothin or cephapirin. For oral therapy, cephalexin or cephradine can be used. The "second-generation" cephalosporins cefamandole, cefuroxime, cefuroxime axetil, cefonicid, ceforanide, cefotetan, and cefoxitin are more active than the first-generation drugs against gram-negative bacteria. Cefuroxime and cefamandole are active against ampicillin-resistant strains of H. influenzae, but cefamandole has been associated with prothrombin deficiency and occasional bleeding. Cefoxitin and cefotetan are active against B. fragilis. The "third-generation" cephalosporins cefotaxime, cefotizoxime, ceftriaxone, cefoperazone, ceftazidime, and ceftazidime have greater activity than the second-generation drugs against enteric gram-negative bacilli. Moxalactam, another "third-generation" cephalosporin, has been associated with serious, sometimes fatal, bleeding disorders, and Medical Letter consultants now advise against its use; in any case, it should not be used to treat infections caused by gram-positive organisms. With the exception of cefoperazone (which can also cause bleeding) and ceftazidime, the activity of all currently available cephalosporins against Pseudomonas aeruginosa is poor or inconsistent (GR Donowitz and GL Mandell, N Engl J Med, 318:490,1988).

4. Not recommended for children.

5. For oral use against penicillinase-producing staphylococci, cloxacillin or dicloxacillin is preferred; for severe infections, a parenteral formulation of methicillin, nafcillin, or oxacillin should be used. Neither ampicillin, amoxicillin, amdinocillin, bacampicillin, cyclacillin, hetacillin, ticarcillin, mezlocillin, azlocillin, nor piperacillin is effective against penicillinase-producing staphylococci. However, the combinations of clavulanic acid with amoxicillin or ticarcillin and of sulbactam with ampicillin are active against these organisms.

6. Occasional strains of coagulase-positive staphylococci and many strains of coagulase-negative staphylococci are resistant to penicillinase-resistant penicillins; these strains are also resistant to cephalosporins and to imipenem.

7. Not approved for this indication by the U.S. Food and Drug Administration.

8. Occasional strains of Group A streptococci and pneumococci may be resistant to erythromycins.

9. In endocarditis, disk sensitivity testing does not provide adequate information; dilution tests for susceptibility should be used to assess bactericidal as well as inhibitory end points. Peak bactericidal activity of the serum against the patient's own organism should be present at a serum dilution of at least 1:8.

10. Routine antimicrobial susceptibility tests may be misleading. Because of high urine concentrations, ampicillin may be effective in urinary tract infections, even when the organism is reported to be "resistant."

11. In patients allergic to penicillin, an erythromycin is preferred for respiratory infections and chloramphenicol is recommended for meningitis. Rare strains of Streptococcus pneumoniae may be relatively resistant or resistant to penicillin; these strains are susceptible to vancomycin.

12. Because of the frequency of serious adverse effects, this drug should be used only for severe infections when less hazardous drugs are ineffective.

13. Tetracyclines are generally not recommended for pregnant women or children less than eight years old.

14. For more details, see The Medical Letter, 30:5,1988.

15. Rifampin is recommended for prophylaxis in close contacts of patients infected by sulfonamide-resistant organisms. Minocycline may also be effective for such prophylaxis but frequently causes vomiting and vertigo. An oral sulfonamide is recommended for prophylaxis in close contacts of patients known to be infected by sulfonamide-sensitive organisms.

16. Sulfonamide-resistant strains are frequent in the USA and sulfonamides should be used only when susceptibility is established by susceptibility tests.

17. Debridement is primary. Large doses of penicillin G are required. Hyperbaric oxygen therapy may be a useful adjunct to surgical debridement in management of the spreading, necrotic type.

18. For prophylaxis, a tetanus toxoid booster and, for some patients, tetanus immune globulin (human) are required.

19. Antibiotic-associated diarrhea or colitis should be treated by discontinuing the implicated antibiotic and avoiding use of antiperistaltic drugs or cor-

Continued

ticosteroids. When C. difficile is involved, vancomycin, metronidazole, or bacitracin should be given by mouth. If oral therapy cannot be used (such as with severe ileus or recent surgery), parenteral metronidazole is preferred.

20. Antitoxin is primary; antimicrobials are used only to halt further toxin production and to prevent the carrier state.

21. The proportion of penicillin-resistant Bacteroides species from the oropharynx has been increasing recently; for patients seriously ill with infections that may be due to these organisms, or where response to penicillin is delayed, clindamycin is preferred.

22. When infection is in the central nervous system, either intravenous metronidazole or chloramphenicol is recommended.

23. In severely ill patients, some Medical Letter consultants would add gentamicin, tobramycin, or amikacin.

24. In severely ill patients, some Medical Letter consultants would add gentamicin, tobramycin, or amikacin (but see footnote 36).

25. Indicated for treatment of urinary tract infections only.

26. For an acute, uncomplicated urinary tract infection, before the infecting organism is known, the drug of first choice is one of the oral soluble sulfonamides, such as sulfisoxazole, or (for E. coli or Proteus mirabilis) ampicillin or amoxicillin or (for Klebsiella) a cephalosporin. Trimethoprim or trimethoprim-sulfamethoxazole is also useful for treatment of urinary tract infections caused by susceptible organisms.

27. In some areas, a fairly high percentage of E. coli strains may be resistant to ampicillin.

28. Large doses (6 grams or more daily) are usually necessary for systemic infections. In severely ill patients, some Medical Letter consultants would add gentamicin, tobramycin, or amikacin.

29. Ampicillin or amoxicillin may be effective in milder cases. Ciprofloxacin[4] or ampicillin is the drug of choice for S. typhi carriers.

30. Most cases of Salmonella gastroenteritis subside spontaneously without antimicrobial therapy. For treatment of Salmonella meningitis, some Medical Letter consultants recommend cefotaxime or ceftriaxone.

31. In severely ill patients, some Medical Letter consultants would add gentamicin or amikacin.

32. In severely ill patients, some Medical Letter consultants would add gentamicin or amikacin (but see footnote 36).

33. Metronidazole is effective for bacterial vaginosis even though it is not active against Gardnerella in vitro. Ampicillin should be used for sepsis.

34. Some strains of H. influenzae are resistant to ampicillin and rare strains are resistant to ampicillin and chloramphenicol. Chloramphenicol (75-100 mg/kg/day IV) plus ampicillin can be used initially for treatment of meningitis in children more than one month old until the organism is identified and its antimicrobial susceptibility is determined. Ampicillin is preferred by some Medical Letter consultants for treatment of organisms known to be susceptible.

35. Rifampin should be added only for patients who do not respond to erythromycin alone or in severely immunocompromised patients.

36. Neither gentamicin, tobramycin, netilmicin, nor amikacin should be mixed in the same bottle with carbenicillin, ticarcillin, mezlocillin, piperacillin, or azlocillin for intravenous administration. In high concentrations or in patients with renal failure, carbenicillin or ticarcillin may inactivate the aminoglycosides.

37. Seriously ill patients should be treated with both tetracycline and chloramphenicol.

38. Antibiotic therapy is an adjunct to and not a substitute for prompt fluid and electrolyte replacement.

39. Susceptibility tests should be performed by appropriate reference laboratories, but antituberculosis drugs may be effective in vivo even when in vitro tests show resistance. Some isolates may require vigorous chemotherapy using multiple drugs.

40. Rifampin should be used concurrently with other drugs to prevent emergence of resistance. It is always included in treatment regimens for isoniazid-resistant organisms and is generally used together with isoniazid in the treatment of cavitary and far-advanced pulmonary tuberculosis as well as for extrapulmonary infections. For initial treatment of uncomplicated pulmonary and extrapulmonary tuberculosis, many clinicians add pyrazinamide to INH and rifampin for the first two months of a 6 month course of therapy. Alternatively, INH and rifampin can be given alone for 9 months.

41. An investigational drug in the USA.

42. Most infections are self-limited without drug treatment.

43. For treatment of early infection in non-pregnant adults, tetracycline is preferred; for fully developed infection with arthritis or meningitis, intravenous penicillin G or ceftriaxone is preferred.

Immunobiologics and Drugs Distributed by Centers for Disease Control

THE CENTERS FOR DISEASE CONTROL (CDC) distribute about 17 special immunobiologic agents and drugs through the Division of Host Factors, Center for Infectious Diseases (CID). These products fall into 4 categories: 1) antitoxins, 2) immune globulins (human) and immune plasmas, 3) vaccines and toxoids, and 4) drugs for parasitic diseases (See Table 1).

The CDC Drug Service dispenses an immunobiologic agent or drug to a requesting physician for administration to a patient whose situation or condition calls for its use (eg, hazardous environmental exposure, clinical syndrome). Appropriate information regarding indications/contraindications, dosages, routes and frequencies of administration, expected adverse reactions, toxicity, and other general data are included in the package inserts with all drugs and biological agents released from the CDC. The consent forms for the IND products are available upon request.

Request for drugs or biologicals may be made by calling the Division of Host Factors, Monday through Friday, 8 AM to 4:30 PM (eastern time) at (404) 329-3356 or 329-3670. The telephone number after working hours, holidays and weekends is (404) 329-2888.

Table 1. Agents Available from CDC

PRODUCT	INDICATIONS
DRUGS	
Bithionol (Lorothidol®)	Paragonimiasis, *Fasciola hepatica.*
Dehydroemetine	Amebiasis.
Diloxanide Furoate (Furamide®)	Intestinal amebiasis.
Melarsoprol (Mel B, Arsobal®)	African tripanosomiasis.
Quinine Dihydrochloride (parenteral)	Life-threatening pernicious malaria.
Rifabutin (ansamycin)	*Mycobacterium avium* complex disease.
Sodium Antimony Gluconate (Pentostam®)	Leishmaniasis.
Suramin (Bayer 205, Antrypol®)	African tripanosomiasis; onchocerciasis.
IMMMUNOBIOLOGICS	
Antitoxins	
Botulism Equine Antitoxin (ABE)	Botulism.
Diphtheria Equine Antitoxin	Diphtheria.
Immune Globulins (Human)	
Vaccinia Immune Globulin	Smallpox.
Western Equine Encephalitis Immune Globulin	Western equine encephalitis exposure (eg, laboratory accident).
Toxoids and Vaccines	
Anthrax Vaccine, Adsorbed	Workers at high risk.
Botulinum Toxoid Pentavalent	Laboratory personnel.
Japanese Encephalitis Vaccine	Travelers to high-risk areas.
Smallpox Vaccine	Laboratory personnel.

Table 2. VZIG Regional Distribution Centers

Massachusetts: Massachusetts Public Health Biologics Laboratories. (617) 522-3700
Maine: American Red Cross Blood Services. (617) 731-2130 or (207) 775-2367
Connecticut: American Red Cross Blood Services. (203) 678-2730
Vermont, New Hampshire: American Red Cross Blood Services. (802) 658-6400
Rhode Island: Rhode Island Blood Center. (401) 863-8368
New Jersey, New York: The Greater New York Blood Program. (212) 570-3067 or (212) 570-3068 (night)
New York: American Red Cross Blood Services. (518) 449-5020 or (518) 462-7461 or (518) 462-6964 (night) or American Red Cross Blood Services, Greater Buffalo Chapter. (716) 886-7500 or American Red Cross Blood Services Rochester Region. (716) 461-9800 or American Red Cross Blood Services Syracuse Region. (315) 425-1647
Delaware, Pennsylvania, Southern New Jersey: American Red Cross Blood Services. (215) 299-4110
Maryland: American Red Cross Blood Services. (301) 467-9905
Virginia: American Red Cross Blood Services. (804) 446-7708 or Richmond Metropolitan Blood Service. (804) 359-5100
Washington, D.C., Maryland, Virginia, West Virginia: American Red Cross Blood Services. (202) 728-6426
Georgia: American Red Cross Blood Services. (404) 881-9800 or (404) 881-6752 (night)
North Carolina: American Red Cross Blood Services. (704) 376-1661
South Carolina: American Red Cross Blood Services. (803) 256-2301
Florida: South Florida Blood Service. (305) 326-8888 or American Red Cross Blood Services. (904) 255-5444
Alabama, Mississippi: American Red Cross Blood Services. (205) 322-5661
Indiana: American Red Cross Blood Services. (219) 482-3781
Michigan: American Red Cross Blood Services. (313) 494-2715 or American Red Cross Blood Services. (313) 232-1176 or American Red Cross Blood Services. (517) 484-7461
Ohio: American Red Cross Blood Services. (216) 781-1800 or American Red Cross. (614) 253-7981
Wisconsin, Iowa, North Dakota, South Dakota: The Blood Center of S.E. Wisconsin. (414) 933-5000
Wisconsin: American Red Cross Blood Services Badger Region. (608) 255-0021
Minnesota: American Red Cross Blood Services. (612) 291-6789 or (612) 291-6767 (night)
Northern Illinois (Chicago): American Red Cross Blood Services. (312) 440-2222
Arkansas, Kansas, Kentucky, Missouri, Southern Illinois: American Red Cross Blood Services. (314) 658-2000 or (314) 658-2136 (night)
Nebraska: American Red Cross Blood Services. (402) 341-2723
Tennessee: American Red Cross Blood Services. (615) 327-1931, ext. 315
Louisiana, Oklahoma, Texas: Gulf Coast Regional Blood Center. (713) 791-6250 or American Red Cross Blood Services. (817) 776-8754 or American Red Cross Blood Services. (817) 322-8686
Colorado, New Mexico: United Blood Services. (505) 247-9831
Arizona: American Red Cross Blood Services. (602) 623-0541
Hawaii, Southern California: American Red Cross Blood Services. (213) 739-5200
Nevada, Utah, Wyoming, Northern California: American Red Cross Blood Services, (408) 292-1626
Alaska, Montana, Oregon: American Red Cross Blood Services. (503) 243-5286
Idaho: American Red Cross Blood Services. (208) 342-4500
Washington: Puget Sound Blood Center. (206) 292-6525
Canada: Canadian Red Cross Blood Transfusion Service. (416) 923-6692
Puerto Rico: American Red Cross Servicio de Sangre Capitulo. (809) 759-7979
Central and South America: South Florida Community Blood Center, 1676 N.W. Ninth Ave., Miami, FL 33142. (305) 326-8888
All other countries: American Red Cross Blood Services Northeast Region, 60 Kendrick St., Needham, MA 02194. (617) 449-0773 or American Red Cross Blood Services, 812 Huntington Avenue, Boston, MA 02115. (617) 731-2130

8:08 ANTHELMINTICS

General References: 1-3

Class Instructions. Purgation, enemas or special dietary restrictions are unnecessary with this drug, which may be taken with food or beverages. To avoid reinfestation with pinworms, the perianal area should be washed thoroughly each morning. Nightclothes, undergarments and bedclothes should be changed and washed daily. Wash hands and under fingernails thoroughly after bowel movements and before eating. Treat all family members simultaneously and clean bedroom and bathroom floors thoroughly at the end of the course of treatment. In order to demonstrate a cure, no eggs must be found in the anal area at least 5 weeks after the end of treatment.

Mebendazole

Vermox®

Pharmacology. Inhibits glucose uptake in the parasite with no effect on blood sugar concentrations in the host.

Administration and Adult Dose. PO for pinworms 100 mg in a single dose. PO for roundworms, whipworms and hookworms 100 mg bid for 3 days; if infestation persists 3 weeks later, repeat treatment.

Pediatric Dose. PO (over 2 yr) same as adult dose.

Dosage Forms. Chew Tab 100 mg.

Patient Instructions. Chew tablets before swallowing. See also Class Instructions.

Pharmacokinetics. *Fate.* Almost all eliminated unchanged in the feces, but up to 10% may be recovered in the urine 24 to 48 hr after a dose, primarily as the decarboxylated metabolite.[4]

Adverse Reactions. Occasional abdominal pain and diarrhea in cases of massive infestation and expulsion of worms.

Precautions. Pregnancy.

Parameters to Monitor. When treating whipworm, a stool sample for egg count should be taken 3 weeks after treatment to detect frequent (about 30%) persistent infestation requiring retreatment.[5,6]

Notes. This is the agent of choice for whipworm, producing about 70% cure-rate with single treatment; 90-100% cure-rate with roundworms, hookworms and pinworms.[7,8] Particularly useful in mixed infestations. Nonstaining.

Niclosamide

Niclocide®

Pharmacology. Inhibition of glucose uptake in the parasite without effect on host cells is the proposed mechanism of action.

Administration and Adult Dose. PO for beef, fish or pork tapeworm 2 g as a single dose. PO for dwarf tapeworm, 2 g/day for 7 days.

Pediatric Dose. PO for beef, fish or pork tapeworm (11-34 kg) 1 g as a single dose; (over 34 kg) 1.5 g as a single dose. PO for dwarf tapeworm initial dose as above, then one-half initial dose daily for 6 days.

Dosage Forms. **Chew Tab** 500 mg.

Patient Instructions. Chew tablets thoroughly and swallow with a small amount of water. Do not eat until 2 hr after the dose.

Pharmacokinetics. *Fate.* Minimal absorption from the GI tract.

Adverse Reactions. Up to 10% of patients may experience mild abdominal pain and bloating.

Precautions. Pregnancy.

Notes. Drug of choice for tapeworm infestation. Alternative to praziquantel for *H. nana* infestation.

Piperazine Citrate   Various

Pharmacology. Paralyzes the parasite by blocking response of the neuromuscular junction to acetylcholine, allowing the worm to be expelled by peristalsis.

Administration and Adult Dose. **PO for roundworms** 75 mg/kg/day to maximum of 3.5 g/day for 2 days. Doses are expressed as hexahydrate equivalent.

Pediatric Dose. **PO for roundworms** same as adult dose in mg/kg.

Dosage Forms. **Syrup** 100 mg/ml; **Tab** 500 mg; **Wafer** 500 mg (strengths expressed as hexahydrate equivalent).

Patient Instructions. See Class Instructions.

Pharmacokinetics. *Fate.* 15–75% absorbed and excreted in the urine as changed and unchanged drug.[9]

Adverse Reactions. Rare, except with excessive doses. Nausea, vomiting, diarrhea, headache; other neurological disturbances including vertigo, incoordination, weakness, seizures and coma may occur, especially with pre-existing CNS disorders and impaired renal function.[10]

Precautions. Pregnancy. Use with caution in patients with impaired renal or hepatic function or convulsive disorders.[10]

Notes. Virtually 100% effective for roundworms; no significant effect on hookworms, tapeworms or whipworms. Nonstaining. No clinical differences among salt forms.[11,12]

Praziquantel   Biltricide®

Pharmacology. Praziquantel causes a loss of intracellular calcium, resulting in paralysis and dislodgement of worms from sites of attachment.[3]

Administration and Adult Dose. **PO for schistosomiasis** (*S. haematobium, S. mansoni*) 40 mg/kg as a single dose is usually adequate, but heavy infestations require 60 mg/kg in 3 divided doses at 4–6 hr intervals.[3] (*S. japonicum*) 60 mg/kg in 3 doses at 4–6 hr intervals. **PO for flukes** (eg, fascioliasis, paragonimiasis, clonorchiasis, opisthorchiasis) 75 mg/kg/day in 3 doses for 1-3 days. **PO for tapeworms** 10–25 mg/kg as a single dose. **PO for cysticercosis** 50 mg/kg/day in 3 doses for 14 days.[3]

Pediatric Dose. (Over 4 yr) same as adult dose in mg/kg.

Dosage Forms. Tab 600 mg.

Patient Instructions. Do not chew tablets. This drug may cause dizziness or drowsiness; caution should be used when driving, operating machinery or performing other tasks requiring mental alertness.

Pharmacokinetics. *Fate.* The drug is 80% absorbed orally, but undergoes extensive first-pass metabolism. CSF concentrations are 14-20% of plasma levels. The drug is metabolized and metabolites are excreted primarily in urine.

$t_{1/2}$. 0.8-1.5 hr.

Adverse Reactions. Dizziness, headache and GI distress occur frequently after large doses. Drowsiness occurs frequently due to a structural similarity to benzodiazepines. In patients treated for neurocysticercosis, an inflammatory response, presumably due to dead and dying organisms occurs which is manifested by headache, seizures and increased intracranial pressure.

Contraindications. Ocular cysticercosis.

Precautions. Pregnancy; avoid breast feeding for 72 hr after last dose.

Parameters to Monitor. Observe for CNS toxicity when treating neurocysticercosis.

Notes. Concomitant corticosteroid therapy is recommended for patients treated for neurocysticercosis.

Pyrantel Pamoate   Antiminth®

Pharmacology. A depolarizing neuromuscular blocker that produces spastic paralysis of the parasite with no similar effects on the host after oral use.

Administration and Adult Dose. PO for roundworms, hookworms and pinworms 11 mg/kg, to maximum of 1 g in single dose; for pinworms repeat after 2 week interval. Doses are expressed as base equivalent.

Pediatric Dose. PO (over 1 yr) same as adult dose in mg/kg.

Dosage Forms. Susp 50 mg/ml (strength expressed as base equivalent).

Patient Instructions. See Class Instructions.

Pharmacokinetics. *Fate.* Slight oral absorption with peak plasma levels of 50-130 ng/ml reached within 1-3 hr after an 11 mg/kg dose. Less than 15% of dose is excreted in the urine as parent drug and metabolites.[13]

Adverse Reactions. Rare, nausea, vomiting, headaches and transient AST (SGOT) elevations.[13,14]

Precautions. Pregnancy. Use with caution in patients with impaired liver function.

Notes. Virtually 100% effective for pinworms and roundworms; ineffective for whipworm and *Strongyloides*.

Thiabendazole   Mintezol®

Pharmacology. Proposed to inhibit helminth-specific enzyme, fumarate reductase.

Administration and Adult Dose. **PO for strongyloidiasis** 25 mg/kg bid for 2 days. **PO for cutaneous larva migrans** 25 mg/kg bid for 2–5 days; concomitant topical therapy is also recommended. See Notes. **PO for visceral larva migrans** 25 mg/kg bid for 5 days. **PO for trichinosis** 25 mg/kg bid for 5 days. Dosage for all indications should not exceed 3 g/day.

Pediatric Dose. Same as adult dose in mg/kg.

Dosage Forms. **Susp** 100 mg/ml; **Chew Tab** 500 mg.

Pharmacokinetics. *Fate.* Well absorbed after oral administration. Most of the drug is metabolized to inactive glucuronide or sulfate compounds and excreted in urine within 24 hr.

Adverse Reactions. CNS effects such as dizziness, drowsiness and giddiness occur frequently; nausea and vomiting are also common. Diarrhea, epigastric pain, fever, chills, flushing and headache occur occasionally as do allergic manifestations (eg, pruritus, rash, angioedema). Seizures, leukopenia, lymphadenopathy and liver damage occur rarely.

Precautions. Pregnancy.

Notes. Therapy of disseminated strongyloidiasis should be continued for at least 5 days. Topical therapy using thiabendazole oral suspension for cutaneous larva migrans should be applied qid directly over the end of the larval tunnel in the skin. Systemic corticosteroids may be indicated to reduce inflammation due to dying larvae when the drug is used to treat trichinosis or visceral larva migrans of the eye.

8:12 ANTIBIOTICS

8:12.02 AMINOGLYCOSIDES

General References: 15–21

Aminoglycosides   Various

Pharmacology. Aminocyclitol derivatives which have bactericidal activity against Gram-negative aerobic bacteria via binding to the 30S and 50S ribosomal subunit; anaerobic bacteria are universally resistant, because aminoglycoside transport into cells is oxygen-dependent.[15,16] Dibasic cations (eg, magnesium and calcium) and acidic conditions decrease their in vitro action.[17] Streptomycin and kanamycin have poor activity against some Gram-negative bacteria, especially *Pseudomonas aeruginosa*. Some Gram-positive organisms (eg, streptococci) are relatively resistant to all aminoglycosides; however, in combination with some penicillins or vancomycin, these organisms are often synergistically inhibited or killed.[18] Resistance among Gram-negative organisms is due to transferable R-factor mediated enzymatic inactivation or decreased drug uptake.[18-20] See Notes.

Administration and Adult Dose. **IM or IV by slow intermittent infusion over 30-60 min,** although 15 min infusions are safe. With gentamicin there are some data to indicate that injection over 3–5 min does not increase the risk of toxicity.[21] **Continuous IV infusion** has been used to maintain constant suprainhibitory plasma concentrations; however, studies in experimental infections have shown that toxicity is more frequent and antibacterial effects are lower with continuous infusion compared to intermittent administration.[22,23] **Irrigation of vascularized areas** dosage should not exceed usual parenteral dose. **Intrathecal or intraventricular** administration is usually necessary to achieve therapeutic CSF levels. See Aminoglycosides Comparison Chart.

Dosage Individualization. Individualization is critical because these agents have a low therapeutic index. Use of ideal body weight (IBW) for determining the mg/kg dose appears to be more accurate than dosing on the basis of total body weight (TBW). In morbid obesity, dosage requirement may best be estimated using a dosing weight of IBW + 0.4 (TBW – IBW).[24] Initial and periodic peak and trough plasma drug levels should be determined, particularly in critically ill patients with serious infections or in disease states known to significantly alter aminoglycoside pharmacokinetics (eg, cystic fibrosis, burns or major surgery)[25]—this is unnecessary in less serious infections in patients without significant renal impairment—see Aminoglycosides Comparison Chart.

In renal impairment, the following guidelines may be used to determine initial dosage:[d]

1. Select loading dose in mg/kg (lean body weight or dosing weight as above) to provide peak plasma levels in the range listed below for the desired aminoglycoside.

AMINOGLYCOSIDE[a]	USUAL LOADING DOSES	EXPECTED PEAK PLASMA LEVELS
Tobramycin	1.5–2 mg/kg	4–10 mcg/ml
Gentamicin		
Amikacin	5–7.5 mg/kg	15–30 mcg/ml
Kanamycin		

2. Select maintenance dose (as percentage of chosen loading dose) to continue peak plasma levels indicated above, according to desired dosing interval and the patient's corrected creatinine clearance.

Percentage of Loading Dose Required For Dosage Interval Selected

Cl_{cr} (ML/MIN)	HALF-LIFE[b](HR)	8 HR	12 HR	24 HR
90	3.1	84%	–	–
80	3.4	80	91%	–
70	3.9	76	88	–
60	4.5	71	84	–
50	5.3	65	79	–
40	6.5	57	72	92%
30	8.4	48	63	86
25	9.9	43	57	81
20	11.9	37	50	75
17	13.6	33	46	70
15	15.1	31	42	67
12	17.9	27	37	61
10[c]	20.4	24	34	56
7[c]	25.9	19	28	47
5[c]	31.5	16	23	41
2[c]	46.8	11	16	30
0[c]	69.3	8	11	21

a. Similar levels are expected with netilmicin at doses equal to gentamicin or tobramycin.

b. Alternatively, one-half of the chosen loading dose may be given at an interval approximately equal to the estimated half-life.

c. Dosing for patients with Cl_{cr} less than 10 ml/min should be assisted by measured plasma levels.

d. From reference 26, reproduced with permission.

These guidelines are based on population data; plasma levels in individual patients may deviate significantly from guideline estimates.[27]

Pediatric Dose. See Aminoglycosides Comparison Chart.

Dosage Forms. See Aminoglycosides Comparison Chart.

Patient Instructions. Report any dizziness or sensations of ringing or fullness in the ears.

Pharmacokinetics. *Plasma Levels.* See Aminoglycosides Comparison Chart.

Fate. Absorption after oral or rectal administration is about 0.2-2%; absorption across denuded skin may reach 5%. Irrigation of vascularized areas (eg, peritoneal cavity) results in absorption approximating IM use.[28] IM administration is followed by rapid and complete absorption, with peak plasma levels occurring after 0.5-1.5 hr. IV infusions over 0.5-1 hr produce plasma levels similar to equal IM doses. Binding of aminoglycosides to plasma proteins is low. These agents distribute rapidly into the extracellular fluid compartment with a V_d of about 0.2-0.3 L/kg which is increased by fever, edema, ascites, fluid overload and in neonates.[29] Aminoglycosides accumulate markedly in some tissues, especially the renal cortex, to levels many times those found in the plasma.[29] Levels in the CSF of patients with meningitis generally do not exceed 25% of plasma levels, except in neonates;[29] penetration into the eye is inadequate for treatment of intraocular infections. Penetration into lung tissues and sputum is low and large doses may be necessary to optimally treat pneumonias with relatively insensitive organisms (eg, *Pseudomonas aeruginosa*). Distribution of aminoglycosides into the peritoneal cavity of patients with peritonitis is therapeutically adequate.[29]

Elimination is via glomerular filtration of unchanged drug.[29] After discontinuation, low levels of aminoglycoside can be detected in the urine for several days due to excretion of drug which had accumulated in deep tissue compartments.[29]

$t_{1/2}$. α phase 5-15 min; β phase (adults) about 1.5-3 hr (average 2) with normal renal function (1.5-9 hr in neonates less than 1 week and 3 hr in older infants); may be more variable in certain groups (eg, obstetric and burn patients) despite normal renal function; 50-70 hr in anuria. A prolonged γ elimination phase is observed when concentrations fall to the lower range of detectability, representing egress from deep tissue compartments and subsequent renal elimination;[29] the half-life of this phase ranges from 60-350 hr (usually 150-200). β phase half-life is most important for use in calculating individualized dosage, while the γ phase may account for the gradual rise of plasma levels and apparent increase in half-life with continued therapy, despite stable renal function.[29,30]

Adverse Reactions. Nephrotoxicity, which is manifested by a rise in Cr_s, BUN, aminoglycoside concentrations and appearance of renal tubular casts, enzymes and β_2-microglobulin, occurs in 5-30% of patients, depending on the criteria used and the population studied.[18,29] Depletion of magnesium and other minerals due to increased renal excretion occurs. Duration of therapy, advanced age, *high* initial Cl_{cr}, liver disease, high 1-hr peak plasma level and female sex are risk factors for nephrotoxicity.[31,32] Elevated trough levels are *not* a risk factor, but often a result of nephrotoxicity.[29,31,32] There is no evidence that there are clinically important differences in nephrotoxicity between gentamicin, tobramycin and amikacin.[31-33] Infrequent, but often permanent, vestibular toxicity is reported, usually in association with streptomycin. Subclinical vestibular disturbances can be detected in 40% or more of patients receiving aminoglycosides.[18,29] Early cochlear damage can be detected only by sequential audiometric examination, because hearing loss in conversational frequencies is a sign of advanced auditory impairment. Furthermore, early auditory damage is not as apparent in the elderly or others with pre-existing high-tone deficits. Risk factors for ototoxicity include duration of therapy, bacteremia, high BUN to Cr_s ratio, peak temperature and liver disease.[34] Elevated plasma concentrations are apparently not associated with increased ototoxicity risk, nor does there appear to be any clinically important differences between gentamicin, tobramycin and amikacin.[33,34] Oral aminoglycosides, primarily neomycin, have been associated with a sprue-like malabsorption syndrome.[15] Neuromuscular blockade with respiratory failure is rare, except in predisposed patients—see Precautions.

Precautions. Pregnancy; pre-existing renal impairment; vestibular or cochlear impairment; myasthenia gravis, hypocalcemia, postoperative or other conditions which depress neuromuscular transmission; history of aminoglycoside hypersensitivity reactions. See Drug Interactions chapter.

Parameters to Monitor. Renal function tests before and every 2-3 days during therapy. In patients with pre-existing renal, auditory or vestibular impairment or in patients who receive prolonged, high-dose therapy, obtain baseline and weekly audiograms, and check for tinnitus or vertigo daily, if possible. Audiometry and electronystagmography may be performed in patients able to cooperate. Peak and trough plasma aminoglycoside levels are useful for individualizing dosage and assuring the presence of effective plasma levels. Routine monitoring may not be cost-effective in patients without underlying disease between 3-18 yr of age.[35,36] In neonates or other patients with rapidly changing renal function, obtain plasma drug concentrations initially and every 2-3 days until stable. See Dosage Individualization.

Notes. Of the available aminoglycosides, gentamicin, tobramycin, netilmicin and amikacin are the most clinically useful. **Streptomycin** use is largely restricted to the treatment of enterococcal endocarditis (in combination with penicillin G), tuberculosis, brucellosis, plague and tularemia. **Neomycin** is much more toxic than the other aminoglycosides when given parenterally; it is restricted to oral use for gut sterilization and topical use for minor infections. Resistance among Gram-negative organisms, especially *Pseudomonas aeruginosa,* has limited the use of **kanamycin. Tobramycin** is roughly equivalent to gentamicin therapeutically, although it is about 2-4 times more active against *Pseudomonas aeruginosa* than is gentamicin, and it is often active against gentamicin-resistant *Pseudomonas aeruginosa.* Resistance of Gram-negative bacilli is lowest with amikacin; amikacin use does not appear to result in increased resistance to the drug.[20] Acylampicillins may degrade aminoglycosides in vitro, resulting in artifactually low levels; the extent of degradation is dependent on time, temperature and β-lactam concentration.[29,37] Degradation can occur in vivo in patients with renal insufficiency.[38] Amikacin is the least susceptible aminoglycoside to β-lactam inactivation.[29,37]

Aminoglycosides Comparison Chart

DRUG	DOSAGE FORMS	USUAL ADULT DOSE[a]	PEDIATRIC DOSE[a]	USUAL THERAPEUTIC PLASMA LEVELS (MCG/ML) PEAK[b]	TROUGH
Amikacin Sulfate Amikin®	Inj 50, 250 mg/ml	IM or IV 15–20 mg/kg/day in 2–3 equally divided doses; IT 5–20 mg/day.	IM or IV (less than 1 week) 15–20 mg/kg/day in 2 divided doses q 12 hr; IM or IV (infants over 1 week) 20–25 mg/kg/day in 2–3 divided doses q 8–12 hr; IM or IV (children) same as adult mg/kg dose.	20–35	≤10
Gentamicin Sulfate Garamycin® Various	Inj 10, 40 mg/ml IT Inj 2 mg/ml Ophth Oint 3 mg/g Ophth Soln 3 mg/ml.	IM or IV 5–6 mg/kg/day in 3 equally divided doses q 8 hr; IM or IV for less serious infections[c] 3–5 mg/kg/day in 3 equally divided doses q 8 hr; IT 4–8 mg q 18–24 hr.	IM or IV (less than 1 week) 4–5 mg/kg/day in 2 divided doses q 12 hr; IM or IV (infants over 1 week) 6–7.5 mg/kg/day in 3–4 divided doses q 6–8 hr; IM or IV (children) 6–7.5 mg/kg/day (7–10 mg/kg/day in cystic fibrosis) in 3–4 divided doses q 6–8 hr; IT 1–2 mg q 18–24 hr.	5–12	≤2
Kanamycin Sulfate Kantrex® Various	Cap 500 mg Inj 37.5, 250, 333 mg/ml.	PO 4–8 g/day in 2–4 divided doses; IM or IV 15–20 mg/kg/day in 2–3 equally divided doses; IT 5–20 mg/day.	PO (infants) 50 mg/kg/day in 2–4 divided doses; IM or IV (infants) not well studied, but use amikacin guidelines;	20–30	≤10

Continued

Aminoglycosides Comparison Chart

DRUG	DOSAGE FORMS	USUAL ADULT DOSE[a]	PEDIATRIC DOSE[a]	USUAL THERAPEUTIC PLASMA LEVELS (MCG/ML) PEAK[b]	TROUGH
Netilmicin Sulfate Netromycin®	Inj 100 mg/ml.	IM or IV 3[c]–6.5 mg/kg/day in 2–3 equally divided doses q 8–12 hr.	IM or IV (children) same as adult mg/kg dose. Same as gentamicin.	5–12	≤2
Streptomycin Sulfate Various	Inj 400, 500 mg, 1, 5 g.	IM 15–25 mg/kg/day (usually 1–2 g/day) in 2 equally divided doses q 12 hr; IM for TB 1 g q week.	IM (neonates) 20–30 mg/kg/day in 2 equally divided doses q 12 hr; IM (children) 20–40 mg/kg/day in 2 divided doses q 12 hr.	15–30	≤5
Tobramycin Sulfate Nebcin®	Inj 10, 40 mg/ml.	IM or IV 5–6 mg/kg/day in 3 equally divided doses q 8 hr; IM or IV for less serious infections[a] 3–5 mg/kg/day in 3 equally divided doses q 8 hr; IT 4–8 mg q 18–24 hr.	Same as gentamicin.	5–12	≤2

a. For uncomplicated UTI or mild soft tissue infection.

b. As seen after a 30 min IV infusion or approximately 1 hr after IM administration of a usual adult dose. Uncomplicated UTI may be treated with smaller doses that produce much lower plasma levels; however, serious infections, such as Gram-negative bacteremia, pneumonia or endocarditis may require doses resulting in plasma levels in the higher part of the range. Clinical efficacy appears to increase as the ratio of the peak plasma level to the MIC of the pathogen increases.[39]

c. These doses conform to those used in published clinical trials but higher doses may be necessary in certain patient populations.

8:12.04 ANTIFUNGAL ANTIBIOTICS

General References: 40–42

Amphotericin B

Fungizone®

Pharmacology. A polyene antifungal agent which preferentially binds to fungal cytoplasmic membrane sterols (chiefly ergosterol), increasing the permeability of the membrane. Binds somewhat to human cytoplasmic sterols (chiefly cholesterol), which accounts for a portion of amphotericin's toxicity.

Administration and Adult Dose. IV initial test dose 1 mg by slow infusion advocated by some sources; increase in 5–10 mg/day increments at daily intervals to a maximum of 1.5 mg/kg/day as dictated by severity of infection, clinical response and tolerance of infusion. Dosage should be more rapidly increased to the higher dosages in critically ill patients. During prolonged therapy, the drug may be given every other day.[40-43] **Recommended infusion concentration** is 10 mg/dl of D5W administered over 2–6 hr. Do not mix with electrolyte solutions; protection from light unnecessary if infused in less than 24 hr from time of preparation.[44,45] **Intracavitary for pulmonary aspergilloma** 5–50 mg in D5W daily to 3 times/week.[46] **Intrathecally** 500 mcg in 5 ml CSF 2–3 times a week, or 300 mcg/day in D5W or D10W infused over 1 hr.[43,47] **Bladder irrigation** 15–50 mg/day in 1 L of sterile water as a continuous irrigation over 24 hr.[48]

Dosage Individualization. No dosage alteration necessary with impaired renal function, although further impairment may occur as a result of the amphotericin.[40-43]

Pediatric Dose. IV same as adult dose in mg/kg.

Dosage Forms. Inj 5 mg/ml (when reconstituted); **Top Crm** 30 mg/g; **Top Lot** 30 mg/ml; **Top Oint** 30 mg/g.

Patient Instructions. Patient should be forewarned of expected immediate reactions to infusion. Topical preparations may stain clothes.

Pharmacokinetics. *Fate.* Poor oral and IM absorption. 370–650 mcg/kg/day infused IV over 4–6 hr produces levels of 1.8–3.5 mcg/ml 1 hr after infusion; concentrations of 0.5–1.5 mcg/ml remain 20 hr after infusion discontinued; plasma concentrations are not directly proportional to dose and tend to plateau at doses exceeding 50 mg. With usual doses, trough concentrations on alternate day or daily administration schedules are not significantly different; peaks are generally higher on alternate day schedule. Plasma concentrations represent less than 10% of administered dose; greater than 95% bound to plasma lipoproteins;[15] V_d is about 4 L/kg.[49] High concentrations of drug are found in many tissues, but much of the drug may be biologically inactive because of tissue binding.[50] The drug appears to be stored in the body, very slowly released, metabolized and slowly excreted by the kidneys. Despite slow elimination, plasma concentrations do not increase after repeated administration or in the presence of impaired renal function. When therapy is discontinued, amphotericin and metabolites continue to appear in the urine for 7–8 weeks.[43]

$t_{1/2}$. About 24–48 hr initially, with a terminal phase $t_{1/2}$ of about 15 days; not changed with renal impairment.[49]

Adverse Reactions. Very common during infusion period: fever, chills, headache, anorexia, nausea, vomiting, malaise, pain at infusion site. Severity of reactions may be reduced by premedication with an antipyretic, corticosteroid, antiemetic and addition of phosphate buffer and heparin to solution.[43] Prolonged administration times (greater than 6 hr) may produce more immediate reactions.[43] IV **meperidine** HCl 50 mg rapidly terminates shaking chills in some patients in whom spontaneous disappearance does not occur when the infusion is stopped.[51] **Dantrolene** may also prevent or reduce rigors in patients unresponsive to other measures.[52] With repeated administration: thrombophlebitis, normocytic, normochromic anemia, impaired renal function with distal tubular acidosis, isosthenuria, hypokalemia and hypomagnesemia frequently occur, and are generally reversible, although permanent renal impairment may result, especially if total dose exceeds 4–5 g.[43] Sodium loading may prevent or reverse nephrotoxicity.[53] Potassium supplementation is usually necessary and administration of an alkalinizing potassium salt (bicarbonate, gluconate, etc.) is often useful in preventing the occurrence of hypokalemic acidosis. Mannitol does not appear to provide any protection against renal damage.[43] Rapid infusion has been carried out safely,[43,54] but may produce cardiovascular collapse.[41] Pulmonary reactions characterized by acute dyspnea, hypoxemia and interstitial infiltrates have occurred in patients receiving granulocyte transfusions;[55] infusions of granulocytes and amphotericin B should be separated as far apart as possible. Intrathecal administration can produce peripheral nerve pain, paresthesias, nerve palsies, paraplegia, convulsions and chemical meningitis;[41,47] bladder irrigations containing amphotericin have produced no reported toxicity.[48]

Precautions. Impaired renal function. Safety of use during pregnancy not established despite reports of safe use.

Parameters to Monitor. BUN, serum creatinine or creatinine clearance should be monitored before therapy and at least weekly during therapy; monitor hematocrit, serum and urine electrolytes periodically. Some sources consider temporary drug discontinuation if renal function becomes severely impaired due to the amphotericin (serum creatinine greater than 3.5 mg/dl or BUN greater than 40 mg/dl). Monitor the total dose of amphotericin B; toxicity and perhaps efficacy in some infections may be related to total dose.[43]

Notes. Amphotericin B is very water insoluble; commercial product is a colloidal dispersion in bile salts, buffered with sodium phosphate. Store powder in refrigerator, protect from light. Reconstitute with sterile water for injection *without* a bacteriostatic agent; reconstituted drug is stable for 1 week under refrigeration. The drug is probably removed by in-line filters of less than 1 micron pore size, despite contrary claims; therefore, filtration is not recommended. Necessary dosages and duration of therapy are not established for many diseases.[40] The more water-soluble investigational methyl ester of amphotericin B has been associated with progressive leukoencephalopathy.[56,57] Liposome-encapsulated amphotericin B is less toxic and more efficacious in some animal models; limited studies in humans are promising.[58]

Clotrimazole

Gyne-Lotrimin®, Lotrimin®, Mycelex®, Mycelex-G®

Clotrimazole is an imidazole antifungal agent used for local therapy of fungal infections. The topical formulations are equivalent to other topical antifungals in the treatment of *Candida* or dermatophyte skin infections. For vulvovaginal candidiasis, a 100 mg vaginal tablet is used daily at bedtime for 7 days; alternatively, two 100 mg tablets may be used intravaginally once daily at bedtime for 3 days. Troches of 10 mg are dissolved in the mouth 5 times/day to treat or prevent orotracheal candidiasis. Available as 1% topical cream, lotion and solution; 1% vaginal cream; 100 and 500 mg vaginal tablets and 10 mg troches.

Fluconazole (Investigational - Pfizer)

Fluconazole is an investigational triazole antifungal agent that differs from the imidazoles in that it is more active against yeasts (including *Cryptococcus neoformans*). Its penetration into CSF is good and very preliminary experience as primary treatment and chronic maintenance therapy of cryptococcal meningitis in patients with AIDS has been good. It is being evaluated in both oral and parenteral dosage forms.

Flucytosine   Ancobon®

Pharmacology. Flucytosine (5-FC) is a fluorinated cytosine analogue that appears to be deaminated to the cytotoxic antimetabolite fluorouracil by cytosine deaminase, an enzyme present in fungal, but not human cells.

Administration and Adult Dose. PO 50–150 mg/kg/day in 4 divided doses; the use of higher doses has been suggested in order to prevent the emergence of resistance.

Dosage Individualization. Dosage must be reduced in the presence of impaired renal function.[40,42,59,60] An approximate reduction can be determined by dosing at intervals in hours equal to 4 times the Cr_s in mg/dl. Alternative regimens involving reduced dosage at 6 hr dosing intervals have been recommended. In patients on maintenance hemodialysis q 48–72 hr, may give 20–50 mg/kg after each dialysis.[40,60] May give normal doses to patients with liver disease; however, see Adverse Reactions.

Pediatric Dose. PO same as adult dose in mg/kg.

Dosage Forms. Cap 250, 500 mg.

Patient Instructions. Take the capsules required for a single dose over a 15 min period with food to minimize stomach upset. Close follow-up with the physician is essential.

Pharmacokinetics. *Plasma Levels.* Toxicity most likely over 100 mcg/ml.[40,42,59,61] See also Precautions.

Fate. Rapidly and well absorbed (about 90%) with peak about 1–2 hr after administration of a 500 mg dose to adults averaging 8–12 mcg/ml[61] in patients with normal renal function. Insignificant binding to plasma proteins;[42] V_d is 0.7 L/kg.[60] Widely distributed throughout the body, including the CSF and eye.[42] Eliminated almost entirely (average 90%) in the urine by glomerular filtration of unchanged drug, with urine levels many times greater than plasma levels.[40,60] Low plasma concentrations of fluorouracil have been found in patients taking flucytosine and may be related to hematologic toxicity.[40,42]

$t_{1/2}$. 3–8 hr (average 6); up to 100 hr or greater with renal impairment.[40,42]

Adverse Reactions. Occasional nausea, vomiting, diarrhea, bone marrow depression and elevated liver function tests (usually asymptomatic and rapidly reversible).[40,59] Diarrhea occurs occasionally; ulcerating enteritis occurs rarely.[62]

Precautions. Pregnancy. With severe renal impairment, elimination is highly variable and monitoring of plasma levels is recommended, keeping peak concentrations less than 100 mcg/ml;[40,42] impaired hepatic function; hematologic disorders or history of therapy with myelosuppressive drugs or radiation.

Parameters to Monitor. Before, and frequently during therapy, monitor BUN, serum creatinine, creatinine clearance, full hematology and liver function tests. See also Precautions.

Notes. Certain fungi may develop resistance to the drug during therapy. Flucytosine may be synergistic with amphotericin B, depending on the organism involved; the combination is useful in treating cryptococcal meningitis, and is promising in persistently febrile neutropenic cancer patients with suspected, but undocumented fungal infections.[61,63] Amphotericin B can increase the toxicity of flucytosine by increasing its cellular penetration and impairing its elimination secondary to nephrotoxicity.[15,40,42] Duration of therapy must be guided by severity of infection and response to therapy.

Griseofulvin

Fulvicin P/G®, Fulvicin-U/F®, Grifulvin V®, Grisactin®

Pharmacology. A fungistatic agent concentrated in sensitive organisms and impairing fungal growth by an unknown mechanism which appears to affect mitosis. Very active against most dermatophytes (ringworm fungi); little activity against other yeasts or fungi.

Administration and Adult Dose. PO (microsize) 500 mg–1 g/day in single or 2–4 divided doses; (ultra microsize) 330–660 mg/day in single or 2–4 divided doses. Symptomatic relief usually appears within several days. Lesions of skin not involving the palms, soles or nails usually require 3 weeks of therapy; infections of the palms or soles require 4–8 weeks of therapy; infections of the nails may require 6–12 months of therapy. Continue therapy until lesions clear.[64] See also Notes.

Dosage Individualization. No dosage reduction required for patients with renal disease.

Pediatric Dose. (Over 2 yr) PO (microsize) 11 mg/kg/day in a single or 2–4 divided doses; (ultramicrosize) 7.3 mg/kg/day in a single or 2–4 divided doses. Larger doses may be used initially for severe infections.

Dosage Forms. (Microsize) Cap 125, 250 mg; Susp 25 mg/ml; Tab 250, 500 mg. (Ultramicrosize) Tab 125, 165, 250, 330 mg.

Patient Instructions. Taking dose at noon may increase absorption. Avoid prolonged exposure to direct sunlight while taking this drug. Nausea, vomiting, flushing and faintness may occur if alcohol is taken during therapy with this drug.

Pharmacokinetics. Fate. Considerable individual variation in absorption is experienced with all dosage forms, with an average of 50% absorbed in fasted patients. Fatty meals may increase rate but not extent of absorption.[65] Absorption takes place over 30–40 hr; dissolution of drug appears rate-limiting;[66] 1 g orally in fasted adults produces peak plasma levels at 4–8 hr of 1–2 mcg/ml. The ultramicrosize preparations dispersed in polyethylene glycol are more completely and somewhat more rapidly absorbed allowing a one-third lower dosage. Widely distributed with multicompartment kinetics and a V_d of 1–2 L/kg. Appears in stratum corneum within 8 hr after a single oral dose, due to transport in sweat and other transepidermal fluids.[65] Most of absorbed drug is metabolized by liver to 6-demethylgriseofulvin which is excreted in the urine; about 0.1% appears in the urine as unchanged drug.[65,66]

$t_{1/2}$. Difficult to estimate after oral administration due to prolonged absorption. 9–21 hr (average 17.5 hr) after IV administration.[66]

Adverse Reactions. Headache, nausea and vomiting occasionally occur; may exacerbate acute intermittent porphyria; rare photosensitivity reactions, peripheral neuritis and leukopenia.

Contraindications. Porphyria, hepatocellular failure.

Precautions. Pregnancy.

Parameters to Monitor. Occasional hematologic, hepatic and renal function tests during long-term therapy.

Itraconazole (Investigational - Janssen)

Itraconazole is an investigational triazole antifungal that differs from ketoconazole in that it is more active against certain fungi, notably *Aspergillus, Cryptococcus* and *Sporotrichosis*. Peak concentration after a single oral 100 mg dose is 38 ng/ml; peak concentration is increased 3-4 fold when administered with food. The half-life is 17-24 hr. Adverse reactions are infrequent. More study is required to determine the human tolerance and optimal dosing of this agent.[67]

Ketoconazole   Nizoral®

Pharmacology. Ketoconazole is an imidazole antifungal agent that is more water-soluble than other available agents of this class. It exerts its antifungal effects through inhibiting the synthesis of ergosterol, a fungal cell wall component.

Administration and Adult Dose. PO 200-400 mg 1-3 times/day, depending on severity of infection. **Top** apply once daily.

Dosage Individualization. Limited data suggest that dosage adjustment is unnecessary in patients with hepatic impairment; however, definitive studies are needed. No adjustment in renal dysfunction is necessary.

Pediatric Dose. PO (under 2 yr) not established; (over 2 yr) 3.3-6.6 mg/kg/day in 1-2 divided doses. (The drug is bioavailable when tablets are crushed and mixed in applesauce or juice);[69] doses up to 10 mg/kg/day have been reported.[68] **Top** apply once daily.

Dosage Forms. **Tab** 200 mg; **Susp** 100 mg/5 ml; **Crm** 2%.

Patient Instructions. This drug may be taken with meals if stomach upset occurs. Report symptoms of fatigue, loss of appetite, dark urine or pale stools.

Pharmacokinetics. *Fate.* Bioavailability is approximately 76% and may be dose-dependent. Peak plasma concentrations are 3-4 mcg/ml following a 200 mg dose; bioavailability appears to be decreased 20-40% when administered with food. 93-96% plasma protein bound; V_d is estimated to be 0.36 L/kg. Extensively metabolized by the liver to inactive metabolites; only 2-4% of a dose is excreted unchanged in the urine.[68]

$t_{1/2}$. 8-10 hr.[68]

Adverse Reactions. Generally well tolerated with the most frequent side effects being nausea, vomiting, pruritus and abdominal discomfort. Hepatotoxicity, including massive hepatic necrosis has occurred rarely. Gynecomastia has been reported, which may be caused by reversible ketoconazole-induced suppression of testosterone synthesis.[68] Ketoconazole also blocks cortisol production; however, clinically apparent hypoadrenalism has been noted rarely with clinical use.[70] Irritation, pruritus and stinging may occur with topical use.

Parameters to Monitor. Liver function tests. Prothrombin time if patient is receiving warfarin. Cyclosporine plasma/blood concentrations and Cr_s in patients with bone marrow or renal transplants.

Miconazole
Miconazole Nitrate

Monistat IV®
Monistat-Derm®, Monistat-7®,
Monistat-3®, Micatin®

Miconazole is an imidazole antifungal agent available in topical preparations and as a solubilized preparation in a polyethoxylated castor oil (Cremophor® EL). Due to the serious toxicity (eg, cardiorespiratory arrest, hyponatremia) of the parenteral preparation (most likely due to the vehicle) and data challenging the clinical effectiveness of this agent, parenteral use should be restricted to treating fungal infections known to be resistant to amphotericin B (eg, *Petriellidium boydii*). Phlebitis, pruritus, nausea, vomiting, fever, chills and rash are also frequent side effects of IV miconazole. For vaginal infections, a 7-day course of a 100 mg suppository or 5 g of cream intravaginally once daily at bedtime, or a 3-day course of a 200 mg suppository intravaginally once daily at bedtime can be used. The IV dose is 1.2–3.6 g/day in 3 divided doses, diluted in at least 200 ml of D5W or NS; the dose should be infused over 30–60 min.[71-73] Available as 200 mg ampules (10 mg/ml), 2% topical cream, aerosol, lotion or powder; 2% vaginal cream; and 100 and 200 mg vaginal suppositories.

Nystatin

Mycostatin®, Nilstat®, Various

Nystatin is a polyene antifungal agent similar to amphotericin B, but too toxic for parenteral use. Oral absorption is negligible and there is no absorption through intact skin or mucous membranes. The drug is nontoxic by oral, topical and vaginal routes; allergic sensitization occurs rarely. For oral candidiasis, the dose of the suspension is 400,000–600,000 units qid in adults and 100,000 units qid for newborn infants and 250,000–500,000 units qid in older infants and children for at least 48 hr after oral symptoms have cleared and cultures have returned to normal. The vaginal tablet has been successfully used orally in place of the oral suspension; its slow dissolution allows prolonged contact time. For GI candidiasis the dose is 500,000–1,000,000 units tid orally. For oral candidiasis, nystatin pastilles 200,000–800,000 units 4–5 times/day may be used. For vaginal candidiasis the dose is 100,000 units daily or bid vaginally for 2 weeks. Available as a 100,000 units/ml suspension, 500,000 unit oral tablets, 200,000 unit pastilles, 100,000 unit vaginal tablet and 100,000 units/g topical cream, ointment and powder.

8:12.06 CEPHALOSPORINS

General References 74–86

Cephalosporins

Pharmacology. Cephalosporin antibiotics have broad spectrum activity against many Gram-positive and Gram-negative pathogens. These agents are generally considered to be bactericidal through binding to various penicillin-binding proteins in bacteria, which results in changes in cell wall structure and function.[84] Members of this class are frequently subdivided into "generations" based on their antimicrobial activity (as well as order of introduction into clinical use).

First-generation cephalosporins have activity against Gram-positive bacteria (eg, *Staphylococcus* sp.) as well as a limited, but important, number of species of aerobic Gram-negative bacilli (eg, *E. coli*, *Klebsiella* sp., *Proteus mirabilis*). *Haemophilus influenzae* and most other aerobic Gram-negative bacilli often indigenous to hospitals (eg, *Enterobacter* sp., *Pseudomonas* sp.) are resistant to these drugs. Anaerobic bacteria isolated in the oropharynx are generally susceptible to these agents; however, anaerobes such as *Bacteroides fragilis* are resistant.

The **second-generation cephalosporins** cefamandole, cefonicid, ceforanide and cefuroxime all differ from first-generation agents in their improved activity against *Haemophilus influenzae* and some strains of *Enterobacter* sp., *Providencia* sp. and *Morganella* sp. Cefoxitin and cefotetan, which are actually cephamycins, are notable for their increased activity against anaerobes, including *Bacteroides fragilis*; the other second-generation cephalosporins have poor activity against this organism.

The **third-generation cephalosporins** are notable for their potent activity against many Gram-negative organisms resistant to older agents (eg, *Serratia* sp., *Pseudomonas aeruginosa*). Although grouped together, some agents have better activity against certain organisms (eg, ceftazidime against *Pseudomonas aeruginosa*), and poorer activity against others (eg, moxalactam and ceftazidime against *Staph. aureus*).

Resistance to cephalosporins is mediated by β-lactamase, reduction in outer cell wall membrane permeability and alteration of the affinity of these agents for penicillin-binding proteins. In addition, many agents are capable of inducing the production of a chromosomal β-lactamase which may result in resistance to the inducing agent as well as to other β-lactams; this phenomenon has been associated with some clinical treatment failures.[84]

Administration and Adult Dose. See Cephalosporins Comparison Chart.

Dosage Individualization. Most agents are excreted unchanged in urine to some extent, requiring dosage modification in varying degrees of renal dysfunction; notable exceptions are ceftriaxone and cefoperazone. Adjustment of dosage is required in patients with concomitant hepatic and renal dysfunction for all agents (see Cephalosporins Comparison Chart).

Pharmacokinetics. Some of the greatest differences between agents reside in their pharmacokinetic properties. Of note is the improved CSF penetration of certain newer agents over the first-generation agents. Therapeutic CSF concentrations are achieved with cefuroxime, cefotaxime, moxalactam, ceftriaxone and ceftazidime; these agents have proven efficacy in the treatment of meningitis due to susceptible organisms in adults and children.[76,81,83] Adequate CSF concentrations of ceftizoxime and cefoperazone have also been observed, although their use in the treatment of meningitis is less well established.[76,81] See Cephalosporins Comparison Chart.

Adverse Reactions. Most cephalosporins are generally well tolerated, although a few agents have unique adverse reactions. Hypersensitivity reactions may occur in approximately 10% of patients known to be allergic to penicillin; thus, these agents should not be administered to patients with a history of an immediate reaction to penicillin.[91] All agents with a methylthiotetrazole (MTT) moiety in the three position of the cephem nucleus may produce a disulfiram-like reaction in some patients upon ingestion of alcohol-containing beverages.[85] Some of these agents (moxalactam, cefoperazone and cefamandole) are associated with bleeding secondary to hypoprothrombinemia, which is corrected or prevented by vitamin K administration;[88] although controversial, the mechanism of this reaction appears to involve inhibition of enzymatic reactions requiring vitamin K in the activation of prothrombin precursors by methylthiotetrazole.[92] Thus, cautious use (and perhaps even avoidance in view of the availability of other agents with similar antimicrobial activity) of agents with the MTT side chain is recommended in patients with poor oral intake and critical illness. Administration of vitamin K and monitoring of the prothrombin time is indicated with these agents. Particular caution is advised for moxalactam because this agent further impairs hemostasis through an antiplatelet effect. Periodic monitoring of the bleeding time in patients receiving moderate to high doses of this agent is also warranted.[88] Positive direct Coombs' tests occur frequently, but hemolysis is rare. Development of resistance during treatment of infections due to *Enterobacter* sp., *Serratia* sp., and *Pseudomonas aeruginosa* has occurred in patients treated with these agents.[76,81,84,89]

Precautions. Penicillin allergy. Use agents with MTT side chain with caution in patients with underlying bleeding diathesis, poor oral intake or critical illness. Use with caution in renal impairment. See Drug Interactions chapter.

Parameters to Monitor. Prothrombin time (2–3 times/week) with agents having MTT side chain, particularly when using large doses; monitor bleeding time with moxalactam and with high doses of other agents having MTT side chain. Antimicrobial susceptibility tests for development of resistance in patients relapsing during therapy. Monitor renal function tests initially and periodically during high-dose regimens or when used concurrently with nephrotoxic agents.

Cefazolin Sodium Ancef®, Kefzol®, Various

Pharmacology. Cefazolin is a first-generation cephalosporin with activity against most Gram-positive aerobic organisms (eg, *Staphylococcus aureus*) and some Gram-negative bacilli (eg, *E. coli, Klebsiella* sp.).

Administration and Adult Dose. IM or IV 250 mg–1 g q 6–12 hr, to maximum of 6 g/day. IM or IV for surgical prophylaxis 1 g 30–60 min prior to surgery and 500 mg–1 g q 6–8 hr for up to 24 hr.

Dosage Individualization. Dosage should be reduced for patients with impaired renal function, although recommendations vary considerably.[74,75,82] With severe renal failure, may give a loading dose followed by 10–25% of the usual daily dose q 24 hr.[82] The effect of hemodialysis is variable.[74] No adjustment is necessary for patients with liver disease.

Pediatric Dose. IV (newborn and premature infants) 20 mg/kg q 12 hr. IM or IV (over 1 month) 1.25 g/M^2/day or 25–50 mg/kg/day in 3–4 divided doses, to maximum of 100 mg/kg/day.

Dosage Forms. Inj 250, 500 mg, 1, 5, 10 g.

Pharmacokinetics. Fate. 500 mg IM produces a peak concentration of about 30–40 mcg/ml at 30 min; 1 g IV given over 20 min produces a postinfusion concentration of 110–140 mcg/ml.[74,75,86] 75–85% bound to plasma proteins;[79] V_d is about 10 L/1.73 M^2.[79] Widely distributed throughout the body with high free levels in many tissues and cavities; CSF concentrations are undetectable or subtherapeutic.[74,75,82,90] Negligible metabolism, with virtually 100% urinary excretion via filtration and secretion of unchanged drug.[74,79,82,86]

$t_{1/2}$. 1.6–2 hr; 20–70 hr with severe renal impairment.[74,86]

Adverse Reactions. Infrequent except for various allergic reactions occurring in about 5% of patients. With excessive doses, especially in renal

Adults: he usual dosage is 1 or 2 g IV or IM every 12 hours for 5 to 10 days. Determine proper dosage and route of administration by the condition of the patient, severity of the infection and susceptibility of the causative organism.

General Cefotetan Dosage Guidelines		
Type of Infection	Daily Dose	Frequency and Route
Urinary Tract	1 to 4 g	500 mg every 12 hours IV or IM 1 or 2 g every 24 hours IV or IM 1 or 2 g every 12 hours IV or IM
Other Sites	2 to 4 g	1 or 2 g every 12 hours IV or IM
Severe	4 g	2 g every 12 hours IV
Life-threatening	6 g†	3 g every 12 hours IV

† Maximum daily dosage should not exceed 6 g.

ophylaxis: To prevent postoperative infection in clean contaminated or potentially contaminated surgery in adults, give a single 1 or 2 g IV dose 30 to 60 minutes prior to surgery. In patients undergoing cesarean section, give the dose as soon as the umbilical cord is clamped.

nal function impairment: Reduce the dosage schedule using the following guidelines:

Cefotetan Dosage in Renal Impairment		
Ccr (ml/min)	Dose	Frequency
> 30	Usual Recommended Dose††	Every 12 hours
10-30	Usual Recommended Dose††	Every 24 hours
< 10	Usual Recommended Dose††	Every 48 hours

†† Dose determined by the type and severity of infection, and susceptibility of the causative organism

impairment, neurotoxicity may occur manifested as CNS irritation with delirium, seizures and coma which may be fatal.[87] Also, false positive direct Coombs' reactions and very rare coagulopathy[88] have been observed after high doses in uremic patients. Significant nephrotoxicity not reported with cefazolin;[82] generally well tolerated by IM or IV route.[80,82]

Precautions. Use with caution in patients with a history of severe allergic reaction (ie, anaphylaxis, hives, angioneurotic edema) to penicillin;[91] renal impairment.

Parameters to Monitor. Renal function tests initially and repeated periodically if receiving high-dose regimen or nephrotoxic agents concomitantly.

Notes. See Cephalosporins Comparison Chart.

Cefotaxime Sodium   Claforan®

Pharmacology. Cefotaxime is a third-generation cephalosporin with markedly increased activity against Gram-negative organisms resistant to first- and second-generation cephalosporins (eg, *Enterobacter* sp., *Serratia* sp.). Although also somewhat more active against *Pseudomonas aeruginosa*, its activity is inferior to that of ceftazidime. Its desacetyl metabolite also has activity against certain organisms and may have a synergistic effect with the parent compound against some bacteria.[111] Gram-positive activity is somewhat inferior to cefazolin.

Administration and Adult Dose. IM or IV 250 mg-2 g q 4-12 hr, to a maximum of 12 g/day. Usual dosage is 1-2 g q 8-12 hr.

Dosage Individualization. Reduce dose 50% for patients with Cl_{cr} less than 20 ml/min to avoid accumulation of metabolites.[76,78,93]

Pediatric Dose. IV (neonates up to 1 week) 50 mg/kg q 12 hr; (neonates 1-4 weeks) 50 mg/kg q 8 hr; (infants and children up to 50 kg) IM or IV 50-180 mg/kg/day in 4-6 divided doses.

Dosage Forms. Inj 1, 2, 10 g.

Pharmacokinetics. Fate. 1 g IV produces a peak plasma level of 40 mcg/ml. CSF concentrations range from 0.3-44 mcg/ml and are bactericidal for many bacteria. V_d is 18-33 L/1.73 M^2.[79] About 50% of a dose is metabolized to the active metabolite desacetylcefotaxime (DACM). Peak DACM plasma levels are about 10 mcg/ml after a 1 g dose. DACM is excreted both unchanged and as 2 inactive lactone metabolites.[75,76,78,93]

$t_{1/2}$. See Cephalosporins Comparison Chart. Half-life is about two-fold greater in patients with cirrhosis.[93]

Adverse Reactions. Well tolerated, with no coagulopathies reported.[76,81,93] See also Cephalosporins monograph.

Precautions. See Cephalosporins monograph.

Parameters to Monitor. See Cephalosporins monograph.

Notes. See Cephalosporins Comparison Chart.

Cefoxitin Sodium   Mefoxin®

Pharmacology. Cefoxitin is a parenteral cephamycin structurally similar to cephalosporins. Because of its greater stability to certain β-lactamases, it has greater activity against some Gram-negative bacteria than cefazolin (eg,

E. coli) and superior activity against *Bacteroides fragilis* and other anaerobic bacteria. Gram-positive activity is less than that of cefazolin.[89]

Administration and Adult Dose. **IM or IV** 1–2 g q 6–8 hr. **IM or IV for surgical prophylaxis** 1–2 g 30–60 min prior to surgery, then 1–2 g q 6–8 hr for up to 24 hr.

Dosage Individualization. Reduce dose if Cl_{cr} is less than 50 ml/min. For Cl_{cr} less than 10 ml/min, give 1 g q 12–48 hr.

Pediatric Dose. **IV** (under 3 months) not recommended; (over 3 months) 13–27 mg/kg q 4 hr or 20–40 mg/kg q 6 hr.

Dosage Forms. See Cephalosporins Comparison Chart.

Pharmacokinetics. *Fate.* IM 500 mg results in peak plasma concentrations of about 11 mcg/ml in 20 min. V_d is 7.7–8.1 L.[79,94] CSF concentrations are therapeutic only with concomitant probenecid administration.[90] Less than 5% of a dose is recovered as the descarbamylcefoxitin metabolite;[75,86] the remainder is excreted primarily as unchanged cefoxitin in the urine.[94]

$t_{1/2}$. See Cephalosporins Comparison Chart.

Adverse Reactions. Coagulopathy is rare, although a recent study identified cefoxitin as a risk factor in one group of hospitalized patients.[95] See also Cephalosporins monograph.

Precautions. See Cephalosporins monograph.

Parameters to Monitor. See Cephalosporins monograph.

Notes. See Cephalosporins Comparison Chart.

Cefuroxime Sodium   Zinacef®
Cefuroxime Axetil   Ceftin®

Pharmacology. Cefuroxime is a second-generation cephalosporin with greater activity than cefazolin against *H. influenzae*, (including β-lactamase producing strains) and some species of *Enterobacter*, *Proteus* and *Morganella*. Its activity against anaerobes is similar to that of first-generation cephalosporins.[96,97]

Administration and Adult Dose. **IM or IV** 750 mg–1.5 g q 6–8 hr. **IV for surgical prophylaxis** 1.5 g 1 hr prior to or at induction of anesthesia, then **IM or IV** 750 mg q 8 hr for up to 24 hr (for open heart surgery 1.5 g q 12 hr to a total of 6 g). **PO** 125–500 mg q 12 hr.

Dosage Individualization. Reduce dose when Cl_{cr} is less than 20 ml/min. With Cl_{cr} between 10–20 ml/min, give the usual dose twice daily; when less than 10 ml/min, give full dose once daily.[96-98]

Pediatric Dose. **IM or IV** (under 3 months) 10–33 mg/kg q 8 hr or 15–50 mg/kg q 12 hr; (3 months and over) 12–60 mg/kg q 6 hr or 17–80 mg/kg q 8 hr. **PO** 20 mg/kg q 6–8 hr; may be given in applesauce.[99]

Dosage Forms. See Cephalosporins Comparison Chart.

Pharmacokinetics. *Fate.* IM 750 mg results in average peak plasma levels of 27 mcg/ml in 0.5–1 hr.[96] V_d is 11–16 L.[79,96] CSF concentrations are adequate for treatment of meningitis due to certain organisms.[96,97] Over 95% of a dose is excreted unchanged in urine.

$t_{1/2}$. See Cephalosporins Comparison Chart. Half-life 5.4 hr during peritoneal dialysis.[98]

Adverse Reactions.   Coagulopathy not reported. See also Cephalosporins monograph.

Precautions. See Cephalosporins monograph.

Parameters to Monitor. See Cephalosporins monograph.

Notes. See Cephalosporins Comparison Chart.

Cephalosporins Comparison Chart[a]

DRUG	DOSAGE FORMS	ADULT DOSE	PEAK PLASMA LEVELS (MCG/ML) [b]	PERCENT PROTEIN BOUND	HALF-LIFE (HOURS) NORMAL	HALF-LIFE (HOURS) ANURIC	PERCENT EXCRETED UNCHANGED IN URINE[c]	COMMENTS
FIRST GENERATION								
Cefadroxil Duricef®	Cap 500 mg Susp 125, 250, 500 mg/5 ml Tab 1 g.	PO 500 mg– 1 g q 12–24 hr.	12–16	20	1–2	15–20	90	Spectrum similar to cefazolin.
Cefazolin Sodium Ancef® Kefzol® Various	Inj 250, 500 mg, 1, 5, 10 g.	IM or IV 250 mg– 1 g q 6–12 hr.	80–110	75–85	1.5–2.0	20–70	>95	See monograph.
Cephalexin Keflex® Keflet® Various	Cap 250, 500 mg Drp 100 mg/ml Susp 125, 250 mg/5 ml Tab 250, 500 mg, 1 g.	PO 250 mg–1 g q 6 hr.	10–20	5–15	0.5–1.0	20–40	85–95	Oral absorption is almost complete; spectrum similar to cefazolin.
Cephalothin Sodium Keflin® Seffin® Various	Inj 1, 2, 4, 10, 20 g.	IV 500 mg–1 g q 4–6 hr; IM not recommended.	15–30	65–80	0.5–0.85	2–2.9	60–70	Spectrum similar to cefazolin.

Continued

Cephalosporins Comparison Chart[a]

DRUG	DOSAGE FORMS	ADULT DOSE	PEAK PLASMA LEVELS (MCG/ML) [b]	PERCENT PROTEIN BOUND	HALF-LIFE (HOURS) NORMAL	HALF-LIFE (HOURS) ANURIC	PERCENT EXCRETED UNCHANGED IN URINE[c]	COMMENTS
Cephapirin Sodium Cefadyl® Various	Inj 500 mg, 1, 2, 4, 20 g.	IM or IV 500 mg– 1 g q 4–6 hr.	10–20	45–50	0.3–0.7	1.5–2.4	60	Very similar to cephalothin.
Cephradine Anspor® Velosef® Various	Cap 250, 500 mg Susp 125, 250 mg/5 ml Tab 1 g Inj 250, 500 mg, 1, 2, 4 g.	PO 250 mg–1 g q 6 hr; IM or IV 500 mg– 1 g q 4–6 hr.	10–20 (PO) 15–30 (IV)	5–20	0.7–0.9	↑	80–95	Oral form comparable to cephalexin; spectrum similar to cefazolin.
SECOND GENERATION								
Cefaclor Ceclor®	Cap 250, 500 mg Susp 125, 250 mg/5 ml.	PO 250 mg– 1 g q 6–8 hr.	10–15	22–26	0.5–1	2.3–2.8	60–85	Spectrum similar to cefazolin, but includes some ampicillin-resistant *H. influenzae.*
Cefamandole Naftate Mandol®	Inj 500 mg, 1, 2, 10 g.	IM or IV 500 mg–1 g q 4–8 hr.	80–90	67–74	0.7–1.2	11–18	65–85	MTT side chain. Spectrum similar to cefuroxime.
Cefixime Investigational - Lederle	—	PO.	4.9	37	3.1	11.5	16	More active than cefuroxime or Continued

Cephalosporins Comparison Chart[a]

DRUG	DOSAGE FORMS	ADULT DOSE	PEAK PLASMA LEVELS (MCG/ML)[b]	PERCENT PROTEIN BOUND	HALF-LIFE (HOURS) NORMAL	HALF-LIFE (HOURS) ANURIC	PERCENT EXCRETED UNCHANGED IN URINE[c]	COMMENTS
								cefaclor against *H. influenzae*.
Cefmetazole Investigational - Upjohn	Inj.	—	77	<30	1.1–1.4	15	70–92	MTT side chain; spectrum similar to cefoxitin.
Cefonicid Sodium Monocid®	Inj 500 mg, 1, 10 g.	IM or IV 500 mg–2 g/day as a single dose.	220 (IV bolus)	83–98[d]	4	70	98	Relatively poor activity against *Staphylococcus*. Unbound drug levels are low and excreted rapidly due to saturable protein binding.
Ceforanide Precef®	Inj 500 mg, 1, 10 g.	IM or IV 500 mg– 1 g q 12 hr.	92	81	3	19	90	Spectrum similar to cefonicid.
Cefotetan Disodium Cefotan®	Inj 1, 2 g.	IM or IV 500 mg–2 g q 12 hr.	140–180 (IV bolus)	85	3–4	13–35	60–90	MTT side chain; spectrum similar to cefoxitin.
Cefotiam Hydrochloride	Inj.	—	44	40	0.8	↑	47–56	Spectrum similar to cefamandole.

Continued

Cephalosporins Comparison Chart[a]

DRUG	DOSAGE FORMS	ADULT DOSE	PEAK PLASMA LEVELS (MCG/ML) [b]	PERCENT PROTEIN BOUND	HALF-LIFE (HOURS) NORMAL	HALF-LIFE (HOURS) ANURIC	PERCENT EXCRETED UNCHANGED IN URINE[c]	COMMENTS
Investigational - Ciba-Geigy								
Cefoxitin Sodium Mefoxin®	Inj 1, 2, 10 g.	IV 1–2 g q 6–8 hr.	30–50	65–80	0.7–1	20	85–90	See Monograph.
Cefuroxime Sodium Zinacef®	Inj 750 mg, 1.5 g.	IM or IV 750 mg–1.5 g q 6–8 hr.	140 (IV bolus)	33	1.7	18	85–95	See Monograph.
Cefuroxime Axetil Ceftin®	Tab 125, 250, 500 mg.	PO 125–500 mg bid.	3.6 (PO)					
THIRD GENERATION								
Cefoperazone Sodium Cefobid®	Inj 1, 2 g.	IM or IV 8–12 g/day in 2–4 divided doses.	125	85–95	1.6–2.1	2.2	15–30	MTT side chain.
Cefotaxime Sodium Claforan®	Inj 1, 2, 10 g.	IM or IV 1–2 g 6–12 hr.	40	37	0.8–1.2	1.4–3.6	40–55	See Monograph.
Desacetyl-cefotaxime			1–65	—	1.5	↑	15–25	

Continued

Cephalosporins Comparison Chart[a]

DRUG	DOSAGE FORMS	ADULT DOSE	PEAK PLASMA LEVELS (MCG/ML)[b]	PERCENT PROTEIN BOUND	HALF-LIFE (HOURS) NORMAL	HALF-LIFE (HOURS) ANURIC	PERCENT EXCRETED UNCHANGED IN URINE[c]	COMMENTS
Ceftazidime Fortaz® Tazicef® Tazidime®	Inj 500 mg 1, 2, 6 g.	IM or IV 1-3 g q 8-12 hr.	80	17	1.5	25-34	70	Best activity against *Pseudomonas aeruginosa.* See Monograph.
Ceftizoxime Sodium Cefizox®	Inj 1, 2 g.	IM or IV 1-2 g q 8-12 hr.	75-90	31	1.4-1.7	24-36	85-95	Spectrum similar to cefotaxime except slightly more active against anaerobes.
Ceftriaxone Disodium Rocephin®	Inj 250, 500 mg 1, 2, 10 g.	IM or IV 500 mg-2 g/day as a single dose; IM for gonorrhea 250 mg once.	145	83-96[e]	6.5-8.6	12, but variable	45-65	Spectrum similar to cefotaxime. Reduce dose with concurrent renal and hepatic dysfunction.
Moxalactam Disodium Moxam®	Inj 1, 2, 10 g.	IM or IV 1-2 g q 8-12 hr.	60-70	50	2-2.5	20-40	60-80	MTT side chain; best activity against anaerobes.

a. From references 74-82, 94, 96-110.
b. Peak plasma concentrations following administration of a 500 mg oral dose or 1 g IV infusion over 30 minutes, except as noted.
c. Represents excretion of unchanged drug in normals.
d. Range of reported concentrations.
e. Concentration-dependent.

8:12.07 MISCELLANEOUS β-LACTAM ANTIBIOTICS

Aztreonam   Azactam®

Aztreonam is a monobactam with activity against most Gram-negative aerobic bacteria including *Pseudomonas aeruginosa*, but is inactive against Gram-positive bacteria and anaerobes. Peak plasma levels of 164 and 255 mcg/ml occur after 30 min IV infusion of 1 and 2 g, respectively. With inflamed meninges, CSF levels range from 0.8–16 mcg/ml 1–4 hr after a 2 g IV dose, but experience in treating meningitis is limited. The drug has a V_d of about 0.17 L/kg and is 56–60% plasma protein bound; 60–70% is excreted in urine unchanged. Half-life is 1.5–2 hr, increasing to 6 hr in renal failure and 3.2 hr in alcoholic cirrhosis. Adverse effects of aztreonam are minimal. Cross-allergenicity between aztreonam and other β-lactams is low and it has been used safely in penicillin- or cephalosporin-allergic patients. The usual adult dose is IM or IV 500 mg–2 g q 6–12 hr, to a maximum of 8 g/day, depending on severity and site of infection. The maintenance dose should be reduced by one-half with a Cl_{cr} between 10–30 ml/min and by three-fourths with a Cl_{cr} less than 10 ml/min. One-eighth of the initial dose should be given after hemodialysis. Safety and efficacy is not established in children, but a dose of 30 mg/kg q 6–8 hr IV has been used successfully in children with serious Gram-negative infections.[112-117] Available as injection 500 mg, 1 and 2 g.

Imipenem and Cilastatin Sodium   Primaxin®

Pharmacology. Imipenem is a carbapenem with an extremely broad spectrum against many aerobic and anaerobic Gram-positive and Gram-negative bacterial pathogens. The commercial preparation contains an equal amount of cilastatin, a renal dehydropeptidase inhibitor that has no antimicrobial activity, but prevents imipenem's metabolism by proximal tubular kidney cells, thus increasing urinary imipenem concentrations and possibly decreasing nephrotoxicity.[118,119] See Notes.

Administration and Adult Dose. IV 1–4 g/day in 3 or 4 divided doses. Infuse 250–500 mg doses over 15–30 min, 1 g doses over 40–60 min; slow rate if nausea develops.

Dosage Individualization. Reduce doses with renal insufficiency as follows: Cl_{cr} 30–70 ml/min, give three-fourths the usual dosage; Cl_{cr} 20–30 ml/min, give one-half the usual dosage; below 20 ml/min, give one-fourth the usual dosage. Give a supplemental dose following hemodialysis.

Pediatric Dose. (Under 12 yr) safety and efficacy not established, but IV 25 mg/kg (of imipenem) q 6 hr has been successfully used.[119]

Dosage Forms. Inj 250 mg imipenem/250 mg cilastatin, 500 mg imipenem/500 mg cilastatin.

Pharmacokinetics. *Fate.* Peak plasma imipenem concentrations are 22 and 52 mcg/ml after 30-min infusions of 500 mg and 1 g, respectively; levels are below 1 mcg/ml at 6 hr.[118,120,121] CSF levels range from 0.5–11 mcg/ml with inflamed meninges and appear to be adequate to treat meningitis, but experience in treating meningitis is limited.[118,119] Imipenem V_d is 0.26 L/kg; 20% plasma protein bound.[118,119,121] Probenecid increases imipenem plasma levels and prolongs its half-life.[118] About 70% of imipenem is excreted unchanged in urine when given with cilastatin, with the remainder excreted as metabolite; cilastatin is excreted 90% unchanged in urine.[118-120]

$t_{1/2}$. (Imipenem) 1 hr; 3–4 hr in renal failure. (Cilastatin) 1 hr; 17 hr in renal failure.[119,122,123]

Adverse Reactions. Nausea and vomiting, sometimes associated with hypotension or diaphoresis occur, particularly with high doses and rapid infusion. Rashes occur occasionally and cross-allergenicity with penicillins has been documented. Convulsions have occurred, primarily in the elderly, those with underlying CNS disease, with overdosage in patients with renal failure, or with other predisposing factors.[118,119,124]

Precautions. Use with caution in patients with a history of seizures or who are predisposed. Adjust dosage carefully in renal impairment. Imipenem may cause allergic reactions in patients with a history of anaphylaxis to penicillin.[117]

Parameters to Monitor. Obtain renal function tests periodically.

Notes. Used alone, emergence of resistance during treatment of *Pseudomonas aeruginosa* infections occurs frequently. Addition of an aminoglycoside may prevent development of resistance, but produces in vitro synergism only infrequently.[118] Antagonism, probably due to β-lactamase induction by imipenem, routinely occurs when combined with another β-lactam (eg, broad-spectrum penicillin).[118]

Vials may be reconstituted into a suspension using 10 ml of the infusion solution and then further diluted by transferring the suspension into the infusion container; alternatively, the powder in the 120 ml vials can be diluted initially with 100 ml of solution. The initial dilution must be shaken well to ensure suspension/solution. Do not inject the suspension. The resulting solution ranges from colorless to yellow. Reconstituted solutions are stable in dextrose-containing solutions for 4 hr at room temperature and 24 hr under refrigeration, and in normal saline for 10 hr at room temperature and 48 hr under refrigeration.

8:12.08 CHLORAMPHENICOL

General References: 15, 130

Chloramphenicol and Salts

Chloromycetin®,
Various

Pharmacology. A broad-spectrum bacteriostatic antibiotic particularly useful against ampicillin-resistant *Haemophilus influenzae,* salmonella and most anaerobic organisms. Inhibits protein synthesis by binding the 50S ribosomal subunit; may be bactericidal against some bacteria. Resistance occurs due to impermeability of the cell wall or bacterial elaboration of an R-factor mediated acetyltransferase.

Administration and Adult Dose. PO or IV 50–100 mg/kg/day depending on severity, location and organism; divide into 4 doses. **IM not recommended.**

Dosage Individualization. Reduce dose with impaired liver function as guided by plasma levels; no alteration necessary in impaired renal function.[15,125]

Pediatric Dose. PO or IV (newborn to 2 weeks) 25 mg/kg/day in 1–4 divided doses; (over 2 weeks) 50 mg/kg/day in 4 divided doses; may double dose for a short time in severe infections. These regimens produce unpredictable levels and plasma level monitoring is recommended.[125] **IM not recommended.**

Dosage Forms. Cap (as base) 50, 100, 250 mg; Susp (as palmitate) 30 mg/ml; Inj (as sodium succinate) 250 mg/ml, 1 g (100 mg/ml when reconstituted); **Ophth Oint** 10 mg/g; **Ophth Soln** 5 mg/ml; **Otic Soln** 5 mg/ml; **Top Crm** 10 mg/g (expressed as chloramphenicol base).

Patient Instructions. This drug should be taken with a full glass of water on an empty stomach (1 hr before or 2 hr after meals) for best absorption. Sore throat, fever or oral lesions may be an early sign of a severe, but rare, blood disorder and should be reported immediately.

Pharmacokinetics. *Plasma Levels.* Levels over 25 mcg/ml are associated with bone marrow depression; over 50–100 mcg/ml with gray syndrome. See Adverse Reactions.

Fate. Well absorbed orally (90–100%), with peak plasma levels averaging 12 mcg/ml after administration of 1 g to normal adults. Suspension (palmitate ester) must be hydrolyzed before absorption; in newborns, infants and children, hydrolysis may be inadequate and absorption delayed and unreliable.[126] 1 g IV produces levels of 5–12 mcg/ml 1 hr after administration to normal adults. In infants and young children, hydrolysis of succinate to the active form may be slow and incomplete.[125] IM administration may produce plasma levels of active drug which are 50% lower than the equivalent oral dose and is therefore not recommended for treating severe infections. The drug attains therapeutic levels in most body cavities, the eye and CSF; it is 50% plasma protein bound; V_d is about 1 L/kg.[127] 90% of an oral dose is eliminated by glucuronidation in the liver followed by excretion in the urine; the remainder is excreted in the urine unchanged.[127] The rate of glucuronidation and renal elimination is greatly reduced in neonates.[126] 6.5–80% of succinate may be excreted unhydrolyzed.[125] Urine concentrations may be inadequate to treat UTI, especially in patients with moderately to severely impaired renal function.[128] A small amount (2–4%) of a dose appears in the bile and feces, mostly as the glucuronide.

$t_{1/2}$. 1.5–3 hr in healthy adults; 3.2–4.3 hr in anuria.[125] Extremely prolonged and variable in neonates, infants and young children.[125] Unpredictable in patients with impaired liver function. Some normal patients and patients with impaired renal function exhibit impaired free drug elimination.[125,127,129]

Adverse Reactions. Plasma levels greater than 25 mcg/ml frequently produce reversible bone marrow depression[15,125] with reticulocytopenia, decreased hemoglobin, increased serum iron and iron-binding globulin saturation, thrombocytopenia and mild leukopenia. The drug inhibits iron uptake by bone marrow and anemic patients do not respond to iron or vitamin B_{12} therapy while receiving chloramphenicol.[131] This anemia most often follows parenteral therapy, large doses, long duration of therapy or impaired drug elimination. Complete recovery usually occurs within 1–2 weeks after drug discontinuation.[132] Aplastic anemia is rare (1/40,000–1/100,000), but generally fatal. It is not dose-related and can occur long after a short course of oral or parenteral therapy.[15,130] Fatal cardiovascular-respiratory collapse (gray syndrome) may develop in neonates given excessive doses. This syndrome is associated with plasma levels above 50–100 mcg/ml.[126] A similar syndrome has been reported in children and adults given large overdoses.[15,125]

Contraindications. Trivial infections; uses other than those for which it is indicated (eg, colds, influenza, infections of the throat); prophylactic use.

Precautions. Pregnancy; lactation. Use with caution in patients with liver disease (especially cirrhosis, ascites and jaundice), pre-existing hematologic disorders or patients receiving other bone marrow depressants. May cause hemolytic episodes in patients with G-6-PD deficiency; observe dosing recommendations closely in neonates and infants.

Parameters to Monitor. CBC, with platelet and reticulocyte counts before and frequently during therapy; serum iron and iron-binding globulin saturation may also be useful. Liver and renal function tests before and occasionally during therapy.

8:12.12 ERYTHROMYCINS

General References: 15, 133

Erythromycin and Salts

Various

Pharmacology. A bacteriostatic macrolide antibiotic with a spectrum similar to penicillin G; also active against *Mycoplasma pneumoniae* and *Legionella pneumophila*.[134] Acts by binding to the 50S ribosomal subunit, inhibiting protein synthesis. Gram-positive organisms develop resistance via R-factor mediated alteration of the binding site. Gram-negative organisms are resistant due to cell wall impermeability.

Administration and Adult Dose. See Erythromycins Comparison Chart.

Dosage Individualization. Dosage adjustment is probably unnecessary in renal impairment.[135]

Pediatric Dose. See Erythromycins Comparison Chart.

Dosage Forms. See Erythromycins Comparison Chart.

Patient Instructions. This drug should be taken with a full glass of water on an empty stomach (1 hr before or 2 hr after meals) for optimum absorption; refrigerate suspension and suppositories.

Pharmacokinetics. *Fate.* Oral absorption varies widely with the salt and dosage form (see Erythromycins Comparison Chart), with peak plasma concentrations occurring anywhere from 30 min (suspension) to 4 hr (coated tablet) after administration. However, enteric-coated erythromycin base tablets, stearate tablets and estolate capsules produce equivalent erythromycin plasma levels when administered to fasting subjects. Food or restricted water intake (ie, 20 ml or less) with a dose dramatically lowers the absorption of the stearate form only. V_d is 0.5-0.6 L/kg; 75-90% plasma protein bound.[136] Widely distributed into most tissues, cavities and body fluids except the brain and CSF (even with meningeal inflammation). Partially metabolized in the liver; excreted primarily as unchanged erythromycin with high concentrations in the bile and feces. Only 12-15% of IV dose is excreted unchanged in urine.[136]

$t_{1/2}$. About 1-1.5 hr; 5-6 hr in anuric patients, based on minimal data.[15,136]

Adverse Reactions. Occasional GI distress, IM form is very painful, despite local anesthetic (butamben) in product, and may produce sterile abscesses. IV administration frequently produces pain, venous irritation and phlebitis. Rare, but potentially serious, reversible intrahepatic cholestatic jaundice is seen with the estolate and ethylsuccinate forms, usually in adults after 10-14 days of therapy, although it may occur after the first dose if there is a history of previous use. Prodrome includes malaise, nausea, vomiting, fever and abdominal pain (which may be severe and misdiagnosed as acute surgical abdomen). Symptoms resolve in 1-2 weeks, while serum enzymes return to normal over several months.[15,137] Transient tinnitus and deafness occur rarely.[137]

Contraindications. IM form contraindicated in patients with hypersensitivity to local anesthetics of the para-aminobenzoic acid type (eg, procaine); hepatic dysfunction (estolate and ethylsuccinate forms).

Precautions. Pregnancy. Use with caution in patients with liver disease (impaired excretion).

Parameters to Monitor. Liver function tests in patients who experience prodromal symptoms (see Adverse Reactions) while receiving estolate or ethylsuccinate form; check daily for vein irritation and phlebitis in patients receiving IV forms.

Notes. Avoid injectable forms if at all possible. Erythromycin is more active in an alkaline environment.[15]

Roxithromycin (Investigational - Hoechst)

Roxithromycin is a macrolide analogue which is similar to erythromycin in its in vitro spectrum, but is slightly less potent. The pharmacokinetic disposition of roxithromycin appears to be more favorable in that the elimination half-life is approximately 4 hr. Clinical experience to date is limited, but would appear to suggest that the drug is effective and well tolerated in the treatment of infections normally managed with erythromycin. Dosage used investigationally is 150 mg twice daily.[138]

Erythromycins Comparison Chart

DRUG	DOSAGE FORMS	ADULT DOSE	PEDIATRIC DOSE[a]	COMMENTS[b]
Erythromycin Base E-Mycin® Ery-Tab® Ilotycin® Various	EC Tab 250, 333, 500 mg Tab (buffered) 250, 500 mg Supp 125 mg.	PO 1 g/day in 2–4 doses, to maximum of 4 g/day.	PO 30–50 mg/kg/day in 4 divided doses; may double if severe infection.	Food interferes with absorption except for E-Mycin® and Ery-Tab®; highly susceptible to gastric acid hydrolysis; rectal suppository is very irritating—avoid use.
Erythromycin Estolate Ilosone®	Cap 125, 250 mg Drp 100 mg/ml Susp 125, 250 mg/5 ml (reconstituted) Chew Tab 125, 250 mg Tab 500 mg.	PO 250–500 mg q 6 hr, to maximum of 4 g/day.	PO 30–50 mg/kg/day in 4 divided doses.	PO well absorbed; unaffected by food and highly resistant to gastric acid hydrolysis; absorbed as propionate ester which predominates in plasma (8:1) and may be less active;[139] rare intrahepatic cholestatic jaundice.
Erythromycin Ethylsuccinate E.E.S.® Pediamycin®	Drp 40 mg/ml Susp 200, 400 mg/5 ml Chew Tab 200 mg Tab (coated) 400 mg Inj (IM only) 50 mg/ml.[c]	PO 400 mg q 6 hr, to maximum of 4 g/day; Deep IM 100 mg q 4–8 hr or 5–8 mg/kg/day in divided doses.	PO 30–50 mg/kg/day in 4 divided doses; may double in severe infection; IM (over 13.6 kg) 50 mg q 4–6 hr or 12 mg/kg/day in divided doses.	Absorbed better than base; intermediate susceptibility to gastric acid hydrolysis. Absorbed as ester which predominates in plasma (3:1) and may be less active. IM very painful—avoid use. Rare intrahepatic cholestatic jaundice.

Continued

Erythromycins Comparison Chart

DRUG	DOSAGE FORMS	ADULT DOSE	PEDIATRIC DOSE[a]	COMMENTS[b]
Erythromycin Gluceptate Ilotycin®	Inj (IV only) 250, 500 mg, 1 g.	IV 15–20 mg/kg/day in 4 divided doses, to maximum of 4 g/day.	IV same as adult dose in 2–4 divided doses; may double in severe infection.	Painful; phlebitis frequent; avoid use if possible. Infuse over at least 30 min.
Erythromycin Lactobionate Erythrocin® Various	Inj (IV only) 500 mg, 1 g.			Absorption about equal to ethylsuccinate, although food interferes significantly with absorption. Hydrolyzed to free base before absorption.
Erythromycin Stearate Erythrocin® Various	Tab (film coated) 125, 250, 500 mg.	PO 1 g/day in 2 or 4 doses, to maximum of 4 g/day.	PO 30–50 mg/kg/day in 4 divided doses; may double in severe infection.	

a. In newborns, limited data are available for erythromycin estolate only, suggesting an oral dose of 40 mg/kg/day in 2–4 divided doses.[139]
b. Despite differences in oral absorption, no clinical studies have shown any salt to be clearly superior in any particular therapeutic use.
c. Contains 2% butamben (butyl aminobenzoate) as a local anesthetic.

8:12.16 PENICILLINS

General References: 15, 141–143

Amdinocillin
Coactin®
Amdinocillin Pivoxil
Coactabs®

Amdinocillin (formerly mecillinam) is an amdinopenicillin that is unique in its affinity for penicillin-binding protein 2 of Gram-negative bacteria. It has limited antibacterial activity, but when combined with other β-lactam antibiotics in vitro, a synergistic effect occurs. The spectrum of side effects is similar to other penicillins. Peak plasma concentrations following a 10 mg/kg IV dose are 34–80 mcg/ml, which decline with a half-life of approximately 50 min. Adult dose with another β-lactam is IV 10 mg/kg q 6 hr.[140] The dose for uncomplicated UTI is 200 mg PO q 8 hr for 3 days; for complicated UTI, 400 mg PO q 8 hr for 10 days. Available as 500 mg and 1 g injection and 200 mg tablets.

Amoxicillin
Amoxil®, Larotid®, Polymox®

Amoxicillin differs from ampicillin in the presence of a hydroxyl group on the amino side chain. It has activity essentially identical to ampicillin. However, it is completely absorbed, with about 85% bioavailability due to a small first-pass effect. Plasma levels are greater than those seen after equivalent doses of ampicillin; post-absorptive pharmacokinetics are identical to ampicillin. Adverse effects are similar to ampicillin, although diarrhea is much less frequent with amoxicillin. Oral dosage for adults is 250–500 mg q 8 hr, to maximum of 6 g/day (1 g q 4 hr); for children 20–40 mg/kg/day orally in 3 equally divided doses q 8 hr.[143] See Ampicillin Derivatives Comparison Chart.

Amoxicillin and Potassium Clavulanate   Augmentin®

Clavulanic acid is a potent inhibitor of plasmid-mediated β-lactamases, including those produced by H. influenzae, S. aureus, N. gonorrhoeae, and certain Gram-negative bacilli (eg, E. coli). Thus, when combined with certain other β-lactam antibiotics, the combination is very active against many bacteria resistant to the β-lactam alone. Clavulanic acid has weak antibacterial activity alone. Peak plasma clavulanate level is 2.6 mcg/ml 40–60 min following an oral dose of amoxicillin 250 mg/clavulanate 125 mg. Amoxicillin pharmacokinetics are not affected by clavulanic acid. Clavulanic acid half-life is approximately 60 min. Adverse effects of this preparation include those of amoxicillin; however, diarrhea is more frequent with the combination and is dependent on the dose of clavulanate. Nausea may occur less frequently when this preparation is administered with food.[155,156] See Ampicillin Derivatives Comparison Chart.

Ampicillin
Various

Pharmacology. A semisynthetic penicillin having greater activity than penicillin G against Gram-negative organisms; generally less active against Gram-positive organisms, except enterococci. Mechanism of action similar

Ampicillin Derivatives Comparison Chart

DRUG	DOSAGE FORMS	ADULT DOSE	PEAK PLASMA LEVELS^a (MCG/ML)	PERCENT BIOAVAILABILITY^b	PERCENT GI SIDE EFFECTS^c	COMMENTS
Ampicillin Various **Ampicillin Sodium** Various	Cap 250, 500 mg; Drp 100 mg/ml (reconstituted) Susp 125, 250, 500 mg/5 ml (reconstituted) Inj 125, 250, 500 mg, 1, 2, 10 g.	PO 250-500 mg q 6 hr; IM or IV 0.25-2 g q 6 hr, to maximum of 8-14 g/day.	2-6	30-70	10-20	Recent bioavailability studies have tended to support the higher end of the range.
Ampicillin and Sulbactam Unasyn®	Inj ampicillin 1 g plus sulbactam 500 mg/vial, ampicillin 2 g plus sulbactam 1 g/vial.	IM or IV 1.5-3 g of the combination q 6-8 hr.	58 (ampicillin) 30 (sulbactam)	—	2 (IV)	Active against ampicillin-resistant bacteria such as S. aureus, B. fragilis and β-lactamase-producing Enterobacteriaceae.
Bacampicillin Hydrochloride Spectrobid®	Tab 400 mg (278 mg ampicillin) Susp 125 mg/5 ml (reconstituted).	PO 400-800 mg q 12 hr; PO for gonorrhea 1.6 g plus probenecid 1...	10-15	80-90	3-6	Essentially equivalent to amoxicillin in effica...

to penicillin G. Inactivated by staphylococcal β-lactamase, as well as β-lactamase-producing *H. influenzae.*

Administration and Adult Dose. **PO for mild to moderate infections** 250-500 mg q 6 hr. **IM or IV for mild to moderate infections** 250-500 mg q 6 hr. **IM or IV for severe infections** (eg, meningitis) 150-200 mg/kg/day to maximum of 8-14 g in 6-8 divided doses. **PO for uncomplicated gonorrhea** 3.5 g taken simultaneously with 1 g probenecid.

Dosage Individualization. Except when using large doses for severe infections, dosage adjustment is necessary only with Cl_{cr} less than 10-15 ml/min, whereupon the dosing interval may be doubled.[135,144] No adjustment necessary for liver disease.[145]

Pediatric Dose. **PO** (under 20 kg) 50-100 mg/kg/day in divided doses; **PO** (over 20 kg) or **IV** (over 40 kg) generally same as adult dose, to maximum of 400 mg/kg/day.

Dosage Forms. **Cap** 250, 500 mg; **Drp** 100 mg/ml (reconstituted): **Susp** 125, 250, 500 mg/5 ml (reconstituted); **Inj** 125, 250, 500 mg, 1, 2, 10 g. Strengths are expressed as ampicillin equivalent.

Patient Instructions. This drug should be taken with a full glass of water on an empty stomach (1 hr before or 2 hr after meals) for best absorption. Refrigerate suspension after reconstitution and discard after 14 days.

Pharmacokinetics. *Fate.* Oral forms are 20-70% (average 50) absorbed in the fasting state; food may significantly delay oral absorption. A 500 mg dose produces a peak of about 2-6 mcg/ml 1-2 hr after oral administration to normal adults.[146-148] 500 mg IM produces a peak of 8 mcg/ml at 1 hr.[144] V_d is about 0.3 L/kg in healthy adults and 0.85 L/kg in cirrhotic adults;[145] 15-25% plasma protein bound.[142] The drug attains therapeutic levels in joints, serosal cavities, and very high levels in the biliary tree (without obstruction), kidney tissue and urine (unless severe renal impairment); therapeutic CSF levels only in the presence of meningitis.[141] Approximately 90% of parenteral dose is excreted unchanged in the urine within 24 hr.[141,144]

$t_{1/2}$. About 1.1-1.3 hr;[141] 2 hr in neonates; 8-20 hr in anuric patients;[141,144] may increase to 1.9 hr in chronic liver disease.[145]

Adverse Reactions. Skin rashes are frequent (7-10%); many of these are erythematous, maculopapular rashes which are 2-3 times more frequent in patients with hyperuricemia taking allopurinol and extremely frequent (50-100%) in patients with mononucleosis or certain lymphomas; many of these rashes are suspected to be nonallergic in nature.[149] Nausea and vomiting occasionally occur after oral administration; diarrhea is frequent. Very rarely associated with interstitial nephritis.[150] Very large doses can produce classic penicillin encephalopathy.[151] See also Penicillin G Salts.

Contraindications. See Penicillin G Salts.

Precautions. See Penicillin G Salts.

Parameters to Monitor. Initial and periodic renal function tests with prolonged use or high doses.

Notes. Since IV preparation is very unstable in D5W, use within 1 hr of admixture; stable for 24 hr in sterile water or normal saline. Oral suspension stable for 7 days at room temperature and 14 days under refrigeration. See Ampicillin Derivatives Comparison Chart.

Ampicillin Sodium and Sulbactam Sodium   Unasyn®

Sulbactam is a β-lactamase inhibitor similar to clavulanic acid. Like clavulanate, it has weak antibacterial activity. Following a 15 min IV infusion of ampicillin 2 g/sulbactam 1 g, peak plasma concentrations of ampicillin and sulbactam exceed 94 and 41 mcg/ml, respectively. Sulbactam half-life is about 1 hr; ampicillin pharmacokinetics are unaltered with concomitant sulbactam administration. Adverse reactions include diarrhea, particularly when administered orally.[152-154] See Ampicillin Derivatives Comparison Chart.

DRUG	DOSAGE FORMS	ADULT DOSE	PEAK PLASMA LEVELS[a] (MCG/ML)	PERCENT BIOAVAILABILITY[b]	PERCENT GI SIDE EFFECTS[c]	COMMENTS
Amoxicillin Amoxil® Larotid® Polymox® Various	Cap 250, 500 mg, Chew Tab 125, 250 mg Drp 50 mg/ml (reconstituted) Susp 125, 250 mg/5 ml (reconstituted).	PO 250-500 mg q 8 hr, to maximum of 6 g/day.	6-8	80-90	4-5	In vitro activity essentially equivalent to ampicillin; small volumes of water lower bioavailability, while food has little effect.
Amoxicillin and Clavulanate Augmentin®	Chew Tab amoxicillin 125 mg plus clavulanate 31.25 mg, amoxicillin 250 mg plus clavulanate 62.5 mg Susp amoxicillin 125 mg plus clavulanate 31.25 mg/5 ml, amoxicillin 250 mg plus clavulanate 62.5 mg/5 ml Tab amoxicillin 250, 500 mg plus clavulanate 125 mg.	PO "250"-"500" tab q 8 hr.	4-4.5 (amoxicillin) 2.5-3.5 (clavulanate)	80-90	10	Do not substitute two "250" mg tablets for "500" mg dose.

Continued

Ampicillin Derivatives Comparison Chart

DRUG	DOSAGE FORMS	ADULT DOSE	PEAK PLASMA LEVELS[a] (MCG/ML)	PERCENT BIOAVAILABILITY[b]	PERCENT GI SIDE EFFECTS[c]	COMMENTS
Cyclacillin Cyclapen®	Susp 125, 250 mg/5 ml (reconstituted) Tab 250, 500 mg.	PO 250-500 mg q 6 hr.	10-15	50-70	5-10	Very rapidly eliminated ($t_{1/2}$ = 0.5-0.6 hr); inferior in vitro activity.

a. Peak plasma concentrations following administration of a 500 mg (ampicillin equivalent) oral dose or IV dose. For amoxicillin/clavulanate, 250 mg/125 mg oral dose; for ampicillin/sulbactam, 1 g/500 mg IV dose.

b. Maximum theoretical bioavailability is about 90% (ie, about 10% is removed by the liver during the first pass).[147]

c. Diarrhea is the most frequent GI side effect with ampicillin; upper GI side effects (eg, nausea, vomiting, dyspepsia) are less common and equally frequent with ampicillin, amoxicillin and bacampicillin. [142,153,154]

Carbenicillin Disodium
Carbenicillin Indanyl Sodium

Geopen®, Pyopen®

Geocillin®

Carbenicillin is a broad-spectrum carboxypenicillin with activity similar to that of ampicillin against the Enterobacteriaceae, plus increased activity against *Pseudomonas aeruginosa* and some strains of *Serratia* and *Proteus*. However, it is less active than ticarcillin, azlocillin, mezlocillin and piperacillin against these bacteria. Its pharmacokinetic properties following parenteral administration are similar to those of ticarcillin. Peak plasma concentrations following a 382 mg oral dose of the indanyl ester are approximately 6 mcg/ml; urinary concentrations are much higher (greater than 100 mcg/ml). Use of the oral preparation is limited to treatment of infections of the urinary tract. Because of its lower activity, high sodium content and large antiplatelet effect, the parenteral preparation has been largely replaced by newer agents.[157] See Acylampicillins Comparison Chart.

Ticarcillin Disodium

Ticar®

Pharmacology. A semisynthetic penicillin with activity similar to carbenicillin, but 2–4 times as active against *Pseudomonas aeruginosa*, while slightly less active against Gram-positive organisms.

Administration and Adult Dose. **IV for serious systemic infections** 200–300 mg/kg/day (about 18–24 g/day) in 4–6 divided doses; **IV for complicated UTI** 150–200 mg/kg/day in 4–6 divided doses; **IM or IV for uncomplicated UTI** 50–100 mg/kg/day in divided doses. **IM** maximum dose not more than 2 g per injection.

Dosage Individualization. Carefully adjust dose in renal impairment. In anuria give no more than 2 g q 12 hr after a 3 g loading dose with 3 g after each dialysis. When liver function is also impaired, give only 2 g q 24 hr.

Pediatric Dose. **IV for serious systemic infection** (neonates under 2 kg) 75 mg/kg q 12 hr for the first week and 75 mg/kg q 8 hr thereafter; (neonates over 2 kg) 75 mg/kg q 8 hr for the first week and 100 mg/kg q 8 hr thereafter.

Dosage Forms. See Acylampicillins Comparison Chart.

Pharmacokinetics. *Fate.* Negligible oral absorption. IM 1 g produces a peak plasma level of 22–33 mcg/ml at 0.5–2 hr after administration.[158] IV 2 g infused over 30 min produces a plasma level of about 175 mcg/ml at the end of the infusion.[158] V_d is about 0.2–0.25 L/kg, slightly larger than carbenicillin; about 55–65% bound to plasma proteins.[158] Widely distributed similar to carbenicillin with CSF levels about 6% of simultaneous plasma levels with normal meninges; 39% in patients with meningitis. A total of 90–95% of a dose is recovered in the urine within 24 hr, 10–14% as penicilloic acid and the remainder as unchanged drug.[158]

$t_{1/2}$. 72–77 min in normal adults; 15–16 hr in patients with severely impaired renal function; about 30 hr in patients with simultaneous hepatic and renal failure.[158,159] In neonates (under 2 kg and less than 7 days of age) 3.5–5.6 hr; infants (1–8 weeks) 1.3–2 hr; children (5–13 yr) 0.9 hr.[158]

Adverse Reactions. Ticarcillin and carbenicillin cause a dose-related inhibition of platelet aggregation; bleeding episodes in patients receiving high doses for prolonged periods have been reported.[88] High sodium content may result in fluid retention in some patients. Ticarcillin and carbenicillin may also cause hypokalemia. See Acylampicillins Comparison Chart.

Contraindications. See Penicillin G.

Precautions. See Penicillin G Salts.

Parameters to Monitor.   Serum electrolytes (eg, potassium) 2–3 times/week. Bleeding times in critically ill patients periodically.

Notes.   Efficacy of ticarcillin in most infections is equivalent to carbenicillin. Used almost exclusively in combination with an aminoglycoside for systemic infections. Sodium content is 5.2–6.5 mEq/g. See Acylampicillins Comparison Chart. The combination of ticarcillin and clavulanic acid (Timentin®) has increased activity against anaerobes and *S. aureus*, but activity against *Pseudomonas aeruginosa* is not improved over ticarcillin alone.

Acylampicillins Comparison Chart[a]

DRUG	DOSAGE FORMS	ADULT DOSE	PEAK PLASMA LEVELS (MCG/ML)[b]	SODIUM CONTENT (MEQ/GRAM)	HALF-LIFE (HOURS) NORMAL	HALF-LIFE (HOURS) ANURIC	PERCENT EXCRETED UNCHANGED IN URINE	COMMENTS
Azlocillin Azlin®	Inj 2, 3, 4 g.	IV or IM 3–4 g q 4–6 hr.	214	2.2	0.9–1.5	6.2	60–75	Marked dose-dependent pharmacokinetics.
Carbenicillin Various	Inj 1, 2, 5 g.	IV or IM 3–5 g q 4–6 hr.	175	4.7	1–1.4	10–15	90–100	Potent antiplatelet effect.
Mezlocillin Mezlin®	Inj 1, 2, 3, 4 g.	IV or IM 3–4 g q 4–6 hr.	263	1.8	0.6–1	2.6	33–55	Moderate dose-dependent pharmacokinetics. Lowest antiplatelet effect of group.
Piperacillin Pipracil®	Inj 2, 3, 4, 40 g.	IV or IM 3–4 g q 4–6 hr.	244	1.8	0.6–1	3.6	50–90	Moderate dose-dependency.
Ticarcillin Ticar®	Inj 1, 3, 6, 20 g.	IV or IM 1–4 g q 4–6 hr.	324	5.2	1–1.2	5	80–90	See monograph.
Ticarcillin and Clavulanate Timentin®	Inj 3.1 g (3 g Ticarcillin plus 100 mg Clavulanate).	IV 3.1 g q 4–8 hr.	8 (clavulanate)	4.7	1	2	50	See Ticarcillin Notes.

a. From references 159–162.
b. Represents peak plasma level after a 4 g dose infused over 30 min, except for ticarcillin for which a 3 g dose is shown.

Cloxacillin Sodium

Cloxapen®, Tegopen®, Various

Pharmacology. A narrow-spectrum semisynthetic penicillin resistant to staphylococcal penicillinase. Otherwise, Gram-positive activity is less than other penicillins and Gram-negative activity is negligible.

Administration and Adult Dose. **PO** 250–500 mg q 6 hr; 2–4 times higher doses may be used for severe infections (but a parenteral anti-staphylococcal agent is preferred in such cases).

Dosage Individualization. Dosage is unaltered in patients with renal impairment.[135]

Pediatric Dose. (Infants) no data. **PO** (under 20 kg) 50–100 mg/kg/day in 4 divided doses; 2–4 times higher doses may be used in severe infections. **PO** (over 20 kg) same as adult dose.

Dosage Forms. **Cap** 250, 500 mg; **Soln** 125 mg/5 ml (reconstituted).

Patient Instructions. Oral forms should be taken with a full glass of water on an empty stomach (1 hr before or 2 hr after meals) for best absorption; refrigerate solution.

Pharmacokinetics. *Fate.* 50% absorbed orally, with peak of 7.2 mcg/ml at 1 hr after administration of a 500 mg dose.[163] V_d is about 0.14 L/kg.[164] Significant metabolism; 75% of absorbed drug is excreted unchanged in the urine.[141,157]

$t_{1/2}$. 30 min;[164] 50 min with severe renal impairment.[135]

Adverse Reactions. See Penicillin G Salts.

Contraindications. See Penicillin G Salts.

Precautions. See Penicillin G Salts.

Notes. For treatment of penicillin G-resistant staphylococcal infections only; see Antistaphylococcal Penicillins Comparison Chart.

Nafcillin Sodium

Nafcil®, Nallpen®, Unipen®

Pharmacology. Nafcillin is a semisynthetic derivative of penicillin that is resistant to staphylococcal β-lactamase. Its antibacterial activity is similar to that of methicillin and oxacillin.

Administration and Adult Dose. **IM** 500 mg–1 g q 4–6 hr; limit to 500 mg/dose, if possible. **IV** 500 mg–2 g q 4–6 hr. **PO** 250 mg–1 g q 4–6 hr.

Pediatric Dose. **IV** 50–150 mg/kg/day in 4–6 divided doses. **PO** 50–100 mg/kg/day in 4 divided doses.

Dosage Forms. See Antistaphylococcal Penicillins Comparison Chart.

Pharmacokinetics. *Fate.* 1 g IM results in a peak level of 8 mcg/ml in 1 hr. Oral absorption is variable and erratic. Approximately 90% plasma protein bound; V_d is low. CSF levels are adequate for treatment of meningitis due to most strains of susceptible *S. aureus* in the presence of meningeal inflammation.[165] Primary route of excretion is the biliary tract.[141]

$t_{1/2}$. 0.5–1 hr;[142,166] 1.2 hr in renal impairment.[135]

Adverse Reactions. Neutropenia reported in up to 40% of patients receiving prolonged, high-dose therapy.[167,168] Extravasation may cause deep tissue necrosis, occasionally necessitating multiple surgical procedures involving skin grafting; tissue injury may be avoided by infiltrating hyaluronidase around the site of extravasation.[169] Interstitial nephritis, which frequently occurs with methicillin, is relatively rare with nafcillin.[170] See also Penicillin G Salts.

Contraindications. See Penicillin G Salts.

Precautions. Extravasation of IV infusions should be avoided. See also Penicillin G Salts.

Parameters to Monitor. Periodic WBC count with prolonged and/or high dose therapy.

Antistaphylococcal Penicillins Comparison Chart

DRUG	DOSAGE FORMS	ADULT DOSE	PEAK PLASMA LEVELS (MCG/ML)[a]	PERCENT BIO-AVAILABILITY[b]	PERCENT PROTEIN BINDING	HALF-LIFE (HOURS) NORMAL	HALF-LIFE (HOURS) ANURIC[c]	PERCENT EXCRETED UNCHANGED IN URINE[d]
Cloxacillin Sodium Tegopen® Various	Cap 250, 500 mg Soln 125 mg/5 ml (reconstituted).	PO 250 mg–1 g q 6 hr; may double in severe infection.	7 (PO)	50	94	0.5	0.8	75
Dicloxacillin Sodium Dynapen® Various	Cap 125, 250, 500 mg Susp 62.5 mg/5 ml (reconstituted).	PO 250 mg–1 g q 6 hr; may double in severe infection.	12.4 (PO)	74	96	0.7–0.8	1–2	70
Methicillin[e] **Sodium** Staphcillin® Various	Inj 1, 4, 6 g.	IM or IV 500 mg–2 g q 4–6 hr; may give double or more IV dose in severe infection.	60 (IV)	—	30–50	0.4–0.5	4	70–75
Nafcillin Sodium Unipen®	Cap 250 mg Soln 250 mg/5 ml (reconstituted) Tab 500 mg Inj 500 mg, 1, 2, 4 g.	PO 250 mg–1 g q 4–6 hr; IM 500 mg q 4–6 hr; IV 500 mg–2 g q 4 hr.	3.4 (PO) 20–40 (IV)	50	90	0.5–1	1.2	30–40[f]

Continued

Antistaphylococcal Penicillins Comparison Chart

DRUG	DOSAGE FORMS	ADULT DOSE	PEAK PLASMA LEVELS (MCG/ML)[a]	PERCENT BIO-AVAILABILITY[b]	PERCENT PROTEIN BINDING	HALF-LIFE(HOURS)		PERCENT EXCRETED UNCHANGED IN URINE[d]
						NORMAL	ANURIC[c]	
Oxacillin Sodium[g] Bactocill® Prostaphlin®	Cap 250, 500 mg Soln 250 mg/5 ml (reconstituted) Inj 250, 500 mg, 1, 2, 4 g.	PO 500 mg–1 g q 4–6 hr; IM or IV 250 mg– 2 g q 4–6 hr.	2.5 (PO) 40 (IV)	33	90	0.4–0.7	0.5–1	55[f]

a. Peak plasma concentrations following administration of a 500 mg oral dose or a 1 g IV infusion over 5 minutes.
b. Some studies indicate much lower values for oral absorption of dicloxacillin and nafcillin. Values shown are the best estimates in the opinion of author.
c. Concomitant renal and hepatic dysfunction can greatly increase half-life with these agents.
d. Represents excretion of unchanged drug in urine after parenteral administration or as percent of absorbed oral dose.
e. Methicillin is associated with a dose-related, apparently allergic, interstitial nephritis which is much more common than with other agents in this chart.
f. Significant biliary excretion with concentrations in bile many times plasma concentrations.
g. Adverse reactions include rare interstitial nephritis and cholestatic hepatitis.[171]

Penicillin G Benzathine   Bicillin® L-A, Permapen®

Pharmacology. A very insoluble suspension of benzathine and penicillin G producing low, but prolonged, plasma penicillin levels which limit its use to infections caused by highly susceptible organisms. See Penicillin G Salts.

Administration and Adult Dose. IM only for group A streptococcal upper respiratory infection 1.2 million units as a single injection. **IM for prophylaxis of post-streptococcal rheumatic fever or glomerulonephritis** 1.2 million units once a month or 600,000 units twice a month. **IM for early syphilis (less than a year in duration)** 2.4 million units as a single injection. **IM for syphilis of more than a year in duration** 2.4 million units weekly for 3 successive weeks (7.2 million units total).[172]

Pediatric Dose. IM only for group A streptococcal upper respiratory infection (under 27 kg) 300,000–600,000 units; (over 27 kg) 900,000 units as a single injection. **IM for the prophylaxis of post-streptococcal rheumatic fever or glomerulonephritis** 1.2 million units once a month or 600,000 units twice a month. **IM for congenital syphilis with normal CSF** (under 2 yr) 50,000 units/kg as a single injection.

Dosage Forms. Inj (IM only) 300,000, 600,000 units/ml.

Pharmacokinetics. *Fate.* Very slowly absorbed from the injection site; hydrolyzed in the bloodstream to produce free penicillin G. 600,000 units IM in adults results in an average plasma penicillin concentration of 0.063 mcg/ml.[173] Mean concentration in children following 600,000 or 1.2 million units is 0.15 mcg/ml.[163] In newborns receiving 50,000 units/kg, mean peak concentrations are 1.05–1.23 mcg/ml.[173] A single 1.2 million unit injection results in detectable plasma penicillin levels in adults for an average of 27 days.[173] Distribution and elimination follow the same patterns as penicillin G.[141]

Adverse Reactions. The Jarisch-Herxheimer reaction, an acute febrile reaction presumably due to the release of endotoxin from killed treponemes, frequently occurs in patients treated for early syphilis. The reaction occurs within 24 hr of injection and subsides within 24 hr. Inadvertent intravenous administration of the drug has resulted in cardiac arrest and death. Extensive tissue damage has occurred following inadvertent intra-arterial injection.[173] See also Penicillin G Salts.

Contraindications. See Penicillin G Salts.

Precautions. Hypersensitivity reactions may be prolonged due to slow drug absorption. Prior to IM injection, the plunger should be pulled back and cartridge examined to determine if needle is in a blood vessel. See also Penicillin G Salts.

Penicillin G Procaine   Various

Pharmacology. A relatively insoluble suspension of procaine and penicillin G that dissolves slowly at the site of injection providing prolonged low plasma penicillin levels. See Penicillin G Salts.

Administration and Adult Dose. IM for uncomplicated gonorrhea 4.8 million units in at least 2 divided doses injected at different sites during one visit, together with 1 g probenecid orally. **IM for neurosyphilis** 2.4 million units/day plus probenecid PO 500 mg qid for 10 days, followed by benzathine penicillin G 2.4 million units IM every week for 3 doses.[172] **IM for uncomplicated pneumococcal pneumonia** 600,000–1.2 million units/day.[172]

Pediatric Dose. **IM only for congenital syphilis with abnormal CSF** 50,000 units/kg/day for a minimum of 10 days. **IM for uncomplicated gonorrhea** (less than 45 kg) 100,000 units/kg/day in 2 divided doses, with 25 mg/kg probenecid orally (maximum 1 g).[172]

Dosage Forms. **Inj (IM only)** 300,000, 500,000, 600,000 units/ml.

Pharmacokinetics. *Fate.* Absorbed slowly from the injection site. Hydrolyzed in the plasma to produce peak penicillin G levels of approximately 0.9 mcg/ml 2 hr after the administration of 300,000 units to normal adults; plasma levels fall to 0.13 mcg/ml after 24 hr. Distribution and elimination follow the same patterns as penicillin G.[141]

Adverse Reactions. Similar to penicillin G benzathine. Acute psychotic reactions (known as "pseudoanaphylactic" reactions) and characterized by acute anxiety, hallucinations, confusion and palpitations with or without cardiovascular collapse are reported occasionally. The cause is unknown, although some cases have been documented as being associated with inadvertent IV administration.[175,176] Partially degraded suspensions of the preparation, resulting in higher levels of free procaine, have also been implicated.[174]

Contraindications. See Penicillin G Salts.

Precautions. See Penicillin G Salts.

Penicillin G Salts   Various

Pharmacology. A β-lactam antibiotic with activity against most Gram-positive organisms and some Gram-negative organisms, notably *Neisseria* sp. Acts by interfering with late stages of bacterial cell wall synthesis; resistance is primarily due to bacterial elaboration of β-lactamases, although some organisms have impermeable outer cell wall layers.

Administration and Adult Dose. **PO** 250-500 mg (400,000-800,000 units) q 6 hr for mild to moderate infections. **IV** 2-24 million units/day in 4-12 divided doses, depending on infection. **IM not recommended** (very painful); use benzathine or procaine salt form as indicated.

Dosage Individualization. With usual oral doses no dosage adjustment is required in patients with impaired renal function; however, in treating more severe infections with larger IV doses, careful adjustment is necessary. In anuric patients, give no more than 3 million units/day.[176]

Pediatric Dose. **PO** (under 12 yr) 25,000-90,000 units/kg/day in 3-6 divided doses; **PO** (over 12 yr) same as adult dose. **IV** 100,000-250,000 units/kg/day in 6 divided doses.

Dosage Forms. **Susp/Syrup** (as potassium salt) 200,000, 250,000, 400,000 units/5 ml (reconstituted); **Tab** (as potassium salt) 200,000, 250,000, 400,000, 500,000, 800,000 units; **Inj** (as potassium salt) 200,000, 500,000, 1, 5, 10, 20 million units; **Inj** (as sodium salt) 5 million units.

Patient Instructions. This (oral) drug should be taken with a full glass of water on an empty stomach (1 hr before or 2 hr after meals) for best absorption; refrigerate solution.

Pharmacokinetics. *Fate.* Only 15-30% orally absorbed due to its high susceptibility to gastric acid hydrolysis; peak concentrations of 1.5-2.7 mcg/ml occur 0.5-1 hr after administration of 500 mg.[141] Widely distributed in body tissues, fluids and cavities, with biliary levels up to 10 times plasma levels. 30-60% plasma protein bound.[141] Penetration into CSF is poor, even with inflamed meninges; however, large parenteral doses (greater than 20 million units/day) adequately treat meningitis due to susceptible organisms. 80–85% of absorbed dose is excreted unchanged in the urine.[141]

$t_{1/2}$. 30–40 min; 7–10 hr in patients with renal failure;[135] 20–30 hr in patients with hepatic and renal failure.[141]

Adverse Reactions. Occasional nausea or diarrhea after usual oral doses. CNS toxicity may occur with massive IV doses (60–100 million units/ day) or excessive doses in combination with impaired renal function (usually greater than 10–20 million units/day in anuric patients); characterized by confusion, drowsiness and myoclonus which may progress to convulsions and result in death. Large doses of the sodium salt form may result in hypernatremia and fluid overload with pulmonary edema, especially in patients with impaired renal function or congestive heart failure. Large doses of the potassium salt form may result in hyperkalemia, especially in patients with impaired renal function and with rapid infusions. Occasional positive Coombs' reactions with rare hemolytic anemia have been reported after large IV doses. Interstitial nephritis has been rarely reported following large IV doses.[15] Hypersensitivity reactions (primarily rashes) occur with a 1–10% frequency. Most serious hypersensitivity reactions follow injection rather than oral administration.[177]

Contraindications. History of anaphylactic, accelerated (eg, hives) or serum sickness reaction to previous penicillin administration. See Notes.

Precautions. Use caution in patients with a history of penicillin or cephalosporin hypersensitivity reactions, atopic predisposition (eg, asthma), impaired renal function (hence neonates and geriatric patients), impaired cardiac function or pre-existing seizure disorder.

Parameters to Monitor. Initial renal function tests when using high doses. During prolonged high-dose therapy, periodic renal function tests and serum electrolytes.

Notes. 250 mg equals 400,000 units of penicillin G. Penicillin V potassium is preferred to penicillin G potassium for oral administration, due to more complete and reliable absorption.[141] Skin testing with penicilloyl-polylysine (PPL, Pre-Pen®) and microdeterminant mixture (MDM) can help determine the likelihood of serious reactions to penicillin in penicillin-allergic individuals. Availability of MDM is limited; it is locally available in small amounts only at larger medical centers. Desensitization may be attempted (rarely) in patients with life-threatening infections that are likely to be responsive only to penicillin, but this is a dangerous procedure and many alternative antibiotics are available.[177]

Penicillin V   Various

Pharmacology. A phenoxymethyl derivative of penicillin that is more acid stable than penicillin G. Spectrum and mechanism of action are the same as penicillin G, although penicillin V is 2–4 times less active against sensitive organisms.[15]

Administration and Adult Dose. **PO for mild to moderate infections** 250–500 mg q 6 hr; parenteral penicillin is preferred for more serious infections.

Dosage Individualization. No dosage adjustment is required for patients with impaired renal function with recommended doses.

Pediatric Dose. **PO** (infants and children under 12 yr) 15–50 mg/kg/day in 3–4 divided doses; (over 12 yr) same as adult dose.

Dosage Forms. **Soln/Susp** 125, 250 mg/5 ml (reconstituted); **Tab** 125, 250, 500 mg.

Patient Instructions. This drug should be taken with a full glass of water on an empty stomach (1 hr before or 2 hr after meals) for best absorption; refrigerate solution after reconstitution.

Pharmacokinetics. *Fate.* Average oral absorption of potassium salt form is 60%. Peak plasma levels are between 3–8 mcg/ml following a 500 mg oral dose. Probably distributed in the body in a fashion similar to penicillin G, although no data available; 80% plasma protein bound.[141] Extensively metabolized (about 50%), with products eliminated primarily in the urine. About 50% of absorbed dose is excreted unchanged.[141,178]

$t_{1/2}$. 30 min in normal adults;[15] no other data available, although impaired renal function should not greatly prolong half-life unless liver function is simultaneously impaired.

Adverse Reactions. Nausea and diarrhea are infrequent with usual doses. Hypersensitivity reactions similar to those following oral penicillin G occur. See also Penicillin G Salts.

Contraindications. See Penicillin G Salts.

Precautions. See Penicillin G Salts.

Notes. 250 mg equals approximately 400,000 units of penicillin V base or potassium salt.

8:12.24 TETRACYCLINES

General References: 179–181

Doxycycline and Salts

Vibramycin®

Pharmacology. Somewhat more active than other tetracyclines against anaerobes and facultative Gram-negative bacilli. See Tetracycline.

Administration and Adult Dose. PO 100 mg q 12 hr for one day, followed by 50–100 mg/day in 1–2 doses; **PO for prophylaxis against travelers' diarrhea** 200 mg en route, then 100 mg/day;[182] **PO for uncomplicated gonorrhea** 100 mg bid for 7 days; **PO for primary and secondary syphilis** 100 mg tid for at least 10 days. IV 200 mg in 1–2 divided doses for 1 day, followed by 100–200 mg/day, infused at a concentration of 0.1–1 mg/ml over 1–4 hr; double maintenance dose in severe infections. **Not for SC or IM use.**

Dosage Individualization. No dosage adjustment necessary in renal impairment.[179]

Pediatric Dose. **Not recommended under 8 yr.** PO (under 45 kg) 2.2 mg/kg q 12 hr for 1 day followed by 2.2 ng/kg/day in 1–2 divided doses; (over 45 kg) same as adult dose. IV (under 45 kg) 4.4 mg/kg in 1–2 divided doses for 1 day followed by 2.2–4.4 mg/kg/day in 1–2 divided doses; (over 45 kg) same as adult dose.

Dosage Forms. **Cap** (as hyclate) 50, 100 mg; **Susp** (as monohydrate) 25 mg/5 ml (reconstituted); **Syrup** (as calcium) 50 mg/5 ml; **Tab** (as hyclate) 50, 100 mg; **Inj** (as hyclate) 100, 200 mg.

Patient Instructions. This (oral) drug should be taken with a full glass of water on an empty stomach, but if stomach upset occurs, it may be taken with food or milk, but not antacids or iron products. Avoid prolonged exposure to direct sunlight while taking this drug.

Pharmacokinetics. *Onset and Duration.* Duration of protection against travelers' diarrhea is about 1 week after discontinuation.[182]

Fate. Virtually 100% orally absorbed producing a peak of 3 mcg/ml at 2-4 hr after administration of a 200 mg dose;[15] antacids and iron may significantly impair oral absorption, although food has little effect.[181] V_d is about 0.7 L/kg; about 60-90% plasma protein bound.[15,180] Widely distributed in the body, penetrating most cavities including CSF (12-20% of plasma levels). About 35-57% is excreted unchanged in the urine in normal adults; remainder is eliminated in feces via intestinal and biliary secretion.[179,183]

$t_{1/2}$. 12-20 hr (average 15) in normal adults; 17-25 hr in severe renal impairment.[183]

Adverse Reactions. IV administration frequently produces phlebitis. In contrast to other tetracyclines, doxycycline is not significantly antianabolic and will not further increase azotemia in renal failure. Although oral doxycycline causes less alteration of intestinal flora than other tetracyclines, it may cause nausea and diarrhea with equal frequency. Binds to calcium in teeth and bones, which may cause discoloration of teeth in children, especially during growth; although doxycycline has a lower potential for this effect than most other tetracyclines.[15] Occasional phototoxic skin reactions may occur.[15,179]

Contraindications. Severe hepatic dysfunction.

Precautions. Pregnancy. Oral iron lowers plasma levels, even of IV doxycycline, by binding the drug after its secretion into intestine and increasing fecal elimination.[179]

Parameters to Monitor. Check for signs of phlebitis daily during IV use.

Notes. Doxycycline is the tetracycline of choice for extrarenal infection in the presence of renal impairment, although tetracyclines are the drugs of choice for very few infections.[179,181] Each vial contains 480 mg of ascorbic acid per 100 mg of doxycycline hyclate for injection. See Tetracyclines Comparison Chart.

Tetracycline and Salts   Various

Pharmacology. A broad-spectrum bacteriostatic antibiotic which inhibits protein synthesis at the 30S ribosomal subunit. Many bacteria have developed resistance by an R-factor-mediated enzyme, changes in ribosomal binding characteristics or changes in cell wall permeability.

Administration and Adult Dose. PO 250-500 mg q 6-12 hr, between meals; **IV (not recommended)** 250-500 mg q 12 hr, to maximum of 250 mg q 6 hr. **Ophth Susp for trachoma** 2 drops in each eye bid-qid for 1-2 months or longer; **Ophth Susp for acute bacterial infection** 1-2 drops in affected eye 2-6 times/day; **Ophth Oint** 1/2 inch ribbon to affected eye q 3-4 hr; **Top Oint** apply a small amount to affected area bid-tid. **IM not recommended.**

Pediatric Dose. Not recommended under 8 yr. PO 25-50 mg/kg/day in 2-4 divided doses between meals; **IV (not recommended)** 12 mg/kg/day to maximum of 20 mg/kg/day in 2 divided doses. **Ophth** same as adult dose; **Top** same as adult dose. **IM not recommended.**

Dosage Forms. **Cap** 100, 250, 500 mg; **Susp** 125 mg/5 ml; **Syrup** 125 mg/5 ml; **Tab** 250, 500 mg; **Inj (IM)** 100, 250 mg; **Inj (IV)** 250, 500 mg; **Ophth Oint** 1%; **Ophth Susp** 1%; **Top Oint** 3%. Strengths are expressed as hydrochloride equivalent.

Patient Instructions. This (oral) drug should be taken with a full glass of water on an empty stomach (1 hr before or 2 hr after meals) for best absorption. Do not take within 1 hr of dairy products, antacids (except sodium bicarbonate) or iron products.

Pharmacokinetics. *Fate.* About 75% absorbed orally; however, marked differences in bioavailability have been documented, although no significant differences in absorption reported among the different salts. IM injections are poorly absorbed, producing peak levels significantly lower than after oral administration. V_d is about 1.5 L/kg; 36-65% plasma protein bound.[15,180] Widely distributed in the body, including significant biliary concentrations and low CSF concentrations. About 60% of the absorbed dose appears unchanged in the urine.[15,179]

$t_{1/2}$. 9-11 hr (average 10); up to 100 hr with severe renal impairment.[179,183]

Adverse Reactions. IM injections are very irritating and painful; IV injections frequently cause phlebitis; oral administration produces bowel flora alterations and GI complaints which are dose-related. Antianabolic effect may produce elevation in BUN, hyperphosphatemia and acidosis in patients with pre-existing renal impairment. Binds to calcium in teeth and bones, which may cause mottling and discoloration of teeth in children, especially with repeated courses during growth;[15,180] this may also occur as a result of in utero exposure. Acute, extensive, fatty infiltration of the liver with pancreatitis, acidosis and nonoliguric renal failure has occurred rarely; but, these reactions are more frequently reported after IV administration of large doses (greater than 1.5 g/day) in the presence of renal impairment, especially in pregnant or malnourished individuals. They are frequently fatal.[15,179]

Contraindications. Renal impairment.

Precautions. Pregnancy. Use with caution in patients with liver impairment. Do *not* repeat courses in children under 8 yr.

Parameters to Monitor. Initial renal function tests; liver function tests if liver toxicity likely to occur (parenteral administration, high doses and/or pregnancy). Check for signs of phlebitis daily during IV administration.

Notes. Rarely the drug of choice.[179] Each vial of tetracycline hydrochloride or phosphate complex for injection contains from 250 mg-1 + g of ascorbic acid depending on the manufacturer and the amount of tetracycline. See Tetracyclines Comparison Chart.

Tetracyclines Comparison Chart

DRUG	DOSAGE FORMS	ADULT DOSE	PERCENT ORAL ABSORP- TION	AVERAGE HALF-LIFE (HOURS)	PERCENT UNCHANGED IN URINE	COMMENTS
Demeclocycline Hydrochloride Declomycin®	Cap 150 mg Tab (coated) 150, 300 mg.	PO 600 mg/day in 2-4 divided doses.	66	15	42	Most phototoxic tetracycline; causes nephrogenic diabetes insipidus rarely.
Doxycycline Calcium Doxycycline Hyclate Doxycycline Monohydrate Vibramycin® Various	Cap (as hyclate) 50, 100 mg Susp (as monohydrate) 25 mg/5 ml Syrup (as calcium) 50 mg/5 ml Tab (as hyclate) 50, 100 mg Inj (as hyclate) 100, 200 mg.	PO 100 mg q 12 hr for 1 day, then 50–100 mg/day in 1–2 divided doses; IV 200 mg in 1–2 divided doses for 1 day, then 100–200 mg/day.	90–100	12–20	35–40	Safest in renal failure due to its lack of accumulation and lack of antianabolic effects.
Minocycline Hydrochloride Minocin®	Cap 50, 100 mg Susp 50 mg/5 ml Tab 50, 100 mg Inj (IV only) 100 mg.	PO or IV 200 mg initially, then 100 mg q 12 hr.	95–100	13–17	5–10	Very frequent transient vestibular toxicity.

Continued

Tetracyclines Comparison Chart

DRUG	DOSAGE FORMS	ADULT DOSE	PERCENT ORAL ABSORP-TION	AVERAGE HALF-LIFE (HOURS)	PERCENT UNCHANGED IN URINE	COMMENTS
Oxytetracycline Various **Oxytetracycline Hydrochloride Oxytetracycline Calcium** Various	Cap (as HCl) 250 mg Tab (coated) 250 mg Inj (IV only, as HCl) 250, 500 mg.	PO 250–500 mg q 6 hr; IV 250–500 mg q 6–12 hr to a maximum of 2 g/day.	58	9	70	
Tetracycline Various **Tetracycline Hydrochloride** Various **Tetracycline PO₄ Complex** Tetrex®	Cap (as HCl) 100, 250, 500 mg Cap (as phosphate complex) 250, 500 mg Susp 125 mg/5 ml Syrup 125 mg/5 ml Tab (as HCl) 250, 500 mg Inj (IM only, as HCl) 100, 250 mg Inj (IV only, as HCl) 250, 500 mg.	PO 250–500 mg q 6–12 hr; IV 250–500 mg q 6–12 hr to a maximum of 2 g/day.	75	10	60	IM preparations contain procaine and should not be used IV; IM not recommended due to pain and low plasma levels.

8:12.28 MISCELLANEOUS ANTIBIOTICS

Clindamycin Salts

Cleocin®, Various

Pharmacology. A semisynthetic 7-chloro, 7-deoxylincomycin derivative which is very active against most Gram-positive organisms except enterococci and *Clostridium difficile*. Gram-negative aerobes are highly resistant, while most anaerobes are very sensitive. Inhibits bacterial protein synthesis by binding to the 50S ribosomal subunit; bactericidal or bacteriostatic depending on the concentration, organism and inoculum.[184]

Administration and Adult Dose. PO 150–450 mg q 6 hr; IM or IV 600 mg–2.7 g/day in 2–4 divided doses, to maximum of 4.8 g/day. Single IM doses greater than 600 mg not recommended; infuse IV no faster than 30 mg/min. **Top for acne** apply bid.

Dosage Individualization. Dosage adjustment is unnecessary in renal impairment[185,186] or cirrhosis,[187,188] although the effect of acute liver disease is unknown.[187]

Pediatric Dose. PO (under 10 kg) give no less than 37.5 mg q 8 hr; (over 10 kg) 8–25 mg/kg/day in 3–4 divided doses; IM or IV (under 1 month) 15–20 mg/kg/day in 3–4 divided doses; the lower dose may be adequate for premature infants; (over 1 month) 15–40 mg/kg/day in 3–4 divided doses (not less than 300 mg/day in severe infection, regardless of weight).

Dosage Forms. Cap (as hydrochloride) 75, 150, 300 mg; Soln (as palmitate) 75 mg/5 ml (reconstituted); Inj (as phosphate) 150 mg/ml; Top Soln (as phosphate) 1%; Top Gel (as phosphate) 1%.

Patient Instructions. Report any severe diarrhea immediately and do not take antidiarrheal medication. Do *not* refrigerate the reconstituted oral solution, because it will thicken.

Pharmacokinetics. *Fate.* Absorption is nearly complete and is the same from the capsule or the solution; food may delay, but not decrease, absorption.[15,189] The palmitate and phosphate esters are absorbed intact and rapidly hydrolyzed to the active base. Unhydrolyzed phosphate ester usually constitutes less than 20% of the total peak plasma level after parenteral clindamycin, but may increase to 40% in patients with impaired renal function.[185] A 500 mg oral dose produces a peak plasma level of 5–6 mcg/ml in 1 hr.[189] A 300 mg IM dose produces a peak level of 5–6 mcg/ml 1–2 hr post-injection.[185,186,190] A 600 mg IV dose infused over 30 min produces a peak plasma level of 10 mcg/ml.[15] The drug is widely distributed throughout the body except the CSF.[186,190] V_d is about 0.6 L/kg; 80–94% plasma protein bound.[187] There is significant hepatic metabolism, and excretion of active forms in the bile.[186,190,191] 5–10% of the absorbed dose is recovered as unchanged drug and active metabolites in the urine within 24 hr.[186,187,190]

$t_{1/2}$. 1.5–4 hr (average 2.5);[15,186] unchanged or slightly increased in severe renal disease;[185,186] may be increased or unchanged in liver disease.[187,188]

Adverse Reactions. After oral administration, anorexia, nausea, vomiting, cramps and diarrhea occur frequently.[15,192] Oral, and rarely, parenteral clindamycin may cause severe, sometimes fatal, pseudomembranous colitis (PMC) which may be clinically indistinguishable at onset from non-PMC diarrhea.[15,193] Symptoms usually appear 2–9 days after initiation of therapy. PMC has been reported after topical administration.[194] Clindamycin-associated PMC is secondary to overgrowth of toxin-producing *Clostridium difficile*.[193,195] PMC is terminated in many patients by discontinuing clindamycin immediately; however, if diarrhea is severe or does not improve promptly after discontinuation, treat with vancomycin or metronidazole.[193] The value of corticosteroids, cholestyramine and anti-spasmodics in the management of clindamycin-associated diarrhea and PMC has not been established.[193,196] Antidiarrheals such as diphenoxylate may worsen PMC and should *not* be used.

Precautions. Pregnancy; lactation. Use with caution in neonates under 4 weeks of age, and in patients with liver disease. Discontinue *immediately* if significant diarrhea occurs. Drug accumulation may occur in patients with severe concomitant hepatic and renal dysfunction, however, data are lacking.

Parameters to Monitor. Observe for changes in bowel frequency.

Notes. Oral solution is stable for 2 weeks at room temperature following reconstitution; do not refrigerate.

Colistimethate Sodium   Coly-Mycin M®

Colistimethate is the methane sulfonate salt of colistin (polymyxin E), a polypeptide antibacterial similar to polymyxin B. The drug is rarely used due to the availability of broad spectrum β-lactam compounds and aminoglycosides, as well as significant toxicity. The only indication for its use is serious infection due to aerobic Gram-negative bacilli (particularly *Pseudomonas aeruginosa*) resistant to all other antimicrobial agents. IV dosage is 2.5–5 mg/kg/day in 2–4 equally divided doses. Dosage must be reduced in renal insufficiency, although specific guidelines are not available. One suggestion is to administer 2.5 mg/kg to anuric patients as a loading dose followed by 1.5 mg/kg q 5–7 days.[15] Available as powder for reconstitution equivalent to 150 mg colistin.

Polymyxin B Sulfate   Aerosporin®, Various

This polypeptide antibacterial is similar to colistimethate with regard to mechanism of action, pharmacology and toxicity. It is rarely used systemically due to questionable efficacy, significant toxicity and the availability of broad spectrum β-lactam compounds and aminoglycosides. The drug is found in numerous topical formulations, including those used in the eye and the ear. IV dosage is 1.5–2.5 mg/kg/day in 2 equally divided doses. Intrathecal dose for meningitis is 5 mg daily or every other day. Although dosage adjustment is necessary in renal failure, accurate guidelines are not available. One suggestion is 2.5 mg/kg initially followed by 1 mg/kg q 5–7 days in anuria.[15] Available as 50 mg (500,000 units) powder for reconstitution.

Spectinomycin Dihydrochloride   Trobicin®

This nonaminoglycosidic aminocyclitol is active against a wide variety of Gram-negative bacteria, but is used almost exclusively in the treatment of infections due to penicillinase-producing *N. gonorrhoeae* (PPNG). The pharmacokinetic characteristics of the drug are similar to kanamycin and amikacin. Adverse effects after single doses are limited to pain at the injection site, transient dizziness and nausea. The drug has no activity against *T. pallidum*; therefore, it cannot eradicate syphilis. Pharyngeal gonococcal infection responds poorly to the drug. It is given as a single 2 g IM dose.[172,197] Available as 2 and 4 g injection.

Teicoplanin (Investigational - Merrell-Dow)

Teicoplanin is a glycopeptide antibiotic which resembles vancomycin in spectrum of activity and mode of action (inhibition of cell wall synthesis). Teicoplanin appears to be slightly more active in vitro than vancomycin against staphylococci and streptococci, but may be less rapidly bactericidal. The pharmacokinetics of the drug are complex, fitting to a 3-compartment model. Terminal elimination half-life is approximately 40 hours and $V_{d\ ss}$ is 0.84 L/kg. Total body clearance is estimated to be 1.1 L/hr/70 kg body weight. Urinary recovery is approximately 50% in 4 days. Adverse effects reported thus far have been limited to local irritation at the injection site and rash. Clinical data comparing vancomycin and teicoplanin are limited but appear to indicate that teicoplanin may be somewhat less effective, but doses used may have been too low. Dosage utilized thus far is 200 mg given as a slow IV bolus injection once a day.[198-200]

Vancomycin Hydrochloride   Vancocin®, Various

Pharmacology. Binds irreversibly to cell wall of many Gram-positive cocci and bacilli, including *C. difficile* and methicillin-resistant *Staph. aureus*; inhibits cell wall synthesis in a manner slightly different from β-lactam antimicrobials. Most Gram-negative bacteria are resistant.

Administration and Adult Dose. PO for staphylococcal enterocolitis 2 g/day in 2-4 divided doses. **PO for antibiotic-associated colitis** 125-500 mg q 6 hr for 7-10 days; retreat with a longer course if relapse occurs.[201] **IV** 20-30 mg/kg/day (usually 2 g/day) in 2-4 divided doses as a dilute infusion over 30-60 min. **Not for IM use.**

Dosage Individualization. Adjust dosage carefully in renal impairment; clearance is directly related to Cl_{cr}.[202] Anuric patients on hemodialysis have been given the usual dose q 7-14 days with good results,[202-204] although one source recommends a loading dose of 15 mg/kg followed by 1.9 mg/kg/day.[205] Monitor plasma concentrations. Dosage adjustment is unnecessary in liver disease.

Pediatric Dose. PO or IV (neonate) 12-15 mg/kg/day; (older infants and children) 40 mg/kg/day in 2-4 divided doses.

Dosage Forms. Cap 125, 250 mg; **Pwdr** 1, 10 g; **Inj** 500 mg.

Patient Instructions. Report pain at infusion site, dizziness, fullness or ringing in ears with IV use; nausea or vomiting with oral use.

Pharmacokinetics. *Plasma Levels.* Therapeutic range not well defined, but ototoxicity is likely with peaks over 80 mcg/ml and possible with peaks of 25-50 mcg/ml; therapeutic peaks are 20-40 mcg/ml; troughs over 13-32 mcg/ml may be associated with ototoxicity and over 30 mcg/ml with nephrotoxicity.[202]

Fate. Oral absorption negligible. Fecal concentrations during therapy with PO 500 mg q 6 hr reach 3 mg/g.[206] 500 mg IV produces plasma levels of 6-10 mcg/ml in 1 hr. V_c is 0.1-0.15 L/kg; V_{dss} is 0.4-0.9 L/kg; plasma protein binding variously reported as 10-30% and 44-82%.[202] Widely distributed, except to the CSF. Negligible metabolism or biliary excretion; 80-90% is excreted in the urine unchanged within 24 hr.[202]

$t_{1/2}$. α-phase 0.5-1 hr; β-phase 3-9 hr, 6-10 days with renal impairment. No change with hepatic disease.[202-204,207]

Adverse Reactions. Chills, fever, nausea, phlebitis may occur, especially with direct injection of undiluted drug (not recommended). Rapid infusion may cause transient systolic hypotension.[205,208] The "red man" or "red neck" syndrome of erythema, pruritus and localized edema occurring with too rapid infusion is probably due to histamine release with the first dose of the drug and should not occur with subsequent doses. Extravasation causes local tissue necrosis. Ototoxicity (auditory and vestibular) and possibly nephrotoxicity occur with excessive plasma concentrations; usually reversible upon discontinuation. Eosinophilia, neutropenia and urticarial rashes have been reported frequently. Side effects of vancomycin may not be as prevalent today as in the past, perhaps due to changes in the manufacturing process which eliminated some impurities.[209]

Precautions. Pregnancy. Use with caution in patients with impaired renal function, pre-existing hearing loss or those receiving other ototoxic or nephrotoxic agents.

Parameters to Monitor. With IV use, obtain initial renal function tests and repeat frequently during therapy; serial audiometry should be performed if patient is over 60 yr or has decreased renal function. With decreased renal function, plasma concentrations should be monitored. Check for signs of phlebitis daily.

Notes. An alternative agent for treatment or prophylaxis of staphylococcal or streptococcal infections when a less toxic agent is inappropriate (eg, penicillin or cephalosporin allergy, or resistant organisms) or has not produced an adequate therapeutic response. Oral drug of choice for antibiotic-associated colitis refractory to conservative management (ie, discontinue offending agent, fluid/electrolyte replacement); however, metronidazole may be equally effective and is much less expensive.[193]

8:16 ANTITUBERCULOSIS AGENTS

(SEE ALSO STREPTOMYCIN 8:12.02)

General References: 210

Ethambutol Hydrochloride   Myambutol®

Pharmacology. A synthetic tuberculostatic which acts by an unknown mechanism, possibly as an RNA antimetabolite; its activity is restricted to mycobacteria. Primary resistance among mycobacteria is rare, but resistance occurs rapidly if used alone.

Administration and Adult Dose. PO for treatment of tuberculosis 15 mg/kg/day for a total of 18-24 months in combination with rifampin or isoniazid.[210] Alternatively, 50 mg/kg twice weekly.[210]

Dosage Individualization. Dosage should be decreased in severe renal impairment; exact guidelines are not established, but one source recommends 8-10 mg/kg/day in severe renal impairment.[212]

Pediatric Dose. (Under 5 yr) not recommended; (5 yr and over) same as adult dose.[210]

Dosage Forms. Tab 100, 400 mg.

Patient Instructions. Report any changes in vision.

Pharmacokinetics. _Fate._ About 80% absorbed orally with 15 mg/kg producing peak plasma concentrations of 4-6 mcg/ml at 2-4 hr after the dose.[211] The distribution of ethambutol is largely unknown, although low therapeutic concentrations appear in the CSF in the presence of inflamed meninges. Disposition is complex and multicompartmental with a prolonged (5 hr) initial distribution phase.[211] V_d is about 1.5-4 L/kg;[212] 20-30% plasma protein bound.[211] Of the absorbed dose, nearly 100% is recovered in the urine within 24 hr, with 80% as unchanged ethambutol.[212]

$t_{1/2}$. 4-6 hr in normal adults.[211] In anuric patients, reported half-life values range from 7-32 hr,[212] although the upper end of this range appears most likely.

Adverse Reactions. Optic neuritis is rare with doses less than 25 mg/kg/day, but may be more frequent in the presence of impaired renal function. It appears over several months, usually as blurred vision, color blindness and restriction of visual fields. It is usually completely reversible over weeks to months with prompt drug discontinuation, although defective color vision may persist for prolonged periods and permanent impairment of vision may occur if the drug is not promptly discontinued.[213,214] Hyperuricemia due to impaired urinary excretion of uric acid may occur.

Contraindications. Optic neuritis.

Precautions. Pregnancy. Use with caution in patients with impaired renal function.

Parameters to Monitor. Initial renal function tests. With prolonged therapy at dosages greater than 15 mg/kg/day, or if pre-existing renal impairment or visual loss, periodic visual acuity and color discrimination testing is advised.

Isoniazid   Various

Pharmacology. A synthetic hydrazine derivative of isonicotinic acid which inhibits the synthesis of mycolic acid, a component of mycobacterial cell wall; it probably has other unknown actions. Activity is limited to mycobacteria; tuberculostatic or tuberculocidal depending on concentration and reproductive rate of the organism. Primary resistance is uncommon, but resistance can develop rapidly if used alone in active tuberculosis; resistance is uncommon in preventive therapy.

Administration and Adult Dose. **PO for prophylaxis of tuberculosis** 5 mg/kg/day (usually 300 mg) as a single daily dose, to maximum of 300 mg/day, given as a single agent for 1 yr — see Notes. **PO for treatment of tuberculosis** same dose as above, but combine with at least one other antitubercular agent for 18-24 months. Course may be shortened to 9 months if isoniazid (INH) is combined with rifampin 600 mg/day;[210] or use these same doses for 2-8 weeks, followed by INH 15 mg/kg and rifampin 600 mg twice weekly for a total of 9-12 months.[210] **IM or IV** (rarely used) same as oral dose.

Dosage Individualization. Acetylator phenotype has not been evaluated as a parameter for dosage individualization; however, some sources recommend a dose of 150-200 mg/day in slow acetylators with renal impairment.[15,215]

Pediatric Dose. **PO for prophylaxis of tuberculosis** 10 mg/kg/day as a single daily dose, to maximum of 300 mg/day, given as a single agent for 1 year.[216] **PO for treatment of pulmonary tuberculosis** 10-15 mg/kg/day for 9 months. Alternatively after daily use for 2-8 weeks, **PO intermittently** 20-40 mg/kg twice weekly with rifampin 10-20 mg/kg twice weekly.[210]

Dosage Forms. **Tab** 50, 100, 300 mg; **Inj** 100 mg/ml.

Patient Instructions. Report any burning, tingling or numbness in the extremities, unusual malaise, fever, dark urine or yellowing of eyes.

Pharmacokinetics. *Fate.* Rapid and nearly complete oral absorption with peak plasma concentrations of 1–5 mcg/ml 1 hr after a 5 mg/kg dose.[216] Widely distributed in the body tissues including the CSF of normal patients and those with meningitis. V_d is 0.6–0.7 L/kg in adults and 0.97 L/kg in children;[215,217] 15% plasma protein bound.[216] Eliminated primarily by acetylation in the liver to inactive metabolites which are excreted in the urine. Specific pattern of elimination depends on acetylator phenotype of the individual.[217]

$t_{1/2}$. (Rapid acetylators) 0.5–1.5 hr; (slow acetylators) 2–4 hr. 4 hr with renal impairment;[215,218] increased to 6.7 hr in patients with liver disease.[219]

Adverse Reactions. Pyridoxine-responsive peripheral neuropathy can occur, especially in alcoholics, diabetics, renal failure, malnourished patients, slow acetylators and with doses greater than 5 mg/kg/day.[220] Subclinical hepatitis is frequent (10–20%) and characterized by usually asymptomatic elevation of AST (SGOT) and ALT (SGPT) which may return to normal despite continued therapy; it may be more common with combined INH-rifampin therapy.[221] Clinical hepatitis is rare, but is strikingly related to age (rising to 2–3% in 50–65 year old patients). Rare cases of massive liver atrophy resulting in death usually appear in association with alcoholism or pre-existing liver disease; most severe cases occur within the first 6 months.[222,223] With acute overdosage (usually 6–10 g), INH may produce severe CNS toxicity including coma and seizures as well as hypotension, acidosis and occasionally death.[224]

Contraindications. Acute or chronic liver disease, previous INH-associated hepatitis.

Precautions. Pregnancy; lactation. Use with caution in daily users of alcohol, elderly patients and those with a slow acetylator phenotype.

Parameters to Monitor. Question for prodromal signs of hepatitis (eg, fever, malaise) and signs of peripheral neuropathy (eg, burning, tingling, numbness) monthly during therapy. Baseline and monthly AST and ALT are recommended only in high risk groups (those over 35 yr, daily alcohol users, and those with a history of liver dysfunction);[225] although, they are not predictive of clinical hepatitis.[226]

Notes. It is generally recommended that all patients receive INH for prophylaxis of tuberculosis who have had a positive reaction to intermediate strength Purified Protein Derivative (PPD 5 Tuberculin Units) and who: (1) are household contacts of patients with active tuberculosis; or (2) converted their PPD to positive within the past 12–24 months; or (3) have radiologic evidence of inactive tuberculosis or a history of inadequately treated active tuberculosis; or (4) are receiving prolonged treatment with corticosteroids or immunosuppressants (although the need for prophylaxis in this group has been questioned);[227] or (5) have leukemia, Hodgkin's disease, diabetes mellitus, silicosis or have undergone a subtotal or total gastrectomy.[220] Most sources suggest that the use of INH prophylaxis in patients older than 35 yr should be further restricted due to the increased risk of fatal hepatotoxicity.[225,228]

To prevent peripheral neuropathy, adults receiving large doses of INH (10 mg/kg/day or more) and those who are predisposed to peripheral neuritis (eg, alcoholics) should receive **pyridoxine** in a dose of 50 mg/day. Pyridoxine IV in a dose equal to the estimated amount of INH ingested is recommended for acute INH overdose.[224,229]

Rifampin

Rimactane®, Rifadin®

Pharmacology. A synthetic rifamycin B derivative; highly active against mycobacteria, most Gram-positive bacteria and some Gram-negative bacteria, most notably, *Neisseria meningitidis.* Inhibits the action of DNA-dependent RNA polymerase. Primary resistance is uncommon, but resistance can develop rapidly if used alone.

Administration and Adult Dose. PO for treatment of tuberculosis 600 mg/day as a single daily dose in combination with at least one other antitubercular agent — see Isoniazid; **PO for prophylaxis of meningococcal meningitis** 600 mg bid for 2 days.[230,231]

Dosage Individualization. No dosage adjustment is necessary in patients with impaired renal function; accumulation would be expected in patients with hepatic dysfunction or biliary obstruction, but dosage guidelines for use in patients with these conditions are not available.

Pediatric Dose. PO for treatment of tuberculosis (over 5 yr) 10–20 mg/kg/day as a single daily dose, to maximum of 600 mg/day, in combination with at least one other antitubercular agent.[210] **PO for prophylaxis of meningococcal meningitis** (less than 1 yr) 5 mg/kg bid for 2 days; (1–12 yr) 10 mg/kg bid, to maximum of 600 mg bid, for 2 days.[230,231]

Dosage Forms. Cap 150, 300 mg.

Patient Instructions. This medication should be taken with a full glass of water on an empty stomach (1 hr before or 2 hr after meals) for best absorption. It is important to take this medication regularly as directed, because inconsistent dosing may increase its toxicity. May cause harmless red-orange discoloration of sweat, saliva, feces and urine.

Pharmacokinetics. *Fate.* 100% absorbed orally, with a 600 mg dose producing a peak plasma concentration of approximately 10 mcg/ml 1–3 hr after administration.[232] Food delays absorption, but does not affect overall bioavailability.[232,233] First-pass hepatic extraction is substantial, but saturated with doses greater than 300–450 mg; thus, larger doses produce disproportionate plasma levels.[232] Widely distributed throughout the body; however, significant amounts appear in the CSF only in the presence of inflamed meninges.[232,234] About 80% plasma protein bound.[232] Eliminated primarily by deacetylation in the liver to a partially active metabolite which is extensively enterohepatically recirculated, producing very high biliary concentrations.[232,235] About 50–60% of a dose is eventually excreted in the feces. Urinary excretion is variable and appears to increase with the dose. At usual doses, 12–15% is excreted unchanged in the urine.[232]

$t_{1/2}$. 1.5–5 hr (average 2.8).[232] Half-life increases with higher doses, but may become shorter over the first few weeks of treatment. It is not changed by renal impairment, but is increased unpredictably by liver disease or biliary obstruction.[219,235]

Adverse Reactions. Adverse reactions are more frequent and severe with intermittent, high-dose administration. GI symptoms are frequent. Acute, reversible renal failure, characterized as tubular damage with interstitial nephritis, sometimes appearing with concomitant hepatic failure has been reported rarely, especially in association with intermittent administration.[15,225] Subclinical hepatitis may be frequent (up to 18%), while clinical hepatitis is rare, but apparently more common with pre-existing liver disease or alcoholism; the effect of INH co-administration on the frequency of hepatitis is unclear.[221] Competition with bile for biliary excretion may produce jaundice, especially with pre-existing liver disease.[236] Intermittent therapy is also associated with thrombocytopenia and a flu-like syndrome (ie, fever, joint pain, muscle cramps). Rifampin affects cellular immunity, impairing skin-test reactivity in about 50% of recipients.[237]

Contraindications. Previous rifampin-associated hepatitis.

Precautions. Pregnancy; lactation. Use with caution in daily users of alcohol and those with pre-existing liver disease.

Parameters to Monitor. Question for prodromal signs of hepatitis (eg, fever, malaise). Baseline and monthly AST (SGOT) and ALT (SGPT) have been recommended, especially for patients with factors predisposing to hepatotoxicity from rifampin (eg, alcoholism, pre-existing liver disease), although they are not predictive of clinical hepatitis in the absence of symptomatology.

Second-Line Antituberculosis Agents Comparison Chart[a,b]

DRUG	DOSAGE FORMS	ADULT DOSE	HALF-LIFE (HOURS) NORMAL	HALF-LIFE (HOURS) ANURIA	PERCENT EXCRETED UNCHANGED IN URINE	MAJOR ADVERSE EFFECTS
Aminosalicylic Acid Salts Various	Tab 500 mg, 1 g Tab (coated) 500 mg Pwdr 4.18, 454 g.	PO 8–12 g/day in 2–4 divided doses (as the acid).	1	—	20	GI intolerance; hepatitis; lupus-like syndrome.
Capreomycin Sulfate Capastat®	Inj 1 g.	IM 15–20 mg/kg/day (usually 1 g) for 60–120 days, then 1 g 2–3 days/week.	2.5	↑	50–60	Nephrotoxicity; ototoxicity.
Cycloserine Seromycin®	Cap 250 mg.	PO 15 mg/kg/day (usually 500 mg) in 2 divided doses, to maximum of 1 g/day.	10	↑	60–70	CNS (drowsiness, dizziness, headache, depression, rare seizures and psychosis).
Ethionamide Trecator-SC®	Tab 250 mg.	PO 10–15 mg/kg/day (usually 500–750 mg) as a single daily dose, to maximum of 1 g/day.	3	—	1–5	GI intolerance; hepatitis; CNS (drowsiness, dizziness, headache, depression, rare seizures).
Kanamycin Sulfate Kantrex®	Inj 37.5, 250, 333 mg/ml.	IM 15 mg/kg/day (usually 1 g/day) 5–7 days/week.	2–3	80–90	90	Nephrotoxicity; ototoxicity.

Continued

Second-Line Antituberculosis Agents Comparison Chart[a,b]

DRUG	DOSAGE FORMS	ADULT DOSE	HALF-LIFE (HOURS)		PERCENT EXCRETED UNCHANGED IN URINE	MAJOR ADVERSE EFFECTS
			NORMAL	ANURIA		
Pyrazinamide	Tab 500 mg.	PO 20-35 mg/kg/day in 3-4 divided doses, to maximum of 3 g/day.	9-10	↑	4-14	Hepatitis; hyperuricemia.
Streptomycin Sulfate Various	Inj 1, 5 g.	IM 1 g 2-3 times/week.	5	↑	40	Vestibular toxicity.

a. Adapted from references 15, 225, 238, 239.
b. Use only in combination with other effective antituberculars.
c. Potassium salt contains 81%, and sodium salt contains 73% aminosalicylic acid; increase dose accordingly.

8:18 ANTIVIRALS

(SEE ALSO AMANTADINE 92:00)

Acyclovir   Zovirax®

Pharmacology. Acyclovir is an acyclic nucleoside analogue of guanosine. Acyclovir is selectively phosphorylated by the herpes-coded deoxynucleoside kinase to its monophosphate form. Cellular enzymes then convert the monophosphate to the active antiviral acyclovir triphosphate. This drug inhibits viral DNA synthesis; incorporation of acyclovir into viral DNA results in termination of the chain. Acyclovir has potent activity against Herpes simplex I and II (HSV), and also Herpes zoster [Varicella zoster (VZV)]. Activity against cytomegalovirus and Epstein-Barr virus has not been found to be clinically useful.[240,241] See Notes.

Administration and Adult Dose. IV for severe localized HSV infection 5 mg/kg tid for 5-7 days; **IV for VZV infection** 5-10 mg/kg tid; **IV for HSV encephalitis** 10 mg/kg tid. Dilute to 50-250 ml and infuse over 60 min. Maintain urine volume of 500 ml/24 hr for each gram of acyclovir administered. **PO for treatment of primary or recurrent genital HSV infection** 1 g/day for 5-10 days. **PO for prevention of recurrent genital HSV infection** 600 mg-1 g/day in 3-5 divided doses.[242] **Top for initial genital herpes genitalis and limited nonlife-threatening mucocutaneous Herpes simplex infections in immunocompromised patients** 0.5 inch ribbon to cover 4 square inch affected skin area q 3 hr, 6 times/day for 7 days.

Dosage Individualization. Reduce parenteral and oral dosage in renal insufficiency as follows: Cl_{cr} over 50 ml/min, no dosage adjustment is necessary; Cl_{cr} 25-50 ml/min, give the usual dose q 12 hr; Cl_{cr} 10-25 ml/min, give the usual dose q 24 hr; Cl_{cr} 0-10 ml/min, give one-half of the usual dose q 24 hr. For patients on hemodialysis, the usual daily dosage should be given after dialysis.

Pediatric Dose. IV (neonates) dosage not established; (13 months-11 yr) 750 mg/M^2 in 3 divided doses for HSV infection.

Dosage Forms. Cap 200 mg; Inj 500 mg; Oint 5%.

Patient Instructions. Use a finger cot or latex glove when applying the ointment to avoid autoinoculation.

Pharmacokinetics. *Fate.* Oral bioavailability averages 20%; average time to peak concentration is 2 hr; mean peak steady-state levels range from 2.5-5.9 μM (0.56-1.3 mcg/ml) with oral doses of 200-600 mg. Mean peak steady-state levels after IV range from 22.6-104.8 μM (5.1-23.6 mcg/ml) for doses of 2.5-15 mg/kg.[241] Biphasic decay, with V_d of 0.7 L/kg. CSF concentration is 25-70% of simultaneous plasma level;[241] 86-91.5% excreted unchanged in urine. Remainder is metabolized to 9-carboxy-methoxymethyl-guanine. Renal clearance is 75-80% of total clearance and is significantly reduced by concomitant probenecid.[241]

$t_{1/2}$. Approximately 3 hr in adult patients with normal renal function, increasing to nearly 20 hr in end-stage renal disease. Half-life on dialysis is 5.7 hr; half-life in neonates is about 4 hr.[240]

Adverse Reactions. Nephrotoxicity thought to be due to precipitation of acyclovir crystals in the nephron occurs in about 10% of patients if drug is given by bolus (<10 min) injection. Phlebitis at injection site occurs occasionally with IV infusion due to high pH (9-11) of product. Other side effects reported are CNS toxicity (eg, headache, lethargy, tremulousness, delirium, seizures), nausea, vomiting and skin rash.[240-242] CNS toxicity has occurred primarily in patients with underlying neurologic disease and may not be primarily due to the drug. Topical application to Herpes lesions may be painful.

Precautions. Use with caution in renal impairment, dehydration and preexisting neurologic disorders.

Parameters to Monitor. Monitor renal function and injection site for signs of phlebitis daily. Carefully monitor patients with underlying neurologic diseases for evidence of neurotoxicity. See Adverse Reactions.

Notes. Although vidarabine has been the treatment of choice for HSV encephalitis, acyclovir is at least as effective and is less toxic.[243] Acyclovir-resistant strains of virus have been isolated from patients after treatment. However these mutants, which are deficient in thymidine kinase, are significantly less virulent than sensitive strains.[244]

Vidarabine   Vira-A®

Vidarabine is a poorly soluble analogue of adenine deoxyriboside which is active primarily against herpes viruses. Vidarabine and its active major metabolite are phosphorylated in cells and inhibit both viral and cellular DNA polymerase. The drug is also effective in the treatment of Herpes zoster (shingles) in immunosuppressed patients, but is ineffective for the treatment of CMV infection. Adverse effects with IV administration are primarily related to dose and include encephalopathy, thrombocytopenia and leukopenia. Nausea and vomiting occur in about 10% of patients given IV vidarabine. IV vidarabine is being displaced by IV acyclovir which has been shown to be as effective, is much easier to administer and is less toxic. The IV dose for Herpes simplex encephalitis is 15 mg/kg/day by continuous infusion over 12–24 hr. The concentration should not exceed 450 mg/L and the infusion should be administered using an inline filter of 0.45 microns or less. The IV dosage should be reduced with renal or liver disease, but specific guidelines are not available. The ophthalmic ointment (0.5 inch or 1 cm ribbon) is placed into the lower conjunctival sac every 3 hr (5 times/day) for herpes keratoconjunctivitis.[245,246] Available as 30 mg/g ophthalmic ointment and a 200 mg/ml solution for IV injection.

Zidovudine   Retrovir®

Zidovudine (formerly azidothymidine, AZT) is a synthetic thymidine analogue which inhibits DNA synthesis in the human immunodeficiency virus (HIV). Zidovudine is incorporated into viral DNA by intracellular DNA polymerase (reverse transcriptase). HIV reverse transcriptase is about 100 times more susceptible to zidovudine than human DNA polymerase. Zidovudine is about 50% absorbed from the GI tract. Hepatic metabolism and renal excretion both contribute to an elimination half-life of about 1 hr. Adverse effects include severe anemia due to marrow suppression in 50% of AIDS patients and granulocytopenia or thrombocytopenia necessitating discontinuation of therapy in 5% of patients. Headache is also a frequent complaint. In a controlled trial, zidovudine was significantly more effective than placebo in preventing mortality among patients with AIDS or ARC. Patients taking the drug gained more weight and had fewer opportunistic infections than those on placebo. Dosage is PO 200 mg q 4 hr. This should be reduced if anemia develops, but efficacy of the lower doses is not established.[247] Available as 100 mg capsules.

8:22 QUINOLONES

General References: 248

Ciprofloxacin

Cipro®

Pharmacology. Ciprofloxacin is a fluoroquinolone that differs from older quinolones (eg, nalidixic acid) in its potent activity against many Gram-positive and Gram-negative bacteria. Its mechanism of action involves inhibition of bacterial DNA-gyrase, an enzyme responsible for the unwinding of DNA for transcription and subsequent supercoiling of DNA for packaging into chromosomal subunits. It is highly active against *Enterobacteriaceae*, with MICs often less than 0.1 mcg/ml. It is also very active against many strains of *Pseudomonas aeruginosa* and *Staphylococcus* sp. with a MIC_{90} of 0.5–1 mcg/ml. It has poor activity against streptococci and anaerobes.[210]

Administration and Adult Dose. PO 250–750 mg q 12 hr.

Dosage Individualization. Reduce dose by one-half or double the dosing interval when Cl_{cr} is less than 30 ml/min; special dosage adjustment in patients with cystic fibrosis and the elderly is not necessary.[249]

Pediatric Dose. Not recommended.

Dosage Forms. See Fluoroquinolones Comparison Chart.

Patient Instructions. This drug may be taken with food to minimize stomach upset. Avoid antacid use during treatment with ciprofloxacin.

Pharmacokinetics. *Fate.* Approximately 70% absorbed orally; food decreases the rate, but not extent of absorption; antacids significantly decrease the extent of absorption.[248-250] Peak plasma concentrations are 2.6–3 mcg/ml following a 750 mg oral dose; a 200 mg IV dose infused over 30 min results in a peak concentration of about 3.2 mcg/ml.[249] V_d averages 2 L/kg.[249,251] Less than 30% plasma protein bound.[249] Ciprofloxacin attains very high concentrations in many body fluids and tissues, most notably urine, prostate and pulmonary mucosa. CSF concentrations are less than 1 mcg/ml; experience with the drug in the treatment of meningitis is very limited. 45–60% of a parenteral dose is recovered unchanged in urine; the remainder is excreted as four metabolites or eliminated in feces.[248,249]

$t_{1/2}$. 3.5–5 hr; 5–13 hr in severe renal failure.[249]

Adverse Reactions. GI intolerance (nausea, vomiting, diarrhea, abdominal discomfort) and CNS effects (usually limited to mild dizziness, restlessness and headaches) and skin rashes occur occasionally.[248,252]

Precautions. Pregnancy; children. Magnesium- and aluminum-containing antacids markedly reduce oral absorption. Theophylline clearance may be slightly reduced in some patients receiving ciprofloxacin.[211] Probenecid may increase ciprofloxacin plasma levels. The solubility of ciprofloxacin is reduced at higher pH values; thus, alkalinization of the urine should be avoided.

Parameters to Monitor. Monitor plasma theophylline levels closely in patients receiving a theophylline-containing preparation.

Norfloxacin

Noroxin®

Norfloxacin, a fluoroquinolone antibiotic, is generally less active against bacteria than ciprofloxacin. Peak plasma levels following the maximum recommended oral doses of 400 mg are 1.4–1.6 mcg/ml, with a half-life of

3-4 hr. Unlike ciprofloxacin, use of norfloxacin is limited to the treatment or prophylaxis of infections in the genitourinary or GI tracts. The usual dose is 400 mg bid; with a Cl_{cr} less than 30 ml/min, the dose is 400 mg once daily.[248,249] Available as 400 mg tablets. See Fluoroquinolones Comparison Chart.

Fluoroquinolones Comparison Chart[a]

DRUG	DOSAGE FORMS	ADULT DOSE	ORAL BIO-AVAILABILITY (PERCENT)	PEAK PLASMA LEVELS (MCG/ML) [b]	PERCENT PROTEIN BOUND	HALF-LIFE (HOURS) NORMAL	HALF-LIFE (HOURS) ANURIC	PERCENT EXCRETED UNCHANGED IN URINE
Ciprofloxacin Cipro®	Tab 250, 500, 750 mg.	PO 250–750 mg q 12 hr.	60–80	2.6–3 (PO 750 mg)	30[c]	3.5–5	5–13	40–60
Enoxacin Comprecin® (Investigational - Warner-Lambert)	—	PO or IV 200–800 mg q 12 hr.	79–90	3.7–4.2 (PO 600 mg)	18	4–6	↑	40
Fleroxacin (Investigational - Roche)	—	—	—	5.6 (PO 400 mg)	27	12	↑	59
Norfloxacin Noroxin®	Tab 400 mg.	PO 200–400 mg q 12 hr.	75 (estimated)	1.4–1.6 (PO 400 mg)	15	3–7	3–9	30
Ofloxacin (Investigational - Ortho)	—	—	81–94	6.7–8.1 (PO 600 mg)	30[c]	3.5–5.5	10–50	90
Pefloxacin (Investigational - Rhone-Poulenc)	—	—	>90	3.3–4.1 (PO 400 mg)	30[c]	8–12	11–15	10–15

a. From references 248–251, 253.
b. Peak plasma concentrations following administration of the dose shown in parentheses.
c. Percent protein bound value is an approximation.

8:24 SULFONAMIDES

General References: 254, 255

Sulfamethoxazole and Trimethoprim

Bactrim®, Septra®, Various

Pharmacology. A combination which provides sequential and synergistic inhibition of bacterial folate synthesis. Sulfamethoxazole (SMZ) acts similarly to other sulfonamides (see Sulfisoxazole) while trimethoprim (TMP) acts at a later step to inhibit the enzymatic reduction of dihydrofolic acid to tetrahydrofolic acid. TMP binds selectively to bacterial dihydrofolic acid reductase (50,000 times more avidly than to the comparable human enzyme). The combination is active against many bacteria except anaerobes, *Ps. aeruginosa* and many *S. faecalis*. It is also highly active and effective against the protozoa, *Pneumocystis carinii*. The most important determinant of efficacy is usually the level of susceptibility to TMP. The basic mechanisms of resistance to SMZ and TMP are similar to sulfisoxazole, although resistance is very uncommon with the combination.[254,255]

Administration and Adult Dose. PO for UTI 800 mg of SMZ and 160 mg of TMP q 12 hr for 10–14 days. **PO for prophylaxis of recurrent UTI** 200 mg of SMZ and 40 mg of TMP at bedtime 3 times weekly.[254] **PO for shigellosis** 800 mg of SMZ and 160 mg of TMP q 12 hr for 5 days.[255] **IV for severe Gram-negative infections or shigellosis** 40–50 mg/kg/day of SMZ and 8–10 mg/kg/day of TMP, in 2–4 equally divided doses, q 6–12 hr for 5 days for shigellosis and up to 14 days for severe UTI. **PO or IV for** *Pneumocystis carinii* **pneumonia** 100 (PO) or 75 (IV) mg/kg/day of SMZ and 20 (PO) or 15 (IV) mg/kg/day of TMP, in 2–4 equally divided doses, for up to 14 days.[256] **PO for** *Pneumocystis carinii* **infection prophylaxis** 20 mg/kg/day of SMZ and 4 mg/kg/day of TMP in 2 equally divided doses.[254,255] See Notes.

Dosage Individualization. Dosage should be reduced in patients with severe renal impairment. No dosage adjustment is necessary for patients with Cl_{cr} greater than 30 ml/min.[254,255,257] For UTI in patients with Cl_{cr} less than 30 ml/min, give normal dosage for 1–6 doses. For patients with Cl_{cr} between 10–30 ml/min, follow with ½ usual dose; with Cl_{cr} less than 10 ml/min, follow with ¼–½ usual dose,[254,255] although this probably does not produce effective urinary concentrations, and some authorities advocate full dosage.[258] For systemic infections treated with higher doses, monitor plasma levels.

Pediatric Dose. PO for UTI or shigellosis (2 months–12 yr) 40 mg/kg/day of SMZ and 8 mg/kg/day of TMP (Susp 1 ml/kg/day) in 2 equally divided doses; (over 12 yr) same as adult dose; **PO for otitis media** same as UTI. **IV for severe Gram-negative infection or shigellosis** (2 months and over) same as adult mg/kg dose. **PO or IV for** *Pneumocystis carinii* **pneumonia** (2 months and over) same as adult mg/kg dose. **PO for** *Pneumocystis carinii* **infection prophylaxis** (2 months and over) same as adult mg/kg dose.

Dosage Forms. Susp 40 mg/ml of SMZ and 8 mg/ml of TMP; Tab 400 mg of SMZ and 80 mg of TMP, 800 mg of SMZ and 160 mg of TMP; Inj 80 mg/ml of SMZ and 16 mg/ml of TMP.

Patient Instructions. This medication should be taken with a full 8 ounce glass of water on an empty stomach (1 hr before or 2 hr after meals) for best absorption. Drink several additional glasses of water daily, unless directed otherwise.

Pharmacokinetics. *Plasma Levels.* Trimethoprim levels above 5 mcg/ml may be required in *P. carinii* pneumonia.[256]

Fate. SMZ and TMP are 90-100% absorbed orally.[259] In normal adults, peak plasma concentrations of 20-50 mcg/ml of SMZ and 0.9-1.9 mcg/ml of TMP occur about 1-4 hr after administration of 800 mg of SMZ and 160 mg of TMP.[259] An additional 10-20 mcg/ml of SMZ exists in the plasma as inactive metabolites.[257] IV infusion over 1 hr of 800 mg of SMZ and 160 mg of TMP in adults produces peak plasma levels of 46.3 mcg/ml of SMZ and 3.4 mcg/ml of TMP.[260] SMZ and TMP are widely distributed in the body, although TMP is much more widely distributed due to its higher lipophilicity; TMP is 45% plasma protein bound and has a V_d of 1-2 L/kg.[259] SMZ has a V_d of 0.36 L/kg and is 60% plasma protein bound.[254,259] TMP concentrations in various tissues and fluids (including the prostate, bile and sputum) are several times greater than concomitant plasma concentrations. CSF concentrations in normal adults are approximately 50% of plasma concentrations. SMZ usually appears in much lower concentrations in body tissues and fluids.[254,259,260] SMZ undergoes extensive liver metabolism, producing N^4-acetylated and N^4-glucuronidated derivatives; 85% is excreted in the urine within 24-72 hr, 10-30% as unchanged drug. Nearly all TMP is excreted in the urine within 24-72 hr, 50-75% as unchanged drug. The pharmacokinetics of these drugs are essentially unchanged when given in combination.[257,259] The pH of the urine influences renal excretion of these compounds, but does not significantly alter overall elimination.[255,257]

$t_{1/2}$. Approximately 8-11 hr (average 9) for SMZ in normal adults; 6-15 hr for TMP in normal adults.[254,255,260] Increased in the presence of severe renal failure (20-30 hr or more) for TMP; 18-24 hr for SMZ in anuria.

Adverse Reactions. Blood dyscrasias (primarily thrombocytopenia, leukopenia, megaloblastic anemia and hemolytic anemia in patients with G-6-PD deficiency) have been reported in association with SMZ and TMP, although they are probably no more common than with SMZ alone.[254,255] In usual doses, TMP does not affect plasma folate levels as determined by radioisotopic techniques,[261] although effects on folate metabolism may be more significant in patients with pre-existing folate depletion (eg, alcoholics, the elderly, pregnant or malnourished patients).[254] Calcium leucovorin reverses antifolate effects without interfering with antimicrobial action.[254,256] It appears that SMZ and TMP compete for tubular excretion with creatinine and reduce the Cl_{cr} in some patients, although glomerular filtration is maintained.[262] May cause jaundice and kernicterus in neonates, and rashes and other hypersensitivity reactions similar to those caused by other sulfonamides.[254,255] In patients with AIDS, adverse effects unrelated to folate suppression such as fever, rash, and leukopenia, as well as thrombocytopenia, occur frequently.[263]

Contraindications. Pregnancy; infants under 2 months; megaloblastic anemia due to folate deficiency.

Precautions. Lactation; history of hypersensitivity reaction to sulfonamide derivatives; G-6-PD deficiency; impaired renal or hepatic function.

Parameters to Monitor. Baseline and periodic CBC for patients on long-term or high-dose treatment.

Notes. The efficacy and safety of SMZ and TMP has been demonstrated in numerous other infectious conditions (eg, chronic UTI, chronic bronchitis, sepsis, enteric fever, prostatitis, endocarditis, meningitis and gonorrhea) and is considered an effective alternative to conventional therapy in most cases.[254,255,264] Efficacy of SMZ and TMP in the treatment of *Pneumocystis carinii* pneumonitis is equivalent to pentamidine which makes the combination the therapy of choice due to its increased safety.[254,256] However, the combination appears to be more toxic than pentamidine in patients with AIDS.[263] SMZ is available as a single agent (Gantanol® **Susp** 100 mg/ml; **Tab** 500 mg) and is similar to sulfisoxazole in effectiveness. TMP is available as a single agent (Trimpex® **Tab** 100 mg) and has been shown to be effective in acute UTI.[265,266] It has a potential advantage in patients with allergy or toxicity attributed to the sulfonamide;[265,267] however, the relative potential for the single agent to permit the development of resistance is unsettled.[268]

Sulfasalazine

Azulfidine®, Various

Pharmacology. Sulfasalazine (SS) is a conjugate of sulfapyridine (SP) and 5-aminosalicylic acid (5-ASA). 5-ASA has anti-inflammatory activity which includes potent inhibition of prostaglandin synthesis; this probably accounts for the usefulness of SS in inflammatory bowel disease. SP does not contribute to the anti-inflammatory effect of SS.[269]

Administration and Adult Dose. PO for initial therapy of inflammatory bowel disease 3–4 g/day in equally divided doses. Starting with doses of 1–2 g/day may decrease GI side effects. PO for maintenance therapy 2 g/day in divided doses. Doses up to 8 g/day have been used, but doses over 4 g/day are associated with increased frequency of side effects. Regimens for desensitization of allergic patients have also been reported.[269]

Pediatric Dose. (Under 2 yr) not recommended; (over 2 yr) PO for initial therapy of inflammatory bowel disease 40–60 mg/kg/day in 4 equally divided doses. PO for maintenance therapy 30 mg/kg/day in 4 equally divided doses.

Dosage Forms. EC Tab 500 mg; Susp 250 mg/5 ml; Tab 500 mg.

Patient Instructions. Take each dose after meals or with food, and drink at least 1 full glass of water with each dose; drink several additional glasses of water daily. This medication must be taken continually to be effective. Report any nausea, vomiting, excessive change in appetite, abrupt change in character or volume of stools, or skin rashes.

Pharmacokinetics. *Onset and Duration.* Maximum effect in 1–2 weeks; duration 8–12 hr following a dose.

Plasma Levels. Sulfapyridine levels over 50 mcg/ml are associated with increased toxicity and are most likely in slow acetylators.[270-272] Therapeutic effect is related to 5-ASA levels in the bowel.[269]

Fate. SS is about 30% absorbed from the small intestine, but is almost completely secreted unchanged in the bile.[273] It is then metabolized in the large bowel, probably by intestinal bacteria, to SP and 5-ASA. Most of SP is absorbed from the colon, metabolized by the liver and excreted in the urine; slow acetylators have higher plasma SP concentrations. 5-ASA is eliminated in the feces. After an oral dose of SS, about 91% of SP is recovered in the urine in 3 days as SP, SP metabolites and small amounts of SS.[273,274]

$t_{1/2}$. (SP) 5–13 hr, depending on acetylator phenotype.[269]

Adverse Reactions. Anorexia, nausea, vomiting, epigastric pain and headache occur frequently, especially with high doses and plasma SP levels;[270,271,274,276] reversible oligospermia occurs frequently in males.[275] Skin rash is reported occasionally; hemolytic anemia and leukopenia occur rarely. Impairment of dietary folate absorption has been reported.[277]

Contraindications. Intestinal tract obstruction; history of sulfonamide or salicylate allergy; porphyria.

Precautions. Pregnancy (despite promising reports of safety).[278] Use with caution in renal impairment, slow acetylators or G-6-PD deficiency.

Parameters to Monitor. Observe patient for therapeutic response (decrease in crampy diarrhea) and toxicity (headache, anorexia, epigastric pain, nausea). Obtain baseline and periodic WBC and reticulocyte counts. Plasma SP levels may be useful in monitoring for toxicity.[270,271,274]

Notes. Sulfasalazine, often in combination with an oral and/or rectal corticosteroid, is most effective in ulcerative colitis with a lower degree of efficacy in Crohn's disease.[269] Occasionally the enteric coated tablet may appear whole in the stool; if this occurs, the patient should be switched to the uncoated form. A number of preparations of 5-ASA (**mesalamine**) have been formulated to deliver the drug to the large bowel, avoiding systemic absorption.[279] Mesalamine is available as a 4 g/60 ml enema (Rowasa®) useful for distal ulcerative colitis in a maintenance dose of 4 g/day rectally at bedtime.

Sulfisoxazole and Salts   Gantrisin®, Various

Pharmacology. A synthetic analogue of para-aminobenzoic acid (PABA) which competitively inhibits the synthesis of dihydropteric acid (an inactive folic acid precursor) from PABA in micro-organisms. Bacteriostatic against many bacteria, although acquired resistance has narrowed the indications primarily to lower UTI. Resistance can occur due to bacterial mutation which reduces the affinity of the folic acid synthesizing enzyme for sulfonamide or which increases bacterial production of PABA. Resistance also results from decreased cell permeability, which may be R-factor mediated and transferred among microbial populations.[15]

Administration and Adult Dose. PO (as sulfisoxazole or sulfisoxazole acetyl) 4–8 g/day in 4–6 divided doses; **Vag** 250–500 mg (2.5–5 g of **Crm** 10%) bid. **Ophth Soln** 1–2 drops to affected eye q 2–3 hr; **Ophth Oint** small amount to affected eye 1–3 times/day and hs.

Dosage Individualization. Most sources recommend that the dosing interval be extended to 18–24 hr[135,280] or that the drug be avoided[281] in patients with severely impaired renal function. However, the degree of accumulation and risk of toxicity is probably quite small, and full doses may be necessary to achieve therapeutic levels in the urinary tract.[135]

Pediatric Dose. PO (over 2 months) (as sulfisoxazole or sulfisoxazole acetyl) 150 mg/kg/day in 4–6 equally divided doses; **PO** do not exceed 6 g/day. **Ophth Soln** 1–2 drops to affected eye q 2–3 hr; **Ophth Oint** small amount to affected eye 1–3 times/day and hs.

Dosage Forms. **Susp** (as acetyl) 100 mg/ml; **Syrup** (as acetyl) 100 mg/ml; **Tab** 500 mg; **Ophth Oint** (as diolamine) 4%; **Ophth Soln** (as diolamine) 4%; **Vag Crm** 10%.

Patient Instructions. Oral forms should be taken with a full 8 ounce glass of water on an empty stomach (1 hr before or 2 hr after meals) for best absorption. Drink several additional glasses of water daily, unless directed otherwise.

Pharmacokinetics. *Fate.* Nearly 100% absorbed orally, with peak plasma concentrations of approximately 10–15 mcg/ml at 2–4 hr after a 2 g dose.[281-283] Sulfisoxazole acetyl form is deacetylated in the GI tract and absorbed as free sulfisoxazole; it produces a delayed and lower peak plasma concentration.[282] V_d is 0.16 L/kg; about 85–90% plasma protein bound.[283] Distribution is largely restricted to extracellular space, with low concentrations in many tissues and fluids; CSF concentrations equal 10–50% of plasma concentrations; fetal plasma concentrations equal 50% of maternal concentrations.[15,282] Extensive liver metabolism to N^4-acetylated derivative. Approximately 95% of a single dose is excreted in the urine within 24 hr, 40–60% as unchanged active drug.[15,281-283]

$t_{1/2}$. In normal adults 5–7 hr (average 6); approximately 11 hr with severe renal impairment.[15,135,281] Alkalinization of the urine decreases the half-life to 4.4 hr in normal adults.[281]

Adverse Reactions.   Reactions are infrequent, but include blood dyscrasias (primarily thrombocytopenia and leukopenia and hemolytic anemia in patients with G-6-PD deficiency) and hypersensitivity reactions. Jaundice and kernicterus can occur in neonates due to displacement of bilirubin from albumin binding sites. Nephrotoxicity due to crystalluria is unlikely due to the high solubility of sulfisoxazole, although in patients with renal failure the accumulation of the less soluble acetylated metabolite may increase this risk.[15,281,282]

Contraindications.   Pregnancy at term; lactation; infants under 2 months.

Precautions.   Pregnancy; history of hypersensitivity reaction to sulfonamide derivatives; G-6-PD deficiency; impaired renal or hepatic function.

Parameters to Monitor.   Baseline and periodic CBC and urinalysis for patients on long-term or high-dose treatment.

Notes.   Drug of choice in acute, uncomplicated UTI in females; development of resistance limits its usefulness in the treatment of recurrent or persistent infections.

8:36 URINARY ANTI-INFECTIVES

Methenamine Hippurate   Hiprex®, Urex®
Methenamine Mandelate   Mandelamine®

Methenamine is converted to ammonia and formaldehyde in acidic urine (pH < 6) and is, therefore, a weak urinary antiseptic. These drugs are used primarily for prevention of recurrent UTI, but more effective agents (eg, sulfamethoxazole-trimethoprim) are available. Adverse effects are primarily GI distress and occasional skin rash. Moderate to severe renal insufficiency precludes the use of methenamine, because inadequate concentrations are achieved in urine. PO dosage is 1 g bid as hippurate or 1 g qid as mandelate. Pediatric dose is one-half of adult dose. Patients must usually take at least 4 g/day of ascorbic acid to adequately acidify urine, but this may not be effective due to patient's diet and/or presence of urea-splitting organisms (eg, *Proteus* sp).[284-287] Available as (hippurate) 1 g tablet; (mandelate) 500 mg, 1 g packets of granules; 250, 500 mg/5 ml suspension; and 250, 500 mg, 1 g tablets.

Nitrofurantoin   Furadantin®, Macrodantin®,
                                                    Various

Nitrofurantoin is active against most bacteria which cause urinary tract infections, except *Pseudomonas aeruginosa* and most *Proteus* sp. The drug is used primarily to prevent recurrent UTI, but is also effective in the treatment of uncomplicated UTI. Plasma and extra-urinary tissue concentrations are subtherapeutic. Adverse effects are primarily GI upset and are dose-related; use of macrocrystalline form and administration with food may minimize GI distress. Hypersensitivity reactions, such as rash, occur only rarely. Acute allergic pneumonitis is reversible with discontinuation of therapy. Chronic interstitial pulmonary fibrosis also occurs occasionally and may be irreversible. Ascending polyneuropathy associated with prolonged high-dose therapy or use of the drug in renal failure is only slowly reversible. Intravascular hemolysis may occur in patients with severe G-6-PD deficiency. Although mutagenic in mammalian cells, there is no clinical evidence of carcinogenicity or teratogenicity. Adult dose is usually PO 50–100 mg tid-qid or PO 50–100 mg at bedtime for chronic suppression.[288-291] Pediatric dose is 5–7 mg/kg/day in 4 divided doses. Available as 25, 50, 100 mg capsules; 5 mg/ml suspension and 50, 100 mg tablets.

8:40 MISCELLANEOUS ANTI-INFECTIVES

Clofazimine   Lamprene®

Clofazimine is a phenazine dye approved for treating leprosy and used in atypical *Mycobacterium* infections. The drug is about 50% bioavailable; it accumulates in fatty tissues and the reticuloendothelial system and is eliminated with a half-life of about 70 days. Bodily secretions, skin, conjunctivae, urine and feces, may turn red to brownish black; skin discoloration may take months to years to disappear after stopping the drug. Dose-related GI pain, nausea, vomiting and diarrhea may occur due to crystalline deposits in GI tissue. Eosinophilic enteritis and anticholinergic symptoms may also occur. The usual dose is 100 mg/day with food for leprosy and *M. avium* complex infections; doses up to 200 mg/day are used for erythema nodosum leprosum.[310,311] Available as 50 and 100 mg capsules.

Metronidazole   Flagyl®

Pharmacology. A nitroimidazole with activity against *T. vaginalis* (trichomoniasis), *E. histolytica* (amebiasis) and *Giardia lamblia* (giardiasis), and is bactericidal against nearly all obligate anaerobic bacteria, including *Bacteroides fragilis*. It is essentially inactive against aerobic and microaerophilic bacteria. Reduced by a nitroreductase enzyme within sensitive organisms to highly reactive intermediates which disrupt DNA and inhibit nucleic acid synthesis.

Administration and Adult Dose. **PO for trichomoniasis** 2 g as a single dose or in 2 doses in the same day, or 500 mg bid for 5 days, or 250 mg tid for 7 days.[292,293] **PO for symptomatic intestinal amebiasis (amebic dysentery)** 750 mg tid for 5–10 days. **PO for extraintestinal amebiasis** 750 mg tid for 5–10 days;[292] some practitioners include a drug effective against the intestinal cyst form, because occasional failures with metronidazole therapy have been reported — see Notes. **PO or IV for anaerobic infections** 15 mg/kg (usually 1 g) initially, followed by 7.5 mg/kg (usually 500 mg) q 6 hr to maximum of 4 g/day. Infuse each IV dose over 1 hr. **PO for giardiasis** 250 mg bid-tid for 7–10 days or 2 g/day as a single dose for 3 days;[292,294] see Notes. **PO for "nonspecific" vaginitis due to G. vaginalis** 500 mg bid for 7 days.[294] **PO for antibiotic-associated colitis** 250–500 mg tid-qid for 7–10 days.[193]

Dosage Individualization. Dose is not altered with impaired renal function.[294,295] Patients with severe hepatic disease metabolize metronidazole slowly, with resultant accumulation of metronidazole and its metabolites in the plasma. For such patients, doses below those usually recommended should be administered cautiously, although specific guidelines are not available; close monitoring of plasma metronidazole levels as well as signs of toxicity is recommended.

Pediatric Dose. **PO for amebic dysentery or extraintestinal amebiasis** 35–50 mg/kg/day in 3 divided doses for 5–10 days, to maximum of 2.4 g/day. **PO for giardiasis** 25 mg/kg/day in 2–3 divided doses for 7–10 days, to maximum of 750 mg/day.[297] See Notes.

Dosage Forms. **Tab** 250, 500 mg; **Inj** 500 mg.

Patient Instructions. This drug may be taken with food to minimize stomach upset. It may occasionally cause a harmless dark coloration of the urine and metallic taste in mouth. Nausea, vomiting, flushing and faintness may occur if alcohol is taken during therapy with this drug.

Pharmacokinetics. *Fate.* Very well absorbed orally, with 250 and 500 mg producing peak concentrations of 5 and 12 mcg/ml, respectively, at 1–2 hr in adults.[293,298] IV infusions over 1 hr produce plasma levels similar to those seen after equivalent PO doses. IV 7.5 mg/kg q 6 hr produces steady-state peak and trough levels of 24 and 19 mcg/ml, respectively.[292] V_d is 0.6–0.8 L/kg (ie, about equal to total body water); 10–20% plasma protein bound;[293] wide distribution with therapeutic levels in many tissues, including abscesses, bile, bone and CSF.[294,299] Extensively metabolized in the liver by hydroxylation, oxidation and glucuronide formation; 44–80% excreted in the urine in 24 hr, about 8–20% as unchanged drug.[293,300]

$t_{1/2}$. 6–8 hr in adults;[293,298,300] not increased with impaired renal function;[294] prolonged variably with severe hepatic impairment.

Adverse Effects. Metallic taste in mouth and GI complaints may be frequent with high doses. Occasional dizziness, vertigo and paresthesias have been reported with very high doses. Reversible mild neutropenia reported occasionally.[292,294,295,301] Reversible, rare, but severe peripheral neuropathy may occur with high doses given over prolonged periods. Antibiotic-associated colitis has been reported rarely with oral metronidazole.[302,303] The IV preparation is associated occasionally with phlebitis at the infusion site. Experimental production of tumors in some rodent species and mutations in bacteria have raised serious concern regarding potential carcinogenicity; to date, mammalian testing and human epidemiologic research have not detected a significant risk, although further data are needed.[294,301]

Contraindications. First trimester of pregnancy, although there is no direct evidence of teratogenicity in humans or animals.[292,294]

Precautions. Pregnancy; active CNS disease or neutropenia.

Parameters to Monitor. Before and after the completion of any lengthy or repeated courses of therapy, monitor WBC count.[294]

Notes. Therapy of amebiasis with metronidazole alone is somewhat controversial. For *asymptomatic* patients passing cyst forms of the parasite, metronidazole is not useful; **PO iodoquinol** 650 mg tid for 20 days has been effective in only 60–70% of such cases; and **PO diloxanide furoate** (Furamide®) 500 mg tid for 10 days is 80–85% effective — see Immunobiologics and Drugs Distributed by CDC, Table 1, page 312. For *symptomatic* patients with amebic dysentery or extra-intestinal amebiasis, **IM emetine hydrochloride** 1 mg/kg/day in 1–2 divided doses for 7 days, to maximum of 60 mg/day has been successful, usually in combination with **PO chloroquine phosphate** 10 mg/kg/day in 2 divided doses for 2–3 weeks, to maximum of 500 mg/day. **IM or SC dehydroemetine** 1–1.5 mg/kg/day for 10 days appears to be as effective as emetine and may have less cardiac toxicity[296] — see Immunobiologics and Drugs Distributed by CDC, Table 1, page 312.

The treatment of *asymptomatic* trichomoniasis is controversial. Signs of endocervical inflammation or erosion on physical exam are considered an indication for treatment. Also, most practitioners choose to treat asymptomatic male consorts, because lack of such treatment may be a cause of treatment failure or recurrent infection of the female partner.[292,294,301]

For the treatment of giardiasis, metronidazole appears to be about as effective as **PO quinacrine hydrochloride** (Atabrine®) 100 mg tid for 7 days.[294] Metronidazole has also been effective in chronic and active Crohn's disease and in Crohn's patients with refractory perineal disease.[312]

Proper reconstitution of the IV preparation is important. IV metronidazole reacts with aluminum; aluminum needles should not be used. First, reconstitute with 4.4 ml of sterile water (preserved or nonpreserved). Then dilute dose in normal saline, D5W or lactated Ringer's to a final concentration of no more than 8 mg/ml. Finally, neutralize with 5 mEq of sodium bicarbonate for each 500 mg of drug. Do not refrigerate neutralized solution. Also available as prepared, stabilized solution (Flagyl I.V. RTU® or metronidazole Redi-Infusion®).

Pentamidine Isethionate   Pentam–300®

Pharmacology. Pentamidine is an aromatic diamidine used in the treatment of trypanosomiasis and *Pneumocystis carinii* pneumonia. The mechanism by which pentamidine kills *P. carinii* is unclear, but may be inhibition of dihydrofolate reductase or glucose metabolism.[304]

Administration and Adult Dose. IV (preferred) or IM 4 mg/kg/day as a single dose for 2–3 weeks; infuse IV over 60 min. **Inhal for *P. carinii* pneumonia** (investigational) 600 mg in 6 ml sterile water via special nebulizer daily (usually only 200–400 mg is actually inhaled) for treatment; used less frequently for prophylaxis, but optimal dosage and duration are not established.[311] See Notes.

Dosage Individualization. Dosage adjustment does not appear to be necessary in renal impairment.

Pediatric Dose. Same as adult dose.

Dosage Forms. Inj (as isethionate) 300 mg.

Pharmacokinetics. *Plasma Levels.* No clinical correlations with plasma levels are known.

Fate. Peak plasma levels of 0.5–3 mcg/ml have been observed after 4 mg/kg IV infusion. Widespread distribution into tissues with highest concentrations found in spleen, liver, kidneys and adrenals.[305] Less than 10% of a dose is excreted unchanged in urine.

$t_{1/2}$. 15–20 min for plasma elimination, but urinary excretion half-life is 5.1 days. This suggests rapid tissue uptake with slow release and subsequent urinary excretion. No data on effects of renal or liver impairment.

Adverse Reactions. Nephrotoxicity in up to 24% of patients and hypoglycemia (at least 5–10%) occur frequently. Fever, rash, leukopenia and liver damage also occur occasionally. Hyperglycemia and insulin-dependent diabetes mellitus have been reported. IM injection frequently produces pain and abscess formation at the injection site.[306-308] Hypotension, especially with IV administration, occurs occasionally.

Precautions. Use with caution in diabetes mellitus.

Parameters to Monitor. Obtain serum glucose, Cr_s, BUN, liver function tests, electrolytes, CBC and platelet count daily. Monitor blood pressure after administration.

Notes. Solutions in 5% dextrose are stable at room temperature for 24 hr at concentrations of 1–2.5 mg/ml. Although trimethoprim-sulfamethoxazole is believed to be the therapy of choice for *P. carinii* pneumonia, the high frequency of adverse effects in patients with AIDS leads some authorities to prefer pentamidine.[306,307] Concomitant therapy with both pentamidine and trimethoprim-sulfamethoxazole appears to offer no clinical benefit and may be additively toxic.[309]

References, 8:00 Anti-Infective Agents

1. Marr JJ. Antiparasitic agents. In: Mandell GL, Douglas RG, Bennett JE, eds. Principles and practice of infectious diseases, 2nd ed. New York. John Wiley and Sons. 1985:286-301.

2. Pratt WB, Fekety R. Chemotherapy of helminthic diseases. In: The antimicrobial drugs. New York. Oxford University Press. 1986:414-48.

3. Brandt JRA, Kumar V, Geerts S. Praziquantel. In: Peterson PK, Verhoef J, eds. The antimicrobial agents annual 1. Amsterdam. Elsevier. 1986:287-94.

4. Brugmans JP, Thienpont DC, van Wijngaarden I et al. Mebendazole in enterobiasis: radiochemical and pilot clinical study in 1,278 subjects. JAMA 1971;217:313-6.

5. Miller MJ, Krupp IM, Little MD et al. Mebendazole: an effective anthelmintic for trichuriasis and enterobiasis. JAMA 1974;230:1412-4.

6. Wolfe MS, Wershing JM. Mebendazole: treatment of trichuriasis and ascariasis in Bahamian children. JAMA 1974;230:1408-11.

7. Chavarria AP, Swartzwelder JC, Villarejos VM et al. Mebendazole, an effective broad-spectrum anthelmintic. Am J Trop Med Hyg 1973;22:592-5.

8. Sargent RG, Savory AM, Mina A et al. A clinical evaluation of mebendazole in the treatment of trichuriasis. Am J Trop Med Hyg 1974;23:375-7.

9. Hanna S, Tang A. Human urinary excretion of piperazine citrate from syrup formulations. J. Pharm Sci 1973;62:2024-5.

10. Parsons AC. Piperazine neurotoxicity: ''worm wobble.'' Br Med J 1971;4:792.

11. Goodwin LG, Standen OD. Treatment of ascariasis with various salts of piperazine. Br Med J 1958;1:131-3.

12. Rogers EW. Excretion of piperazine salts in urine. Br Med J 1958;1:136-7.

13. Pitts NE, Migliardi JR. Antiminth (pyrantel pamoate): the clinical evaluation of a new broad-spectrum anthelmintic. Clin Pediatr 1974;13:87-94.

14. Bumbalo TS, Fugazzotto DJ, Wyczalek JV. Treatment of enterobiasis with pyrantel pamoate. Am J Trop Med Hyg 1969;18:50-2.

15. Mandell GL, Douglas RG, Bennett JE, eds. Principles and practice of infectious diseases. 2nd ed. New York: John Wiley & Sons, 1985.

16. DeTorres OH. A closer look at aminoglycosides. Clin Ther 1981;3:399-412.

17. Medeiros AA, O'Brien TF, Wacker WEC et al. Effect of salt concentration on the apparent in vitro susceptibility of Pseudomonas and other gram-negative bacilli to gentamicin. J Infect Dis 1971;124(Suppl.):S59-64.

18. Eliopoulos GM, Moellering RC Jr. In: Remington JS, Swartz MN (eds). A critical comparison of new aminoglycosidic aminocyclitol antibiotics. Current Clinical Topics in Infectious Diseases, vol IV. New York: McGraw-Hill, 1983.

19. Mayer KH. Review of epidemic aminoglycoside resistance worldwide. Am J Med 1986;80:(Suppl. 6B):56-64.

20. Young LS, Hindler J. Aminoglycoside resistance: a worldwide perspective. Am J Med 1986;80(Suppl. 6B):15-21.

21. Pechere J-O, Dugal R. Clinical pharmacokinetics of aminoglycoside antibiotics. Clin Pharmacokinet 1979;4:170-99.

22. Zinner SH, Dudley MN, Blaser J. In vitro models for the study of combination therapy in neutropenic patients. Am J Med 1986;80(Suppl. 6B):156-60.

23. Powell SH, Thompson WL, Luthe MA et al. Once-daily vs. continuous aminoglycoside dosing: efficacy and toxicity in animal and clinical studies of gentamicin, netilmicin, and tobramycin. J Infect Dis 1983;147:918-32.

24. Bauer LA, Blouin RA, Griffen WO et al. Amikacin pharmacokinetics in morbidly obese patients. Am J Hosp Pharm 1980;37:519-22.

25. Yee GC, Evans WB. Reappraisal of guidelines for pharmacokinetic monitoring of aminoglycosides. Pharmacotherapy 1981;1:55-75.

26. Sarubbi FA, Hull JH. Amikacin serum concentrations, prediction of levels and dosage guidelines. Ann Intern Med 1978;89:612-8.

27. Lesar TS, Rotschafer JC, Strand LM et al. Gentamicin dosing errors with 4 commonly used nomograms. JAMA 1982;248:119-23.

28. Walshe JJ, Morse GD, Janicke DM et al. Crossover pharmacokinetic analysis comparing intravenous and intraperitoneal administration of tobramycin. J Infect Dis 1986;153:796-9.

29. Evans WE, Schentag JJ, Jusko WJ, eds. Applied pharmacokinetics: principles of therapeutic drug monitoring, 2nd ed. Spokane, Applied Therapeutics. 1986.

30. Blaser J, Ruttimann, Bhend H et al. Increase in amikacin half-life during treatment of patients with renal insufficiency. Antimicrob Agents Chemother 1983;23:888-91.

31. Moore RD, Smith CR, Lipsky JJ et al. Risk factors for nephrotoxicity in patients treated with aminoglycosides. Ann Intern Med 1984;100:352-7.

32. Sawyers CL, Moore RD, Lerner SA et al. A model for predicting nephrotoxicity in patients treated with aminoglycosides. J Infect Dis 1986;153:1062-8.

33. Evans DA, Buring J, Mayrent S et al. Qualitative overview of randomized trials of aminoglycosides. Am J Med 1986;80(Suppl. 6B):39-43.

34. Moore RD, Smith CR, Leitman PS. Risk factors for the development of auditory toxicity in patients receiving aminoglycosides. J Infect Dis 1984;149:23-30.

35. Green TP, Mirkin BL, Peterson PK et al. Tobramycin serum level monitoring in young patients with normal renal function. Clin Pharmacokinet 1984;9:457-68.

36. Massey KL, Hendeles L, Neims A. Identification of children in which routine aminoglycoside serum concentration monitoring is not cost-effective. J Pediatr 1986;109:897-901.

37. Pickering LK, Rutherford I. Effect of concentration and time upon inactivation of tobramycin, gentamicin, netilmicin, and amikacin by azlocillin, carbenicillin, mecillinam, mezlocillin, and piperacillin. J Pharmacol Exper Ther 1981;217:345-9.

38. Chow MSS, Quintiliani R, Nightingale CH. In vivo inactivation of tobramycin by ticarcillin. JAMA 1982;247:658-9.

39. Moore RD, Leitman PS, Smith CR. Clinical response to aminoglycoside therapy: implication of the ratio of the peak concentration to MIC. J Infect Dis 1987;155:93-9.

40. Medoff G, Kobayashi GS. Strategies in the treatment of systemic fungal infections. N Engl J Med 1980;302:145-55.

41. Bennett JE. Chemotherapy of systemic mycoses. N Engl J Med 1974;290:30-2, 320-3.

42. Graybill JR, Craven PC. Antifungal agents used in systemic mycosis: activity and therapeutic use. Drugs 1983;25:41-62.

43. Maddox MS, Barriere SL. A review of complications of amphotericin-B therapy; recommendations for prevention and management. Drug Intell Clin Pharm 1980;14:177-81.

44. Gotz VP, Mar DD, Roche JJ. Compatibility of amphotericin B with drugs used to reduce adverse reactions. Am J Hosp Pharm 1981;38:378-9.

45. Jurgens RW, DeLuca PP, Papadimitriou D. Compatibility of amphotericin B with certain large-volume parenterals. Am J Hosp Pharm 1981;38:377-8.

46. Hargis JL, Bone RC, Stewart J et al. Intracavitary amphotericin B in the treatment of symptomatic pulmonary aspergillomas. Am J Med 1980;68:389-94.

47. Alazraki NP, Fierer J, Halpern SE et al. Use of a hyperbaric solution for administration of intrathecal amphotericin B. N Engl J Med 1974;290:641-6.

48. Dudley MN, Barriere SL. Antimicrobial irrigations in the prevention and treatment of catheter-related urinary tract infections. Am J Hosp Pharm 1981;38:59-65.

49. Atkinson AJ, Bennett JE. Amphotericin B pharmacokinetics in humans. Antimicrob Agents Chemother 1978;13:271-6.

50. Christiansen KJ, Bernard EM, Gold JWM et al. Distribution and activity of amphotericin B in humans. J Infect Dis 1985;152:1037-43.

51. Burks LC, Aisner J, Fortner CL et al. Meperidine for the treatment of shaking chills and fever. Arch Intern Med 1980;140:483-4.

52. Gross MH, Fulkerson WJ, Moore JO. Prevention of amphotericin B-induced rigors by dantrolene. Arch Intern Med 1986;146:1587-8.

53. Heidemann HT, Gerkens JF, Spickard WA et al. Amphotericin B nephrotoxicity in humans decreased by salt repletion. Am J Med 1983;75:476-81.

54. Tarala RA, Smith JD. Cryptococcosis treated by rapid infusion of amphotericin B. Br Med J 1980;2:28.

55. Wright DG, Robichaud KJ, Pizzo PA et al. Lethal pulmonary reactions associated with the combined use of amphotericin B and leukocyte transfusions. N Engl J Med 1981;304:1185-9.

56. Hoeprich PD. Amphotericin B methyl ester and leukoencephalopathy: the other side of the coin. J Infect Dis 1982;146:173-6.

57. Ellis WG, Sobel RA, Nielsen SL. Leukoencephalopathy in patients treated with amphotericin B methyl ester. J Infect Dis 1982;146:125-37.

58. Lopez-Berestein G, Fainstein V, Hopfer R et al. Liposomal amphotericin B for the treatment of systemic fungal infections in patients with cancer: a preliminary study. J Infect Dis 1985;151:704-10.

59. Steer PL, Marks MI, Klite PD et al. 5-fluorocytosine: an oral antifungal compound. Ann Intern Med 1972;76:15-22.

60. Cutler RE, Blair AD, Kelly MR. Flucytosine kinetics in subjects with normal and impaired renal function. Clin Pharmacol Ther 1978;24:333-42.

61. Bennett JE, Dismukes WE, Duma RJ et al. A comparison of amphotericin B alone and combined with flucytosine in the treatment of cryptococcal meningitis. N Engl J Med 1979;301:126-31.

62. White CA, Traube J. Ulcerating enteritis associated with flucytosine therapy. Gastroenterology 1982;83:1127-9.

63. Horn R, Wong B, Kiehn TE et al. Fungemia in a cancer hospital: changing frequency, earlier onset, and results of therapy. Rev Infect Dis 1985;7:646-55.

64. Goldman L. Griseofulvin. Med Clin North Am 1970;54:1339-45.

65. Epstein WL, Shah V, Riegelman S. Dermatopharmacology of griseofulvin. Cutis 1975;15:271-5.

66. Rowland M, Riegelman S, Epstein WL. Absorption kinetics of griseofulvin in man. J Pharm Sci 1968;57:984-9.

67. Van Cautern H, Heykants J, De Coster R et al. Itraconazole: pharmacokinetic studies in animals and humans. Rev Infect Dis 1987;9:(Suppl. 1):S43-6.

68. Van Tyle JH. Ketoconazole: mechanism of action, spectrum of activity, pharmacokinetics, drug interactions, adverse reactions, and therapeutic use. Pharmacotherapy 1984;4:343-73.

69. Ginsburg CM, McCracken GH Jr., Olsen K. Pharmacology of ketoconazole suspension in infants and children. Antimicrob Agents Chemother 1983;23:787-9.

70. Pont A, Williams PL, Loose DS et al. Ketoconazole blocks adrenal steroid synthesis. Ann Intern Med 1982;97:370-2.

71. Fainstein V, Bodey GP. Cardiorespiratory toxicity due to miconazole. Ann Intern Med 1980;93:432-3.

72. Heel RC, Brogden RN, Pakes GE et al. Miconazole: a preliminary review of its therapeutic efficacy in systemic fungal infections. Drugs 1980;19:7-30.

73. Bennett JE, Remington JS. Miconazole in cryptococcosis and systemic candidiasis: a word of caution. Ann Intern Med 1981;94:708-9.

74. Nightingale CH, Greene DS, Quintiliani R. Pharmacokinetics and clinical use of cephalosporin antibiotics. J Pharm Sci 1975;64:1899-927.

75. Plaisance KI, Nightingale CH. Pharmacology of cephalosporins. In: Queener SF, Webber JA, and Queener SW, eds. Beta-lactam antibiotics for clinical use. New York. Marcel Dekker. 1986;285-347.

76. Barriere SL, Flaherty JF. Third-generation cephalosporins: a critical evaluation. Clin Pharm 1984;3:351-73.

77. Brogard JM, Comte F. Pharmacokinetics of the new cephalosporins. Antibiot Chemother 1982;31:145-210.

78. Neu HC. The pharmacokinetics of new cephalosporins: significance in clinical practice. Bull NY Acad Sci 1984;60:327-39.

79. Dudley MN, Nightingale CH. Effects of protein binding on the pharmacology of cephalosporins. In: Neu HC, ed. New beta-lactam antibiotics: a review from chemistry to clinical efficacy of the new cephalosporins. Philadelphia. Francis Clarke Wood Institute for the History of Medicine, 1982:227-39.

80. Murray BE, Moellering RC. Cephalosporins. Ann Rev Med 1981;32:559-81.

81. Neu HC. The new beta-lactamase-stable cephalosporins. Ann Intern Med 1982;97:408-19.

82. Quintiliani R, Nightingale CH. Cefazolin. Ann Intern Med 1978;89(part 1):650-6.

83. Marsh TD. The cephalosporin antibiotics. II. First- and second-generation agents. Infect Control 1984;5:577-82.

84. Sanders CC, Sanders WE Jr. Microbial resistance to newer generation beta-lactam antibiotics: clinical and laboratory implications. J Infect Dis 1985;151:399-406.

85. Uri JV, Parks DB. Disulfiram-like reactions to certain cephalosporins. Ther Drug Monit 1983;5:219-24.

86. Brogard JM, Comte F, Pinget M. Pharmacokinetics of cephalosporin antibiotics. Antibiot Chemother 1978;25:123-62.

87. Gardner ME, Fritz WL, Hyland RN. Antibiotic induced seizures: a case attributed to cefazolin and a review of the literature. Drug Intell Clin Pharm 1978;12:268-71.

88. Babiak LM, Rybak MJ. Hematological effects associated with beta-lactam use. Drug Intell Clin Pharm 1986;20:833-6.

89. Sanders CV, Greenberg RN, Marier RL. Cefamandole and cefoxitin. Ann Intern Med 1985;103:70-8.

90. Landesman SH, Corrado ML, Shah PM et al. Past and current roles for cephalosporin antibiotics in treatment of meningitis. Am J Med 1981;71:693-703.

91. Petz LD. Immunologic cross-reactivity between penicillins and cephalosporins: a review. J Infect Dis 1978;137(Suppl):S74-9.

92. Barza M, Furie B, Brown AE et al. Defects in vitamin K-dependent carboxylation associated with moxalactam treatment. J Infect Dis 1986;153:166-9.

93. Dudley MN, Barriere SL. Cefotaxime: microbiology, pharmacology, and clinical use. Clin Pharm 1982;1:114-24.

94. Carver P, Quintiliani R, Nightingale CH. Comparative pharmacokinetic study of cefotetan and cefoxitin in healthy volunteers. Infect Surg 1986 (April Suppl.):11-4.

95. Brown RB, Klar J, Lemeshow S et al. Enhanced bleeding with cefoxitin or moxalactam. Arch Intern Med 1986;146:2159-64.

96. Smith BR, LeFrock JL. Cefuroxime: antibacterial activity, pharmacology, and clinical efficacy. Ther Drug Monit 1983;5:149-60.

97. Gold B, Rodriguez WJ. Cefuroxime: mechanism of action, antimicrobial activity, pharmacokinetics, clinical applications, adverse reactions and therapeutic indications. Pharmacotherapy 1983;3:82-100.

98. Bundtzen RW, Toothaker RD, Nielson OS et al. Pharmacokinetics of cefuroxime in normal and impaired renal function: comparison of high-pressure liquid chromatography and microbiological assays. Antimicrob Agents Chemother 1981;19:443-9.

99. Ginsburg CM, McCracken GH Jr., Petruska M et al. Pharmacokinetics and bactericidal activity of cefuroxime. Antimicrob Agents Chemother 1985;28:504-7.

100. Derry JE. Evaluation of cefaclor. Am J Hosp Pharm 1981;38:54-8.

101. Bergman HD. Cefaclor. Drug Intell Clin Pharm 1980;14:11-6.

102. Neu HC, Srinivasan S. Pharmacology of ceftizoxime compared to that of cefamandole. Antimicrob Agents Chemother 1981;20:366-9.

103. Ward A, Richards DM. Cefotetan: a review of its antibacterial activity, pharmacokinetic properties and therapeutic use. Drugs 1985;30:382-426.

104. Dudley MN, Quintiliani R, Nightingale CH. Review of cefonicid, a long-acting cephalosporin. Clin Pharm 1984;3:23-32.

105. Dudley MN, Shyu W-C, Nightingale CH et al. Effect of saturable serum protein binding on the pharmacokinetics of unbound cefonicid in humans. Antimicrob Agents Chemother 1986;30:565-9.

106. Polk RE, Kline BJ, Markowitz SM. Cefazolin and moxalactam pharmacokinetics after simultaneous intravenous infusion. Antimicrob Agents Chemother 1981;20:576-9.

107. Guay DRP, Meatherall RC, Harding GK et al. Pharmacokinetics of cefixime (CL 284,635; FK 027) in healthy subjects and patients with renal insufficiency. Antimicrob Agents Chemother 1986;30:485-90.

108. Stoeckel K. McNamara PJ, Brandt R et al. Effects of concentration dependent plasma protein binding on ceftriaxone kinetics. Clin Pharmacol Ther 1981;29:650-7.

109. Barriere SL, Mills J. Ceforanide: antibacterial activity, pharmacology, and clinical efficacy. Pharmacotherapy 1982;2:322-7.

110. Garzone P, Lyon J, Yu VL. Third-generation and investigational cephalosporins. (2 parts). Drug Intell Clin Pharm 1983;17:507-15;615-22.

111. Chin N-X, Neu HC. Cefotaxime and desacetylcefotaxime: an example of advantages of antimicrobial metabolism. Diagn Microbiol Infect Dis 1984;2:21S-31S.

112. Brogden RN, Heel RC. Aztreonam: a review of its antibacterial activity, pharmacokinetic properties, and therapeutic uses. Drugs 1986;31:96-130.

113. Adkinson NF, Saxon A, Spence MR et al. Cross-allergenicity and immunogenicity of aztreonam. Rev Infect Dis 1985;7:S613-21.

114. Fillastre JP, Leroy A, Bandoin L et al. Pharmacokinetics of azetreonam in patients with chronic renal failure. Clin Pharmacokinet 1985;10:191-200.

115. Modai J, Vittecoq D, Decazes JM et al. Penetration of aztreonam into cerebrospinal fluid of patients with bacterial meningitis. Antimicrob Agents Chemother 1986;78(Suppl 2a):19-26.

116. Stutman HR, Chartland SA, Tolentino T et al. Aztreonam therapy for serious gram-negative infections in children. Am J Dis Child 1986;140:1147-51.

117. Saxon A, moderator. Immediate hypersensitivity reactions to beta-lactam antibiotics. Ann Intern Med 1987;107:204-15.

118. Barza M. Imipenem: first of a new class of beta-lactam antibiotics. Ann Intern Med 1985;105:552-60.

119. Pastel DA. Imipenem-cilastatin sodium, a broad spectrum carbapenem antibiotic. Clin Pharm 1986;5:719-36.

120. Norrby SR, Rogers J, Ferber F et al. Disposition of radiolabeled imipenem and cilastatin in normal human volunteers. Antimicrob Agents Chemother 1984;26:707-14.

121. Drusano GL, Standiford HC. Pharmacokinetic profile of imipenem-cilastatin in normal volunteers. Am J Med 1985;78(Suppl. 6A):47-53.

122. Verpooten GA, Verbist L, Butinx AP et al. Pharmacokinetics of imipenem (thienamycin-formamidine) and the renal dehydropeptidase inhibitor cilastatin sodium in patients with renal failure. Br J Clin Pharmacol 1984;18:183-93.

123. Gibson TP, Demetriades JL, Bland JA. Imipenem-cilastatin: pharmacokinetic profile in renal insufficiency. Am J Med 1985;78(Suppl. 6A):54-61.

124. Calandra GB, Brown KR, Grad LC et al. Review of adverse experiences and tolerability in the first 2,516 patients treated with imipenem-cilastatin. Am J Med 1985;78(Suppl. 6A):73-8.

125. Powell DA, Nahata MC. Chloramphenicol: new perspectives on an old drug. Drug Intell Clin Pharm 1982;16:295-300.

126. Weiss CF, Glazko AJ, Weston JK. Chloramphenicol in the newborn infant: a physiologic explanation of its toxicity when given in excessive doses. N Engl J Med 1960;262:787-94.

127. Koup JR, Lau AH, Brodsky B et al. Chloramphenicol pharmacokinetics in hospitalized patients. Antimicrob Agents Chemother 1979;15:651-7.

128. Lindberg AA, Nilsson LH, Bucht H et al. Concentration of chloramphenicol in the urine and blood in relation to renal function. Br Med J 1966;3:724-8.

129. Suhrland LG, Weisberger AS. Delayed clearance of chloramphenicol from serum in patients with hematologic toxicity. Blood 1969;34:466-71.

130. Marks MI, LaFerriere C. Chloramphenicol: recent developments and clinical indications. Clin Pharm 1982;1:315-20.

131. Saidi P, Wallerstein RO, Aggeler PM. Effect of chloramphenicol on erythropoiesis. J Lab Clin Med 1961;57:247-56.

132. Scott JL, Finegold SM, Belkin GA et al. A controlled double-blind study of the hematologic toxicity of chloramphenicol. N Engl J Med 1965;272:1138-42.

133. Washington JA, Wilson WR. Erythromycin: a microbial and clinical perspective after 30 years of clinical use (2 parts). Mayo Clin Proc 1985;60:189-203, 271-8.

134. Miller AC. Erythromycin in legionaires' disease: a re-appraisal. J Antimicrob Chemother 1981;7:217-22.

135. Bennett WM, Aronoff GR, Morrison G et al. Drug prescribing in renal failure: dosing guidelines in adults. Am J Kidney Dis 1983;3:155-93.

136. Griffith RS. Pharmacology of erythromycin in adults. Pediatr Infec Dis 1986;5:130-40.

137. Eichenwald HF. Adverse reactions to erythromycin. Pediatr Infec Dis 1986;5:147-50.

138. Rolston KVI, LeBlanc B, Ho DH. In vitro activity of RU-28965, a new macrolide, compared to that of erythromycin. J Antimicrob Chemother 1986;17:161-4.

139. Ginsburg CM. Pharmacology of erythromycin in infants and children. Pediatr Infec Dis 1986;5:124-9.

140. Gambertoglio JG, Barriere SL, Lin ET et al. Amdinocillin pharmacokinetics-simultaneous infusion with cephalothin and cerebrospinal fluid penetration. Am J Med 1983;(Aug 23 Suppl):54-9.

141. Barza M, Weinstein L. Pharmacokinetics of the penicillins in man. Clin Pharmacokinet 1976;1:297-308.

142. Wright AJ, Wilkowske CJ. The penicillins. Mayo Clin Proc 1983;58:21-32.

143. Neu HC. Amoxicillin. Ann Intern Med 1979;90:356-60.

144. Jusko WJ, Lewis GP, Schmitt GW. Ampicillin and hetacillin pharmacokinetics in normal and anephric subjects. Clin Pharmacol Ther 1973;14:90-9.

145. Lewis GP, Jusko WJ. Pharmacokinetics of ampicillin in cirrhosis. Clin Pharmacol Ther 1975;18:475-84.

146. Sjovall J, Magni L, Bergan T. Pharmacokinetics of bacampicillin compared with those of ampicillin, pivampicillin and amoxycillin. Antimicrob Agents Chemother 1978;13:90-6.

147. Ehrnebro M, Nilsson S-O, Boreus LO. Pharmacokinetics of ampicillin and its prodrugs bacampicillin and pivampicillin in man. J Pharmacokinet Biopharm 1979;7:429-51.

148. Eshelman FN, Spyker DA. Pharmacokinetics of amoxicillin and ampicillin: crossover study of the effect of food. Antimicrob Agents Chemother 1978;14:539-43.

149. Kagan BM. Ampicillin rash. West J Med 1977;126:333-5.

150. Appel GB, Neu HC. The nephrotoxicity of antimicrobial agents. N Engl J Med 1977;296:663-70, 722-8, 784-7.

151. Nicholls PJ. Neurotoxicity of penicillin. J Antimicrob Chemother 1980;6:161-5.

152. Foulds G. Pharmacokinetics of sulbactam/ampicillin in humans: a review. Rev Infect Dis 1986;8(Suppl. 5):S503-11.

153. Hartley S, Wise R. A 3-way crossover study to compare the pharmacokinetics and acceptability of sultamicillin at 2 dose levels with that of ampicillin. J Antimicrob Chemother 1986;10:49-55.

154. Lees L, Milsen JA, Knirsch AK et al. Sulbactam plus ampicillin: Interim review of efficacy and safety for therapeutic and prophylactic use. Rev Infect Dis 1986;8(Suppl. 5):S644-50.

155. Stein GE, Gurwith MJ. Amoxicillin-potassium clavulanate, a beta-lactamase-resistant antibiotic combination. Clin Pharm 1984;3:591-9.

156. Brogden RN, Carmine A, Heel RC et al. Amoxicillin/clavulanic acid: a review of its antibacterial activity, pharmacokinetics, and therapeutic use. Drugs 1981;22:337-62.

157. Knirsch AK, Hobbs DC, Korst JJ. Pharmacokinetics, toleration, and safety of indanyl carbenicillin in man. J Infect Dis 1973;127(Suppl):S105-8.

158. Brogden RN, Heel RC, Speight TM et al. Ticarcillin: a review of its pharmacological properties and therapeutic efficacy. Drugs 1980;20:325-52.

159. Jungbluth GL, Cooper DL, Doyle GD et al. Pharmacokinetics of ticarcillin and clavulanic acid (Timentin) in relation to renal function. Antimicrob Agents Chemother 1986;30:896-900.

160. Drusano GL, Schimpf SC, Hewitt WL. The acyampicillins: mezlocillin, piperacillin, and azlocillin. Rev Infect Dis 1984;6:13-32.

161. Bergan T. Overview of acylureidopenicillin pharmacokinetics. Scand J Infect Dis 1981;29(Suppl):33-48.

162. Eliopoulos GM, Moellering RC Jr. Azlocillin, mezlocillin, and piperacillin: new broad-spectrum penicillins. Ann Intern Med 1982;97:755-60.

163. Bass JW, Bruhn FW, Merritt WT et al. Comparison of oral penicillinase-resistant penicillins: contrasts between agents and assays. South Med J 1982;75:408-10.

164. Nauta EH, Mattie H. Dicloxacillin and cloxacillin: pharmacokinetics in healthy and hemodialysis subjects. Clin Pharmacol Ther 1976;20:98-108.

165. Kane JG, Parker RH, Jordan GW et al. Nafcillin concentrations in cerebrospinal fluid during treatment of staphylococcal infections. Ann Intern Med 1977;87:309-11.

166. Kind AC, Tupasi TE, Standiford HC et al. Mechanisms responsible for plasma levels of nafcillin lower than those of oxacillin. Arch Intern Med 1970;125:685-90.

167. Nahata MC, DeBolt SL, Powell DA. Adverse effects of methicillin, nafcillin, and oxacillin in pediatric patients. Dev Pharmacol Ther 1982;4:117-23.

168. Korzeniowski O, Sande MA, and the Endocarditis Study Group. Combination antibiotic therapy for S. aureus endocarditis in patients addicted to parenteral drugs and in non-addicts. Ann Intern Med 1982;97:496-503.

169. Zenk KE, Dungy CI, Greene GR. Nafcillin extravasation injury. Am J Dis Child 1981;35:1113-4.

170. Barriere SL, Conte JE Jr. Absence of nafcillin-associated nephritis. West J Med 1980;133:472-7.

171. Bruckstein AH, Attia AA. Oxacillin hepatitis. Am J Med 1978;64:519-22.

172. Center for Disease Control. STD treatment guidelines 1985. Morbid Mortal Wkly Rep 1985;34:75s-108s.

173. Peter G, Dudley MN. Clinical pharmacology of benzathine penicillin G. Pediatr Infect Dis 1985;4:586-91.

174. Green RL, Lewis JE, Kraus SJ et al. Elevated plasma procaine concentrations after administration of procaine penicillin G. N Engl J Med 1974;291:223-6.

175. Bradberry JC, Owens J. Acute psychotic reaction to procaine penicillin. Am J Hosp Pharm 1975;32:411-3.

176. Bryan CS, Stone WJ. ''Comparably massive'' penicillin G therapy in renal failure. Ann Intern Med 1975;82:189-95.

177. Levitz R, Mendolson LM. Managing patients with a history of penicillin allergy. Infect Surg 1982;1:18-25.

178. Josefsson K, Bergan T. Pharmacokinetics of phenoxymethylpenicillin in volunteers. Chemotherapy (Basel) 1982;28:241-6.

179. Barza M, Schiefe RT. Antimicrobial spectrum, pharmacology and therapeutic use of antibiotics part 1: tetracyclines. Am J Hosp Pharm 1977;34:49-57.

180. Baptista RJ, Harvie RJ, Guen R. The tetracyclines: an overview. US Pharmacist 1979;4:33-44.

181. Siegel D. Tetracyclines: new look at old antibiotic. NY State J Med 1978;78:950-5, 1115-20.

182. Sack DA, Kaminsky DC, Sack RB et al. Prophylactic doxycycline for travelers' diarrhea: results of a prospective double-blind study of Peace Corps volunteers in Kenya. N Engl J Med 1978;298:758-63.

183. Heaney D, Eknoyan G. Minocycline and doxycycline kinetics in chronic renal failure. Clin Pharmacol Ther 1978;24:233-9.

184. Leigh DA. Antibacterial activity and pharmacokinetics of clindamycin. J Antimicrob Chemother 1981;7(Suppl A):3-9.

185. Roberts AP, Eastwood JB, Gower PE et al. Serum and plasma concentrations of clindamycin following a single intramuscular injection of clindamycin phosphate in maintenance haemodialysis patients and normal subjects. Eur J Clin Pharmacol 1978;14:435-9.

186. Rimmer DMD, Sales JEL. Lincomycin and clindamycin. Antibiot Chemother 1978;25:204-16.

187. Avant GR, Schenker S, Alford RH. The effect of cirrhosis on the disposition and elimination of clindamycin. Am J Dig Dis 1975;20:223-30.

188. Hinthorn DR, Baker LH, Romig DA et al. Use of clindamycin in patients with liver disease. Antimicrob Agents Chemother 1976;9:498-501.

189. DeHaan RM, Vanden Bosch WD, Metzler CM. Clindamycin serum concentrations after administration of clindamycin palmitate with food. J Clin Pharmacol 1972;12:205-11.

190. DeHaan RM, Metzler CM. Schelienberg D et al. Pharmacokinetic studies of clindamycin phosphate. J Clin Pharmacol 1973;13:190-209.

191. Brown RB, Martyak SN, Barza M et al. Penetration of clindamycin phosphate into the abnormal human biliary tract. Ann Intern Med 1976;84:168-70.

192. Swartzberg JE, Maresca RM, Remington JS. Gastrointestinal side effects associated with clindamycin. Arch Intern Med 1976;136:876-9.

193. Gross MH. Management of antibiotic-associated pseudomembranous colitis. Clin Pharm 1985;4:304-10.

194. Milstone EB, McDonald AJ. Scholhamer CF. Pseudomembranous colitis after topical application of clindamycin. Arch Dermatol 1981;117:154-5.

195. Borriello SP, Larson HE. Antibiotic and pseudomembranous colitis. J Antimicrob Chemother 1981;7(Suppl A):53-62.

196. Anon. Antibiotic colitis—new cause, new treatment. Med Lett Drugs Ther 1979;21:97-8.

197. McCormack WM, Finland M. Spectinomycin. Ann Intern Med 1976;84:712-6.

198. Tuazon CU, Miller H. Comparative in vitro activities of teichomycin and vancomycin alone and in combination with rifampin and aminoglycosides against staphylococci and enterococci. Antimicrob Agents Chemother 1984;25:411-2.

199. Traina GL, Bonati M. Pharmacokinetics of teicoplanin in man after intravenous administration. J Pharmacokinet Biopharm 1984;12:119-27.

200. Glupczynski Y, Lagast H, Van der Auwera P et al. Clinical evaluation of teicoplanin for therapy of severe infections caused by gram-positive bacteria. Antimicrob Agents Chemother 1986;29:52-7.

201. Bartlett JG, Tedesco FJ, Shull S et al. Symptomatic relapse after oral vancomycin therapy of antibiotic associated pseudomembranous colitis. Gastroenterology 1980;78:431-4.

202. Matzke GR, Zhanel GG, Guay DRP. Clinical pharmacokinetics of vancomycin. Clin Pharmacokinet 1986;11:257-82.

203. Eykyn S, Phillips I, Evans J. Vancomycin for staphylococcal shunt site infections in patients on regular haemodialysis. Br Med J 1970;3:80-2.

204. Morris AJ, Bilinsky RT. Prevention of staphylococcal shunt infections by continuous vancomycin prophylaxis. Am J Med Sci 1971;262:87-92.

205. Moellering RC, Krogstad DJ, Greenblatt DJ. Vancomycin therapy in patients with impaired renal function: a nomogram for dosage. Ann Intern Med 1981;94:343-6.

206. Tedesco F, Markham R, Gurwith M et al. Oral vancomycin for antibiotic-associated pseudomembranous colitis. Lancet 1978;2:226-8.

207. Nielsen HE, Hansen HE, Korsager B et al. Renal excretion of vancomycin in kidney disease. Acta Med Scand 1975;197:261-4.

208. Newfield P, Roizen MF. Hazards of rapid administration of vancomycin. Ann Intern Med 1979;91:581.

209. Farber BF, Moellering RC. Retrospective study of the toxicity of preparations of vancomycin from 1974-1981. Antimicrob Agents Chemother 1983;23:138-41.

210. Snider DE, Cohn DL, Davidson PT et al. Standard therapy for tuberculosis—1985. Chest 1985;87(Suppl):117S-24S.

211. Lee CS, Gambertoglio JG, Brater DC et al. Kinetics of oral ethambutol in the normal subject. Clin Pharmacol Ther 1977;22:615-21.

212. Lee CS, Brater DC, Gambertoglio JG et al. Disposition kinetics of ethambutol in man. J Pharmacokinet Biopharm 1980;8:335-46.

213. Leibold JC. The ocular toxicity of ethambutol and its relation to dose. Ann NY Acad Sci 1966;135:904-9.

214. Holdiness MR. Neurological manifestations and toxicities of the antituberculosis drugs: a review. Med Toxicol 1987;2:33-51.

215. Gold CH, Buchanan N, Tringham V et al. Isoniazid pharmacokinetics in patients in chronic renal failure. Clin Nephrol 1976;6:365-9.

216. Chow MSS, Ronfeld RA. Pharmacokinetic data and drug monitoring: I. antibiotics and antiarrhythmics. J Clin Pharmacol 1975;15:405-18.

217. Kergueris MF, Bourin M, Larousse C. Pharmacokinetics of isoniazid: influence of age. Eur J Clin Pharmacol 1986;30:335-40.

218. Bowersox DW, Winterbauer RH, Stewart GL et al. Isoniazid dosage in patients with renal failure. N Engl J Med 1973;289:84-7.

219. Acocella G, Bonollo L, Garimoldi M et al. Kinetics of rifampicin and isoniazid administered alone and in combination to normal subjects and patients with liver disease. Gut 1972;13:47-53.

220. Bailey WC, Byrd RB, Glassroth JL et al. Preventive treatment of tuberculosis. Chest 1985;87(Suppl):128S-32S.

221. Gronhagen-Riska C, Hellstrom P-E, Froseth B. Predisposing factors in hepatitis induced by isoniazaid-rifampin treatment of tuberculosis. Am Rev Respir Dis 1978;118:461-6.

222. Kopanoff DE, Snider DE, Caras GJ. Isoniazid-related hepatitis: a US Public Health Service cooperative surveillance study. Am Rev Respir Dis 1978;117:991-1001.

223. Bernstein RE. Isoniazid hepatotoxicity and acetylation during tuberculosis chemoprophylaxis. Am Rev Respir Dis 1980;121:429-30.

224. Sievers ML, Herrier RN. Treatment of acute isoniazid toxicity. Am J Hosp Pharm 1975;32:202-6.

225. Glassroth J, Robins AG, Snider DE. Tuberculosis in the 1980s. N Engl J Med 1980;302:1441-50.

226. Byrd RB, Horn BR, Solomon DA et al. Toxic effects of isoniazid in tuberculosis chemoprophylaxis: role of biochemical monitoring in 1,000 patients. JAMA 1979;241:1239-41.

227. Schatz M, Patterson R, Kloner R et al. The prevalence of tuberculosis and positive tuberculin skin tests in a steroid-treated asthmatic population. Ann Intern Med 1976;84:261-5.

228. Dash LA, Comstock GW, Flynn JPG. Isoniazid preventive therapy: retrospect and prospect. Am Rev Respir Dis 1980;121:1039-44.

229. Wason S, Lacouture PG, Lovejoy FH. Single high-dose pyridoxine treatment for isoniazid overdose. JAMA 1981;246:1102-4.

230. Jacobson JA, Fraser DW. A simplified approach to meningococcal disease prophylaxis. JAMA 1976;236:1053-4.

231. Anon. Preventing spread of meningococcal disease. Med Lett Drugs Ther 1981;23:37-8.

232. Acocella G. Clinical pharmacokinetics of rifampicin. Clin Pharmacokinet 1978;3:108-27.

233. Siegler DI, Bryant M, Burley DM et al. Effect of meals on rifampicin absorption. Lancet 1974;2:197-8.

234. Sippel JE, Mikhail IA, Girgis NI et al. Rifampin concentrations in cerebrospinal fluid of patients with tuberculous meningitis. Am Rev Respir Dis 1974;109:579-80.

235. Curci G, Claar E, Bergamini N et al. Studies on blood serum levels of rifampicin in patients with normal and impaired liver function. Chemotherapy 1973;19:197-205.

236. Capelle P, Dhumeaux D, Mora M et al. Effect of rifampicin on liver function in man. Gut 1972;13:366-71.

237. Gupta S, Grieco MH, Siegel I. Suppression of T-lymphocyte rosettes by rifampin: studies in normals and patients with tuberculosis. Ann Intern Med 1975;82:484-8.

238. Black HR, Griffith RS, Peabody AM. Absorption, excretion and metabolism of capreomycin in normal and diseased states. Ann NY Acad Sci 1966;135:974-82.

239. American Thoracic Society. Guidelines for short-course tuberculosis chemotherapy. Am Rev Resp Dis 1980;121:429-30.

240. Laskin OL. Acyclovir, pharmacology and clinical experience. Arch Intern Med 1984;144:1241-6.

241. Hopefl AW. The clinical use of intravenous acyclovir. Drug Intell Clin Pharm 1983;17:623-8.

242. True BL, Carter BL. Update on acyclovir: oral therapy for herpesvirus infections. Clin Pharm 1984;3:607-13.

243. Whitley RJ, Alford CA, Hirsch MS et al. Vidarabine versus acyclovir therapy in Herpes simplex encephalitis. N Engl J Med 1986;314:144-9.

244. McLaren C, Chen MS, Ghazzouli I et al. Drug resistance patterns of Herpes simplex virus isolates from patients treated with acyclovir. Antimicrob Agents Chemother 1985;28:740-4.

245. Whitley R, Alford C, Hess F et al. Vidarabine: a preliminary review of its pharmacological properties and therapeutic use. Drugs 1980;20:267-82.

246. Whitley RJ. Soong S-J, Hirsch MS et al. Herpes simplex encephalitis: vidarabine therapy and diagnostic

problems. N Engl J Med 1981;304:313-8.

247. Yarchoan R, Broder S. Development of antiretroviral therapy for the acquired immunodeficiency syndrome and related disorders. N Engl J Med 1987;316:557-64.

248. Hooper DC, Wolfson JS. The fluoroquinolones: pharmacology, clinical uses and toxicities in humans. Antimicrob Agents Chemother 1985;28:716-21.

249. Dudley MN. Pharmacokinetic and pharmacodynamic properties of new fluoroquinolone antibiotics. Hosp Formul 1987;22(Suppl A):9-15.

250. Drusano GL, Standiford HC, Plaisance K et al. Absolute oral bioavailability of ciprofloxacin. Antimicrob Agents Chemother 1986;30:444-6.

251. Dudley MN, Mandler HD, Ericson J et al. Pharmacokinetics and pharmacodynamics of intravenous ciprofloxacin: studies in vivo and in an in vitro dynamic model. Am J Med 1987;82(Suppl 4A):363-8.

252. Ball AP. Ciprofloxacin: an overview of adverse experiences. J Antimicrob Chemother 1986;18(Suppl. D):187-93.

253. Holmes B, Brogden RN, Richard DM. Norfloxacin: a review of its antibacterial activity, pharmacokinetic properties, and therapeutic use. Drugs 1985;30:482-513.

254. Rubin RH, Swartz MN. Trimethoprim-sulfamethoxazole. N Engl J Med 1980;303:426-32.

255. Gleckman R, Alvarez S, Joubert DW. Drug therapy reviews: trimethoprim-sulfamethoxazole. Am J Hosp Pharm 1979;36:893-906.

256. Winston DJ, Lau WK, Gale RP et al. Trimethoprim-sulfamethoxazole for the treatment of Pneumocystis carinii pneumonia. Ann Intern Med 1980;92:762-9.

257. Bergan T, Brodwall EK, Vik-Mo H et al. Pharmacokinetics of sulfadiazine, sulfamethoxazole and trimethoprim in patients with varying renal function. Infection 1979;7(Suppl 4):S382-6.

258. Bennett WM, Craven R. Urinary tract infections in patients with severe renal disease: treatment with ampicillin and trimethoprim sulfamethoxazole. JAMA 1976;236:946-8.

259. Reeves DS, Wilkinson PJ. The pharmacokinetics of trimethoprim and trimethoprim/sulfonamide combinations, including penetration into body tissues. Infection 1979;7(Suppl 4):S330-41.

260. Grose WE, Bodey GP, Loo TL. Clinical pharmacology of intravenously administered trimethoprim-sulfamethoxazole. Antimicrob Agents Chemother 1979;15:447-51.

261. Bateson MC, Hayes JPLA, Pendahrker P. Cotrimoxazole and folate metabolism. Lancet 1976;2:339-40.

262. Kainer G, Rosenberg AR. Effect of co-trimoxazole on the glomerular filtration rate of healthy adults. Chemotherapy (Basel) 1981;27:229-32.

263. Gordin FM, Simon GL, Wofsy CB et al. Adverse reactions to trimethoprim-sulfamethoxazole in patients with the acquired immunodeficiency syndrome. Ann Intern Med 1984;100:495-9.

264. Sattler FR, Remington JS. Intravenous sulfamethoxazole and trimethoprim for serious gram-negative bacillary infection. Arch Intern Med 1983;143:1709-12.

265. Vree TB, Hekster YA, Damsma JE et al. Renal excretion of sulfamethoxazole and its metabolite N4-acetylsulfamethoxazole in patients with impaired kidney function. Ther Drug Monit 1981;3:129-35.

266. Trimethoprim study group. Comparison of trimethoprim at three dosage levels with co-trimoxazole in the treatment of acute symptomatic urinary tract infection in general practice. J Antimicrob Chemother 1981;7:179-83.

267. Friesen WT, Hekster YA, Vree TB. Trimethoprim: clinical use and pharmacokinetics. Drug Intell Clin Pharm 1981;15:325-30.

268. Guerrant RL, Wood SJ, Krongaard L et al. Resistance among fecal flora of patients taking sulfamethoxazole-trimethoprim or trimethoprim alone. Antimicrob Agents Chemother 1981;19:33-8.

269. Watkinson G, Sulphasalazine: a review of 40 years' experience. Drugs 1986;32(Suppl 1):1-11.

270. Singleton JW, Law DH, Kelley ML et al. National cooperative Crohns' disease study: adverse reactions to study drugs. Gastroenterology 1979;77:870-82.

271. Goldman P, Peppercorn MA. Sulfasalazine. N Engl J Med 1975;293:20-3.

272. Das K, Dubin R. Clinical pharmacokinetics of sulfasalazine. Clin Pharmacokinet 1976;1:406-25.

273. Das KM, Chowdhury J, Zapp B et al. Small bowel absorption of sulfasalazine and its hepatic metabolism in human beings, cats, and rats. Gastroenterology 1979;77:280-4.

274. Das KM, Eastwood MA, McManus JPA et al. Adverse reactions during salicylazosulfapyridine therapy and the relation with drug metabolism and acetylator phenotype. N Engl J Med 1973;289:491-5.

275. Birnie GG, McLeod TIF, Watkinson G. Incidence of sulfasalazine-induced male infertility. Gut 1981;22:452-5.

276. Klotz U, Maier K, Fischer C et al. Therapeutic efficacy of sulfasalazine and its metabolites in patients with ulcerative colitis and Crohn's disease. N Engl J Med 1980;303:1499-1502.

277. Halsted CH, Gandhi G, Tamura T. Sulfasalazine inhibits the absorption of folates in ulcerative colitis. N Engl J Med 1981;305:1513-7.

278. Mogadam M, Dobbins WO, Korelitz BI et al. Pregnancy in inflammatory bowel disease: effect of sulfasalazine and corticosteroids on fetal outcome. Gastroenterology 1981;80:72-6.

279. Friedman G. Sulfasalazine and new analogues. Am J Gastroenterol 1986;81:141-4.

280. Appel GB, Neu HC. The nephrotoxicity of antimicrobial agents (parts 1, 2, 3). N Engl J Med 1977;296:663-70, 722-8, 784-7.

281. Jackson EA, McLeod DC. Pharmacokinetics and dosing of antimicrobial agents in renal impairment. part II Am J Hosp Pharm 1974;31:137-48.

282. Weinstein L, Madoff MA, Samet CM. The sulfonamides. N Engl J Med 1960;263:793-800, 842-9, 900-7.

283. Chow MSS, Ronfeld RA. Pharmacokinetic data and drug monitoring. 1. antibiotics and antiarrhythmics. J Clin Pharmacol 1975;13:405-18.

284. Hamilton-Miller JMT, Brumfitt W. Methenamine and its salts as urinary tract antiseptics: variables affecting the antibacterial activity of formaldehyde, mandelic acid and hippuric acid in vitro. Invest Urol 1977;14:287-91.

285. Vainrub B, Musher DM. Lack of effect of methenamine in suppression of, or prophylaxis against, chronic urinary tract infection. Antimicrob Agents Chemother 1977;12:625-9.

286. McLeod DC, Nahata MC. Methenamine therapy and urinary acidification with ascorbic acid and cranberry juice. Am J Hosp Pharm 1978;35:654. Letter.

287. Kalowski S, Nanra RS, Friedman A et al. Controlled trial comparing co-trimoxazole and methenamine hippurate in the prevention of recurrent urinary tract infections. Med J Aust 1975;1:585-7.

288. Gleckman R, Alvarez S, Joubert DW. Drug therapy reviews: nitrofurantoin. Am J Hosp Pharm 1979;36:342-51.

289. Holmberg L, Boman G, Bottiger LE et al. Adverse reactions to nitrofurantoin. Analysis of 921 reports. Am J Med 1980;69:733-8.

290. Koch-Weser J, Sidel VW, Dexter M et al. Adverse reactions to sulfisoxazole, sulfamethoxazole, and nitrofurantoin. Arch Intern Med 1971;399-404.

291. Toole JF, Parrish ML. Nitrofurantoin polyneuropathy. Neurology 1973;23:554-9.

292. Finegold SM. Metronidazole. Ann Intern Med 1980;93:585-7.

293. Amon I, Amon K, Huller H. Pharmacokinetics and therapeutic efficacy of metronidazole at different dosages. Int J Clin Pharmacol 1978;16:384-6.

294. Goldman P. Metronidazole. N Engl J Med 1980;303:1212-8.

295. Brogden RN, Heel RC, Speight TM et al. Metronidazole in anaerobic infections: a review of its activity, pharmacokinetics and therapeutic use. Drugs 1978;16:387-417.

296. Krogstad DJ, Spencer HC, Healy GR. Current concepts in parsitology: amebiasis. N Engl J Med 1978;298:262-5.

297. Wolfe MS. Giardiasis. JAMA 1975:233;1362-5.

298. Bergan T, Bjerke PEM, Fausa O. Pharmacokinetics of metronidazole in patients with enteric disease compared to normal volunteers. Chemotherapy 1981;27:233-8.

299. Warner JF, Perkins RL, Cordero L. Metronidazole therapy of anaerobic bacteremia, meningitis, and brain abscess. Arch Intern Med 1979;139:167-9.

300. Nilsson-Ehle I, Ursing B, Nilsson-Ehle P. Liquid chromatographic assay for metronidazole and tinidazole: pharmacokinetic and metabolic studies in human subjects. Antimicrob Agents Chemother 1981;19:754-60.

301. Goldman P. Metronidazole: proven benefits and potential risks. Johns Hopkins Med J 1980;147:1-9.

302. Saginur R, Hawley CR, Bartlett JG. Colitis associated with metronidazole therapy. J Infect Dis 1980;141:772-4.

303. Thomson G, Clark AH, Hare K et al. Pseudomembranous colitis after treatment with metronidazole. Br Med J 1981;282:864-5.

304. Sands M, Kron MA, Brown RB. Pentamidine: a review. Rev Infect Dis 1985;7:625-34.

305. Bernard EM, Donnelly HJ, Maher MP et al. Use of a new bioassay to study pentamidine pharmacokinetics. J Infect Dis 1985;152:750-4

306. Drake S, Lampasona V, Nicks HL et al. Pentamidine isethionate in the treatment of Pneumocystis carinii pneumonia. Clin Pharm 1985;4:507-16.

307. Gordin FM, Simon GL, Wofsy CB et al. Adverse reactions to trimethoprim-sulfamethoxazole in patients with the acquired immunodeficiency syndrome. Ann Intern Med 1984;100:495-9.

308. Stahl-Bayliss CM, Kalman CM, Laskin OL. Pentamidine-induced hypoglycemia in patients with the acquired immune deficiency syndrome. Clin Pharmacol Ther 1986;39:271-5.

309. Haverkos HW. Assessment of therapy for Pneumocystis carinii pneumonia. PCP therapy project group. Am J Med 1984;76:501-8.

310. Anon. Clofazimine for leprosy and *Mycobacterium avium* complex reactions. Med Lett Drugs Ther 1987;29:77-8.

311. Montgomery AB, Debs RJ, Luce JM et al. Aerosolized pentamidine as sole therapy for *Pneumocystis carinii* pneumonia in patients with acquired immunodeficiency syndrome. Lancet 1987;2:480-3.

10:00 ANTINEOPLASTIC AGENTS

General References: 1-4

Introduction

THE AGENTS INCLUDED IN THIS SECTION are those having widespread use in cancer chemotherapy. The list is not exhaustive, however, and many agents with therapeutic importance in small patient populations are not included.

Cancer chemotherapeutic agents as a class are the most toxic drugs in use. Adverse reactions listed represent those most likely to occur with the usual doses and methods of use; infrequent, but serious reactions are also listed. Information on the dosing of these drugs has largely been determined empirically, and clinical investigations are continually being performed to find safer and more effective dosage regimens. Thus, doses in this section should only be considered as guidelines based on the most widely accepted usage at the time of this writing.

Because space does not permit in-depth discussions of the toxicity, dosing and other aspects of these drugs, the reader should become familiar with specific agents before initiating treatment. References are provided in this section for more detailed information concerning the proper and safe use of these agents. If specific investigational protocols are available, these may also provide information that is unavailable in other sources, especially with regard to dosage and dosing regimens.

Class Instructions. This drug is very potent and some side effects can be expected to occur with its use. Be sure that you understand the possible dangers as well as the possible benefits of the drug before you begin to take it.

(Cytotoxic Agents). Because this drug can decrease your body's ability to fight infections, any signs of infection such as fever, shaking chills or sore throat should be reported immediately. Unusual bruising or bleeding, shortness of breath, or painful or burning urination should also be reported. The use of aspirin-containing products should be avoided, and alcohol should be avoided or used in moderation. Nausea, vomiting or hair loss may sometimes occur with this drug. The severity of these effects depends on the individual, the dose and other drugs that may be given at the same time. This drug may cause temporary or sometimes permanent sterility in men and women. It may also cause birth defects if the father is taking the drug at the time of conception or if the mother is taking it any time during pregnancy.[2] If you are breast feeding, this drug may appear in the milk and cause problems in your baby; therefore, an alternate form of feeding your baby should be used.

Alkylating Agents, Oral

Busulfan	Myleran®
Chlorambucil	Leukeran®
Melphalan	Alkeran®

Pharmacology. Water soluble compounds which alkylate DNA, forming a variety of covalent cross-links. The drugs are polyfunctional and may form more than one covalent bond to susceptible cell constituents (typically the N^7 position of guanine). Cell cycle phase-nonspecific and chemically stable enough for oral absorption before significant alkylator activation occurs.

Administration, Dose and Dosage Forms.

	BUSULFAN	CHLORAMBUCIL	MELPHALAN
Administration	PO.	PO.	PO; IV (investigational).
Adult Dose	Up to 8 mg/day (usually 1–3 mg/day).	0.1–0.2 mg/kg/day for 1 day; or 6–12 mg/day maintenance; or 0.4 mg/kg q 2–4 weeks.[5]	0.25 mg/kg/day for 4 days; or 2–4 mg/day maintenance.
Pediatric Dose	—	—	—
Dosage Forms	Tab 2 mg.	Tab 2 mg.	Tab 2 mg Inj 100 mg (investigational).

Dosage Individualization. Melphalan elimination is significantly correlated with the glomerular filtration rate.[6] Studies in nephrectomized animals demonstrate markedly increased myelotoxicity with unadjusted melphalan doses. Thus, one group currently recommends a 50% decrease in the melphalan dose for BUN > 30 mg/dl or Cr_s > 1.5 mg/dl.[6]

Patient Instructions. See Class Instructions.

Pharmacokinetics.

	BUSULFAN	CHLORAMBUCIL	MELPHALAN[7,8]
Fate.			
Absorption	Reported by manufacturer to be well absorbed orally.	Oral bioavailability is about 70–80% by radiolabeled drug studies;[9] further reduced by 10–20% if ingested with food.[10]	Oral absorption erratic and incomplete; some patients show no levels after standard doses.
Distribution	Homogeneous; good ascites penetration; exact V_d not known; binds extensively to proteins.	V_d 0.14–0.24 L/kg.[9]	V_d 0.5–0.6 L/kg.
Metabolism	Extensively metabolized, major fraction as methanesulfonic acid.	Rapid metabolism to a number of inactive metabolites.	Not actively metabolized; spontaneous chemical degradation to mono- and dihydroxy products.
Excretion	No intact drug found in urine; however, metabolites are renally excreted.	< 1% unchanged drug in urine over 24 hr.	24-hr urinary excretion only 10–15% of a dose.
$t_{1/2}$.	Rapid plasma clearance—90% of dose after 3 min.	2 hr (intact drug); 2.5 hr (major metabolite, aminophenylacetic acid).	IV administration: $t_{1/2\alpha}$ 8 min $t_{1/2\beta}$ 108 min. Oral administration: terminal $t_{1/2}$ 90 min.

Adverse Reactions. Dose-limiting toxicity for this group is typically myelosuppression, with nadirs of 14–21 days for leukopenia and thrombocytopenia after pulse dosing; daily administration results in chronic low indices with cumulative effects. Not uncommonly, blood counts continue to drop after drug discontinuation; fatal pancytopenias are reported. Therefore, routine hematologic assessments are important with chronic daily dosing regimens. There may be some selectivity for different normal cell lines by these drugs; busulfan and perhaps chlorambucil selectively depress granulocytes, relatively sparing platelets and lymphoid elements. The nadir for melphalan can be prolonged (4–6 weeks); continuous administration frequently leads to severe myelosuppression (especially platelets) continuing after the drug is discontinued. Nausea and vomiting are rare with chronic dosing, although large single doses can be strongly emetogenic. Pulmonary fibrosis can occur with all these drugs, especially busulfan; symptoms include cough, dyspnea and fever, while histopathologic changes include bilateral fibrosis. High-dose corticosteroids may help early evolving pulmonary disease due to melphalan and chlorambucil, but "busulfan lung" is usually fatal within 6 months of diagnosis.[11-13] Busulfan frequently causes hyperpigmentation (especially of intertriginous areas) and broad suppression of testicular, ovarian and adrenal function (occasionally leading to Addisonian crisis). Chronic daily administration of these drugs predisposes patients to drug-induced carcinogenesis, often heralded by preleukemic pancytopenias culminating in acute myelocytic leukemias. Allergic hypersensitivity reported, especially with melphalan. With prolonged use, sterility occurs with all alkylators; females appear more sensitive than males.

Contraindications.   Documented hypersensitivity; inadequate marrow reserve.

Precautions.   See Dosage Individualization for melphalan use in renal impairment.

Parameters to Monitor.   Routine (at least monthly) WBC and platelet counts; reduce dosage at first sign of significant myelosuppression (ie, WBC < 2,500–3,500/cu mm or platelets < 60,000–100,000/cu mm). Conversely, patients receiving oral melphalan should be assessed for evidence of mild to moderate myelotoxicity to ensure that some absorption is occurring.

Amsacrine (Investigational - Bristol)   Amsidine®
Amsacrine Gluconate (Investigational - Parke-Davis)   Amsidyl®

Amsacrine is an intercalator-like antineoplastic derived from an acridine dye. Preliminary studies indicate primary hepatic metabolism with a half-life of 2.5 hr. Major toxicities are dose-related leukopenia and thrombocytopenia; rarely, cardiac arrest occurs if hypokalemia is present. It has some activity against nonlymphocytic leukemia at doses of 75–90 mg/M^2/day for 5–7 days and solid tumors at 120 mg/M^2 once q 3–4 weeks. Each dose is diluted in 500 ml of D5W (only) to minimize phlebitis. Caution should be used in preparing solutions to avoid inhalation of the powder or contact with skin; wear mask and rubber gloves during preparation. Use only a glass syringe to prepare, because of possible inactivation by plastic.[14,15] Available from NCI.

Anthracycline Agents

Daunorubicin Hydrochloride   Cerubidine®
Doxorubicin Hydrochloride   Adriamycin® RDF

Pharmacology.   Daunorubicin (daunomycin) and doxorubicin (hydroxy-daunomycin) are tetracyclic amino sugar-linked antibiotics which are actively taken up by cells and concentrated in the nucleus; intercalation or fitting between DNA base pairs occurs (which impairs DNA synthesis). Other biochemical lesions produced include quinone moiety-generated production of oxygen and hydroxyl free radicals with lipid peroxidation of plasma membranes, mitochondrial membranes and direct free radical DNA denaturation. Both agents are primarily cell cycle phase-nonspecific, but with slightly greater activity in late S or G$_2$ phase cells.

Administration, Dose and Dosage Forms.

	DAUNORUBICIN	DOXORUBICIN
Administration	IV push, infusion.	IV push, infusion.
	Both compounds are extremely toxic if inadvertently extravasated; very careful IV technique is mandatory.	

Continued

Administration, Dose and Dosage Forms.

	DAUNORUBICIN	DOXORUBICIN
Adult Dose	30–60 mg/M^2/day for 1–3 days; generally not repeated more often than q 3 weeks.	60–90 mg/M^2 for 1 dose or 20–30 mg/M^2/day for 3 days; generally not repeated more often than q 3 weeks. Alternatively, 20 mg/M^2/week.
Pediatric Dose	Same as adult dose.	Same as adult dose.
Cumulative Dose Limits[b]	550 mg/M^2, up to 850 mg/M^2.	550 mg/M^2; 400 mg/M^2 with prior chest irradiation.[a]
Dosage Forms	Inj 20 mg.	Inj 10, 20, 50, 150 mg.

a. Low weekly doses or continuous 96-hr infusion[16] appear to be less toxic and may allow attainment of greater cumulative doses (> 550 mg/M^2).[16,17]

b. Attainment of maximal cumulative dose generally precludes continued use, despite evidence of continuing drug response; however, some patients may continue to respond without development of cardiomyopathy.[18]

Patient Instructions. Immediately report any change in sensation (eg, stinging) at injection site during infusion; this may be an early sign of infiltration. See also Class Instructions.

Pharmacokinetics.

Fate.
Absorption — Extensively degraded to inactive aglycone in GI tract.

Distribution — Both drugs enter cells rapidly, with subsequent concentration in the nucleus. Tissue concentrations are highest in lung, kidney, spleen, small intestine and liver; insignificant amounts are found in the CNS. Avid tissue binding is probably responsible for prolonged terminal half-lives and V_d of 500–600 L/M^2.

Metabolism — Both drugs are extensively metabolized, initially to active alcohol metabolites; further metabolized by liver microsomes to inactive aglycones and demethylated glucuronide and sulfate conjugates.[19]

	DAUNORUBICIN	DOXORUBICIN
Excretion		
Biliary	20–30% of a dose.	40–60% of a dose.
Urinary	14–23% as unchanged drug and metabolites (primarily daunorubicinol).	5–10% as metabolites over 5 days.[20]
$t_{1/2}$	α 45 min β 18.5 hr (daunorubicinol $t_{1/2}$ 27 hr).[21]	α 30 min β 3 hr γ 17 hr (32 hr for metabolites).[20]

Dosage Individualization. Cumulative doses of both agents must be reduced in patients with prior irradiation of the cardiac chest region. Doxorubicin requires no dosage adjustment for severe renal impairment, while with daunorubicin theoretically 75% of the dose would be recommended in severe renal impairment. Doxorubicin doses, however, *must* be substantially reduced with severe hepatic dysfunction:[20]

SERUM BILIRUBIN (MG/DL)	% OF DOXORUBICIN DOSE RECOMMENDED
≤ 1.2	100 (no reduction)
1.2–3	50
> 3	25 (75% reduction)

Adverse Reactions.   Myelosuppression, affecting both platelets and WBCs, constitutes the major acute dose-limiting side effect. Typical nadirs range from 9–14 days, with recovery nearly complete within 3 weeks of administration. Stomatitis, nausea and vomiting are dose-dependent and frequent; prophylactic antiemetics are often helpful. Alopecia usually occurs; during low-dose adjuvant chemotherapy administration, regional scalp hypothermia may decrease hair loss. Severe, protracted ulceration and necrosis can occur with inadvertent perivenous infiltration of either drug; partially effective local antidotes include topical DMSO and icepacking. Large evolving lesions necessitate early plastic surgery consultation. Chronic anthracycline use can lead to severe and often fatal cardiomyopathy — see Cumulative Dose Limits; symptoms are nonspecific and indicative of advanced CHF such as shortness of breath, edema and fatigue. The frequency is low (overall 2.2%),[22] when total dose limits are observed and may be lower when monthly doses are given over several days or by continuous infusion. During drug infusion, various nonspecific EKG changes may occur; these do *not* imply an increased risk of cardiotoxicity. Graded endomyocardial biopsy and graded radionuclide angiography have proved most effective for assessment of the emergence of severe cardiomyopathy. Other reactions include transient erythema and phlebitis during administration and a radiation-synergy phenomenon involving heightened tissue reactions in concurrently or previously irradiated tissues, especially the esophagus (avoid by spacing weeks apart). Urine remains red for 1–2 days after administration.

Contraindications.   Pre-existing bone marrow suppression (WBCs < 3,000/cu mm; platelets < 120,000/cu mm); myocardial infarction in previous 6 months; history of CHF.

Precautions.   Careful administration technique is mandatory to avoid extravasation and tissue necrosis. A number of conditions or other drugs may interact with the anthracyclines: vinca alkaloids (cross-resistance); amphotericin B (increased drug uptake); phenobarbital (increased rate of aglycone production); hepatocellular disease or cirrhosis (slowed production of alcohol metabolites). Most of these drug interactions have only been studied in vitro and require clinical confirmation.

Parameters to Monitor.   Pretreatment and at least monthly WBC and platelet counts. General cardiac status and serial radionuclide scans of the heart in high-risk patients.

Notes.   Both drugs are compatible with usual IV solutions; incompatible with $NaHCO_3$ and fluorouracil. IV push doses are best reconstituted with NS or D5W; avoid sterile water. Such reconstitutions are stable for prolonged periods and can withstand freezing and thawing. Doxorubicin is widely effective in numerous solid tumors, such as ovarian, thyroid and gastric carcinomas, sarcomas and cancer of the breast as well as hematologic malignancies, such as the lymphomas and leukemias.[23] Daunorubicin's activity is limited primarily to acute myelogenous leukemia (AML).

Asparaginase

Elspar®

Pharmacology. A macromolecular protein, isolated from *E. coli* and other bacteria, which hydrolyzes the essential amino acid asparagine in the plasma, thus depriving susceptible lymphocyte-derived malignancies of a necessary element for protein synthesis. Cell cycle G_1 phase-specific.

Administration and Adult Dose. IV or preferably IM for combination therapy of acute leukemia 200 IU/kg/day for 28 days;[24] or 1,000–6,000 IU/M^2/day for 5 days;[25] or 20,000 IU/M^2/week.[26]

Pediatric Dose. IV or preferably IM 1,000–6,000 IU/M^2/day for 5 days,[25,27] up to 20,000 IU/M^2/week.

Dosage Forms. Inj 10,000 IU vial. A 10,000 IU/2 ml vial of *Erwinia* asparaginase (investigational) is available from National Cancer Institute (NSC 106977) for use in patients allergic to *E. coli* preparation.

Patient Instructions. Asparaginase often causes allergic reactions which can occasionally be life-threatening. This drug may also alter blood sugar and might aggravate diabetes mellitus. Report any abdominal pain immediately. See also Class Instructions.

Pharmacokinetics. *Fate.* IV and IM produce equivalent plasma levels. Negligible distribution out of the vascular compartment with minimal urinary and biliary excretion. Clearance is probably immune-mediated. Asparaginase remains detectable in plasma 13–22 days after administration.[29]

$t_{1/2}$. α phase 4–9 hr; β phase 1.4–1.8 days.[29]

Adverse Reactions. Moderate to severe nondose-related hypersensitivity reactions occur in about 20–35% of patients (IM use may reduce and/or delay allergic complications); prophylactic antihistamines may sometimes be helpful. Usually not emetogenic or myelotoxic, but can transiently lower blood sugar followed by a pancreatitis-induced hyperglycemia. Elevated serum cholesterol, severely elevated hepatic enzymes, steatosis and depressed clotting factors (especially profound for fibrinogen) and decreased albumin synthesis may occur. Lethargy and somnolence occur, which may be more frequent in adults.[28] Fatal hyperthermia has been reported.

Contraindications. Anaphylaxis to commercial *E. coli* preparation (use *Erwinia* preparation); severe pancreatitis or history of pancreatitis.

Precautions. Onset of abdominal pain, serum amylase elevation, any changes in mental status or severe elevation of prothrombin time require drug discontinuation. Some elevations of liver function tests should be anticipated. Anaphylaxis can occur with any dose and facilities for treatment should be at hand. Intradermal scratch tests and desensitization procedures are not reliably predictive or preventive for anaphylaxis.[24,29]

Parameters to Monitor. Hepatic enzymes, amylase and prothrombin time routinely and all vital signs upon administration.

Notes. Reconstitute with normal saline or D5W (2 ml maximum for IM use); stable at least 24 hr; do not filter.

Azacitidine (Investigational - Upjohn)

Mylosar®

Azacitidine is a pyrimidine antimetabolite used in refractory acute myelocytic leukemia. Most of a dose is eliminated in the urine as metabolites. The short terminal half-life (3.5–4.2 hr) and the cell cycle S phase-specific action each mandate continuous drug infusion or multiple

SC doses for maximal efficacy. Primary toxicities are myelosuppression, primarily leukopenia (10-day nadir) and moderate to severe nausea and vomiting. Rarer toxicities include neurologic muscle pain and weakness, transient fever, rhabdomyolysis and renal tubular damage with occasionally profound hypophosphatemia. Severe hepatic failure and coma have occurred in patients with metastatic liver involvement. It is given IV in doses of 150–400 mg/M^2/day for 5–10 days as a continuous infusion, or by SC injections. Ringer's lactate (RL) is the only diluent recommended (stable only 6 hr in RL).[30] Available from NCI.

Bleomycin Sulfate   Blenoxane®

Pharmacology. A mixture of 13 glycopeptide fractions produced by *Streptomyces verticillus*. Antineoplastic effects include single and double strand DNA scission, producing excision of thymine bases, possibly mediated through binding with ferric iron and subsequent production of highly reactive hydroxyl and •O_2 radicals. Cell cycle phase-specific with maximal activity occurring in the G_2 (premitotic) phase of cell division.[31]

Administration and Adult Dose. **IM test dose** 1–2 units may be useful in malignant lymphoma patients to assess exaggerated hyperpyrexic response. If no reaction occurs in 2–4 hr, give regular dose. **SC, IM or IV** 10–20 units/M^2 1–2 times/week.[31] **IV continuous infusion** 15–20 units/day for 4–5 days.[32] Experimental evidence in animals favors continuous administration to lessen pulmonary toxicity and maximize cell kill. A total lifetime dose limit of 400 units is recommended to avoid pulmonary fibrosis. **Intracavitary for pleural effusion** 15–240 units.[33]

Dosage Individualization. Significant dose reduction has been recommended in renal impairment:[34]

SERUM CREATININE (MG/DL)	% OF DOSE RECOMMENDED
2.5–4.0	25 (75% reduction)
4.0–6.0	20
6.0–10.0	5–10 (90–95% reduction)

Pediatric Dose. **SC, IM or IV** 10–20 units/M^2 1–2 times/week in combination regimens. **IV continuous infusion** 15–20 units/M^2/day for 4–5 days, usually as a single agent.

Dosage Forms. **Inj** 15 units.

Patient Instructions. Report any coughing, shortness of breath or wheezing. Skin rashes, shaking chills or transient high fever may occur following administration. Hyperpigmentation of skin fold areas, scars, pressure areas or sites of trauma may occur. See also Class Instructions.

Pharmacokinetics. *Fate.* Poorly absorbed topically; roughly one-half of intracavitary-administered drug may be systemically available. Following an IV dose of about 15 units/M^2, plasma levels of 10–1,000 micro-units/ml are obtained.[32] Steady-state levels during continuous infusion of 20 units/day are 50–200 micro-units/ml.[35] 50–60% of a dose is recovered in the urine (20–40% as active drug). Tissue inactivation is mediated by specific bleomycin-hydrolase, an enzyme observed to be low in skin and lung, the two main toxicity targets of the drug.[32,35]

$t_{1/2}$. α phase 24 min; β phase 2–4 hr.[32,35]

Adverse Reactions. Acute fever and a cutaneous, generalized erythema with edema, eventually leading to hyperpigmentation and skin thickening are frequent. Chronically, the most serious toxicity is pulmonary fibrosis manifested by dry cough, rales, dyspnea and bilateral infiltrates. Pulmonary function studies show hypoxemia and reduced CO diffusing capacity. Pulmonary toxicity is usually not noted below 150 units/M^2, increasing to 55% at doses above 283 units/M^2 and 66% at 360 units/$M^{2;36}$ life-threatening pulmonary fibrosis is rare if dosage limits are observed. Prior chest radiotherapy, age over 70 yr and hyperoxic ventilation predispose patients to toxicity. About 1% of bleomycin-treated patients die from pulmonary fibrosis. Low-dose hypersensitivity pneumonitis which may be responsive to corticosteroids also occurs.[37]

Precautions. Use with extreme caution in patients with renal or pulmonary disease, in those with lymphoma and in those over 70 yr.

Parameters to Monitor. Calculate cumulative dose at each treatment. Monitor temperature initially, especially in lymphoma patients. Assess renal function prior to dosing. Pulmonary damage is best monitored with CO diffusing capacity and forced vital capacity; specific serial pulmonary function studies have been suggested during therapy. Characteristic x-ray findings include changes suggestive of progressive bilateral fibrosis.

Notes. 1 mg of bleomycin equals 1 unit of activity. Reconstituted solution is stable for 1 month under refrigeration and 2 weeks at room temperature. Incompatible with divalent cations (especially copper), ascorbic acid and compounds with sulfhydryl groups. Vinca alkaloids, which are known to arrest cells at the G_2-M junction, experimentally enhance bleomycin cell kill (bleomycin following vinca by 6–24 hr).[38]

Cyclophosphamide   Cytoxan®, Various

Pharmacology. Inactive in vitro and must be enzymatically activated in the liver to yield both active alkylating compounds and toxic metabolites.[39] Cell cycle phase-nonspecific.

Administration and Adult Dose. IV (usually) or PO in high-dose intermittent regimens maximum of 40–50 mg/kg given once or over 2–5 days, repeat q 2–4 weeks — these doses are not well tolerated orally. IV 10–15 mg/kg q 7–10 days or 3–5 mg/kg twice weekly. IV doses may be given in any convenient volume of all common IV solutions. **Continuous daily dosing PO** 1–5 mg/kg/day. Continuous doses must be individualized to patient reponse.

Dosage Individualization. No dosage alteration appears necessary in renal impairment, because differences in toxicity between normals and patients with renal failure have not been reported.[40]

Pediatric Dose. Same as adult dose.

Dosage Forms. Tab 25, 50 mg; Inj 100, 200, 500 mg, 1 g.

Patient Instructions. Drink 2–3 quarts of fluids daily (1–2 quarts in smaller children) and urinate frequently; oral doses should *not* be taken at bedtime. Report any blood in the urine. See also Class Instructions.

Pharmacokinetics. *Fate.* Oral absorption averages 97%. Metabolized to active compounds (including the highly toxic nonalkylating aldehyde, acrolein, and the principal alkylator, phosphoramide mustard) primarily in hepatic microsomal mixed-function oxidase. Alkylating metabolites are 50% plasma protein bound; V_d is about 0.7 L/kg.[41] Renal elimination accounts for 22% of drug and 60% of metabolites,[41,42] with a mean renal clearance of 0.66 L/hr of unchanged drug.[43] Elimination is linear over a wide range of doses.[39]

$t_{1/2}$. (Plasma alkylating activity) 6.5–8 + hr, slightly longer in patients on allopurinol or those previously exposed to cyclophosphamide.[41,44]

Adverse Reactions. Nausea, vomiting and alopecia are frequent. Dose-limiting toxicity is myelosuppression with a WBC nadir of about 10 days; platelets are also suppressed, perhaps to a lesser extent. Transient, reversible blurred vision occurs occasionally. The drug is locally nonirritating. Renally eliminated active metabolites occasionally cause sterile hemorrhagic cystitis which may resolve slowly, often leading to a fibrotic, contracted bladder. Bladder epithelial changes range from minimal to frank neoplasia. An early sign of cystitis is microscopic hematuria which can lead to frank hemorrhage. Prophylactic hydration is recommended; N-acetylcysteine (Mucomyst®) bladder irrigations may have antidotal activity. Rarely, bladder dysplasia can lead to bladder cancer after very high doses or with concurrent or prior bladder radiation. Cross-allergenicity with other alkylators, such as mechlorethamine, may occur. Ovarian and testicular function may be permanently lost following high-dose, long-term therapy. Rare reactions include a high-dose fatal cardiomyopathy, "allergic" interstitial pneumonitis and a transient condition similar to SIADH which is preventable with vigorous isotonic hydration.

Contraindications. Previous life-threatening hypersensitivity to cyclophosphamide; significant leukopenia and thrombocytopenia; hemorrhagic cystitis; pulmonary toxicity due to prior alkylator therapy; tumor cell infiltration of bone marrow.

Precautions. Pregnancy. Consider dosage reduction or discontinuation of drug in patients who develop infections; use with caution in impaired renal or hepatic function. Concomitant cimetidine may reduce drug clearance and enhance myelotoxicity.

Parameters to Monitor. Prior to induction therapy dosing, the patient should be assessed for adequate numbers of WBCs (generally > 3,500/cu mm and platelets > 120,000/cu mm). With chronic dosing, these counts should be assessed at least monthly. Monitor closely for hematuria, especially if patient has received a large cumulative dose.

Notes. Do not dilute with benzyl alcohol-preserved solutions. Dissolution of powder is quite slow; vigorous shaking and/or slight warming may hasten dissolution. Diluted solution is stable for 24 hr at room temperature and 6 days under refrigeration. Widely used in both hematologic and solid malignancies and as an immunosuppressant in a variety of autoimmune disorders.

Cytarabine

Cytosar®

Pharmacology. Cytarabine (cytosine arabinoside, Ara-C) is an arabinose sugar analogue of the natural pyrimidine nucleoside cytidine. Cytarabine is cell cycle S phase-specific with activity markedly enhanced by continuous administration over several days.

Administration and Adult Dose. IV for remission induction 100–150 mg/M^2/day as a continuous infusion for 5–10 days.[45] Experimental therapy has successfully used induction doses of up to 3 g/M^2 q 12 hr as a 2-hr infusion for 4–12 doses in refractory AML.[46] SC for remission induction 100 mg/M^2 q 12 hr for 5–10 days. SC for remission maintenance 70–100 mg/M^2/day for 5 days in 4 divided doses. Intrathecal 70 mg/M^2 (usually 100 mg) 1–2 times weekly, diluted with nonpreserved isotonic solutions only (eg, normal saline, D5W, Ringer's lactate).[47] See Notes.

Pediatric Dose. IV or SC same as adult dose. Intrathecal (3 yr or older) 70 mg/M^2, diluted as above, repeated no more often than q 3-5 days; (2-3 yr) reduce dose by 1/6; (1-2 yr) reduce dose by 1/3; (< 1 yr) reduce dose by 1/2.

Dosage Forms. Inj 100, 500 mg.

Patient Instructions. See Class Instructions.

Pharmacokinetics. *Plasma Levels.* 0.05-0.1 mcg/ml necessary for cytotoxic effects;[48] this is similar to reported "therapeutic" levels of 0.1-0.4 mcg/ml produced by 60-min continuous infusion of 17-80 mg.[49] Plasma levels up to 1 mM (240 mcg/ml) are achieved with high-dose regimens.

Fate. Not systemically bioavailable following oral absorption. After injection, there is a large interpatient variation in plasma levels attained as measured by various assay techniques.[50] It is widely distributed and deactivated by cytidine deaminase, primarily in the liver. The deamination product, uracil arabinoside (Ara-U), is inactive and rapidly excreted in the urine; 24 hr after injection, 72% of the dose is recovered in the urine as Ara-U, only 8% as unchanged drug.[51] The CSF to plasma ratio is 0.1 with slow elimination from the CSF due to low CNS deaminating activity; however, to attain therapeutic CSF concentrations following standard IV doses, intrathecal injections are required. Up to 14% of plasma levels are attained in the CNS with high-dose therapy.[52] Tear concentrations are also detectable after high-dose therapy. About 13% plasma protein bound; reported V$_d$ is quite variable: 20-270 L[49] and 70-760 L.[50]

$t_{1/2}$. α phase 1.6-12 min; β phase 9-111 min.[49,51] Following intrathecal administration, CNS half-life of 2-11 hr has been reported.[53]

Adverse Reactions. Principal side effect is dose-related myelosuppression with a leukopenic nadir of 3-11 days and a thrombocytopenic nadir of 12-14 days; megaloblastosis is typically noted in the recovering bone marrow and in the rare cases in which anemia develops. Mild to moderate nausea and vomiting are frequent; prophylactic anti-emetics are often suppressive. Mild oral ulceration occurs occasionally. A flu-like syndrome is occasionally produced, manifested by arthralgias, fever and sometimes rash. Hepatic enzyme elevation is rare, even with 3 g/M^2 doses; one instance of SIADH reported with this large dose.[46] Ocular toxicity occurs frequently with high-dose therapy; typically, conjunctival injection and central punctate corneal opacities occur.[54] Irreversible cerebellar toxicity (ataxia, cognitive dysfunction) is a risk after cumulative doses of 30 g/M^2 or greater.[55]

Intrathecal toxicities are dose-related and include transient headaches and vomiting.[47] Seizures and paraplegia are very rare and involve high-dose, closely spaced treatments.

Precautions. Significant myelosuppression is *not* a contraindication, because marrow hypoplasia with complete suppression of the leukemic clone is the desired clinical endpoint; however, extensive supportive facilities must be available during therapy, including WBC and platelet transfusion capability.

Parameters to Monitor. Routine WBC and platelet counts; RBC indices.

Notes. Physically incompatible with sodium methotrexate and fluorouracil; avoid direct admixture. Chemically stable in solution for up to 7 days at room temperature. Intrathecal doses should *not* be diluted with bacteriostatic diluents. Patients may be taught sterile technique for self-dosing of SC drug for remission maintenance. The use of small reconstitution volumes (1 ml/100 mg) and rotation of injection sites should be observed. Clinical activity is limited primarily to selected hematologic malignancies (eg, AML, ALL, DHL).

Dacarbazine

DTIC-Dome®

Dacarbazine is an imidazole analogue of a purine precursor that alkylates DNA via several azo-metabolites in primarily a cell cycle phase-nonspecific fashion. It is used in malignant melanoma with about a 10–20% objective response rate. The drug is extensively metabolized, some microsomally mediated (50% by N-demethylation); it is 5% plasma protein bound with 30–45% of a dose excreted unchanged in the urine. The drug has an α half-life of 35 min and a β half-life of about 5 hr; in one patient with renal and hepatic dysfunction, the terminal half-life increased to 7.2 hr. Nausea and vomiting, which are occasionally severe, occur almost invariably; these may decrease in severity with successive courses of therapy. Dose- and duration-dependent mutagenicity, teratogenicity and sterility have been reported. Pain on injection also occurs. The dose-limiting toxicity is myelosuppression with a leukopenic nadir at 21–25 days. Rarely, a flu-like syndrome of myalgia, fever and malaise occurs within 1 week of drug administration. Dacarbazine should be used with caution in patients with pre-existing bone marrow aplasia. The drug is light-sensitive and exposure to light should be minimized after reconstitution; acute toxicity may be increased with exposure to sunlight. The reconstituted solution is clear to pale yellow and is stable for 8 hr after reconstitution at room temperature; pink discoloration denotes drug decomposition. The drug is administered IV as a single dose of up to 850 mg/M^2, repeated in 3–4 weeks. Alternatively, it may be given in doses of up to 250 mg/M^2/day for 5 days and repeated in 3–4 weeks. The dose should be reduced in renal and/or hepatic impairment.[56,57] Available as 100 and 200 mg injection.

Dactinomycin

Cosmegen®

Dactinomycin (actinomycin D) is a tricyclic, peptide-containing antibiotic which acts as an intercalator of DNA, resulting in decreased mRNA synthesis in a phase-nonspecific fashion. It is used in the treatment of sarcomas and choriocarcinoma. About 30% of the drug is recovered from the feces and urine after 1 week; there is no CNS penetration and it is probably concentrated in the bile. The terminal half-life is over 36 hr. Nausea, vomiting, mucositis, diarrhea and reversible alopecia occur frequently. Dose- and duration-dependent hepatotoxicity and genotoxic effects have been reported. Severe ulceration occurs if the drug is extravasated. The dose-limiting toxicity is myelosuppression with a leukopenic nadir at 7–10 days. Rarely, radiation "recall" occurs. Dactinomycin should be reconstituted with preservative-free diluents. It is bound by cellulose filters, so in-line filtration should be avoided. The adult dose is 2 mg/week IV or 500 mcg/day for up to 5 days, repeated at 3–4 week intervals. In children, the dose is 450 mcg/M^2/day, to a maximum of 500 mcg/day, for up to 5 days; the course is repeated in 3 weeks. The dose should be reduced in presence of hepatobiliary dysfunction.[58,59] Available as a 0.5 mg injection.

Estramustine Phosphate

Emcyt®

Pharmacology.   Estramustine is a conjugate of nor-nitrogen mustard linked by a carbamate bond to the 3-position of the steroidal nucleus of estradiol. The phosphorylation at position 17 adds water solubility. It was originally thought to act as a hormonally directed alkylating agent, but later studies suggest alternate activities that impair mitotic spindle formation.

Dephosphorylated estradiol and estrone metabolites produce typical estrogenic effects.[60]

Administration and Adult Dose. PO for prostatic carcinoma 14 mg/kg/day in 3–4 divided doses.

Dosage Individualization. Diabetic and hypertensive patients may require increased doses of insulin or antihypertensives due to estrogenic effects.

Dosage Forms. Cap 140 mg.

Patient Instructions. This drug should be taken on an empty stomach; particularly avoid taking with milk.

Pharmacokinetics. *Fate.* Readily dephosphorylated during absorption to estradiol and estrone congeners. Milk reduces oral bioavailability.

Adverse Reactions. The major side effects are due to estrogenic actions. These include cardiovascular effects (frequent edema, occasional leg cramps or thrombophlebitis and rare pulmonary embolism and infarction), gastrointestinal effects (frequent nausea without vomiting, diarrhea and occasional anorexia), and very frequent gynecomastia. Laboratory abnormalities are minimal; notably, no consistent hematologic suppression and only mild increases in AST (SGOT) or LDH in about 30% of patients.[60]

Contraindications. Thrombophlebitis or thromboembolic conditions (except when tumor is the cause).

Precautions. Pregnancy. Use with caution in patients with severe underlying cardiovascular diseases. Poorly controlled CHF can also be exacerbated by estrogen-induced fluid retention. Insulin-dependent diabetics and patients on antihypertensive medications may have increased medication requirements for these diseases.

Parameters to Monitor. Responses in prostate cancer are predominantly subjective, including reduced pain and less urinary retention. Objective responses can be followed with serial acid phosphatase determinations. For toxicity, attention to cardiovascular or thromboembolic signs and symptoms is important.

Notes. Estramustine phosphate is principally used in the palliative treatment of advanced prostate cancer. Objective response rates of 20–30% are common and the drug can be safely combined with other cytotoxic agents.[60]

Fluorouracil   Various

Pharmacology. Fluorouracil (5-fluorouracil, 5-FU) is a fluorinated antimetabolite of the DNA pyrimidine precursor uracil. It inhibits thymidine formation, thereby blocking DNA synthesis. Some fluorouracil may be incorporated into RNA, inhibiting subsequent protein synthesis. Cell cycle S phase-specific.

Administration and Adult Dose. Rapid IV 15 mg/kg/week for 4 weeks, followed by 20 mg/kg/week until severe toxicity develops. Drug is stopped until resolution is complete, then resumed at 5 mg/kg/week.[61] **IV "loading course"** 12 mg/kg (800 mg maximum) as a single dose daily for 4 days, then 12–15 mg/kg/week is recommended by manufacturer; however, it has been associated with severe, life-threatening bone marrow toxicity.[62] **IV continuous infusion** 1–2 g/day for up to 5 days has been used by special treatment centers; continuous infusion does not consistently increase antitumor efficacy, but does appear to lessen hematologic toxicity.[63] **PO** doses are associated with very low bioavailability and short clinical response. **Intra-arterial, intraperitoneal and intracavitary** administration have also been used. **Top for neoplastic keratoses** apply daily for 1-2 weeks, applied as a thin layer with gloved hand or nonmetal applicator. Skin response progresses sequentially through erythema, vesiculation, erosion, ulceration, necrosis and finally regranulation. Treatment is usually stopped once erosion is evident to allow healing to occur over the next 1-2 months. **Vag for condylomata acuminata** 1/3 applicatorful (1.5 g) of 5% cream once/week hs for 10 weeks.[135]

Pediatric Dose. Generally indicated for adult malignancies, although theoretically, equivalent mg/kg doses could be used in children.

Dosage Forms. **Inj** 50 mg/ml; **Top Crm** 5%; **Top Soln** 2, 5%.

Patient Instructions. Avoid prolonged exposure to strong sunlight; report any severe sores in the mouth immediately. See also Class Instructions.

Pharmacokinetics. *Fate.* Oral doses are erratically and incompletely absorbed with bioavailability of 50-80%, worsened by mixing with acidic fruit juices.[64] V_d is about 25-35 L/kg with drug diffusing to effusions and CSF (peak CSF levels of 6-8 x 10^{-8} M after a 15 mg/kg IV bolus). Extensively and rapidly metabolized, primarily in the liver, to a variety of inactive metabolites which are renally excreted. Up to 15% of drug is renally excreted unchanged, 90% within 6 hr of administration. Fluoroacetate and citrate metabolites found in the CSF are believed to mediate rare CNS toxicities.

$t_{1/2}$. α phase about 8 min; β phase 12-37 min.[65]

Adverse Reactions. Dose-limiting toxicity is myelosuppression (when given by bolus injection) with leukopenic and thrombocytopenic nadirs at 7-14 days. Severe stomatitis 5-8 days after therapy can herald severe impending myelosuppression; this is unpredictably seen with large bolus doses (> 12 mg/kg). Oral dosing increases severity of the frequent mild diarrhea. GI ulceration is occasionally severe, although acute nausea and vomiting are usually mild. Cutaneous toxicities include mild to moderate alopecia, hyperpigmentation of skin and veins, and rashes which are often worsened by sunlight. Excessive lacrimation is frequent; occasionally tear duct fibrosis develops. Rare toxicities involve CNS dysfunction manifested by ataxia, confusion, visual disturbances and headaches. Very rarely, cardiotoxicity has been reported.

Contraindications. Pre-existing severe myelosuppression (WBC < 2,000/cu mm, platelet count < 100,000/cu mm).

Precautions. Concurrent allopurinol appears to block one activation pathway, thereby reducing fluorouracil hematologic toxicity. Fluorouracil can inhibit the antipurine effects of methotrexate. The clinical significance of these two interactions is unclear.

Parameters to Monitor. Pretreatment and monthly assessment of bone marrow function, particularly WBC and platelet counts. In the weeks following dosing, observe for severe stomatitis which may herald life-threatening myelosuppression.

Notes. If precipitate is noted in ampule, gently warm in a water bath and/or vigorously shake to redissolve. Fluorouracil is physically incompatible with diazepam, doxorubicin, cytarabine and methotrexate injections. Mild to moderate activity in GI tract tumors and in breast cancer; topical application of cream is often curative in superficial skin cancers.

Hexamethylmelamine (Investigational - NCI)

Hexamethylmelamine may act as an antimetabolite to inhibit DNA and RNA synthesis; metabolites may also have alkylating activity. It is used in combination chemotherapy of ovarian, cervical and lung cancers. Hexamethylmelamine is N-demethylated to pentamethylmelamine by hepatic microsomal enzymes. Over 50% of a dose is renally excreted in 24 hr. Oral absorption is incomplete and erratic, and may be dose-dependent. Nausea, vomiting and abdominal cramps may be dose-limiting in some patients. Neurotoxic effects are frequent, including agitation, hallucinations and confusion; these are reversible and amenable to dosage reduction. Leukopenia and thrombocytopenia are typically mild. Oral dosage ranges from 4–12 mg/kg/day in 4 divided doses for periods up to 3–6 weeks. Use of a single dose at night may lessen acute toxicity. **Pentamethylmelamine** is a water-soluble (injectable) derivative now also in clinical trials.[66]

Interferon Alpha
Alfa-2a
Alfa-2b

Roferon®

Intron®-A

Pharmacology. Alpha interferons are natural product, single chain proteins. Alfa-2a has a lysine at positon 23, alfa-2b, an arginine. Interferons bind to specific membrane receptors and are then taken up intracellularly to affect diverse cellular functions. These include cell membrane alterations (eg, enhanced antigen expression), cell cycle blockade at the G_1-S portion, enhanced antiviral enzyme synthesis (eg, $2'-5'$ oligo-adenylate synthetase with resultant products which destroy double and single stranded viral RNAs), and immunomodulatory activity [eg, increased activity of natural killer (NK) lymphocytes and phagocytic macrophages].

Administration and Adult Dose. IM or SC 2 million IU/M^2/day or 3 times/week; IV infusion regimens are undergoing experimental testing at markedly reduced total dosage. Experimental regimens include intravesically 50–200 million IU over 2 hr q week for 8 weeks; and intraperitoneally up to 5 million IU/week for up to 4 months.

Pediatric Dose. Not recommended in children under 18 yr.

Dosage Forms. (Alfa-2a) **Inj** 3, 18 million IU; (alfa-2b) **Inj** 3, 5, 10, 25 million IU.

Patient Instructions. *Patients must be instructed in aseptic technique and SC injection technique.* Rotate SC injection sites. Acetaminophen is preferred to reduce frequent "flu-like" symptoms which usually decrease with continued therapy.

Pharmacokinetics. Fate. 100% bioavailable after IM or SC administration, with an absorption half-life of about 6 hr. IM or SC doses of 10 million IU produce peak plasma levels of 100–200 IU/ml within 4 hr; the same dose IV produces peak plasma levels of 500–600 IU/ml within 15–30 min. The majority of a dose is thought to be metabolized, with none filtered or secreted by the kidney.[69,70]

$t_{1/2}$. α phase 0.11 hr; β phase 2 hr after IV or IM, 3 hr after SC.[69,70]

Adverse Reactions. The most frequent reactions include fever to 38–39° C, chills, arthralgias, headache, malaise and myalgias (the "flu-like" syndrome). These reactions are more severe upon initiation of therapy and are ameliorated by acetaminophen or dosage reduction. Anorexia and nausea without vomiting are also frequent. In large doses (generally over 1 million IU) hematologic suppression (eg, mild thrombocytopenia, leukopenia) occurs, as does slight elevation of hepatic enzymes [AST (SGOT), LDH, alkaline phosphatase] and mild hypertension, occasionally associated with tachycardia. Very high doses (30 million IU or greater) are associated with somnolence, dizziness and confusion. Mild erythema and pruritus at the injection site can also occur. Interferons are not mutagenic nor carcinogenic in standard animal or in vitro models.

Contraindications. Severe hypersensitivity.

Precautions. Pregnancy; lactation. Use with caution in patients with cardiovascular disease, seizure disorder, hepatic or renal impairment. Proper hydration during therapy may help lessen hypotensive reactions. Neutralizing serum antibodies can form after prolonged interferon dosing. This has been associated with reduced toxicities and antitumor effects. It may be more common with the alfa 2a preparation.[71]

Notes. A clear dose-response relationship is established for toxicity, but not for antitumor effectiveness. Alpha interferons have activity in reducing the symptomatology of hairy cell leukemia; hematologic response rates of 80-90% are possible in this disease. Other cancers responsive to alpha interferon include renal cell cancer (10-30% partial response rate); acute leukemias (15-30% response rates) and the nonblastic phase of chronic myelogenous leukemia (40-60% response rate).

Interleukin-2 (Investigational - Cetus)　　　Proleukin®

Pharmacology. Interleukin-2 (IL-2) is a lymphokine protein produced by normal peripheral blood lymphocytes. It binds to T-lymphocyte receptors and induces a mitogen response. It also induces the production of cytotoxic lymphocytes (LAK cells) which have been shown to have antitumor activity. The pharmaceutical product is a nonglycosylated IL-2 molecule produced by recombinant DNA techniques.[72,136]

Administration and Adult Dose. IV bolus in phase I studies (with or without adoptive cellular therapy) doses up to 100,000 units/kg (or 0.033 mg/kg of protein) have been given q 8 hr for 5 days. **IV infusion** up to 2 million units/M^2 (0.67 mg/M^2) infused over 6 hr have been given.[73,136]

Dosage Individualization. Interpatient IL-2 pharmacokinetic differences are not known; however, dosage reduction is required if severe cardiovascular collapse or pulmonary insufficiency occurs.

Dosage Forms. Inj 1, 5 mg (investigational; 1 mg = 3 million units).

Pharmacokinetics. *Fate.* Limited human data indicate that the drug undergoes biphasic elimination after IV administration. As in animals, the kidney is believed to be the major organ of elimination in man via active metabolism.[74]

$t_{1/2}$. α phase 5-7 min; β phase 30-120 min.[74]

Adverse Reactions. When combined with adoptive cellular therapy [reinfused lymphokine-activated killer (LAK) cells], immediate fever and chills result; indomethacin orally or meperidine IM or IV 25-50 mg may lessen these. More severe cardiovascular toxicities include fluid retention (over 10% of body weight) and pulmonary interstitial edema. Hypotension requiring treatment has occurred, usually 2-4 hr after an IV bolus, in patients receiving doses of 0.33 mg/M^2 or more. Frequently, nausea, vomiting, diarrhea, rash, pruritus and nasal congestion occur. Abnormal laboratory findings include frequent increased Cr_s, eosinophilia and thrombocytopenia.[73] Increased serum transaminases and bilirubin occur occasionally; hepatic dysfunction occurs rarely. Myocardial ischemia may also occur and fatal infarction has been reported. "Capillary leak syndrome" may occur and requires close monitoring of fluid balance.[73,136]

Precautions. IL-2 has produced severe cardiopulmonary toxicity and must be cautiously used in any patient with a history of cardiac insufficiency from any cause. Patients must also be in good general physical condition in order to tolerate the hypotension and pulmonary edema which can complicate high-dose IL-2 therapy. Glucocorticoids block all IL-2 actions.

Parameters to Monitor. Monitor blood pressure, cardiac output and fluid balance closely.

Notes. IL-2 combined with a patient's LAK cells has produced short-term partial responses (up to 30%) in patients with advanced solid tumors including melanoma, colon cancer and renal cell cancer.[73] In larger multigroup trials, lower response rates of 10–15% have been noted. The contribution of the LAK cells to the therapeutic outcome is not established.

Leuprolide Acetate   Lupron®

Pharmacology.   Leuprolide is a synthetic nonapeptide of human gonadotropin-releasing hormone. A *d*-amino acid and other substitutions lead to prolonged activity by impairing enzymatic destruction. Actions include marked suppression of gonadal steroid levels with resultant inhibition of hormone-dependent tissue growth. Following an initial brief stimulation, chronic leuprolide administration inhibits gonadotropin release which suppresses steroidogenesis in both ovarian and testicular tissues.

Administration and Adult Dose. SC for prostatic carcinoma 1 mg/day.

Dosage Forms. Inj 5 mg/ml.

Patient Instructions. *Patient must be taught aseptic technique and SC injection technique.* Rotate SC injection sites frequently. Disease flare (increased bone pain, urinary retention) can briefly occur with initiation of therapy. Store vial under refrigeration, but do not freeze.

Pharmacokinetics. Fate. Inactive orally; bioavailability of SC and IV doses is reportedly comparable. No information on human distribution, metabolism or excretion is available.

$t_{1/2}$. 3 hr.

Adverse Reactions. About one-half of patients with prostatic carcinoma receiving leuprolide experience hot flashes. However, more serious estrogenic effects (eg, gynecomastia, breast tenderness, nausea, vomiting, edema and thrombosis/phlebitis) occur much less frequently.[67] Patients allergic to benzyl alcohol may experience irritation at the SC injection site. Less than 3% of patients experience any hematologic, hepatic, cardiovascular, renal, respiratory, musculoskeletal or neurologic adverse reactions.

Precautions. Benzyl alcohol hypersensitivity; potential urinary tract obstruction upon therapy initiation.

Parameters to Monitor. Responses can be monitored by measuring (decreased) plasma levels of both testosterone and acid phosphatase. These should be measured 2 weeks after initiation and monthly thereafter.

Notes. Leuprolide is indicated in the palliative management of advanced prostatic cancer. Most responses are not complete and require 8–12 weeks of therapy for adequate evaluation.

Mechlorethamine Hydrochloride   Mustargen®

Pharmacology. Mechlorethamine (nitrogen mustard, HN_2) is a prototype bischloroethylamine, polyfunctional alkylating agent. In solution, the compound readily ionizes to an active form which can alkylate at a number of nucleophilic protein sites, principally the N^7 position of guanine in both DNA and RNA. This action is cell cycle phase-nonspecific.

Administration and Adult Dose. **IV for Hodgkin's disease** (in the classical "MOPP" regimen) 6 mg/M^2 by careful push on days 1 and 8 of a monthly treatment cycle.[75] Vein irritation and sclerosis occur in exposed veins; therefore, it is common to begin venipunctures low on the limb and move up serially, and to administer mechlorethamine last in a combination drug sequence. **IV as a single agent** up to 0.4 mg/kg as a single monthly dose. **Top for mycosis fungoides and psoriasis** 10 mg/60 ml of water, applied to the affected body areas 1-2 times/day.[76]

Pediatric Dose. **IV** same as adult dose.

Dosage Forms. **Inj** 10 mg.

Patient Instructions. See Class Instructions.

Pharmacokinetics. *Fate.* Chemical cyclization occurs in vivo to form positively charged carbonium ions which rapidly react with various cellular components; unchanged drug cannot be detected in the blood within minutes of administration. Less than 0.01% of unchanged drug is recovered in the urine; however, up to 50% of radioactively labeled products may be found in urine within 24 hr.[77]

Adverse Reactions. The major dose-limiting toxicity is myelosuppression: leukopenic nadir 6-8 days, thrombocytopenic nadir 10-16 days. Extravasation causes delayed and protracted (months) ulceration and necrosis; a 1/6 M sodium thiosulfate solution (4 ml of 10% sodium thiosulfate plus 6 ml sterile water) and copious flushing with water may be used as topical antidotes to lessen serious tissue damage. Nausea and vomiting within the first 3 hr are severe and, rarely, may last over 1 day. Primary reproductive failure and alopecia are frequent in both males and females. IV or topical use can cause maculopapular rashes and sometimes severe sensitivity reactions (anaphylaxis and occasional cross-reactivity with other alkylating agents).

Contraindications. Prior severe hypersensitivity reactions; pre-existing profound myelosuppression; infection.

Precautions. Patients with lymphomas (especially "bulky" lymphomas) should receive prophylactic allopurinol 2-3 days prior to therapy to prevent hyperuricemia and urate nephropathy following massive tumor lysis. Every effort should be made to avoid topical contact with this highly vesicant drug (except during topical therapy).

Parameters to Monitor. Pretreatment and at least monthly assessment of bone marrow function, particularly WBC and platelet counts.

Notes. Mechlorethamine is a powerful vesicant and should be prepared with great caution. Use mask and rubber gloves during preparation and avoid inhalation of dust and vapors, or contact with skin and mucous membranes, especially the eyes. Injection should be used within 1 hr of preparation; topical solution and ointment are stable for 1 month under refrigeration.[78] Because of its extreme acute toxicity, use is limited primarily to malignant lymphomas[75] and topically in mycosis fungoides, a cutaneous non-Hodgkin's lymphoma.[79]

Methotrexate   Mexate®, Various

Pharmacology. Methotrexate (MTX) is a folic acid analogue which binds to dihydrofolate reductase, blocking formation of the DNA nucleotide thymidine; purine synthesis is also inhibited. Most active in S phase.

Administration and Adult Dose. *Single Agent Therapy:* **IM, IV or PO for choriocarcinoma** 15–30 mg/day for 5 days, repeated q 1–2 weeks for 3–5 courses; **IM for mycosis fungoides** 50 mg once weekly or 25 mg twice weekly; **IM, IV or PO for head and neck cancer** 25–50 mg/M^2 once weekly (watch for cumulative myelosuppression with continued dosing on this regimen); **Intrathecal for meningeal leukemia** 12 mg/M^2 in a preservative-free, isotonic diluent (eg, Elliott's B solution, patient's own CSF or D5LR); **IV high-dose therapy** (1–3 g/M^2) with leucovorin rescue should be used only by experts in major research centers; **IM or PO for psoriasis** maintenance 5–10 mg initially then **IM, IV or PO** 10–25 mg/week, to maximum of 50 mg/week, depending on clinical response; chronic daily dosing results in increased hepatotoxicity compared to weekly oral or parenteral doses.

Combined Modality Therapy: **for acute lymphocytic leukemia** various schedules are reported for remission-maintenance therapy: **IM or IV** 30 mg/M^2 twice weekly, or 7.5 mg/kg/day for 5 days, or **PO** 2.5 mg/kg/day for 2 weeks; repeat at monthly intervals. **IM, IV or PO for Burkitt's lymphoma** 0.625–2.5 mg/kg/day for 1–2 weeks, then off drug for 7–10 days; **IM or IV for breast cancer** (combined with cyclophosphamide and fluorouracil) 40 mg/M^2 on days 1 and 8, repeat monthly.[80]

Dosage Individualization. Patients with any "third space" fluids (eg, ascites, pleural effusions) should receive reduced doses due to drug retention and slow release of drug from these compartments.[81] Reduce dosage in renal impairment as follows:[82,83]

CREATININE CLEARANCE (ML/MIN)	% OF DOSAGE RECOMMENDED
> 50	60–100% (0–40% reduction)
10–50	30–50% (50–70% reduction)
< 10	15% (85% reduction)

Pediatric Dose. **IM or IV for remission maintenance** same as adult dose for acute lymphoblastic leukemia. **Intrathecally for meningeal cancer** use age-adjusted dosing rather than mg/M^2 dose.[84]

AGE (YR)	IT DOSE (MG)
> 3	12
2–3	10
1–2	8
< 1	6

Dosage Forms. **Tab** 2.5 mg; **Inj** (as sodium) 2.5, 25 mg/ml (preserved solution); 20, 25, 50, 100, 250 mg (nonpreserved powder).

Patient Instructions. See Class Instructions.

Pharmacokinetics. *Plasma Levels.* Following high-dose therapy, a threshold for bone marrow and mucosal toxicity is approximately 1×10^{-6} M 48 hr after dosing. To prevent toxicity, plasma levels should be kept below 10^{-5} M at 24 hr, 5×10^{-7} M at 48 hr and 5×10^{-8} M at 72 hr.[85]

Fate. PO and IM absorption are rapid, peaking at 1–2 and 0.1–1 hr, respectively. Oral bioavailability averages 30%.[83] Following intrathecal administration, the drug slowly diffuses into the bloodstream. About 60–70% is plasma protein bound; V_d is 0.5–1 L/kg. Over 90% of a dose is excreted in the urine, 90% unchanged, after IV administration. Methotrexate solubility is markedly enhanced in acidic urine.

$t_{1/2}$. α phase 0.75 min; β phase 2–4 hr.[86]

Adverse Reactions.   Nearly all reactions are dose- and duration-related. The primary toxicity is hematologic suppression, principally leukopenia with the nadir at 7–14 days depending upon the administration schedule (more prolonged with daily dosing). Thrombocytopenia and macrocytic anemia, dose-related nephrotoxicity and ocular irritation occur also. Mucosal ulcerations of the mouth and tongue, and diarrhea may occasionally become severe within 1–3 weeks after administration, sometimes heralding severe myelotoxicity. Mild to moderate nausea and vomiting just after dosing occur occasionally and erythematous rashes have been reported. Leukoencephalopathy occurs rarely with either IV or intrathecal use. Other toxicities following intrathecal use include nausea and vomiting, meningismus, paresthesias and, rarely, convulsions. Chronic daily dosing in psoriasis has led to hepatocellular damage including fibrotic liver changes and atrophy of the liver; the frequency may be lower with larger intermittent doses.

Contraindications.   Pregnancy; severe renal or hepatic dysfunction; psoriasis patients with pre-existing bone marrow depression.

Precautions.   Renal function must be adequate prior to administration of this drug. Concomitant vinca alkaloids (vincristine or vinblastine) can impair methotrexate elimination from the CSF; similarly, probenecid diminishes renal elimination. Both interactions augment the biological effects of a given dose of methotrexate. Asparaginase given 1 week prior to or 24 hr after methotrexate appears to reduce methotrexate hematologic toxicities.

Parameters to Monitor.   Monitoring should include pretreatment and periodic hepatic, renal and bone marrow function (including WBCs, platelets and RBCs). High doses should be followed with 24 hr and/or 48 hr plasma levels and institution of appropriate leucovorin rescue. The urine should also be alkalinized prior to high doses to enhance methotrexate solubility.

Notes.   Reconstitute lyophilized forms with normal saline, D5W or Elliott's B solution (for intrathecal use). Reconstituted solutions are chemically stable for 7 days at room temperature. Physically incompatible with fluorouracil, prednisolone sodium phosphate and cytarabine. Clinically useful in a variety of hematologic and solid tumors as well as nonmalignant hyperplastic conditions such as psoriasis. If overdosage occurs, the antidote is **calcium leucovorin** (citrovorum factor) which can be given IV or IM in methotrexate-equivalent doses up to 75 mg q 6 hr for 4 doses. A delay of greater than 36 hr lessens the chance of rescue.

Mitomycin   Mutamycin®

Mitomycin (mitomycin-C) is an antibiotic that contains quinone, urethane and aziridine groups. It is activated chemically and metabolically to a variety of alkylator moieties; it is cell cycle phase-nonspecific, but maximum efficacy is in the G_1 and S phases. Mitomycin is used primarily in GI tract tumors and bladder cancers. Following IV doses of 15 mg/M², the peak plasma level is about 1 mg/ml. The drug is eliminated primarily by hepatic metabolism with about 20% hepatic extraction and 10–30% recovery of intact drug in the urine. Clearance is 0.3–0.4 L/hr/kg. The drug has an α half-life of 5–10 min after IV injection and β half-life of 46 min. Nausea, vomiting, diarrhea, alopecia and nephrotoxicity occur frequently. Dose- and duration-dependent mutagenicity, teratogenicity and sterility have been reported.

The dose-limiting toxicities are myelosuppression with a long leukopenic nadir of 3-4 weeks, thrombocytopenia and anemia, all of which may be cumulative. The patient should be monitored carefully for delayed and prolonged myelosuppression. Severe ulceration may occur if the drug is extravasated. Interstitial pneumonia, for which corticosteroids are helpful, occurs rarely. Mitomycin is contraindicated in patients with pre-existing myelosuppression or anemia. As a single agent, mitomycin is given IV in a single dose of 20 mg/M^2 repeated q 6 weeks if hematologic toxicity has resolved. In combination regimens, it is given in doses of 5-10 mg/M^2, repeated in 4-6 weeks. Up to 60 mg/week may be given intravesically in bladder cancer.[87-89] Available as 5 and 20 mg injections.

Mitoxantrone   Novantrone®

Pharmacology. A substituted salt of a planar ring anthracene. The drug binds to DNA by intercalation, producing DNA strand breaks; DNA synthesis is impaired in a cell cycle phase-nonspecific fashion.[90]

Administration and Adult Dose. IV for solid tumors 12 mg/M^2 q 4 weeks or 5 mg/M^2/week for 3 weeks. **IV for leukemia** 10-12 mg/M^2/day for 3 days.

Dosage Individualization. Doses must be reduced by approximately 30-50% in patients with abnormal hepatobiliary function and/or significant third-space fluid accumulations.[91] Reduced doses are also required in patients with poor bone marrow reserve. No dosage alteration is required with renal function impairment.

Pediatric Dose. IV for leukemia up to 8 mg/M^2/week for 3 weeks or up to 18 mg/M^2 q 4 weeks.

Dosage Forms. Inj 2 mg/ml.

Patient Instructions. This drug may turn your urine green due to the dark blue drug color. See also Class Instructions.

Pharmacokinetics. Fate. Drug is over 95% plasma protein bound and exhibits prolonged retention in tissues. Some liver metabolism to glucuronyl and glutathione conjugates occurs. Urinary recovery is less than 8% of a dose; the majority is eliminated in the bile; fecal recovery averages 18% of a dose over 5 days.[91]

$t_{1/2}$. α phase 14 min; β phase 1.1 hr; γ phase 38-43 hr.[90,91]

Adverse Reactions. Myelosuppression, principally granulocytopenia (nadir at 10-14 days), occurs and is most severe in heavily pretreated or irradiated patients. Mild to moderate nausea and vomiting occur; mucositis, which is dose-limiting, occurs only with weekly regimens. A low frequency of CHF reported, most often after prior anthracycline therapy. Cumulative cardiotoxicity limits are not well known, but may approach 100 mg/M^2 with prior anthracyclines and 160 mg/M^2 without.[90] Alopecia is minimal.

Precautions. Dosage adjustment may be necessary in patients previously treated with marrow suppressant or cardiotoxic agents. Doses should also be reduced in patients with poor hepatobiliary function.

Parameters to Monitor. Pretreatment serum bilirubin; cardiac function assessment in patients with prior anthracycline therapy or severe pre-existing cardiovascular disease. Monitor absolute granulocyte levels prior to each dose; nadir counts 7-10 days after the dose are optional.

Notes. Mitoxantrone is not a vesicant.

Nitrosoureas
Carmustine
Lomustine

BiCNU®
CeeNU®

Pharmacology. Carmustine (BCNU) and lomustine (CCNU) are highly lipid soluble drugs which are metabolized to active alkylating and carbamoylating moieties. Several key cellular enzymatic steps are inhibited, including those involving DNA polymerase and RNA protein synthesis. There is typically only partial cross-resistance to classical alkylators. The nitrosoureas are cell cycle phase-nonspecific and even have significant activity on G_0 (resting phase) cells.

Administration, Dose and Dosage Forms.

	CARMUSTINE	LOMUSTINE
Administration	IV in 100–200 ml D5W over 15–45 min.	PO only.
Adult Dose	75–100 mg/M^2/day for 1–2 days or 200 mg/M^2 as single dose, or 80 mg/M^2/day for 3 days,[92] repeat at 6–8 week intervals.	100–130 mg/M^2 as single dose, repeat at 6–8 week intervals.
Pediatric Dose	Same as adult dose.	—
Dosage Forms	Inj 100 mg (with alcohol diluent).	Cap 100 mg (2)* + 40 mg (2) + 10 mg (2).

*Commercial packet totals 300 mg.

Dosage Individualization. Elderly patients or those with heavily pretreated bone marrows should receive 50–75% of the recommended dose and/or lengthened treatment intervals (8 weeks minimum). Lomustine absorption is rapid; thus, vomiting 45 or more minutes after ingestion does not require redosing.

Patient Instructions. Lomustine should be taken on an empty stomach. See also Class Instructions.

Pharmacokinetics.

	CARMUSTINE	LOMUSTINE
Fate.		
Absorption	—	Complete after 30 min.[93]
Distribution	Both drugs are diffusely distributed with decreasing relative concentrations in spleen, liver and ovaries; both achieve substantial penetration into CNS with simultaneous CSF levels of > 50% of plasma for intact carmustine and metabolites[94] and > 30% for intact lomustine and metabolites;[93] enterohepatic cycling of active metabolites is possible and may explain subsequent peaks in nitrosourea plasma levels at 1 and 4 hr.	
Metabolism	Both drugs are rapidly and extensively metabolized (par-	

Continued

Pharmacokinetics.

	CARMUSTINE	LOMUSTINE
	tially by liver microsomal enzymes) to a number of active products which have long plasma half-lives compared to the parent compounds.	
Excretion	30% urinary drug recovery as metabolites after 24 hr, 65% after 96 hr.[94]	50% urinary drug recovery as metabolites after 12 hr, 60% after 48 hr; less than 5% fecal excretion.[93]
$t_{1/2}$.	Intact drug 5 min; biological effect 15–30 min; metabolites, slow decay over 3–4 days.[94]	Intact drug 15 min; cyclohexyl and carbonyl metabolites: α phase 4–5 hr, β phase 30–50 hr; chloroethyl metabolite 72 hr.[93]

Adverse Reactions. Major dose-limiting toxicity is delayed and potentially cumulative myelosuppression; nadirs are unusually prolonged with leukopenia at approximately 35 days and thrombocytopenia at about 30 days. Thus, doses are not repeated more often than q 6 weeks.[95] Nausea and vomiting are frequent; prophylactic phenothiazine antiemetics are moderately effective. Carmustine frequently causes severe pain at injection site and venospasm which may be reduced by slow, dilute infusions. Both drugs may transiently raise liver enzymes; nephrotoxicity is consistently reported following cumulative doses of 1,500 mg/M^2 or more. Pulmonary fibrosis is also reported, usually following cumulative doses over 1,000 mg/M^{2};[96] variant carmustine-induced pulmonary fibrosis, highly responsive to early drug discontinuation and corticosteroids, has been reported.[97] Other rare toxicities include CNS effects (eg, confusion, lethargy, ataxia), stomatitis and alopecia. In animal models, the nitrosoureas are highly carcinogenic and several clinical cases of leukemia after nitrosourea therapy have been reported.

Contraindications.   Demonstrated hypersensitivity; significant pre-existing myelosuppression.

Precautions. Pregnancy. Clinical resistance to carmustine and perhaps other nitrosoureas is significantly reduced by concomitant amphotericin B administration. Experimentally in rats, carmustine, lomustine and the investigational drug **semustine** are cleared much more rapidly (with reduced antitumor activity) by pretreatment with phenobarbital, which stimulates microsomal enzymes. Conversely, cimetidine can impair metabolism and increase nitrosourea myelotoxicity.

Notes. Carmustine should be stored under refrigeration; appearance of an oily film in the vial is evidence of decomposition, and such vials should be discarded. Carmustine is incompatible with sodium bicarbonate. **Semustine** is an oral investigational methyl derivative of lomustine with no advantages over presently available agents; it is available from NCI.

Platinum-Containing Analogues
Cisplatin   Platinol®

Pharmacology. A planar coordinate dichlorodiammino compound of platinum in the + II valence state. Aquated in vivo to a positively charged species that can attack nucleophilic sites in DNA such as purine and pyrimidine bases. Action is cell cycle phase-nonspecific.

Administration and Adult Dose. IV bolus or continuous infusion (usually with aggressive hydration) single doses up to 120 mg/M^2 have been used.[98] Einhorn testicular cancer regimen calls for 20 mg/M^2/day for 5 days.[99] See Notes.

Dosage Individualization. Reduce dosage in renal impairment; specific dose reduction guidelines have not been established.

Pediatric Dose. IV maximum single dose 100 mg/M^2 q 2-3 weeks; IV 10-20 mg/M^2/day for 4-5 days, repeat q 3-4 weeks.

Dosage Forms. Inj 10, 50 mg.

Patient Instructions. Be prepared for severe nausea and vomiting following drug administration. See also Class Instructions.

Pharmacokinetics. *Plasma Levels.* In vitro cell culture data suggest cytotoxicity at levels of 50 mcg/ml for 1 hr or 5 mcg/ml for 8 hr.
   Fate. Peak plasma levels of free platinum following a 100 mg/M^2 bolus are about 3.4 mcg/ml when given with mannitol (12.5 g) and 2.7 mcg/ml without mannitol.[100] Over 90% of platinum is protein bound to RBCs, albumin and pre-albumin. Freely distributed to most organs including kidneys, liver, skin and lungs; minimal accumulation in CSF only after repeated doses. Cumulative 24-hr urinary excretion of platinum is 20% with mannitol, 40% without.
   $t_{1/2}$. Free platinum 48 min (without mannitol); 59 min (with mannitol). Terminal $t_{1/2}$ 58-73 hr, probably reflecting slow release of protein-bound drug.[101]

Adverse Reactions. Primary toxicity is weakly dose-related nephrotoxicity. Major acute toxicity is severe and often prolonged (days) nausea and vomiting, which may be managed with aggressive prophylaxis using butyrophenones (eg, droperidol), metoclopramide or high-dose corticosteroids. Ototoxicity, total dose-related hypomagnesemia and cumulative severe peripheral neuropathy are reported. Slight leukopenia, thrombocytopenia and frequent anemia occur. Very rare toxicities include transient cortical dysfunction (blindness) and hypersensitivity (including anaphylaxis).

Contraindications. Marked renal insufficiency (Cr_s over 1.5-2 mg/dl); myelosuppression; hearing impairment. Anaphylaxis; however, some patients experiencing prior anaphylaxis have been successfully retreated with cisplatin and concomitant antihistamines, epinephrine and corticosteroids.

Precautions. Use cautiously in renal impairment and with other nephrotoxic drugs, especially aminoglycosides.[102] Assure adequate hydration prior to administration. Both furosemide and mannitol are used to decrease platinum nephrotoxicity, although each apparently retards free platinum elimination.

Parameters to Monitor. Assess renal function prior to each dose (eg, serial BUN and/or Cr_s) and serum magnesium levels periodically.

Notes. Reconstitute with sterile water; may then be mixed in saline-containing solutions; stable for 24 hr in mannitol. Do not expose solution to metals (eg, metal drippers or cannulae), because platinum may rapidly plate onto these surfaces. Hydrate the patient with at least one liter of a saline-containing solution with 20 mEq of KCl and 3 g of $MgSO_4$/L.[103]

Carboplatin (Investigational - Bristol)   Paraplatin®

Carboplatin is a platinum II analogue which is a diamine 1, 1- cyclobutane dicarboxylate derivative. It has a much higher solubility than cisplatin (17 mg/ml vs 1 mg/ml) with reduced protein binding and is therefore more readily excreted in the urine (55–75% in 24 hr). Free platinum half-lives are α phase 87 min and β phase 354 min. Carboplatin is slowly activated in vivo and has relatively low frequencies of nephrotoxicity, nausea and vomiting compared to cisplatin; ototoxicity, neurotoxicity and renal magnesium wasting are virtually absent. Myelosuppression, principally thrombocytopenia, is more prevalent than with cisplatin. Clinical uses of carboplatin are similar to cisplatin. Doses average 400 mg/M^2 IV once monthly without hydration.[104,105]

Iproplatin (Investigational - Bristol)

Iproplatin is a platinum +IV isopropylamine derivative. Cumulative urinary platinum excretion is about 60%. Renal magnesium wasting does not occur. The drug has a toxicity profile intermediate between cisplatin and carboplatin with both neurotoxicity and myelotoxicity reported. Thrombocytopenia appears to be the dose-limiting toxicity following the maximally tolerated monthly dose of 300 mg/M^2 IV.[106]

Plicamycin   Mithracin®

Plicamycin (mithramycin) is a complex, polycyclic, sugar-linked antibiotic that acts by DNA binding in a cell cycle phase-nonspecific fashion; it also has a separate calcium-lowering effect. It is used in testicular cancer and to control hypercalcemia due to malignancy. The metabolic fate of the drug is unknown, but 40% of radioactivity from a radiolabeled dose appears in the urine and the drug penetrates well into the CNS. Mild to moderate myelosuppression with a leukopenic nadir at 7–12 days, nausea and vomiting occur frequently. Dose- and duration-dependent nephrotoxicity (increased Cr$_s$ and proteinuria), hepatotoxicity [increased LDH and AST (SGOT)], mutagenicity, teratogenicity and sterility have been reported. The dose-limiting toxicity is a hemorrhagic tendency characterized by decreased platelet count and responsiveness, and depressed clotting factor synthesis. Rarely, stomatitis, progressive skin thickening and hyperpigmentation occur. The drug is contraindicated in patients with pre-existing bleeding diatheses, hypocalcemia, or, severe renal or hepatic dysfunction. It should be used cautiously, if at all, with other drugs affecting platelet function (eg, aspirin). The dose for testicular tumors is 25–30 mcg/kg/day for up to 5 days, repeated in 4 weeks if toxicity has resolved. For hypercalcemia, a dose of 25 mcg/kg/day is given for 3–4 days. The dose should be reduced by 25–50% in moderate to severe renal impairment.[107,108] Available as a 2.5 mg injection. Note: dosage is in micrograms.

Podophyllotoxins
Etoposide   VePesid®

Pharmacology. Etoposide (VP-16) is a substituted epipodophyllotoxin derivative from the May apple plant. The major cytotoxic activity is cell cycle phase-specific for G$_2$ and involves the induction of DNA strand breaks by inhibiting DNA topoisomerase II enzymes.

Administration and Adult Dose. IV bolus 200-250 mg/M² once weekly, or 70 mg/M²/day for 5 days, or **IV continuous infusion** 125 mg/M²/day for 5 days.[109] **PO for small cell lung cancer** 2 times the IV dose, rounded to the nearest 50 mg.

Dosage Individualization. With Cl_{cr} of 20 ml/min or less, give 75% of standard dose; reduced doses are also required if severe bone marrow compromise is present. No dosage reduction is necessary with altered hepatobiliary function.

Dosage Forms. Inj 100 mg/5 ml; **Cap** 50 mg.

Patient Instructions. See Class Instructions.

Pharmacokinetics. *Fate.* Oral bioavailability is 50% (range 37-67) with large inter- and intrapatient variability. Less than 10% of a dose penetrates into the CNS. 30-40% is eliminated in urine; about 70% of this is unchanged. Up to 16% of a dose may be eliminated in bile. Inactive metabolites include the hydroxyacid and cis-lactones. V_{dss} is 10-20 L/M²; Cl is 1.1-1.7 L/hr/M².[109]

$t_{1/2}$. 6-11 hr.[109]

Adverse Reactions. Myelosuppression occurs with a nadir at 7-10 days (longer with daily regimens), principally affecting the granulocytes, but also affecting platelets with a nadir at 9-16 days. Mild mucositis, alopecia, nausea and vomiting can occur. Diarrhea is more frequent with oral doses. Hypotension occurs rarely with rapid IV bolus injections. Anaphylactic reactions and possible synergistic neuropathies with vincristine and/or cardiomyopathy with anthracyclines have been reported. There is one report of radiation recall skin injury in 13 of 23 patients with small cell lung cancer.[110]

Precautions. Pregnancy; decrease dose in severe renal dysfunction; avoid rapid IV bolus injection.

Parameters to Monitor. Peripheral granulocyte counts should be obtained immediately prior to dosing on repetitive courses. Nadir counts (1-2 weeks after dosing) are optional.

Notes. Etoposide is indicated in the combination treatment of small cell carcinoma of the lung and refractory nonseminomatous testicular cancer. The drug is also active in lymphomas and in acute leukemias (both lymphoblastic and myeloblastic varieties). Etoposide is not a vesicant. Store capsules under refrigeration.

Teniposide (Investigational - Bristol)   Vumon®

Teniposide is an investigational podophyllum derivative which possesses cell cycle S and G_2 phase-specific cytotoxic activities similar to etoposide. Teniposide is over 90% plasma protein bound and is eliminated much more slowly than etoposide. Teniposide half-lives are α phase 45 min, β phase 4 hr and γ phase 11-30 hr (average 20); 40% of a dose is eliminated in the feces; CSF drug levels are high (27% of plasma levels). The dose-limiting side effect of teniposide is myelosuppression with the leukopenic nadir at 10-14 days. Nausea and vomiting are typically mild (more severe after oral etoposide). Hypotension is reported with rapid drug infusions. Rarely, severe hypersensitivity reactions (including anaphylaxis), alopecia and chemical phlebitis during infusion occur. Teniposide has clinical activity primarily in lymphomas and in pediatric acute leukemias in IV doses of 100 mg/M²/week or 50 mg/M²/day for 5 days, up to 165 mg/M² twice weekly.[111,112] Available as a 50 mg/ml injection (investigational).

Procarbazine Hydrochloride
Matulane®

Procarbazine is an N-methyl hydrazine derivative that undergoes auto-oxidation and microsomal activation to form several alkylating species, including H_2O_2, •OH and •O_2 (superoxide) free radicals. It is cell cycle S phase-specific and used in Hodgkin's and non-Hodgkin's lymphomas and in brain tumors. The drug is rapidly and completely absorbed after oral administration; CNS levels are equal to plasma after 0.5–1.5 hr. Procarbazine is 70% recovered in the urine primarily as an acid metabolite with less than 5% excreted unchanged. Frequent CNS side effects include paresthesias, dizziness, headache, ataxia, nightmares, depression and hallucinations (in up to 30% of patients). Mild to moderate nausea and vomiting occur, but tolerance usually develops rapidly. Dose- and duration-dependent mutagenicity, teratogenicity and sterility have been reported frequently. The dose-limiting toxicity is myelosuppression with a pancytopenic nadir at 2–3 weeks. Rare side effects include a flu-like syndrome, allergic pneumonitis and rash. Procarbazine is contraindicated in patients with *severe* hypersensitivity to the drug or pre-existing bone marrow aplasia. Concomitant use with MAO inhibitors, alcohol, heterocyclic antidepressants, sympathomimetics or tyramine-containing foods should be avoided. Microsomal enzyme-inducing drugs may augment procarbazine cytotoxicity. Procarbazine potentiates barbiturates, narcotics and other hepatically metabolized drugs. Periodic evaluations of neurological status and monthly CBCs may be useful. Procarbazine is given orally in doses of 50–200 mg/M^2/day for 10–25 days, repeated in 3–4 weeks. The dose should be calculated based on ideal body weight and reduced for a BUN over 40 mg/dl, Cr$_s$ over 2 mg/dl or serum bilirubin over 3 mg/dl.[113] Available as 50 mg capsules.

Purine Analogues
Azathioprine
Imuran®
Mercaptopurine
Purinethol®
Thioguanine
Thioguanine

Pharmacology. Azathioprine, mercaptopurine (6-MP) and thioguanine (6-TG) are thiolated purines that act as antimetabolites following metabolic activation to the nucleotide forms (phosphorylated ribose sugar attachment). Subsequently, purine biosynthesis is interrupted at a number of enzymatic sites, including the conversion of inosinic acid to adenine- or xanthine-based ribosides. DNA and RNA synthesis is halted in a cell cycle S phase-specific fashion.

Administration, Dose and Dosage Forms.

	AZATHIOPRINE	MERCAPTOPURINE	THIOGUANINE
Administration	PO, IV.	PO, IV (investigational).	PO, IV (investigational).
Adult Dose Initial:	3–5 mg/kg/day.	500 mg/M^2/day for 5 days.	—
Maintenance:	1–2 mg/kg/day.	80–100 mg/M^2/day.	2–3 mg/kg/day.

Continued

Administration, Dose and Dosage Forms.

	AZATHIOPRINE	MERCAPTOPURINE	THIOGUANINE
Pediatric Dose Initial:	3–5 mg/kg for 1 dose.	500 mg/M^2/day for 5 days.	—
Maintenance:	1–2 mg/kg/day.	70 mg/M^2/day.	2–3 mg/kg/day.
Dosage Forms	Tab 50 mg Inj 100 mg.	Tab 50 mg Inj 500 mg (investigational).	Tab 40 mg Inj 75 mg (investigational).

Dosage Individualization. Purine antimetabolite toxicities are not consistently increased in patients with renal failure.[114,115] See Precautions.

Patient Instructions. To maximize absorption, these drugs should not be taken with meals. Nausea and vomiting are rare with usual doses. See also Class Instructions.

Pharmacokinetics.

	AZATHIOPRINE	MERCAPTOPURINE	THIOGUANINE
Fate.			
Absorption	Unknown.	16% (range 5–37).[116]	Unknown.
Distribution	Approximately 30% plasma protein bound; freely distributed throughout the body including placental transfer; CSF/plasma ratios: 0.19–0.27 for mercaptopurine, 0.16 for thioguanine.		
Metabolism	Rapid conversion to mercaptopurine; this is not altered in renal failure.	Metabolized extensively by xanthine oxidase, also methylated to active metabolite and sulfated to inactive thiouric acid.	Predominantly eliminated by methylation to inactive metabolites.
$t_{1/2}$.	IV azathioprine: 12.5 min; mercaptopurine after PO azathioprine: ½–4 hr (1 hr onset).	36–90 min.	α phase 15 min; β phase 11 hr.

Adverse Reactions. The dose-limiting toxicity is myelosuppression (leukopenia and thrombocytopenia). Mild to moderate mucositis occurs with large doses, but nausea and vomiting are rare with low daily maintenance doses. Predominantly cholestatic liver toxicities are reported rarely with long-term therapy. Significant crystalluria with hematuria reported with large IV mercaptopurine doses.[117] Restrictive lung disease is also described with azathioprine, which reverses upon drug discontinuation. A variety of rashes have also been described with this class of agents. Chronic immunosuppressive therapy with any of these agents exposes patients to a significant risk of carcinogenesis; CNS lymphomas and acute myeloid leukemia are the most frequent malignancies.[119]

Contraindications. Significant or impending severe bone marrow depression.

Precautions. Pregnancy. Patients on allopurinol *must* receive substantially reduced doses of oral mercaptopurine or azathioprine (1/4–1/3 the normal dose), to avoid life-threatening myelosuppression. Thioguanine is primarily inactivated by methylation; thus, no dosage reduction is necessary with concomitant allopurinol.

Parameters to Monitor. WBC and platelet counts and total bilirubin at least monthly.

Notes. Azathioprine is also used for severe rheumatoid arthritis.

Streptozocin   Zanosar®

Streptozocin (streptozotocin) is a glucose-containing nitrosourea. It has some selective cytotoxic activity in insulinomas and malignant carcinoid and is active to a lesser extent in other adenocarcinomas of the GI tract. The drug inhibits DNA synthesis via inhibition of pyrimidine biosynthesis and blockade of key enzymatic sites in gluconeogenesis pathways. It is cell cycle phase-nonspecific. The drug is rapidly and extensively metabolized (unchanged drug half-life is 35 min) and only 10–20% is renally excreted unchanged. It is highly lipophilic, achieving good CNS penetration. Streptozocin and metabolites have a short distribution phase ($t_{1/2}$ 6 min) followed by possibly two elimination phases representing active metabolites ($t_{1/2\ \beta}$ 3.5 hr, $t_{1/2\ \gamma}$ 40 hr). Common acute toxicities include nausea, vomiting and phlebitis; carefully avoid extravasation. The drug is only mildly myelotoxic, but is extremely nephrotoxic. Signs of streptozocin nephrotoxicity include various renal tubular defects as well as proteinuria; adequate hydration may offer some protection. It also selectively destroys pancreatic beta cells. The drug is administered IV 1–1.5 g/M^2/week or 500 mg/M^2/day for 5 days, repeated every 6 weeks.[120] Available as Inj 1 g.

Tamoxifen Citrate   Nolvadex®, Various

Pharmacology. Synthetic nonsteroidal anti-estrogen which binds to cytosol and/or nuclear estrogen receptor (ER) proteins in hormonally sensitive organs including the breast, prostate, uterus and ovary.[121] The tamoxifen-receptor complex binds to chromatin in the cell nucleus wherein estrogen-dependent growth-stimulatory mRNA synthesis is halted.

Administration and Adult Dose. PO 10–20 mg/M^2/day in 2 divided doses (usually 20 mg bid in premenopausal patients and 10 mg bid in postmenopausal patients). To rapidly achieve steady-state levels, an initial 2-week course of 40 mg/M^2 bid, followed by the standard maintenance dose has been recommended.[122]

Dosage Forms. Tab 10 mg.

Patient Instructions. Lactation may occur while on tamoxifen. In premenopausal patients the chance of becoming pregnant is increased and mechanical contraceptive use should be instituted. See also Class Instructions.

Pharmacokinetics. *Onset and Duration.* Therapeutic levels attained with 10–20 mg/M^2/day in 7 or more days, versus 3 hr after the loading dose regimen of 40 mg/M^2 or more bid.[122] There is no long-term antitumor effect after drug discontinuation.

Plasma Levels. There does not appear to be a direct relationship between levels and response or time to response, but all responders have tamoxifen levels over 180 ng/ml at the time of remission.

Fate. Well absorbed orally with a peak level of 42 ng/ml (12 ng/ml is N-desmethyl metabolite) achieved 3–4 hr after a 20 mg dose.[123] Initially, the N-desmethyl concentration is only 50% of the tamoxifen level, but after 21 days the 2 fractions are roughly equal. With low-dose continuous therapy, mean steady-state tamoxifen levels of 260 ng/ml or more are achieved after 16 weeks. Following absorption, tamoxifen is slowly, but extensively metabolized, mainly to N-desmethyltamoxifen which is equally antiestrogenic to tamoxifen. Neither is readily conjugated and both undergo hepatic hydroxylation and conjugation followed by elimination into the bile and feces; levels are measurable for up to 6 weeks after drug discontinuation.[122]

$t_{1/2}$. (Tamoxifen) 4 days; (N-desmethyltamoxifen) 9 days.[123] With chronic dosing, these half-lives increase slightly.[122]

Adverse Reactions. Well tolerated, producing rare myelosuppression (usually in heavily pretreated patients). Menopausal symptomatology, including hot flashes, nausea and rarely vomiting, is produced in one-third of patients. Menstrual difficulties include irregularity, vaginal bleeding and pruritus vulvae. A serious disease "flare" is infrequently seen during initial therapy involving hypercalcemia and an increase in bone or soft tissue pain;[124] this often subsides even with continued therapy and may indicate early tumor response. Retinopathy has occurred only after very large doses (over 120 mg/day for 1 yr).[125]

Precautions. Pregnancy. Use with caution in patients with pre-existing leukopenia and thrombocytopenia.

Notes. The response rate in breast cancer is about 50–70% in estrogen receptor (ER) positive patients, whereas the rate in ER negative patients is only about 5–10%.[126]

Thiotepa   Various

Thiotepa (TESPA, TSPA) is a thiophosphoramide compound that is slowly hydrolyzed to release ethyleneimine moieties that alkylate DNA. It is used systemically in the treatment of breast cancer, intracavitarily for bladder or pleural disease and intrathecally for CNS disease. Thiotepa is metabolized primarily to TEPA. The total body clearance is 8.5 L/hr/M^2, with 15% recovered in the urine as TEPA in 24 hr. It has an α half-life of 7.5 min and a β half-life of 109 min. Mild nausea and vomiting occur frequently. The dose-limiting toxicity is myelosuppression (both granulocytes and platelets). Myelosuppression can occur after intravesicular or intrapleural administration. Anaphylaxis occurs rarely and mutagenicity, teratogenicity and sterility have been reported. Thiotepa can be administered IV, IM or SC in a dose of 0.5 mg/kg monthly or 6 mg/M^2/day for 4 days. The dosage by all routes should be reduced with pre-existing bone marrow suppression. The intracavitary dose is 60 mg and the intrathecal dose is 10 mg/M^2.[127] Available as a 15 mg injection.

Tumor Necrosis Factor (Investigational - Genentech)

Pharmacology. Tumor necrosis factor (TNF) is a protein obtained from BCG or lipopolysaccharide-stimulated macrophags. The recombinant product (rTNF) binds specifically to cellular receptors of several tumor cell lines. It subsequently induces necrosis by an unknown mechanism, possibly involving lysosomes. Early studies show an ischemic necrosis pattern in solid tumors such as fibrosarcoma.[128]

Administration and Adult Dose. IV **bolus** 200-300 mcg/M^2 every other day has been used in preliminary phase I trials.[129]

Dosage Forms. **Inj** 0.3 mg protein (about 10 units/mg).

Pharmacokinetics. *Fate.* In early human trials, plasma levels of 100 units/ml appear achievable. Biphasic elimination after IV administration.[129]
 t$_{1/2}$. α phase 2 min; β phase 31 min.[129]

Adverse Reactions. Fever and chills occur very frequently; nausea and vomiting occur in about one-half of patients. Malaise, fatigue and headache occur in about one-third of patients. Elevations in AST (SGOT), alkaline phosphatase and serum triglycerides also occur in about one-third of patients; however, cholesterol and LDL are not elevated. The peripheral WBC count drops precipitously (by 80–95%), but transiently after rTNF. Mild to moderate hypotension occurs with high doses.[129,130]

Precautions. Use cautiously in patients with poor bone marrow reserve and in those with pre-existing hepatic function abnormalities. Cachectic or malnourished patients are probably poor candidates for rTNF, because of its inhibitory effects on lipid utilization.

Parameters to Monitor. Obtain peripheral WBC counts prior to therapy and weekly thereafter. Hepatic enzymes and serum triglycerides should probably be obtained with each course of therapy and monthly. Monitor the patient's weight as an index of nutritional status and drug-induced cachexia.

Vinca Alkaloids
Vinblastine Sulfate   Velban®, Various
Vincristine Sulfate   Oncovin®, Various
Vindesine Sulfate (Investigational - Lilly)
                 Eldisine®

Pharmacology. Periwinkle plant-derived antimitotic agents; cytotoxic activity is related to specific binding to the microtubule protein tubulin, blocking formation of the mitotic spindle apparatus necessary for cell division. The vincas are lethal at high concentrations and at lower concentrations dividing cells are arrested in metaphase. Occasionally, vincas may be used to synchronize tumor cell populations for subsequent treatment by G$_2$-M phase-specific agents such as bleomycin.

Administration, Dose and Dosage Forms.

	VINBLASTINE	VINCRISTINE	VINDESINE
Administration	IV push, infusion.	IV push.	IV push, infusion.
Adult Dose	IV push 4–12 mg/M^2 as a single agent, at weekly or greater intervals; or 1.5–1.7 mg/M^2/day for 5 days as a continuous infusion.[131]	0.4–1.4 mg/M^2/week (2 mg typical single dose limit).	IV push 3 mg/M^2 q 1–2 weeks; or 1.5 mg/M^2/day for 5–7 days as a continuous infusion.[132]

Continued

Administration, Dose and Dosage Forms.

	VINBLASTINE	VINCRISTINE	VINDESINE
Pediatric Dose	IV push 4–10 mg/M^2, at weekly or greater intervals.	1.4–2 mg/M^2/week (2 mg typical single dose limit).	IV push 4 mg/M^2 q 1–2 weeks.
Dosage Forms	Inj 10 mg.	Inj 1 mg/ml.	Inj 5 mg.

Dosage Individualization.   Vinblastine and vindesine may require substantial (75%) dose reduction in heavily pretreated patients (drugs, radiation therapy). All the vinca alkaloids are extensively eliminated in the bile and doses must be reduced by approximately 50–75% in the presence of severe hepatobiliary dysfunction.

Patient Instructions.   See Class Instructions.

Pharmacokinetics.

Fate.

Distribution	Pharmacokinetic patterns can be described by a three compartment open model: an initial short phase with rapid tissue uptake (V_d approximating total body water) and a long terminal phase of about 1 day with a large V_d reflecting slow drug release from tissue binding sites. Vincas do not effectively penetrate the CNS or other fatty tissues and achieve highest levels in liver, gallbladder and spleen. See also $t_{1/2}$.
Metabolism	Approximately 50% of renally and fecally excreted products are closely related metabolites. An example is the formation of desacetyl vinblastine (which is more active on a weight basis than vinblastine) following either vindesine or vinblastine.
Excretion	The vinca alkaloids appear to be eliminated primarily in the bile and feces, some in the urine.

	VINBLASTINE	VINCRISTINE	VINDESINE
Urine (cumulative)	– 33% (72 hr)	10% (24 hr) 13% (72 hr)	13% (24 hr) 19% (72 hr)
Feces (cumulative)	– 21% (72 hr)	33% (24 hr) 67% (72 hr)	– –
Pharmacokinetic Parameters[133,134]			
V_c (L/kg)	0.7	0.33	0.054
V_d area (L/kg)	27.3	8.4	8.8
$t_{1/2}$.			
$t_{1/2}$ α (hr)	0.062	0.077	0.037
$t_{1/2}$ β (hr)	0.164	2.3	0.9
$t_{1/2}$ γ (hr)	25	85	24

Adverse Reactions.   Myelosuppression is the dose-limiting toxicity for vinblastine and vindesine with the leukopenic nadir at 4–10 days; unless patients have been heavily pretreated (ie, with drugs or radiation), recovery from leukopenia is rather prompt, sometimes facilitating weekly or semimonthly dosing. Significant thrombocytopenia is rare and with vindesine the platelet count may actually increase; defective erythropoiesis is also reported for vindesine. The major toxicity of vincristine is peripheral neuropathy manifested by paresthesias, constipation, jaw pain, diminished deep tendon reflexes and, rarely, bladder atony or paralytic ileus. These slowly resolve over a month and necessitate substantial dose reduction if present at the time of dosing. Seizures and ocular toxicity presenting as diplopia or ptosis occur rarely. Mild laxatives may be useful for constipation. The vincas are extremely toxic if inadvertently extravasated; hyaluronidase (150 units/3 ml) may be effective as a local antidote. Infrequently, nausea and vomiting can occur, along with transiently severe pain in tumor masses (with vinblastine or vindesine). Alopecia is common with all agents.

Contraindications. (Vinblastine.) Severe bone marrow compromise from prior therapy. (Vincristine.) Severe peripheral nervous system effects from prior doses, particularly paralytic ileus; demyelinating form of Charcot-Marie-Tooth Syndrome.

Precautions. Pregnancy. Use with caution in patients with neurologic deficiencies or hepatic disease. Vinca administration (especially vincristine) has been associated with increased cellular retention of methotrexate (increased even in CNS tissues).

Parameters to Monitor. (Vinblastine and vindesine) pretreatment and at least monthly WBC and hemoglobin/hematocrit assessments; (vincristine) serial peripheral neurologic assessments; (all vincas) biliary function prior to dosing and making dosage adjustments for impaired hepatobiliary status.

Notes. Protect these drugs from light and store under refrigeration. Useful in hematologic neoplasms (primarily nonmyelotoxic vincristine) and in solid tumors (primarily vinblastine).

References, 10:00 Antineoplastic Agents

1. Dorr RT, Fritz WL, comps. Cancer chemotherapy handbook. New York: Elsevier, 1980.
2. Rieche K. Carcinogenicity of antineoplastic agents in man. Cancer Treat Rev 1984;11:39-67.
3. Pratt WB, Rudden RW, comps. The anticancer drugs. New York: Oxford University Press, 1979.
4. Haskell CM, ed. Cancer treatment. Philadelphia: WB Saunders, 1980.
5. Sawitsky A, Rai KR, Glidewell O et al. Comparison of daily versus intermittent chlorambucil and prednisone therapy in the treatment of patients with chronic lymphocytic leukemia. Blood 1977;50:1049-59.
6. Adair CG, Bridges JM, Desai ZR. Renal function in the elimination of oral melphalan in patients with multiple myeloma. Cancer Chemother Pharmacol 1986;17:185-8.
7. Alberts DS, Chang SY, Chen H-SG et al. Oral melphalan kinetics. Clin Pharmacol Ther 1979;26:737-45.
8. Alberts DS, Chang SY, Chen H-SG et al. Kinetics of intravenous melphalan. Clin Pharmacol Ther 1979;26:73-80.
9. McLean A, Woods RL, Catovsky D et al. Pharmacokinetics and metabolism of chlorambucil in patients with malignant disease. Cancer Treat Rev 1979;6(Suppl): 33-42.
10. Adair CG, Bridges JM,, Desai ZR. Can food affect the bioavailability of chlorambucil in patients with haemotological malignancies. Cancer Chemother Pharmacol 1986;17:99-102.
11. Taetle R, Dickman PS, Feldman PS. Pulmonary histopathologic changes associated with melphalan therapy. Cancer 1978;42:1239-46.
12. Heard BE, Cooke RA. Busulfan lung. Thorax 1968;23:187-93.
13. Lane SD, Besa EC, Justh G et al. Fatal interstitial pneumonitis following high-dose intermittent chlorambucil therapy for chronic lymphocytic leukemia. Cancer 1981;47:32-6.
14. Issell BF. Amsacrine (AMSA). Cancer Treat Rev 1980;7:73-83.
15. Omura GA, Winton EF, Vogler WR et al. Phase II study of amsacrine (m-AMSA) gluconate in refractory adult acute leukemia. Proc Am Assoc Cancer Res 1982;23:112. Abstract.
16. Legha SS, Benjamin RS, Mackay B et al. Reduction of doxorubicin cardiotoxicity by prolonged continuous intravenous infusion. Ann Intern Med 1982;96:133-9.
17. Weiss AJ, Metter GE, Fletcher WS et al. Studies on adriamycin using a weekly regimen demonstrating its clinical effectiveness and lack of cardiac toxicity. Cancer Treat Rep 1976;60:813-22.
18. Von Hoff DD, Rozencweig M, Layard M et al. Daunomycin-induced cardiotoxicity in children and adults: a review of 110 cases. Am J Med 1977;62:200-8.
19. Bachur NR. Adriamycin (NSC-123127) pharmacology. Cancer Chemother Rep (part 3)1975;6:153-8.

20. Benjamin RS, Wiernik PH, Bachur NR. Adriamycin chemotherapy — efficacy, safety, and pharmacologic basis of an intermittent single high-dosage schedule. Cancer 1974;33:19-27.

21. Huffman DH, Benjamin RS, Bachur NR. Daunorubicin metabolism in acute nonlymphocytic leukemia. Clin Pharmacol Ther 1972;13:895-905.

22. Von Hoff DD, Layard MW, Basa P et al. Risk factors for doxorubicin-induced congestive heart failure. Ann Intern Med 1979;91:710-7.

23. Blum RH, Carter SK. Adriamycin: a new anticancer drug with significant clinical activity. Ann Intern Med 1974;80:249-59.

24. Clarkson B, Krakoff I, Burchenal J et al. Clinical results of treatment with E. coli l-asparaginase in adults with leukemia, lymphoma, and solid tumors. Cancer 1970;25:279-305.

25. Sutow WW, George S, Lowman JT et al. Evaluation of dose and schedule of l-asparaginase in multidrug therapy of childhood leukemia. Med Pediatr Oncol 1976;2:387-95.

26. Pratt CB, Simone JV, Zee P et al. Comparison of daily versus weekly l-asparaginase for the treatment of childhood acute leukemia. J Pediatr 1970;77:474-83.

27. Nesbit M, Chard R, Evans A et al. Evaluation of intramuscular versus intravenous administration of l-asparaginase in childhood leukemia. Am J Pediatr Hematol Oncol 1979;1:9-13.

28. Haskell CM, Canellos GP, Leventhal BG et al. L-asparaginase: therapeutic and toxic effects in patients with neoplastic disease. N Engl J Med 1969;281:1028-35.

29. Ohnuma T, Holland JF, Freeman A et al. Biochemical and pharmacological studies with asparaginase in man. Cancer Res 1970;30:2297-305.

30. Von Hoff DD, Slavik M, Muggia FM. 5-Azacytidine: a new anticancer drug with effectiveness in acute myelogenous leukemia. Ann Intern Med 1976;85:237-45.

31. Bennett JM, Reich SD. Bleomycin. Ann Intern Med 1979;90:945-8.

32. Alberts DS, Chen H-SG, Liu R et al. Bleomycin pharmacokinetics in man. Cancer Chemother Pharmacol 1978;1:177-81.

33. Paladine W, Cunningham TJ, Sponzo R et al. Intracavitary bleomycin in the management of malignant effusions. Cancer 1976;38:1903-8.

34. Crooke ST, Comis RL, Einhorn LH et al. Effects of variations in renal function on the clinical pharmacology of bleomycin administered as an IV bolus. Cancer Treat Rep 1977;61:1631-6.

35. Kramer WG, Feldman S, Broughton A et al. The pharmacokinetics of bleomycin in man. J Clin Pharmacol 1978;18:346-52.

36. Sostman HD, Matthay RA, Putnam CE. Cytotoxic drug-induced lung disease. Am J Med 1977;62:608-15.

37. Yagoda A, Mukherji B, Young C et al. Bleomycin, an antitumor antibiotic: clinical experience in 274 patients. Ann Intern Med 1972;77:861-70.

38. Samuels ML, Johnson DE, Holoye PY. Continuous intravenous bleomycin (NSC-125066) therapy with vinblastine (NSC-49842) in stage III testicular neoplasia. Cancer Chemother Pharmacol 1975;59 (part 1):563-70.

39. Brock N, Gross R, Hohorst H-J et al. Activation of cyclophosphamide in man and animals. Cancer 1971;6:1512-29.

40. Grochow LB, Colvin M. Clinical pharmacokinetics of cyclophosphamide. Clin Pharmacokinet 1979;4:380-94.

41. Bagley CM, Bostick FW, DeVita VT. Clinical pharmacology of cyclophosphamide. Cancer Res 1973;33:226-33.

42. Mouridsen HT, Jacobsen E. Pharmacokinetics of cyclophosphamide in renal failure. Acta Pharmacol Toxicol 1975;36:409-14.

43. Cohen JL, Jao JY, Jusko WJ. Pharmacokinetics of cyclophosphamide in man. Br J Clin Pharmacol 1971;43:667-80.

44. Juma FD, Rogers HJ, Trounce JR. Pharmacokinetics of cyclophosphamide and alkylating activity in man after intravenous and oral administration. Br J Clin Pharmacol 1979;8:209-17.

45. Southwest Oncology Group. Cytarabine for acute leukemia in adults. Arch Intern Med 1974;133:251-9.

46. Rudnick SA, Cadman EC, Capizzi RL et al. High dose cytosine arabinoside (HDARAC) in refractory acute leukemia. Cancer 1979;44:1189-93.

47. Band PR, Holland JF, Bernard J et al. Treatment of central nervous system leukemia with intrathecal cytosine arabinoside. Cancer 1973;32:744-58.

48. Wan SH, Huffman DH, Azarnoff DL et al. Pharmacokinetics of 1-β-D-arabinofuranosylcytosine in humans. Cancer Res 1974;34:392-7.

49. van Prooijen R, van der Kleijn E, Haanen C. Pharmacokinetics of cytosine arabinoside in acute myeloid leukemia. Clin Pharmacol Ther 1977;21:744-50.

50. Harris AL, Potter C, Bunch C et al. Pharmacokinetics of cytosine arabinoside in patients with acute myeloid leukaemia. Br J Clin Pharmacol 1979;8:219-27.

51. Ho DHW, Frei E. Clinical pharmacology of 1-β-D-arabinofuranosylcytosine. Clin Pharmacol Ther 1971;12:944-54.

52. Pommier Y, Pochat L, Marie J-P et al. High-dose cytarabine in acute leukemia: toxicity and pharmacokinetics. Cancer Treat Rep 1983;67:371-3.

53. Chabner BA, Myers CE, Oliverio VT. Clinical pharmacology of anticancer drugs. Semin Oncol 1977;4:165-91.

54. Ritch PS, Hansen RM, Heuer DK. Ocular toxicity from high-dose cytosine arabinoside. Cancer 1983;51:430-2.

55. Lazarus HM, Herzig RH, Herzig GP et al. Central nervous system toxicity of high-dose systemic cytosine arabinoside. Cancer 1981;48:2577-82.

56. Carter SK, Friedman MA. 5-(3,3-dimethyl-l-triazeno)-imidazole-4-carboxamide(DTIC, DIC, NSC-45388)—a new antitumor agent with activity against malignant melanoma. Eur J Cancer 1972;8:85-92.

57. Loo TL, Housholder GE, Gerulath AH et al. Mechanism of action and pharmacology studies with DTIC (NSC-45388). Cancer Treat Rep 1976;60:149-52.

58. Frei E. The clinical use of actinomycin. Cancer Chemother Rep 1974;58:49-54.

59. Tattersall MHN, Sodergren JE, Sengupta SK et al. Pharmacokinetics of actinomycin D in patients with malignant melanoma. Clin Pharmacol Ther 1975;17:701-8.

60. Hauser AR, Merryman R. Estramustine phosphate sodium. Drug Intell Clin Pharm 1984;18:368-74.

61. Jacobs EM, Reeves WJ, Wood DA et al. Treatment of cancer with weekly 5-fluorouracil; study by the Western cooperative Cancer Chemotherapy Group (WCCCG). Cancer 1971;27:1302-5.

62. Horton J, Olson KB, Sullivan J et al. 5-Fluorouracil in cancer: an improved regimen. Ann Intern Med 1970;73:897-900.

63. Seifert P, Baker LH, Reed ML et al. Comparison of continuously infused 5-fluorouracil with bolus injection in treatment of patients with colorectal adenocarcinoma. Cancer 1975;36:123-8.

64. Cohen JL, Irwin LE, Marshall GJ et al. Clinical pharmacology of oral and intravenous 5-fluorouracil (NSC-19893). Cancer Chemother Rep 1974;58 (part 1):723-31.

65. Kirkwood JM, Ensminger W, Rosowsky A et al. Comparison of pharmacokinetics of 5-fluorouracil and 5-fluorouracil with concurrent thymidine infusions in a phase I trial. Cancer Res 1980;40:107-13.

66. Legha SS, Slavik M, Carter SK. Hexamethylmelamine: an evaluation of its role in the therapy of cancer. Cancer 1976;38:27-35.

67. Leuprolide Study Group. Leuprolide versus diethylstilbestrol for metastatic prostate cancer. N Engl J Med 1984;311:1281-6.

68. Goldstein D, Laszlo J. Interferon therapy in cancer: from imaginon to interferon. Cancer Res 1986;46:4315-29.

69. Spiegel RJ. Intron A (interferon alfa-2b): clinical overview. Cancer Treat Rev 1985;12(Suppl B):5-16.

70. Wills RJ,, Dennis S, Spiegel HE et al. Interferon kinetics and adverse reactions after intravenous, intramuscular, and subcutaneous injection. Clin Pharmacol Ther 1984;35:722-7.

71. Quesada JR, Rios A, Swanson D et al. Antitumor activity of recombinant-derived interferon alpha in metastatic renal cell carcinoma. J Clin Oncol 1985;3:1522-8.

72. Konrad M, Childs A, Bradley EC. The pharmacology of recombinant IL-2 in rabbits. Proc Am Assoc Cancer Res 1985;26:302. Abstract.

73. Rosenberg SA, Lotze MT. Muul LM et al. Observations on the systemic administration of autologous lymphokine-activated killer cells and recombinant interleukin-2 to patients with metastatic cancer. N Engl J Med 1985;313:1485-92.

74. Lotze MT, Frana LW, Sharrow SO et al. In vivo administration of purified human interleukin 2. I. Half-life and immunologic effects of the Jurkat cell line-derived interleukin 2. J Immunol 1985;134:157-66.

75. DeVita VT, Serpick AA, Carbone PP. Combination chemotherapy in the treatment of advanced Hodgkin's disease. Ann Intern Med 1970;73:881-95.

76. Taylor JR, Halprin KM. Topical use of mechlorethamine in the treatment of psoriasis. Arch Dermatol 1972;106:362-4.

77. Gilman AG, Goodman LS, Rall TW et al, eds. Goodman and Gilman's the pharmacological basis of therapeutics. 7th ed. New York: Macmillan, 1985.

78. Taylor JR, Halprin KM, Levine V et al. Mechlorethamine hydrochloride solutions and ointment. Arch Dermatol 1980;116:783-5.

79. Van Scott EJ, Kalmanson JD. Complete remissions of mycosis fungoides lymphoma induced by topical nitrogen mustard (HN2). Cancer 1973;32:18-30.

80. Bonadonna G, Brusamolino E, Valagussa P et al. Combination chemotherapy as an adjuvant treatment in operable breast cancer. N Engl J Med 1976;294:405-10.

81. Evans WE, Pratt CB. Effect of pleural effusion on high-dose methotrexate kinetics. Clin Pharmacol Ther 1979;24:68-72.

82. Values were derived using the nomogram of Rowland M, Tozer TN. Clinical pharmacokinetics: concepts and applications. Philadelphia: Lea and Febiger 1980:233.

83. Campbell MA, Perrier DG, Dorr RT et al. Methotrexate: bioavailability and pharmacokinetics. Cancer Treat Rep 1985;69:833-8.

84. Bleyer WA. Clinical pharmacology of intrathecal methotrexate II. An improved dosage regimen derived from age-related pharmacokinetics. Cancer Treat Rep 1977;61:1419-25.

85. Isacoff WH, Morrison PF, Aroesty J et al. Pharmacokinetics of high-dose methotrexate with citrovorum factor rescue. Cancer Treat Rep 1977;61:1665-74.

86. Shen DD, Azarnoff DL. Clinical pharmacokinetics of methotrexate. Clin Pharmacokinet 1978;3:1-13.

87. Crooke ST, Bradner WT. Mitomycin C: a review. Cancer Treat Rev 1976;3:121-39.

88. DeFuria MD, Bracken RB, Johnson DE et al. Phase I-II study of mitomycin C topical therapy for low-grade, low-stage transitional cell carcinoma of the bladder; an interim report. Cancer Treat Rep 1980;64:225-30.

89. Buice RG, Niell HB, Sidho P et al. Pharmacokinetics of mitomycin C in non-oat cell carcinoma of the lung. Cancer Chemother Pharmacol 1984;13:1-4.

90. Shenkenberg TD, Von Hoff DD. Mitoxantrone: a new anticancer drug with significant clinical activity. Ann Intern Med 1986;105:67-81.

91. Savaraj N, Lu K, Manuel V et al. Pharmacology of mitoxantrone in cancer patients. Cancer Chemother Pharmacol 1982;8:113-7.

92. Fewer D, Wilson CB, Boldrey EB et al. The chemotherapy of brain tumors. JAMA 1972;222:549-52.

93. Sponzo RW, De Vita VT, Oliverio VT. Physiologic disposition of 1-(2-chloroethyl)-3-cyclohexyl-1-nitrosourea (CCNU) and 1-(2-chloroethyl)-3-(4-methyl cyclohexyl)-1-nitrosourea (MeCCNU) in man. Cancer 1973;31:1154-9.

94. De Vita VT, Carbone PP, Owens A et al. Clinical trials with 1,3-bis(2-chloroethyl)-1-nitrosourea, NSC-409962. Cancer Res 1965;25:1876-81.

95. Oliverio VT. Toxicology and pharmacology of the nitrosoureas. Cancer Chemother Rep 1973;4(part 3):13-20.

96. Aronin PA, Mahaley MS, Rudnick SA et al. Prediction of BCNU pulmonary toxicity in patients with malignant gliomas. N Engl J Med 1980;303:183-8.

97. Durant JR, Norgard MJ, Murad TM et al. Pulmonary toxicity associated with bischloroethylnitrosourea (BCNU). Ann Intern Med 1979;90:191-4.

98. Prestayko AW, D'Aoust JC, Issell BF et al. Cisplatin (cis-diamminedichloroplatinum II). Cancer Treat Rev 1979;6:17-39.

99. Einhorn LH, Donahue J. Cis-diamminedichloroplatinum, vinblastine, and bleomycin combination chemotherapy in disseminated testicular cancer. Ann Intern Med 1977;87:293-8.

100. Belt RJ, Himmelstein KJ, Patton TF et al. Pharmacokinetics of non-protein-bound platinum species following administration of cis-dichlorodiammineplatinum (II). Cancer Treat Rep 1979;63:1515-21

101. DeConti RC, Toftness BR, Lange RC et al. Clinical and pharmacological studies with cis-diamminedichloroplatinum (II). Cancer Res 1973;33:1310-5.

102. Gonzalez-Vitale JC, Hayes DM, Cvitkovic E et al. Acute renal failure after cis-dichlorodiammineplatinum (II) and gentamicin-cephalothin therapies. Cancer Treat Rep 1978;62:693-8.

103. Macaulay VM, Begent RHJ, Phillips ME et al. Prophylaxis against hypomagnesemia induced by cisplatinum combination therapy. Cancer Chemother Pharmacol 1982;9:179-81.

104. Calvert AH, Harland SJ, Newell DR et al. Early clinical studies with cis-diammine-1,1-cyclobutane dicarboxylate platinum(II). Cancer Chemother Pharmacol 1982;9:140-7.

105. Harland SJ, Newell DR, Siddik ZH et al. Pharmacokinetics of cis-diammine-1,1-cyclobutane dicarboxylate platinum(II) in patients with normal and impaired renal function. Cancer Res 1984;44:1693-7.

106. Sessa C, Cavalli F, Kaye S et al. Phase II study of iproplatin (CHIP) in advanced epithelial ovarian carcinoma. Proc Am Soc Clin Oncol 1986;5:123.

107. Slayton RE, Schnider BI, Elias E et al. New approach to the treatment of hypercalcemia; the effect of short-term treatment with mithramycin. Clin Pharmacol Ther 1971;12:833-47.

108. Kennedy BJ. Metabolic and toxic effects of mithramycin during tumor therapy. Am J Med 1970;49:494-503.

109. O'Dwyer PJ, Leyland-Jones B, Alonso MT et al. Etoposide (VP-16-213): current status of an active anticancer drug. N Engl J Med 1985;312:692-700.

110. Giever RJ, Heusinkveld RS, Manning MR et al. Enhanced radiation reaction following combination chemotherapy for small cell carcinoma of the lung, possibly secondary to VP16-213. Int J Radiat Oncol Biol Phys 1982;8:921-3.

111. Allen LM, Creaven PJ. Comparison of the human pharmacokinetics of VM-26 and VP-16, two antineoplastic epipodophyllotoxin glucopyranoside derivatives, Eur J Cancer 1975;11:697-707.

112. Rozencweig M, VonHoff DD, Henney JE et al. VM-26 and VP 16-213: a comparative analysis. Cancer 1977;40:334-42.

113. Spivack SD. Procarbazine. Ann Intern Med 1974;81:795-800.

114. Lin S-N, Jessup K, Floyd M et al. Quantitation of plasma azathioprine and 6-mercaptopurine levels in renal transplant patients. Transplantation 1980;29:290-4.

115. Bach JF, Dardenne M. The metabolism of azathioprine in renal failure. Transplantation 1971;12:253-9.

116. Zimm S, Collins JM, Riccardi R et al. Variable bioavailability of oral mercaptopurine. N Engl J Med 1983;308:1005-9.

117. Duttera MJ, Carolla RL, Gallelli JF et al. Hematuria and crystalluria after high-dose 6-mercaptopurine administration. N Engl J Med 1972;287:292-4.

118. Sloth K, Thomsen AC. Acute renal insufficiency during treatment with azathioprine. Acta Med Scand 1971;189:145-8.

119. Penn I, Starzl TE. A summary of the status of de novo cancer in transplant recipients. Transplant Proc 1972;4:719-32.

120. Schein PS, O'Connell MJ, Blom J et al. Clinical antitumor activity and toxicity of streptozotocin (NSC-85998). Cancer 1974;34:993-1000.

121. Patterson JS, Battersby LA. Tamoxifen: an overview of recent studies in the field of oncology. Cancer Treat Rep 1980;64:775-8.

122. Fabian C, Sternson L, Barnett M. Clinical pharmacology of tamoxifen in patients with breast cancer: comparison of traditional and loading dose schedules. Cancer Treat Rep 1980;64:765-74.

123. Adam HK, Patterson JS, Kemp JV. Studies on the metabolism and pharmacokinetics of tamoxifen in normal volunteers. Cancer Treat Rep 1980;64:761-4.

124. Plotkin D, Lechner JJ, Jung WE et al. Tamoxifen flare in advanced breast cancer. JAMA 1978;240:2644-6.

125. Beck M, Mills PV. Ocular assessment of patients treated with tamoxifen. Cancer Treat Rep 1979;63:1833-4.

126. Lippman ME, Allegra JC. Receptors in breast cancer: estrogen receptor and endocrine therapy of breast cancer. N Engl J Med 1978;299:930-3.

127. Cohen BE, Egorin MJ, Kohlhepp E et al. Human plasma pharmacokinetics and urinary excretion of thiotepa and its metabolites. Cancer Treat Rep 1986;70:859-64.

128. Carswell EA, Old LJ, Kassel RL et al. An endotoxin-induced serum factor that causes necrosis of tumors. Proc Natl Acad Sci 1975;12:3666-70.

129. Khan A, Pardue A, Aleman C et al. Phase I clinical trial with recombinant tumor necrosis factor (TNF). Proc Am Assoc Clin Oncol 1986;5:226. Abstract.

130. Blick MB, Sherwin SA, Rosenblum MG et al. A phase I trial of recombinant tumor necrosis factor (rTNF) in cancer patients. Proc Am Assoc Clin Oncol 1986;5:14. Abstract.

131. Yap H-Y, Blumenschein GR, Keating MJ et al. Vinblastine given as a continuous 5-day infusion in the treatment of refractory advanced breast cancer. Cancer Treat Rep 1980;64:279-83.

132. Bodey GP, Yap H-Y, Yap B-S et al. Continuous infusion vindesine in solid tumors. Cancer Treat Rev 1980;7(Suppl):39-45.

133. Owellen RJ, Root MA, Hains FO. Pharmacokinetics of vindesine and vincristine in humans. Cancer Res 1977;37:2603-7.

134. Nelson RL, Dyke RW, Root MA. Comparative pharmacokinetics of vindesine, vincristine and vinblastine in patients with cancer. Cancer Treat Rev 1980;7(Suppl):17-24.

135. Krebs H-B. Treatment of vaginal condylomata acuminata by weekly topical application of 5-fluorouracil. Obstet Gynecol 1987;70:68-71.

136. Anon. Interleukin-2. Med Lett Drugs Ther 1987;29:88-9.

12:00 AUTONOMIC DRUGS

12:04 PARASYMPATHOMIMETIC (CHOLINERGIC) AGENTS

Physostigmine Salicylate   Antilirium®

Pharmacology. A centrally active reversible cholinesterase inhibitor most commonly used in the management of severe overdoses of drugs with anticholinergic properties, including heterocyclic antidepressants.

Administration and Adult Dose. IV as a therapeutic trial in anticholinergic overdose 2 mg (no faster than 1 mg/min), may repeat in 10–30 min to a maximum total dose of 4 mg; lowest effective dose may be repeated as needed (usually q 30–60 min).[1] **IM or IV for post anesthesia care** 0.5–1 mg (if IV, no faster than 1 mg/min), may repeat q 10–30 min.

Pediatric Dose. IV as a therapeutic trial in anticholinergic overdose 0.5 mg (no faster than 0.5 mg/min), may repeat q 5–10 min as needed.[1]

Dosage Forms. Inj 1 mg/ml.

Pharmacokinetics. *Onset and Duration.* Onset rapid; peak 5–10 min;[2] duration variable from 30–60 min[3,4] to no more than 4 hr.[5]
Fate. Rapidly metabolized by cholinesterase to inactive products.[6]

Adverse Reactions. Dose-related salivation, urination, emesis, defecation, bronchospasm, increased pulmonary secretions, bradycardia and hypotension may occur.[1-3] Onset of these symptoms requires reduction of dose or drug discontinuation. Asystole[7] and convulsions[2] have been reported when physostigmine has been used in the treatment of heterocyclic antidepressant overdose.

Contraindications. Asthma; gangrene; diabetes; cardiovascular disease; intestinal or urinary obstruction.

Precautions. Rapid IV injection should be avoided to reduce the possibility of bradycardia and convulsions.

Parameters to Monitor. Anticholinergic symptoms; symptoms of cholinergic excess; level of consciousness; heart rate.

Notes. Physostigmine should not be given in all heterocyclic antidepressant overdoses, rather only those with severe or life-threatening anticholinergic signs such as hallucinations, coma with respiratory depression, uncontrollable seizures or severe hypertension. Physostigmine excess can be countered with 0.5 mg atropine per 1 mg of physostigmine administered.[3]

12:08 ANTICHOLINERGIC AGENTS

12:08.04 ANTIPARKINSONIAN AGENTS

General References: 8

Class Instructions. These drugs may cause constipation, difficult or painful urination, dry mouth, blurred vision or drowsiness. Until the extent of these latter effects is known, caution should be used when driving, operating machinery or performing other tasks requiring mental alertness. Avoid excessive concurrent use of alcohol and other drugs which cause drowsiness. Becoming overheated during exercise or hot weather may result in heat stroke.

Benztropine Mesylate   Cogentin®

Pharmacology. A synthetic competitive antagonist of acetylcholine. In Parkinson's disease, the drug reduces the relative excess of cholinergic activity in the basal ganglia that develops due to absolute dopamine deficiency in this area.

Administration and Adult Dose. **PO, IM or IV for Parkinson's disease** 0.5–1 mg/day initially, increase in 0.5 mg/day increments q 5–6 days to effective dose, to maximum of 6 mg/day. Usual maintenance dose is 1–2 mg/day in 2–3 divided doses. **PO, IM or IV for drug-induced extrapyramidal disorders** 1–4 mg/day in 1 or 2 doses.

Pediatric Dose. Contraindicated under 3 yr.

Dosage Forms. **Tab** 0.5, 1, 2 mg; **Inj** 1 mg/ml.

Patient Instructions. See Class Instructions.

Adverse Reactions. The most frequent adverse effects are dose-related and include dry mouth, blurred vision, nausea, drowsiness, constipation, nervousness, decreased sweating and urinary retention. Occasionally, skin rash and visual hallucinations occur. Confusional states and impairment of recent memory are occasionally observed with use of high doses and in patients with underlying dementia.[8] Rarely, paralytic ileus occurs.

Contraindications. Children under 3 yr; narrow angle glaucoma.

Precautions. Pregnancy. Use with caution in hot weather or during exercise and in patients with tachyarrhythmias, prostatic hypertrophy, open angle glaucoma or obstructive diseases of the GI tract. Carefully observe patients given concomitant phenothiazines and/or heterocyclic antidepressants, because intensification of mental symptoms may occur to the point of toxic psychosis. Abrupt withdrawal of the drug in patients with parkinsonism may result in rebound of symptoms.

Parameters to Monitor. Monitor intra-ocular pressure periodically.

Notes. Anticholinergic agents are considered useful for the initial treatment of mild symptoms in patients with Parkinson's disease. Modest improvements of 10–25% in parkinsonian symptoms are reported.[8] The drug does not alleviate the symptoms of tardive dyskinesia.

Trihexyphenidyl Hydrochloride   Artane®, Various

Pharmacology. See Benztropine Mesylate.

Administration and Adult Dose. **PO for Parkinson's disease** 1 mg/day initially, increase in 2 mg/day increments q 3–5 days to effective dose, to maximum of 12–15 mg/day. Usual maintenance dose is 6–10 mg/day in 3–4 divided doses. SR caps may be given bid when the maintenance dose is determined. **PO for drug-induced extrapyramidal disorders** 1 mg initially, increase in 1 mg increments q few hours until symptoms are controlled. Usual dose is 5–15 mg/day in 3–4 divided doses.

Dosage Forms. **Elxr** 2 mg/5 ml; **SR Cap** 5 mg; **Tab** 2, 5 mg.

Patient Instructions. See Class Instructions.

Pharmacokinetics. *Onset and Duration.* Oral peak 1.5 hr.[9]
$t_{1/2}$. 1.3–8.7 hr (average 3.7).[9]

Adverse Reactions. See Benztropine Mesylate.

Contraindications. Narrow angle glaucoma.

Precautions. See Benztropine Mesylate.

Parameters to Monitor. See Benztropine Mesylate.

Notes. See Benztropine Mesylate.

12:08.08 ANTIMUSCARINICS/ANTISPASMODICS

General References: 10–12

Class Instructions. These drugs may cause dry mouth, constipation, blurring of vision, or drowsiness. Until the extent of these latter effects is known, caution should be used when driving, operating machinery, or performing other tasks requiring mental alertness. Avoid excessive concurrent use of alcohol and other drugs which cause drowsiness.

Atropine Sulfate   Various

Pharmacology. A competitive antagonist of acetylcholine at peripheral muscarinic and central receptors, causing an increase in heart rate and decreased salivary secretion, GI motility, sweating, urinary bladder contractability and bronchodilation.

Administration and Adult Dose. PO, SC, IM or IV for GI anticholinergic effect 400–600 mcg qid (with meals and at bedtime); SC, IM or IV for preanesthetic medication 300–600 mcg about one hr before induction. Inhal as a bronchodilator 0.025–0.05 mg/kg q 4–6 hr diluted to 2–3 ml with NS and delivered by compressed air nebulizer.

Pediatric Dose. PO or SC for general use 10 mcg/kg q 4–6 hr. Inhal as a bronchodilator 0.05–0.075 mg/kg q 4–6 hr diluted to 2–3 ml with NS and delivered by compressed air nebulizer.

Dosage Forms. Tab 0.4 mg; Hyp Tab 0.3, 0.4, 0.6 mg; Inj 0.3, 0.4, 0.5, 0.6, 1, 1.3 mg/ml; Inhal Soln 1, 2.5 mg/0.5 ml; Ophth Soln 5, 10 mg/ml. See Notes.

Patient Instructions. See Class Instructions.

Pharmacokinetics. *Onset and Duration.* (Inhal) onset 3–5 min; peak 1–2 hr; duration 3–6 hr, dose-dependent.

Fate. Rapidly absorbed from GI tract; significant, but inconsistent absorption following inhalation.[13] Approximately 60% excreted unchanged in urine; the remainder is metabolized.[14]

$t_{1/2}$. 3–4 hr in healthy volunteers;[14] may be greater in infants and elderly.

Adverse Reactions. Toxic effects are dose-related and frequent, especially in children. Atropine may accumulate and produce systemic effects with multiple dosing by inhalation in the elderly.[13] The following may occur in adults: at 0.5 mg—slight dryness of nose and mouth, bradycardia, inhibition of sweating (may lead to fever); at 1 mg—definite dryness of nose and mouth, thirst, acceleration of heart (possibly preceded by slowing), slight mydriasis; 2 mg—marked dry mouth, tachycardia, palpitation, mydriasis, slight blurring of near vision, flushed and dry skin; 5 mg—increase in above symptoms, plus speech disturbance, swallowing difficulty, headache, hot and dry skin, restlessness with asthenia; greater than 10 mg—above symptoms in the extreme, ataxia, excitement, disorientation, hallucinations, delirium and coma.

Contraindications. Acute angle glaucoma; adhesions (synechiae) between the iris and lens of the eye; obstructive disease of GI tract; obstructive uropathy; intestinal atony of elderly or debilitated patients; megacolon complicating ulcerative colitis; hiatal hernia with reflux esophagitis; unstable cardiovascular status in acute hemorrhage; tachycardia; myasthenia gravis.

Precautions. Pregnancy. Patients over 40 yr, particularly those with any severe heart disease, hypertension, ulcerative colitis, ileus, chronic lung disease, hyperthyroidism, autonomic neuropathy, hepatic or renal disease, or prostatic hypertrophy (these latter patients may experience urinary hesitancy, and should micturate at time of administration). Overdosage may cause a curare-like action.

Notes. As an inhaled bronchodilator, atropine is less potent than the β_2-adrenergic agents, but may produce useful additive bronchodilation with these drugs during acute asthma attacks.[11,12,15] Atropine may be combined directly with these drugs in the nebulizer. Ophthalmic atropine solutions (without methylcellulose or similar agents) may be used in the nebulizer.

Ipratropium Bromide   Atrovent®

Pharmacology. A competitive antagonist of acetylcholine at peripheral muscarinic receptors, but not centrally due to its quaternary structure.[12] Used primarily as a bronchodilator in asthma and COPD.

Administration and Adult Dose. Inhal for bronchospasm of COPD (including chronic bronchitis) 36 mcg (2 inhalations) qid by metered-dose inhaler to a maximum of 216 mcg (12 inhalations)/day.[13]

Pediatric Dose. Safety and efficacy not established. Inhal 18–36 mcg q 6–8 hr by metered-dose inhaler or 250 mcg q 6–8 hr by powered nebulizer has been used.[12]

Dosage Forms. Inhal 18 mcg/inhalation (200 doses/inhaler).

Patient Instructions. Shake inhaler prior to use, place mouthpiece in the mouth making sure the teeth and tongue are not in the way. Then actuate the device during a *slow* deep inhalation and hold breath for 5–10 seconds. Wait at least 1 min between inhalations. Temporary blurring of vision may occur if sprayed into eyes.

Pharmacokinetics. *Onset and Duration.* Onset 3 min; peak 1–2 hr;[10,11] duration 4–6 hr, depending on intensity of response.[11,12]

   Fate. Only 32% or less orally absorbed and less than 5% of inhaled dose is absorbed.[11] Metabolized to 8 metabolites which are excreted in the urine and bile.

   $t_{1/2}$. 2–4 hr.[11]

Adverse Reactions. Dryness of the mouth. Due to quaternary nature of molecule, usual systemic anticholinergic side effects are absent.[11,12]

Precautions. Use with caution in narrow-angle glaucoma, prostatic hypertrophy or bladder neck obstruction.

Notes. Anticholinergics appear to be more potent bronchodilators than β_2-adrenergics in bronchitis and emphysema, but less potent in asthma.[12] Anticholinergics produce an additive bronchodilation with β_2-adrenergic agents.[12]

12:12 SYMPATHOMIMETIC (ADRENERGIC) AGENTS

General References, Antiasthmatic: 16, 17
Shock: 18, 19

Class Instructions. Anti-asthmatic inhalers. Attach mouthpiece (to slow rate of inhalation and thereby increase penetration into airways) to spacer device. To use inhaler, tilt head up and place mouthpiece extension into mouth. While breathing normally, release one dose of aerosolized medication, inhale, remove inhaler from mouth and hold breath for 5 seconds. Do not exceed prescribed dose. Report if symptoms do not completely clear or the inhaler is required more than prescribed. Clean mouthpiece weekly with hot water and soap. Store away from heat and direct sunlight. Bronchodilators may cause nervousness, tremors (especially with terbutaline or albuterol) or rapid heart rate. Report if these effects continue after dosage reduction, or if chest pain, dizziness or headache occur, or if asthmatic symptoms are not relieved.

Dobutamine Hydrochloride   Dobutrex®

Pharmacology. A synthetic sympathomimetic amine that exerts complex cardiovascular actions. These actions consist of significant direct β_1-agonist activity and, at low doses, only slight agonist effect on β_2- and α-adrenergic receptors; this specificity is dose-dependent and is lost at high doses. At low doses, it increases myocardial contractility without significantly increasing heart rate. Unlike dopamine, dobutamine does not release stored catecholamines, nor does it have any effect on dopaminergic receptors.[20-22]

Administration and Adult Dose. **IV for inotropic support, by infusion only** (in any nonalkaline IV fluid), 2.5 mcg/kg/min initially, increasing gradually in increments of 2.5 mcg/kg/min up to 20 mcg/kg/min, titrating to desired response in each patient. Most patients can be maintained on 10 mcg/kg/min or less. Although infusions up to 40 mcg/kg/min have been used, doses over 20 mcg/kg/min should be used with caution because of increased risks of tachycardia and tachydysrhythmias.[23]

Pediatric Dose. Safety and efficacy not established; however, limited experience with IV infusions of 2 and 7.7 mcg/kg/min indicates that the drug may be safe.[24]

Dosage Forms. Inj 250 mg.

Pharmacokinetics. *Onset and Duration.* Onset 1–2 min; peak within 10 min; duration less than 10 min.
   Fate. Eliminated primarily in the liver to inactive glucuronide conjugates and 3-O-methyldobutamine.[23]
   $t_{1/2}$. About 2 min.[23]

Adverse Reactions. Ventricular dysrhythmias may occur (although less likely than with other catecholamines). Some increases in heart rate or systolic blood pressure occur occasionally, but marked increases are uncommon; reduction of dosage usually reverses these effects rapidly. Patients with atrial fibrillation may be at risk of developing rapid ventricular responses, because dobutamine facilitates A-V conduction. Nausea, headache, angina and shortness of breath are occasionally noted.

Contraindications. Idiopathic hypertrophic subaortic stenosis.

Precautions. Correct hypovolemia before using in patients who are hypotensive. Use with caution in patients receiving cyclopropane or halogenated hydrocarbon anesthesia. Although most cases of extravasation cause no signs of tissue damage, at least one case of dermal necrosis following extravasation of a 2.5 mcg/kg/min infusion has been reported.

Parameters to Monitor. Heart rate, arterial blood pressure, urine output, pulmonary capillary wedge pressure, cardiac index, EKG for ectopic activity and infusion rate of solution.

Notes. Physically incompatible with sodium bicarbonate and other alkaline solutions. Reconstituted solution is stable for 48 hr under refrigeration and 6 hr at room temperature.

Dobutamine Dilution Guide

AMOUNT ADDED		VOLUME	
MG	VOLUME (RECONSTITUTED)	OF DILUENT	FINAL CONCENTRATION
250	1 vial (20 ml)	1000 ml	250 mcg/ml*
250	1 vial (20 ml)	500 ml	500 mcg/ml*
250	1 vial (20 ml)	250 ml	1000 mcg/ml*

*Recommended concentrations, but concentrations up to 5 mg/ml have been used.

Dopamine Hydrochloride Dopastat®, Intropin®, Various

Pharmacology. A catecholamine which acts directly on peripheral dopaminergic receptors to produce renal and mesenteric vasodilation as well as on β_1- and α-adrenergic receptors. Additionally, it acts indirectly by releasing norepinephrine from sympathetic nerve storage sites. Dosage ranges are approximately as follows: dopaminergic 0.5–2 mcg/kg/min, β_1 1–10 mcg/kg/min, α 10+ mcg/kg/min.[22,25,26]

Administration and Adult Dose. IV for shock, by infusion only (in any nonalkaline IV fluid) 2–5 mcg/kg/min initially, increasing gradually in increments of 5–10 mcg/kg/min up to 20–50 mcg/kg/min, titrating dosage to desired response in each patient. Most patients can be maintained on 20 mcg/kg/min or less. Doses over 50 mcg/kg/min should be used only with careful monitoring of urinary output. IV for chronic refractory congestive heart failure 0.5–1 mcg/kg/min initially, increasing gradually until increases in urine flow, diastolic blood pressure or heart rate are observed. Most patients respond to 1–3 mcg/kg/min.[25,27]

Pediatric Dose. Safety and efficacy not established; however, limited experience with IV infusions of 0.3–25 mcg/kg/min indicates that the drug may be efficacious and safe.[28]

Dosage Forms. Inj 40, 80, 160 mg/ml.

Pharmacokinetics. *Onset and Duration.* Onset 2–4 min;[29] duration less than 10 min.

Fate. 75% metabolized to homovanillic acid (HVA) and other metabolites; 25% metabolized to norepinephrine and excreted in urine as HVA and metabolites of HVA and norepinephrine; very little is excreted as unchanged dopamine.[30]

Adverse Reactions. Ventricular arrhythmias may occur (although less likely than with other catecholamines); reduce dose if increased number of ventricular ectopic beats occurs. Hypotension at low infusion rates indicates that rate should be rapidly increased; hypertension may occur at high infusion rates. Nausea, vomiting and angina pectoris are occasionally seen. Gangrene of the extremities has occurred in patients with profound shock given large doses of dopamine for long periods of time.

Contraindications.   Pheochromocytoma; presence of uncorrected tachyarrhythmias or ventricular fibrillation.

Precautions. Correct hypovolemia before using in patients with shock. If increased diastolic pressure, decreased pulse pressure or decreased urine flow occurs, decrease infusion rate and observe patient for signs of excessive vasoconstriction. Use with caution in patients with occlusive vascular disease, and extreme caution in patients receiving cyclopropane or halogenated hydrocarbon anesthesia. Avoid extravasation of solution; however, if it occurs, the area may be infiltrated with 5–10 mg of phentolamine diluted in 10–15 ml normal saline.

Parameters to Monitor. In shock, closely monitor heart rate, pulmonary capillary wedge pressure, cardiac index, arterial blood pressure, arterial blood gases, acid-base balance, toe temperature, urine output, infusion rate of solution and for signs of vasoconstriction or extravasation (eg, blanching).[31]

Notes. Physically incompatible with sodium bicarbonate or other alkaline solutions.

Dopamine Dilution Guide

AMOUNT ADDED		VOLUME	FINAL
MG	VOLUME	OF DILUENT	CONCENTRATION
200	5 ml (1 amp-40 mg/ml)	250 ml	800 mcg/ml*
200	5 ml (1 amp-40 mg/ml)	500 ml	400 mcg/ml*
400	5 ml (1 amp-80 mg/ml)	500 ml	800 mcg/ml*
800	10 ml (1 amp-160 mg/ml)	500 ml	1600 mcg/ml

*Recommended concentrations, but concentrations up to 3.2 mg/ml have been used.

Epinephrine and Salts   Adrenalin®, Medihaler-Epi®, Sus-Phrine®, Various

Pharmacology. Stimulates α- (vasoconstriction, pressor effects), β_1- (increased myocardial contractility and conduction), and β_2-adrenergic (bronchodilation and vasodilation) receptors. Used for reversible bronchospasm, anaphylactic reactions, laryngeal edema (croup) and open-angle glaucoma.

Administration and Adult Dose. SC for anaphylaxis 0.3–0.5 mg (0.3–0.5 ml of 1:1000 aqueous solution), may repeat q 10–15 min,[32] to maximum of 1 mg/dose and 5 mg/day; **SC for asthma,** same dose as above, may repeat q 20 min for 3 doses, then q 4 hr prn. **SC aqueous suspension for asthma** 0.5–1.5 mg (0.1–0.3 ml of 1:200 or 0.2–0.6 ml of 1:400), may repeat with 0.5–1.5 mg no sooner than q 6 hr. **Inhal (metered dose) not recommended** because of low efficacy and ultra-short duration of action; β_2 selective agonists (eg, terbutaline, albuterol) are preferred. See also Medical Emergencies chapter.

Pediatric Dose. SC for anaphylaxis or asthma 0.01 mg/kg/dose, to maximum of 0.5 mg/dose of 1:1000 aqueous solution, may repeat q 15 min for 3 doses. **SC aqueous suspension for asthma** (1 month to 12 yr) 0.005 ml/kg/dose of 1:200, to maximum of 0.15 ml/dose for children 30 kg or less, may repeat q 6 hr. **Inhal for croup** 0.5 ml of 2.25% racemic aqueous solution in 3.5 ml of NS q 1–2 hr prn by nebulizer.[33]

Dosage Forms. Inhal (bitartrate/HCl) 0.16, 0.2, 0.27 mg free base/inhal; Inhal Soln (racemic) 1, 2.25%; Inj (aqueous solution as HCl) 1 mg/ml (1:1000), 0.1 mg/ml (1:10,000), 0.01 mg/ml (1:100,000); Inj (aqueous suspension as free base) 5 mg/ml (1:200).

Patient Instructions. See Class Instructions.

Pharmacokinetics. *Onset and Duration.* Onset SC (aqueous solution or suspension) 3–10 min; inhal peak 3–5 min; duration SC (aqueous suspension) up to 6–10 hr,[34] (aqueous solution) 0.5–2 hr; inhal 15–60 min.

   Fate. Oral drug rapidly inactivated in GI tract. Parenteral action terminated by uptake into adrenergic neurons. Metabolism is by MAO and COMT.[6,34]

Adverse Reactions.   Dose-related restlessness, anxiety, tremor, weakness, dizziness, headache, palpitations and hypertension. Anginal pain may occur when coronary insufficiency is present. Cardiac arrhythmias, cerebral hemorrhage from a sharp rise in blood pressure from overdose, and elevation of blood glucose.[6] Local necrosis from repeated injections and tolerance with prolonged use may occur.

Contraindications. Intra-arterial administration is not recommended due to marked vasoconstriction; use with local anesthetics in fingers or toes; during general anesthesia with halogenated hydrocarbons or cyclopropane;[6] α-adrenergic blocker-induced (including phenothiazines) hypotension; cerebral arteriosclerosis; organic heart disease; narrow-angle glaucoma; shock.

Precautions. Pregnancy. Allow sufficient time to elapse before changing to another systemic sympathomimetic agent. Use with caution in the elderly and in patients with cardiovascular disease, hypertension, diabetes or hyperthyroidism; and in psychoneurotic patients. Avoid use with drugs that sensitize the heart to arrhythmias. IM injection may produce local tissue necrosis.

Parameters to Monitor. Blood pressure, heart rate, relief of asthmatic or allergic symptoms.

Notes. Do not use solution if it is brown in color or contains a precipitate. Protect solution from light. Suspension provides a sustained effect; shake suspension well prior to use. Nonprescription inhalers have only a transient effect because of their low dose.[16] They should be used only by patients who have infrequent symptoms (less than once/week) and obtain total relief of symptoms from administration of two inhalations. Parenteral administration offers no advantage over inhalation for the treatment of acute bronchospasm.[35]

Isoproterenol Salts — Anti-Asthmatic Uses

Isuprel®, Medihaler-Iso®, Various

Pharmacology. A nonspecific β-adrenergic agonist used as a bronchodilator. β-agonist effect may result from increased cyclic AMP by activation of adenyl cyclase.

Administration and Adult Dose. **Inhal by metered dose** (both HCl and sulfate) 1–2 inhalations with 1–5 min between inhalations, may repeat up to 5 times/day; **Inhal by hand bulb nebulizer** 6–12 inhalations of 0.25% solution up to 5 times/day; **Inhal for severe acute bronchospasm nebulized by compressed air or oxygen** 2.5 ml of a 0.1% solution (dilute 0.5 ml of 1:200 in 2 ml NS) over 15–20 min, repeat q 1–2 hr prn under medical supervision. **IV, PO, SL** not recommended.

Pediatric Dose. **Inhal by metered dose** (both HCl and sulfate) 1–2 inhalations q 4–6 hr; **Inhal for acute bronchospasm nebulized by compressed air or oxygen** 0.05–0.1 mg/kg up to adult dose, diluted to 2–3 ml in NS q 2–4 hr under medical supervision. **IV for life-threatening asthma** (only in ICU with cardiac monitoring) 0.1 mcg/kg/min, increase in 0.1 mcg/kg/min increments at 15 min intervals based on response or to heart rate of 180–200 beats/min.[35] **PO, SL** not recommended.

Dosage Forms. Inhal (metered dose) 0.08, 0.120, 0.131 mg/inhal; **Inhal Soln** 0.25, 0.5, 1%; **Inj** 0.2 mg/ml. **SL Tab** not recommended.[16] Isoproterenol is formulated as the hydrochloride or sulfate salt.

Patient Instructions. See Class Instructions. Seek medical attention immediately if you need to use inhaler excessively.

Pharmacokinetics. *Onset and Duration.* Onset Inhal within 2 min; peak effect 3–5 min.[36] Duration—see Sympathomimetic Bronchodilators Comparison Chart.
    Fate. Poorly and irregularly absorbed after PO or SL administration.[37] After aerosol use, 80% excreted in urine as sulfate conjugate, because most of the dose is deposited in the oropharynx, swallowed and metabolized in the gut. Less than 4% of the overall dose is metabolized by COMT to 3-O-methyl isoproterenol, but a large portion of the dose reaching the lung is metabolized to this substance, which is a weak β-adrenergic blocker.[38]

Adverse Reactions.   Dose-related tachycardia, palpitations, nervousness, nausea and vomiting may occur.

Contraindications.   Pre-existing cardiac arrhythmias associated with tachycardia.

Precautions.   Use with caution in patients with coronary insufficiency. Deaths have been associated with overuse of aerosol. Limit use to no more than 6 doses/day (except under medical supervision). See Notes.

Parameters to Monitor.   Question patient concerning number of inhalations per day, relief of symptoms and duration of benefit.

Notes.   Useful for pulmonary function testing because of rapid onset. Isuprel® Compound Elixir is an irrational formulation; the drug is degraded in the gut. Addition of phenylephrine (Duo-Medihaler®) does not improve efficacy. Deaths associated with excessive use of inhaler are most likely due to acute deterioration of lung function and delay in seeking medical attention.

Isoproterenol Hydrochloride— Cardiac Uses

Isuprel®, Various

Pharmacology.   A direct acting, nonspecific β-adrenergic agonist whose primary cardiovascular actions are on the heart (inotropic and chronotropic) and skeletal muscle vasculature (vasodilation).

Administration and Adult Dose. IV for shock, by infusion in 5% dextrose only titrate dosage to desired response in each patient or to heart rate of no more than 130 beats/min.[18] Usual dosage range is 0.05–0.2 mcg/kg/min (usually 1–4 mcg/min).[18,19] Rates of over 30 mcg/min have been used in advanced states of shock. See also Medical Emergencies chapter.

Pediatric Dose. IV for shock, by infusion in 5% dextrose only begin at 0.1 mcg/kg/min, titrating to response. Infusions of up to 2.7 mcg/kg/min have been used in status asthmaticus without significant toxicity.[39]

Dosage Forms.   Inj 200 mcg/ml (1:5000).

Pharmacokinetics. *Onset and Duration.*   SL onset variable, up to 30 min; duration 1–2 hr.[34,37] IV onset immediate; duration 8 min with low dose, up to 50 min with large doses.[40]

Fate. After oral administration, drug is rapidly and extensively metabolized to inactive sulfate conjugate, probably in the intestine. After IV administration, 50% is excreted unchanged in the urine, 25–35% metabolized by COMT to 3-O-methyl metabolite which is then excreted unchanged or as sulfate conjugate. The 3-O-methyl metabolite is a weak β-blocker, but has a short half-life. Termination of drug activity appears to be by uptake into adrenergic neurons rather than by metabolism.[40]

Adverse Reactions. Flushing of face, sweating, mild tremors, nervousness, headache, tachycardia with palpitations can occur. Anginal pain in patients with angina pectoris has been reported.

Contraindications. Tachycardia caused by digitalis intoxication; patients with pre-existing arrhythmias associated with tachycardia (except ventricular tachycardias and arrhythmias that require isoproterenol's inotropic effect for therapy).

Precautions. Correct hypovolemia before use in patients with shock. Do not administer simultaneously with epinephrine. Use with caution, and in carefully adjusted doses, in patients with coronary insufficiency, hyperthyroidism or sensitivity to sympathomimetics. Doses sufficient to raise the heart rate above 130 beats/min may induce ventricular arrhythmias.

Parameters to Monitor. When used in situations other than resuscitation from cardiac arrest, closely monitor EKG, heart rate, pulmonary capillary wedge pressure, cardiac index, arterial blood pressure, arterial blood gases, acid-base balance, urine output and infusion rate of solution; may be advisable to slow, or temporarily stop infusion if heart rate exceeds 100 beats/min.

Notes. Physically incompatible with sodium bicarbonate or other alkaline solutions.

Isoproterenol Dilution Guide

AMOUNT ADDED		VOLUME OF	
MG	VOLUME	5% DEXTROSE	FINAL CONCENTRATION
1	5 ml (1:5000)	500 ml	2 mcg/ml (1:500,000)*
2	10 ml (1:5000)	500 ml	4 mcg/ml (1:250,000)

*Recommended concentration, but concentrations of 10 times this have been used.

Norepinephrine Bitartrate   Levophed®

Pharmacology. A catecholamine which directly stimulates β_1- and α-adrenergic receptors. It has little action on β_2-receptors.

Administration and Adult Dose. *IV for shock, by infusion only* (in any nonalkaline IV fluid) 8–12 mcg of base/min initially, adjusting rate to maintain a systolic blood pressure of about 80–100 mm Hg (but no more than 40 mm Hg below pre-existing systolic pressure); average maintenance dosage ranges from 2–4 mcg of base/min.

Pediatric Dose. *IV for shock, by infusion only* 2 mcg/M²/min initially, titrating to desired blood pressure, to maximum of 6 mcg/M²/min.

Dosage Forms. *Inj* 1 mg (of levarterenol base)/ml.

Pharmacokinetics. *Onset and Duration.* Onset rapid; duration 1–2 min after discontinuing infusion.[34]

Fate. After oral administration, drug is rapidly inactivated in GI tract. IV action is terminated by uptake into adrenergic neurons; drug is metabolized primarily by COMT, and to a lesser extent by MAO, to inactive metabolites and their conjugates.[34,37]

Adverse Reactions. Dose-related hypertension (sometimes indicated by headache), reflex bradycardia, increased peripheral vascular resistance and decreased cardiac output. Volume depletion may occur if fluid is not replaced.

Contraindications. Hypotension secondary to uncorrected blood volume deficit; mesenteric or peripheral vascular thrombosis, unless drug is lifesaving; cyclopropane or halogenated hydrocarbon anesthesia.

Precautions. Use with caution in patients receiving MAO inhibitors or heterocyclic antidepressants (may cause profound hypertension). Administer into a large vein (antecubetal or femoral preferred) to avoid necrosis secondary to vasoconstriction; avoid the leg veins in elderly patients or in those with occlusive vascular diseases. Avoid extravasation of solution; however, if it occurs, the area may be infiltrated with 5–10 mg of phentolamine diluted in 10 ml of NS.

Parameters to Monitor. In shock, closely monitor heart rate, pulmonary capillary wedge pressure, cardiac index, arterial blood pressure, arterial blood gases, acid-base balance, urine output, infusion rate of solution and for signs of vasoconstriction or extravasation (eg, blanching).

Notes. Do not use solution if it has a brown color or precipitate. 2 mg of norepinephrine bitartrate = 1 mg norepinephrine base.

Norepinephrine Dilution Guide

AMOUNT ADDED		VOLUME OF	FINAL
MG (BASE)	VOLUME	5% DEXTROSE	CONCENTRATION
2 mg	2 ml	500 ml	4 mcg/ml*
4 mg	4 ml	500 ml	8 mcg/ml*
8 mg	8 ml	500 ml	16 mcg/ml†

*Recommended pediatric concentration.
†Recommended adult concentration.

Pseudoephedrine Hydrochloride   Sudafed®, Various

Pharmacology. An indirect acting agent that stimulates α-, β_1- and β_2-adrenergic receptors via release of endogenous adrenergic amines.

Administration and Adult Dose. PO 60–120 mg qid prn;[41] **PO SR Cap/Tab** 120 mg q 8–12 hr.

Pediatric Dose. PO 120–240 mg/day divided into 4 doses for rapid release products and into 2-3 doses for slow release. Do not give SR 120 mg to patients under 12 yr.[41]

Dosage Forms. **SR Cap** 120 mg; **Syrup** 15, 30 mg/5 ml; **Tab** 30, 60 mg; **SR Tab** (as sulfate) 120 mg.

Patient Instructions. Take last dose a few hours before bedtime if insomnia occurs with bedtime administration.

Pharmacokinetics. *Onset and Duration.* Onset within 30 min on empty stomach, within 1 hr for SR dosage form; duration 3 hr or longer, 8–12 hr for SR dosage form.[42,43]

 Fate. Partly metabolized to inactive metabolite(s) and 6% metabolized to active metabolite, norpseudoephedrine.[44] 45–90% excreted unchanged in urine depending on urinary pH and flow.[44]

$t_{1/2}$. Average 7 hr; urinary flow and pH dependent: 9–16 hr at pH 8; 5–8 hr at pH 5.5–6; 3–6 hr at pH 5.[44,45]

Adverse Reactions. Mild transient nervousness, insomnia, irritability or headache. Usually negligible pressor effect in normotensive patients.

Contraindications. Severe hypertension; coronary artery disease; MAO inhibitor therapy.

Precautions. Use with caution in patients with hypertension, diabetes mellitus, ischemic heart disease, increased intraocular pressure or prostatic hypertrophy. Elderly patients may be particularly sensitive to CNS effects. If use is necessary in infants with phenylketonuria, reduce dose to avoid possible increased agitation.[46]

Parameters to Monitor. Nasal stuffiness, blood pressure, CNS stimulation.

Notes. Used primarily for decongestion of nasal mucosa and eustachian tubes.[42,47] Combination with an antihistamine may provide additive benefit in seasonal allergic rhinitis, because antihistamines do not relieve nasal stuffiness.[48,49]

Terbutaline Sulfate   Brethaire®, Brethine®, Bricanyl®

Pharmacology. A selective β_2-adrenergic agonist which produces bronchodilation, vasodilation, uterine relaxation, skeletal muscle stimulation, peripheral vasodilation and tachycardia.[50-52]

Administration and Adult Dose. **Inhal for asthma by metered dose** 1–3 inhalations with 1–5 min between inhalations q 4–6 hr prn and just before exercise.[50,53,54] **Inhal for severe acute bronchospasm nebulized by compressed air or oxygen** 5–7 mg undiluted q 4–6 hr prn; q 1–2 hr under medical supervision.[53,54] **PO for asthma** 5 mg q 6–8 hr, increase as tolerated. **SC for asthma** 0.25–0.5 mg q 2–6 hr prn. **IV for life-threatening asthma** (only in ICU with cardiac monitoring) 10 mcg/kg over 10 min initially, then 0.1 mcg/kg/min; increase in 0.1 mcg/kg/min increments q 15 min based on response and heart rate.[55]

Pediatric Dose. Not FDA approved in children under 12 yr; however, these doses have been used in children over 4 months of age. **Inhal for asthma by metered dose** 1–2 inhalations q 4–6 hr and just before exercise. **Inhal for severe bronchospasm nebulized by compressed air or oxygen** 0.1–0.3 mg/kg q 4–6 hr prn; q 1–2 hr under medical supervision.[53,55] **PO for asthma** 0.075 mg/kg q 6–8 hr, increase in 0.025 mg/kg increments as tolerated. **SC for asthma** 0.01 mg/kg up to 0.25 mg q 2–6 hr prn. **IV for life-threatening asthma** (only in ICU with cardiac monitoring) same as adult dose.

Dosage Forms. **Inhal** 0.2 mg/inhalation, (300 doses/inhaler); **Inj** 1 mg/ml; **Tab** 2.5, 5 mg.

Patient Instructions. (Metered-dose aerosol). Shake thoroughly, place mouthpiece between teeth, actuate device during a *very slow* deep breath, hold breath 5–10 seconds, and wait at least 1 minute before next dose.[50,53] Do not use more frequently than prescribed without medical advice.

Pharmacokinetics. *Onset and Duration.* (Inhal) onset within 5 min, peak 15–30 min; (PO) onset 30–60 min, peak 2–3 hr; (SC) onset 5 min, peak 30 min. Duration—see Sympathomimetic Bronchodilators Comparison Chart.

Fate. 50% absorbed orally; first-pass metabolism by sulfate conjugation results in a systemic availability of 10–30%.[53,56] 1–10% of an inhaled dose is absorbed. Peak plasma concentrations occur 2–4 hr after an oral dose. 65% excreted unchanged in urine, the rest is conjugated to sulfate and glucuronide by the liver.

$t_{1/2}$. 3–4 hr.[53,54,56]

Adverse Reactions. Dose-related reflex tachycardia from peripheral vasodilation and from direct stimulation of cardiac β_2-receptors.[52,54] Tremor, palpitations and nausea are other dose-related effects that are significantly reduced with aerosol administration. All β_2-agonists lower serum potassium concentrations. Pulmonary edema reported with IV use for tocolysis.[54,56]

Precautions. Pregnancy; cardiac arrhythmias (particularly in patients taking theophylline), diabetes.

Parameters to Monitor. Asthma symptoms, pulmonary function (FEV_1, PEFR) and heart rate.

Notes. Injectable solution diluent is NS, so it may be nebulized undiluted by compressed air or oxygen. Duration of action is dependent on the dose, dosage form and clinical condition; following inhalation, duration for prevention of exercise-induced asthma is only 2–4 hr, whereas duration of bronchodilation is 4–6 hr. Inhaled β_2-adrenergics are the treatment of choice for exercise-induced asthma.

Sympathomimetic Agents for Hemodynamic Support Comparison Chart[a]

DRUG	INJECTABLE DOSAGE FORMS	ADRENERGIC RECEPTOR SELECTIVITY					TOTAL PERIPHERAL RESISTANCE	CARDIAC OUTPUT
		INOTROPIC ACTIVITY (β_1)	CHRONO-TROPIC ACTIVITY (β_1)	VASO-DILATION (β_2)	VASO-CONSTRICTION (a)			
Phenylephrine[b] Neo-Synephrine®	10 mg/ml (1%).	0	0[c]	0	+++++	↑	↑	↓
Norepinephrine[d] Levophed®	1 mg (base)/ml.	++	++[c]	0	++++	↑	↑	0/↓
Epinephrine Adrenalin® Various	1 mg/ml (1:1000) 0.1 mg/ml (1:10,000) 0.01 mg/ml (1:100,000).	+++	+++	++	++++	↓	↑	↑
Dopamine Intropin® Various	40, 80, 160 mg/ml.	++	+/++[e]	++	+/++	↓/↑[e]	↑	↑
Dobutamine Dobutrex®	250 mg/vial.	++	0/+[e]	+	0/+[e]	↓	↑	↑
Isoproterenol Isuprel® Various	200 mcg/ml (1:5000).	++++	++++	+++++	0	↓	↑	↑

Continued

Sympathomimetic Agents for Hemodynamic Support Comparison Chart[a]

DRUG	INJECTABLE DOSAGE FORMS	ADRENERGIC RECEPTOR SELECTIVITY				TOTAL PERIPHERAL RESISTANCE	CARDIAC OUTPUT
		INOTROPIC ACTIVITY (β_1)	CHRONO-TROPIC ACTIVITY (β_1)	VASO-DILATION (β_2)	VASO-CONSTRICTION (α)		
Phentolamine[f] Regitine®	5 mg/ml.	—	g	—	—	↓	↑

Key. +++++ = Pronounced effect; + = Minimal effect; 0 = No effect; ↓ = Decreased; ↑ = Increased.
  a. This table compares only a few of the many factors important in the treatment of shock. Consult references 18, 19 and 27 for a complete guide. Cross-table comparisons of the adrenergic selectivity properties between this table and the Sympathomimetic Bronchodilators Comparison Chart cannot be made for the following reasons: (1) the rating scale of this table reflects a finer degree of differentiation of effects (hence 0-5+ vs. 0-4+); (2) the routes of administration are different; and (3) vascular β_2-receptors appear to respond slightly differently from bronchiolar β_2-receptors.
  b. Only use is to ↑ BP to reflexly ↑ vagal tone in paroxysmal supraventricular tachycardias.
  c. Decrease in heart rate may result from reflex mechanisms.
  d. Primarily used to increase peripheral vascular resistance in volume-repleted hypotensive patients.
  e. Dose-dependent.
  f. α-adrenergic blocking agent; useful in severe vasoconstriction (ie, extravasation of norepinephrine or dopamine).
  g. Increase in heart rate may result from reflex and direct mechanisms.

Sympathomimetic Bronchodilators Comparison Chart[a,b]

DRUG	DOSAGE FORMS	DOSAGE ADULT	DOSAGE PEDIATRIC[c]	β-ADRENERGIC RECEPTOR SELECTIVITY[d] β₁	β₂[d]	RELATIVE β₂ POTENCY[e]	DURATION[f]
Albuterol Proventil® Ventolin®	Inhal (soln) 0.5%, (unit dose) 0.083%; (metered dose) 0.09 mg/inhalation; SR Tab 4 mg; Syrup 2 mg/5 ml; Tab 2, 4 mg.	Inhal (soln) 2.5–5 mg in 2–3 ml NS by nebulizer; (metered dose) 1–2 inhalations q 4–6 hr prn and prior to exercise; PO 2–4 mg q 6–8 hr.	Inhal (soln) 0.05–0.15 mg/kg in 2–3 ml NS q 2–6 hr by nebulizer; (metered dose) 1–2 inhalations q 4–6 hr prn and prior to exercise; PO 0.1–0.2 mg/kg q 6–8 hr.	±	++++	5	Inhal 2–6 hr. PO 4–8 hr.
Bitolterol[g] Tornalate®	Inhal (metered dose) 0.37 mg/inhalation.	Inhal 1–3 inhalations q 4–6 hr prn.	Inhal 1–2 inhalations q 4–6 hr prn.	±	++++	5	Inhal 2–6 hr.
Epinephrine Adrenalin® Various	Inhal (soln) 1%, 2.25% (racemic); Inj 1 mg/ml.	See Monograph		+++	+++	5	Inhal 15–60 min. SC 0.5–2 hr.
Epinephrine Aq Suspension Sus-Phrine®	Inj 5 mg/ml.	SC 0.5–1.5 mg q 6–10 hr.	SC 0.005 ml/kg q 6–10 hr.	+++	+++	5	SC 6–10 hr.

Continued

Sympathomimetic Bronchodilators Comparison Chart[a,b]

DRUG	DOSAGE FORMS	DOSAGE ADULT	DOSAGE PEDIATRIC[c]	β-ADRENERGIC RECEPTOR SELECTIVITY[d] β_1	β-ADRENERGIC RECEPTOR SELECTIVITY[d] β_2[d]	RELATIVE β_2 POTENCY[e]	DURATION[f]
Fenoterol Berotec® (Investigational - Boehringer Ingelheim)	Inhal (metered dose) 0.16 mg/inhalation.	Inhal 1-2 inhalations q 4-6 hr prn; PO 5-10 mg q 6-8 hr.	—	+	+ + + +	5	Inhal 2-6 hr. PO 4-8 hr.
Isoetharine Bronkometer® Bronkosol® Various	Inhal (soln) 0.1, 0.125, 0.2, 0.25, 0.5, 1%; (metered dose) 0.34 mg/inhalation.	Inhal (soln) 5-10 mg diluted 1:3 in NS q 2-4 hr prn; (metered dose) 1-2 inhalations q 4-6 hr prn.	Inhal (soln) 0.1-0.2 mg/kg q 2-4 hr prn; (metered dose) 1-2 inhalations q 4-6 hr prn.	+ +	+ + +	1.7	Inhal 1-2 hr.
Isoproterenol Isuprel® Various	Inhal (soln) 0.25, 0.5, 1%; (metered dose) various 80-131 mcg/inhalation; Inj 0.2 mg/ml.	See Monograph		+ + + +	+ + + +	10	Inhal 1-2 hr.

Continued

Sympathomimetic Bronchodilators Comparison Chart[a,b]

DRUG	DOSAGE FORMS	DOSAGE ADULT	DOSAGE PEDIATRIC[c]	β-ADRENERGIC RECEPTOR SELECTIVITY[d] β₁	β₂[d]	RELATIVE β₂ POTENCY[e]	DURATION[f]
Metaproterenol Alupent® Metaprel® Various	Inhal (soln) 0.4% (unit dose 10 mg), 0.6% (unit dose 15 mg), 5%; (metered dose) 0.65 mg/inhalation; Syrup 10 mg/5 ml; Tab 10, 20 mg.	Inhal (soln) 15 mg q 2–4 hr prn (q 1–2 hr under medical supervision); (metered dose) 1–3 inhalations q 4–6 hr prn and prior to exercise; PO 20 mg 4–6 times/day.	Inhal (soln) 0.25–0.5 mg/kg up to 15 mg q 2–4 hr prn; (metered dose) 1–2 inhalations prn and prior to exercise; PO 0.5 mg/kg q 4–6 hr, increase by 0.25 mg/kg as tolerated.	++	++	1	Inhal 2–3 hr. PO 4–6 hr.
Pirbuterol Maxair®	Inhal (metered dose) 0.2 mg/inhalation.	Inhal 1–2 inhalations q 4–6 hr.	—	±	++++	3	Inhal 5 hr.
Terbutaline Brethaire® Brethine® Bricanyl®	Inhal (metered dose) 0.2 mg/inhalation; Inj 1 mg/ml; Tab 2.5, 5 mg.	Inhal 1–3 inhalations q 4–6 hr prn; 5–7 mg undiluted by nebulizer q 4–6 hr prn;[h] SC 0.25–0.5 mg q 2–6 hr prn;	Inhal 1–2 inhalations q 4–6 hr prn; 0.1–0.3 mg/kg q 4–6 hr prn (q 1–2 hr under medical supervision);[h] SC 0.01 mg/kg up	±	++++	2.5	Inhal 2–6 hr. PO 4–8 hr. SC 2–4 hr.

Continued

Sympathomimetic Bronchodilators Comparison Chart[a,b]

| DRUG | DOSAGE FORMS | DOSAGE | | β-ADRENERGIC RECEPTOR SELECTIVITY[d] | | RELATIVE β₂ POTENCY[e] | DURATION[f] |
		ADULT	PEDIATRIC[c]	β₁	β₂[d]		
		PO 5 mg q 6–8 hr.	to 0.25 mg q 2–6 hr prn; PO 0.075 mg/kg q 6–8 hr.				

a. From references 50–57.
b. See footnote "a", in Sympathomimetic Agents for Hemodynamic Support Comparison Chart.
c. Isoproterenol and isoetharine are the only metered-dose aerosols approved by the FDA for use in children under 12 yr.
d. β_2-selectivity does not equate to bronchoselectivity; β_2-stimulation produces reflex tachycardia from vasodilation as well as stimulation of cardiac β_2-receptors.
e. Equimolar potency relative to metaproterenol; larger numbers indicate more potent compounds.
f. Duration is dependent on dose, dosage form and clinical situation; values are based on single-dose studies; tolerance from continuous administration can result in a 50% decrease in duration.
g. Bitolterol is a prodrug converted in the body to colterol, the active drug, which is more potent than isoproterenol; the relative potency value is due to incomplete conversion.
h. Use injectable solution; not an FDA approved use.

12:16 SYMPATHOLYTIC (ADRENERGIC BLOCKING) AGENTS

General References: 58

Ergotamine Tartrate   Ergomar®, Ergostat®

Pharmacology. An ergot alkaloid with α-adrenergic blocking properties in the peripheral and central nervous systems. It is also a uterine stimulant via its tryptaminergic and α-blocking activity. Mechanism in migraine is thought to be vasoconstriction of cranial blood vessels, with concomitant decrease in the amplitude of pulsations.

Administration and Adult Dose. **PO for migraine** 1–2 mg initially, then 1 mg each half hr prn, to maximum of 6 mg/day or 10 mg/week; **Inhal** one inhalation (0.36 mg) initially, then q 5+ min, to maximum of 6 inhalations/day or 15 inhalations/week; **PR** 2 mg initially, may repeat in 1 hr prn to maximum of 4 mg/attack or 10 mg/week; **SL** not recommended.

Pediatric Dose. Safety and efficacy not established.

Dosage Forms. **Inhal** 9 mg/ml; **SL Tab** 2 mg; **Tab** 1 mg with caffeine 100 mg (Cafergot®, various); **Supp** 2 mg with caffeine 100 mg (Cafergot®, Wygraine®).

Patient Instructions. Initiate therapy at first signs of attack. Take only as directed and do not exceed specified dosages.

Pharmacokinetics. *Onset and Duration.* Onset averages up to 5 hr orally,[58] 1–3 hr after rectal and 15–30 min after inhalation.[59]

Plasma Levels. 0.2 ng/ml or greater may be therapeutic;[59] a high frequency of adverse reactions has been associated with levels above 1.8 ng/ml.[60]

Fate. Oral bioavailability is poor due to first-pass effect; the effects of caffeine on absorption is unclear. Bioavailability is low and variable after inhalation. SL bioavailability is very poor, while rectal absorption appears to be good.[59,61] Peak plasma levels after 2 mg orally with 100 mg caffeine average 21.4 pg/ml, while an equal dose rectally produces a peak of 454 pg/ml.[61] The drug is extensively metabolized in the liver with 90+ % of metabolites excreted in the bile. After IV, V_d is 1.85 L/kg; Cl is 0.68 L/hr/kg.[59]

$t_{1/2}$. 1.86 hr IV;[59] 3.35 hr rectally.[61]

Adverse Reactions. Frequently nausea, vomiting, diarrhea, dizziness, weakness in legs, coldness and muscle pains in extremities and numbness or tingling of fingers and toes occur; occasional headache, precordial distress and pain and transient tachycardia or bradycardia occur; rarely, gangrene or serious cardiovascular effects have been reported. Rebound headaches can occur during chronic use, possibly leading to escalation of dosage by patient.

Contraindications. Pregnancy; occlusive or peripheral vascular disease; coronary artery disease; hypertension; hepatic or renal impairment; sepsis; severe pruritus; malnutrition.

Precautions. Avoid overdosing or prolonged administration due to the potential for ergotism and gangrene.

Notes. The stimulant action of preparations containing caffeine (eg, Cafergot®) may keep patients from the beneficial effect of sleep. Calcium antagonists (eg, verapamil, nimodipine) and β-adrenergic blocking agents (eg, propranolol) are useful in migraine prophylaxis.[62-64]

References, 12:00 Autonomic Drugs

1. Anon. Physostigmine for tricyclic antidepressant overdosage. Med Lett Drugs Ther 1980;22:55.

2. Newton RW. Physostigmine salicylate in the treatment of tricyclic antidepressant overdosage. JAMA 1975;231:941-3.

3. Rumack BH. Anticholinergic poisoning: treatment with physostigmine. Pediatrics 1973;52:449-51.

4. Burks JS, Walker JE, Rumack BH et al. Tricyclic antidepressant poisoning: reversal of coma, choreoathetosis and myoclonus by physostigmine. JAMA 1974;230:1405-7.

5. Snyder BD, Blonde L, McWhirter WR. Reversal of amitriptyline intoxication by physostigmine. JAMA 1974;230:1433-4.

6. Gilman AG, Goodman LS, Rall TW et al, eds. Goodman and Gilman's the pharmacological basis of therapeutics, 7th ed. New York: Macmillan, 1985:110-29.

7. Pentel P, Peterson CD. Asystole complicating physostigmine treatment of tricyclic antidepressant overdose. Ann Emerg Med 1980;9:588-90.

8. Quinn NP. Anti-parkinsonian drugs today. Drugs 1984;28:236-62.

9. Burke RE, Fahn S. Pharmacokinetics of trihexyphenidyl after short-term and long-term administration to dystonic patients. Ann Neurol 1985;18:35-40.

10. Rebuck AS, Chapman KR, Braude AC. Anticholinergic therapy of asthma. Chest 1982;82 (Suppl):55S-7S.

11. Pakes GE, Brogden RN, Heel RC et al. Ipratropium bromide: a review of its pharmacological properties and therapeutic efficacy in asthma and chronic bronchitis. Drugs 1980;20:237-66.

12. Gross NJ, Skorodin MS. Anticholinergic, antimuscarinic bronchodilators. Am Rev Respir Dis 1984;129:856-70.

13. Kradjan WA, Smallridge RC, Davis R et al. Atropine serum concentrations after multiple inhaled doses of atropine sulfate. Clin Pharmacol Ther 1985;38:12-5.

14. Hinderling PH, Gundert-Remy U, Schmidlin O. Integrated pharmacokinetics and pharmacodynamics of atropine in healthy humans I: pharmacokinetics. J Pharm Sci 1985;74:703-10.

15. Karpel JP, Appel D, Breidbart D et al. A comparison of atropine sulfate and metaproterenol sulfate in the emergency treatment of asthma. Am Rev Respir Dis 1986;133:727-9.

16. Iafrate RP, Massey KL, Hendeles L. Current concepts in clinical therapeutics: asthma. Clin Pharm 1986;5:206-27.

17. Ahrens RC, Hendeles L, Weinberger M. The clinical pharmacology of drugs used in the treatment of asthma. In: Yaffe SJ, ed. Pediatric pharmacology: therapeutic principles in practice. New York: Grune & Stratton, 1980:233-80.

18. Tarazi RC. Sympathomimetic agents in the treatment of shock. Ann Intern Med 1974;81:364-71.

19. Weil MH, Shubin H, Carlson R. Treatment of circulatory shock: use of sympathomimetic and related vasoactive agents. JAMA 1975;231:1280-6.

20. Leier CV, Heban PT, Huss P et al. Comparative systemic and regional hemodynamic effects of dopamine and dobutamine in patients with cardiomyopathic heart failure. Circulation 1978;58:466-75.

21. Anon. Dobutamine (Dobutrex). Med Lett Drugs Ther 1979;21:15-6.

22. Colucci WS, Wright RF, Braunwald E. New positive inotropic agents in the treatment of congestive heart failure (2 parts). N Engl J Med 1986;314:290-9, 349-58.

23. Sonnenblick EH, Frishman WH, LeJemtel TH. Dobutamine: a new synthetic cardioactive sympathetic amine. N Engl J Med 1979;300:17-22.

24. Driscoll DJ, Gillette DC, Duff DF et al. Hemodynamic effects of dobutamine in children. Am J Cardiol 1979;43:581-5.

25. Goldberg LI. Dopamine—clinical uses of an endogenous catecholamine. N Engl J Med 1974;291:707-10.

26. Dasta JF, Kirby MG. Pharmacology and therapeutic use of low-dose dopamine. Pharmacotherapy 1986;6:304-10.

27. Rosenblum R. Physiologic basis for the therapeutic use of catecholamines. Am Heart J 1974;87:527-30.

28. Driscoll DJ, Gillette PC, McNamara DG. The use of dopamine in children. J Pediatr 1978;92:309-14.

29. Allwood MJ et al. Peripheral vascular effects of noradrenaline, isopropylnoradrenaline and dopamine. Br Med Bull 1963;19:132-6.

30. Goodall McC, Alton H. Metabolism of 3-hydroxytyramine (dopamine) in human subjects. Biochem Pharmacol 1968;17:905-14.

31. Ruiz CE, Weil MH, Carlson RW. Treatment of circulatory shock with dopamine. JAMA 1979;242:165-8.

32. Kelly JF, Patterson R. The treatment of anaphylaxis. Ration Drug Ther 1973;7(11):1-5.

33. Newth CJL. Acute epiglottitis and croup. In: Nussbaum E, ed. Pediatric intensive care. Mount Kisco: Futura, 1984:277-98.

34. McEvoy GK, ed. American Hospital Formulary Service, Drug Information '87. Bethesda. American Society of Hospital Pharmacists. 1987.

35. Sybert A, Weiss EB. Status asthmaticus. In: Weiss EB, Segal MS, Stein M, eds. Bronchial asthma: mechanisms and therapeutics. 2nd ed. Boston: Little, Brown, 1985:808-43.

36. Holmes TH, Morgan B. A comparative clinical trial of metaproterenol and isoproterenol as bronchodilator aerosols. Clin Pharmacol Ther 1968;9:615-24.

37. Reynolds JEF, ed. Martindale, the extra pharmacopoeia. 28th edition. London: The Pharmaceutical Press, 1982.

38. Blackwell EW, Briant RH, Conolly ME et al. Metabolism of isoprenaline after aerosol and direct intrabronchial administration in man and dog. Br J Pharmacol 1974;50:587-91.

39. Wood DW, Downes JJ, Scheinkopf H et al. Intravenous isoproterenol in the management of respiratory failure in childhood status asthmaticus. J Allergy Clin Immunol 1972;50:75-81.

40. Conolly ME, Davies DS, Dollery CT et al. Metabolism of isoprenaline in dog and man. Br J Pharmacol 1972;46:458-72.

41. Hendeles L, Weinberger M, Wong L. Medical management of noninfectious rhinitis. Am J Hosp Pharm 1980;37:1496-1504.

42. Roth RP, Cantekin EI, Bluestone CD et al. Nasal decongestant activity of pseudoephedrine. Ann Otol Rhinol Laryngol 1977;86:235-42.

43. Hamilton LH, Chobanian SL, Cato A et al. A study of sustained action pseudoephedrine in allergic rhinitis. Ann Allergy 1982;48:87-92.

44. Brater DC, Kaojarern S, Benet LZ et al. Renal excretion of pseudoephedrine. Clin Pharmacol Ther 1980;28:690-4.

45. Kuntzman RG, Tsai I, Brant L et al. The influence of urinary pH on the plasma half-life of pseudoephedrine in man and dog and a sensitive assay for its determination in human plasma. Clin Pharmacol Ther 1971;12:62-7.

46. Spielberg SP, Schulman JD. A possible reaction to pseudoephedrine in a patient with phenylketonuria. J Pediatr 1977;90:1026.

47. Anon. Establishment of a monograph for OTC cold, cough, allergy, bronchodilator and antiasthmatic products. Fed Regist 1976;41:38312-424.

48. Empey DW, Bye C, Hodder M et al. A double-blind crossover trial of pseudoephedrine and triprolidine, alone and in combination, for the treatment of allergic rhinitis. Ann Allergy 1975;34:41-6.

49. Connell JT. A novel method to assess antihistamine and decongestant efficacy. Ann Allergy 1979;42:278-85.

50. Nelson HS. Beta-adrenergic therapy. In: Middleton E, Reed CE, Ellis EF, eds. Allergy: principles and practice. 2nd ed. St. Louis: CV Mosby;1983:511-27.

51. Webb-Johnson DC, Andrews JL. Bronchodilator therapy (first of 2 parts). N Engl J Med 1977;297:476-82.

52. Kelly HW. Controversies in asthma therapy with theophylline and the β_2-adrenergic agonists. Clin Pharm 1984;3:386-95.

53. Kelly HW. New β_2-adrenergic agonist aerosols. Clin Pharm 1985;4:393-403.

54. Tashkin DP, Jenne JW. Alpha and beta adrenergic agents. In: Weiss EB, Segal MS, Stein M, eds. Bronchial asthma: mechanisms and therapeutics. 2nd ed. Boston: Little, Brown;1985:604-39.

55. Kelly HW, Murphy SA, Jenne JW. Appendix. In: Jenne JW, Murphy SA, eds. Drug therapy for asthma: research and clinical practice. New York: Marcel Dekker;1986.

56. Nyberg L, Wood C, eds. Advances in terbutaline pharmacokinetics. Eur J Respir Dis 1984;65(Suppl 134):9-240.

57. Nelson HS. Adrenergic therapy of bronchial asthma. J Allergy Clin Immunol 1986;77:771-85.

58. Gilman AG, Goodman LS, Rall TW et al, eds. Goodman and Gilman's the pharmacological basis of therapeutics, 7th ed. New York: Macmillan, 1985.

59. Perrin VL. Clinical pharmacokinetics of ergotamine in migraine and cluster headache. Clin Pharmacokinet 1985;10:334-52.

60. Orton DA, Richardson RJ. Ergotamine absorption and toxicity. Postgrad Med J 1982;58:6-11.

61. Sanders SW, Haering N, Mosberg H et al. Pharmacokinetics of ergotamine in healthy volunteers following oral and rectal dosing. Eur J Clin Pharmacol 1986;30:331-4.

62. Anon. Propranolol for prevention of migraine headaches. Med Lett Drugs Ther 1979;21:77-8.

63. Behan PO, Reid M. Propranolol in the treatment of migraine. Practitioner 1980;224:201-4.

64. Meyer JS. Calcium channel blockers in the treatment of vascular headaches. Ration Drug Ther 1985;19(Mar):1-4.

20:00 BLOOD FORMATION AND COAGULATION

20:04 ANTIANEMIA DRUGS

20:04.04 IRON PREPARATIONS

General References: 1, 2

Ferrous Salts   Various

Pharmacology. Ferrous salts are soluble forms of iron, an essential nutrient which functions primarily as the oxygen-binding core of heme in red blood cells (as hemoglobin), muscles (as myoglobin) and the respiratory enzyme, cytochrome C.

Administration and Adult Dose. PO 2–3 mg/kg/day of elemental iron in divided doses.[3] See Ferrous Salts Comparison Chart for usual dosage ranges for individual salts. Dose-related adverse effects may be decreased by using suboptimal dosages, by increasing the daily dose gradually, or by administering with a small amount of food (although this latter method reduces absorption). After hemoglobin is normalized, oral therapy should continue for approximately 3 months to replenish iron stores.

Dosage Individualization. Iron requirement during pregnancy is approximately twice that of the normal, nonpregnant woman due to an expanding blood volume and the demands of the fetus and placenta. A prophylactic dose of 30–60 mg/day elemental iron during the second and third trimesters has been recommended to prevent depletion of maternal iron stores. Iron deficient patients may need higher doses.[4,5]

Pediatric Dose. **PO for prophylaxis** 1 mg/kg/day of elemental iron in single or divided doses. **PO for treatment** 4-6 mg/kg/day of elemental iron in 3 divided doses.

Dosage Forms. See Ferrous Salts Comparison Chart.

Patient Instructions. This drug should be taken with a full glass of water on an empty stomach (1 hr before or 2 hr after meals) for best absorption. If gastric distress or nausea occurs, a small quantity of food may be taken with the drug, but do not take with antacids because absorption will be decreased. Stools will probably become black. Keep out of the reach of children.

Pharmacokinetics. *Onset and Duration.* Response to equivalent amounts of oral or parenteral therapy is essentially the same. Reticulocytes increase within 3-7 days and reach a peak of 5-15% about the tenth day, and an initially rapid increase in hemoglobin occurs in 2 weeks.[6] Three to six months of therapy are generally required for restoration of iron stores.[1]

Plasma Levels. 50-150 mcg/dl. A decrease in the transferrin saturation (serum iron ÷ total iron binding capacity x 100) is an indication of pre-anemic iron deficiency. A transferrin saturation less than 16% indicates probable iron deficiency.[1] In overdosage, toxicity may occur at levels greater than 350 mcg/dl. Chelation therapy is indicated at levels greater than 500 mcg/dl and possibly with levels over 350 mcg/dl if the patient is symptomatic.

Fate. Iron is absorbed primarily from the duodenum at a rate dependent on the amount of iron in storage sites. About 10% of dietary iron is absorbed in normal subjects, 20% in iron deficient patients and as much as 70% of medicinal iron during marked iron deficiency or increased erythropoiesis. In the plasma, iron is oxidized to the ferric state, combined with transferrin, and either utilized or stored as ferritin (mostly in the reticuloendothelial system and hepatocytes). The average loss in the healthy adult male is about 1 mg/day. Gastrointestinal loss of extravasated red cells, iron in bile and exfoliated mucosal cells accounts for two-thirds of this iron. The other third is lost in the skin and urine. Menstruating women have an additional loss of about 0.5 mg/day.

Adverse Reactions. Occasional GI irritation, constipation, diarrhea, and stained teeth (liquid preparations only — dilute and use a drinking straw).

Contraindications. Hemochromatosis, hemosiderosis and hemolytic anemias in which no true iron deficiency exists.

Precautions. Use with caution in patients with peptic ulcer, regional enteritis or ulcerative colitis. Serious acute poisoning (which can be fatal) occurs frequently in children: doses as low as 20 mg/kg of elemental iron can cause toxicity.[7] Food and antacids significantly impair the absorption of iron.

Parameters to Monitor. Periodic reticulocyte count, hemoglobin and hematocrit—see Onset and Duration.

Notes. Ferrous salts are used in prevention and treatment of iron deficiency anemias. Such anemias occur most frequently with exceptional blood losses (eg, pathological bleeding, menstruation) and during periods of rapid growth (eg, infancy, adolescence, pregnancy). Iron is ineffective in hemoglobin disturbances not caused by iron deficiency. Concurrent administration of high doses of ascorbic acid may enhance absorption (particularly when given with sustained-release formulations), but cost/benefit may not warrant its use. Wide variation in dissolution and absorption exists among sustained-release and enteric-coated products, and the frequency of adverse effects, while negligible, probably reflects the small amount of ionic iron available for absorption due to transport of the iron past the duodenum and proximal jejunum.[8]

Iron Dextran Injection

Imferon®, Various

Pharmacology. See Ferrous Salts. The overall response to parenteral iron is not significantly different from orally administered iron, and therefore, iron dextran is indicated *only* when oral iron therapy is determined to be ineffective or impossible.

Administration and Adult Dose. The total cumulative amount required for restoration of hemoglobin and body stores of iron can be approximated from the formula:

$0.66 \times$ body weight in kg

$$\times \left(100 - \frac{\text{patient's hemoglobin in g/dl} \times 100}{14.8} \right)$$

= total mg iron to be injected.

To calculate dose in ml, divide the result by 50. The requirements for infants weighing 13.6 kg (30 lb) or less are 80% of the amount calculated from the formula. **Deep IM** (in upper outer quadrant of buttock using Z-track technique) 25 mg (0.5 ml) test dose the first day, then, if no adverse reaction occurs, proceed to administer (until the total calculated amount is reached) a daily dose not to exceed 25 mg (0.5 ml) for infants under 4.5 kg, 50 mg (1 ml) for children under 9 kg, 100 mg (2 ml) for all others. **Slow IV** test dose of 25 mg (0.5 ml) the first day, then, if no adverse reaction occurs, proceed (until the total calculated amount is reached) by daily increments over 2-3 days, to maximum daily dose of 100 mg. **Total dose IV infusion** the total calculated dose of iron dextran is diluted in 200-250 ml of normal saline (dextrose solutions cause increased local phlebitis) and infused (after a 25 mg test dose is delivered over 5 min) over a period of 1-2 hr.[9] This method is *not* FDA approved and is discouraged by the manufacturers.

Pediatric Dose. See Administration and Adult Dose.

Dosage Forms. 50 mg elemental iron/ml. **Inj for IM or IV use** (contains no preservative) 2, 5 ml ampule. **Inj for IM use only** (contains 0.5% phenol as preservative) 10 ml vial.

Pharmacokinetics. *Onset and Duration.* Hematological response is equivalent to oral therapy, although total body stores of iron are replaced when the above dosage regimens are used.

Fate. Following IV administration, the inert complex is gradually cleared from the plasma by the reticuloendothelial cells of the liver, spleen and bone marrow; in doses greater than 500 mg the clearance rate is 10-20 mg/hr. The iron dextran is then dissociated and released as free ferric iron (at a rate controlled by the serum iron level), which combines with transferrin and is incorporated into hemoglobin within the bone marrow.[9,10]

$t_{1/2}.$ 6 hr with doses less than 500 mg;[10] 2.3-3 days with larger doses.[11]

Adverse Reactions. Immediate anaphylactoid reactions, which may be life threatening, occur rarely. Delayed systemic reactions resembling serum sickness and starting within 4-48 hr after injection are characterized by lymphadenopathy, myalgia, arthralgia, fever and headache. IM injections are associated with variable degrees of soreness and inflammation at the injection site and with brown skin discoloration at the injection site. Hypotension and peripheral vascular "flushing" are seen with too rapid IV administration.

Contraindications.   Anemias other than iron deficiency anemia; hemochromatosis; hemosiderosis; subcutaneous administration.

Precautions.   Pregnancy. Use with extreme caution in the presence of serious liver impairment. Patients with rheumatoid arthritis may have an acute exacerbation or reactivation of joint pain and swelling following IV administration. History of allergies and/or asthma. Epinephrine should be immediately available.

Parameters to Monitor.   See Ferrous Salts.

Ferrous Salts Comparison Chart

DRUG	SOLID DOSAGE FORMS[a]	ADULT DOSE (CAP OR TAB/DAY)	ELEMENTAL IRON/CAP OR TAB (PERCENT)	(MG FE)	OTHER DOSAGE FORMS[a]
Ferrous Fumarate	SR Tab 324 mg	1-2	33	106	Drp 45 mg/0.6 ml Susp 100 mg/5 ml.
	SR Cap 325 mg	1-2	33	107	
	Tab (Chewable) 100 mg	1-4	33	33	
	Tab 63, 195, 200 mg	1-4	33	20,64,66	
	Tab 300, 324, 325 mg.	1-2	33	99,106,107	
Ferrous Gluconate	Cap 86, 325, 435 mg	3-6	12	10,39,52	Elxr 300, 325 mg/5 ml.
	Tab 300, 320, 325 mg.	3-6	12	36,38,39	
Ferrous Sulfate Exsiccated	Cap 190 mg	3	30	57	
	SR Cap 159 mg	1-2	30	47	
	SR Tab 160 mg	1-2	30	48	
	Tab 200 mg.	3-4	30	60	

Continued

Ferrous Salts Comparison Chart

DRUG	SOLID DOSAGE FORMS[a]	ADULT DOSE (CAP OR TAB/DAY)	ELEMENTAL IRON/CAP OR TAB (PERCENT)	(MG FE)	OTHER DOSAGE FORMS[a]
Ferrous Sulfate Hydrous	SR Cap/Tab Various	—	20	—	Drp 75 mg/0.6 ml Elxr 195 mg/4 ml
	Tab 195 mg	3-6	20	39	Elxr 220 mg/5 ml Soln 125 mg/ml
	Tab 300, 325 mg.	3	20	60,65	Syrup 90 mg/5 ml.

a. Doses listed represent total iron salt, not elemental iron.

20:12 COAGULANTS AND ANTICOAGULANTS

20:12.04 ANTICOAGULANTS

General References: 12-14

Class Instructions. These drugs are potentially harmful when taken with nonprescription or prescription drugs. Consult the physician or pharmacist when considering the use of other medications, particularly aspirin-containing products.

Dihydroergotamine Mesylate and Heparin Sodium

Embolex®

This combination product is approved for use in the prevention of postoperative deep venous thrombosis and pulmonary embolism in patients undergoing abdominal, thoracic or pelvic surgery. The dihydroergotamine (DHE) component is included because of its relatively selective constrictive effect on venous capacitance vessels. This effect supposedly increases venous return, minimizing venous stasis. The combination product produces a greater reduction in venous thrombosis than the same amount of heparin alone. However, as with other ergot alkaloids, DHE may cause arterial spasm, severely limiting its use in patients with cardiovascular disease (eg, coronary disease with angina, recent MI, hypertension). In addition, the combination product is associated with more frequent adverse reactions than heparin alone, including nausea, vomiting, chest pain and rash. Several studies evaluating low-dose heparin alone versus placebo have demonstrated efficacy similar to that reported with the DHE/heparin combination. Because of its contraindications and side effects, this product may have limited clinical utility. The dosage is 2500-5000 units DHE/heparin SC administered 2 hr preoperatively and q 12 hr for 5-7 days.[15-18] Embolex® contains 5000 units heparin sodium, 0.5 mg dihydroergotamine mesylate, and 7.46 mg lidocaine HCl per 0.7 ml ampule.

Heparin Calcium
Heparin Sodium

Calciparine®
Various

Pharmacology. A heterogeneous group of mucopolysaccharides derived from the mast cells of animal tissues. It binds with antithrombin III, accelerating the rate at which antithrombin III neutralizes *activated forms* of factors XII, XI, IX, X, VII, and II. It is active in vitro and in vivo.

Administration and Adult Dose. Express dose in units only; dose must be individually titrated to desired effect (usually 1.5-2.5 times control clotting test used).[19-21] **IV for thrombophlebitis** (continuous infusion) 50-100 units/kg initially, then 10-15 units/kg/hr; (intermittent) 75-125 units/kg q 4 hr. **IV for pulmonary embolus** (continuous infusion) 50-100 units/kg initially, then 25 units/kg/hr; alternatively, 5000 units initially, then 1000 units/hr; (intermittent) 75-125 units/kg q 4 hr.[20,22,23] Duration of therapy for thrombophlebitis or pulmonary embolus is 7-10 days, followed by oral anticoagulation (preferably initiated during the first 24 hr of heparin therapy).[20,35] **SC for thrombophlebitis or pulmonary embolus** 10,000-20,000 units initially (preceded by a 5000 unit IV loading dose), then 8000-10,000 units q 8 hr or 15,000-20,000 units q 12 hr. **SC for prophylaxis of deep vein thrombosis (low-dose)** 5000 units 2 hr before surgery, repeated q 8-12 hr until patient is ambulatory.[24,25] **IV for heparin lock flush** inject sufficient solution (of 10 or 100 units/ml) into injection hub to fill the entire set after each heparin lock use. Some institutions reserve the 100 units/ml solution for flushing triple lumen catheters.

Dosage Individualization. Patients with pulmonary embolus seem to require larger heparin doses than patients with thrombophlebitis.[21,23] There is no good evidence that renal or liver disease significantly affect dosage considerations.[26] However, uremia may cause a hemostatic defect increasing the risk of hemorrhage.[20] See Precautions.

Pediatric Dose. Same as adult dose in units/kg.

Dosage Forms. **Inj** (sodium) 1000, 2500, 5000, 7500, 10,000, 15,000, 20,000, 40,000 units/ml; **Inj** (calcium) 5000 units/0.2 ml; **Heparin Lock Flush** (sodium) 10, 100 units/ml.

Patient Instructions. See Class Instructions.

Pharmacokinetics. *Onset and Duration.* Onset immediate after IV administration.
  Fate. No biotransformation in plasma or liver, nor any renal excretory mechanism has been identified as primarily responsible for heparin elimination; transfer and storage in reticuloendothelial cells has been suggested.[20,26] V_d is 70 ml/kg (approximates plasma volume).
  $t_{1/2}$. (Pharmacologic) 93 min (deep venous thrombosis); 52 min (pulmonary embolus).[27] Half-life appears to be dose-related; higher doses lead to increased half-life and decreased clearance.[23,26]

Adverse Reactions. Hemorrhage. Thrombocytopenia is thought to be more common with heparin derived from bovine lung, although recent studies suggest little difference and an overall decline in the prevalence.[28-30] It is speculated that the decline may be due to improved manufacturing techniques and reduced therapy duration.[28] Osteoporosis may occur with doses of 15,000 units/day or more for 6 months or longer.[20]

Contraindications. Active bleeding; thrombocytopenia; threatened abortion; subacute bacterial endocarditis; suspected intracranial hemorrhage; regional or lumbar block anesthesia; severe hypotension; shock; and after eye, brain or spinal cord surgery.

Precautions. Risk factors for hemorrhage may include IM injections, trauma, recent surgery, women over 60 yr, malignancy, peptic ulcer disease, potential bleeding sites and acquired or congenital hemostatic defects.[20,21]

Parameters to Monitor. Baseline values for APTT or ACT, PT, hematocrit and platelet count. Obtain APTT or ACT (therapeutic range 1.5-2.5 times control) 3-4 times (or until therapeutic range is achieved) on day 1, and at least daily thereafter. Platelets and hematocrit every other day; signs of bleeding (melena, hematuria, ecchymosis, hematemesis, epistaxis) daily.[20]

Notes. Continuous IV infusion may cause a lower frequency of bleeding complications than intermittent IV administration.[20,31] Questionable efficacy in reducing mortality and reinfarction in acute MI; current treatment practices (eg, coronary care units, early ambulation) may have reduced the need for or benefit from full-dose anticoagulation.[32-34] Some authors recommend the use of low-dose heparin following acute MI to reduce the risk of pulmonary embolism.[34] Bovine lung heparin has a greater effect on platelet aggregation and a higher affinity for antithrombin III binding than porcine intestinal mucosa heparin.[28,29] The clinical importance of these findings is unclear.

Warfarin Sodium   Coumadin®, Panwarfin®

Pharmacology. Warfarin prevents the conversion of vitamin K back to its active form from the vitamin K epoxide. This impairs formation of the vitamin K-dependent clotting factors VII, IX, X, II (prothrombin) and protein C (a physiologic anticoagulant). The S warfarin enantiomer appears to be a more potent anticoagulant than R warfarin.[46]

Administration and Adult Dose. PO or IV 2–10 mg/day, titrating dose to 1.5 to 2.5 times control prothrombin time (PT). Less intense warfarin therapy (1.3 times PT control value with Simplastin®) is as effective as conventional therapy in treating proximal-vein thrombosis with a lower risk of hemorrhage.[20] See Notes.

Dosage Individualization. Large variability in response requires that dosage be carefully individualized in all patients. Patients with liver disease, CHF, hyperthyroidism, or fever and the elderly may be particularly sensitive to warfarin. Renal failure does not enhance the hypoprothombinemic response to warfarin; however, these patients may have compromised hemostatic mechanisms which predispose to bleeding.[36]

Dosage Forms. **Tab** 2, 2.5, 5, 7.5, 10 mg; **Inj** 50 mg.

Patient Instructions. See Class Instructions.

Pharmacokinetics. *Onset and Duration.* Peak PT effect 36–72 hr;[37] at least 5–7 days of warfarin therapy are required before full therapeutic effect is achieved.[38] Duration after discontinuation is dependent on resynthesis of vitamin K-dependent clotting factors II, VII, IX and X (about 4–5 days).

Fate. Completely absorbed orally; well absorbed following small bowel resection;[39] greater than 97% plasma protein bound.[40,41] Undergoes oxidative biotransformation in the liver, producing warfarin alcohols which have some minor anticoagulant activity.[42,43] Warfarin enantiomers are metabolized by different routes. Less than 1% is excreted unchanged in the urine.[40]

$t_{1/2}$. Average 42 hr,[44] unchanged in acute hepatic disease.[45] Enantiomer half-lives: R warfarin 20–70 hr; S warfarin 18–34 hr.[46]

Adverse Reactions. Hemorrhage (especially when PT is greater than 2.5 times control);[39,47] rarely necrosis of the skin, purple-toe syndrome.

Contraindications. Pregnancy; hemorrhagic tendencies; blood dyscrasias; surgery or trauma; severe hepatic or renal disease; disturbances of intestinal flora; severe hypertension.

Precautions. Many drug interactions. Avoid IM injections due to risk of hematoma formation. Several other factors may influence response: diet, travel and environment. Monitor patients with liver disease, CHF, hyperthyroidism or fever especially carefully.

Parameters to Monitor. PT daily while hospitalized, then weekly to monthly to monitor therapeutic effect; hematocrit, stool guaiac, urinalysis (for hematuria) for toxicity. Also observe for ecchymosis, hemoptysis and epistaxis.

Notes. Loading dose has no therapeutic advantage and may be unsafe due to excessive depression of factor VII.[20,48] Phytonadione (vitamin K_1) begins to restore the PT toward normal within 4–8 hr, although large doses may subsequently induce a resistance to anticoagulant effect lasting one or more weeks.[49]

Antiplatelet Drugs

THE USE OF ANTICOAGULANTS has been found useful in preventing venous thrombosis. They are, however, less effective in preventing arterial thrombosis, possibly because of differences in factors leading to the formation of venous and arterial thrombi. Venous thrombi contain primarily fibrin in combination with some platelet aggregates. Also, the amount of platelets adhering to venous walls is limited. On the other hand, a platelet nidus plays the major role in the formation of arterial thrombi and thrombi which form on prosthetic surfaces. These considerations have led to the investigation of drugs affecting platelet function as an approach to the prevention of thrombosis.

Agents offering the most promise are reviewed in the following summary. These agents act by various mechanisms to inhibit platelet function. Aspirin inhibits cyclo-oxygenase, reducing the formation of thromboxane (proaggregant) from platelets and prostacyclin (antaggregant) from the vessel wall. Low doses of aspirin have been recommended in an attempt to inhibit thromboxane formation while minimizing effects on prostacyclin. However, there have been no studies which clearly demonstrate a clinical benefit over standard doses (1300 mg/day) of aspirin. Sulfinpyrazone appears to reversibly inhibit cyclo-oxygenase, while dipyridamole prolongs shortened platelet survival and inhibits aggregation by blocking phosphodiesterase. Investigational agents include **ticlopidine** (Syntex) which may affect the first phase of platelet aggregation by inhibiting various aggregating stimuli; **dazoxiben** (Pfizer), **dazmegrel** (Pfizer), **OKY-046** and **CGS 13080** which selectively inhibit thromboxane synthetase; and **BM 13.177** which antagonizes thromboxane receptors.

Antiplatelet Drug Therapy Summary

INDICATION	DRUG, DOSAGE AND COMMENTS
Acute Myocardial Infarction	**Aspirin** 325–975 mg/day. A reduction of mortality and reinfarction may occur, especially when instituted early after MI.[50-52] When used for primary prevention, aspirin 325 mg every other day has been demonstrated to reduce nonfatal and fatal MI by 47%, but not the overall death rate.[81]
	Aspirin 975 mg/day plus **dipyridamole** 225 mg/day have a greater influence on mortality than aspirin alone or placebo, especially when initiated early after MI.[53] PARIS II demonstrated a 25% reduction in cardiac death and nonfatal MI compared to placebo. Differences in total mortality and coronary mortality were not statistically significant.[50]
	Sulfinpyrazone 800 mg/day. The ART study claiming effectiveness in preventing sudden death has been criticized for inconsistent classification and exclusion of data.[54,55] Continued

Antiplatelet Drug Therapy Summary

INDICATION	DRUG, DOSAGE AND COMMENTS
	ARIS demonstrated significant reductions in reinfarctions and thromboembolic events.[56] No difference in cardiac deaths was observed.
Angina, Unstable	**Aspirin** 325–1300 mg/day. A statistically significant reduction in death and nonfatal MI (30–51%) was observed in these patients compared to placebo.[57,58]
	Aspirin 1300 mg/day plus **sulfinpyrazone** 800 mg/day. No additional benefit over aspirin alone.[58]
	Sulfinpyrazone 800 mg/day. No benefit over placebo.[58]
	Ticlopidine 500 mg/day (investigational). A significant reduction in angina and ST-segment depression was demonstrated in a study of 10 patients.[59]
AV Shunts	**Aspirin** 160 mg/day. May be more effective than higher doses in preventing thrombosis because of its potential to block thromboxane synthesis while minimizing effect on vascular prostacyclin.[60] See Introduction.
	Sulfinpyrazone 600 mg/day. Demonstrated benefit in reducing thrombosis.[50]
Coronary Artery Bypass Operation	**Aspirin** 100 mg/day. A reduction in occlusion rate over placebo has been demonstrated; however, sample size was small and the occlusion rate in the placebo group was very high.[61]
	Dipyridamole 100 mg qid for 2 days prior to operation, 100 mg on the day of operation at 6 AM and 1 hr after surgery, then 75 mg plus **aspirin** 325 mg 7 hr post-op and tid thereafter for 1 year. A benefit over placebo in reducing early and late vein graft occlusion has been demonstrated.[62,63]
Heart Valves	**Aspirin** 1000 mg/day or **dipyridamole** 400 mg/day with conventional oral anticoagulant therapy. These are more effective than oral anticoagulant therapy alone; however, the aspirin combination is associated with a high risk of GI hemorrhage.[50,51]
	Aspirin 1–3 g/day plus **dipyridamole** 100–450 mg/day. An uncontrolled trial showed this combination to be more effective than placebo.[52] Some investigators recommend this combination for patients unable to tolerate oral anticoagulant therapy.[51] Antiplatelet agents alone are not as effective as oral anticoagulants alone.[50-52]
Stroke and TIA	**Aspirin** 1300 mg/day. Several studies demonstrated a significantly reduced risk of TIA, stroke and death, primarily in males, although

Continued

Antiplatelet Drug Therapy Summary

INDICATION	DRUG, DOSAGE AND COMMENTS
	most studies show a favorable trend in females.[50,52,64]
	Aspirin 1300 mg/day plus **sulfinpyrazone** or **dipyridamole.** No additional benefit has been demonstrated over aspirin alone.[50,64]

20:40 THROMBOLYTIC AGENTS

General References: 65-68

Alteplase   Activase®

Pharmacology. Alteplase (tissue-type plasminogen activator; t-PA) is a fibrinolytic protein from the endothelial lining of blood vessels produced commercially by recombinant DNA technology. It has a high affinity for fibrin, allowing plasminogen to be activated directly on the fibrin surface. Plasmin formed remains bound to the fibrin clot, minimizing systemic effects.[77-80]

Administration and Adult Dose. IV infusion for post-MI clot lysis 60 mg over 1 hr (6–10 mg in the first 1–2 min), then 20 mg/hr for 2 hr to a total of 100 mg. Begin as soon as possible after acute MI symptoms.

Dosage Forms. Inj 20, 50 mg.

Pharmacokinetics. *Onset and Duration.* Duration is several hours due to binding to fibrin.
    Fate. Metabolized rapidly by the liver, presumably to its constituent amino acids.[80] Cl is 33–41 L/hr.
    $t_{1/2}$. 5–8 min.[77]

Adverse Reactions. Bleeding from GI and GU tracts and ecchymoses occur occasionally; less frequently retroperitoneal or gingival bleeding or epistaxis occur. Superficial bleeding from trauma sites may also occur.

Contraindications. Active internal bleeding; history of CVA; recent (within 2 months) intracranial or intraspinal surgery or trauma; intracranial neoplasm, AV malformation or aneurysm; bleeding diathesis; severe uncontrolled hypertension.

Precautions. Use with caution in the following: recent (within 10 days) major surgery, trauma, GI or GU bleeding; cerebrovascular disease; systolic blood pressure of 180 mm Hg or above, diastolic of 110 mm Hg or above; high likelihood of left heart thrombus; acute pericarditis; subacute bacterial endocarditis; hemostatic defects; significant liver dysfunction; pregnancy; hemorrhagic ophthalmic conditions; septic thrombophlebitis; age over 75 yr; concurrent oral anticoagulants. Avoid IM injections and noncompressible arterial punctures; minimize arterial and venous punctures and excessive patient handling. Stop immediately if severe bleeding or anaphylactoid reaction occurs.

Notes. More effective than IV streptokinase in reperfusing of occluded coronary arteries, with a lower risk of bleeding.[79,80]

Streptokinase   Kabikinase®, Streptase®

Pharmacology. A bacterial protein derived from group C β-hemolytic streptococci. Acts indirectly, forming a streptokinase-plasminogen activator complex which activates other plasminogen, converting it to the proteolytic enzyme plasmin. Plasmin then hydrolyzes fibrin, fibrinogen, factors V, VIII, II, complement and kallikreinogen.

Administration and Adult Dose. IV for post-MI clot lysis 1.5 million IU within 60 minutes. **Intracoronary infusion for post-MI clot lysis** 20,000 IU bolus followed by 2000 IU/min for 60 min.[70,71,75,76] **IV for pulmonary embolism, DVT, arterial thrombosis or embolism** 250,000 IU over 30 min, followed by 100,000 IU/hr for 24-72 hr (72 hr if DVT suspected). Institute heparin therapy — see Parameters to Monitor. **For arteriovenous cannula occlusion** slowly instill 250,000 IU in 2 ml solution into each occluded limb of cannula; clamp for 2 hr, aspirate contents and flush with NS. **Selective intra-arterial infusion** (investigational) 5000 IU/hr for 5-16 hr.[69]

Dosage Individualization. The recommended fixed dosage schedule results in sufficient activation of plasminogen in 95% of patients.[65] An increase in dosage is sometimes necessary in patients with high titer antistreptokinase antibodies (eg, recent streptococcal infection or recent treatment with streptokinase).

Pediatric Dose. Safety and efficacy not established.

Dosage Forms. Inj 250,000, 600,000, 750,000, 1.5 million IU.

Pharmacokinetics. *Onset and Duration.* Onset of fibrinolytic activity immediately following IV loading dose; peak occurs 6-8 hr into the infusion; duration 8-24 hr following discontinuation of the infusion.[72]

Fate. Plasma clearance results, in part, from formation of an antigen-antibody complex which remains soluble and is rapidly removed. It is postulated that the reticuloendothelial system also contributes to clearance.[73]

$t_{1/2}$. α phase averages 18 min and is related to antigen-antibody formation, β phase averages 83 min and appears to be related to clearance by the reticuloendothelial system.[73]

Adverse Reactions. Surface bleeding complications occur frequently and are primarily related to invasive procedures (eg, venous cutdowns, arterial punctures and sites of surgical intervention). Severe internal bleeding is reported occasionally; however, its prevalence is no greater than with standard anticoagulant therapy. Rarely, cerebral hemorrhage occurs. Occasional allergic reactions include fever, urticaria, itching, flushing and musculoskeletal pain. Anaphylactoid reactions occur rarely with the preparations now in use.[66]

Contraindications. Active internal bleeding or cerebrovascular accident within the last 2 months; intracranial or intraspinal surgery; intracranial neoplasm.

Precautions. Major relative contraindications include major surgery within the last 10 days, recent serious GI bleeding, recent trauma and severe hypertension. Minor relative contraindications are bacterial endocarditis, severe hepatic or renal disease, pregnancy, diabetic hemorrhagic retinopathy, likelihood of a left heart thrombus and age greater than 75 yr.[66] Avoid IM injections and drugs that affect clotting and platelet function.

Parameters to Monitor. Monitor thrombin time, activated partial thromboplastin time or prothrombin time to detect activation of the fibrinolytic system, performed 3-4 hr after initiating therapy and q 12 hr throughout treatment.[66,67] No correlation has been made between clotting test results and likelihood of hemorrhage or efficacy;[68] however, prolongation of the thrombin time to 2-5 times normal control value has been recommended.[67] Institute anticoagulant therapy with heparin after completion of the thrombolytic infusion. When the coagulation test being used no longer exceeds twice normal control (usually 3-4 hr after discontinuation of the thrombolytic agent) heparin therapy is initiated without a loading dose.[66]

Notes. Recommended only for treatment of thrombosis involving the popliteal vein or deep veins of the thigh and pelvis, and for patients in whom pulmonary emboli has caused obstruction of blood flow to one or more lung segments or when clinical shock is present.[66] The effectiveness of thrombolytic therapy is markedly diminished in patients with thrombosis of more than 5 days duration.[65] Thrombolytic therapy may help prevent venous valvular damage and the development of venous hypertension.[66,74] Low-dose streptokinase by selective intra-arterial infusion has been used successfully to treat arterial occlusion, while minimizing hemorrhagic complications.[69] Streptokinase by selective intracoronary artery infusion administered within 4-6 hr of acute myocardial infarction has been shown to lower morbidity and mortality.[71,75,76]

Urokinase   Abbokinase®

Urokinase is a proteolytic enzyme produced by renal parenchymal cells that acts to directly convert plasminogen to plasmin with effects similar to streptokinase. Side effects are similar to streptokinase, although allergic reactions occur much less frequently. It is administered IV as a 4400 IU/kg loading dose over 10 min, followed by 4400 IU/kg/hr for 12 hr. It may be given by selective intracoronary infusion 6000 IU/min for up to 2 hr. For IV catheter clearance, attach a 1 ml tuberculin syringe filled with 5000 IU reconstituted solution (Open-Cath®) and slowly inject an amount equal to the catheter volume; aspirate and repeat q 5 min as necessary. If not successful, allow urokinase to remain in the catheter for 30-60 min before attempting to aspirate. Available as injection 5000 and 250,000 IU vials.

References, 20:00 Blood Formation and Coagulation

1. Dallman PR. Iron deficiency: diagnosis and treatment. West J Med 1981;134:496-505.

2. Hamstra RD, Block MH, Schocket AL. Intravenous iron dextran in clinical medicine. JAMA 1980;243:1726-31.

3. Camitta BM, Nathan DG. Anemia in adolescence: 1. disturbances of iron balance. Postgrad Med 1975;57:143-6.

4. Trace elements—Iron. In: Committee on Dietary Allowances. National Research Council. Recommended dietary allowances. 9th ed. Washington, DC: National Academy of Sciences, 1980:137-43.

5. Berkowitz RL, Coustan DR. Mochizuki TK, eds. Handbook for prescribing medications during pregnancy. Boston: Little, Brown, 1981:240-42.

6. Gilman AG, Goodman LS, Rall TW, eds. Goodman and Gilman's the pharmacological basis of therapeutics. 7th ed. New York: Macmillan, 1985.

7. Rumack BH, ed. Iron management. In: Poisindex. Denver: Micromedex, 1987.

8. Middleton EJ, et al. Studies on the absorption of orally administered iron from sustained-release preparations. N Engl J Med 1966;274:136-9.

9. Hanson DB, Hendeles L. Guide to total dose intravenous iron dextran therapy. Am J Hosp Pharm 1974;31:592-5.

10. McEvoy GK, ed. American hospital formulary service. Washington, DC: American Society of Hospital Pharmacists, 1959-87.

11. Wood JK, Milner PFA, Pathak UN. The metabolism of iron-dextran given as a total-dose infusion to iron deficient Jamaican subjects. Br J Haematol 1968;14:119-29.

12. Thomas DP. Heparin in the prophylaxis and treatment of venous thromboembolism. Semin Hematol 1978;15:1-17.

13. Wessler S, Gitel SN. Heparin: new concepts relevant to clinical use. Blood 1979;53:525-44.

14. Fenech A, Douglas AS. Individualization of oral anticoagulant therapy. Drugs 1979;18:48-57.

15. The Multicenter Trial Committee. Dihydroergotamine-heparin prophylaxis of postoperative deep vein thrombosis. JAMA 1984;251:2960-6.

16. The Multicenter Trial Committee. Prophylactic efficacy of low-dose dihydroergotamine and heparin in postoperative deep venous thrombosis following intra-abdominal operations. J Vasc Surg 1984;1:608-16.

17. Hayes AC, Baker WH. Heparin prophylaxis trials of venous thrombosis: a critical review. Semin Thromb Hemostas 1985;11:222-6.

18. Barone JA, Raia JJ, Levy DB. Combination of dihydroergotamine mesylate and heparin sodium with lidocaine HCl: pharmacokinetics, mechanism of action, clinical efficacy, and adverse effects. Pharmacotherapy 1986;6:3S-11S.

19. Basu D, Gallus A, Hirsh J et al. A prospective study of the value of monitoring heparin treatment with the activated partial thromboplastin time. N Engl J Med 1972;287:324-7.

20. Carter BL, Jones ME, Waickman LA. Pathophysiology and treatment of deep-vein thrombosis and pulmonary embolism. Clin Pharm 1985;4:279-96.

21. Coon WW. Some recent developments in the pharmacology of heparin. J Clin Pharmacol 1979;19:337-49.

22. Salzman EW, Deykin D, Shapiro RM et al. Management of heparin therapy: controlled prospective trial. N Engl J Med 1975;292:1046-50.

23. Simon TL, Hyers TM, Gaston JP et al. Heparin pharmacokinetics: increased requirements in pulmonary embolism. Br J Haematol 1978;39:111-20.

24. Gallus AS, Hirsh J, Tuttle RJ et al. Small subcutaneous doses of heparin in prevention of venous thrombosis. N Engl J Med 1973;288:545-51.

25. Gallus AS, Hirsh J, O'Brien SE et al. Prevention of venous thrombosis with small, subcutaneous doses of heparin. JAMA 1976;235:1980-2.

26. Estes JW. Clinical pharmacokinetics of heparin. Clin Pharmacokinet 1980;5:204-20.

27. Hirsh J, van Aken WG, Gallus AS et al. Heparin kinetics in venous thrombosis and pulmonary embolism. Circulation 1976;53:691-5.

28. Bailey RT, Ursick JA, Heim KL et al. Heparin-associated thrombocytopenia: a prospective comparison of bovine lung heparin, manufactured by a new process, and porcine intestinal heparin. Drug Intell Clin Pharm 1986;20:374-8.

29. Green D, Martin GJ, Shoichet SH et al. Thrombocytopenia in a prospective, randomized, double-blind trial of bovine and porcine heparin. Am J Med Sci 1984;288:60-4.

30. Bell WR, Royall RM. Heparin-associated thrombocytopenia: a comparison of three heparin preparations. N Engl J Med 1980;303:902-7.

31. Glazier RL, Crowell EB. Randomized prospective trial of continuous vs intermittent heparin therapy. JAMA 1976;236:1365-7.

32. Goldman L, Feinstein AR. Anticoagulants and myocardial infarction. Ann Intern Med 1979;90:92-4.

33. Selzer A. Use of anticoagulant agents in acute myocardial infarction: statistics or clinical judgment? Am J Cardiol 1978;41:1315-7.

34. Goldberg RJ, Gore JM, Dalen JE. The role of anticoagulant therapy in acute myocardial infarction. Am Heart J 1984;108:1387-93.

35. Kruchoski ME, Emory CE. Initiating heparin and warfarin therapy concurrently. Hosp Pharm 1986;21:174.

36. O'Reilly RA, Aggeler PM. Determinants of the response to oral anticoagulant drugs in man. Pharmacol Rev 1970;22:35-96.

37. Nagashima R, O'Reilly RA, Levy G. Kinetics of pharmacologic effects in man: the anticoagulant action of warfarin. Clin Pharmacol Ther 1969;10:22-35.

38. Kazmier FJ, Spittell JA, Thompson JJ et al. Effect of oral anticoagulants on factors VII, IX, X, and II. Arch Intern Med 1965;115:667-73.

39. Lutomski DM, LaFrance RJ, Bower RH et al. Warfarin absorption after massive small bowel resection. Am J Gastroenterol 1985;80:99-102.

40. O'Reilly RA, Aggeler PM, Leong LS. Studies on the coumarin anticoagulant drugs: a comparison of the pharmacodynamics of dicumarol and warfarin in man. Thrombosis et Diathesis Haemorrhagica 1964;11:1-22.

41. Bachmann K, Shapiro R. Protein binding of coumarin anticoagulants in disease states. Clin Pharmacokinet 1977;2:110-26.

42. Yacobi A, Udall JA, Levy G. Serum protein binding as a determinant of warfarin body clearance and anticoagulant effect. Clin Pharmacol Ther 1976;19:552-8.

43. Lewis RJ, Trager WF, Robinson A et al. Warfarin metabolites: the anticoagulant activity and pharmacology of warfarin alcohols. J Lab Clin Med 1973;81:925-31.

44. O'Reilly RA, Aggeler PM, Leong LS. Studies on the coumarin anticoagulant drugs: the pharmacodynamics of warfarin in man. J Clin Invest 1963;42:1542-51.

45. Williams RL, Schary WL, Blaschke TF et al. Influence of acute viral hepatitis on disposition and pharmacologic effect of warfarin. Clin Pharmacol Ther 1976;20:90-7.

46. Breckenridge A, Orme M, Wesseling H et al. Pharmacokinetics and pharmacodynamics of the enantiomers of warfarin in man. Clin Pharmacol Ther 1974;15:424-30.

47. Levine MN, Raskob G, Hirsh J. Risk of haemorrhage associated with long term anticoagulant therapy. Drugs 1985;30:444-60.

48. O'Reilly RA, Aggeler PM. Studies on coumarin anticoagulant drugs. Initiation of warfarin therapy without a loading dose. Circulation 1968;38:169-77.

49. Deykin D. Warfarin therapy (second of two parts). N Engl J Med 1970;283:801-3.

50. de Gaetano G, Cerletti C, Dejana E et al. Current issues in thrombosis prevention with antiplatelet drugs. Drugs 1986;31:517-49.

51. Chesebro JH, Steele PM, Fuster V. Platelet-inhibitor therapy in cardiovascular disease. Effective defense against thromboembolism. Postgrad Med 1985;78:48-70.

52. Hirsh J. The clinical role of antiplatelet agents. Drug Ther 1981;6:63-70.

53. The Persantine-Aspirin Reinfarction Study Research Group. Persantine and aspirin in coronary heart disease. Circulation 1980;62:449-61.

54. The Anturane Reinfarction Trial Research Group. Sulfinpyrazone in the prevention of cardiac death after myocardial infarction. N Engl J Med 1978;298:289-95.

55. The FDA's Critique of the Anturane Reinfarction Trial. N Engl J Med 1980;303:1488-92.

56. Anturan Reinfarction Italian Study. Sulphinpyrazone in post-myocardial infarction. Lancet 1982;1:237-42.

57. Lewis JD, Davis JW, Archibald DG et al. Protective effects of aspirin against acute myocardial infarction and death in men with unstable angina. Results of a Veterans Administration cooperative study. N Engl J Med 1983;309:396-403.

58. Cairns JA, Gent M, Singer J et al. Aspirin, sulfinpyrazone, or both in unstable angina. Result of a Canadian multicenter trial. N Engl J Med 1985;313:1369-75.

59. Weintraub M, Evans P. Ticlopidine: an inhibitor of platelet aggregation currently under investigation. Hosp Formul 1984;19:649-54.

60. Harter HR, Burch JW, Majerus PW et al. Prevention of thrombosis in patients on hemodialysis by low-dose aspirin. N Engl J Med 1979;301:577-9.

61. Lorenz RL, Schacky CV, Weber M et al. Improved aortocoronary bypass patency by low-dose aspirin (100 mg daily). Effects on platelet aggregation and thromboxane formation. Lancet 1984;1:1261-4.

62. Chesebro JH, Clements IP, Fuster V et al. A platelet-inhibitor-drug trial in coronary-artery bypass operations. N Engl J Med 1982;307:73-8.

63. Chesebro JH et al. Effect of dipyridamole and aspirin on late vein-graft patency after coronary bypass operations. N Engl J Med 1984;310:209-14.

64. The Canadian Cooperative Study Group. A randomized trial of aspirin and sulfinpyrazone in threatened stroke. N Engl J Med 1978;299:53-9.

65. Marder VJ. The use of thrombolytic agents: choice of patient, drug administration, laboratory monitoring. Ann Intern Med 1979;90:802-8.

66. Sherry S, Bell WR, Duckert H et al. Thrombolytic therapy in thrombosis: a National Institutes of Health consensus development conference. Ann Intern Med 1980;93:141-4.

67. Bell WR, Meek AG. Guidelines for the use of thrombolytic agents. N Engl J Med 1979;301:1266-70.

68. Verstraete M. Biochemical and clinical aspects of thrombolysis. Semin Hematol 1978;15:35-54.

69. Katzen BT, van Breda A. Low dose streptokinase in the treatment of arterial occlusions. AJR 1981;136:1171-8.

70. Mathey DG, Kuck K-H, Tilsner V et al. Nonsurgical coronary artery recanalization in acute transumural myocardial infarction. Circulation 1981;63:489-99.

71. Natarajan N, Karlekar K, Turkevich D et al. Intracoronary streptokinase therapy in the coronary care unit for acute myocardial infarction. Clin Cardiol 1984;7:583-7.

72. Fletcher AP, Alkjaersig N, Sherry S. The maintenance of a sustained thrombolytic state in man. I. Induction and effects. J Clin Invest 1959;38:1096-110.

73. Fletcher AP, Alkjaersig N, Sherry S. The clearance of heterologous protein from the circulation of normal and immunized man. J Clin Invest 1958;37:1306-15.

74. Arnesen H, Hoiseth A, Ly B. Streptokinase or heparin in the treatment of deep vein thrombosis. Acta Med Scand 1982;211:65-8.

75. Kennedy JW, Ritchie JL, Davis KB et al. The Western Washington randomized trial of intracoronary streptokinase in acute myocardial infarction. N Engl J Med 1985;312:1073-8.

76. Kennedy JW, Gensini GG, Timmis GC et al. Acute myocardial infarction treated with intracoronary streptokinase: a report of the Society for Cardiac Angiography. Am J Cardiol 1985;55:871-7.

77. Collen D. Tissue-type plasminogen activator: therapeutic potential in thrombotic disease states. Drugs 1986;31:1-5.

78. Jaffe AS, Sobel BE. Thrombolysis with tissue-plasminogen activator in acute myocardial infarction: potentials and pitfalls. JAMA 1986;255:237-9.

79. The TIMI Study Group. The thrombolysis in myocardial infarction (TIMI) trial. N Engl J Med 1985;312:932-6.

80. Crabbe SJ, Cloninger CC. Tissue plasminogen activator: a new thrombolytic agent. Clin Pharm 1987;6:373-86.

81. The Steering Committee of the Physicians' Health Study Research Group. Preliminary report: findings from the aspirin component of the ongoing physicians' health study. N Engl J Med 1988;318:262-4.

24:00 CARDIOVASCULAR DRUGS

24:04 CARDIAC DRUGS

General References: 1-6

Amiodarone Hydrochloride   Cordarone®

Pharmacology. Amiodarone is a type III antiarrhythmic agent which prolongs the effective refractory period of atrial and ventricular tissue. It also decreases sinus rate and slows conduction through the AV node by noncompetitive adrenergic blockade. The antiarrhythmic actions may be due to interruption of re-entrant substrate or abolition of premature beats which trigger re-entry.[7,8]

Administration and Adult Dose. PO loading dose 800–1600 mg/day for 1-3 weeks. **Maintenance dose** 200–600 mg/day (usually 400 mg/day). Some suggest a 600–1000 mg/day priming dose for 1–2 months after the initial loading period and prior to maintenance therapy.

Pediatric Dose. Safety and efficacy not established.

Dosage Forms. Tab 200 mg.

Patient Instructions. Report any shortness of breath, tiredness, abdominal discomfort or visual abnormalities. Avoid intense sunlight; use sunscreen.

Pharmacokinetics. **_Onset and Duration._** Onset variable from several days to a month; full effect may not occur for 2–5 months.[9]

Plasma Levels. 1–2.5 mcg/ml is proposed, although the therapeutic range is not well established.[10] Desethylamiodarone accumulates to plasma levels similar to or greater than the parent drug.

Fate. Oral absorption is erratic and incomplete; bioavailability is 22–88% (average 50).[9,11,12] V_d ranges from 70–150 L/kg; 95–98% plasma protein bound.[9,11] Amiodarone is primarily hepatically eliminated with at least one active metabolite, desethylamiodarone. No unchanged amiodarone or desethylamiodarone is found in urine.[9,11]

_$t_{1/2}$._ α phase 4–12 hr; β phase 15–100 days (average 30). Similar half-life for desethylamiodarone.[9,12]

Adverse Reactions. Corneal microdeposits occur in virtually all patients; however, visual disturbances are reported in only about 5%.[7,13] Neurologic effects include tremor, ataxia, paresthesias and nightmares which may be due to drug-induced neurolipidosis.[14] Anorexia and/or constipation occur frequently. Transient elevations in hepatic enzymes occur in over 50% of patients, but clinical hepatitis is infrequent.[15,16] Photosensitivity may occur and a blue-grey skin pigmentation (sometimes irreversible) develops in 2–4% of patients.[7,16] Hypothyroidism (low T_3 syndrome) or hyperthyroidism may occur.[17,18] Proximal muscle weakness and myopathy have been reported. Symptomatic pulmonary fibrosis has been reported in 1–6% of patients. Pulmonary symptoms usually improve upon drug discontinuation, but death due to this side effect has been reported.[7,10,16] Pulmonary fibrosis is probably not immunologic in etiology and seems to occur more often in patients with underlying lung disease.[17,19] Aggravation of ventricular tachycardia and drug-induced torsades de pointes may occur.[20] Severe sinus bradycardia (requiring a pacemaker) or AV block has been reported occasionally.

Contraindications. Sick sinus syndrome or second or third degree heart block in the absence of a ventricular pacemaker; long QT syndrome.

Precautions. Amiodarone increases digoxin, quinidine and procainamide plasma levels and potentiates warfarin's anticoagulant effects; initial dose of warfarin should be reduced by one-half. Electrophysiologic studies may not predict long-term efficacy of amiodarone.[7,21] Because of its side effects, amiodarone should be reserved for life-threatening arrhythmias refractory to other antiarrhythmics. Amiodarone should be initiated *only* during hospitalization.

Parameters to Monitor. Daily EKG should be monitored during loading phase for heart rate, PR, QRS and QT duration. Baseline and periodic thyroid function tests and liver enzymes (especially if symptoms present). Obtain baseline pulmonary function tests; repeat if pulmonary symptoms arise. Some suggest baseline and periodic ophthalmologic (slit-lamp) examinations.

Amrinone Lactate   Inocor®

Pharmacology. Amrinone improves cardiac output by vasodilatory and positive inotropic actions. The ultimate mechanism(s) responsible for these properties is unknown, but seems to involve altered calcium availability and increased intracellular cyclic AMP concentrations, possibly by the inhibition of phosphodiesterase.[22-24]

Administration and Adult Dose. **IV loading dose** 0.5-1 mg/kg (usually 0.75 mg/kg) over 2-3 min, may repeat in 30 min based on response. **IV maintenance dose by continuous infusion** 5-10 mcg/kg/min.

Pediatric Dose. Safety and efficacy not established.

Dosage Forms. Inj 5 mg/ml.

Pharmacokinetics. ***Onset and Duration.*** IV onset 2-5 min after bolus, peak 10 min, duration 60-90 min.[24,25]

Plasma Levels. 1.5-4 mcg/ml is associated with therapeutic response. Although a correlation exists between amrinone levels and increased cardiac output, their clinical usefulness is questionable.[22,26]

Fate. Over 90% absorbed orally. 20-50% plasma protein bound; V_d is 1.3-1.7 L/kg. The drug is eliminated primarily by hepatic metabolism, with 10-40% excreted in urine unchanged.[27]

$t_{1/2}$. α phase 1-5 min; β phase 2-4 hr in normals, possibly longer in patients with CHF.[22,26]

Adverse Reactions. A dose-dependent, asymptomatic thrombocytopenia may occur. Platelet counts return to normal within 2-4 days of discontinuing therapy; in some cases, this side effect may be reversible when dosage is maintained or reduced.[28] Nausea and vomiting are frequent with oral administration, but unusual with IV.[24] Occasional side effects include nephrogenic diabetes insipidus, liver enzyme elevation, fever, taste disturbances, flu-like syndrome, rash[29] and aggravation of underlying arrhythmias.[30]

Contraindications. Hypertrophic obstructive cardiomyopathy.

Precautions. Use concomitant antiplatelet agents with caution. One study suggests a decreased survival rate in patients on long-term amrinone therapy.[30]

Parameters to Monitor. Continuous electrocardiography and frequent vital signs. Pulmonary capillary wedge pressure and cardiac output by flow-directed, balloon tipped catheter is necessary in seriously ill patients for adequate dosage titration.

Notes. Do not dilute with dextrose-containing solutions.

Bretylium Tosylate   Bretylol®, Various

Pharmacology. A type III antiarrhythmic with actions thought to be due to an initial catecholamine release and subsequent catecholamine depletion and/or direct effect independent of the adrenergic nervous system.[31] Direct actions may be mediated by blockade of potassium channels. Bretylium causes an initial increase in blood pressure, heart rate and myocardial contractility (catecholamine release) followed by hypotension (neuronal blockade).[32] Its greatest usefulness is in severe ventricular tachyarrhythmias resistant to other antiarrhythmics. Bretylium can be effective for ventricular fibrillation, but is usually ineffective against ventricular tachycardia.[33,34]

Administration and Adult Dose. IV 5 mg/kg push with additional dose of 10 mg/kg if no response. Maintenance can be given as IM or IV (over 8 min or more) 5-10 mg/kg q 6 hr or an IV infusion of 1-2 mg/min.

Dosage Individualization. In renal impairment, lower doses may be required.[35] A nomogram for dosing in renal insufficiency has been described.[36]

Pediatric Dose. Safety and efficacy not established.

Dosage Forms. Inj 50 mg/ml.

Pharmacokinetics. *Onset and Duration.* IV onset may be delayed by 20–60 min after administration; myocardial levels peak in 1.5–6 hr.[33] Duration is usually 6–12 hr after a single dose.[37] Due to persistent myocardial levels, duration after multiple doses may be much longer.[38]

Fate. A quaternary ammonium compound absorbed only 15–20% after oral administration.[37] One study estimated V_d to be 8.2 L/kg;[40] not bound to plasma proteins.[42] After IV dosing, bretylium is primarily cleared renally, with about 70–85% excreted in the urine unchanged.[39,40] Disposition is probably route- and concentration-dependent.[41]

$t_{1/2}$. α phase about 25 min; β phase 5.5–13.5 hr.[39-42] $t_{1/2}$ reported to average 33.4 hr in renal insufficiency.[36]

Adverse Reactions. Hypotension (usually orthostatic) via adrenergic blockade is most common. The drop in mean arterial pressure is usually not more than 20 mm Hg; however, sometimes it can be severe, necessitating drug discontinuation.[43] Nausea and vomiting may occur after rapid IV administration.[43]

Contraindications. Suspected digitalis-induced ventricular tachycardia (may increase the rate of ventricular tachycardia or the likelihood of ventricular fibrillation).[44]

Precautions. Use with caution if hypotension exists prior to administration.[32] Keep patients supine until tolerance to hypotension develops. Prolonged effects may occur and dosage reduction in patients with impaired renal function may be required.

Parameters to Monitor. Close monitoring of blood pressure and constant EKG monitoring is required.

Notes. **Bethanidine** (Tenathan® - Robins) **clofilium** (Lilly) and **meobentine** (Rhythmatine®-BW) are investigational agents similar to bretylium.[33,34]

Digitoxin

Crystodigin®, Various

Pharmacology. See Digoxin.

Administration and Adult Dose. PO or IV loading dose 0.8–1.4 mg in divided doses over 12–24 hr at intervals of 6–8 hr;[45] alternatively, 10–15 mcg/kg loading dose in divided doses. **Daily maintenance dose** 10% of total digitalizing dose.

Dosage Individualization. Unlike digoxin, no significant maintenance dosage changes are needed in patients with impaired renal function.[46]

Pediatric Dose. PO or IV digitalizing dose (premature and newborn) 22 mcg/kg; (2 weeks–1 yr) 45 mcg/kg; (1–2 yr) 40 mcg/kg; (over 2 yr) 30 mcg/kg. Give loading dose in divided doses over 12–24 hr at intervals of 6–8 hr. **Daily maintenance dose** 10% of total digitalizing dose.

Dosage Forms. Elxr 50 mcg/ml; **Soln** 20 mcg/drop; **Tab** 0.05, 0.1, 0.15, 0.2 mg; **Inj** 0.2, 0.25 mg/ml.

Patient Instructions. See Digoxin.

Pharmacokinetics. *Onset and Duration.* IV onset 25–120 min; IV peak 4–12 hr;[48] somewhat slower with oral dosing.

Plasma Levels. Therapeutic 15–30 ng/ml; toxic, greater than 35 ng/ml. Considerable overlap exists between toxic and therapeutic ranges.

Fate. Definitive data unavailable, but probably well absorbed with approximately 70% absorbed from the small bowel and 15% from the stomach.[49,50] About 14% of the absorbed drug is enterohepatically recycled.[50] Because greater than 90% is plasma protein bound, V_d is less than that of digoxin, being approximately 0.6 L/kg.[50] Eliminated primarily by hepatic metabolism; 30–50% is excreted in urine and feces as unchanged drug.[49] About 8% of daily losses of digitoxin are due to metabolic conversion to digoxin; however, even in severe renal dysfunction, accumulation of digoxin is not significant.[45]

$t_{1/2}$. α phase 1–2 hr; β phase 2.4–16.4 days (average 7.6).[50]

Adverse Reactions. See Digoxin.

Precautions. See Digoxin.

Parameters to Monitor. See Digoxin.

Digoxin

Lanoxin®, Various

Pharmacology. Digitalis glycosides exert positive inotropic effects through improvement of availability of calcium to myocardial contractile elements, thereby increasing cardiac output in heart failure. Antiarrhythmic actions of digitalis glycosides are primarily due to an increase in AV nodal refractory period via increased vagal tone, sympathetic withdrawal and direct mechanisms.[51] Additionally, digitalis exerts a moderate direct vasoconstrictor action on arterial and venous smooth muscle.[52]

Administration and Adult Dose. IV loading dose 10–15 mcg/kg in divided doses over 12–24 hr at intervals of 6–8 hr.[53] PO dose should be adjusted for percent oral absorption (see Fate). Usually, 0.5 mg is given initially, then 0.25 mg q 6 hr until desired effect or total digitalizing dose is achieved. **Maintenance dose** = (total body stores) × (% lost/day), where total body stores is the original calculated loading dose and % lost/day is 14 + (Cl_{cr} ÷ 5). Usual maintenance doses range from 0.125 to 0.5 mg/day.[53] A dosing nomogram has also been described.[54] **IM not recommended.**[55]

Dosage Individualization. Decrease loading and maintenance dose in renal impairment. Base dosage on ideal body weight in obese individuals.

Pediatric Dose. Total digitalizing dose (TDD) (premature newborn) IV 20 mcg/kg; (full-term newborn) IV 30–50 mcg/kg; (1–24 months) PO 60–80 mcg/kg or IV 40–60 mcg/kg; (2–10 yr) PO 40–60 mcg/kg or IV 20–40 mcg/kg; (over 10 yr) PO or IV 0.75–1.25 mg. Give 1/2 TDD initially, then 1/4 TDD q 6–8 hr twice. **Maintenance dose** (under 10 yr) IV 20–30% of TDD/day in 2 divided doses; PO dose is 1.3 times IV dose. Premature infants may require lower maintenance doses.[47] Base all doses on ideal body weight.

Dosage Forms. Elxr 50 mcg/ml; Tab 0.125, 0.25, 0.375, 0.5 mg; Inj 0.25 mg/ml; Caps 0.05, 0.1, 0.2 mg.

Patient Instructions. Report feelings of tiredness, appetite loss, nausea, abdominal discomfort or visual disturbances such as hazy vision, light sensitivity, spots or halos and red-green blindness.[56]

Pharmacokinetics. *Onset and Duration.* IV onset 14–30 min; peak 1.5–5 hr;[48] somewhat slower with oral dosing.

Plasma Levels. Therapeutic 0.5–2 ng/ml; toxic, greater than 3 ng/ml. Considerable overlap exists between therapeutic and toxic ranges.[57] Signs or symptoms of digitalis toxicity may be evident below 3 ng/ml, especially if other risk factors are present.[57] Digoxin concentrations (digitalis-like immunoreactive substance) have been detected in patients with renal failure, neonates, pregnant women, and those with severe liver disease not receiving digitalis glycosides.[58] Obtain blood samples for digoxin levels at least 6–8 hr after a dose to allow central and tissue compartment equilibration.

Fate. Oral absorption is 60–75% from tablets; 85% from elixir; 95% from capsules.[59] Differences in tablet dissolution rates and altered bioavailability for various brands have been reported.[60] Enterohepatic recycling of digoxin may be as high as 30%.[61] V_d is 7–8 L/kg, dependent on renal function; protein binding to albumin is 20–30%.[59] Excreted 60–80% unchanged in the urine in normal patients.[59] Active metabolites include digitoxigenin, bisdigitoxoside, digoxigenin monodigitoxoside and dihydrodigoxin.[59]

$t_{1/2}$. α phase 0.5–1 hr; β phase 1.6 days;[59] β phase 3.5–4.5 days in anephric patients.[53]

Adverse Reactions. Arrhythmias, listed in decreasing prevalence, are premature ventricular beats, second and third degree heart block, AV junctional tachycardia, atrial tachycardia with block, ventricular tachycardia and SA nodal block.[62] GI symptoms include abdominal discomfort, anorexia, nausea and vomiting. CNS side effects occur frequently, yet are nonspecific, such as weakness, lethargy, disorientation, agitation and nervousness. Visual disturbances are common, and include blurred vision, yellow or green tinting, flickering lights or halos or red-green color blindness. Hallucinations and psychosis have been reported. Rare reactions include gynecomastia, hypersensitivity and thrombocytopenia.[56]

Treatment of severe/life threatening digitalis (digoxin or digitoxin) toxicity should include IV digoxin-specific antibodies (Digibind®).[63] About 40 mg (one vial) of digoxin-specific Fab fragments will bind 0.6 mg of the glycoside. Exact dosage can be calculated based upon estimated total body stores.

Contraindications. Hypertrophic obstructive cardiomyopathy, except for supraventricular arrhythmias;[64] suspected digitalis intoxication; second or third degree heart block in the absence of mechanical pacing; atrial fibrillation with accessory AV pathway.

Precautions. Electrolyte abnormalities predisposing to digitalis toxicity include hypokalemia, hypomagnesemia and hypercalcemia. Hypothyroidism may reduce digoxin requirements due to lower V_d and clearance.[59] Direct current cardioversion carries little risk in the absence of digitalis toxicity.[63] Use with caution in patients with pulmonary disease, because hypoxia may sensitize the myocardium to arrhythmias and increase the risk of toxicity.[65] Serious bradyarrhythmias may occur with sick sinus syndrome, but controversy exists concerning the significance of its effects on the SA node.[66] Digitalis glycosides may increase infarct size in the nonfailing heart.[67] Quinidine may cause an increase in both digitoxin[68] and digoxin[69] levels.

Parameters to Monitor. Digitalis plasma levels need only be obtained when compliance, effectiveness or systemic availability is questioned or toxicity is suspected — see Plasma Levels.[70,71] Heart rate, EKG for digitalis-induced arrhythmias, subjective complaints of toxicity, renal function (BUN, Cr_s), serum electrolytes (especially potassium) frequently initially, then every 1–2 months when stabilized.

Diltiazem Hydrochloride   Cardizem®

Pharmacology. A calcium channel blocking agent that decreases heart rate, prolongs AV nodal conduction and decreases arteriolar and coronary vascular tone. It also has negative inotropic properties.[72,73]

Administration and Adult Dose. PO for angina 30–60 mg q 6–8 hr. Higher dosages up to 360 mg/day may be required for symptomatic relief of angina.[74] PO for hypertension usually 320 mg/day using SR capsule; doses of 120–480 mg/day have been used.

Dosage Individualization. Patients with liver disease may require lower dosages; titrate to clinical response.

Pediatric Dose. Safety and efficacy not established.

Dosage Forms. Tab 30, 60, 90, 120 mg; **SR Cap** 90, 120, 160 mg.

Patient Instructions. Report dizziness, swelling or shortness of breath.

Pharmacokinetics. *Onset and Duration.* PO onset 0.5-3 hr; duration 6-10 hr,[75,76] 24 hr with SR cap for hypertension.

   Plasma Levels. Levels over 95 ng/ml are necessary to cause hemodynamic changes, but their clinical usefulness is questionable.[77] Levels of desacetyldiltiazem are similar to diltiazem.[78]

   Fate. Oral bioavailability is about 40% with the first dose, but up to 90% with chronic therapy, probably due to saturation of the elimination pathway.[78] 80-85% plasma protein bound; V_d is 3-5 L/kg (average 3.8).[78,79] Enterohepatic recycling occurs.[78] Almost entirely metabolized by the liver, with only 1-3% excreted unchanged in urine. One metabolite, desacetyldiltiazem, has 40-50% the activity of diltiazem. Metabolites are excreted primarily in the feces.[79]

   $t_{1/2}$. α phase 2-5 min; β phase 3-6 hr (average 4.9).[75,76,78] β phase for desacetyldiltiazem 5-7 hr (average 6.1).[78]

Adverse Reactions. Frequency of side effects may be dose-related.[79,80] Hypotension, flushing, dizziness and edema occur occasionally. Sinus bradycardia and AV block have been reported, sometimes in association with concomitant propranolol.[80] Worsening of CHF may occur in patients with underlying left ventricular dysfunction. Hepatitis occurs rarely.

Contraindications. Second or third degree block or sick sinus syndrome in the absence of a ventricular pacemaker; symptomatic hypotension or severe CHF; atrial fibrillation with accessory AV pathway.

Precautions. Caution with concomitant use of β blockers in patients with underlying CHF, especially with poor left ventricular function.[79] Cimetidine, propranolol and possibly ranitidine may increase diltiazem plasma levels.[80,81]

Parameters to Monitor. Blood pressure, heart rate and EKG, especially when initiating therapy. Observe for symptoms of hypotension and CHF. Serial treadmill exercise tests can be performed to assess efficacy in angina. Maintain diary to document number of SL nitroglycerin used and chest pain episodes.

Disopyramide Phosphate

Norpace®, Norpace® CR, Various

Pharmacology. Disopyramide qualitatively has the same electrophysiological actions as procainamide and quinidine.[82] It causes an increase in systemic vascular resistance through a vasoconstrictor action;[83] additionally, it may exert a profound negative inotropic effect[84] and has significant anticholinergic properties systemically and on the heart. Disopyramide's isomers have stereoselective pharmacologic actions.[85]

Administration and Adult Dose. PO loading dose 300-400 mg. **PO maintenance dose** 400-800 mg/day to a maximum of 1.6 g/day. Large maintenance doses such as 1.2-1.6 g/day should be reserved for patients with resistant arrhythmias such as recurrent ventricular tachycardia. Give daily dosage in 4 equally divided portions q 6 hr with non-SR cap, or in 2 equally divided portions q 12 hr with SR cap.

Dosage Individualization. In patients less than 50 kg, or with hepatic disease or moderate renal insufficiency (Cl_{cr} over 35 ml/min), load with 150-200 mg, then give 400 mg/day in 2 or 4 divided doses, depending on the dosage form used. In patients with severe renal insufficiency, give maintenance doses as follows (non-SR cap):

CREATININE CLEARANCE	DAILY MAINTENANCE DOSAGE
20-35 ml/min	300 mg
5-20 ml/min	200 mg
1-5 ml/min	100 mg

Initial daily dose in patients with hepatic disease is about 4.4 mg/kg/day.[86]

Pediatric Dose. PO (under 1 yr) 10-30 mg/kg/day; (1-4 yr) 10-20 mg/kg/day; (4-12 yr) 10-15 mg/kg/day; (12-18 yr) 6-15 mg/kg/day. See Notes.

Dosage Forms. Cap 100, 150 mg; SR Cap 100, 150 mg. See Notes.

Patient Instructions. Report any symptoms such as difficulty in urination, constipation, blurred vision or dry mouth. Shortness of breath, weight gain or edema should also be reported.

Pharmacokinetics. *Onset and Duration.* PO onset within 1 hr. Duration varies with individual differences in drug disposition, but is usually 6-12 hr.

Plasma Levels. Usual range is 2-4 mcg/ml[88] with toxicity more likely over 4 mcg/ml. However, levels of 7 mcg/ml or greater may be required occasionally in some resistant ventricular dysrhythmias.[89] Therapeutic range of unbound drug is 0.5-2 mcg/ml.[86] Monitoring unbound concentrations eliminates variability due to concentration-dependent disposition.[86,87]

Fate. Oral absorption is rapid; systemic availability is 80-90%.[87,90,91] V_d is about 0.8-1.5 L/kg in normal subjects.[92] The percent of unbound drug in plasma varies from 19-46% over a plasma concentration range of 2-8 mcg/ml[94,95] and is also age-dependent.[87] About 50% excreted unchanged in the urine.[92] The major metabolite is a mono-N-dealkylated form that possesses weak antiarrhythmic activity and appears in the urine.[93,94]

$t_{1/2}$. α phase 2-4 min (IV);[94] β phase is concentration-dependent. $t_{1/2}$ β ranges from 4.4-8.2 hr in normals;[92] prolonged with renal dysfunction, ranging from 11-17 hr.[87]

Adverse Reactions. The most important adverse reactions include dry mouth, urinary retention, blurred vision and constipation. These anticholinergic side effects are dose-related, may occur in up to 70% of patients and result in drug discontinuation in about 20%.[96] Occasionally disopyramide causes hypotension, probably by its negative inotropic action.[93] Exacerbation of CHF is most prevalent in patients with left ventricular dysfunction.[84] Through its vagolytic action, it may cause sinus tachycardia. Severe bradycardia, AV nodal block, or asystole may occur, especially in patients with SA or AV nodal disease.[97] Torsades de pointes, similar to quinidine syncope, has been reported.[98] Disopyramide may occasionally cause nausea, vomiting or rash; rarely, hepatic cholestasis, psychosis, peripheral neuropathy or hypoglycemia occur.

Contraindications. History of disopyramide-induced heart block or serious ventricular arrhythmias; second or third degree heart block in the absence of a ventricular pacemaker; long QT syndrome; severe CHF or cardiogenic shock.

Precautions. In atrial fibrillation or flutter, digitalis or propranolol should be given prior to disopyramide to block the AV node. Use very cautiously in patients with CHF, because of negative inotropic and vasoconstrictive actions.[83,84] May worsen sick sinus syndrome, or aggravate underlying ventricular arrhythmias. If possible, other antiarrhythmics should be used in patients with prostatic hypertrophy or pre-existing urinary retention. Disopyramide may exacerbate glaucoma or myasthenia gravis. Disopyramide should probably be initiated during hospitalization.

Parameters to Monitor. Because of concentration-dependent protein binding, total drug levels unreliably reflect active drug concentration and monitoring unbound drug concentrations is preferable. Plasma levels and symptoms or signs of toxicity should be closely monitored in patients with altered states of drug disposition such as renal dysfunction. Daily EKG should be observed for QT, QRS or PR prolongation. Obtain frequent vital signs initially for evidence of adverse hemodynamic effects (ie, CHF), and less frequently when a maintenance dose is attained. Question the patient about anticholinergic manifestations, such as urinary and visual abnormalities.

Notes. A 1-10 mg/ml suspension in cherry syrup is stable for 1 month under refrigeration in amber bottle.

Encainide Hydrochloride   Enkaid®

Encainide is a type Ic antiarrhythmic agent with electrophysiologic actions similar to flecainide. Encainide is variably absorbed with bioavailability ranging from 7-82% (average 42). The peak plasma concentration occurs 0.5-2 hr after oral administration. Encainide's metabolism is genetically determined, with most patients hepatically metabolizing the drug to two major active metabolites, O-demethylencainide (ODE) and 3-methoxydemethyl encainide (MODE). Plasma concentrations of the metabolites exceed that of the parent compound and both are more active than the parent compound. β-phase half-lives are 1-2 hr for encainide, 3-4 hr for ODE and 6-12 hr for MODE. Less than 10% of patients metabolize encainide slowly, with a half-life of 6-11 hr and eliminate the drug unchanged in urine. Encainide has proarrhythmic actions in some patients and can aggravate pre-existing ventricular arrhythmias. The most frequent side effects are neurologic and include blurred vision, dizziness, headache, tremor and ataxia. Dosage in adults is begun at 25 mg q 8 hr and adjusted at 3-5 day intervals to 35 mg q 8 hr and then to 50 mg q 8 hr, if necessary. Doses greater than 200 mg/day require hospitalization of the patient. Available as 25, 35 and 50 mg capsules.[99-101]

Esmolol Hydrochloride   Brevibloc®

Esmolol is an ultrashort acting, cardioselective (β_1) adrenergic blocking agent. It is effective in controlling ventricular response in patients with atrial fibrillation and other supraventricular tachycardias and in slowing heart rate in patients with sinus tachycardia associated with acute MI or cardiac surgery. The drug may also be effective in perioperative hypertension. α-half-life is about 2 min; V_d is 2-5 L/kg (average 3.5). Esmolol is rapidly hydrolyzed by plasma and blood esterases resulting in an elimination half-life of about 9 min. Esmolol is metabolized to a metabolite with very weak, clinically insignificant β-blocking activity and small amounts of methanol. No unchanged esmolol appears in the urine. Effective plasma levels are about 1-1.5 mcg/ml; concurrent IV morphine use may increase plasma levels by 46%. Side effect profile is similar to other β_1-selective β-blockers. Particularly frequent is dose-related hypotension; IV site phlebitis occurs occasionally. Dilute injection to a final concentration of 10 mg/ml. The IV loading dose is 500 mcg/kg/min for 1 min, then 50 mcg/kg/min. IV loading dose may be repeated as often as q 5 min with a concomitant increase of infusion rate in 50 mcg/kg/min increments, titrated to ventricular response, heart rate and/or blood pressure. Most patients respond to infusions of 150–200 mcg/kg/min. Once desired end-point is obtained, infusion rate may be lowered in 25–50 mcg/kg/min increments at 5–10 min intervals. Infusions up to 48 hr in duration appear to be well tolerated. Available as 250 mg/ml injection. **Flestolol** (Du Pont) is another ultrashort acting β-blocker with a half-life of about 6 min.[102,103]

Flecainide Acetate   Tambocor®

Pharmacology. Flecainide is a type Ic antiarrhythmic that differs from other type I agents by its effects on repolarization (see Electrophysiologic Actions of Antiarrhythmics Comparison Chart) and its binding characteristics to the sodium channel.[104] It can decrease cardiac output by a negative inotropic action.

Administration and Adult Dose. PO for ventricular arrhythmias 100 mg q 12 hr initially, then increase in increments of 50 mg q 12 hr every 4–7 days until desired response. Usual maintenance doses are 100–200 mg q 12 hr for ventricular tachycardia (maximum 400 mg/day).

Dosage Individualization. Some suggest an initial dose of 50 mg q 12 hr in patients with CHF.[105] Lower maintenance dosage requirements are expected in patients with CHF, liver disease or renal insufficiency. In these patients one may begin with 50–100 mg q 12 hr and cautiously increase dose as required with the aid of plasma levels.[105]

Pediatric Dose. Safety and efficacy not established.

Dosage Forms. Tab 100, 150 mg.

Patient Instructions. Report any symptoms of dizziness or visual disturbances. Report symptoms of worsening shortness of breath or exercise intolerance.

Pharmacokinetics. *Onset and Duration.* Onset 1–6 hr (average 3); duration 12–30 hr.[105]

Plasma Levels. 200–1000 ng/ml for suppression of ventricular ectopy.[104,106]

Fate. Oral bioavailability is 90–100%.[106,107] 37–50% plasma protein bound, but may be higher (61%) post-MI due to increases in α_1-acid glycoprotein.[105] V_d is 8–10 L/kg;[105] Cl decreases in CHF, renal failure and liver disease. The drug is hepatically metabolized to two major active, but clinically insignificant metabolites.[104,106,107]

$t_{1/2}$. α phase 3–8 min; β phase 7–23 hr (average 14). β phase is about 20 hr with ventricular ectopy; 14–26 hr (average 19) with CHF; 17 hr with a Cl_{cr} of 10–30 ml/min and up to 26 hr with a Cl_{cr} below 10 ml/min.[104,106]

Adverse Reactions. Neurological side effects, which include dizziness and visual abnormalities, occur frequently. Nausea and headache may also occur.[108] Flecainide has proarrhythmic effects which may result in new sustained ventricular tachycardia or aggravation of underlying ventricular arrhythmias. These reactions are associated with high plasma levels, left ventricular dysfunction and recent administration of type Ia antiarrhythmics.[104,109] Flecainide-induced ventricular tachycardia may be unresponsive to cardioversion or pacing, but may respond to lidocaine therapy.[109,110] Aggravation of underlying conduction disturbances may also occur. Exacerbation of heart failure in patients with underlying left ventricular dysfunction has been reported.[111]

Contraindications. Second or third degree AV block or bifasicular block in the absence of a ventricular pacemaker; severe CHF.

Precautions. Cimetidine and amiodarone may increase flecainide plasma concentrations; flecainide slightly elevates plasma digoxin levels. Use with caution in patients with sick sinus syndrome and in combination with other negative inotropes such as disopyramide or propranolol or following recent therapy with type Ia agents. Flecainide may increase pacemaker capture threshold. Because of pro-arrhythmic and negative inotropic actions, some clinicians reserve flecainide for the treatment of life-threatening ventricular arrhythmias such as symptomatic nonsustained or sustained ventricular tachycardia.

Parameters to Monitor. Frequent EKG (continuous electrocardiography preferable) when therapy initiated, then periodically on an ambulatory basis. Obtain a baseline evaluation of left ventricular function prior to starting flecainide. Obtain periodic plasma levels once an individual's effective level is determined. Observe closely for neurologic toxicities and CHF symptoms when initiating therapy.

Notes. Flecainide can be effective for some supraventricular tachycardias (although not approved for this use).

Lidocaine Hydrochloride   Xylocaine®, Various

Pharmacology. Electrophysiological actions differ in healthy and diseased cardiac tissues—see Electrophysiologic Actions of Antiarrhythmics Comparison Chart.[112,113] Most antiarrhythmic activity is due to frequency-dependent blockade of the fast sodium channel in Purkinje fibers.[113] It also has a slight negative inotropic action. Used in the acute treatment of ventricular arrhythmias associated with myocardial infarction or digitalis intoxication. Effectiveness in the treatment of supraventricular arrhythmias is limited.

Administration and Adult Dose. **IV loading dose for ventricular tachycardia or fibrillation** 100 mg (1-1.5 mg/kg) over 1 min; if ineffective, may repeat with 50-100 mg q 5-10 min, to maximum of 300 mg.[114] **IV maintenance** 2-4 mg/min infusion.[114] **IV for post-MI prophylaxis of primary ventricular fibrillation** 100 mg followed by infusion of 3 mg/min[115] or 100 mg followed by 50 mg in 10-15 min and a continuous infusion of 2 mg/min. **IM for prehospital, post-MI, arrhythmia prophylaxis** 300-400 mg.[116] **PO not recommended.**

Dosage Individualization. In CHF, use one-half of IV loading doses.[114] In liver disease or CHF, initial maintenance infusion is 1 mg/min with maximum of 2-3 mg/min.[114] In myocardial infarction without CHF, maintenance infusion rate may have to be decreased by 30-50% in 24 hr;[114] however, empiric dosage alterations in MI are not recommended due to increases in α_1-acid glycoprotein and lidocaine binding.[117]

Pediatric Dose. **IV loading dose** 1 mg/kg, may repeat q 5-10 min, to maximum of 3-4.5 mg/kg/hr. **IV maintenance** 20-50 mcg/kg/min infusion.[47]

Dosage Forms. Inj 10, 20, 40, 100 mg/ml.

Patient Instructions. Report minor side effects such as drowsiness, perioral numbness or tingling, dizziness or nausea, during maintenance infusion.

Pharmacokinetics. *Onset and Duration.* IV onset immediate; duration after initial IV bolus is 10-20 min.[118] IM onset 10 min; duration 3 hr.[118]

Plasma Levels. Therapeutic 1.5-6.4 mcg/ml (total);[115] 0.5-1.5 mcg/ml (unbound).[117] Toxic reactions are more likely at total concentrations over 5 mcg/ml.[114] See Adverse Reactions.

Fate. Lidocaine is well absorbed orally; however, a large hepatic first-pass effect limits systemic availability to about 35%.[119] About 70% plasma protein bound;[114] V_d is about 1.3 L/kg in normals, 0.9 L/kg in CHF.[120] Clearance is decreased in CHF, liver disease and long-term infusion.[114,120,123] Primarily metabolized in the liver with less than 10% excreted unchanged in the urine.[120] Major metabolites, monoethylglycinexylidide (MEGX) and glycinexylidide (GX) both possess neurotoxic[121] and antiarrhythmic[122] actions. Accumulation of these metabolites in renal impairment or prolonged infusions may contribute to lidocaine toxicity.

$t_{1/2}$. α phase about 8 min,[118,120] β phase 80-108 min.[114,120] IM absorption half-life 12-28 min.[114] β phase in CHF or liver disease may be prolonged (about 5.5 hr and 6.6 hr, respectively).[114,120] Elimination half-life of total lidocaine increases to an average of 3.2 hr, 24 hr after MI without CHF;[124] the rise in total lidocaine half-life is greater than that of unbound lidocaine.[125]

Adverse Reactions. Level-related neurological side effects include dizziness, nausea, drowsiness, speech disturbances, perioral numbness, muscle twitching, confusion, vertigo or tinnitus and usually occur at plasma levels greater than 5 mcg/ml;[114,126] serious toxicities occurring at plasma levels greater than 9 mcg/ml include psychosis, seizures and respiratory depression.[114,126] Sinus arrest or severe bradycardia is associated with sinus node disease, toxic drug levels or concomitant therapy with other antiarrhythmics.[126] Complete AV block may occur, especially in patients with pre-existing bifasicular bundle branch block, AV nodal block or inferior wall MI.[126,127]

Contraindications. History of hypersensitivity to any amide-type local anesthetic (rare); second or third degree heart block unless the site of block can be localized to the AV node itself[126] or ventricular pacemaker is functional; severe sinus node dysfunction.

Precautions. Propranolol may decrease lidocaine clearance so that close monitoring is necessary with concomitant administration of these two agents. Cimetidine may decrease lidocaine clearance, but empiric dosage reduction with concomitant cimetidine is not recommended.[128] Caution in patients with atrial fibrillation and accessory AV pathway.

Parameters to Monitor. Plasma levels and signs or symptoms of toxicity should be closely monitored in patients with altered drug disposition such as heart failure, hepatic disease, acute MI or prolonged IV infusion (greater than 24 hr). Monitoring unbound levels is preferable post-MI. Minor subjective and objective toxicities are extremely important because they are often subtle and may forecast more serious toxicities (ie, seizures). Continuously observe EKG for therapeutic and/or toxic actions. Monitor vital signs such as blood pressure, heart rate and respirations frequently.

Notes. Pirmenol (Parke-Davis) is an investigational agent with both quinidine- and lidocaine-like properties.[129]

Lorcainide Hydrochloride (Investigational - Janssen)

Lorcainide is a type Ic antiarrhythmic with electrophysiologic actions similar to flecainide. Bioavailability is poor and probably dose-related, ranging from 5-65% after a single dose. Bioavailability increases with chronic therapy, probably due to saturable first-pass metabolism. About 70% plasma protein bound. Lorcainide is primarily hepatically eliminated with less than 3% excreted in the urine unchanged. An active metabolite, norlorcainide, is present in higher plasma concentrations than the parent compound. β-phase half-life of lorcainide is about 7–12 hr (average 9); β-phase half-life of norlorcainide is about 26 hr. Side effects are primarily neurologic and include insomnia, nightmares, visual disturbances and paresthesias. Oral dosage is 100–300 mg q 12 hr.[99,130,131]

Mexiletine Hydrochloride   Mexitil®

Pharmacology. Mexiletine has electrophysiological actions similar to lidocaine and tocainide.[132] Depression of conduction is accentuated in ischemic/hypoxic tissue.[133] It is used in the treatment of ventricular arrhythmias; effectiveness in supraventricular tachycardias is limited. Slight negative inotropic action.

Administration and Adult Dose. PO loading dose 400–600 mg; PO maintenance dose 200–300 mg q 8 hr, to a maximum of 400 mg q 8 hr.

Dosage Individualization. Although firm guidelines are unavailable, it seems prudent to reduce maintenance dose by 30–50% in patients with hepatic disease or severe CHF.[134] Dosage may also need to be decreased with Cl_{cr} below 10 ml/min.[135]

Pediatric Dose. PO 15–25 mg/kg/day;[136] however, safety and efficacy not well established.

Dosage Forms. Cap 100, 150, 200, 250 mg.

Patient Instructions. Report numbness, drowsiness, dizziness or tingling. Nausea or loss of appetite may occur and may be reduced by taking the drug with food. Report any abnormal bruising.

Pharmacokinetics. *Onset and Duration.* PO onset 1–4 hr (average 2); duration 8–16 hr.
   Plasma Levels. 0.5–2 mcg/ml, although not well correlated with therapeutic or toxic effects.[137]
   Fate. Oral bioavailability 80–90% and (unlike lidocaine) mexiletine undergoes less than 10% first-pass hepatic elimination.[138,139] Absorption can be incomplete in MI patients receiving narcotic analgesics.[137,138] About 70% plasma protein bound; V_d large and variable, ranging from 5–12 L/kg. Cl decreases in both CHF and liver disease.[138] Predominantly metabolized by the liver with 10–20% excreted unchanged in urine, depending on urinary pH.[137,138,140]
   $t_{1/2}$. α phase 3–12 min;[141] β phase 6–12 hr.[139,141] β phase averages 16 hr in severe renal dysfunction,[135] 15 hr in CHF with or without MI,[142,143] and may be prolonged in cirrhosis.

Adverse Reactions. Neurologic toxicities include tremor, ataxia, drowsiness, confusion, paresthesias and, potentially, psychosis or seizures. Minor CNS side effects may occur in up to 40% of patients.[134,144] Nausea, vomiting and anorexia are frequent. Mexiletine may aggravate underlying ventricular arrhythmias or conduction disturbances. Thrombocytopenia has been reported.[144] Mexiletine is an ether analogue of lidocaine so there should not be cross-sensitivity between mexiletine and tocainide or lidocaine.[145]

Contraindications. Second or third degree AV block in the absence of a ventricular pacemaker.

Precautions. Mexiletine may accelerate ventricular response in patients with atrial fibrillation or flutter. Worsening of sick sinus syndrome may occur.

Parameters to Monitor. Frequent EKG when therapy is initiated, then periodically on an ambulatory basis. Obtain periodic plasma levels once an individual's effective level is determined.[134] Observe closely for neurologic toxicities when initiating therapy.

Notes. The efficacy of mexiletine for ventricular ectopy or ventricular tachycardia can be increased by the addition of a type Ia agent such as procainamide or quinidine.[146] **Moricizine** (Ethmozine® -Du Pont) is an investigational agent with electrophysiologic actions similar to the type Ib drugs.[147]

Milrinone   Coratrope®

Milrinone is an inotrope that is a bipyridine derivative similar in structure to amrinone. It decreases vascular resistance and increases contractility by mechanisms different from digitalis glycosides or adrenergic agents (possibly by phosphodiesterase inhibition). Milrinone appears to be 10-20 times more potent than amrinone. The drug is well absorbed with bioavailability ranging from 75-90%. Hemodynamic actions peak 1-2 hr after oral administration and last for 2-4 hr. Milrinone is primarily eliminated by renal clearance (80%) and V_d is about 0.3 L/kg. Elimination half-life ranges from 1-2.5 hr. Unlike oral amrinone, therapy with milrinone usually does not result in thrombocytopenia or GI intolerance. Milrinone may aggravate ventricular arrhythmias. Also, long-term milrinone may adversely affect survival in patients with severe CHF. The effects of this agent on ventricular rhythm and prognosis require further study. Oral dose is initiated at 2.5-5 mg q 6 hr and titrated to clinical response; doses as high as 50 mg/day have been used. Dosage may need reduction in renal insufficiency.[148-153]

Nifedipine   Adalat®, Procardia®

Pharmacology. A calcium channel blocking agent which has potent vasodilating properties (arterial and coronary). Reflex increase in sympathetic tone (in response to vasodilation) counteracts the direct depressant effects on SA and AV nodal conduction. This renders nifedipine ineffective in the treatment of supraventricular tachycardias. Used for vasospastic and chronic stable angina, in the treatment of hypertension, and as an unloading agent in CHF.[72,154]

Administration and Adult Dose. PO 10-20 mg tid, increased to a usual maximum of 20-30 mg tid-qid. Dosages over 180 mg/day are not recommended. **PO for severe hypertension** 10 mg, may repeat in 20 min.[155]

Dosage Individualization. Patients with liver disease may require lower dosages; titrate to clinical response.

Pediatric Dose. Safety and efficacy not established.

Dosage Forms. Cap 10, 20 mg.

Patient Instructions. Report flushing, edema, dizziness or increased frequency of chest discomfort.

Pharmacokinetics. *Onset and Duration.* PO onset 0.5-2 hr; duration 4-8 hr. PO (punctured capsule) onset 10-30 min; duration 3-4 hr.[155]
   Plasma Levels. (Therapeutic) above 90 ng/ml, although clinical utility is questionable.[154]
   Fate. Bioavailability is 45-65%;[154,156] first-pass hepatic elimination is 30-50%; 92-98% plasma protein bound; V_d 0.6-1.5 L/kg.[154,156] Almost all

excreted by hepatic metabolism with only traces of unchanged drug excreted in urine.[154]

$t_{1/2}$. α phase 4-7 min; β phase 1-4 hr (average 2).[154,156]

Adverse Reactions. Most side effects relate to vasodilatory actions and occur frequently; symptoms include dizziness (with or without hypotension), flushing and headache.[80] Edema occurs frequently and is related to venous pooling and usually not exacerbation of CHF.[80] Nifedipine can paradoxically worsen anginal chest pain, possibly due to a reflex increase in sympathetic tone or redistribution of coronary blood flow away from ischemic areas.[154] Acute, reversible renal failure may occur in patients with chronic renal insufficiency;[158] rare reactions include hepatitis and hyperglycemia.[80]

Contraindications. Symptomatic hypotension.

Precautions. Caution in unstable angina pectoris when used as a single agent (without a β-blocker). Nifedipine may increase quinidine levels.[157] Nifedipine has an antiplatelet action and may increase bleeding time.[159] Caution in obstructive cardiomyopathy; may worsen symptoms.

Parameters to Monitor. Blood pressure and heart rate, especially when initiating therapy. Observe for symptoms of hypotension and edema. Serial treadmill exercise tests can be performed to assess efficacy. Maintain a diary to document the number of SL nitroglycerin used and chest pain episodes.

Notes.   Other potential uses for nifedipine include migraine prophylaxis,[160] achalasia and Raynaud's phenomenon.

Procainamide Hydrochloride   Procan®, Procan-SR®, Pronestyl®, Various

Pharmacology. Class I antiarrhythmic that alters normal and ischemic Purkinje action potential in a fashion similar to quinidine. It may decrease systemic blood pressure by causing peripheral ganglionic blockade;[161] it also possesses weak anticholinergic action and a slight negative inotropic action.

Administration and Adult Dose. PO loading dose 1 g over 2 hr in 2 divided doses. **PO maintenance dose** 1-9 g/day in 4-6 divided doses.[162] **SR** may be given q 6-8 hr. **IV loading dose** 1-2.5 g at a rate no greater than 20 mg/min.[163,164] **IV maintenance dose** 1.5-5 mg/min (20-80 mcg/kg/min) infusion.[164] **Intermittent IV or IM** 1-9 g/day in 4-6 divided doses.

Dosage Individualization. Maintenance dose should be reduced in liver disease and in the aged. In renal insufficiency, procainamide and its active metabolite accumulate, necessitating lower maintenance doses.[165] Previous information suggested decreasing loading and maintenance doses in CHF and MI.[166] Recent data imply no need for dosage reduction in these diseases.[167,168]

Pediatric Dose. Safety and efficacy not well established. **PO** 15-50 mg/kg/day in 4-8 divided doses, to maximum of 4 g/day; **IV loading dose** 3-6 mg/kg/dose to 100 mg over 5 min, repeated to maximum of 1 g. **IV maintenance dose** 20-80 mcg/kg/min infusion. **IM maintenance dose** 20-30 mg/kg/day in 4-6 divided doses, to maximum of 4 g/day.[47]

Dosage Forms. Cap, Tab 250, 375, 500 mg; SR Tab 250, 500, 750 mg; Inj 100, 500 mg/ml.

Patient Instructions. Report any symptoms such as nausea, vomiting, fever, sore throat, joint pain, rash, chest or abdominal pain or shortness of breath.

Pharmacokinetics. *Onset and Duration.* PO onset within 1 hr; SR preparation is somewhat slower. IM onset within 1 hr; IV immediate. Duration is usually 3-6 hr.

Plasma Levels. Therapeutic range is 4-10 mcg/ml;[163] toxicity is more likely at plasma levels greater than 12 mcg/ml.[169] In some arrhythmias (eg, recurrent ventricular tachycardia), levels of 20 mcg/ml or greater may be required for prevention of arrhythmias with average effective levels of 13 mcg/ml.[162] Effective plasma levels of NAPA are 15-25 mcg/ml, with the toxic range overlapping with the therapeutic range.[170]

Fate. Oral absorption is 75-95%;[171] V_d is about 2 L/kg in normals[171] and 1.5-2 L/kg in CHF;[166,167] approximately 15% bound to plasma proteins.[171] About 50% excreted in the urine as unchanged drug; the remainder is metabolized, mostly to active N-acetylprocainamide (NAPA) by the liver, with smaller amounts excreted as p-aminobenzoic acid.[166] The total quantity of NAPA produced is dependent on liver function and acetylator phenotype.[166]

$t_{1/2}$. (Procainamide) α phase about 6 min;[172] β phase in normals 2.5-4.7 hr (average 3.5).[172] $t_{1/2}$ in renal dysfunction 5.3-20.7 hr with anephric patients averaging 10.1 hr.[173] (NAPA) 4.3-15.1 hr (average 7);[170] may be as long as several days in renal failure.[165,170]

Adverse Reactions. Hypotension may occur, especially after rapid IV administration. Severe bradycardia, AV nodal block or asystole have been reported.[174,175] Procainamide can aggravate underlying ventricular arrhythmias and cause torsades de pointes.[176] GI symptoms occur frequently and include nausea and vomiting; drug fever and dermatological reactions may also occur.[175] Agranulocytosis is rare, but potentially fatal.[177] It is controversial whether or not the SR product carries a higher risk of neutropenia than the fast release preparation.[178,179] About 50-80% of patients develop a positive antinuclear antibody (ANA) with 30-50% developing SLE symptoms; genetically slow acetylators more rapidly develop positive ANA and SLE symptoms.[180] Common symptoms or signs are rash, arthralgias, fever, pericarditis and pleuritis. Although drug cessation usually reverses these symptoms in about 2 weeks, some patients have prolonged manifestations and for others the SLE syndrome may be initially life-threatening.[180] Hepatitis has been reported.[181]

Contraindications. History of procainamide-induced SLE; second or third degree heart block in the absence of a ventricular pacemaker; long QT syndrome or severe sinus node dysfunction.

Precautions. In atrial fibrillation or flutter, procainamide may paradoxically increase ventricular rate; digitalis, propranolol or verapamil should be given before procainamide in these situations to block the AV node. Procainamide may worsen symptoms of sick sinus syndrome;[182] it may also exacerbate myasthenia gravis. Procainamide should probably be started during hospitalization.

Parameters to Monitor. Plasma levels and symptoms or signs of toxicity should be monitored in patients with suspected altered drug disposition such as hepatic disease or renal dysfunction. EKG should be monitored continuously (with IV) or daily (with PO) for QRS, QT or PR prolongation. Blood pressure should be monitored frequently when therapy is initiated (especially with IV), and less frequently when a maintenance dose is established. Periodically monitor WBC counts and signs of infection for the development of drug-induced agranulocytosis. Observe closely for symptoms of drug-induced SLE.

Notes. Procan-SR® is a wax matrix formulation; the matrix may appear in the stool, but this does not imply a lack of bioavailability.

Propranolol Hydrochloride

Inderal®, Various

Pharmacology. A nonselective β-adrenergic blocker used in arrhythmias, hypertension and angina pectoris. Antiarrhythmic mechanism is due to decreased AV nodal conduction in supraventricular tachycardias and blockade of catecholamine-induced dysrhythmias.[183] Antihypertensive mechanism is unknown, but contributing factors are a CNS mechanism, renin blockade and decreases in myocardial contractility and cardiac output.[184] Propranolol also lowers myocardial oxygen demand by decreasing contractility and heart rate, which symptomatically alleviates anginal pain and increases exercise tolerance in coronary artery disease.[185] See Beta-Adrenergic Blocking Agents Comparison Chart.

Administration and Adult Dose. PO 10–20 mg q 6 hr initially, increasing gradually to desired effects. In hypertension, over 1 g/day has been used; however, consider adding another agent if 480 mg/day is ineffective.[186] In angina pectoris, dose is titrated to pain relief and exercise evidence of β-blockade (bradycardia). The endpoint for dosing in acute arrhythmias is return to sinus rhythm or ventricular rate less than 100 beats/min and hemodynamic stability (in atrial fibrillation or flutter). Twice daily dosing has been shown effective in angina pectoris[187] and hypertension.[188] Administer SR Cap in same daily dosage once or twice daily (not indicated for MI). **PO for post-MI prophylaxis** 180–240 mg/day in 2–3 divided doses. **IV slow push** 1 mg q 5 min, to maximum of 0.15 mg/kg; some authors recommend that the first dose be given over 2–10 min.[188,189]

Dosage Individualization. Therapeutic endpoints may be achieved with lower doses in hypothyroidism or liver disease; patients with thyrotoxicosis require higher doses to achieve desired effect.[190]

Pediatric Dose. PO 0.5–1 mg/kg/day in 3–4 divided doses, to maximum of 60 mg/day. **IV slow push** 0.01–0.1 mg/kg/dose up to 1 mg, may repeat in 6–8 hr.[47]

Dosage Forms. Soln 4, 8, 80 mg/ml; Susp 10 mg/ml; Tab 10, 20, 40, 60, 80, 90 mg; SR Cap 60, 80, 120, 160 mg; Inj 1 mg/ml.

Patient Instructions. Report any symptoms such as shortness of breath, swelling, wheezing, fatigue, depression, nightmares or inability to concentrate. Do not stop therapy abruptly.

Pharmacokinetics. *Onset and Duration.* PO onset variable; duration varies from 6 to at least 12 hr.[186,187,190]

Plasma Levels. No definite relationship between plasma concentrations and therapeutic effect in the treatment of arrhythmias, angina pectoris or hypertension. β-blockade is associated with plasma concentrations greater than 100 ng/ml.[191]

Fate. Rapidly and completely absorbed after oral administration; however, a large hepatic first-pass effect occurs, limiting systemic availability to between 20–40%.[190-192] First-pass elimination is saturable with an oral dose greater than about 30 mg.[191] V_d is approximately 4–6 L/kg;[192,193] about 90% bound to albumin and other plasma proteins.[190] Unlike most other drugs, displacement from plasma proteins increases elimination half-life and V_d due to high tissue affinity (nonrestrictive elimination).[194] Only 1–4% of a dose is excreted in the urine as unchanged drug.[190] An active metabolite, 4-hydroxypropranolol is formed after oral, but not IV administration.[190]

$t_{1/2}$. α phase about 10 min;[195] β phase after a single PO dose is approximately 3 hr. With chronic oral therapy, β phase is 4–6 hr; however, it may be as long as 10–20 hr in patients with liver disease.[195]

Adverse Reactions. Adverse effects are usually not dose-related.[196] May cause occasional life-threatening reactions with initial (especially IV) dosing; acute heart failure with pulmonary edema and hypotension, or symptomatic bradycardia and heart block may occur.[196] Acute drug cessation in patients with coronary artery disease may precipitate unstable angina pectoris or MI.[197] May precipitate hypoglycemia, but probably more important in diabetics is its ability to mask hypoglycemic symptoms.[198] May exacerbate symptoms of peripheral vascular disease or Raynaud's disease. β-blockers may exacerbate previously stable asthma or chronic airway obstruction by causing bronchospasm,[196] or renal dysfunction by further depressing GFR.[199] Depression or, less often, psychotic changes may occur, probably more often with the lipophilic β-blockers.[196]

Contraindications. Severe obstructive pulmonary disease, asthma or active allergic rhinitis; cardiogenic shock or severe heart failure; second or third degree heart block; brittle diabetes; history of hypoglycemic episodes; severe sinus node disease; concomitant MAO inhibitor therapy.

Precautions. In coronary artery disease, discontinue drug by tapering the dose over 4–7 days. Use cautiously in patients with Prinzmetal's vasospastic angina to prevent worsening of chest pain.[200] Caution should be used in peripheral vascular disease or heart failure. May worsen atrial fibrillation associated with accessory AV pathway. Concurrent digitalis therapy may lessen the β-blocker exacerbation of heart failure.

Parameters to Monitor. During IV administration, blood pressure and pulse must be taken q 5 min with constant EKG monitoring for signs of AV nodal block (lengthened PR interval) or bradycardia. Vital signs should be evaluated routinely for hemodynamic endpoints (eg, blood pressure in hypertension and heart rate or pressure-rate product in angina pectoris). Question the patient about subjective complaints such as nightmares or fatigue. When a patient at risk for adverse reactions is first given propranolol, signs and symptoms of toxicity must be searched out (eg, heart failure—shortness of breath or edema; bronchospasm—wheezing or shortness of breath; diabetes—blood glucose; peripheral vascular disease—painful or cold extremities).

Notes. Propranolol may be beneficial for treatment of symptomatic hypertrophic obstructive cardiomyopathy by increasing end-diastolic volume, producing ventricular relaxation and relieving ventricular outflow obstruction.[64] If a β-blocker must be used in lung disease, β_1-selective agents cause alterations in pulmonary function that are more easily reversed by bronchodilators; these agents are probably a better choice than propranolol or other nonselective β-blockers.[201]

Quinidine Sulfate   Various
Quinidine Gluconate   Duraquin®, Quinaglute®

Pharmacology. A class I antiarrhythmic which slows conduction velocity, prolongs effective refractory period and decreases automaticity of normal and diseased fibers — see Electrophysiologic Actions of Antiarrhythmics Comparison Chart.[161] Cellular mechanism appears to be frequency-dependent blockade of the fast sodium channel.[202] AV nodal conduction may be increased reflexly through vasodilation, attributed to peripheral α-adrenergic blockade or vagolytic action. Slight negative inotropic action may be clinically significant.

Administration and Adult Dose. **PO loading dose** (sulfate salt) 200 mg q 2 hr for 5-6 doses; **maintenance dose** 200-600 mg q 6-8 hr. **SR products** gluconate salt may be given q 12 hr and polygalacturonate may be given q 8 hr.[203] **IV** (as gluconate) 5-8 mg/kg (3.75-6 mg/kg in CHF) at a rate of 0.3 mg/kg/min. **IM not recommended.** See Notes.

Dosage Individualization. The elderly (over 60 yr) and patients with liver disease or heart failure are likely to have decreased clearance and lower initial doses are recommended.[204] After an initial dosage regimen is selected, maintenance doses should be adjusted based on side effects, therapeutic response and plasma levels.

Pediatric Dose. PO (gluconate salt) 15-60 mg/kg/day in 4 divided doses. **IV and IM not recommended.**[47]

Dosage Forms. **Tab** (sulfate salt) 100, 200, 300 mg; (polygalacturonate salt) 275 mg; **SR Tab** (gluconate salt) 324, 330 mg; (sulfate salt) 300 mg; **Inj** (sulfate salt) 200 mg/ml; (gluconate salt) 80 mg/ml. See Notes.

Patient Instructions. Report any symptoms such as blurred vision, dizziness, tinnitus, diarrhea, abnormal bleeding or bruising, rash or fainting episodes.

Pharmacokinetics. *Onset and Duration.* PO onset of sulfate within 1 hr, and SR gluconate and polygalacturonate salts 2-4 hr. IM onset within 1 hr; IV is immediate. Duration 6-8 hr;[205] SR gluconate 12 hr.

Plasma Levels. Therapeutic range about 2-6 mcg/ml depending on assay. Toxicity is more likely with plasma levels greater than 6 mcg/ml.[206]

Fate. Oral sulfate and gluconate are about 70-80% bioavailable[203,207] with significant first-pass elimination;[204] IM absorption is incomplete.[205] V_d is 2-3 L/kg,[204,205] lower in patients with CHF (1.3-2.3 L/kg);[210] 70-90% bound to plasma proteins.[205,209] Primarily metabolized in the liver to two active metabolites: 3-hydroxyquinidine and 2'-oxoquinidinone.[208] 10-20% of the dose is excreted unchanged in the urine.[209]

$t_{1/2}$. α phase about 7 min; β phase in normals 6-8 hr.[205,209] In heart failure, clearance is decreased and V_d smaller than normal, such that elimination half-life remains about the same.[210] Half-life in alcoholic cirrhosis is prolonged to 8-10 hr.[211]

Adverse Reactions. Cinchonism may occur at high quinidine levels; symptom complex includes tinnitus, blurred vision, headache and nausea; may progress in severe cases to delirium and psychosis. Hypotension may occur, especially after IV administration. Quinidine may aggravate underlying ventricular arrhythmias or heart failure. Non-dose-related syncope, attributed to the occurrence of drug-induced ventricular tachycardia, fibrillation or torsade de pointes may occur in 1-8% of patients.[212-214] Asystole or AV nodal block has been reported. Nausea or vomiting may occur. Diarrhea, which may occur in as many as 30% of patients receiving quinidine, may be treated with aluminum hydroxide gel or by using the polygalacturonate salt.[215,216] Idiosyncratic reactions include hepatitis, drug fever, rare anaphylactoid reactions, SLE, thrombocytopenia and hemolytic anemia. IM use may cause pain and muscle damage.[205]

Contraindications. History of past immunological reaction to quinidine or quinine; previous occurrence of quinidine syncope; second or third degree heart block in the absence of a ventricular pacemaker; severe sinus node dysfunction or long QT syndromes.

Precautions. In atrial fibrillation or flutter, quinidine may increase AV nodal conduction and ventricular rate so that digitalis, propranolol or verapamil should be given first, in an attempt to block AV nodal conduction. Quinidine may exacerbate myasthenia gravis. Quinidine should only be initiated during hospitalization.[213,214] Care should be taken with concurrent digitalis and quinidine therapy as quinidine increases digoxin or digitoxin plasma levels.

Parameters to Monitor. Plasma levels and signs or symptoms of toxicity should be monitored in patients with altered drug disposition such as CHF or liver disease. EKG, observing for QT, QRS or PR prolongation; blood pressure (especially with IV) should be monitored frequently when therapy is initiated. These may be done less frequently when a maintenance dose is determined. Other parameters, such as platelet count, liver enzymes and hematocrit should be routinely monitored only if idiosyncratic reactions are suspected.

Notes. Dosage adjustment should be made when switching from one salt form to another; sulfate salt contains 83% quinidine, gluconate 62% and polygalacturonate 60%. The gluconate and polygalacturonate forms are slowly dissociating salts of quinidine. **Propafenone** (Knoll) is an investigational agent with quinidine-like, β-blocker and calcium blocker actions.[217]

Tocainide Hydrochloride   Tonocard®

Pharmacology. Tocainide has electrophysiological actions similar to lidocaine and mexiletine. Depression of conduction is accentuated in ischemic/hypoxic tissue. Antiarrhythmic actions are somewhat stereodependent.[218] It is used in the treatment of ventricular arrhythmias, but its effectiveness in supraventricular tachycardias is limited. It has a slight negative inotropic action. There seems to be a concordance of response (and nonresponse) between tocainide and lidocaine.[219]

Administration and Adult Dose. PO loading dose 600 mg, then 400 mg 2 hr later.[220] **Maintenance dose** 400 mg q 8 hr initially; usual maintenance dosage is 1.2-2.4 g/day in 2 or 3 divided doses q 8-12 hr. **PO for lidocaine to tocainide conversion** 600 mg q 6 hr for 3 doses, then 600 mg q 12 hr; discontinue lidocaine infusion at the time of the second oral dose of tocainide.[221]

Dosage Individualization. Reduce initial maintenance dose by 50% in severe liver disease, by 25% in patients with Cl_{cr} of 10-30 ml/min and by 50% in patients with Cl_{cr} below 10 ml/min.[220] Loading and maintenance doses may have to be slightly reduced in CHF, but more data are needed.[222]

Pediatric Dose. Safety and efficacy not established.

Dosage Forms. Tab 400, 600 mg.

Patient Instructions. Report any symptoms of numbness, drowsiness, dizziness or tingling. Nausea or loss of appetite may occur and may be reduced by taking the drug with food. Report sore throat, mouth sores, fever or abnormal bruising.

Pharmacokinetics. *Onset and Duration.* PO onset 1-2 hr (delayed by food); duration 12-24 hr.
   Plasma Levels. 3-10 mcg/ml, although not well correlated with therapeutic or toxic effects.[218]
   Fate. Oral bioavailability is 90-100% with negligible first-pass metabolism.[218,220,223] About 5-10% plasma protein bound;[223] V_d 2-3 L/kg, slightly lower in CHF.[220,222] About 40-50% of the drug is excreted unchanged in urine and 50-60% is hepatically eliminated.[218,220,221] Renal clearance is dependent on urine pH; hepatic metabolism is probably stereoselective.[218]
   $t_{1/2}$. α phase 5-10 min;[223] β phase 9-15 hr. β phase 14-19 hr with ventricular arrhythmias or CHF;[218,221] and 14-34 hr in renal insufficiency.[224]

Adverse Reactions. Neurologic toxicities which include tremor, ataxia, drowsiness, confusion and paresthesias are frequent (30-50%). Psychosis and seizures have been reported. The neurologic toxicities of lidocaine and tocainide may be additive.[225] Nausea, vomiting and anorexia also occur frequently. Tocainide may exacerbate underlying ventricular arrhythmias or conduction disturbances. Agranulocytosis has been reported in about 0.18% of patients.[218] Pulmonary fibrosis or interstitial pneumonitis occurs in 0.03% of patients.[221] Rash and fever may occur, with cross-sensitivity between lidocaine and tocainide possible.[145]

Contraindications. Second or third degree AV block in the absence of a ventricular pacemaker.

Precautions. Tocainide may accelerate ventricular response in patients with atrial fibrillation or flutter. Worsening of sick sinus syndrome may occur.

Parameters to Monitor. Monitor EKG frequently when therapy is initiated, then periodically on an ambulatory basis. Obtain periodic plasma levels once an individual's effective level is determined. Observe closely for neurologic toxicities when initiating therapy. WBC counts should be performed frequently, particularly during the first several weeks of therapy.[218]

Notes. Because of reports of bone marrow toxicity and hypersensitivity reactions, the indications for tocainide have been restricted in the United Kingdom to patients with life-threatening ventricular arrhythmias refractory to other therapies.[218]

Verapamil Hydrochloride   Calan®, Isoptin®, Various

Pharmacology. A slow channel (calcium-dependent) blocking agent that prolongs AV nodal conduction.[226] It is used to convert re-entrant supraventricular tachycardias and to slow ventricular rate in atrial fibrillation or flutter.[227] Because it decreases contractility and arteriolar resistance, it is used in angina caused by coronary obstruction or vasospasm. Verapamil is also effective in the treatment of hypertension, hypertrophic obstructive cardiomyopathy and migraine prophylaxis.

Administration and Adult Dose. IV for supraventricular arrhythmias 5–10 mg (0.075–0.15 mg/kg) over at least 2 min (3 min in elderly), may repeat with 10 mg (0.15 mg/kg) in 30 min if arrhythmia is not terminated or desired endpoint is not achieved. **IV constant infusion** 5–10 mg/hr.[228] **PO for angina** 80 mg tid-qid initially, increasing at daily (for unstable angina) or weekly intervals to usual maintenance dose of 320–480 mg/day. **PO for hypertension** usually 240 mg/day using SR tablet; SR doses of 120 mg/day to 240 mg bid have been used.

Dosage Individualization. Dose may need to be decreased in patients with liver disease.[229,230]

Pediatric Dose. IV (under 1 yr) 0.1–0.2 mg/kg (usually 0.75–2 mg) over 2 min initially, may repeat with same dose in 30 min if initial response inadequate; (1–15 yr) 0.1–0.3 mg/kg, to maximum of 5 mg (usually 2–5 mg) over 2 min initially, may repeat with same dose to maximum of 10 mg in 30 min if initial response inadequate.[47]

Dosage Forms. Tab 40, 80, 120 mg; SR Tab 240 mg; Inj 2.5 mg/ml.

Patient Instructions. Take SR tablets with food.

Pharmacokinetics. *Onset and Duration.* IV onset immediate; hemodynamic duration 20 min.[231] PO electrophysiologic effect lasts for up to 6 hr,[232] while maximum effects in angina are apparent during the first 24–48 hr of therapy.

Plasma Levels. 50–400 ng/ml, although therapeutic range is not well established.

Fate. Although well absorbed orally, only 10–30% is bioavailable due to extensive first-pass elimination; bioavailability increases in liver disease.[229,230] Peak plasma levels occur 1–2 hr after administration of the immediate-release tablets and 5.2 hr (fasting) or 7.7 hr (with food) after the sustained-release tablet. V_d is 2.5–4.7 L/kg and increases in liver disease.[233] About 90–95% plasma protein bound.[230,231] Verapamil has stereospecific pharmacology and pharmacokinetics.[234] L-Verapamil is a more potent AV nodal blocking agent, but undergoes greater first-pass metabolism.[234] Norverapamil is an active metabolite.[5]

$t_{1/2}$. (Verapamil) α phase 5–30 min; β phase 2.5–8 hr;[230,233] may increase during chronic use. (Norverapamil) 4–10 hr.[235]

Adverse Reactions. Constipation is a frequent side effect. CHF may occur in patients with left ventricular dysfunction. Major hemodynamic side effects (eg, severe hypotension) and conduction abnormalities (eg, symptomatic bradycardia or asystole) have been reported; these reactions usually occur when the patient is concurrently receiving a β-blocker.[5] IV calcium (10–20 ml of a 10% solution) and/or isoproterenol may, in part, reverse these adverse effects.[5] The use of IV calcium prior to verapamil may prevent hypotension without abolishing the antiarrhythmic actions.[236]

Contraindications. Concomitant IV β-blocker administration; shock or severely hypotensive states; second or third degree AV nodal block; sick sinus syndrome, unless functioning ventricular pacemaker is in place; hypotension or heart failure unless due to supraventricular tachyarrhythmias amenable to verapamil therapy; atrial fibrillation and an accessory AV pathway.

Precautions. May increase serum digoxin concentrations. Use with caution in combination with oral β-blockers and poor left ventricular function.

Parameters to Monitor. Blood pressure readings and constant EKG monitoring should be observed during IV administration. Particular attention should be paid to signs and symptoms of heart failure and hypotension. The EKG should also be monitored for PR prolongation and bradycardia.

Notes. Verapamil has been successfully used for prophylaxis of vascular headaches.[160]

Beta-Adrenergic Blocking Agents Comparison Chart[a]

DRUG	DOSAGE FORMS	CARDIO-SELECTIVITY	BETA HALF-LIFE (HOURS)	EXCRETED UNCHANGED IN URINE	PROTEIN BINDING	APPROVED USES	STARTING DOSE	MAXIMUM DOSE
Acebutolol[b] Sectral®	Cap 200 mg.	+	3-4 (diacetolol) 8-13	30-40%	25%	Hypertension Arrhythmias.	400 mg/day.	1.2 g/day.
Atenolol Tenormin®	Tab 50, 100 mg.	+ (up to 100 mg)	6-7	85%	10%	Hypertension.	50 mg/day.	200 mg/day.
Betaxolol[c] Kerlone® (Investiga-tional - Searle)	—	+	16.6	15%	—	Hypertension (Investigational).	20 mg/day.	—
Esmolol Brevibloc®	Inj 250 mg/ml.	+	9 min	0%	55%	Supraventricular tachychardia.	25-50 mcg/kg/min.	300 mcg/kg/min.
Labetalol[d] Trandate® Normodyne®	Tab 100, 200, 300 mg.	0	6-8	5%	50%	Hypertension.	200 mg/day.	2.4 g/day.
Metoprolol Lopressor®	Tab 50, 100 mg Inj 1 mg/ml.	+ (up to 100 mg)	3-7	39%	10%	Hypertension Acute MI.	100 mg/day.	450 mg/day.
Nadolol Corgard®	Tab 20, 40, 80, 120 mg.	0	17-24	70%	25%	Hypertension Angina pectoris.	40 mg/day.	320 mg/day.

Continued

Beta-Adrenergic Blocking Agents Comparison Chart[a]

DRUG	DOSAGE FORMS	CARDIO-SELECTIVITY	BETA HALF-LIFE (HOURS)	EXCRETED UNCHANGED IN URINE	PROTEIN BINDING	APPROVED USES	STARTING DOSE	MAXIMUM DOSE
Pindolol[b] Visken®	Tab 5, 10 mg.	0	3–4	40%	57%	Hypertension.	20 mg/day.	60 mg/day.
Propranolol Inderal® Various	See Monograph.	0	3–6	1%	90%	Hypertension Angina pectoris Arrhythmias. Post MI-prophylaxis.	40–80 mg/day. 180 mg/day.	480 mg/day. 240 mg/day.
Sotalol[e] Betapace® (Investigational - Bristol)	—	0	7–15	>75%	0%	—	80 mg/day.	640 mg/day.
Timolol[c] Blocadren®	Tab 10, 20 mg.	0	4–5	20%	<10%	Hypertension. Post-MI prophylaxis.	20 mg/day. 20 mg/day.	60 mg/day. 20 mg/day.
Carteolol[b] Cartrol® (Investigational - Abbott)	—	—	6–11	60%	15%	—	15 mg/day.	60 mg/day.

a. From references 102, 237–246 and 473.
b. Pindolol, acebutolol and carteolol have intrinsic agonist activity.
c. Betaxolol is also available as Betoptic® ophthalmic drops 0.5% and timolol is also available as Timoptic® ophthalmic drops 0.25 and 0.5% for treatment of glaucoma.
d. Labetalol has potent alpha blocking actions.
e. Sotalol also has antiarrhythmic properties.

Calcium Channel Blocking Agents Comparison Chart[a]

DRUG	CONTRAC-TILITY	HEART RATE	AV NODAL CONDUCTION	VASCULAR RESISTANCE	QT DURATION
Bepridil[b,f] Vasocor® (Investigational - McNeil)	↓	↓	↓	↓	↑
Cinnarizine[c,f] (Investigational - Janssen)	0	0	0	↓	0
Diltiazem[d] Cardizem®	↓	↓	↓	↓	0
Felodipine[e,f] (Investigational - MSD)	0/↑	0/↑	0/↑	↓↓	0
Flunarizine[c,f] (Investigational - Janssen)	0	0	0	↓	0
Gallopamil[d,f] (Investigational)	↓↓	↓	↓↓	↓	0
Lidoflazine[b,f] Clinium® (Investigational - McNeil)	0	0	0	↓	↑
Nicardipine[e,f] Cardene®	0/↑	0/↑	0/↑	↓↓	0
Nifedipine[e] Adalat® Procardia®	0/↑	0/↑	0/↑	↓↓	0
Niludipine[e,f] (Investigational)	0/↑	0/↑	0/↑	↓↓	0
Nimodipine[e,f] Nimotop® (Investigational - Miles)	0/↑	0/↑	0/↑	↓↓	0
Nisoldipine[e,f] (Investigational - Miles)	0/↑	0/↑	0/↑	↓↓	0
Nitrendipine[e,f] Baypress® (Investigational - Miles)	0/↑	0/↑	0/↑	↓↓	0
Perhexiline[b,f] Pexid® (Investigational - Merrell Dow)	0	↓	0	↓	↑

Continued

Calcium Channel Blocking Agents Comparison Chart[a]

DRUG	CONTRAC-TILITY	HEART RATE	AV NODAL CONDUCTION	VASCULAR RESISTANCE	QT DURATION
Prenylamine[b,f] (Investigational)	0	0	0	↓↓	↑
Tiapamil[d,f] (Investigational - Roche)	↓↓	↓	↓↓	↓	0
Verapamil[d] Calan® Isoptin®	↓↓	↓	↓↓	↓	0

a. From reference 247.
b. Complex pharmacology with probable sodium channel blockade (quinidine-like).
c. Selective vascular actions.
d. Vascular and electrophysiologic actions.
e. Predominantly vascular actions.
f. Investigational.

Electrophysiologic Actions of Antiarrhythmics Comparison Chart

CLASS[a,b]	DRUG	CONDUCTION VELOCITY	REFRACTORY PERIOD	AUTOMATICITY	AV NODAL CONDUCTION	REFERENCES
Ia (Fast Channel Blockers)	**Disopyramide**	↓↓	↑↑	↓↓	↑	82
	Procainamide	↓↓	↑↑	↓↓	↑/↓	161,164
	Quinidine	↓↓	↑↑	↓↓	↑/↓	161,164
Ib	**Lidocaine** Normal Tissue	0	↓	↓	0	112,248
	Ischemic Tissue	↓↓	↑	↓↓	0	
	Mexiletine	0	↓	↓	0	132,133,138
	Phenytoin Normal Tissue	0	↓	↓	↑	249,250
	Ischemic Tissue	↓↓	↑	↓↓	↑	
	Tocainide	0	↓	↓	0	218,221
Ic	**Encainide**	↓↓	0	↓	0	131
	Flecainide	↓↓	0	↓	0	104,105

Continued

Electrophysiologic Actions of Antiarrhythmics Comparison Chart

CLASS[a,b]	DRUG	CONDUCTION VELOCITY	REFRACTORY PERIOD	AUTOMATICITY	AV NODAL CONDUCTION	REFERENCES
II (Beta Blockers)	Propranolol[c]	↓	↓ (acute) ↑ (chronic)	↓	↓↓	132,183
III	Amiodarone	0/↓	↑↑	0	↓	7,8
	Bretylium	0	↑↑	↑/0	↑/0	31
	Sotalol[d]	0	↑	0	↓	473
IV (Slow Channel Blockers)	Diltiazem	0	0	0	↓	82,85
	Verapamil	0	0	0	↓↓	226

Key: ↑ = increase, ↓ = decrease, 0 = minimal or no effect, ↑/↓ = variable.

a. Classification system from references 5 and 132.
b. Type I agents are subdivided into Ia, Ib and Ic based upon their actions on repolarization in normal ventricular tissue and their binding characteristics to the sodium channel: type Ia prolongs repolarization; type Ib shortens repolarization; type Ic, no change in repolarization.
c. When due to sympathetic stimulation.
d. Sotalol also has class II or β-adrenergic blocking activity.

24:06 ANTILIPEMIC AGENTS

General References: 251-254

Cholestyramine Resin

Cholybar®, Questran®

Pharmacology. An anion exchange resin which binds with bile acids in the intestine to form an insoluble complex that is excreted in the feces. The loss of bile acids leads to an increased catabolism of cholesterol to form new bile acids, resulting in decreased plasma low-density lipoprotein (LDL) and cholesterol levels.

Administration and Adult Dose. **PO for hypercholesterolemia** 12-16 g/day initially, adjust incrementally to maximum of 16-32 g/day, in 2-4 divided doses, preferably just before meals.[251,255] **PO for pruritus of cholestasis** 4 g tid-qid. Dosages are expressed in terms of anhydrous resin (444 mg of anhydrous resin are contained in 1 g of powder).

Dosage Individualization. Decrease dose or discontinue in patients with constipation, because impaction may occur. See Adverse Reactions.

Pediatric Dose. PO (over 6 yr) 80 mg/kg tid.[256]

Dosage Forms. **Pwdr** 4 g resin/9 g packet; 378 g can; **Chew Bar** 4 g.

Patient Instructions. Do not take this drug in dry form; mix with moisturized pulpy fruit (applesauce, crushed pineapple), highly fluid soups or at least 120 ml of liquid—allow to stand for 1-2 min before stirring. Take thyroid preparations 4-6 hr before or after cholestyramine; take other oral medications at least 1 hr before or 4-6 hr after cholestyramine.

Pharmacokinetics. *Onset and Duration.* Onset 1-4 weeks for the maximal lipid lowering effect; plasma lipids return to pretreatment levels 2-4 weeks after drug discontinuation.[256]

Fate. Not absorbed from GI tract.

Adverse Reactions. Constipation (often controlled with increased dietary fiber or stool softeners) occurs in 10-20% of patients, especially the elderly; occasionally nausea, vomiting, flatulence, diarrhea, steatorrhea (at high doses), abdominal distention and cramps occur. Large doses (above 24 g/day) may result in malabsorption of fat-soluble vitamins; osteomalacia and hemorrhagic diatheses have been reported with cholestyramine impairment of vitamin D and K absorption, respectively. Folic acid deficiency, hyperchloremic acidosis and GI obstruction have been reported in children and/or small patients.[253,254]

Precautions. Pregnancy. Constipation. Discontinue if significant elevation in plasma triglycerides occurs. Binds several drugs (particularly acidic drugs) and may interfere with GI absorption of fat-soluble vitamins; initiation or discontinuation can be hazardous if potentially toxic resin-bound drugs (eg, digitoxin) have been titrated to a maintenance level.

Parameters to Monitor. Plasma cholesterol and triglycerides q 2 weeks initially, then approximately q 3 months; children should have periodic hemoglobin and plasma folic acid determinations.

Notes. Cholestyramine is indicated for type II hyperlipoproteinemias; it reduces LDL cholesterol 15-30%; VLDL may increase or remain unchanged. Recent studies demonstrate that long-term use significantly lowers total and LDL cholesterol and may reduce the risk of coronary heart disease;[257-259] however, it is unclear whether the reduction in CHD can be extrapolated beyond the study group.[253] Concurrent use with niacin or clofibrate may be indicated in certain patients (eg, patients with sustained triglyceride elevations).[253,260,261] In a recent test,[262] cholestyramine-vehicle combinations were preferred over colestipol-vehicle combinations in terms of taste, texture and smell. Long-term use of cholestyramine appears to effectively reduce plasma cholesterol in children with familial hypercholesterolemia.[263] Contrary to prior reports, a recent study found concurrent use with neomycin no more effective than cholestyramine alone.[264] Resins may be useful in treating diarrhea associated with ileal resection,[265] for treating refractory diarrhea associated with pseudomembranous colitis,[266] and as adjunctive treatment for digitoxin intoxication[267] (although most clinicians believe that it is not useful when cardiac glycoside toxicity is life-threatening).[256]

Clofibrate   Atromid-S®, Various

Clofibrate presumably interrupts cholesterol biosynthesis prior to mevalonate formation, increases triglyceride and VLDL clearance and increases biliary excretion of neutral sterols. This results in significant reduction of VLDL and triglycerides, with variable effects on LDL. Clofibrate is indicated for type IIb (combined with other drugs), III, IV or V hyperlipoproteinemias. The drug is completely absorbed orally and rapidly hydrolyzed to the active metabolite chlorophenoxyisobutyric acid (CPIB), which attains peak plasma concentrations in 3–6 hr. CPIB is over 90% plasma protein bound and is eliminated in the urine, 40–70% as glucuronide.[268] CPIB half-life is 10–25 hr, which increases 2- to 6-fold in renal impairment.[268,269] Triglycerides decrease within 2–5 days of drug use, with maximal response occurring within 3 weeks; lipids return to pretreatment levels 2–3 weeks after drug discontinuation.[256] Occasionally nausea, vomiting, diarrhea and GI distress occur with clofibrate use and, less frequently or rarely, skin reactions, headache, drowsiness, dizziness, weakness, weight gain, alopecia, peptic ulcer reactivation, leukopenia, anemia, renal dysfunction, elevated AST (SGOT)/ALT (SGPT) levels, impotence and decreased libido in men are reported. Creatine phosphokinase levels may increase, and acute myositis with flu-like symptoms may occur, especially with co-existing renal disease. The Coronary Drug Project[270] also reported a high frequency of thromboembolism, angina, intermittent claudication and cardiac arrhythmia. Because of a reported twofold increase in the prevalence of cholelithiasis and cholecystitis, and increased rate of overall mortality and a higher mortality from noncardiovascular causes,[270,271] clofibrate is no longer considered a drug of choice; however, it has a role as an alternative agent alone or in combination with other drugs.[252,253] Its use should probably be limited to patients with severe hypertriglyceridemia that poses a danger of acute pancreatitis and is unresponsive to gemfibrozil, or to patients with familial dyslipoproteinemia, who have a high risk of atherosclerotic complications.[300] Clofibrate is contraindicated during pregnancy and lactation, and in the presence of clinically significant hepatic or renal dysfunction or primary biliary cirrhosis; safety and efficacy has not been established for use in children. The manufacturer recommends drug discontinuation in the following instances: several months prior to planned pregnancy; if lipid response is inadequate after 3 months; or if hepatic function test results increase steadily or excessively. Caution should be used with concurrent oral anticoagulant therapy. Plasma lipids should be monitored every 2 weeks initially, then every 1–3 months. Periodic CBC, liver function test and CPK determinations should be made. Although there is no evidence that clofibrate has a long-term effect in decreasing fatal myocardial infarction (MI), there is a reported 25% decrease in nonfatal MI.[271] Clofibrate dosage is usually 1.5–2 g/day in 2–4 divided doses, which may be taken with food or milk to minimize stomach upset. The drug is available as 500 mg capsules. Gemfibrozil, a fibric acid derivative like clofibrate, is probably the preferred agent due to a lower prevalence of adverse effects and somewhat greater effectiveness in lowering VLDL and plasma triglycerides and in increasing high-density lipoprotein (HDL).[253,272]

Colestipol Hydrochloride

Colestid®

Pharmacology. An anion exchange resin with a mechanism of action similar to cholestyramine.

Administration and Adult Dose. PO for hypercholesterolemia 15-30 g/day, in 2-4 divided doses, preferably just before meals.

Dosage Individualization. Decrease dose or discontinue in patients with constipation, because impaction may occur. See Adverse Reactions.

Pediatric Dose. PO 10-20 g/day, or 500 mg/kg/day, in 2-4 divided doses (other dosages are also used).[256]

Dosage Forms. Granules 5 g packet, 500 g bottle.

Patient Instructions. Do not take this drug in dry form; mix with moisturized pulpy fruit (applesauce, crushed pineapple), highly fluid soups or at least 120 ml of liquid—stir until completely mixed (will not dissolve). Take thyroid preparations 4-6 hr before or after colestipol; take other oral medications at least 1 hr before or 4-6 hr after colestipol.

Pharmacokinetics. See Cholestyramine.

Adverse Reactions. See Cholestyramine.

Contraindications. See Cholestyramine.

Precautions. See Cholestyramine.

Parameters to Monitor. See Cholestyramine.

Notes. Colestipol is indicated for type II hyperlipoproteinemias; it reduces LDL cholesterol 15-30%; VLDL may increase or remain unchanged. Effectiveness may be enhanced in certain patients by concurrent use with niacin or clofibrate.[273-275] In a recent test,[262] cholestyramine-vehicle combinations were preferred over colestipol-vehicle combinations in terms of taste, texture and smell. See also Cholestyramine.

Gemfibrozil

Lopid®

Pharmacology. Gemfibrozil is a fibric acid derivative structurally and pharmacologically related to clofibrate. In addition, it inhibits the secretion of VLDL which may enhance its effectiveness.[272]

Administration and Adult Dose. PO 900-1500 mg/day (usually 1200 mg) in 2 divided doses given 30 min before the morning and evening meal.

Pediatric Dose. Safety and efficacy not established in children under 18 yr.

Dosage Forms. Cap 300 mg; Tab 600 mg.

Pharmacokinetics. *Onset and Duration.* Plasma triglyceride and total cholesterol usually decrease maximally within 4-12 weeks; lipids return to pretreatment levels 6-8 weeks after drug discontinuation.[256]

Fate. Rapidly and completely absorbed orally and metabolized in the liver to 4 major metabolites which further undergo conjugation; about 95% of drug is plasma protein bound. Peak plasma concentrations are attained within 1-2 hr. Approximately 70% is excreted in urine as conjugated and unchanged drug (principally) and metabolites.[256,284]

$t_{1/2}$. 1.5 hr after a single dose; 1.3 hr after multiple doses.[256,284]

Adverse Reactions. Although side effects are similar to those seen with clofibrate, it appears that the prevalence is lower.[253] Occasional skin reactions and GI effects (including abdominal and epigastric pain, diarrhea, nausea, vomiting, flatulence) occur. Also, headache, blurred vision, dizziness, fatigue, muscle pains, leukopenia, anemia, eosinophilia and liver function test elevations have been reported. Gemfibrozil's potential to cause gallstones approaches that of clofibrate.

Contraindications. Hepatic (including primary biliary cirrhosis) or severe renal dysfunction, and pre-existing gallbladder disease.

Precautions. Lactation, pregnancy and prior to planned pregnancy. Discontinue use after 3 months if lipid response is inadequate; discontinue if liver function test results increase steadily or excessively. The dose of concurrent oral anticoagulants should be reduced; the doses of insulin and oral hypoglycemics may have to be increased during gemfibrozil therapy.[256,284] Because of the increased prevalence of serious morbidity and mortality associated with the use of clofibrate,[270,271] the possibility that such findings may also apply to use of gemfibrozil should be considered.[256]

Parameters to Monitor. Determine plasma lipids every few weeks initially, then approximately every 3 months. Periodic CBC and liver function tests are recommended.

Notes. Gemfibrozil is indicated for type IIb and in high risk patients with type III, IV or V hyperlipoproteinemia. VLDL and triglyceride concentrations are lowered 40–57%,[272,282-284] with a variable effect on LDL—generally, LDL cholesterol is decreased during treatment of type II disorders and increased in type IV or V disorders.[256] Gemfibrozil significantly inceases HDL cholesterol, an action possibly beneficial to slowing the atherosclerotic process. Compared with clofibrate, gemfibrozil is somewhat more effective in lowering VLDL and plasma triglycerides and in increasing HDL.[272] A recent five-year study in middle-aged men with primary dyslipidemia showed gemfibrozil therapy to decrease the incidence of coronary heart disease.[283]

Lovastatin   Mevacor®

Pharmacology. Lovastatin (formerly mevinolin) acts primarily via competitive inhibition of HMG-CoA reductase, which catalyzes the rate-limiting step in cholesterol synthesis.

Administration and Adult Dose. PO 20 mg/day with the evening meal initially, increasing at intervals of 4 or more weeks to a maximum of 80 mg/day in single or divided doses. Those with an initial serum cholesterol over 300 mg/dl on diet may be started at 40 mg/day.

Dosage Individualization. No dosage alteration necessary in renal impairment.

Pediatric Dose. Safety and efficacy not established. One 6 year-old was treated with one-half the adult dose.[278]

Dosage Forms. Tab 20 mg.

Patient Instructions. Avoid excessive concurrent use of alcohol. Promptly report any unexplained muscle pain or tenderness, especially if accompanied by malaise or fever.

Pharmacokinetics. *Onset and Duration.* Onset 3 days, maximum effect in 2–4 weeks. LDL cholesterol returns to pretreatment levels 3–4 weeks after discontinuation.[288,289]

   Fate. Not well studied, but apparently only about 5% bioavailability due to first-pass metabolism. Hydrolyzed to a very active β-hydroxyacid and other less active metabolites. Peak active metabolite levels occur 2–4 hr after a dose. Lovastatin and the β-hydroxyacid are over 95% plasma protein bound. 10% of a radiolabelled oral dose appears in urine and 83% in feces.[279]

Adverse Reactions. Lovastatin is generally well tolerated, but long-term safety is not established. Occasional GI effects include constipation, diarrhea, dyspepsia, flatulence, abdominal cramps and nausea. Occasionally, marked persistent elevations in AST(SGOT) and ALT(SGPT) occur during long-term therapy, usually 3-12 months after initiation of therapy. Frequent mild elevations in noncardiac CPK levels, myalgia and, occasionally, myositis have been reported. Headache, skin rash or dizziness reported occasionally. Lens opacities have been reported, but causality is not established.

Contraindications. Pregnancy; lactation; active liver disease or unexplained persistent elevations in serum aminotransferases (transaminases).

Precautions. Use with caution in patients who consume substantial quantities of alcohol and/or have a history of liver disease. Discontinue if markedly elevated CPK levels or myositis occur, or if hepatic enzyme elevations persist above 3 times normal. Consider withholding the drug in those with any risk factor for renal failure secondary to rhabdomyolysis.

Parameters to Monitor. Liver function tests q 4-6 weeks for the first 15 months and periodically thereafter. Baseline and annual slit lamp ophthalmologic examination.

Notes. Plasma total cholesterol levels fall by 23-32% and LDL cholesterol by 24-45%. HDL cholesterol may increase by up to 16% while VLDL and serum triglycerides may fall slightly.[276,277,285,286,289] Lovastatin is additive with the bile acid sequestering resins (ie, cholestyramine, colestipol).[287,290] It may be effective in type III hyperlipidemia.[280] **Simvastatin** (formerly synvinolin; Zocor® - MSD) and **pravastatin** (Squibb) are investigational drugs with similar activity.[253,281]

Niacin   Various

Pharmacology. In pharmacologic doses, niacin may reduce the release of free fatty acids to the liver and inhibit hepatic secretion of lipoproteins, leading to decreased triglyceride and VLDL synthesis and subsequent reduced formation of LDL.

Administration and Adult Dose. PO for hyperlipoproteinemia 100 mg tid initially, increasing in 300 mg/day increments q 4-7 days to maintenance dose of 1-2 g tid, to maximum of 3 g tid.[256,292] Administration of 300 mg aspirin 30 min before dose may decrease flushing.[260]

Pediatric Dose. Safety and efficacy not established.

Patient Instructions. This drug may be taken with food or milk to minimize stomach upset. Transient flushing, itching or headache may occur.

Dosage Forms. Tab 20, 25, 50, 100, 500 mg; **Inj** 100 mg/ml; **Elxr** 10 mg/ml. SR products not recommended.

Pharmacokinetics. *Onset and Duration.* (Decrease in plasma triglycerides and cholesterol) onset within 2 weeks; lipids return to pretreatment levels 2-6 weeks after drug discontinuation.[256]

Plasma Levels. Measurable pharmacologic effects occur at 0.1-0.2 mcg/ml; a therapeutic range of 0.5-1 mcg/ml has been suggested.[268]

Fate. Rapidly absorbed from GI tract, with peak plasma concentrations attained in 20–70 min (average 45). One-third of drug is excreted unchanged in urine.[268]

$t_{1/2}$. About 45 min.[268]

Adverse Reactions.   Frequent dose-related cutaneous flushing and pruritus occurs initially, with tolerance developing in 1–2 weeks. Occasionally, transient headache, dry eyes, nausea, vomiting and diarrhea occur. Glucose intolerance, hyperuricemia, gouty attacks and elevated liver function tests occur occasionally. An increased frequency of atrial fibrillation and other arrhythmias has been reported.[270] Hepatotoxicity, usually cholestasis, occasionally with jaundice may occur and is more likely with SR forms.[254]

Contraindications.   Active peptic ulcer; hepatic dysfunction.

Precautions.   Pregnancy; lactation. Use with caution, if at all, in patients with gallbladder disease, or prior history of liver disease, diabetes, hyperuricemia or peptic ulcer. Due to the higher incidence of arrhythmias reported,[270] use with caution in patients with coronary heart disease. One source states that, generally, niacin should not be used in patients with angina. May potentiate hypotensive effect of ganglionic blocking antihypertensive agents.

Parameters to Monitor.   Plasma lipids every 2 weeks initially, then every 1–3 months. Signs of the development of arrhythmias; perform liver function test, blood glucose and serum uric acid determinations periodically.

Notes.   Decreases VLDL and LDL (triglycerides 26%, cholesterol 10%)[270] and increases HDL. Indicated for hypertriglyceridemia, mixed hyperlipidemia, and hypercholesterolemia (combined with other drugs).[274,275,293] Coronary heart disease patients taking niacin had a decrease in nonfatal myocardial infarctions,[270] and, for several years after that study, a lower mortality rate.[294] **Niacinamide** (nicotinamide) is a closely related vitamin, but it has no hypolipoproteinemic effect.

Probucol

Lorelco®

Probucol is thought to inhibit early stages of cholesterol synthesis and increase fecal bile acids. It is moderately effective in the treatment of type II hyperlipoproteinemia, reducing plasma cholesterol 10–15% and over 23% after 2 years of treatment; it also decreases LDL cholesterol 6–11%, HDL cholesterol 9–26% and apoprotein A-1; VLDL is unaffected. The significance of these latter effects, particularly the reduction in HDL, is unknown. Reduction in plasma cholesterol occurs within 2–4 weeks and maximum effects occur in 1–3 months. Adverse effects are minimal, with diarrhea, nausea, anorexia and other GI disturbances predominating; transient eosinophilia, abnormal elevations in laboratory test [serum aminotransferases (transaminases), alkaline phosphatase, creatine phosphokinase, bilirubin, uric acid, blood urea nitrogen and blood glucose] values and prolongation of the QT interval have been reported. Although less than 10% is absorbed, the drug accumulates in adipose tissue and may persist in the blood for over six months after being discontinued; for this reason, the manufacturer cautions against becoming pregnant for at least six months after discontinuation. Safety of use for children, during pregnancy or lactation is not established and use of the drug is not recommended. The manufacturer also recommends against the use of probucol with clofibrate (and presumably gemfibrozil), because of little therapeutic additive effect and the possibility of pronounced lowering of HDL-cholesterol.[256,295-299] Dosage is 500 mg bid, taken with morning and evening meals. It is available as 250 mg tablets.

Hyperlipoproteinemias: Classification and Treatment[a,b]

TYPE:	I	IIa	IIb	III	IV	V
PREVALENCE:	RARE	COMMON	COMMON	UNCOMMON	COMMON	UNCOMMON
Plasma Lipoprotein Pattern[c]	↑Chylomicrons	↑LDL (β)	↑LDL (β) ↑VLDL (pre-β)	↑Abnormal ILDL ↑VLDL (β) Remnants	↑VLDL (pre-β)	↑Chylomicrons ↑VLDL (pre-β)
Plasma Lipids	→Sl↑Cholesterol ↑Triglycerides	↑Cholesterol	↑Cholesterol Sl↑Triglycerides	↑Cholesterol ↑Triglycerides	→Sl↑Cholesterol ↑Triglycerides	Sl↑Cholesterol ↑Triglycerides
Drug(s) of Choice	None	Cholestyramine or Colestipol	Niacin	Niacin	Niacin	Gemfibrozil or Niacin
Alternate Drug(s)	None	Lovastatin; Lovastatin, Niacin or Probucol combined with a resin	Gemfibrozil; Niacin, Gemfibrozil or Clofibrate combined with a resin	Gemfibrozil or Clofibrate	Gemfibrozil or Clofibrate	Clofibrate

Key: LDL = low-density lipoproteins; VLDL = very low-density lipoproteins; ILDL = intermediate low-density lipoproteins; →Sl↑ = normal or slightly elevated.
a. Dietary treatment is the basic treatment for all types of hyperlipoproteinemias. In secondary hyperlipoproteinemias, the primary cause should be treated specifically. Drugs are a supplement to dietary control. See *Circulation* 1984;69:1065A-90A 'or dietary recommendations.
b. Information in table derived from references 251-253, 293 and 300.
c. Classified by density. Letters in parentheses refer to corresponding lipoprotein pattern in electrophoretic mobility classification system.

24:08 HYPOTENSIVE AGENTS

(SEE ALSO BETA-ADRENERGIC BLOCKING AGENTS 24:04, CALCIUM CHANNEL BLOCKING AGENTS 24:04, and DIURETICS 40:28)

General Reference: 301

Class Instructions. This medication can control hypertension, but it will not cure the disease. Long-term compliance is necessary to control hypertension and prevent damage to several body systems. Do not start or stop taking medications or adjust the dose without medical supervision, and avoid running out of your medications. Some prescription and non-prescription medications may interact with your medications for hypertension; make sure that your physician and pharmacist know the names of any other medications you are taking regularly.

This drug may cause drowsiness. Until the extent of this effect is known, caution should be used when driving, operating machinery or performing other tasks requiring mental alertness. Avoid excessive concurrent use of alcohol and other drugs which cause drowsiness. This drug may also cause faintness or dizziness, especially on rising suddenly, standing for prolonged periods or after exertion or alcohol intake. If this occurs, sit or lie down immediately.

Captopril

Capoten®

Pharmacology. Captopril is a competitive inhibitor of angiotensin-converting enzyme (ACE) which is responsible for converting angiotensin I to angiotensin II. Angiotensin II is a potent endogenous vasopressor which has additional effects on blood pressure homeostatic mechanisms by stimulating release of aldosterone and enhancing activity of the sympathetic nervous system. The clinical significance of associated reductions in bradykinin inactivation and subsequent increases in vasodilator prostaglandin synthesis remains unclear.[302] ACE inhibitors produce both acute and sustained reductions in blood pressure by decreasing total peripheral resistance.

Administration and Adult Dose. PO for mild to moderate hypertension 12.5 mg tid;[304,305] bid dosing may be as effective as tid.[306] PO for severe hypertension 25 mg bid-tid initially, increasing to 50 mg bid-tid after 1–2 weeks if blood pressure control is inadequate. Concomitant dietary sodium restriction may enhance the hypotensive effect. If response after an additional 1–2 weeks is not satisfactory, a low dose of a thiazide diuretic should be added (eg, hydrochlorothiazide 12.5 mg/day). Addition of a thiazide diuretic may be quite effective in nonresponding black patients.[303] With continued unsatisfactory response, the diuretic dose may be increased at 1–2 week intervals until the maximal antihypertensive dose is achieved. If control remains inadequate, the captopril dose may be increased to 100 mg bid-tid and, if necessary, to 150 mg bid-tid to a maximum of 450 mg/day. PO for congestive heart failure 25 mg tid initially, increased to 50 mg tid if response is inadequate; usual dosage range is 50–100 mg tid to a maximum of 450 mg/day.

Dosage Individualization. In renal failure the initial dose for hypertension should be reduced or the dosing interval lengthened to avoid an excessive hypotensive response. When titrating the dose upward, smaller increments should be used in addition to longer adjustment intervals. If a diuretic is required, a loop diuretic should be used. In CHF, reduce the initial dose to 6.25–12.5 mg tid if the patient has been vigorously treated with diuretics or may be hyponatremic or hypovolemic due to salt restriction.

Pediatric Dose. Safety and efficacy not established.

Dosage Forms. **Tab** 12.5, 25, 50, 100 mg.

Patient Instructions. Doses should be taken at least one hour prior to meals. Potassium supplements or salt substitutes should be used with caution and only on medical advice. Report any indication of infection, such as sore throat or fever, development of progressive swelling, or severe vomiting or diarrhea. Report occurrence of skin rash, abnormal taste or persistent dry cough. Excessive exercise and perspiration should be avoided. See also Class Instructions.

Pharmacokinetics. *Onset and Duration.* PO onset 15 min (may be less SL), peak 2–5 hr, duration 13 + hr during continuous dosing.[305,307]

Plasma Levels. No reliable correlation between plasma levels and therapeutic or toxic effects.

Fate. Bioavailability from radiolabeled doses is about 62%.[308] Peak plasma levels occur about 0.75 hr following an oral dose. About 30% plasma protein bound.[309] V_c is 0.22 ± 0.02 L/kg; $V_{d\ beta}$ is 2 ± 0.09 L/kg; V_{dss} is 0.7 $\pm$ 0.08 L/kg.[308] About 24% of an oral dose is excreted in the urine as unchanged captopril in 24 hr.[308] Metabolized to captopril disulfide which can link with endogenous thiol compounds, the disulfide may form a pool of potentially active drug because this disulfide can be reconverted to active captopril in vivo.[310] Total body clearance in renal dysfunction decreases with Cl_{cr}: 0.76 L/hr/kg in normals; 0.31 L/hr/kg in mild renal dysfunction; and 0.096 L/hr/kg in dialysis patients interdialysis.[308,311]

$t_{1/2}$. 1.93 hr $\pm$ 0.20 SD.[308]

Adverse Reactions. During early studies many side effects were reported which now appear to have been due to the use of higher than necessary doses and patient populations with a high frequency of renal dysfunction. The use of the lower doses now recommended and dosage adjustment in renal failure has resulted in a lower frequency of adverse effects in recent studies; rash and dysgeusia, although still frequent, have also declined. Maculopapular and morbilliform rashes are the most frequent and are sometimes accompanied by fever, pruritus and eosinophilia. Dosage reduction usually results in resolution of the rash. Dysgeusia is characterized by a diminution or loss of taste which is self-limiting, resolving in 2–3 months despite continued treatment. Proteinuria occurs in 3.5% of patients with renal impairment on doses greater than 150 mg/day, but is 0.2% in individuals with normal renal function on less than 150 mg/day.[312] Onset is usually after the third month of treatment.[313] Occasionally patients develop a persistent dry cough. Hypotension on initiation of therapy and reversible renal dysfunction occur occasionally. Neutropenia occurs rarely in normal hypertensives, increasing to 0.5% in patients with Cr_s over 2 mg/dl and 7.2% in azotemic patients with collagen vascular diseases.[312] Laryngeal edema with some deaths have been reported following the first dose.

Precautions. Patients on dietary salt restriction, diuretic therapy, or dialysis (salt/volume depletion) should be monitored for hypotensive episodes following the initial dose. If possible, patients should discontinue salt restricted diets and diuretics one week prior to treatment. Use with caution in patients having an increased risk of developing neutropenia or agranulocytosis due to the presence of impaired renal function, autoimmune or collagen vascular disorders (especially SLE), or drugs altering WBC or immune function. Elevation in Cr_s and BUN may occur in patients with renal artery stenosis, necessitating a reduction in dose or discontinuation of diuretic therapy. Discontinuation of captopril may be necessary in some cases.[314,315] Hypotension responsive to circulatory volume expansion may occur during surgical procedures. Use with caution with diuretics, sympatholytic agents, agents stimulating renin secretion, potassium supplements and potassium sparing diuretics.

Parameters to Monitor. Monitor blood pressure response regularly. Cr_s and BUN initially to determine potential risk for adverse effects and dosage adjustment, then periodically. Serum potassium, WBC count with differential q 2 weeks for the first three months, then periodically in renally impaired patients, or if signs of infection occur. Periodic urinary protein estimates (morning urines) by dipstick in patients with renal impairment.

Clonidine Hydrochloride   Catapres®, Catapres-TTS®, Various

Pharmacology. Clonidine binds to central postsynaptic α_2-adrenergic receptors in the region of the nucleus tractus solitarius, vasomotor center and vagal nucleus. Stimulation of these receptors activates an inhibitory neuron, reducing peripheral sympathetic outflow, producing a decrease in vasomotor tone and heart rate, and resulting in vagal reflex-mediated reduction in heart rate.[316]

Administration and Adult Dose. PO for hypertension 0.1 mg bid initially, increasing in 0.1–0.2 mg/day increments at 1–2 week intervals until control is achieved. The usual dosage range is 0.2–0.8 mg/day in divided doses to a usual maximum of 1.2 mg/day; doses up to 2.4 mg/day have been used rarely. **SR patch for hypertension** initially apply one #1 (0.1 mg/24 hr) patch weekly; dose may be increased weekly up to a #3 patch that delivers 0.3 mg/24 hr. Most responders require a patch delivering either 0.1 or 0.2 mg/24 hr.[317] PO for opiate withdrawal 16–17 mcg/kg/day, usually about 0.1–0.2 mg tid and 0.2 mg hs, individually adjusted to minimize withdrawal symptoms and clonidine side effects (eg, dry mouth, sedation, hypotension). Monitor patients daily and decrease opiate dose rapidly. Once opiate is stopped, taper clonidine dose daily in 0.1–0.2 mg/day increments. Limit course of clonidine to 3–4 weeks.[318,319] See Notes.

Pediatric Dose. Safety and efficacy not established.

Dosage Individualization. Renal impairment may require dosage adjustment. At Cl_{cr} of 10 ml/min or less, one group recommends that 50–75% of the usual dose be administered.[320]

Dosage Forms. Tab 0.1, 0.2, 0.3 mg; SR Patch 0.1, 0.2, 0.3 mg/24 hr.

Patient Instructions. Do not abruptly discontinue this drug because this may result in a rapid increase in blood pressure and possible cardiac arrhythmias.[321,322] Transdermal patches should be applied weekly at bedtime to a clean, hairless area of the upper, outer arm or chest that is free of irritations, abrasions, scars or callouses. Do not touch the adhesive surface of the patch. Rotate patch application sites weekly. See also Class Instructions.

Pharmacokinetics. *Onset and Duration.* (Hypertension) PO onset 30–60 min; peak 2–4 hr;[323] manufacturer lists the duration as 6–8 hr; however, several studies show that bid dosing is usually effective.[323-325] Transdermally, maximal reduction in blood pressure occurs in 2–3 days; response remains similar throughout the 7-day application period and decreases slowly over 2 days following removal.[326] (Opiate withdrawal) PO peak 2 hr; duration 4–6 hr; antiwithdrawal effects appear to be limited to 3–4 weeks.[318]

Plasma Levels. 0.3-2.0 ng/ml.[327]

Fate. About 75% of dose absorbed orally;[328] V_{dss} ranges from 2.1-3.9 L/kg.[328,329] Metabolized in liver with drug and metabolites excreted in the urine; 38% of absorbed drug is excreted unchanged within 24 hr. Transdermally, therapeutic plasma levels are reached in 2-3 days, remaining in this range for the 7-day application period and up to 11 total days.[330] Application of a replacement patch does not significantly alter plasma levels. Fluctuation in plasma levels with patches is minimal compared to tablets.[326]

$t_{1/2}$. α phase 2.2-28.7 min (average 10.8);[328] β phase 7.4-12.7 hr in single-dose studies,[329,331-333] up to 16.4 hr ± 4.8 SD after multiple doses.[331] Transdermal half-life of 17-20 hr reflects transdermal absorption rate.[330]

Adverse Reactions. Dry mouth, drowsiness, constipation, dizziness, fatigue and headache occur frequently; anorexia, parotid pain, Raynaud's phenomenon, impotence, vivid dreams or nightmares, insomnia and anxiety are occasional. Dry mouth and sedation are reduced in intensity with transdermal use.[334] Allergic contact dermatitis occurs frequently with transdermal patches and is an indication to discontinue the patch.[335] Abrupt discontinuation of oral doses over 0.4 mg/day regularly causes increased pulse rate and blood pressure; the hypertension is increased by concomitant β-blocker use.

Precautions. Use with caution in cerebrovascular disease, coronary insufficiency, recent myocardial infarction or chronic renal dysfunction.

Parameters to Monitor. Blood pressure; patient compliance.

Notes. Clonidine has been used investigationally to suppress symptoms of withdrawal of opiates; however, it is most effective as a "bridge" between opiates and narcotic antagonist (ie, naltrexone) therapy. Clonidine does not suppress opiate withdrawal insomnia, so a sedative-hypnotic at bedtime should be given concomitantly. **Lofexidine** (Merrell Dow) is related to clonidine with equivalent antiwithdrawal effects, but causing less sedation and hypotensive effects.[318,319] Clonidine also appears to be effective in reducing craving and other symptoms associated with alcohol and tobacco withdrawal.[319] Clonidine has been used in the treatment of various psychiatric disorders such as mania, anxiety, panic and schizophrenia; it may have efficacy in the treatment of antipsychotic-induced tardive dyskinesia.[319] Clonidine also appears to be effective in the treatment of menopausal flushing.[336]

Diazoxide   Hyperstat®, Proglycem®, Various

Pharmacology. A nondiuretic thiazide that reduces total peripheral resistance via direct relaxation of arteriolar smooth muscle. It also increases blood glucose by inhibiting insulin release and by other mechanisms.

Administration and Adult Dose. IV for hypertension 1-3 mg/kg to a maximum single dose of 150 mg, administered in 30 seconds or less; may repeat q 5-15 min until diastolic pressure is reduced to 100 mm Hg or less. Repeat q 4-24 hr as needed to maintain blood pressure reduction. A slow infusion of 15 mg/min, to a total dose of 5 mg/kg is also effective and may avoid excessive reduction of blood pressure. The infusion may be stopped when an adequate hypotensive response has been achieved.[337] See Notes. **PO for hypoglycemia** 1 mg/kg q 8 hr initially, then titrate to response. Usual maintenance dose is 3-8 mg/kg/day in 2-3 doses.

Dosage Individualization. Pregnant women and patients with renal dysfunction may require much lower initial doses and careful titration of maintenance doses to avoid hypotension.[338-340]

Pediatric Dose. IV for hypertension 5 mg/kg (or 175 mg/M^2). PO for hypoglycemia (infants and neonates) 3.3 mg/kg q 8 hr initially, then titrate to response. Usual maintenance dose is 8–15 mg/kg/day in 2–3 doses.

Dosage Forms. (Hyperstat®) Inj 15 mg/ml; (Proglycem®) Cap 50, 100 mg; Susp 50 mg/ml.

Patient Instructions. See Class Instructions.

Pharmacokinetics. *Onset and Duration.* (Hypertension) onset 1–2 min; peak 2–3 min; duration 4–12 hr.[341] (Hypoglycemia) onset 1 hr; duration 8 hr.

   Plasma Levels. No correlation between elimination phase plasma levels and hypotensive effect.[342]

   Fate. Absorbed orally; V_d is 210 ml/kg with normal renal function and 200–290 ml/kg in renal failure;[343] 94% plasma protein bound (84% in renal failure)[338] with binding inversely related to plasma concentration.[342] Metabolized by oxidation and conjugation with sulfate, with 19–22% excreted unchanged in urine.[343] See Notes.

   $t_{1/2}$. β phase 10–72 hr; 20–53 hr in renal failure.[343]

Adverse Reactions. Sodium and water retention and hyperglycemia are frequent with repeated use. Hyperuricemia occurs; however, reports of gout are lacking. Occasionally hypotension, possibly leading to symptoms of myocardial or cerebral ischemia, occurs.

Contraindications. Allergy to thiazides or other sulfonamides; hypertension secondary to arteriovenous shunt or coarctation of the aorta; aortic aneurism.

Precautions. Extravasation should be avoided due to the alkalinity of the solution. Hyperglycemia may occasionally require treatment. Renal failure may enhance the hyperglycemic effects.[344] Antihypertensive effects may be enhanced by recent use of methyldopa or reserpine or by the use of other direct-acting vasodilators such as hydralazine, minoxidil, nitroprusside, nitrates or papaverine.

Parameters to Monitor. Periodic serum uric acid level with prolonged use. (Hypertension) Frequent measurements of blood pressure until stable, then hourly; blood glucose levels with repeated doses, especially in patients with diabetes mellitus and/or renal failure. (Hypoglycemia) Frequent blood glucose levels initially and periodically after stabilization occurs in several days. Observe for signs of edema.

Notes. It was previously thought that IV administration had to be rapid to avoid a loss of hypotensive effect due to extensive protein binding. A recent study indicates that diazoxide has a greater affinity for arterial wall binding sites than serum albumin, resulting in an effective free fraction of 65% rather than in the range of 5%.[345]

Enalapril Maleate/Enalaprilat   Vasotec®

Pharmacology. Enalapril is a prodrug rapidly converted to its active metabolite, enalaprilat, by ester hydrolysis in the liver. Enalaprilat is an ACE inhibitor. See Captopril.

Administration and Adult Dose. PO for hypertension 2.5–5 mg/day initially; usual dosage range is 10–40 mg/day given in 1–2 doses. Bid dosing may be necessary in some individuals to achieve good 24 hr blood pressure control. A diuretic may be added if blood pressure control is inadequate with enalapril alone. PO for CHF 2.5 mg/day initially, titrate up to 10 mg bid. IV for hypertension 1.25 mg (0.625 mg if patient on diuretic) q 6 hr over 5 min.

Dosage Individualization. With a Cl_{cr} under 30 ml/min or a Cr_s over 3 mg/dl the initial dose should be reduced to 2.5 mg/day. Patients receiving diuretics prior to initiating enalapril should stop diuretic therapy for 2–3 days before enalapril is started, or the initial dose should be reduced to 2.5 mg/day.

Pediatric Dose. Safety and efficacy not established.

Dosage Forms. **Tab** (enalapril) 5, 10, 20 mg; **Inj** (enalaprilat) 1.25 mg/ml.

Patient Instructions. Potassium supplements or salt substitutes should be used with caution and only on medical advice. Avoid excessive dietary sodium restriction which could predispose to hypotension, or excessive sodium intake which could counteract the effect of enalapril. Report any of the following: swelling of face, eyes, lips, tongue, or difficulty in breathing (indicative of angioedema); lightheadedness or syncope (hypotension); excessive fluid losses due to perspiration, vomiting, or diarrhea which can precipitate hypotension; sore throat or fever (possibly indicative of neutropenia). See also Class Instructions.

Pharmacokinetics. *Onset and Duration.* Onset 1 hr; peak 3.5–8 hr; duration, by 24 hr the antihypertensive effect is about 50% of maximum.[346] The onset of action and maximal hemodynamic response correspond to the appearance of enalaprilat in plasma and its peak plasma levels.[347]

Plasma Levels. (Enalaprilat) 10 ng/ml produces near maximal suppression of ACE activity.

Fate. Oral bioavailability ranges from 53 to 73% and is not altered by meals.[348-350] About 94% of dose is converted to enalaprilat and there is essentially no additional metabolism.[349] Enalaprilat has an accumulation half-life of approximately 11 hr.[351] Urinary excretion accounts for 61% and fecal excretion accounts for 33% following a 10 mg oral dose.[349] Renal clearance of enalaprilat is 9.5 L/hr (range 5.8 to 15.4), which indicates renal tubular secretion.[349] Plasma enalaprilat levels accumulate with progressive renal dysfunction.[352]

$t_{1/2}.$ (Enalaprilat) 35 hr in normals, increased in CHF.[349,353]

Adverse Reactions. Headache, dizziness, fatigue and rash occur frequently. Hypotension is most likely in volume depleted or CHF patients. Cough, orthostatic effects and nausea occur occasionally. Azotemia is most likely to occur in patients with renal artery stenosis on concomitant diuretic therapy.[354,355] Dysgeusia, neutropenia, angioedema or proteinuria occur rarely.[356]

Precautions. See Captopril.

Parameters to Monitor. See Captopril.

Guanabenz Acetate   Wytensin®

Pharmacology. Guanabenz is a central α_2-adrenergic receptor agonist, structurally and pharmacologically similar to clonidine.

Administration and Adult Dose. PO for hypertension 4 mg bid initially; may be increased in 4–8 mg/day increments q 1–2 weeks to a maximum of 32 mg bid.

Pediatric Dose. Safety and efficacy not established.

Dosage Forms. Tab 4, 8, 16 mg.

Patient Instructions. Do not discontinue therapy abruptly or a rapid increase in blood pressure, anxiety, insomnia and palpitations may occur. See also Class Instructions.

Pharmacokinetics. *Onset and Duration.* Onset within 60 min; peak 2–4 hr; effect wanes by 6–8 hr and approaches baseline 12 hr after a single dose.

Plasma Levels. No therapeutic range established.

Fate. Bioavailability is about 75%; 90% plasma protein bound. The time of peak plasma level (3 hr) corresponds to peak antihypertensive effect. Peak plasma levels of unchanged guanabenz are 2.5 and 2.9 ng/ml with 16 and 32 mg doses, respectively. Only 1.4% of drug appears unchanged in the urine; hepatic hydroxylation followed by glucuronidation is the primary route of elimination. Primary metabolite, *E-p*-hydroxyguanabenz is inactive; renal clearance is 5.4–7.9 L/hr following 16 and 32 mg doses.[357]

$t_{1/2}$. 12–14 hr.[357]

Adverse Reactions. Drowsiness or sedation are frequent and dose-related. Dry mouth, dizziness and weakness also occur occasionally. Chest pain, edema, arrhythmias, palpitations, and sleep disturbances have been reported.

Precautions. Use with caution in conjunction with other sedating medications and in patients with severe coronary insufficiency, recent myocardial infarction, cerebrovascular disease, hepatic or renal dysfunction.

Parameters to Monitor. Monitor blood pressure response regularly.

Guanadrel Sulfate   Hylorel®

Guanadrel is a peripheral adrenergic neuron-blocking agent which is pharmacologically similar to guanethidine. Its antihypertensive activity is equivalent to that of guanethidine, but it has a faster onset and shorter duration of action. Onset of action is 30–120 min (average 77), peak 4–6 hr, duration 14 hr. The drug is 20% plasma protein bound; 85% is eliminated in urine in 24 hr, 40% unchanged, with an elimination half-life of 10 hr. Adverse reactions include frequent orthostatic hypotension and diarrhea; drowsiness; occasional fluid and water retention, ejaculation disturbances, impotence, limb aches and cramps and syncope. See Guanethidine Sulfate for contraindications and precautions. The initial oral dose is 5 mg bid; the usual dosage range is 20–75 mg bid; higher doses may require tid or qid dosing; maximum daily dosage is 400 mg. Doses should be carefully titrated.[358,359] Available as 10 and 25 mg tablets.

Guanethidine Sulfate   Ismelin®

Pharmacology. Guanethidine is a ganglionic blocking agent whose long-term antihypertensive action is due to a reduction in total peripheral resistance produced by norepinephrine depletion from presynaptic storage granules and an inhibition of action potential-induced release of norepinephrine.

Administration and Adult Dose. PO in ambulatory patients 10 mg/day initially, increasing daily dose in 10–25 mg/day increments at 5–7 day intervals, based on patient response. **PO in hospitalized patients** 25–50 mg/day initially, increasing dose in 25–50 mg/day increments daily or every other day as indicated. Doses may be given once daily.

Pediatric Dose. PO 0.2 mg/kg/day or 6 mg/M^2/day initially as a single oral dose, increasing q 7–10 days by the same amount as the initial dose. Final dose may be 5–8 times the starting dose.

Dosage Forms. Tab 10, 25 mg.

Patient Instructions. Avoid the use of nonprescription products containing ephedrine, phenylpropanolamine or pseudoephedrine. See also Class Instructions (the cautions regarding orthostatic hypotension and its precipitating factors should be emphasized).

Pharmacokinetics. *Onset and Duration.* Maximum hypotensive response may not occur for up to 14 days after initiating or changing dose.

Plasma Levels. Adrenergic blockade at 8 ng/ml or greater.[360]

Fate. Bioavailability 3–27% in one study[361] and 43% in another (although this may include metabolites formed before entry into systemic circulation).[362] Metabolized to inactive metabolites and excreted in urine as unchanged drug and metabolites.

$t_{1/2}$. α phase 1.5 days; β phase 4.1–7.7 days.[363]

Adverse Reactions. Frequently postural or exertional hypotension (producing symptoms of dizziness, weakness, lassitude or syncope), bradycardia, impotence, inhibition of ejaculation and diarrhea occur. Occasionally fluid retention and edema (possibly progressing to CHF) occur.

Contraindications. Known or suspected pheochromocytoma; frank CHF not due to hypertension; use with MAO inhibitors.

Precautions. May potentially aggravate asthma. Use with caution in renal dysfunction (because renal function may decrease with a fall in blood pressure), coronary heart disease, recent MI, cerebrovascular disease, encephalopathy or peptic ulcer disease. Amphetamines and cocaine block neuronal guanethidine uptake and inhibit its effects. Drugs used in surgical anesthesia may enhance the hypotensive action of guanethidine, possibly leading to cardiovascular collapse.

Parameters to Monitor. Blood pressure routinely.

Guanfacine Hydrochloride   Tenex®

Guanfacine is a central α_2-adrenergic receptor agonist pharmacologically similar to clonidine. In equipotent doses, guanfacine is equivalent to clonidine in antihypertensive activity alone or in combination with a diuretic. It has a bioavailability of 100%; V_d is 300 L. 80% of the dose is eliminated in the urine; of this amount 28% is unchanged drug. Therapeutic plasma levels are 5–10 ng/ml. Sedation, dry mouth and dizziness occur occasionally. Abrupt discontinuation can result in a rise in blood pressure which is apparently delayed (4th day) due to the drug's long half-life of 14–17 hr; it occurs less frequently than with clonidine. Dosage is initiated at 1 mg/day at bedtime. The dose can be increased in 1 mg/day increments at 3–4 week intervals. Doses over 3 mg/day are associated with increased adverse reactions; most patients can be maintained on a dose of 1 mg/day.[364-368] Available as 1 mg tablets.

Hydralazine Hydrochloride   Apresoline®, Various

Pharmacology. Hydralazine is a vasodilator that reduces total peripheral resistance through a direct relaxation of arterial smooth muscle. Hydralazine may produce its direct relaxation by preventing release of bound calcium from intracellular storage sites.[369] A reflex increase in heart rate, cardiac output, plasma renin activity, and sodium and water retention can attenuate its antihypertensive action; therefore, long-term regimens using hydralazine should include a diuretic and a sympatholytic agent.

Administration and Adult Dose. PO 10 mg qid initially, increasing dose during the first week to 25 mg qid; in the second and subsequent weeks the dose may be increased to 50 mg qid, to maximum of 200–300 mg/day. In slow acetylators, the risk of drug-induced SLE may be reduced by limiting the total daily dose to 100 mg.[370] Several studies indicate that bid dosing is as effective as qid.[371,372] **IM or IV** 10–40 mg prn.

Pediatric Dose. **PO** 0.75 mg/kg/day, or 25 mg/M[2]/day initially, in 4 divided doses; the dose may be titrated to 10 times the initial dose over a period of 3–4 weeks. **IM or IV** 1.7–3.5 mg/kg/day or 50–100 mg/M[2]/day in 4–6 divided doses as needed for continued control of blood pressure.

Dosage Forms. **Tab** 10, 25, 50, 100 mg; **Inj** 20 mg/ml.

Patient Instructions. This drug may cause headache, dizziness or palpitations; report if these symptoms are persistent. Report symptoms (of drug-induced systemic lupus erythematosus) such as fever, joint pains and generalized malaise. Take each dose at a fixed time in relation to meals, because food may reduce the response.[373] See also Class Instructions.

Pharmacokinetics. *Onset and Duration.* PO onset 1 hr; duration (following 300 mg/day) a minimum of 30 hr is required for mean arterial pressure to return to 50% of baseline value.[371] IV onset 10–20 min, IM onset 20–40 min; duration for both 3–8 hr.[374]

Plasma Levels. Hypotensive effect is directly related to the plasma concentration of hydralazine; however, no therapeutic or toxic ranges are established.[375]

Fate. Bioavailability depends on acetylator phenotype and is only 6.6% in fast acetylators and 39.3% in slow acetylators, probably due to extensive first-pass acetylation.[376] Taking hydralazine after meals can reduce peak hydralazine levels and vasodepressor response.[373] V_d ranges from 4.2–8.2 L/kg in fast acetylators and 4.2–7.3 L/kg in slow acetylators.[377-379] The drug is extensively metabolized in the liver by acetylation; the acetylation rate is genetically determined. About 11–14% excreted unchanged in the urine after IV and 2–4% after PO dosing;[380] metabolites are excreted in urine.

$t_{1/2}$. β phase 0.34–2.3 hr (independent of acetylator phenotype); renal impairment may increase half-life to 3.8–15.8 hr.[381] The discrepancy between half-life and duration of action has been attributed to arteriolar binding.

Adverse Reactions. Headache, tachycardia, palpitations, anorexia, nausea and vomiting, diarrhea and angina pectoris occur frequently. Occasionally peripheral neuropathy, dizziness, blood dyscrasias, depression, nasal congestion and flushing occur. A syndrome similar to SLE with joint pain and skin rash has been reported, but kidney damage rarely occurs. The overall frequency of SLE was approximately 6.7% in 281 patients during a period of 51 months; daily doses were shown to affect the frequency, with none at 50 mg/day, 5.4% at 100 mg/day, and 10.4% at 200 mg/day. Women had a higher overall frequency than men (11.6 compared with 2.8%), and women taking 200 mg/day had a 19.4% rate.[370] There are a few reports of immune complex glomerulonephritis in individuals with hydralazine-induced SLE.[382-384]

Contraindications. Coronary artery disease; mitral valvular rheumatic disease.

Precautions. Hypotensive effects may be additive when combined with other parenteral antihypertensive agents such as diazoxide.

Parameters to Monitor. Blood pressure. Baseline and periodic CBC and ANA titers, renal function (Cr_s, BUN), especially if the patient relates symptoms of drug-induced SLE.

Lisinopril

Prinivil®, Zestril®

Lisinopril is an ACE inhibitor (see Captopril) which is the lysine analogue of enalaprilat. Peak effect occurs at 6–8 hr and serum half-life is 12 hr or more. Initial dose for hypertension is 10 mg/day; the usual dosage range is 20–40 mg/day as a single dose. Lower doses should be used in the elderly and those taking diuretics. Doses of 2.5–20 mg/day have been used in CHF.[469,470] Available as 5, 10 and 20 mg tablets.

Methyldopa
Methyldopate Hydrochloride

Aldomet®, Various

Pharmacology. The antihypertensive action of methyldopa is thought to be mediated through stimulation of central α_2-adrenergic receptors in a manner similar to clonidine. Stimulation is due to the metabolites α-methyldopamine, α-methylnorepinephrine and possibly α-methyl-epinephrine.

Administration and Adult Dose. PO 250 mg bid-tid initially, increased every few days to maximum of 2–3 g/day in 2–4 divided doses. There is some evidence that a single daily dose at bedtime is effective in some patients.[385] IV usual dose is 250–500 mg q 6 hr to maximum of 1 g q 6 hr.

Dosage Individualization. The dosing interval may have to be extended to 12–24 hr when Cl_{cr} is less than 10 ml/min.[386]

Pediatric Dose. PO 10 mg/kg/day in 2–4 doses initially, to maximum of 65 mg/kg/day or 3 g/day, whichever is less. IV 20–40 mg/kg/day divided into 4 doses q 6 hr, to maximum of 65 mg/kg/day or 3 g/day, whichever is less.

Dosage Forms. Susp 250 mg/5 ml; Tab 125, 250, 500 mg; Inj 250 mg/5 ml.

Patient Instructions. Report changes in mood (depression), loss of appetite, jaundice, abdominal pain or unexplained fevers and arthralgias. See also Class Instructions.

Pharmacokinetics. *Onset and Duration.* PO gradual onset occurring within 6 hr.[387] IV onset 2–3 hr, maximum 3–5 hr; duration 6–12 hr.[374]

   Fate. Oral bioavailability is low and variable, 7.9–61.5% (average 25) in one study[388] and average 32% in another,[389] probably due to extensive first-pass metabolism to 3-O-methyldopa. Peak plasma levels occur in 2–4 hr.[369,388] IV bioavailability is similar to oral, apparently because a significant portion of the methyldopate ester is not hydrolyzed to methyldopa.[390] 10–15% plasma protein bound.[391] V_d is 0.28–1.4 L/kg (average 0.69). The drug is excreted in the urine as metabolites, sulfate conjugate and as unchanged drug, with 64% excreted unchanged after IV and 18% after PO dose.[388]

   $t_{1/2}$. α phase 0.53 hr;[389] β phase 90–130 min (average 106).[388]

Adverse Reactions. Somewhat dose-related reactions include weight gain, drowsiness, nasal congestion and dizziness frequently. Positive Coombs' test occurs in 5–25%; however, less than 1% develop hemolytic anemia. Occasionally indigestion, depression, diarrhea, nightmares, impotence, ejaculatory failure and orthostatic hypotension occur.[392] Rarely hemolytic anemia, hepatitis, drug fever and lupus-like syndrome occur.

Contraindications. Active hepatic disease, such as acute hepatitis or active cirrhosis; liver dysfunction associated with previous methyldopa therapy.

Precautions. Use with caution in any patient with a history of prior hepatic disease.

Parameters to Monitor. Obtain CBC, direct Coombs' test and liver function tests initially to establish baseline values. Periodically obtain CBC (to monitor for hemolytic anemia and blood dyscrasias) and liver function tests during therapy.

Minoxidil   Loniten®, Rogaine®, Various

Pharmacology. Minoxidil is a potent vasodilator that acts by direct relaxation of arteriolar smooth muscle, resulting in a reduction of total peripheral resistance. The subsequent decrease in blood pressure leads to a reflex sympathetic activation, producing an increase in heart rate, cardiac output and renin secretion. Redistribution of renal blood flow also leads to sodium and water retention. Because these factors may attenuate the antihypertensive response, minoxidil should be administered with a sympatholytic agent and a diuretic (often, a loop diuretic is required). Topically, minoxidil stimulates hair growth in some individuals.

Administration and Adult Dose. PO for hypertension 5 mg/day initially, increase in 5–10 mg/day increments q 3 days; usual dosage range 10–40 mg/day, to maximum of 100 mg/day. If a single dose reduces supine blood pressure by more than 30 mm Hg, the total daily dose should be divided into 2 equal doses. **Top for male pattern baldness** 1 ml bid to affected area of scalp.

Pediatric Dose. PO for hypertension 0.2 mg/kg initially as a single daily dose, increased in 50–100% increments q 3 days; usual dosage range is 0.25–1 mg/kg/day, to maximum of 50 mg/day.

Dosage Forms. Tab 2.5, 10 mg (Loniten®). **Top** 2% (Rogaine®).

Patient Instructions. Report any of the following side effects: 20 beat/min increase in resting heart rate; rapid weight gain of more than 5 lbs or the development of edema; respiratory difficulty; development or worsening of chest pain (that may indicate myocardial ischemia); dizziness; lightheadedness; or fainting. See also Class Instructions.

Pharmacokinetics. *Onset and Duration.* PO onset 30 min; peak 4–8 hr in one study and 7–11 hr in another; duration 2–5 days.[393,394] Top onset 4 or more months; duration, relapse may occur 3–4 months after discontinuation.

    Fate. About 97% of a C^{14}-labeled dose is recovered from the urine over a 4-day period;[395] however, this may not reflect the amount of unchanged drug reaching the systemic circulation. Protein binding is negligible; V_d values reported vary widely and range from 99–826 L (average 200) in one study, to 542 L ± 186 SD in another.[393,395] The drug is extensively metabolized to glucuronic acid conjugates and more polar metabolites. In the first 24 hr, 9.8 ± 7% of the dose is excreted unchanged in the urine.[395]

    $t_{1/2}$. 1.4 hr.[394]

Adverse Reactions. Frequently sodium and water retention, tachycardia, hypertrichosis and reversible EKG T wave changes.[396] Occasionally angina pectoris, CHF and pericardial effusion, sometimes leading to tamponade, occur.[397] Minor dermatologic reactions may occur after topical administration.

Contraindications. Pheochromocytoma.

Precautions. Degenerative myocardial lesions reported in dogs, but have not been demonstrated in man.[398] The addition of minoxidil to pre-existing guanethidine therapy may result in significant orthostatic hypotension; if possible, discontinue guanethidine 5 days prior to starting minoxidil.

Parameters to Monitor. Blood pressure, pulse rate, body weight, cardiac and pulmonary function regularly.

Nitroprusside Sodium   Nipride®, Various

Pharmacology. Nitroprusside is a vasodilator that reduces peripheral vascular resistance (afterload) via direct relaxation of arteriolar smooth muscle and by reducing venous return (preload) by dilation of the venous system.

Administration and Adult Dose. **IV by constant infusion** average rate 3 mcg/kg/min with a range of 0.5–10 mcg/kg/min. Patients receiving other antihypertensive agents can usually be controlled with a smaller dose. Administration rates should be carefully controlled through the use of microdrip regulators or infusion pumps. For prolonged (several days) administration, infusion rates should be kept in the range of 4 mcg/kg/min to avoid cyanide toxicity; the total dose should be kept under 70 mg/kg (during a 14-day period) to avoid thiocyanate toxicity in patients with normal renal function.[399] See Notes.

Dosage Individualization. Start with low infusion rates and carefully titrate upwards in elderly patients.

Pediatric Dose. **IV by constant infusion**—a report of 20 cases indicates that an average dose of 1.4 mcg/kg/min (range 0.5–3.5 mcg/kg/min) is required for adequate blood pressure control.[400]

Dosage Forms. **Inj** 50 mg.

Patient Instructions. See Class Instructions.

Pharmacokinetics. *Onset and Duration.* Onset 30–60 seconds; peak effect 1–2 min; duration 3–5 min.[374]
   Plasma Levels. Therapeutic and toxic nitroprusside levels not established. Thiocyanate levels over 10–12 mg/dl are associated with toxicity.[401]
   Fate. Cyanide is released from nitroprusside following the interaction of the iron in nitroprusside with vascular wall and RBC sulfhydryl groups. Cyanide is then converted to thiocyanate by the liver enzyme rhodanase; thiocyanate and an insignificant amount of unchanged nitroprusside are eliminated in the urine.
   $t_{1/2}$. (Thiocyanate) 2.7 days with normal renal function; 9 days in renal impairment.[402]

Adverse Reactions. Rapid infusion may lead to nausea, retching, diaphoresis, apprehension, headache, restlessness, muscle twitching, retrosternal discomfort, palpitations, dizziness and abdominal pain, which are relieved by decreasing the infusion rate. Thiocyanate is not particularly toxic and accumulates to toxic levels only following long-term treatment with nitroprusside. Accumulation may be potentiated by renal dysfunction. Toxicity may present as fatigue, anorexia, nausea, headaches, disorientation, psychotic behavior or muscle spasms. Cyanide toxicity can develop quickly if large doses are administered rapidly; this seems to occur only in individuals who appear resistant to nitroprusside and subsequently receive high doses in attempts to reduce blood pressure. Toxicity may present as tachypnea, tachycardia, altered consciousness, convulsions or coma.

Contraindications. Increased intracranial pressure;[403] hypertension secondary to arteriovenous shunts or coarctation of the aorta; use as an agent to produce intraoperative controlled hypotension in patients with inadequate cerebral circulation.

Precautions. If an adequate hypotensive response is not achieved after 10 min of infusing a dose of 10 mcg/kg/min the infusion should be stopped, because larger doses increase the risk of cyanide toxicity.[404] Use with caution in renal, hepatic or thyroid disease and in vitamin B_{12} deficiency.

Parameters to Monitor. Blood pressure should be monitored frequently, usually by intra-arterial catheter, due to the rapid onset and dissipation of clinical effect. Plasma cyanide and thiocyanate levels should be monitored daily in patients with renal or hepatic dysfunction. The appearance of unexplained nausea, vomiting and alterations in mental function should be considered signs of potential toxicity until proven otherwise.[405] Metabolic acidosis was once used as a monitoring parameter for cyanide toxicity, but it can develop suddenly and its appearance indicates serious toxicity, so it may not be a good early indicator of impending toxicity.

Notes. Protect from light and discard solution 24 hr after preparation.

Pinacidil (Investigational - Lilly)   Pindac®

Pinacidil is a direct acting arterial vasodilator that is pharmacologically similar to hydralazine. It has no direct stimulant action on the heart, but it may cause reflex tachycardia. It is well absorbed orally and eliminated primarily by metabolism with some renal excretion of unchanged drug; the half-life is 2–4 hr. Fluid retention occurs frequently, and the drug should be given with a diuretic. Tachycardia, T-wave abnormalities, headache, dizziness and palpitations have been reported. The usual oral dosage range is 12.5–25 mg bid.[471,472]

Prazosin Hydrochloride   Minipress®

Pharmacology. Prazosin causes a postsynaptic α_1-adrenergic receptor blockade which produces a decrease in total peripheral resistance. Reflex tachycardia usually observed with traditional α-blockers (eg, phentolamine) is infrequent, because of the absence of presynaptic α-receptor blockade. Thus, norepinephrine in the synapse can stimulate α_2-receptors and inhibit further norepinephrine release.[406]

Administration and Adult Dose. PO for hypertension 1 mg bid-tid initially, increasing slowly based on response. Usual dosage range is 6–15 mg/day, to maximum of 20 mg/day. Doses up to 40 mg/day may produce a response in a few individuals not responding to a lower dose.

Dosage Individualization. Carefully titrate dose in CHF.

Pediatric Dose. Safety and efficacy not established.

Dosage Forms. Cap 1, 2, 5 mg.

Patient Instructions. To minimize the potential danger from first dose syncope, the initial dose should be taken at bedtime and the patient warned against arising suddenly. See also Class Instructions.

Pharmacokinetics. *Onset and Duration.* Onset 1.5 hr after 1.5 mg PO dose.[407] Full antihypertensive response may not be achieved for 2–9 weeks (average 4).[408]

   Fate. About 55–57% oral bioavailability;[409-411] 92–97% plasma protein bound; V_d is 0.45–0.57 L/kg (average 0.51).[412] Cl is 0.24 L/hr/kg ± 0.04 SD in young patients and 0.21 L/hr/kg ± 0.06 SD in the elderly.[411] Metabolized in the liver by demethylation and conjugation; metabolites have about 20% the activity of prazosin; excreted renally as metabolites and 3.4% as unchanged drug.[411]

$t_{1/2}$. α phase 3 min; β phase 0.65 ± 0.08 hr; γ phase 2.6-3 hr, prolonged in CHF to 6.47 ± 4.6 hr.[409,410,412,413]

Adverse Reactions.   Dizziness, headache, drowsiness, weakness, palpitations and nausea occur frequently. Occasionally syncope, tachycardia and abdominal discomfort occur. Priapism occurs rarely.

Precautions.   First-dose syncope usually occurs within 30–90 min of initial dose. With a 1 mg initial dose, the frequency of syncopal episodes is less than 1%.[414] Syncope seems to be more common in patients on low sodium diets and those on diuretics.

Parameters to Monitor.   Blood pressure routinely.

Notes.   Doxazosin (Pfizer) is an investigational agent, pharmacologically similar to prazosin which has similarly been used in both hypertension and CHF.[415]

Reserpine   Various

Reserpine is a hypotensive agent that acts primarily by depleting norepinephrine from postganglionic adrenergic neurons. It is a very weak antihypertensive used alone, but may be effective in mild to moderate hypertension in combination with a diuretic and vasodilator. Its maximum effect occurs after about 3 weeks orally; duration is up to 24 hours, with CNS and cardiovascular effects lasting up to several weeks after chronic oral therapy. The drug is extensively metabolized. Dose-related mental depression occurs in about 10% of patients taking usual antihypertensive doses. Drowsiness, weakness, GI disturbances (eg, abdominal pain, activation of peptic ulcer disease, diarrhea, epigastric distress), nasal congestion, sexual dysfunction and bradycardia occur occasionally. Reserpine is contraindicated in patients with mental depression and suicidal tendencies, during electroconvulsive therapy and in those with active peptic ulcer disease or ulcerative colitis. It must be used with caution in patients with a history of mental depression and patients should be warned to report any symptoms of depression. The adult oral dosage is 0.5 mg/day for 1–2 weeks, followed by a maintenance dose of 0.1-0.25 mg/day in a single dose.[256,416-419] It is available as 0.1, 0.25, 0.5 and 1 mg tablets.

Terazosin Hydrochloride   Hytrin®

Terazosin is a postsynaptic α_1-receptor blocking agent which is structurally and pharmacologically similar to prazosin. Bioavailability is complete and not affected by food. 90–94% plasma protein bound; V_d is 25–30 L; Cl is 4.8 L/hr and renal clearance is 0.6 L/hr. Elimination half-life is between 11.8–13.3 hr in hypertensive patients. The most frequent adverse reactions are dizziness, asthenia, palpitations, dyspnea, nausea and headache. Initial dosage is 1 mg PO at bedtime to avoid syncope. Dosage is slowly increased to a usual range of 1-5 mg/day in a single dose, to a maximum of 20 mg/day.[420-423] Available as 1, 2 and 5 mg tablets.

Drugs For Hypertensive Emergencies Comparison Chart[a]

DRUG	DOSAGE RANGE	ONSET	DURATION	COMMENTS[b,c]
Captopril Capoten®	SL 12.5–25 mg.	5–25 min	2–6 hr	Hypotensive effect is particularly large in patients on a diuretic or in hypertensive crisis. Subsequent doses may be less effective unless given with a diuretic.
Clonidine Catapres®	PO 0.1–0.2 mg initially, then 0.1 mg/hr to a maximum of 0.8 mg.	30–90 min	6–8 hr	Rate of onset slower after a meal; drowsiness or dry mouth can occur. Rebound hypertension is possible.
Diazoxide Hyperstat® I.V.	IV 1–3 mg/kg (up to 150 mg) over 30 seconds; may repeat q 5–15 min.	1–5 min	4–12 hr	Acts rapidly and for a long period; increases cardiac output; requires blood pressure monitoring at hourly intervals.
Hydralazine Apresoline®	IM or IV 5–50 mg q 3–6 hr.	10–40 min	3–8 hr	Not predictably effective; increases cardiac output; many patients may be sensitive to parenteral doses, resulting in excessive hypotension.
Labetalol Normodyne® Trandate®	IV push 20 mg initially, then 40–80 mg q 10–15 min until desired response achieved (average total dose required is 200 mg).	5–10 min	1–8 hr	Hypotensive effect is predictable; contraindicated in CHF, head trauma, intracranial hemorrhage; potential for bradycardia, bronchospasm; often causes marked postural hypotension.

Continued

Drugs For Hypertensive Emergencies Comparison Chart[a]

DRUG	DOSAGE RANGE	ONSET	DURATION	COMMENTS[b,c]
Methyldopa Aldomet®	IV only, 250 mg–1 g q 4–8 hr.	2–3 hr	6–12 hr	Hypotensive response is highly variable; does not affect cardiac output or renal blood flow; slow onset.
Nifedipine Adalat® Procardia®	SL, PO or buccal 10 mg, may repeat in 30 min prn.	1–5 min	2–4 hr	Predictable hypotensive response; puncture capsule and suck on contents or cut capsule and squeeze contents under tongue for SL use; alternatively, bite and swallow. Increases cardiac output; mild flushing, headaches and palpitations may occur; use with caution in patients with severe arteriosclerotic stenosis, may precipitate cerebral ischemic symptoms.
Nitroprusside Sodium Nipride®	IV infusion 100 mg/L at a rate of 0.25–8 mcg/kg/min by continuous infusion using infusion pump. Average dose is 3 mcg/kg/min.	½–1 min	3–5 min	Hypotensive action is predictable and effective; must be given by IV infusion with continuous monitoring of the patient; arterial pressure response adjusted by changing infusion rate; decreases cardiac output; hypotensive effect is enhanced by elevating head of the patient's bed.
Trimethaphan Arfonad®	IV infusion 0.5–5 mg/min using infusion pump.	1–5 min	10 min	Drug of choice for emergency treatment of aortic dissection.

a. Adapted from references 374, 424–428, 467.
b. Reduction of arterial pressure may lead to sodium and fluid retention, thus reducing the antihypertensive effectiveness of these drugs; diuretic drugs should therefore be administered concomitantly during therapy.
c. Consult the drug monograph or product literature for additional information.

24:12 VASODILATING AGENTS

General References: 429–433

Class Instructions. This drug may cause headache, dizziness and/or flushing; alcohol may potentiate these side effects. During an acute angina attack, discontinue activity, assume a sitting position and dissolve 1 tablet under the tongue. Keep tablets in the original container, tightly closed. Patients on chronic therapy should not discontinue these medications abruptly.

Isosorbide Dinitrate   Isordil®, Sorbitrate®, Various

Pharmacology. See Nitroglycerin.

Administration and Adult Dose. **SL Tab for acute anginal attack** 2.5–10 mg q 2–3 hr or prn;[429,432] doses up to 40 mg have been used; **Chew Tab for acute anginal attack** 5 mg initially, then 5–10 mg q 2–3 hr or prn.[429] **PO for prophylaxis of angina and for CHF** 10–60 mg q 4–6 hr, doses up to 120 mg have been used.[429,432-435] **SR products for prophylaxis of angina** 20–40 mg q 6–8 hr, doses up to 80 mg have been used.[436] Dosage must be started low and titrated slowly upward over a period of several days to weeks to patient tolerance or to the desired therapeutic effect. Because of the possibility of tolerance and dependence, patients on long-acting nitrate regimens should be maintained on the lowest effective dosage. Tolerance may be less with bid-tid dosing than with qid.[468] The dose should be slowly tapered if nitrates are discontinued.[437] See Notes.

Dosage Forms. **Cap** 40 mg; **Chew Tab** 5, 10 mg; **SL Tab** 2.5, 5, 10 mg; **SR Cap** 40 mg; **SR Tab** 20, 40 mg; **Tab** 5, 10, 20, 30, 40 mg.

Patient Instructions. See Class Instructions.

Pharmacokinetics. *Onset and Duration.* Onset 5–20 min after SL and Chew Tab administration, 15–45 min after PO administration, up to 4 hr in rare cases or with SR products; peak 15–60 min after SL administration; 45–120 min after PO administration;[432] duration 1–3 hr after SL or Chew Tab, 4–6 hr after PO, 6–8 hr after SR;[429,433] duration claimed to be up to 12 hr after high-dose SR administration.[436,438]

Fate. Extensive first-pass metabolism by liver after oral administration to less active mononitrate metabolites (2-ISMN, 5-ISMN). Larger doses and chronic administration overcome degradation processes with significant increases in plasma concentration of the parent compound and metabolites.[439]

$t_{1/2}$. (Isosorbide dinitrate) 1.1–1.3 hr; (2-ISMN) 1.8 hr; (5-ISMN) 4–4.2 hr.[440]

Adverse Reactions. See Nitroglycerin.

Contraindications. See Nitroglycerin.

Precautions. See Nitroglycerin.

Parameters to Monitor. Observe for headache and other side effects. In angina, monitor frequency of angina. In CHF, monitor hemodynamic and functional measurements.

Notes. Oral nitrates, sometimes in doses greater than recommended by the manufacturer, have been shown to be effective in the prophylaxis of angina pectoris and in the treatment of CHF.[429,439,441-443] See Vasodilators in Heart Failure Comparison Chart.

Nitroglycerin   Various

Pharmacology. An organic nitrate that specifically relaxes vascular smooth muscle. The venous (capacitance) system is affected to a greater degree than the arterial (resistance) system. Venous pooling, decreased venous return to the heart (preload) and decreased arterial resistance (afterload) reduce intracardiac pressures and left ventricular size, thereby decreasing myocardial oxygen consumption and ischemia. In myocardial ischemia, nitrates may improve regional myocardial blood supply, although total coronary flow decreases or remains the same. The various nitrate preparations have the same pharmacological effects and differ only in dose, onset and duration.[429,438]

Administration and Adult Dose. SL Tab for acute anginal attack 150–600 mcg prn; **SL aerosol for acute anginal attack** 400–800 mcg prn, up to 1200 mcg/15 min; **Buccal for acute anginal attack and/or prophylaxis and treatment of angina pectoris or CHF** 1–3 mg q 4–6 hr; **PO for prophylaxis of angina or CHF** 6.5–19.5 mg q 4–6 hr;[432] **Top ointment for prophylaxis and treatment of angina pectoris or CHF** 0.5–2 inches, to maximum of 5 inches q 3–6 hr.[429,432,438] Dosage must be started low and titrated slowly upward over a period of several days to weeks to patient tolerance or to the desired therapeutic effect. **SR Patch for prophylaxis and treatment of angina pectoris** 2.5–15 mg/day, titrated to patient response. **IV for CHF post-MI, angina pectoris, peri-operative blood pressure control or hypotensive anesthesia** 5 mcg/min initially by constant infusion using an infusion pump. Dosage must be titrated to the individual patient's response. Initially increase dose in 5 mcg/min increments q 3–5 min until response noted. If no response occurs at 20 mcg/min, increments of 10 mcg/min and later 20 mcg/min can be used. Once partial blood pressure response occurs, incremental increases should be decreased and intervals increased.[430,431] See Notes.

Dosage Forms. **Buccal Tab** 1, 2, 3 mg; **Oint** 2%; **SL Aerosol** 400 mcg/spray; **SL Tab** 150, 300, 400, 600 mcg; **SR Cap** 2.5, 6.5, 9 mg; **SR Patch** (Deponit®) 5, 10 mg/24 hr; (Nitrodisc®) 5, 7.5, 10 mg/24 hr; (Nitro-Dur® II) 2.5, 5, 7.5, 10, 15 mg/24 hr; (Transderm-Nitro®) 2.5, 5, 10, 15 mg/24 hr; **SR Tab** 2.6, 6.5, 9 mg; **Inj** 0.8, 5, 25 mg/ml.

Patient Instructions. See Class Instructions.

Pharmacokinetics. *Onset and Duration.* Onset immediate after IV, 1–2 min after buccal, 2–5 min after SL, 30–60 min after topical and transdermal administration, 20–45 min after SR Cap and Tab;[432,433] peak 30 min after buccal, 4–8 min after SL, 2–3 hr after topical and transdermal administration, 45–120 min after SR Tab and Caps;[432,433,444] duration 10–30 min after IV and SL, 4–6 hr after buccal, 3–6 hr after topical and oral, and up to 24 hr after transdermal administration.[429,432,433,438]

Fate. Well absorbed sublingually and transcutaneously. V_d is about 200 L; plasma protein binding is 60% for drug and 30–60% for dinitro metabolites. Metabolized in the liver to less active dinitro and inactive mononitro metabolites; extensive first-pass metabolism occurs after oral administration. Larger doses and chronic administration may saturate metabolism and result in increased plasma concentrations of drug and metabolites.[445]

$t_{1/2}$. 1.9–3.3 min (estimated).[432,446,447]

Adverse Reactions. Headache occurs very frequently; occasionally flushing, dizziness, weakness, nausea, vomiting, palpitations, tachycardia and postural hypotension occur. Many of these effects may be minimized by slow upward titration of the dose. Tolerance and dependence may occur with prolonged use. Intolerable skin reactions have occurred in 40% of patients using transdermal patches.[448]

Contraindications. Severe anemia; severe postural hypotension; increased intracranial pressure; purported hypersensitivity or idiosyncrasy to nitroglycerin, nitrates or nitrites. Glaucoma has been stated to be a contraindication, but nitrates can probably be used safely in these patients.[429,445]

Precautions. Some tolerance and cross-tolerance with other nitrates may occur with long-term or excessive use. Use with caution in patients with severe renal or hepatic disease, those with low or normal pulmonary capillary wedge pressure and in those receiving drugs that lower blood pressure.

Parameters to Monitor. Observe for headache and other side effects. In angina, monitor frequency of angina. In CHF, obtain hemodynamic and functional measurements. During IV use, blood pressure and heart rate should be constantly monitored in all patients; pulmonary capillary wedge pressure may also be useful in some patients.

Notes. A burning sensation and localized erythema under the tongue is an indication of potency of SL tablets, but does not always occur with coated or stabilized tablets.[449] Large and unpredictable amounts of nitroglycerin are lost through polyvinyl chloride containers, most IV administration sets and tubing, as well as in certain IV filters.[450,451] The injection should always be diluted in glass containers and administered with the special administration sets provided by the manufacturer; in-line filters should be avoided. Stored in glass containers, the diluted injection is stable for 48 hr at room temperature and 7 days under refrigeration. The special administration set (eg, Tridilset®) has a rather large dead-space and the line should be flushed whenever the concentration of solution is changed. See Vasodilators in Heart Failure Comparison Chart.

Nitroglycerin Dilution Guide

AMOUNT ADDED		VOLUME OF DILUENT	FINAL CONCENTRATION
MG	VOLUME		
8	1 amp (8 mg/ml)	250 ml	32 mcg/ml.
16	2 amps (8 mg/ml)	250 ml	64 mcg/ml.
32	4 amps (8 mg/ml)	250 ml	128 mcg/ml.
50	1 amp (50 mg/ml)	250 ml	200 mcg/ml.
50	1 amp (50 mg/ml)	500 ml	100 mcg/ml.*
100	2 amps (50 mg/ml)	250 ml	400 mcg/ml.†
100	2 amps (50 mg/ml)	500 ml	200 mcg/ml.
200	4 amps (50 mg/ml)	500 ml	400 mcg/ml.†

*Recommended *initial* concentration.
†Recommended *maximum* concentration.

Vasodilators in Heart Failure Comparison Chart[a,b]

DRUG	DOSAGE[c]	DURATION	SITE OF ACTION[d]	HR	MAP	PCWP	CI	SVR
Captopril Capoten®	PO 25–100 mg tid.	hours	A,V	↓	↓	↓	↑	↓
Clonidine[e] Catapres® Various	PO 0.2–0.4 mg q 6–8 hr.	hours	A,V	↓	↓	↓	0	SI↑
Diltiazem Cardizem®	PO 90–120 mg q 8 hr.	hours	A	↓	↓	↓	↑	↓
Enalapril Vasotec®	PO 2.5–20 mg bid.	hours	A,V	↓	↓	↓	↑	↓
Hydralazine Apresoline® Various	PO 50–100 mg q 6–8 hr.	hours	A	0	SI↓	SI↓	↑	↓
Isosorbide Dinitrate Isordil® Sorbitrate® Various	PO 10–60 mg q 4–6 hr.	hours	V,(A)	SI↑/↓	↓	↓	↑/↓	SI↓
Nifedipine Procardia®	PO 10–30 mg q 8 hr.	hours	A	0	↓	0	↑	↓

Continued

Vasodilators in Heart Failure Comparison Chart[a,b]

DRUG	DOSAGE[c]	DURATION	SITE OF ACTION[d]	HR	MAP	PCWP	CI	SVR
Nitroglycerin Various	IV 5–100 mcg/min.	minutes	V,(A)	SI↑/↓	→	→	↑/↓	SI↓
	TOP 2% 0.5–5 inches q 3–6 hr.	hours	V,(A)	SI↑/↓	→	→	↑/↓	SI↓
Nitroprusside Sodium Nipride® Various	IV 15–400 mcg/min.	minutes	A,V	o	SI↓	→	↑	→
Phentolamine Regitine®	IV 0.1–2 mg/min.	minutes	A	SI↑	→	→	↑	→
Prazosin Minipress®	PO 2–7 mg q 6–8 hr.	hours	A,V	o	SI↓	→	↑	→
Trimazosin (Investigational - Pfizer)	PO 50–300 mg q 6–8 hr.	hours	A,V	o	→	→	↑	→

Key: A = arterial; V = venous; HR = heart rate; MAP = mean arterial pressure; PCWP = pulmonary capillary wedge pressure; CI = cardiac index; SVR = systemic vascular resistance; ↑ = increase; ↓ = decrease; SI = slight; o = no change.

a. From references 429–431, 452–466.

b. These agents have been shown to be effective in the acute treatment of congestive heart failure. Long-term therapy with some of these agents is presently being evaluated and should be assessed in individual patients by measurements of functional and hemodynamic performance.

c. Dosages of these agents should be started low and increased gradually with continuous hemodynamic monitoring. To avoid adverse rebound effects, carefully taper the dosages of these drugs if they are to be discontinued. See Nitroglycerin Notes.

d. Predominant site of action. Parentheses denote lesser activity.

e. Clinical role is restricted because of negative inotropic effects.

References, 24:00 Cardiovascular Drugs

1. Singh BN. Rational basis of antiarrhythmic therapy: clinical pharmacology of commonly used antiarrhythmic drugs. Angiology 1978;29:206-42.

2. Surawicz B. Pharmacologic treatment of cardiac arrhythmias: 25 years progress. J Am Coll Cardiol 1983;1:365-81.

3. Harrison DC, Meffin PJ, Winkle RA. Clinical pharmacokinetics of antiarrhythmic drugs. Prog Cardiovasc Dis 1977;20:217-42.

4. Smith TW. Digitalis. N Engl J Med 1988;318:358-65.

5. Singh BN, Collett JT, Chew CYC. New perspectives in the pharmacologic therapy of cardiac arrhythmias. Prog Cardiovasc Dis 1980;22:243-301.

6. Zipes DP, Troup PJ. New antiarrhythmic agents. Am J Cardiol 1978;41:1005-22.

7. Zipes DP, Prystowsky EN, Heger JJ. Amiodarone: electrophysiologic actions, pharmacokinetics and clinical effects. J Am Coll Cardiol 1984;3:1059-71.

8. Singh BN. Amiodarone: historical development and pharmacologic profile. Am Heart J 1983;106:788-97.

9. Latini R, Tognoni G, Kates RE. Clinical pharmacokinetics of amiodarone. Clin Pharmacokinet 1984;9:136-56.

10. Rotmensch HH, Belhassen B, Swanson BN et al. Steady-state serum amiodarone concentrations: relationship with antiarrhythmic efficacy and toxicity. Ann Intern Med 1984;101:462-9.

11. Holt DW, Tucker GT, Jackson PR et al. Amiodarone pharmacokinetics. Am Heart J 1983;106:840-7.

12. Paton DM, Webster DR, Neutze JN. A review of the clinical pharmacokinetics of amiodarone. Meth Find Exp Clin Pharmacol 1984;6:411-9.

13. D'Amico DJ, Kenyon KR, Ruskin JN. Amiodarone keratopathy. Drug-induced lipid storage disease. Arch Ophthalmol 1981;99:257-61.

14. Lemaire JF, Autret A, Biziere K et al. Amiodaron neuropathy: further arguments for human drug-induced neurolipidosis. Eur Neurol 1982;21:65-8.

15. Rigas B, Rosenfeld LE, Barwick KW et al. Amiodarone hepatotoxicity. A clinicopathologic study of five patients. Ann Intern Med 1986;104:348-51.

16. Raeder EA, Podrid PJ, Lown B. Side effects and complications of amiodarone therapy. Am Heart J 1985;109:975-83.

17. Harris L, McKenna WJ, Rowland E et al. Side effects and possible contraindications of amiodarone use. Am Heart J 1983;106:916-21.

18. Jonckheer MH, Blockx P, Broeckaert I et al. 'Low T_3 syndrome' in patients chronically treated with an iodine-containing drug, amiodarone. Clin Endocrinol 1978;9:27-35.

19. Marchlinski FE, Gansler TS, Waxman HL et al. Amiodarone pulmonary toxicity. Ann Intern Med 1982;97:839-45.

20. Sclarovsky S, Lewin RF, Kracoff O et al. Amiodarone-induced polymorphous ventricular tachycardia. Am Heart J 1983;105:6-12.

21. Prystowsky EN, Heger JJ, Miles WM et al. Amiodarone treatment in patients with ventricular arrhythmias. Drugs 1985;29(Suppl 3):47-52.

22. Ward A, Brogden RN, Heel RC et al. Amrinone. A preliminary review of its pharmacological properties and therapeutic use. Drugs 1983;26:468-502.

23. Scholz H. Pharmacological actions of various inotropic agents. Eur Heart J 1983;4(Suppl A):161-72.

24. Wynne J, Braunwald E. New treatment for congestive heart failure: amrinone and milrinone. J Cardiovasc Med 1984;9:393-405.

25. LeJemtel TH, Keung E, Sonnenblick EH et al. Amrinone: a new non-glycosidic, non-adrenergic cardiotonic agent effective in the treatment of intractable myocardial failure in man. Circulation 1979;59:1098-104.

26. Edelson J, LeJemtel TH, Alousi AA et al. Relationship between amrinone plasma concentration and cardiac index. Clin Pharmacol Ther 1981;29:723-8.

27. Rocci ML, Wilson H, Likoff M et al. Amrinone pharmacokinetics after single and steady state doses in patients with chronic cardiac failure. Clin Pharmacol Ther 1983;33:260. Abstract.

28. Weber KT, Andrews V, Janicki JS. Cardiotonic agents in the management of chronic cardiac failure. Am Heart J 1982;103:639-49.

29. Dunkman WB, Wilen MM, Franciosa JA. Adverse effects of long-term amirnone administration in congestive heart failure. Am Heart J 1983;105:861-3.

30. Packer M, Medina N, Yushak M. Hemodynamic and clinical limitations of long-term inotropic therapy with amrinone in patients with severe chronic heart failure. Circulation 1984;70:1038-47.

31. Heissenbuttel RH, Bigger JT. Bretylium tosylate: a newly available antiarrhythmic drug for ventricular arrhythmias. Ann Intern Med 1979;91:229-38.

32. Chatterjee K, Mandel WJ, Vyden JK et al. Cardiovascular effects of bretylium tosylate in acute myocardial infarction. JAMA 1973;223:757-60.

33. Patterson E, Lucchese BR. Bretylium. A prototype for future development of antidysrhythmic agents. Am Heart J 1983;106:426-31.

34. Bauman JL, Gallastegui J, Prechel D et al. Bethanedine sulfate in paroxysmal ventricular tachycardia. Toxicity and antifibrillatory actions. Pharmacotherapy 1986;6:184-92.

35. Adir J, Narang PK, Josselson J et al. Pharmacokinetics of bretylium in renal insufficiency. N Engl J Med 1979;300:1390-1.

36. Adir J, Narang PK, Josselson J. Nomogram for bretylium dosing in renal impairment. Ther Drug Monit 1985;7:265-8.

37. Dollery CT, Emslie-Smith D, McMichael J. Bretylium tosylate in the treatment of hypertension. Lancet 1960;1:296-9.

38. Anderson JL, Patterson E, Conlon M et al. Kinetics of antifibrillatory effects of bretylium: correlation with myocardial drug concentrations. Am J Cardiol 1980;46:583-92.

39. Kuntzman R, Tsai I, Chang R et al. Disposition of bretylium in man and rat. Clin Pharmacol Ther 1970;11:829-37.

40. Narang PK, Adir J, Josselson J et al. Pharmacokinetics of bretylium in man after intravenous administration. J Pharmacokinet Biopharm 1980;8:363-73.

41. Anderson JL, Patterson E, Wagner JG et al. Clinical pharmacokinetics of intravenous and oral bretylium tosylate in survivors of ventricular tachycardia or fibrillation: clinical application of a new assay for bretylium. J Cardiovasc Pharmacol 1981;3:485-99.

42. Anderson JL, Patterson E, Wagner JG et al. Oral and intravenous bretylium disposition. Clin Pharmacol Ther 1980;28:468-78.

43. Koch-Weser J. Bretylium. N Engl J Med 1979;300:473-7.

44. Gillis RA, Clancy MM, Anderson RJ. Deleterious effects of bretylium in cats with digitalis-induced ventricular tachycardia. Circulation 1973;47:974-83.

45. Jelliffe RW, Buell J, Kalaba R et al. An improved method of digitoxin therapy. Ann Intern Med 1970;72:453-64.

46. Rasmussen K, Jervell J, Storstein L et al. Digitoxin kinetics in patients with impaired renal function. Clin Pharmacol Ther 1972;13:6-14.

47. Cole CC, ed. The Harriet Lane handbook. 10th ed. Chicago: Yearbook Medical Publishers, 1984.

48. Smith TW, Haber B. Digitalis (3rd of 4 parts). N Engl J Med 1973;289:1063-72.

49. Gold H, Cattell McK, Modell W et al. Clinical studies on digitoxin with further observations on its use in the single average full dose method of digitalization. J Pharmacol Exp Ther 1944;82:187-95.

50. Perrier D, Mayersohn M, Marcus FI. Clinical pharmacokinetics of digitoxin. Clin Pharmacokinet 1977;2:292-311.

51. Bresnahan JF, Vlietstra RE. Digitalis glycosides. Mayo Clin Proc 1979;54:675-84.

52. Rosen MR, Wit AL, Hoffman BF. Electrophysiology and pharmacology of cardiac arrhythmias. IV. cardiac antiarrhythmic and toxic effects of digitalis. Am Heart J 1975;89:391-9.

53. Jelliffe RW. An improved method of digoxin therapy. Ann Intern Med 1968;69:703-17.

54. Jelliffe RW, Brooker G. A nomogram for digoxin therapy. Am J Med 1974;57:63-8.

55. Steiness E, Svendsen O, Rasmussen F. Plasma digoxin after parenteral administration: local reaction after intramuscular injection. Clin Pharmacol Ther 1974;16:430-3.

56. American Hospital Formulary Service: Current drug therapy: cardiac glycosides. Am J Hosp Pharm 1978;35:1495-507.

57. Doherty JE, de Soyza N, Kane JJ et al. Clinical pharmacokinetics of digitalis glycosides. Prog Cardiovas Dis 1978;21:141-58.

58. Soldin SJ. Digoxin—issues and controversies. Clin Chem 1986;32:5-12.

59. Iisalo E. Clinical pharmacokinetics of digoxin. Clin Pharmacokinet 1977;2:1-16.

60. Sim SK. Digoxin tablets - a review of the bioavailability problems. Am J Hosp Pharm 1976;33:44-8.

61. Caldwell JH, Cline CT. Biliary excretion of digoxin in man. Clin Pharmacol Ther 1976;19:410-5.

62. Ewy GA, Marcus FI, Fillmore SJ et al. Digitalis intoxication - diagnosis, management and prevention. Cardiol Clin 1974;6:153-74.

63. Mann DL, Maisel AS, Atwood JE et al. Absence of cardioversion-induced ventricular arrhythmias in patients with therapeutic digoxin levels. J Am Coll Cardiol 1985;5:882-8.

64. Epstein SE, Henry WL, Clark CE et al. Asymmetric septal hypertrophy. Ann Intern Med 1974;81:650-80.

65. Green LH, Smith TW. The use of digitalis in patients with pulmonary disease. Ann Intern Med 1977;87:459-65.

66. Mason DT, Awan NA. Recent advances in digitalis research. Am J Cardiol 1979;43:1056-9.

67. Maroko PR, Kjekshus JK, Sobel BE et al. Factors influencing infarct size following experimental coronary artery occlusions. Circulation 1971;43:67-82.

68. Fenster PE, Powell JR, Graves PE et al. Digitoxin-quinidine interaction: pharmacokinetic evaluation. Ann Intern Med 1980;93:698-701.

69. Hager WD, Fenster P, Mayersohn M et al. Digoxin-quinidine interaction: pharmacokinetic evaluation. N Engl J Med 1979;300:1238-41.

70. Slaughter RL, Schneider PJ, Visconti JA. Appropriateness of the use of serum digoxin and digitoxin assays. Am J Hosp Pharm 1978;35:1376-9.

71. Weintraub M. Interpretation of the serum digoxin concentration. Clin Pharmacokinet 1977;2:205-19.

72. Spivack C, Ocken S, Frishman WH. Calcium antagonists: clinical use in the treatment of systemic hypertension. Drugs 1983;25:154-77.

73. Hung J-S, Yeh S-J, Lin F-C et al. Usefulness of intravenous diltiazem in predicting subsequent electrophysiologic and clinical responses to oral diltiazem. Am J Cardiol 1984;54:1259-62.

74. Petru MA, Crawford MH, Kennedy GT et al. Long-term efficacy of high-dose diltiazem for chronic stable angina pectoris: 16-month serial studies with placebo controls. Am Heart J 1985;109:99-103.

75. Zelis RF, Kinney EL. The pharmacokinetics of diltiazem in healthy American men. Am J Cardiol 1982;49:529-32.

76. Kinney EL, Moskowitz RM, Zelis R. The pharmacokinetics and pharmacology of oral diltiazem in normal volunteers. J Clin Pharmacol 1981;21:337-42.

77. Joyal M, Pieper J, Cremer K et al. Pharmacodynamic aspects of intravenous diltiazem administration. Am Heart J 1986;111:54-60.

78. Smith MS, Verghese CP, Shand DG et al. Pharmacokinetic and pharmacodynamic effects of diltiazem. Am J Cardiol 1983;51:1369-74.

79. McAuley BJ, Schroeder JS. The use of diltiazem hydrochloride in cardiovascular disorders. Pharmacotherapy 1982;2:121-33.

80. Lewis JG. Adverse reactions to calcium antagonists. Drugs 1983;25:196-222.

81. Winship LC, McKenney JM, Wright JT et al. The effect of ranitidine and cimetidine on single-dose diltiazem pharmacokinetics. Pharmacotherapy 1985;5:16-9.

82. Sasyniuk BI, Kus T. Cellular electrophysiologic changes induced by disopyramide phosphate in normal and in-

farcted hearts. J Int Med Res 1976;4(Suppl 1):20-5.

83. Kotter V, Linderer T, Schroder R. Effects of disopyramide on systemic and coronary hemodynamics and myocardial metabolism in patients with coronary artery disease: comparison with lidocaine. Am J Cardiol 1980;46:469-75.

84. Podrid PJ, Schoeneberger A, Lown B. Congestive heart failure caused by oral disopyramide. N Engl J Med 1980;302:614-7.

85. Kidwell GA, Lima JJ, Schaal SF et al. Hemodynamic and electrophysiologic effects of the enantiomers of disopyramide. Circulation 1985;72(Suppl III):232. Abstract.

86. Lima JJ. Disopyramide. In: Taylor WJ, Caviness MHD, eds. A textbook for the clinical application of therapeutic drug monitoring. Irving, Tx: Abbott Diagnostics, 1986:97-108.

87. Siddoway LA, Woosley RL. Clinical pharmacokinetics of disopyramide. Clin Pharmacokinet 1986;11:214-22.

88. Yu PN. Editorial: disopyramide phosphate (Norpace): a new antiarrhythmic drug. Circulation 1979;59:236-7.

89. Niarchos AP. Disopyramide: serum level and arrhythmia conversion. Am Heart J 1976;92:57-64.

90. Lima JJ, Haughey DB, Leir CV. Disopyramide pharmacokinetics and bioavailability following simultaneous administration of disopyramide and 14C-disopyramide. J Pharmacokinet Biopharm 1984;12:289-313.

91. Dubetz DK, Brown NN, Hooper WD et al. Disopyramide pharmacokinetics and bioavailability. Br J Clin Pharmacol 1978;6:279-81.

92. Hinderling PH, Garrett ER. Pharmacokinetics of the antiarrhythmic diospyramide in healthy humans. J Pharmacokinet Biopharm 1976;4:199-230.

93. Koch-Weser J. Disopyramide. N Engl J Med 1979;300:957-62.

94. Karim A. The pharmacokinetics of Norpace. Angiology 1975;26:85-98.

95. Meffin PJ, Robert EW, Winkle RA et al. Role of concentration-dependent plasma protein binding in disopyramide disposition. J Pharmacokinet Biopharm 1979;7:29-46.

96. Bauman JL, Gallastegui J, Strasberg B et al. Long-term therapy with disopyramide phosphate: side effects and effectiveness. Am Heart J 1986;111:654-60.

97. Warrington SJ, Hamer J. Some cardiovascular problems with disopyramide. Postgrad Med J 1980;56:229-33.

98. Dhuranahar RW, Nademanee K, Goldman AM. Ventricular tachycardia-flutter associated with disopyramide therapy: a report of three cases. Heart Lung 1978;7:783-7.

99. Gillis AM, Kates RE. Clinical pharmacokinetics of the newer antiarrhythmic agents. Clin Pharmacokinet 1984;9:375-403.

100. Pottage A. Clinical profiles of newer class I antiarrhythmic agents — tocainide, mexiletine, encainide, flecainide and lorcainide. Am J Cardiol 1983;52:24C-31C.

101. Winkle RA, Peters F, Kates RE et al. Possible contribution of encainide metabolites to the long-term antiarrhythmic efficacy of encainide. Am J Cardiol 1983;51:1182-8.

102. Angaran DM, Schultz NS, Tschida VH. Esmolol hydrochloride: an ultrashort-acting β-adrenergic blocking agent. Clin Pharm 1986;5:288-303.

103. MacCosbe PE, Katz R, Steinberg J et al. Flestolol—a short-acting beta-blocking agent in acute supraventricular tachyarrhythmia. Drug Intell Clin Pharm 1986;20:457. Abstract.

104. Roden DM, Woosley RL. Flecainide. N Engl J Med 1986;315:36-41.

105. Holmes B, Heel RC. Flecainide. A preliminary review of its pharmacodynamic properties and therapeutic efficacy. Drugs 1985;29:1-33.

106. Conard GJ, Ober RE. Metabolism of flecainide. Am J Cardiol 1984;53:41B-51B.

107. Nappi JM, Anderson JL. Flecainide: a new prototype antiarrhythmic agent. Pharmacotherapy 1985;5:209-21.

108. Smith GH. Flecainide: a new class Ic antidysrhythmic. Drug Intell Clin Pharm 1985;19:703-7.

109. Griffith L, Platia E, Ord S et al. Persistent ventricular tachycardia/fibrillation — a possible adverse interaction between flecainide and class I anti-arrhythmic drugs. J Am Coll Cardiol 1984;3:583. Abstract.

110. Wynn J, Fingerhood M, Keefe D et al. Refractory ventricular tachycardia with flecainide. Am Heart J 1986;112:174-5.

111. Josephson MA, Ikeda N, Singh BN. Effects of flecainide on ventricular function: clinical and experimental correlations. Am J Cardiol 1984;53:95B-100B.

112. Rosen MR, Hoffman BF, Wit AL. Electrophysiology and pharmacology of cardiac arrhythmias. V. cardiac antiarrhythmic effects of lidocaine. Am Heart J 1975;89:526-36.

113. Lazzara R, Hope RR, El-Sherif N et al. Effects of lidocaine on hypoxic and ischemic cardiac cells. Am J Cardiol 1978;41:872-9.

114. Benowitz NL, Meister W. Clinical pharmacokinetics of lignocaine. Clin Pharmacokinet 1978;3:177-201.

115. Lie KI, Wellens HJ, van Capelle FJ et al. Lidocaine in the prevention of primary ventricular fibrillation. N Engl J Med 1974;291:1324-6.

116. Koster RW, Dunning AJ. Intramuscular lidocaine for prevention of lethal arrhythmias in the prehospital phase of acute myocardial infarction. N Engl J Med 1985;313:1105-10.

117. Routledge PA, Stargel WW, Barchowsky A et al. Control of lidocaine therapy: new perspectives. Ther Drug Monit 1982;4:265-70.

118. Rowland M, Thomson PD, Guichard A et al. Disposition kinetics of lidocaine in normal subjects. Ann NY Acad Sci 1971;179:383-98.

119. Boyes RN, Scott DB, Jebson PJ et al. Pharmacokinetics of lidocaine in man. Clin Pharmacol Ther 1971;12:105-16.

120. Thomson PD, Melmon KL, Richardson JA et al. Lidocaine pharmacokinetics in advanced heart failure, liver disease, and renal failure in humans. Ann Intern Med 1973;78:499-508.

121. Blumer J, Strong JM, Atkinson AJ. The convulsant potency of lidocaine and its N-dealkylated metabolites. J Pharmacol Exp Ther 1973;186:31-6.

122. Burney RG, DiFazio CA, Peach MJ et al. Anti-arrhythmic effects of lidocaine metabolites. Am Heart J 1974;88:765-9.

123. Bauer LA, Brown T, Gibaldi M et al. Influence of long-term infusions on lidocaine kinetics. Clin Pharmacol

Ther 1982;31:433-7.

124. LeLorier J, Grenon D, Latour Y et al. Pharmacokinetics of lidocaine after prolonged intravenous infusions in uncomplicated myocardial infarction. Ann Intern Med 1977;87:700-2.

125. Routledge PA, Stargel WW, Wagner GS et al. Increased alpha-1-acid glycoprotein and lidocaine disposition in myocardial infarction. Ann Intern Med 1980;93:701-4.

126. Ribner HS, Isaacs ES, Frishman WH. Lidocaine prophylaxis against ventricular fibrillation in acute myocardial infarction. Prog Cardiovasc Dis 1979;21:287-313.

127. Gupta PK, Lichstein E, Chadda KD. Lidocaine-induced heart block in patients with bundle branch block. Am J Cardiol 1974;33:187-92.

128. Berk SI, Gal P, Bauman JL et al. The effect of oral cimetidine on total and unbound serum lidocaine concentrations in patients with suspected myocardial infarction. Int J Cardiol 1987;14:91-4.

129. Reiter MJ, Pritchett ELC. Investigational antiarrhythmic agents: pirmenol. Clin Cardiol 1984;7:330-4.

130. Keefe DL. Pharmacology of lorcainide. Am J Cardiol 1984;54:18B-21B.

131. Somberg JC. New directions in antiarrhythmic drug therapy. Am J Cardiol 1984;54:8B-17B.

132. Vaughan Wiliams EM. A classification of antiarrhythmic actions reassessed after a decade of new drugs. J Clin Pharmacol 1984;24:129-47.

133. Burke GH, Berman ND. Differential electrophysiologic effects of mexiletine on normal and hypoxic canine Purkinje fibers. Circulation 1982;66(Suppl II):292. Abstract.

134. Bauman JL, Mexiletine. In: Taylor WJ, Caviness MHD eds. A textbook for the clinical application of therapeutic drug monitoring. Irving, TX: Abbott Diagnostics, 1986:125-30.

135. Allaf D, Henrard L, Crochelet L et al. Pharmacokinetics of mexiletine in renal insufficiency. Br J Clin Pharmacol 1982;14:431-5.

136. Holt DW, Walsh AC, Curry PV et al. Paediatric use of mexiletine and disopyramide. Br Med J 1979;4:1476-7.

137. Schrader BJ, Bauman JL. Mexiletine: a new type I antiarrhythmic agent. Drug Intell Clin Pharm 1986;20:255-60.

138. Woosley RL, Wang T, Stone W et al. Pharmacology, electrophysiology, and pharmacokinetics of mexiletine. Am Heart J 1984;107:1058-65.

139. Haselbarth V, Doevendans JE, Wolf M. Kinetics and bioavailability of mexiletine in healthy subjects. Clin Pharmacol Ther 1981;29:729-36.

140. Mitchell BG, Clements JA, Pottage A et al. Mexiletine disposition: individual variation in response to urine acidification and alkalinisation. Br J Clin Pharmacol 1983;16:281-4.

141. Campbell NPS, Kelly JG, Adgey AAJ et al. The clinical pharmacology of mexiletine. Br J Clin Pharmacol 1978;6:103-8.

142. Leahey EB, Giardina EGV, Bigger JT. Effect of ventricular failure on steady state kinetics of mexiletine. Clin Res 1980;239A. Abstract.

143. Pentikainen PJ, Halinen MO, Helin MJ.. Pharmacokinetics of oral mexiletine in patients with acute myocardial infarction. Eur J Clin Pharmacol 1983;25:773-7.

144. Campbell NPS, Pantridge JF, Adgey AAJ. Long-term oral antiarrhythmic therapy with mexiletine. Br Heart J 1978;40:796-801.

145. Duff HJ, Roden DM, Marney S et al. Molecular basis for the antigenicity of lidocaine analogs: tocainide and mexiletine. Am Heart J 1984;107:585-9.

146. Duff HJ, Roden D, Primm RK et al. Mexiletine in the treatment of resistant ventricular arrhythmias: enhancement of efficacy and reduction of dose-related side effects by combination with quinidine. Circulation 1983;67:1124-8.

147. Keefe DLD, Kates RE, Harrison DC. New antiarrhythmic drugs: their place in therapy. Drugs 1981;22:363-400.

148. Hasegawa GR. Milrinone, a new agent for the treatment of congestive heart failure. Clin Pharm 1986;5:201-5.

149. Maskin CS, Sinoway L, Chadwick B et al. Sustained hemodynamic and clinical effects of a new cardiotonic agent, WIN 47203, in patients with severe congestive heart failure. Circulation 1983;67:1065-70.

150. Stroshane RM, Koss RF, Biddlecome CE et al. Oral and intravenous pharmacokinetics of milrinone in human volunteers. J Pharm Sci 1984;73:1438-41.

151. Holmes JR, Kubo SH, Cody RJ et al. Milrinone in congestive heart failure: observations on ambulatory ventricular arrhythmias. Am Heart J 1985;110:800-6.

152. Baim DS, Colucci WS, Monrad ES et al. Survival of patients with severe congestive heart failure treated with oral milrinone. J Am Coll Cardiol 1986;7:661-70.

153. Larsson R, Liedholm H, Andersson KE et al. Pharmacokinetics and effects on blood pressure of a single oral dose of milrinone in healthy subjects and in patients with renal impairment. Eur J Clin Pharmacol 1986;29:549-53.

154. Sorkin EM, Clissold SP, Brogden RN. Nifedipine. A review of its pharmacodynamic and pharmacokinetic properties, and therapeutic efficacy, in ischemic heart disease, hypertension and related cardiovascular disorders. Drugs 1985;30:182-274.

155. Weidmann P, Gerber A, Laederach K. Calcium antagonists in the treatment of hypertension: a critical overview. Yearbook of Medicine 1984:197-234.

156. Foster TS, Hamann SR, Richards VR et al. Nifedipine kinetics and bioavailability after single intravenous and oral doses in normal subjects. J Clin Pharmacol 1983;23:161-70.

157. Green JA, Clementi WA, Porter C et al. Nifedipine-quinidine interaction. Clin Pharm 1983;2:461-5.

158. Diamond JR, Cheung JY, Fang LST. Nifedipine-induced renal dysfunction: alterations in renal hemodynamics. Am J Med 1984;77:905-9.

159. Dale J, Landmark KH, Myhre E. The effects of nifedipine, a calcium antagonist, on platelet function. Am Heart J 1983;105:103-5.

160. Meyer JS. Calcium channel blockers in the treatment of vascular headaches. Ration Drug Ther 1985;19(March):1-4.

161. Hoffman BF, Rosen MR, Wit AL. Electrophysiology and pharmacology of cardiac arrhythmias. VII. cardiac effects of quinidine and procaine amide. B Am Heart J 1975;90:117-22.

162. Greenspan AM, Horowitz LN, Spielman SR et al. Large dose procainamide therapy for ventricular tachyar-

rhythmia. Am J Cardiol 1980;46:453-62.

163. Giardina E-GV, Heissenbuttel RH, Bigger JT. Intermittent intravenous procaine amide to treat ventricular arrhythmias. Ann Intern Med 1973;78:183-93.

164. Hoffman BF, Rosen MR, Wit AL. Electrophysiology and pharmacology of cardiac arrhythmias. VII. cardiac effects of quinidine and procaine amide. Am Heart J 1975;89:804-8.

165. Drayer DE, Lowenthal DT, Woosley RL et al. Cumulation of N-acetylprocainamide, an active metabolite of procainamide, in patients with impaired renal function. Clin Pharmacol Ther 1977;22:63-9.

166. Karlsson E. Clinical pharmacokinetics of procainamide. Clin Pharmacokinet 1978;3:97-107.

167. Kessler KM, Kayden DS, Estes DM et al. Procainamide pharmacokinetics in patients with acute myocardial infarction or congestive heart failure. J Am Coll Cardiol 1986;7:1131-9.

168. Wyman MG, Goldreyer BN, Cannom DS et al. Factors influencing procainamide total body clearance in the immediate postmyocardial infarction period. J Clin Pharmacol 1981;21:20-5.

169. Koch-Weser J. Serum procainamide levels as the therapeutic guides. Clin Pharmacokinet 1977;2:389-402.

170. Connolly SJ, Kates RE. Clinical pharmacokinetics of N-acetylprocainamide. Clin Pharmacokinet 1982;7:206-20.

171. Koch-Weser J, Klein SW. Procainamide dosage schedules, plasma concentrations, and clinical effects. JAMA 1971;215:1454-60.

172. Koch-Weser J. Pharmacokinetics of procainamide in man. Ann NY Acad Sci 1971;179:370-82.

173. Gibson TP, Atkinson AJ, Matusik E et al. Kinetics of procainamide and N-acetylprocainamide in renal failure. Kidney Int 1977;12:422-9.

174. Dhingra RC, Rosen KM. Procainamide and the sinus node. Chest 1979;76:620-1.

175. Lawson DH, Jick H. Adverse reactions to procainamide. Br J Clin Pharmacol 1977;4:507-11.

176. Strasberg B, Sclarovsky S, Erdberg A et al. Procainamide-induced polymorphous ventricular tachycardia. Am J Cardiol 1981;47:1309-14.

177. Prince RA, Brown BT, Jacknowitz AI. Agranulocytosis with procainamide therapy - report of a case. Am J Hosp Pharm 1977;34:1362-5.

178. Meyers DG, Gonzalez ER, Peters LL et al. Severe neutropenia associated with procainamide: comparison of sustained release and conventional preparations. Am Heart J 1985;109:1393-5.

179. Ellrodt AG, Murata GH, Riedinger MS et al. Severe neutropenia associated with sustained-release procainamide. Ann Intern Med 1984;100:197-201.

180. Henningsen NC, Cederberg A, Hanson A et al. Effects of long-term treatment with procaine amide: a prospective study with special regard to ANF and SLE in fast and slow acetylators. Acta Med Scand 1975;198:475-82.

181. Rotmensch HH, Yust I, Siegman-Igra Y et al. Granulomatous hepatitis: a hypersensitivity response to procainamide. Ann Intern Med 1978;89:646-7.

182. Goldberg D, Reiffel JA, Davis JC et al. Electrophysiologic effects of procainamide on sinus function in patients with and without sinus node disease. Am Heart J 1982;103:75-9.

183. Wit AL, Hoffman BF, Rosen MR. Electrophysiology and pharmacology of cardiac arrhythmias. IX. cardiac electrophysiologic effects of beta adrenegic receptor stimulation and blockade. Part C. Am Heart J 1975;90:795-803.

184. Kelly KL. Beta-blockers in hypertension: a review Am J Hosp Pharm 1976;33:1284-90.

185. Frishman W, Silverman R. Clinical pharmacology of the newer beta-adrenergic blocking drugs. part 2. physiologic and metabolic effects. Am Heart J 1979;97:797-807.

186. Berglund G, Andersson O, Hansson L et al. Propranolol given twice daily in hypertension. Acta Med Scand 1973;194:513-5.

187. Thadani U, Parker JO. Propranolol in the treatment of angina pectoris. comparison of duration of action in acute and sustained oral therapy. Circulation 1979;59:571-9.

188. Federman J, Vlietstra RE. Antiarrhythmic drug therapy. Mayo Clin Proc 1979;54:531-42.

189. Woosley RL, Shand DG. Pharmacokinetics of antiarrhythmic drugs. Am J Cardiol 1978;41:986-95.

190. Routledge PA, Shand DG. Clinical pharmacokinetics of propranolol. Clin Pharmacokinet 1979;4:73-90.

191. Nies AS, Shand DG. Clinical pharmacology of propranolol. Circulation 1975;52:6-15.

192. Pieper JA. Beta blockers. In: Taylor WJ, Caviness MHD, eds. A textbook for the clinical application of therapeutic drug monitoring. Irving, TX: Abbott Diagnostics, 1986:149-60.

193. Borgstrom L, Johansson C-G, Larsson H et al. Pharmacokinetics of propranolol. J Pharmacokinet Biopharm 1981;9:419-29.

194. Wilkinson GR, Shand DG. A physiological approach to hepatic drug clearance. Clin Pharmacol Ther 1975;18:377-90.

195. Johnsson G, Regardh CG. Clinical pharmacokinetics of β-adrenoreceptor blocking drugs. Clin Pharmacokinet 1976;1:233-63.

196. Greenblatt DJ, Koch-Weser J. Adverse reactions to β-adrenergic receptor blocking drugs: a report from the Boston collaborative drug surveillance program. Drugs 1974;7:118-29.

197. Miller RR, Olson HG, Amsterdam EA et al. Propranolol-withdrawal rebound phenomenon. N Engl J Med 1975;293:416-8.

198. Waal-Manning HJ. Can β-blockers be used in diabetic patients? Drugs 1979;17:157-60.

199. Bauer JH, Brooks CS. The long-term effect of propranolol therapy on renal function. Am J Med 1979;66:405-10.

200. Luchi RJ, Chahine RA, Raizner AE. Coronary artery spasm. Ann Intern Med 1979;91:441-9.

201. Johnsson G, Use of β-adrenoreceptor blockers in combination with β-stimulators in patients with obstructive lung disease. Drugs 1976;11(Suppl 1):171-7.

202. Conn HL, Luchi RJ. Some cellular and metabolic considerations relating to the action of quinidine as a prototype antiarrhythmic agent. Am J Med 1964;37:685-99.

203. Covinsky JO, Russo J, Kelly KL et al. Relative bioavailability of quinidine gluconate and quinidine sulfate in healthy volunteers. J Clin Pharmacol 1979;19:261-9.

204. Ochs HR, Greenblatt DJ, Woo E. Clinical pharmacokinetics of quinidine. Clin Pharmacokinet 1980;5:150-68.

205. Greenblatt DJ, Pfeifer HJ, Ochs HR et al. Pharmacokinetics of quinidine in humans after intravenous, intramuscular and oral administration. J Pharmacol Exp Ther 1977;202:365-78.

206. Carliner NH, Fisher ML, Crouthamel WG et al. Relation of ventricular premature beat suppression to serum quinidine concentration determined by a new and specific assay. Am Heart J 1980;100:483-9.

207. Guentert TW, Holford NHG, Coates PE et al. Quinidine pharmacokinetics in man: choice of a disposition model and absolute bioavailability studies. J Pharmacokinet Biopharm 1979;7:315-30.

208. Drayer DE, Lowenthal DT, Restivo KM et al. Steady-state serum levels of quinidine and active metabolites in cardiac patients with varying degrees of renal function. Clin Pharmacol Ther 1978;24:31-9.

209. Ueda CT, Hirschfeld DS, Scheinman MM et al. Disposition kinetics of quinidine. Clin Pharmacol Ther 1976;19:30-6.

210. Ueda CT, Dzindzio BS. Quinidine kinetics in congestive heart failure. Clin Pharmacol Ther 1978;23:158-64.

211. Kessler KM, Humphries WC, Black M et al. Quinidine pharmacokinetics in patients with cirrhosis or receiving propranolol. Am Heart J 1978;96:627-35.

212. Reynolds EW, Vander Ark CR. Quinidine syncope and the delayed repolarization syndromes. Mod Concepts Cardiovasc Dis 1976;45:117-22.

213. Bauman JL, Bauernfeind RA, Hoff JV et al. Torsade de pointes due to quinidine: observations in 31 patients. Am Heart J 1984;107:425-30.

214. Roden DM, Woosley RL, Primm RK. Incidence and clinical features of the quinidine-associated long QT syndrome: implications for patient care. Am Heart J 1986;111:1088-93.

215. Romankiewicz JA, Reidenberg M, Drayer D et al. The noninterference of aluminum hydroxide gel with quinidine sulfate absorption: an approach to control quinidine-induced diarrhea. Am Heart J 1978;96:518-20.

216. Gerstenblith T, Katabi G, Stein I et al. Quinidine utilization in cardiac arrhythmias: report of study involving sulfate and polygalacturonate salts. NY State J Med 1966;66:701-6.

217. Connolly SJ, Kates RE, Lebsack CS et al. Clinical pharmacology of propafenone. Circulation 1983;68:589-96.

218. Roden DM, Woosley RL. Tocainide. N Engl J Med 1986;315:41-5.

219. Winkle RA, Mason JW, Harrison DC. Tocainide for drug-resistant ventricular arrhythmias: efficacy, side effects, and lidocaine responsiveness for predicting tocainide success. Am Heart J 1980;100:1031-6.

220. Routledge PA. Tocainide. In: Taylor WJ, Caviness MHD, eds. A textbook for the clinical application of therapeutic drug monitoring. Irving, TX: Abbott Diagnostics, 1986:175-80.

221. Kutalek SP, Morganroth J, Horowitz LN. Tocainide: a new oral antiarrhythmic agent. Ann Intern Med 1985;103:387-91.

222. Mohiuddin SM, Esterbrooks D, Hilleman DE et al. Tocainide kinetics in congestive heart failure. Clin Pharmacol Ther 1983;34:596-603.

223. Holmes B, Brogden RN, Heel RC et al. Tocainide. A review of its pharmacological properties and therapeutic efficacy. Drugs 1983;26:93-123.

224. Braun J, Sorgel F, Engelmaier F et al. Pharmacokinetics of tocainide in patients with severe renal failure. Eur J Clin Pharmacol 1985;28:665-70.

225. Forrence E, Covinsky JO, Mullen C. A seizure induced by concurrent lidocaine-tocainide therapy-is it just a case of additive toxicity? Drug Intell Clin Pharm 1986;20:56-9.

226. Rosen MR, Wit AL, Hoffman BF. Electrophysiology and pharmacology of cardiac arrhythmias. VI. cardiac effects of verapamil. Am Heart J 1975;89:665-73.

227. Stone PH, Antman EM, Muller JE et al. Calcium channel blocking agents in the treatment of cardiovascular disorders. part II: hemodynamic effects and clinical applications. Ann Intern Med 1980;93:886-904.

228. Barbarash RA, Bauman JL, Lukazewski AA et al. Verapamil infusions in the treatment of atrial tachyarrhythmias. Crit Care Med 1986;14:886-8.

229. Kates RE. Calcium antagonists: pharmacokinetic properties. Drugs 1983;25:113-24.

230. Hamann SR, Blouin RA, McAllister RG. Clinical pharmacokinetics of verapamil. Clin Pharmacokinet 1984;9:26-41.

231. Singh BN, Roche AHG. Effects of intravenous verapamil on hemodynamics in patients with heart disease. Am Heart J 1977;94:593-9.

232. Krikler D. Verapamil in cardiology. Eur J Cardiol 1974;2:3-10.

233. McAllister RG, Kirsten EB. The pharmacology of verapamil. IV. Kinetic and dynamic effects after single intravenous and oral doses. Clin Pharmacol Ther 1982;31:418-26.

234. Hoon TJ, Bauman JL, Rodvold KA et al. The pharmacodynamic and pharmacokinetic differences of the D-and L-isomers of verapamil: implications in the treatment of paroxysmal supraventricular tachycardia. Am Heart J 1986;112:396-403.

235. Schwartz JB, Keefe DL, Kirsten E et al. Prolongation of verapamil elimination kinetics during chronic oral administration. Am Heart J 1982;104:198-203.

236. Singh BN. Intravenous calcium and verapamil—when the combination may be indicated. Int J Cardiol 1983;4:281-4.

237. Frishman W. Clinical pharmacology of the new beta-adrenergic blocking drugs. part 9. nadolol: a new long-acting beta-adrenoreceptor blocking drug. Am Heart J 1980;99:124-8.

238. Blanford MF. Nadolol (Corgard®-Squibb). Drug Intell Clin Pharm 1980;14:825-30.

239. Dasta JF. Metoprolol (Lopressor®-Geigy). Drug Intell Clin Pharm 1979;13:320-2.

240. Avery GS, ed. Drug treatment: principles and practice of clinical pharmacology and therapeutics. 2nd ed. New York: ADIS Press, 1980;653-4.

241. Heel RC, Brogden RN, Speight TM et al. Atenolol: a review of its pharmacological properties and therapeutic efficacy in angina pectoris and hypertension. Drugs 1979;17:425-60.

242. Clark BJ. Beta-adrenoceptor-blocking agents: are the pharmacologic differences relevant? Am Heart J 1982;104:334-46.

243. MacCarthy EP, Bloomfield SS. Labetolol. a review of its pharmacology, pharmacokinetics, clinical uses and adverse effects. Pharmacotherapy 1983;3:193-219.

244. Ryan JR. Clinical pharmacology of acebutolol. Am Heart J 1985;109:1131-6.

245. Hasenfub G, Shafer-Korting M, Knauf H et al. Pharmacokinetics of carteolol in relation to renal function. Eur J Clin Pharmacol 1985;29:461-5.

246. Stoll RW, Cavanaugh JH, MacLeod CM. Beta-blocking effect of single oral doses of carteolol. Clin Pharmacol Ther 1981;30:605-10.

247. Singh BN, Baky S, Nademanee K. Second generation calcium antagonists: search for greater selectivity and versatility. Am J Cardiol 1985;55:214B-21B.

248. Kupersmith J, Antman EM, Hoffman BF. In vivo electrophysiological effects of lidocaine in canine acute myocardial infarction. Circ Res 1975;36:84-91.

249. Wit AL, Rosen MR, Hoffman BF. Electrophysiology and pharmacology cardiac arrhythmias. VIII. cardiac effects of diphenylhydantoin. B. Am Heart J 1975;90:397-404.

250. El-Sherif N, Lazzara R. Re-entrant ventricular arrhythmias in the late myocardial infarction period: mechanism of action of diphenylhydantoin. Circulation 1978;57:465-72.

251. Illingworth DR. Lipid-lowering drugs: an overview of indications and optimum therapeutic use. Drugs 1987;33:259-79.

252. Schaefer EJ, Levy RI. Pathogenesis and management of lipoprotein disorders. N Engl J Med 1985;312:1300-10.

253. Perry RS. Contemporary recommendations for evaluating and treating hyperlipidemia. Clin Pharm 1986;5:113-27.

254. Knodel LC, Talbert RL. Adverse effects of hypolipidaemic drugs. Med Toxicol 1987;2:10-32.

255. Blum CB, Havlik RJ, Morganroth J. Cholestyramine: an effective, twice-daily dosage regimen. Ann Intern Med 1976;85:287-9.

256. McEvoy GK, ed. American hospital formulary service/drug information 87. Washington, DC: American Society of Hospital Pharmacists, 1987.

257. Brensike JF, Levy RI, Kelsey SF et al. Effects of therapy with cholestyramine on progression of coronary arteriosclerosis: results of the NHLBI type II coronary intervention study. Circulation 1984;69:313-24.

258. Levy RI, Brensike JF, Epstein SE et al. The influence of changes in lipid values induced by cholestyramine and diet on progression of coronary artery disease: results of the NHLBI type II coronary intervention study. Circulation 1984;69:325-37.

259. NIH Lipid Research Clinics Program. The lipid research clinics coronary primary prevention trial results: (I) reduction in incidence of coronary heart disease; (II) the relationship of reduction in incidence of coronary heart disease to cholesterol lowering. JAMA 1984;251:351-64, 365-74.

260. Anon. Lipid-lowering drugs. Med Lett Drugs Ther 1985;27:74-6.

261. Grundy SM. Modern management of hyperlipidemia. Compr Ther 1984;10(9):46-53.

262. Shaefer MS, Jungnickel PW, Jacobs EW et al. Acceptability of cholestyramine or colestipol combinations with six vehicles. Clin Pharm 1987;6:51-4.

263. West RJ, Lloyd JK, Leonard JV. Long-term follow-up of children with familial hypercholesterolaemia treated with cholestyramine. Lancet 1980;2:873-5.

264. Hoeg JM, Maher MB, Bailey KR et al. Effects of cholestyramine-neomycin treatment on plasma lipoprotein concentrations in type II hyperlipoproteinemia. Am J Cardiol 1985;55:1282-6.

265. Hofmann AF, Poley JR. Cholestyramine treatment of diarrhea associated with ileal resection. N Engl J Med 1969;281:397-402.

266. Burbige EJ, Milligan FD. Pseudomembranous colitis: association with antibiotics and therapy with cholestyramine. JAMA 1975;231:1157-8.

267. Pieroni RE, Fisher JG. Use of cholestyramine resin in digitoxin toxicity. JAMA 1981;245:1939-40.

268. Gugler R. Clinical pharmacokinetics of hypolipidaemic drugs. Clin Pharmacokinet 1978;3:425-39.

269. Gugler R, Kurten JW, Jensen CJ et al. Clofibrate disposition in renal failure and acute and chronic liver disease. Eur J Clin Pharmacol 1979;15:341-7.

270. Coronary Drug Project Research Group. Clofibrate and niacin in coronary heart disease. JAMA 1975;231:360-81.

271. Committee of Principal Investigators. A co-operative trial in the primary prevention of ischaemic heart disease using clofibrate. Br Heart J 1978;40:1069-118.

272. Kesaniemi YA, Grundy SM. Influence of gemfibrozil and clofibrate on metabolism of cholesterol and plasma triglycerides in man. JAMA 1984;251:2241-6.

273. Heel RC, Brogden RN, Pakes GE et al. Colestipol: a review of its pharmacological properties and therapeutic efficacy in patients with hypercholesterolaemia. Drugs 1980;19:161-80.

274. Kane JP, Malloy MJ, Tun P et al. Normalization of low-density-lipoprotein levels in heterozygous familial hypercholesterolemia with a combined drug regimen. N Engl J Med 1981;304:251-8.

275. Illingworth DR, Phillipson BE, Rapp JH et al. Colestipol plus nicotinic acid in treatment of heterozygous familial hypercholesterolaemia. Lancet 1981;1:296-8.

276. Illingworth DR, Sexton GJ. Hypocholesterolemic effects of mevinolin in patients with heterozygous familial hypercholesterolemia. J Clin Invest 1984;74:1972-8.

277. Havel RJ, Hunninghake DB, Illingworth DR et al. Mevinolin in the therapy of familial hypercholesterolemia. Circulation 1987;72(Suppl 3):198.

278. East C, Grundy SM, Bilheimer DW. Normal cholesterol levels with lovastatin (mevinolin) therapy in a child with homozygous familial hypercholesterolemia following liver transplantation. JAMA 1986;256:2843-8.

279. Mevacor product information. Merck Sharpe and Dohme. Aug 1987.

280. East CA, Grundy SM, Bilheimer DW. Preliminary report: treatment of type 3 hyperlipoproteinemia with mevinolin. Metabolism 1986;35:97-8.

281. Mol MJ, Erkelens DW, Leuven JA et al. Effects of synvinolin (MK-733) on plasma lipids in familial hypercholesterolemia. Lancet 1986;2:936-9.

282. Kaukola S, Manninen V, Malkonen M et al. Gemfibrozil in the treatment of dyslipidaemias in middle-aged male survivors of myocardial infarction. Acta Med Scand 1981;209:69-73.

283. Frick MH, Elo O, Haapa K et al. Helsinki heart study: primary-prevention trial with gemfibrozil in middle-aged men with dyslipidemia. N Engl J Med 1987;317:1237-45.

284. Samuel P. Effects of gemfibrozil on serum lipids. Am J Med 1983;74(5A):23-7.

285. Grundy SM, Bilheimer DW. Inhibition of 3-hydroxy-3-methylglutaryl-CoA reductase by mevinolin in familial

hypercholesterolemia heterozygotes: effects on cholesterol balance. Proc Natl Acad Sci 1984;81:2538-42.

286. Hoeg JM, Maher MB, Zech LA et al. Effectiveness of mevinolin on plasma lipoprotein concentrations in type II hyperlipoproteinemia. Am J Cardiol 1986;57:933-9.

287. Illingworth DR. Mevinolin plus colestipol in therapy for severe heterozygous familial hypercholesterolemia. Ann Intern Med 1984;101:598-604.

288. Tobert JA, Bell GD, Birtwell J et al. Cholesterol-lowering effect of mevinolin, an inhibitor of 3-hydroxy-3-methylglutaryl-coenzyme A reductase, in healthy volunteers. J Clin Invest 1982;69:913-9.

289. The Lovastatin Study Group II. Therapeutic response to lovastatin (mevinolin) in nonfamilial hypercholesterolemia: a multicenter study. JAMA 1986;256:2829-34.

290. Vega GL, Grundy SM. Treatment of primary moderate hypercholesterolemia with lovastatin (mevinolin) and colestipol. JAMA 1987;257:33-8.

291. Illingworth DR. Comparative efficacy of once versus twice daily mevinolin in the therapy of familial hypercholesterolemia. Clin Pharmacol Ther 1986;40:338-43.

292. Cathcart-Rake WF, Dujovne CA. The treatment of hyperlipoproteinemias. Ration Drug Ther 1979;13(July):1-4.

293. NIH Consensus Conference. Treatment of hypertriglyceridemia. JAMA 1984;251:1196-200.

294. Canner PL. Mortality in coronary drug project patients during a nine-year post-treatment period. J Am Coll Cardiol 1985;5(2/2/Abstracts):442. Abstract.

295. Heel RC, Brogden RN, Speight TM et al. Probucol: a review of its pharmacological properties and therapeutic use in patients with hypercholesterolaemia. Drugs 1978;15:409-28.

296. Mellies MJ, Gartside PS, Glatfelter L et al. Effects of probucol on plasma cholesterol, high and low density lipoprotein cholesterol, and apolipoproteins A1 and A2 in adults with primary familial hypercholesterolemia. Metabolism 1980;29:956-64.

297. Atmeh RF, Stewart JM, Boag DE et al. The hypolipidemic action of probucol: a study of its effects on high and low density lipoproteins. J Lipid Res 1983;24:588-95.

298. Kesaniemi YA, Grundy SM. Influence of probucol on cholesterol and lipoprotein metabolism in man. J Lipid Res 1984;25:780-90.

299. McCaughan D. The long-term effects of probucol on serum lipid levels. Arch Intern Med 1981;141:1428-32.

300. Anon. Choice of cholesterol-lowering drugs. Med Lett Drugs Ther 1988;30:85-8.

301. Genest J, comp. Hypertension, physiopathology and treatment. 2nd ed. New York: McGraw-Hill, 1986.

302. Mann JFE. Mechanisms of the antihypertensive action of captopril. Contr Nephrol 1984;43:171-81.

303. Veterans Administration Co-operative Study Group on Antihypertensive Agents. Racial differences in response to low-dose captopril are abolished by the addition of hydrochlorothiazide. Br J Clin Pharmacol 1982;14:97S-101S.

304. Veterans Administration Cooperative Study Group on Antihypertensive Agents. Low-dose captopril for the treatment of mild to moderate hypertension. I. Results of a 14-week trial. Arch Intern Med 1984;144:1947-53.

305. Veterans Administration Cooperative Study Group on Antihypertensive Agents. Time course of antihypertensive effect of low-dose captopril in mild to moderate hypertension. Clin Pharmacol Ther 1984;36:307-14.

306. Schuna AA, Schmidt GR, Pitterle ME et al. Managing hypertension with captopril and hydrochlorothiazide using two versus three daily doses. Clin Pharm 1985;4:65-7.

307. Koffer H, Vlasses PH, Ferguson RK et al. Captopril in diuretic-treated hypertensive patients. JAMA 1980;244:2532-5.

308. Duchin KL, Singhvi SM, Willard DA et al. Captopril kinetics. Clin Pharmacol Ther 1982;31:452-8.

309. McKinstry DN, Singhvi SM, Kripalani KJ et al. Disposition and cardiovascular-endocrine effects of an orally active angiotensin-converting enzyme inhibitor, SQ 14,225, in normal subjects. Clin Pharmacol Ther 1978;23:121-2.

310. Migdalof BH, Wong KK, Lan SJ et al. Evidence for dynamic interconversion of captopril and its disulfide metabolites in vivo. Fed Proc 1980;39:757.

311. Duchin KL, Pierides AM, Heald A et al. Elimination kinetics of captopril in patients with renal failure. Kidney Int 1984;25:942-7.

312. Frolich ED, Cooper RA, Lewis EJ. Review of the overall experience of captopril in hypertension. Arch Intern Med 1984;144:1441-4.

313. Groel JT, Tadros SS, Dreslinski GR et al. Long-term antihypertensive therapy with captopril. Hypertension 1983;5(Suppl III):III-145-51.

314. Hricik DE, Browning PJ, Kopelman R et al. Captopril-induced functional renal insufficiency in patients with bilateral renal-artery stenosis or renal-artery stenosis in a solitary kidney. N Engl J Med 1983;308:373-6.

315. Watson AM, Bell GM, Muir AL et al. Captopril/diuretic combinations in severe renovascular disease: a cautionary note. Lancet 1983;2:404-5.

316. Van Zwieten PA, Thoolen MJMC, Timmermans PBMWM. The hypotensive activity and side effects of methyldopa, clonidine, and guanfacine. Hypertension 1984;6(Suppl II):II-28-33.

317. Weber MA, Drayer JIM. Clinical experience with rate-controlled delivery of antihypertensive therapy by a transdermal system. Am Heart J 1984;108:231-6.

318. Washton AM, Resnick RB. Clonidine in opiate withdrawal: review and appraisal of clinical findings. Pharmacotherapy 1981;1:140-6.

319. Bond WS. Psychiatric indications for clonidine: the neuropharmacologic and clinical basis. J Clin Psychopharmacol 1986;6:81-7.

320. Nakagawa S, Yamamoto Y, Koiwaya Y. Ventricular tachycardia induced by clonidine withdrawal. Br Heart J 1985;53:654-8.

321. Peters RW, Hamilton BP, Hamilton J et al. Cardiac arrhythmias after abrupt clonidine withdrawal. Clin Pharmacol Ther 1983;34:435-9.

322. Bennett WM, Muther RS, Parker RA et al. Drug therapy in renal failure: dosing guidelines for adults. Part II. Ann Intern Med 1980;93:286-325.

323. Lilja M, Jounela AJ, Juustila H et al. Antihypertensive effects of clonidine. Clin Pharmacol Ther 1979;25:864-9.

324. Frisk-Holmberg M. The effectiveness of clonidine as an antihypertensive in a two-dose regimen. Acta Med Scand 1980;207:43-5.

325. Jain AK, Ryan JR, Vargas R et al. Efficacy and acceptability of different dosage schedules of clonidine. Clin Pharmacol Ther 1977;21:382-7.

326. Shaw JE. Pharmacokinetics of nitroglycerin and clonidine delivered by the transdermal route. Am Heart J 1984;108:217-23.

327. Frisk-Holmberg M, Paalzow L, Wibell L. Relationship between the cardiovascular effects and steady-state kinetics of clonidine in hypertension. Eur J Clin Pharmacol 1984;26:309-13.

328. Davies DS, Wing LMH, Reid JL et al. Pharmacokinetics and concentration-effect relationships of intravenous and oral clonidine. Clin Pharmacol Ther 1977;21:593-601.

329. Dollery CT, Davies DS, Draffan GH et al. Clinical pharmacology and pharmacokinetics of clonidine. Clin Pharmacol Ther 1976;19:11-7.

330. MacGregor TR, Matzek KM, Keirns JJ et al. Pharmacokinetics of transdermally delivered clonidine. Clin Pharmacol Ther 1985;38:278-84.

331. Wing LMH, Reid JL, Davies DS et al. Pharmacokinetic and concentration-effect relationships of clonidine in essential hypertension. Eur J Clin Pharmacol 1977;12:463-9.

332. Frisk-Holmberg M, Edlund PO, Paalzow L. Pharmacokinetics of clonidine and its relation to the hypotensive effect in patients. Br J Clin Pharmacol 1978;6:227-32.

333. Keranen A, Nykanen S, Taskinen J. Pharmacokinetics and side-effects of clonidine. Eur J Clin Pharmacol 1978;13:97-101.

334. Arndts D, Arndts K. Pharmacokinetic and pharmacodynamics of transdermally administered clonidine. Eur J Clin Pharmacol 1984;26:79-85.

335. Grattan CEH, Kennedy CTC. Allergic contact dermatitis to transdermal clonidine. Contact Dermatitis 1985;12:225-6.

336. Hammar M, Berg G. Clonidine in the treatment of menopausal flushing. Acta Obstet Gynecol Scand 1985;132(Suppl):29-31.

337. Huysmans FTM, Thien T, Koene RA. Acute treatment of hypertension with slow infusion of diazoxide. Arch Intern Med 1983;143:882-4.

338. Pearson RM, Breckenridge AM. Renal function, protein binding and pharmacological response to diazoxide. Br J Clin Pharmacol 1976;3:169-75.

339. O'Malley K, Velasco M, Pruitt A et al. Decreased plasma protein binding of diazoxide in uremia. Clin Pharmacol Ther 1975;18:53-8.

340. Pearson RM. Pharmacokinetics and response to diazoxide in renal failure. Clin Pharmacokinet 1977;2:198-204.

341. Koch-Weser J. Hypertensive emergencies. N Engl J Med 1977;290:211-4.

342. Sellers EM, Koch-Weser J. Influence of intravenous injection rate on protein binding and vascular activity of diazoxide. Ann NY Acad Sci 1973;226:319-32.

343. Sadee W, Segal J, Finn C. Diazoxide urine and plasma levels in humans by stable-isotope dilution-mass fragmentography. J Pharmacokinet Biopharm 1973;1:295-305.

344. Charles MA, Danforth E. Nonketoacidotic hyperglycemia and coma during intravenous diazoxide therapy in uremia. Diabetes 1971;20:501-3.

345. Andreasen F, Botker HE, Christensen JH et al. The biological relevance of the protein binding of diazoxide. Acta Pharmacol Toxicol 1985;57:30-5.

346. Gomez HJ, Cirillo VJ, Jones KH. The clinical pharmacology of enalapril. J Hypertension 1983;1(Suppl 1):65-70.

347. Ferguson RK, Vlasses PH, Swanson BN et al. Effects of enalapril, a new converting enzyme inhibitor, in hypertension. Clin Pharmacol Ther 1982;32:48-53.

348. Irvin JD, Till AE, Vlasses PH et al. Bioavailability of enalapril maleate. Clin Pharmacol Ther 1984;35:248. Abstract.

349. Ulm EH, Hichens M, Gomez HJ et al. Enalapril maleate and a lysine analogue (MK-521): disposition in man. Br J Clin Pharmacol 1982;14:357-62.

350. Swanson BN, Vlasses PH, Ferguson RK et al. Influence of food on the bioavailability of enalapril. J Pharm Sci 1984;73:1655-7.

351. Vlasses PH, Larijani GE, Conner DP et al. Enalapril, a nonsulfhydryl angiotensin-converting enzyme inhibitor. Clin Pharm 1985;4:27-40.

352. Lowenthal DT, Irvin JD, Merrill D et al. The effect of renal function on enalapril kinetics. Clin Pharmacol Ther 1985;38:661-6.

353. Schwartz JB, Taylor A, Abernethy D et al. Pharmacokinetics and pharmacodynamics of enalapril in patients with congestive heart failure and patients with hypertension. J Cardiovasc Pharmacol 1985;7:767-76.

354. Davies RO, Irvin JD, Kramsch DK et al. Enalapril worldwide experience. Am J Med 1984;77(Suppl 2A):23-35.

355. Bender W, La France N, Walker WG. Mechanism of deterioration in renal function in patients with renovascular hypertension treated with enalapril. Hypertension 1984;6(Suppl I):I-193-7.

356. Edwards CRW, Padfield PL. Angiotensin-converting enzyme inhibitors: past, present, and bright future. Lancet 1985;1:30-4.

357. Meacham RH, Emmett M, Kyriakopoulos AA et al. Disposition of C-14-guanabenz in patients with essential hypertension. Clin Pharmacol Ther 1980;27:44-52.

358. Hansson L, Pascual A, Julius S. Comparison of guanadrel and guanethidine. Clin Pharmacol Ther 1973;14:204-8.

359. Chrysant SG, Frohlich ED. Comparison of the antihypertensive effectiveness of guanadrel and guanethidine. Curr Ther Res 1976;19:379-85.

360. Walter IE, Khandelwal J, Falkner F et al. The relationship of plasma guanethidine levels to adrenergic blockade. Clin Pharmacol Ther 1975;18:571-80.

361. McMartin C, Simpson P. The absorption and metabolism of guanethidine in hypertensive patients requiring

different doses of the drug. Clin Pharmacol Ther 1971;12:73-7.

362. Rahn KH, Goldberg LI. Comparison of antihypertensive efficacy, intestinal absorption, and excretion of guanethidine in hypertensive patients. Clin Pharmacol Ther 1969;10:858-66.

363. Hengstmann JH, Falkner FC. Disposition of guanethidine during chronic oral therapy. Eur J Clin Pharmacol 1979;15:121-5.

364. Jain AK, Hiremath A, Michael R et al. Clonidine and guanfacine in hypertension. Clin Pharmacol Ther 1985;37:271-6.

365. Jerie P. Clinical experience with guanfacine in long-term treatment of hypertension. Part I: efficacy and dosage. Br J Clin Pharmacol 1980;10:37S-47S.

366. Frisk-Holmberg M, Wibell L. Concentration-dependent blood pressure effects of guanfacine. Clin Pharmacol Ther 1986;39:169-72.

367. Kirch W, Kohler H, Braun W. Elimination of guanfacine in patients with normal and impaired renal function. Br J Clin Pharmacol 1980;10:33S-5S.

368. Kiechel JR. Pharmacokinetics and metabolism of guanfacine in man: a review. Br J Clin Pharmacol 1980;10:25S-32S.

369. Lipe S, Moulds RFW. Comparison of the effects of endralazine, hydralazine and verapamil on human isolated arteries and veins. Clin Exp Pharmacol Physiol 1982;9:613-20.

370. Cameron HA, Ramsay LE. The lupus syndrome induced by hydralazine: a common complication with low dose treatment. Br Med J 1984;289:410-2.

371. O'Malley K, Segal JL, Israili ZH et al. Duration of hydralazine action in hypertension. Clin Pharmacol Ther 1975;18:581-6.

372. Silas JH, Ramsay LE, Freestone S. Hydralazine once daily in hypertension. Br Med J 1982;284:1602-4.

373. Shepherd AMM, Irvine NA, Ludden TM. Effect of food on blood hydralazine levels and response in hypertension. Clin Pharmacol Ther 1984;36:14-8.

374. Koch-Weser J. Hypertensive emergencies. N Engl J Med 1977;290:211-4.

375. Zacest R, Koch-Weser J. Relation of hydralazine plasma concentration to dosage and hypotensive action. Clin Pharmacol Ther 1972;13:420-5.

376. Shepherd AMM, Ludden TM, McNay JL et al. Hydralazine kinetics after single and repeated oral doses. Clin Pharmacol Ther 1980;28:804-11.

377. Ludden TM, Shepherd AMM, McNay JL et al. Hydralazine kinetics in hypertensive patients after intravenous administration. Clin Pharmacol Ther 1980;28:736-42.

378. Shen DD, Hosler JP, Schroder RL et al. Pharmacokinetics of hydralazine and its acid-labile hydrazone metabolites in relation to acetylator phenotype. J Pharmacokinet Biopharm 1980;8:53-68.

379. Reece PA, Cozamanis I, Zacest R. Kinetics of hydralazine and its main metabolites in slow and fast acetylators. Clin Pharmacol Ther 1980;28:769-78.

380. Talseth T. Studies on hydralazine. III. Bioavailability of hydralazine in man. Eur J Clin Pharmacol 1976;10:395-401.

381. Talseth T. Elimination rate and steady-state concentration in patients with impaired renal function. Eur J Clin Pharmacol 1976;10:311-7.

382. Shapiro KS, Pinn VW, Harrington JT et al. Immune complex glomerulonephritis in hydralazine-induced SLE. Am J Kidney Dis 1984;3:270-4.

383. Naparstek Y, Kopolovic J, Tur-Kaspa R et al. Focal glomerulonephritis in the course of hydralazine-induced lupus syndrome. Arthritis Rheum 1984;27:822-5.

384. Bjorck S, Svalander C, Westberg G. Hydralazine-associated glomerulonephritis. Acta Med Scand 1985;218:261-9.

385. Wright JM, McLeod PJ, McCullough W. Antihypertensive efficacy of a single bedtime dose of methyldopa. Clin Pharmacol Ther 1976;20:733-7.

386. Bennett WM, Muther RS, Parker RA et al. Drug therapy in renal failure: dosing guidelines for adults, part II. Ann Intern Med 1980;93:286-325.

387. Frolich ED. Inhibition of adrenergic function in the treatment of hypertension. Arch Intern Med 1974;133:1033-48.

388. Kwan KC, Foltz EL, Breault GO et al. Pharmacokinetics of methyldopa in man. J Pharmacol Exp Ther 1976;198:264-77.

389. Stenbaek O, Myhre E, Rugstad E et al. Pharmacokinetics of methyldopa in healthy man. Eur J Clin Pharmacol 1977;12:117-23.

390. Walson PD. Metabolic disposition and cardiovascular effects of methyldopa in unanesthetized Rhesus monkeys. J Pharmacol Exp Ther 1975;195:151-8.

391. Myhre E, Rugstad HE, Hansen T. Clinical pharmacokinetics of methyldopa. Clin Pharmacokinet 1982;7:221-33.

392. Johnson P, Kitchin AH, Lowther CP et al. Treatment of hypertension with methyldopa. Br Med J 1966;1:133-7.

393. Lowenthal DT, Onesti G, Mutterperl R et al. Long-term clinical effects, bioavailability, and kinetics of minoxidil in relation to renal function. J Clin Pharmacol 1978;18:500-8.

394. Shen D, O'Malley K, Gibaldi M et al. Pharmacodynamics of minoxidil as a guide for individualizing dosage regimens in hypertension. Clin Pharmacol Ther 1975;17:593-8.

395. Gottlieb TB, Thomas RC, Chidsey CA. Pharmacokinetic studies of minoxidil. Clin Pharmacol Ther 1972;13:436-41.

396. Hall D, Charocopos F, Froer KL et al. ECG changes during long-term minoxidil therapy for severe hypertension. Arch Intern Med 1979;139:790-4.

397. Marquez-Julio A, Uldall PR. Pericardial effusions associated with minoxidil. Lancet 1977;2:816-7.

398. Sobota JT, Martin WB, Carlson RG et al. Minoxidil: right atrial cardiac pathology in animals and in man. Circulation 1980;62:376-87.

399. Vesey CJ, Cole PV. Blood cyanide and thiocyanate concentrations produced by long-term therapy with sodium nitroprusside Br J Anaesth 1985;57:148-55.

400. Gordillo-Paniagua G, Velasquez-Jones L, Martini R et al. Sodium nitroprusside treatment of severe arterial hypertension in children. J Pediatr 1975;87:799-802.

401. AMA Committee on Hypertension. The treatment of malignant hypertension and hypertensive emergencies. JAMA 1974;228(13):1673-9.

402. Schultz V, Bonn R, Kindler J. Kinetics of elimination of thiocyanate in 7 healthy subjects and in 8 subjects with renal failure. Klin Wochenschr 1979;57:243-7.

403. Cottrell JE, Patel K, Turndorf H et al. Intracranial pressure changes induced by sodium nitroprusside in patients with intracranial mass lesions. J Neurosurg 1978;48:329-31.

404. Creiss L, Tremblay NAG, Davies DW. The toxicity of sodium nitroprusside. Can Anaesth Soc J 1976;23:480-5.

405. Rieves RD. Importance of symptoms in recognizing nitroprusside toxicity. South Med J 1984;77:1035-7.

406. Grahm RM, Pettinger WA. Prazosin. N Engl J Med 1979;300:232-6.

407. Dynon MK, Jarrott B, Drummer O et al. Pharmacokinetics of prazosin in normotensive subjects after low oral doses. Clin Pharmacokinet 1980;5:583-90.

408. Stokes GS, Weber MA. Prazosin: preliminary report and comparative studies with other antihypertensive agents. Br Med J 1974;2:298-300.

409. Bateman DN, Hobbs DC, Twomey TM et al. Prazosin, pharmacokinetics and concentration effect. Eur J Clin Pharmacol 1979;16:177-81.

410. Chau NP, Flouvat BL, Le Roux E et al. Prazosin kinetics in essential hypertension. Clin Pharmacol Ther 1980;28:6-11.

411. Vincent J, Meredith PA, Reid JL et al. Clinical pharmacokinetics of prazosin-1985. Clin Pharmacokinet 1985;10:144-54.

412. Jaillon P. Clinical pharmacokinetics of prazosin. Clin Pharmacokinet 1980;5:365-76.

413. Baughman RA, Arnold S, Benet LZ et al. Altered prazosin pharmacokinetics in congestive heart failure. Eur J Clin Pharmacol 1980;17:425-8.

414. Brogden RN, Heel RC, Speight TM et al. Prazosin: a review of its pharmacological properties and therapeutic efficacy in hypertension. Drugs 1977;14:163-97.

415. Weber KT, Kinasewitz GT, West JS et al. Long-term vasodilator therapy with trimazosin in chronic cardiac failure. N Engl J Med 1980;303:242-50.

416. Stitzel RE. The biological fate of reserpine. Pharmacol Rev 1977;28:179-205.

417. Zsoter TT, Johnson GE, DeVeber GA et al. Excretion and metabolism of reserpine in renal failure. Clin Pharmacol Ther 1973;14:325-30.

418. McMahon FG. Management of essential hypertension. Mount Kisco, New York: Futura Publishing, 1978:344-7.

419. Hypertension-Stroke Cooperative Study Group. Effect of antihypertensive treatment on stroke recurrence. JAMA 1974;229:409-18.

420. Sperzel WD, Luther RR, Glassman HN. Clinical trials with terazosin. General methods. Am J Med 1986;80(Suppl 5B):25-9.

421. Chrysant SG. Experience with terazosin administered in combination with other antihypertensive agents. Am J Med 1986;80(Suppl 5B):55-61.

422. Jungers P, Ganeval D, Pertuiset N et al. Influence of renal insufficiency on the pharmacokinetics and pharmacodynamics of terazosin. Am J Med 1986;80(Suppl 5B):94-9.

423. Sonders RC. Pharmacokinetics of terazosin. Am J Med 1986;80(Suppl 5B):20-4.

424. Garcia JY, Vidt DG. Current management of hypertensive emergencies. Drugs 1987;34:263-78.

425. Davidson RC, Bursten SL, Keeley PA et al. Oral nifedipine for the treatment of patients with severe hypertension. Am J Med 1985;79(Suppl 4A):26-30.

426. Bertel O, Conen LD. Treatment of hypertensive emergencies with the calcium blocker nifedipine. Am J Med 1985;79(Suppl 4A):31-5..

427. Burris JF. Hypertensive emergencies. Am Fam Physician 1985;32:97-109.

428. Cressman MD, Vidt DG, Gifford RW et al. Intravenous labetalol in the management of severe hypertension and hypertensive emergencies. Am Heart J 1984;107:980-5.

429. Parker JO. Nitrate therapy in stable angina pectoris. N Engl J Med 1987;316:1635-42.

430. Mason DT, ed. Symposium on vasodilator and inotropic therapy of heart failure. Am J Med 1978;65:101-216.

431. Gould L, Reddy CVR, eds. Vasodilator therapy for cardiac disorders. Mount Kisco N.Y. Futura Pulishing, 1979.

432. Abrams J. Pharmacology of nitroglycerin and long-acting nitrates. Am J Cardiol 1985;56:12A-8A.

433. Abrams J. Nitroglycerin and long-acting nitrates in clinical practice. Am J Med 1983;74(Suppl):85-94.

434. Flugelman MY, Shefer A, Ben-David Y et al. Effect of sustained release isosorbide dinitrate on exercise performance. Cardiology 1985;72:123-8.

435. Tremblay G. High-dose isosorbide dinitrate in management of angina pectoris. Am Heart J 1985;110:280-4.

436. Udhoji VN, Heng MK. Hemodynamic effects of high-dose sustained-action oral isosorbide dinitrate in stable angina. Am J Med 1984;76:234-40.

437. Abrams J. Nitrate tolerance and dependence. Am Heart J 1980;99:113-23.

438. Warren SE, Francis GS. Nitroglycerin and nitrate esters. Am J Med 1978;65:53-62.

439. Sporl-Radun S, Betzien G, Kaufmann B et al. Effects and pharmacokinetics of isosorbide dinitrate in normal man. Eur J Clin Pharmacol 1980;18:237-44.

440. Fung H-L. Pharmacokinetics of nitroglycerin and long-acting nitrate esters. Am J Med 1983;74(Suppl. 6B):13-20.

441. Anon. Oral isosorbide dinitrate for angina. Med Lett Drugs Ther 1979;21:88.

442. Markis JE, Gorlin R, Mills RM et al. Sustained effect of orally administered isosorbide dinitrate on exercise performance of patients with angina pectoris. Am J Cardiol 1979;43:265-71.

443. Aronow WS. Clinical use of nitrates. I. Nitrates as anti-anginal drugs. II. Nitrates in congestive heart failure. Mod Concepts Cardiovasc Dis 1979;48:31-5, 37-42.

444. Parker JO, Vankoughnett KA, Farrell B. Nitroglycerin lingual spray: clinical efficacy and dose-response relation. Am J Cardiol 1986;57:1-5.

445. Abrams J. Pharmacology of nitroglycerin and long-acting nitrates and their usefulness in the treatment of chronic congestive heart failure. In: Gould L, Reddy CVR, eds. Vasodilator therapy for cardiac disorders. Mount Kisco, N.Y.: Futura Publishing, 1979;129-67.

446. Armstrong PW, Armstrong JA, Marks GS. Blood levels after sublingual nitroglycerin. Circulation 1979;59:585-8.

447. Bogaert MG. Clinical pharmacokinetics of organic nitrates. Clin Pharmacokinet 1983;8:410-21.

448. Schrader BJ. Bauman JL, Zeller FP et al. Acceptance of transcutaneous nitroglycerin patches by patients with angina pectoris. Pharmacotherapy 1986;6:83-6.

449. Copelan HW. Burning sensation and potency of nitroglycerin sublingually. JAMA 1972;219:176-9.

450. Baaske DM, Amann AH, Wagenknecht DM et al. Nitroglycerin compatibility with intravenous fluid filters, containers, and administration sets. Am J Hosp Pharm 1980;37:201-5.

451. Amann AH, Baaske DM, Wagenknecht DM. Plastic I.V. container for nitroglycerin. Am J Hosp Pharm 1980;37:618. Letter.

452. Chatterjee K, Parmley WW. The role of vasodilator therapy in heart failure. Prog Cardiovasc Dis 1977;19:301-25.

453. Cohn JN, Franciosa JA. Vasodilator therapy of cardiac failure. N Engl J Med 1977;297:27-31, 254-8.

454. Chatterjee K, Ports TA, Brundage BH et al. Oral hydralazine in chronic heart failure: sustained beneficial hemodynamic effects. Ann Intern Med 1980;92:600-4.

455. Franciosa JA, Cohn JN. Sustained hemodynamic effects without tolerance during long-term isosorbide dinitrate treatment of chronic left ventricular failure. Am J Cardiol 1980;45:648-54.

456. Colucci WS, Wynne J, Holman BL et al. Long-term therapy of heart failure with prazosin: a randomized double blind trial. Am J Cardiol 1980;45:337-44.

457. Orlando JR, Danahy DT, Lurie M et al. Effect of trimazosin on hemodynamics in chronic heart failure. Clin Pharmacol Ther 1978;24:531-6.

458. Ader R, Chatterjee K, Ports T et al. Immediate and sustained hemodynamic and clinical improvement in chronic heart failure by an oral angiotensin-converting enzyme inhibitor. Circulation 1980;61:931-7.

459. Hill NS, Antman EM, Green LH et al. Intravenous nitroglycerin: a review of pharmacology, indications, therapeutic effects and complications. Chest 1981;79:69-76.

460. Awan NA, Mason DT. Oral vasodilator therapy with prazosin in severe congestive heart failure. Am Heart J 1981;101:695-700.

461. Faxon DP, Halperin JL, Creager MA et al. Angiotensin inhibition in severe heart failure: acute central and limb hemodynamic effects of captopril with observations on sustained oral therapy. Am Heart J 1981;101:548-56.

462. Hermiller JB, Magorien RD, Leithe ME et al. Clonidine in congestive heart failure: a vasodilator with negative inotropic effects. Am J Cardiol 1983;51:791-5.

463. Schwartz AB, Chatterjee K. Vasodilator therapy in chronic congestive heart failure. Drugs 1983;26:148-73.

464. Todd PA, Heel RC. Enalapril: a review of its pharmacodynamic and pharmacokinetic properties, and therapeutic use in hypertension and congestive heart failure. Drugs 1986;31:198-248.

465. Walsh RW, Porter CB, Starling MR et al. Beneficial hemodynamic effects of intravenous and oral diltiazem in severe congestive heart failure. J Am Coll Cardiol 1984;3:1044-50.

466. Fifer MA, Colucci WS, Lorell BH et al. Inotropic, vascular and neuroendocrine effects of nifedipine in heart failure: comparison with nitroprusside. J Am Coll Cardiol 1985;5:731-7.

467. Anon. Drugs for hypertensive emergencies. Med Lett Drugs Ther 1987;29:18-20.

468. Parker JO, Farrell B, Lahey KA et al. Effect of intervals between doses on the development of tolerance to isosorbide dinitrate. N Engl J Med 1987;316:1440-4.

469. van Schaik BA, Geyskes GG, Boer P. Lisinopril in hypertensive patients with and without renal failure. Eur J Clin Pharmacol 1987;31:11-6.

470. Karlberg BE, Rosenqvist U. Antihypertensive and hormonal effects of lisinopril, a new angiotensin converting enzyme (ACE) inhibitor in patients with renovascular hypertension. Acta Med Scand 1986;714(Suppl):33-42.

471. Byyny RL, Nies AS, LoVerde ME et al. A double-blind, randomized, controlled trial comparing pinacidil to hydralazine in essential hypertension. Clin Pharmacol Ther 1987;42:50-7.

472. Krusell LR, Christensen CK, Lederballe Pedersen O. Renal effects of pinacidil in hypertensive patients on chronic beta-blocker therapy. Eur J Clin Pharmacol 1986;30:641-7.

473. Singh BN, Nademanee K. Sotalol: a beta blocker with unique antiarrhythmic properties. Am Heart J 1987;114:121-39.

28:00 CENTRAL NERVOUS SYSTEM AGENTS

28:08 ANALGESICS AND ANTIPYRETICS

28:08.4 NONSTEROIDAL ANTI-INFLAMMATORY AGENTS
General References: 29

Aspirin   Various

Pharmacology. An analgesic, antipyretic and anti-inflammatory agent. Anti-inflammatory properties are related to impairment of prostaglandin biosynthesis. Unlike other nonsteroidal anti-inflammatory agents, its anti-platelet effect is irreversible (due to transacetylation of platelet cyclooxygenase) for the life of the platelet (8–11 days). Salicylates without acetyl groups (eg, sodium salicylate) have no useful antiplatelet effect, but retain analgesic, antipyretic and anti-inflammatory activity.[1] Low doses (1–2 g/day) decrease urate excretion while high doses (over 5 g/day) induce uricosuria.[2] See Antiplatelet Drug Therapy Summary, p 463.

Administration and Adult Dose. PO for fever or minor pain 325–975 mg q 4 hr, to maximum of 4 g/day. **PO for rheumatoid arthritis** 3–6 g/day in divided doses. **PO for acute rheumatic fever** 5–8 g/day in 1 g divided doses. **PO for transient ischemic attacks** 1300 mg/day in 2 or 4 divided doses. **PO for myocardial infarction risk reduction** 300–325 mg/day.

Dosage Individualization. Uremia and/or reduced albumin levels are likely to produce higher unbound drug levels which may increase pharmacologic or toxic effects.[3] Salicylate kinetics appear to be highly variable in patients over 70 yr; 50% may be slow eliminators.[4]

Pediatric Dose. PO as an analgesic/antipyretic. See Patient Instructions. 65 mg/kg/day in 4–6 divided doses, to maximum of 3.6 g/day. Alternatively (2–3 yr) 162 mg q 4 hr; (4–5 yr) 243 mg q 4 hr; (6–8 yr) 324 mg q 4 hr; (9–10 yr) 405 mg q 4 hr; (11 yr) 486 mg q 4 hr; (12 yr and over) 648 mg q 4 hr. **PO for juvenile rheumatoid arthritis** 90–130 mg/kg/day in divided doses. **PO for acute rheumatic fever** 100 mg/kg/day in divided doses initially, then 75 mg/kg/day in divided doses for 4–6 weeks. See Precautions.

Dosage Forms. EC Cap 325, 500 mg; **Cap** 325 mg; **Chew Tab** 81 mg; **EC Tab** 325, 500, 650, 975 mg; **SR Tab** 650, 800 mg; **Tab** 65, 81, 325, 500, 650 mg; **Supp** 60, 120, 130, 195, 200, 300, 325, 600, 650, 1200 mg.

Patient Instructions. Children and teenagers should not use this medication for chicken pox or flu symptoms before a physician or pharmacist is consulted about Reye's syndrome, a rare but serious illness. This drug should be taken with food, milk or a full glass of water to minimize stomach upset; report any symptoms of GI ulceration or bleeding.

Pharmacokinetics. *Onset and Duration.* PO onset of analgesia 30 min.[5]
   Plasma Levels. (Salicylate) 200–300 mcg/ml for rheumatic diseases, often accompanied by mild toxic symptoms.[5] "Salicylism" is manifested by tinnitus in the range of 200–400 mcg/ml;[6] severe or fatal toxicity may result from levels over 900 mcg/ml 6 hr after acute ingestion.[7]
   Fate. Rapidly absorbed from GI tract, and rapidly hydrolyzed to salicylic acid (salicylate) which is also pharmacologically active.[5] A single analgesic-antipyretic dose produces peak salicylate levels of 30–60 mcg/ml. About 95% of salicylate is plasma protein bound in normals; 74–83% plasma protein bound in uremia.[3] Protein binding decreases with age probably due to

decreasing albumin.[4] Salicylate is metabolized primarily in the liver to four metabolites (salicyluric acid, phenolic- and acyl- glucuronides, and gentisic acid). In low doses and acidic urine, 5% free salicylate is excreted unchanged in urine, with up to 85% at high doses and alkaline urine.[5,8]

$t_{1/2}$. (Aspirin) 14–20 min;[9] (salicylate) dose-dependent: 2.4 hr with 0.25 g; 5 hr with 1 g; 6.1 hr with 1.3 g; 19 hr with 10–20 g.[10]

Adverse Reactions. See Plasma Levels. Hearing impairment, visual disturbances, nausea and vomiting, and mental confusion are reported. GI upset and occult bleeding are frequent with rare acute hemorrhage from gastric erosion. Rare hepatotoxicity occurs, particularly in children with rheumatic fever or rheumatoid arthritis, and adults with SLE or pre-existing liver disease;[11,12] the syndrome of asthma, angioedema and nasal polyps may be provoked in susceptible patients.[13] Large doses may prolong PT; a single analgesic dose may suppress platelet aggregation leading to prolonged bleeding time.[14]

Precautions. Use with caution in patients with gastric ulcer, bleeding tendencies or hypoprothrombinemia, during anticoagulant therapy or with a history of asthma. Because of the association with Reye's syndrome, the use of salicylates in children with influenza or chickenpox is not recommended.[15,16] Those developing bronchospasm to aspirin may develop a similar reaction to other nonsteroidal anti-inflammatory agents.[13] Sodium salicylate and other nonacetylated salicylates appear to be well tolerated in these patients.[13,17] See Antiplatelet Drug Therapy Summary, p 463.

Parameters to Monitor. Occult GI blood loss should be monitored (periodic hematocrit, stool guaiac) in patients who ingest salicylates regularly. Plasma salicylate level determinations are recommended in the higher dose regimens, due to the wide variation among patients in plasma levels produced. Utilizing tinnitus as an index of maximum salicylate tolerance is *not* recommended in aged patients or those with pre-existing hearing impairment.[6]

Notes. Most buffered formulations do not produce a significant decrease in gastric acidity.[18] Recent evidence suggests that newer enteric coatings allow the use of EC tablets to reduce GI bleeding while maintaining reliable absorption.[19]

Ibuprofen   Advil®, Motrin®, Nuprin®, Various

Pharmacology. A nonsteroidal anti-inflammatory agent with analgesic and antipyretic properties. Effective inhibitor of cyclo-oxygenase; reversibly alters platelet function and prolongs bleeding time.

Administration and Adult Dose. **PO for rheumatoid arthritis and osteoarthritis** 400–800 mg tid–qid, to maximum of 3.2 g/day. **PO for mild to moderate pain** 200–400 mg q 4–6 hr prn. **PO for primary dysmenorrhea** 400 mg q 4 hr prn.

Pediatric Dose. Not recommended in children 14 yr and under.

Dosage Forms. Tab 200, 300, 400, 600, 800 mg.

Patient Instructions. This drug may be taken with a small amount of food, milk or antacid to minimize stomach upset. Report any symptoms of GI ulceration or bleeding, blurred vision or other eye symptoms, skin rash, weight gain or edema. Dizziness may occur; until the extent of this effect is known, use appropriate caution.

Pharmacokinetics. *Plasma Levels.* Plasma concentrations over 200 mcg/ml 1 hr after acute overdosage may be associated with severe toxicity (apnea, metabolic acidosis and coma).[241]

Fate. Rapidly absorbed from GI tract with peak plasma levels of 15-25 mcg/ml attained in 45-90 min following a single 200 mg dose; absorption is slowed after meals and peak plasma levels are about one-half those seen on an empty stomach.[20,242] 99% of drug is plasma protein bound at levels of 20 mcg/ml; metabolized to at least two inactive metabolites; 45-60% of a daily dose is excreted in the urine as metabolites and 8% as unchanged drug.[20]

$t_{1/2}$. 1.9 hr.[21]

Adverse Reactions. Gastric distress, occult blood loss, diarrhea and vomiting, dizziness and skin rash occasionally observed; GI ulceration and fluid retention reported. Rarely, reversible decreased visual acuity and changes in color vision reported; a slight rise in the Ivy bleeding time occurs. Elevation of liver enzymes, lymphopenia, agranulocytosis, aplastic anemia and aseptic meningitis have been reported rarely.[22-24]

Contraindications. Pregnancy; children 14 yr and under; syndrome of nasal polyps, angioedema and bronchospastic reactivity to aspirin or other nonsteroidal anti-inflammatory agents.

Precautions. Use with caution in patients with a history of cardiac decompensation.

Parameters to Monitor. Occult blood loss, visual disturbances and weight gain should be monitored.

Indomethacin   Indocin®, Various

Pharmacology. See Ibuprofen.

Administration and Adult Dose. PO for rheumatoid arthritis, rheumatoid (ankylosing) spondylitis and osteoarthritis of the hip 25 mg bid or tid initially. Increase in 25 mg/day increments at weekly intervals until satisfactory response or to maximum of 150-200 mg/day. Alternatively, **PR** up to 100 mg of the daily dosage may be given hs for persistent night and/or morning stiffness. **PO for acute gouty arthritis** 50 mg tid. Reduce dosage whenever possible to attempt eventual cessation of drug. **SR Cap** 75 mg 1-2 times/day can be substituted for all uses except gouty arthritis, based on non-SR dose. See Notes.

Pediatric Dose. Not recommended in children 14 yr and under.

Dosage Forms. Cap 25, 50 mg; SR Cap 75 mg; Supp 50 mg; Susp 5 mg/ml. See Notes.

Patient Instructions. This drug should be taken with food, milk or an antacid to minimize stomach upset; report any symptoms of GI ulceration or bleeding. Dizziness or headache may occur; until the extent of these effects is known, use appropriate caution. Do not take with aspirin unless directed otherwise.

Pharmacokinetics. Fate. Rapidly and well absorbed from GI tract, with peak plasma levels reached within 2 hr.[25] 97% of drug is plasma protein bound;[26] extensive O-demethylation and N-deacylation to inactive metabolites. 21-42% excreted fecally as metabolites, with about 10-20% excreted unchanged in urine.[26]

$t_{1/2}$. 2.6-11.2 hr.[25]

Adverse Reactions. Frontal lobe headache, drowsiness, dizziness, mental confusion and GI distress are very frequent, especially with doses greater than 100 mg/day; occasional peripheral neuropathy, occult bleeding and peptic ulcer occur. Rarely, pancreatitis, corneal opacities, hepatotoxicity, aplastic anemia, agranulocytosis, thrombocytopenia and allergic reactions are reported.[27] The syndrome of asthma, angioedema and nasal polyps may be provoked in susceptible patients. May aggravate psychiatric disorders, epilepsy or parkinsonism.

Contraindications.   Pregnancy; lactation; children 14 yr and under; history of recurrent or active GI lesions; syndrome of nasal polyps, angioedema and bronchospastic reactivity to aspirin or other nonsteroidal anti-inflammatory agents.

Precautions.   Careful instructions to, and observations of, the patient are essential. Use with great care in the elderly. May mask the signs and symptoms of infection. Blurred vision warrants a thorough ophthalmologic examination. Headache, which persists despite dosage reduction, and corneal deposits and retinal disturbances (including those of the macula) necessitate cessation of drug use.

Parameters to Monitor.   Periodic ophthalmologic examination and CBC during prolonged therapy.

Notes.   The clinical efficacy of indomethacin in the treatment of rheumatoid arthritis has not been impressive in controlled trials and should not generally be used as an alternative to aspirin.[27] Other nonsteroidal anti-inflammatory agents (eg, naproxen, ibuprofen) are preferable due to their proven efficacy and lower toxicity. Also available as inj 1 mg for the treatment of patent ductus arteriosus in neonates.

Naproxen
Naproxen Sodium

Naprosyn®
Anaprox®

Pharmacology.   See Ibuprofen.

Administration and Adult Dose.   **PO for rheumatoid arthritis and osteoarthritis** (naproxen) 250–375 mg bid initially; (naproxen sodium) 275 mg bid or 275 mg q AM and 550 mg q evening initially, to a maximum of 1,500 mg/day for limited periods. If no improvement has occurred after 4 weeks of therapy, other drug therapy should be considered. **PO for acute gout** (naproxen) 750 mg, followed by 250 mg q 8 hr until resolved; (naproxen sodium) 825 mg, followed by 275 mg q 8 hr until resolved. **PO for mild to moderate pain and dysmenorrhea** (naproxen sodium) 550 mg, followed by 275 mg q 6–8 hr.

Pediatric Dose.   **PO for juvenile rheumatoid arthritis** 10 mg/kg/day in 2 divided doses.[28,29]

Dosage Forms.   **Tab** (naproxen) 250, 375, 500 mg; (naproxen sodium) 275, 550 mg; **Susp** (naproxen) 25 mg/ml.

Patient Instructions.   See Ibuprofen.

Pharmacokinetics.   *Plasma Levels.*   Trough concentrations above 50 mcg/ml are associated with response in rheumatoid arthritis.[30]
    Fate.   Readily and completely absorbed orally; more rapid with the sodium salt. 99.6% plasma protein bound at concentrations of 23–49 mcg/ml. About 95% of the drug is excreted in the urine, 10% as unchanged drug and the rest as inactive metabolites. Some enterohepatic recirculation may take place.[31-33] Plasma levels vary considerably between different individuals receiving similar doses. Plasma levels tend to plateau at and above a dose of 250 mg bid. As dosage is increased, binding sites become saturated and more drug is available for renal clearance.[34] Unbound drug

clearance is reduced by about 60% in cirrhosis.[35]

$t_{1/2}$. 12-15 hr.[34]

Adverse Reactions. GI side effects include indigestion, abdominal discomfort, nausea, vomiting and heartburn; these have been generally less frequent than with aspirin or indomethacin. Episodes of GI bleeding have been reported and are at times severe and occasionally fatal. CNS side effects occur occasionally, and include headache, drowsiness, vertigo and tinnitus. Rarely, visual disturbances, thrombocytopenia, agranulocytosis and jaundice occur.[36] Interstitial nephritis and nephrotic syndrome have been reported.[37,38]

Contraindications. Patients exhibiting the syndrome of nasal polyps, angioedema and bronchospasm induced by aspirin or other nonsteroidal anti-inflammatory agents.

Precautions.   Pregnancy. Pre-existing ulcer disease or history of GI bleeding. Because of the high protein binding of naproxen, potential exists for displacement of other highly protein bound drugs such as warfarin, aspirin, sulfonylureas and hydantoins; however, clinically significant interactions have not been reported. GI effects and inhibition of platelet aggregation may be important in predisposing patients receiving anticoagulants to bleeding episodes.

Notes.   Aspirin remains the standard therapy for the treatment of rheumatoid arthritis. Naproxen appears to compare favorably with aspirin in efficacy.[36] Naproxen and/or its metabolites may cause a false elevation in the assay for urinary 17-ketogenic steroids. Measurements of 17-hydroxycorticosteroids are apparently unaltered.

Piroxicam   Feldene®

Piroxicam is an oxicam enolic acid nonsteroidal anti-inflammatory agent chemically and pharmacokinetically distinct from earlier compounds. Piroxicam is effective in patients with rheumatoid arthritis, osteoarthritis and ankylosing spondylitis. The half-life of the drug is about 41 hours which allows a single daily dosage regimen. Piroxicam is 98% plasma protein bound and largely metabolized with only 10% excreted unchanged in the urine. Adverse effects appear to be similar to other available nonsteroidal anti-inflammatory drugs, although some studies suggest that GI complaints and bleeding may be more frequent. Piroxicam appears to be associated with a high frequency of phototoxic cutaneous eruptions. Dosage is usually 20 mg in a single daily dose. Use with caution and at reduced dosage in the elderly. Available as 10 and 20 mg capsules.[39-41]

Nonsteroidal Anti-Inflammatory Agents Comparison Chart[a]

DRUG	DOSAGE FORMS	ADULT DAILY DOSAGE RANGE FOR RHEUMATOID ARTHRITIS	HALF-LIFE (HOURS)	PERCENT PROTEIN BOUND	INTERACTION WITH ORAL ANTICOAGULANTS[b]
ACETIC ACIDS **Diclofenac** Voltaren®	Tab 25, 50, 75 mg.	150–200 mg in 2 divided doses.	1.5	99	Unlikely
Fenclofenac Flenac® (Investigational - Norwich-Eaton)	—	600–1800 mg in 3 divided doses.	30	99	Unknown
Tolmetin Tolectin® Tolectin® DS	Tab 200 mg Cap 400 mg.	1.2–2 g in 3–4 divided doses.	1	99	Unlikely
ANTHRANILIC ACIDS (FENAMATES) **Meclofenamate** Meclomen® Various	Cap 50, 100 mg.	200–400 mg in 3–4 divided doses.	3	high?	Likely
Mefenamic Acid Ponstel®	Cap 250 mg.	250 mg q 6 hr for moderate pain.	3	high?	Likely

Continued

Nonsteroidal Anti-Inflammatory Agents Comparison Chart[a]

DRUG	DOSAGE FORMS	ADULT DAILY DOSAGE RANGE FOR RHEUMATOID ARTHRITIS	HALF-LIFE (HOURS)	PERCENT PROTEIN BOUND	INTERACTION WITH ORAL ANTICOAGULANTS[b]
INDOLE/INDENE ACETIC ACIDS					
Etodolac Ultradol® (Investigational - Ayerst)	—	200–600 mg in 2 divided doses.	7	95	Unknown
Indomethacin Indocin® Various	Cap 25, 50 mg SR Cap 75 mg Susp 5 mg/ml Supp 50 mg.	50–200 mg in 3 divided doses.	7	97	Possible
Sulindac Clinoril®	Tab 150, 200 mg.	300–400 mg in 2 divided doses.	18 (active sulfide metabolite)	93 (sulindac) 98 (sulfide)	Likely
PROPIONIC ACIDS					
Carprofen Rimadyl®	Tab 100, 150 mg.	300 mg in 2 divided doses.	15	99.9	Unknown
Fenbufen Cinopal® (Investigational - Lederle)	—	600–1000 mg in 2 divided doses.	10	99	Unknown

Continued

Nonsteroidal Anti-Inflammatory Agents Comparison Chart[a]

DRUG	DOSAGE FORMS	ADULT DAILY DOSAGE RANGE FOR RHEUMATOID ARTHRITIS	HALF-LIFE (HOURS)	PERCENT PROTEIN BOUND	INTERACTION WITH ORAL ANTICOAGULANTS[b]
Fenoprofen Nalfon®	Cap 200, 300 mg Tab 600 mg.	2.4–3.2 g in 4 divided doses.	2.5	99	Possible
Flurbiprofen Ansaid® (Investigational - Upjohn)	—	150–300 mg in 2–4 divided doses.	3.5	99	Unknown
Ibuprofen Motrin® Various	Tab 200, 300, 400, 600, 800 mg.	1.2–3.2 g in 3–4 divided doses.	1.9	99	Unlikely
Ketoprofen Orudis®	Cap 50, 75 mg.	150–300 mg in 3 divided doses.	2	99	Unknown
Naproxen Anaprox® Naprosyn®	Tab (naproxen sodium) 275, 550 mg Tab (naproxen) 250, 375, 500 mg Susp (naproxen) 25 mg/ml.	500–750 mg in 2 divided doses.	13	99	Unlikely
Oxaprozin Daypro® (Investigational - Wyeth)	—	1.2 g once daily.	40	99	Unlikely

Continued

Nonsteroidal Anti-Inflammatory Agents Comparison Chart[a]

DRUG	DOSAGE FORMS	ADULT DAILY DOSAGE RANGE FOR RHEUMATOID ARTHRITIS	HALF-LIFE (HOURS)	PERCENT PROTEIN BOUND	INTERACTION WITH ORAL ANTICOAGULANTS[b]
Tiaprofenic Acid Surgam® (Investigational - Hoechst-Roussel)	—	600–1200 mg in 3 divided doses.	1.5	98	Unknown
OXICAMS **Piroxicam** Feldene®	Cap 10, 20 mg.	20 mg in 1 or 2 divided doses.	41	98	Possible
PYRAZOLIDINEDIONES **Phenylbutazone** Azolid® Butazolidin® Various	Cap 100 mg Tab 100 mg.	300–400 mg in 3–4 divided doses.	72	99	Very Likely
QUINAZOLINONES **Proquazone** Biarsan® (Investigational - Sandoz)	—	600–900 mg in 3 divided doses.	1.2	98	Unknown

Continued

Nonsteroidal Anti-Inflammatory Agents Comparison Chart[a]

DRUG	DOSAGE FORMS	ADULT DAILY DOSAGE RANGE FOR RHEUMATOID ARTHRITIS	HALF-LIFE (HOURS)	PERCENT PROTEIN BOUND	INTERACTION WITH ORAL ANTICOAGULANTS[b]
SALICYLATES					
Aspirin Various	See Monograph.	3–6 g divided q 4 hr.[c]	2–25 (dose-dependent)	95 (salicylate)	Likely
Choline Magnesium Trisalicylate® Trilisate®	Tab 500, 750 mg, 1 g Liquid 100 mg/ml.	2–3 g in 1 or 2 divided doses.[c]	2–25 (dose-dependent)	95 (salicylate)	Likely
Diflunisal Dolobid®	Tab 250, 500 mg.	500 mg bid for mild-moderate pain.	10	99	Unlikely
Salsalate Disalcid®	Cap 500 mg Tab 500, 750 mg.	3 g in 2 or 3 divided doses.[c]	2–25 (dose-dependent)	95 (salicylate)	Likely

a. Adapted from references 4, 29, 42–47.
b. Refers to alteration in prothrombin time only; all of these agents cause gastritis and, with the exception of the nonacetylated salicylates (eg, choline magnesium trisalicylate, salsalate), interfere with platelet function.
c. Dosage should be guided by plasma salicylate levels; see Aspirin monograph.

28:08.08 OPIATE AGONISTS

Codeine Salts
Various

Pharmacology. Codeine is 3-methoxy morphine and shares the general pharmacologic properties of morphine. See Morphine.

Administration and Adult Dose. PO, SC, IM or IV for analgesia 15-60 mg q 4-6 hr. PO or SC for antitussive action 10-20 mg q 4-6 hr, to maximum of 120 mg/day.

Pediatric Dose. PO, SC or IM for analgesia (1 yr and older) 0.5 mg/kg q 4-6 hr. PO for antitussive action (2-6 yr) 2.5-5 mg q 4-6 hr, to maximum of 30 mg/day; (7-12 yr) 5-10 mg q 4-6 hr, to maximum of 60 mg/day.

Dosage Forms. Tab 15, 30, 60 mg; Hyp Tab 15, 30, 60 mg; Inj 30, 60 mg/ml. Formulated as phosphate or sulfate salt.

Patient Instructions. This drug may cause drowsiness. Until the extent of this effect is known, caution should be used when driving, operating machinery or performing other tasks requiring mental alertness. Avoid excessive concurrent use of alcohol and other drugs which cause drowsiness. Prolonged use of this drug may cause constipation.

Pharmacokinetics. *Onset and Duration.* PO, SC onset 15-30 min; duration 4-6 hr.[48]
   Fate. Well absorbed from GI tract and metabolized in the liver to norcodeine and morphine. A single PO 15 mg dose produces plasma levels of 26-33 ng/ml in 2 hr and 13-22 ng/ml in 5 hr.[49] 7% plasma protein bound.[12] Primarily urinary excretion of inactive forms; 3-16% excreted unchanged in urine.[50]
   $t_{1/2}$. 2.5-3 hr.[51]

Adverse Reactions. Sedation, dizziness, nausea, vomiting, constipation and respiratory depression are most frequent.

Precautions. See Morphine Sulfate for parenteral codeine precautions.

Notes. Low toxicity and potential for addiction.

Meperidine Hydrochloride
Demerol®, Various

Pharmacology. See Morphine.

Administration and Adult Dose. PO, SC or IM for analgesia 50-150 mg (or very slow IV 50-100 mg, preferably diluted) q 3-4 hr prn. Oral doses are about one-half as effective as a parenteral dose.[52] Reduce dosage when given concomitantly with a phenothiazine or other drugs that potentiate the depressant effects of meperidine. See Notes.

Pediatric Dose. PO, SC or IM for analgesia 6 mg/kg/day in 6 divided doses, to maximum of 100 mg/dose. See Notes.

Dosage Forms. Syrup 10 mg/ml; Tab 50, 100 mg; Inj 25, 50, 75, 100 mg/ml.

Pharmacokinetics. *Onset and Duration.* PO onset about 20 min, duration 3 hr;[52] SC or IM onset about 10 min, duration 2-4 hr.[51]
   Plasma Levels. 500-700 ng/ml appear to be required for analgesia.[53]
   Fate. Good absorption by parenteral route; hydrolyzed and also metabolized in the liver to normeperidine (an active metabolite), which is also hydrolyzed. Oral bioavailability is about 56%, increasing to 80-90% in cirrhosis due to decreased first-pass metabolism.[52,53] 60-80% plasma pro-

tein bound, largely to α_1-acid glycoprotein.[53] V_d is 240 L;[54] Cl is about 48–54 L/hr, reduced by 25% in surgical patients and by 50% in cirrhosis.[53] After a single 100 mg IM dose, mean plasma levels of 670 ng/ml and 650 ng/ml are attained in 1 and 2 hr, respectively.[55,56] An average of 2% unchanged drug and 6% (range 1–21%) normeperidine is excreted in urine.[56]

$t_{1/2}$. α phase 12 min, β phase 3.2 hr, increasing to 7 hr in patients with cirrhosis or acute liver disease.[56,57] Normeperidine has a half-life of 14–21 hr in normals, increasing to 35 hr in renal failure.[58]

Adverse Reactions. See Morphine Sulfate. The metabolite normeperidine has excitant effects which may precipitate tremors, myoclonus or seizures. Factors which predispose to seizures include doses greater than 100 mg q 2 hr for greater than 24 hr, renal failure and history of seizures.[58] Local irritation and induration occur with repeated SC injection.

Contraindications. Patients who are taking or have received MAO inhibitors within 14 days.

Precautions. See Morphine Sulfate.

Parameters to Monitor. Signs of respiratory or cardiovascular depression should be monitored.

Notes. 80–100 mg of meperidine by the parenteral route is approximately equivalent to 10 mg of morphine.[59] IM is the preferred route.

Methadone Hydrochloride   Dolophine®, Various

Pharmacology. A synthetic narcotic analgesic qualitatively similar to morphine. Analgesic activity of *l*-methadone is 8–50 times that of the *d* isomer. *d*-Methadone lacks addiction liability, but possesses antitussive activity. Because methadone is a long-acting narcotic agent, it can be substituted for short-acting narcotic agents for maintenance and detoxification. Methadone abstinence syndrome is similar to morphine; however, onset is slower and course more prolonged. See also Morphine Sulfate.

Administration and Adult Dose. IM or SC for pain 2.5–10 mg q 3–4 hr. **PO for pain** 5–15 mg q 4–6 hr. **PO for maintenance and detoxification treatment** 5–20 mg initially, followed by supplementary doses of 5–10 mg if withdrawal is not suppressed or signs reappear. After stabilization, 10–40 mg/day in single (for maintenance) or divided (for detoxification) doses is adequate for most patients. Detoxification by dosage reduction of 20% per day is usually well tolerated in hospitalized patients.[60]

Pediatric Dose. PO or SC for pain 0.7 mg/kg/day or 20 mg/M²/day, in 4–6 divided doses.

Dosage Forms. Tab 5, 10 mg; **Dispersible Tab** 40 mg; **Soln** 1, 2 mg/ml; **Inj** 10 mg/ml.

Pharmacokinetics. *Onset and Duration.* (Analgesia) onset SC or IM 10–20 min, PO 30–60 min; duration PO, SC or IM 4–5 hr after a single dose, may be longer with multiple doses.[60,61]

Plasma Levels. Best rehabilitation in methadone maintenance patients has been associated with plasma levels above 211 ng/ml.[62] There is no good correlation between plasma levels and analgesia.[63]

Fate. About 50% absorbed orally;[59,63] 71–87% plasma protein bound.[63] V_d is about 500 L; Cl is 6–18 L/hr.[64] Following a single dose, 30% is metabolized to form pyrrolidines and pyrrolines which are excreted in urine and bile; 21% is excreted unchanged in the urine.[59,63] Extent of metabolism appears to increase with chronic therapy, resulting in a 15–25% decline in plasma levels after 8–10 days of therapy.[62,63] Urinary methadone excretion is increased by urine acidification.[63]

$t_{1/2}$. α phase 14.3 hr; β phase 54.8 hr, 22.2 hr with chronic administration.[65]

Adverse Reactions. See Morphine Sulfate. Methadone administered frequently and for prolonged periods may have cumulative effects on respiration.[66]

Precautions. See Morphine Sulfate.

Parameters to Monitor. Signs of respiratory or cardiovascular depression should be monitored. During methadone maintenance, monitor for signs of withdrawal which include lacrimation, rhinorrhea, diaphoresis, yawning, restlessness, insomnia, dilated pupils and piloerection.[60]

Notes. For treatment of narcotic addiction in detoxification or maintenance programs, methadone may be dispensed only by approved pharmacies. Maintenance therapy (treatment for longer than 3 weeks) may be undertaken only by approved methadone programs; this does not apply to addicts hospitalized for other medical conditions.

Morphine Sulfate   Various

Pharmacology. Narcotic agents interact with stereospecific opiate receptors in the CNS and other tissues. Analgesia is produced primarily through an alteration in emotional response to pain. The relief of pain is fairly specific; other sensory modalities are essentially unaffected and mental processes are not impaired (unlike anesthetics), except when given in large doses or to unusually susceptible individuals. They also possess antitussive effects, usually at doses less than those required for analgesia.

Administration and Adult Dose. PO for analgesia 8–20 mg q 4 hr or SR Tab 30 mg q 8–12 hr. SC or IM for analgesia 5–15 mg q 4 hr (10 mg/70 kg is optimal initial dose); PR for analgesia 10–20 mg q 4 hr. IV for analgesia 4–10 mg, dilute and inject slowly over 4–5 min period. IV infusion 1–10 mg/hr;[67] some patients with chronic pain may require doses as high as 40–95 or more mg/hr.[68] IV patient-controlled analgesia 1 mg per activation initially with 6–10 min lockout period, both titrated to patient response.[69,70] Epidural for analgesia (unpreserved solution) (intermittent) 5 mg initially, may repeat with 1–2 mg after 1 hr to a maximum of 10 mg/24 hr; (continuous) 2–4 mg/24 hr initially; further doses of 1–2 mg may be given if pain is not relieved initially. Intrathecal for analgesia (unpreserved solution) usually 1/10 of epidural dose.

Dosage Individualization. Reduce initial dose in elderly or debilitated patients.

Pediatric Dose. SC or IM 0.1–0.2 mg/kg/dose, to maximum of 15 mg; may repeat q 4 hr. IV use one-half the IM dose.

Dosage Forms. Soln 2, 4, 20 mg/ml; Supp 5, 10, 20 mg; Tab 10, 15, 30 mg; SR Tab 30 mg; Inj (unpreserved solution) 0.5, 1 mg/ml; (preserved solution) 2, 4, 5, 8, 10, 15 mg/ml.

Pharmacokinetics. *Onset and Duration.* Following single 10 mg SC dose, onset 15–30 min, duration 4–5 hr.[51]

Plasma Levels. It is speculated that moderate analgesia requires plasma levels of at least 50 ng/ml.[71]

Fate. Rapid absorption parenterally with rapid disappearance from plasma, especially after IV administration; inactivated in the liver, primarily by conjugation with glucuronic acid. After an IM dose of 10 mg, peak levels of about 56 ng/ml are reached within 20 min. Well absorbed from GI tract, but first-pass conjugation is so rapid that significant levels of free morphine are not found in either plasma or urine. V_d is 2.12 L/kg in young normals and 1.16 L/kg in elderly patients; Cl is 2.02 L/hr/kg in young normals and 1.66 L/hr/kg in elderly patients.[67] Mostly excreted in urine with 3.4% (oral) and about 9% (parenteral) of dose excreted unchanged.[72,73]

$t_{1/2}$. 2.1–2.9 hr.[72,73]

Adverse Reactions. Respiratory and circulatory depression are major adverse effects, the former occurring with therapeutic doses. Dose-related signs of intoxication include miosis, drowsiness, decreased rate and depth of respiration, bradycardia and hypotension. Sedation, dizziness, nausea, vomiting, sweating and constipation occur frequently. Euphoria, dysphoria, dry mouth, biliary tract spasm, postural hypotension, syncope, tachy- or bradycardia, urinary retention and possible allergic-type reactions are reported occasionally. The majority of allergic-type reactions consist of skin rash, and wheal and flare over a vein which may occur with IV injection; these are due to direct stimulation of histamine release, are not truly allergic and are not a sign of more serious reactions. True allergy is very rare.

Precautions. Use with caution and in reduced dosage when giving concurrently with other CNS depressant drugs. Use with caution in pregnancy; the presence of head injury, other intracranial lesions or pre-existing increase in intracranial pressure; patients having an acute asthmatic attack; the presence of chronic obstructive pulmonary disease or cor pulmonale; decreased respiratory reserve; pre-existing respiratory depression, hypoxia or hypercapnia; patients whose ability to maintain blood pressure is already compromised; patients with atrial flutter or other supraventricular tachycardias; patients with prostatic hypertrophy or urethral stricture; elderly or debilitated patients; and in patients with acute abdominal pain, when administration of drug might obscure the diagnosis or clinical course. Do not administer IV unless a narcotic antagonist and facilities for assisted or controlled respiration are immediately available.

Parameters to Monitor. Signs of respiratory or cardiovascular depression should be monitored.

Notes. Brompton's mixture, which is usually prepared as a combination of morphine and cocaine in an alcohol and syrup base, has been used for many years in the management of chronic pain. Evidence for the superiority of Brompton's or other mixtures over plain morphine solution is questionable.[74,75]

28:08.12 OPIATE PARTIAL AGONISTS

Pentazocine Salts   Talwin®, Talwin® Nx

Pharmacology. A narcotic analgesic with weak opioid antagonist activity. Unlike pure narcotic agonists (and nalbuphine), pentazocine (and butorphanol) increases cardiac workload, making it unacceptable in patients with myocardial infarction.[76] Naloxone is added to tablets to discourage IV abuse. See Notes.

Administration and Adult Dose. PO 50–100 mg q 3–4 hr, to maximum of 600 mg/day; SC or IM (excluding patients in labor) 30–60 mg, or IV 30 mg q 3–4 hr, to maximum of 360 mg/day. Based on duration of analgesic effect, parenteral dosing q 2.5 hr has been recommended.[77]

Pediatric Dose. Not recommended under 12 yr.

Dosage Forms. Tab (hydrochloride) 50 mg with naloxone 0.5 mg (Talwin® Nx); Inj (lactate) 30 mg/ml (Talwin®).

Patient Instructions. This drug may cause dizziness; until the extent of this effect is known, use appropriate caution; report any mental changes.

Pharmacokinetics. *Onset and Duration.* PO onset 15-30 min, duration 3 hr; SC or IM onset 15-20 min, duration 2-3 hr; IV onset 2-3 min, duration 1 hr.[78]

Fate. Well absorbed after parenteral administration; 11-32% of an oral dose is bioavailable, dependent almost entirely on first-pass metabolism.[79] Peak plasma levels are attained in about 2.5 hr (oral), about 45 min (IM) and about 30 min (IV).[80] Extensively metabolized in the liver, but rate of metabolism is highly variable. Data suggest that urban living and/or smoking may increase the rate of metabolism.[81] 60-70% of dose is recovered in urine, of which 3-24% (higher amount in acidic urine and/or after IV use) is unchanged drug.[78,82]

$t_{1/2}$. 2.1 hr (IM).[78]

Adverse Reactions. Sedation, sweating, dizziness, nausea, euphoria and hallucinations are most frequent. Occasionally, insomnia, anxiety, constipation, dry mouth, syncope, visual blurring, flushing, decreased blood pressure and tachycardia are reported. Also, after oral use, rare GI distress, anorexia and vomiting are reported. After parenteral use, diaphoresis, sting on injection, respiratory depression, transient apnea in newborn from use in mother during labor, shock, urinary retention and alterations in uterine contractions during labor occur rarely. Other rarely reported effects include muscle tremor and toxic epidermal necrolysis. Local skin reactions, and ulceration and fibrous myopathy at the injection site have been reported with long-term parenteral use.[77,82]

Precautions. See Morphine. Also, use cautiously in patients with myocardial infarction because pentazocine increases cardiac workload. There are reports of dependence and withdrawal symptoms following extended use.[83]

Notes. Oral pentazocine is about one-third as potent as IM pentazocine[84] and to achieve comparable plasma levels, 75 mg orally is approximately equivalent to 40 mg IM.[78] 30-60 mg parenteral pentazocine is approximately equivalent to 10 mg of morphine and 75-100 mg of meperidine.[83] Effects of pentazocine are antagonized by naloxone only (ie, not by nalorphine or levallorphan). Naloxone is not absorbed orally, but theoretically prevents parenteral abuse of the oral dosage form; however, IV abuse of Talwin® Nx plus tripelennamine has been reported.[85]

Narcotic Analgesics Comparison Chart[a]

DRUG	DOSAGE FORMS	EQUIVALENT IM DOSE[b] (MG)	ORAL/PARENTERAL EFFICACY RATIO	DURATION OF ANALGESIA (HOURS)	CARDIAC WORKLOAD	PARTIAL ANTAGONIST ACTIVITY
Buprenorphine Buprenex®	Inj 0.324 mg/ml.	0.4	—	5.6	—	yes
Butorphanol Stadol®	Inj 1, 2 mg/ml.	2	1/16	3–4	↑	yes
Codeine Various	Inj 30, 60 mg/ml Hyp Tab 15, 30, 60 mg Tab 15, 30, 60 mg.	120 [30]	1/2–2/3	3–6	↓	no
Fentanyl Various	Inj 50 mcg/ml.	0.2	—	1–2	↓	no
Hydromorphone Dilaudid® Various	Inj 1, 2, 3, 4, 10 mg/ml Tab 1, 2, 3, 4 mg/ml Supp 3 mg.	1.5 [1]	1/5	4–5	↓	no
Levorphanol Levo-Dromoran®	Inj 2 mg/ml Tab 2 mg.	2	1/2	4–6	↓	no
Meperidine Demerol® Various	Inj 25, 50, 75, 100 mg/ml Tab 50, 100 mg Syrup 10 mg/ml.	100 [50]	1/3–1/2	2–4	↓	no

Continued

Narcotic Analgesics Comparison Chart[a]

DRUG	DOSAGE FORMS	EQUIVALENT IM DOSE[b] (MG)	ORAL/PARENTERAL EFFICACY RATIO	DURATION OF ANALGESIA (HOURS)	CARDIAC WORKLOAD	PARTIAL ANTAGONIST ACTIVITY
Methadone Dolophine® Various	Inj 10 mg/ml Tab 5, 10 mg Dispersible Tab 40 mg Soln 1, 2 mg/ml.	10 [3]	1/2	3–5	→	no
Morphine Various	Inj 0.5, 1, 2, 4, 5, 8, 10, 15 mg/ml Tab 10, 15, 30 mg Soln 2, 4, 20 mg/ml SR Tab 30 mg Supp 5, 10, 20 mg.	10 [9]	1/6	4–5	→	no
Nalbuphine Nubain® Various	Inj 10, 20 mg/ml.	10	1/6	3–6	→	yes
Oxycodone Roxicodone®	Tab 5 mg Soln 1 mg/ml.	15 [5]	1/2	3–4	→	no
Oxymorphone Numorphan®	Inj 1, 1.5 mg/ml Supp 5 mg.	1	1/6	4–5	→	no

Continued

Narcotic Analgesics Comparison Chart[a]

DRUG	DOSAGE FORMS	EQUIVALENT IM DOSE[b] (MG)	ORAL/PARENTERAL EFFICACY RATIO	DURATION OF ANALGESIA (HOURS)	CARDIAC WORKLOAD	PARTIAL ANTAGONIST ACTIVITY
Pentazocine Talwin® Talwin® Nx	Inj 30 mg/ml Tab 50 mg with naloxone 0.5 mg.	50 [25]	1/3	2–3	↑	yes

a. From references 51, 53, 59, 61, 64, 76, 86–89.
b. Doses in brackets are *oral* doses equivalent to about 30 mg of oral codeine; due to individual variability in bioavailability, equivalent doses may differ between patients.

28:08.92 MISCELLANEOUS ANALGESICS AND ANTIPYRETICS

General References: 90

Acetaminophen

Various

Pharmacology. An analgesic and antipyretic similar to aspirin and other nonsteroidal anti-inflammatory agents. It has the same potency as aspirin in inhibiting brain prostaglandin synthetase, but very little activity as an inhibitor of the peripheral enzyme. This explains the very weak anti-inflammatory action of acetaminophen.[90]

Administration and Adult Dose. PO 325–650 mg q 4–6 hr, to maximum of 3.9 g/day.

Pediatric Dose. 10–15 mg/kg q 4–6 hr, to maximum of 5 doses/day; or (up to 3 months) 40 mg/dose; (4–11 months) 80 mg/dose; (12–23 months) 120 mg/dose; (2–3 yr) 160 mg/dose; (4–5 yr) 240 mg/dose; (6–8 yr) 320 mg/dose; (9–10 yr) 400 mg/dose; (11 yr) 480 mg/dose.

Dosage Forms. **Cap** 325, 500 mg; **Tab** 160, 325, 500, 650 mg; **Drp** 80 mg/0.8 ml, 120 mg/2.5 ml; **Elxr** 120, 160, 325 mg/5 ml; **Syrup** 160 mg/5 ml; **Chew Tab** 80 mg; **Supp** 120, 125, 325, 650 mg; **Wafer** 120 mg.

Pharmacokinetics. *Plasma Levels.* No good correlation has been shown between plasma concentrations and intensity of analgesic action.[90] Plasma concentrations over 200 mcg/ml at 4 hr (or 50 mcg/ml at 12 hr) following acute overdosage are associated with severe hepatic damage, whereas toxicity is unlikely if levels are under 150 mcg/ml at 4 hr (or 30–35 mcg/ml at 12 hr).[91] See Notes.

Fate. Rapidly absorbed from GI tract; less than 50% plasma protein bound. Extensively metabolized in the liver to inactive conjugates of glucuronic and sulfuric acids (saturable), and to a hepatotoxic intermediate metabolite (first-order) by P-450 mixed-function oxidase. The intermediate is detoxified by glutathione (saturable). Only 2–3% is excreted unchanged in urine.[90,92,93]

$t_{1/2}$. 2.75–3.25 hr;[94] increased slightly in chronic hepatic disease.[95] Half-life may exceed 12 hr in acute acetaminophen poisoning.[92,96]

Adverse Reactions. In acute overdosage, potentially fatal hepatic necrosis and possible renal tubular necrosis can occur, but clinical and laboratory evidence of hepatotoxicity may be delayed for several days. (See Plasma Levels).[91] Toxic hepatitis has also been associated with the chronic ingestion of 5–8 g/day for several weeks or 3–4 g/day for a year.[97] Occasionally, erythematous or urticarial skin reactions occur; methemoglobinemia reported rarely.

Precautions. Use with caution in patients with G-6-PD deficiency.

Notes. Acetaminophen does not cause the GI erosion and bleeding associated with aspirin and has no effect on platelet function.[14] Management of acute overdosage includes emesis or gastric lavage, if no more than a few hours have elapsed since ingestion. Administration of activated charcoal is not recommended, because it may interfere with the absorption of **acetylcysteine** which has been used in the treatment of severe acute overdosage. Potentially dangerous acetaminophen levels (see Plasma Levels) can be managed by the administration of 140 mg/kg acetylcysteine diluted 1:3 in cola, grapefruit juice, soft drinks or plain water; follow with 70 mg/kg q 4 hr for 17 doses. If administered within 10–16 hr of ingestion, this therapy may minimize the expected hepatotoxicity.[91]

28:10 OPIATE ANTAGONISTS

Naloxone Hydrochloride   Narcan®, Various

Pharmacology. An allyl derivative of oxymorphone which is a competitive narcotic antagonist. It is essentially free of narcotic agonist properties and is used to reverse the effects of narcotic agonists and drugs with partial agonist properties.

Administration and Adult Dose. **IV (preferred), IM or SC for known or suspected narcotic overdose** 0.4–2 mg initially, may repeat q 2–3 min. If a total of 10 mg has been given and there is no response, the diagnosis of narcotic overdose should be questioned. If the patient responds, additional doses may be repeated prn with the frequency of repeat doses based on clinical evaluation of the patient. **IV infusion** 2 mg in 500 ml D5W or NS can be used for prolonged therapy; administer at a rate adjusted to patient response. **IV for postoperative narcotic depression** 0.1–0.2 mg initially, may repeat q 2–3 min until desired level of reversal is reached. Subsequent doses may be needed if the effect of the narcotic outlasts the action of naloxone. See Notes.

Pediatric Dose. **IV (preferred), IM or SC for known or suspected narcotic overdose** 0.01 mg/kg initially. If the initial response is not satisfactory, then a subsequent dose of 0.1 mg/kg may be given. **IV for postoperative narcotic depression** 0.005–0.01 mg initially, may repeat q 2–3 min until desired level of reversal is reached. **IV (preferred), IM or SC for narcotic depression in neonates** 0.01 mg/kg initially, may repeat q 2–3 min until desired level of reversal is reached.

Dosage Forms. **Inj** 0.02, 0.4, 1 mg/ml.

Pharmacokinetics. *Onset and Duration.* Onset IV within 2–3 min, up to 15 min when given IM or SC; duration variable, but usually 1 hr or less.[98,99]

   Fate. 59–67% metabolized by hepatic conjugation and renal elimination of the conjugated compound.[100]

   $t_{1/2}$. 60–90 min in adults;[101] about 3 hr in neonates.[102]

Precautions. Administration to narcotic-dependent persons (including neonates of dependent mothers) may precipitate acute withdrawal symptoms.

Parameters to Monitor. Respiratory rate, pupil size (may not be useful in mixed drug or narcotic partial agonist overdoses), heart rate, blood pressure, symptoms of acute narcotic withdrawal syndrome.

Notes. Naloxone has been used experimentally for the reversal of septic shock using bolus doses (10–100 mcg/kg)[103] or bolus doses followed by continuous infusion (30 mcg/kg then 30 mcg/kg/hr);[104] however, response is highly variable. Naloxone may only partially antagonize the respiratory depressant effects of **buprenorphine.**

Naltrexone Hydrochloride   Trexan®

Pharmacology. A derivative of oxymorphone which is pharmacologically similar to naloxone but, unlike naloxone, is active when administered orally.

Administration and Adult Dose. **PO for maintenance of a narcotic-free state in detoxified narcotic-dependent patients** 50 mg/day. Some patients may be maintained on 100 mg every other day or 150 mg every third day.

Another successful regimen is 100 mg on Monday and Wednesday and 150 mg on Friday.

Pediatric Dose. Safety and efficacy not established.

Dosage Forms. **Tab** 50 mg.

Patient Instructions. Do not try to reverse the effects of naltrexone by taking large doses of narcotics. Doing so may overcome the antagonist effects of naltrexone and produce acute narcotic overdosage.

Pharmacokinetics. *Onset and Duration.* Duration is dose-related, ranging from 24 hr for 50 mg to 72 hr for 150 mg.
   Fate. Absorption is rapid and nearly complete. There is significant first-pass hepatic metabolism to a less active metabolite (6-β-naltrexol). Ultimately, more than 90% is metabolized.[105,106]
   $t_{1/2}$. (Naltrexone) 4 hr; (6-β-naltrexol) 13 hr in normal adults.[107]

Adverse Reactions. Naltrexone can cause dose-related hepatocellular damage. Hepatotoxicity is associated with doses of 300 mg/day or more given for several weeks.

Contraindications. Current or recent liver disease.

Precautions. To prevent precipitation of acute narcotic withdrawal, patients should be narcotic-free for 7–10 days before receiving naltrexone. If there is a question about the patient's narcotic-free status, a naloxone challenge may be given (IV 0.2 mg, then 0.6 mg 30 seconds later if there is no response to the first dose).

28:12 ANTICONVULSANTS

General References: 108–110

Class Instructions. It is important to take this medication as prescribed to control your seizures. Stopping this drug suddenly may cause an increase in seizures. This medication may cause drowsiness. Until the extent of this effect is known, caution should be used when driving, operating machinery or performing other tasks requiring mental alertness. Avoid concurrent use of alcohol or other drugs which cause drowsiness. Report unusual or bothersome side effects. Contact your physician if you become pregnant.

28:12.04 BARBITURATES

Phenobarbital   Various

Pharmacology. A barbiturate compound that exerts an anticonvulsant effect by suppressing the spread of seizure discharge and increasing the convulsive threshold for electrical and chemical stimulation. See also Phenobarbital 28:24.04.

Administration and Adult Dose. **PO or IM for epilepsy** 30 mg bid-tid initially; increase in 60 mg/day increments q 5 days to effective dose.[108] Usual maintenance dose is 100–300 mg/day or 2–3 mg/kg/day in 2–3 divided doses.[110] **IV for status epilepticus** 250 mg at rate of 60–100 mg/min, may repeat same dose in 30 min if seizures not controlled, to maximum of 20 mg/kg.[111,112] See Adverse Reactions and Notes.

Dosage Individualization. Dosage reduction may be necessary in patients with hepatic cirrhosis.[113] During pregnancy, phenobarbital clearance may increase. During this time and after giving birth, dosage adjustment may be necessary and should be guided by plasma levels and patient status.[114]

Pediatric Dose. **PO or IM for epilepsy** initially, titrate dose to minimize sedation. Usual maintenance dose is 3–5 mg/kg/day in 2–3 divided doses. **IV for status epilepticus** 5 mg/kg at rate of 30 mg/min, may repeat in 20–30 min if seizures not controlled, to maximum of 15 mg/kg.[115] See Adverse Reactions and Notes.

Patient Instructions. See Class Instructions.

Dosage Forms. **Drp** 16 mg/ml; **Elxr** 15, 20 mg/5 ml; **Liquid** 15 mg/5 ml; **Cap** 16 mg; **Tab** 8, 16, 32, 65, 100 mg; **Inj** 30, 60, 65, 130 mg/ml; **Pwdr for Inj** 120 mg.

Pharmacokinetics. **Onset and Duration.** Steady-state plasma levels are attained in 14–21 days.[108,110]

Plasma Levels. (Anticonvulsant) 15–40 mcg/ml; dysarthria, ataxia and nystagmus appear above 40 mcg/ml; stupor and coma can occur at levels exceeding 70 mcg/ml.[108,110]

Fate. Oral bioavailability is 83%; peak plasma level occurs 6–18 hr after oral dose; IM peak in 1–3 hr. V_d is 0.54–1 L/kg; Cl is 0.0038–0.0053 L/hr/kg; 49–58% plasma protein bound. 65% metabolized in liver to p-hydroxy-phenobarbital. 10–30% of drug is excreted unchanged in urine; alkalization of urine increases renal clearance of phenobarbital.[108-110,116,200]

$t_{1/2}$. (Adults) 3–5.8 days; (children) 2–3 days;[108,110,116] 5.4 days in chronic liver disease.

Adverse Reactions. See Plasma Levels. Sedation is frequent, dose-related and tolerance usually develops with chronic administration. Behavioral disturbances and cognitive impairment occur frequently with chronic therapy in children and the elderly.[117] Occasionally, skin rashes or folate deficiency occur. Rarely, megaloblastic anemia, hepatitis, exfoliative dermatitis or Stevens-Johnson syndrome reported. Neonatal hemorrhage has been reported in newborns whose mothers were taking phenobarbital. SC or intra-arterial injection may produce tissue necrosis. IV administration may produce severe respiratory depression and provisions for respiratory support should be made.

Contraindications. History of porphyria or severe respiratory disease where dyspnea or obstruction is present.

Precautions. Pregnancy. Use with caution in patients with severe liver or renal disease. Abrupt withdrawal of the drug in patients with epilepsy may precipitate status epilepticus. See Notes and Barbiturates in Drug Interactions chapter.

Parameters to Monitor. Periodic plasma level monitoring, after attaining steady-state (14–21 days), is useful in evaluating therapeutic efficacy or potential for adverse effects.[109] CBC and liver function tests should be monitored periodically with chronic therapy.

Notes. Barbiturate anticonvulsants may be safely withdrawn from patients with intractable epilepsy who are maintained on appropriate nonbarbiturate anticonvulsants. In one study, no episodes of status epilepticus occurred during barbiturate withdrawal over 2 weeks in inpatients or 3 months in outpatients.[118] In tonic-clonic status epilepticus, phenobarbital is usually considered a third agent after diazepam or lorazepam and phenytoin have failed to control seizures.[112] Considering comparative efficacy and patient tolerability with carbamazepine and phenytoin, phenobarbital is recommended as a secondary choice for single drug therapy of partial (focal or psychomotor) or generalized tonic-clonic (grand mal) seizures.[119] See Anticonvulsants Comparison Chart.

Primidone   Mysoline®, Various

Pharmacology. Primidone (desoxyphenobarbital) is structurally related to the barbiturates. Primidone and its metabolites, phenylethylmalonamide (PEMA) and phenobarbital, all exert anticonvulsant activity. See Phenobarbital.

Administration and Adult Dose. PO for epilepsy 100–125 mg hs initially; increase in 100–125 mg/day increments q 3 days to effective dose, to maximum of 2 g/day. Usual maintenance dose is 250 mg tid-qid.

Pediatric Dose. PO for epilepsy (under 8 yr) 50 mg hs initially; increase by 50 mg in 3 days and thereafter in 100–125 mg/day increments q 3 days to effective dose. Usual maintenance dose is 125–250 mg tid or 10–25 mg/kg/day in 3 divided doses; (8 yr and over) same as adult dose.

Dosage Forms. Susp 50 mg/ml; Tab 50, 250 mg.

Patient Instructions. See Class Instructions.

Pharmacokinetics. *Onset and Duration.* Steady-state plasma levels are attained in 4–7 days.[110]
   Plasma Levels. (Primidone) 6–12 mcg/ml;[110] (PEMA) range not known. See also Phenobarbital.
   Fate. Peak plasma levels occur 3–4 hr after an oral dose.[110] V_d is 0.6–1 L/kg;[108,109] Cl is 0.035–0.052 L/hr/kg;[120] up to 24% plasma protein bound.[109] Metabolized in liver to PEMA and phenobarbital; in patients receiving primidone with other anticonvulsants, 36–45% is converted to PEMA and 4–5% to phenobarbital.[108] Up to 53% of primidone and 81% of PEMA are excreted unchanged in urine.[108,121]
   $t_{1/2}$. (Primidone) 6.5–15.2 hr;[109] (PEMA) 10.8–18.1 hr.[121] See also Phenobarbital.

Adverse Reactions. Nausea, vomiting, dizziness, ataxia and somnolence occur frequently during initial dosing and may become tolerable with dosage reduction.[119] Behavioral disturbances and cognitive impairment occur frequently with chronic therapy in children and the elderly.[117] Occasionally skin rashes, folate deficiency or impotence occur.[108,119] Rarely leukopenia, thrombocytopenia, megaloblastic anemia or lymphadenopathy occur.[108]

Contraindications. History of porphyria.

Precautions. Pregnancy. Use with caution in patients with severe liver or renal disease. Abrupt withdrawal of the drug in patients with epilepsy may precipitate status epilepticus. See Phenobarbital Notes.

Parameters to Monitor. Periodic plasma level monitoring of primidone and phenobarbital, after attaining steady-state (primidone, 4–7 days; phenobarbital, 14–21 days), is useful in evaluating therapeutic efficacy or potential adverse effects.[109] CBC and liver function tests should be monitored periodically with chronic therapy.

Notes. Considering comparative efficacy and good patient tolerance of carbamazepine and phenytoin, primidone is recommended as a secondary choice for single drug therapy of partial (focal or psychomotor) or generalized tonic-clonic (grand mal) seizures.[119] See Anticonvulsants Comparison Chart.

28:12.08 BENZODIAZEPINES

Clonazepam
Klonopin®

Pharmacology. A benzodiazepine anticonvulsant. In animals and humans, clonazepam limits the spread of seizure activity. This effect may be due to benzodiazepine enhancement of the inhibitory neurotransmitter, γ-aminobutyric acid (GABA).

Administration and Adult Dose. PO for epilepsy initial dose should not exceed 0.5 mg tid; increase in 0.5–1 mg/day increments q 3 days to effective dose, to maximum of 20 mg/day.

Pediatric Dose. PO for epilepsy (up to 10 yr or 30 kg) 10–30 mcg/kg/day initially in 2–3 divided doses. Increase in 0.25–0.5 mg/day increments q 3 days to effective dose, to maximum of 0.2 mg/kg/day.

Dosage Forms. Tab 0.5, 1, 2 mg.

Patient Instructions. See Class Instructions.

Pharmacokinetics. *Onset and Duration.* Steady-state plasma levels are attained in 4–8 days.[122] See Notes.

Plasma Levels. 25–75 ng/ml; however, patients having side effects with clonazepam may fall within this same range.[122] Increases in seizure frequency are reported at levels exceeding 100 ng/ml; status epilepticus has been observed at levels exceeding 180 ng/ml.[108]

Fate. Peak plasma level occurs 1–3 hr after an oral dose. V_d is 1.9–4.4 L/kg; Cl is 0.092 L/hr/kg; 47% plasma protein bound. Principal metabolite, 7-aminoclonazepam, is inactive. Up to 2% of drug is excreted unchanged in the urine.[108,109]

$t_{1/2}$. 18–49 hr; usual range 22–36 hr.[108,109]

Adverse Reactions. Drowsiness and ataxia occur frequently and may subside with chronic administration. Behavior disturbances are frequent in children and require dosage reduction.[122] Occasionally, hypersalivation and bronchial hypersecretion occur and may cause respiratory difficulties. Rarely, anemia, leukopenia, thrombocytopenia and respiratory depression occur.

Contraindications. Severe liver disease; acute narrow angle glaucoma.

Precautions. Pregnancy. May increase frequency of generalized tonic-clonic (grand mal) seizures in patients with mixed seizure types. Abrupt withdrawal of the drug in patients with epilepsy may precipitate status epilepticus. Absence status has been reported in patients also receiving valproic acid.

Parameters to Monitor. Periodic plasma level monitoring is of limited value, because of poor correlation between therapeutic and adverse effects and plasma levels.[108] Close attention to changes in patient's seizure frequency is necessary to monitor for therapeutic tolerance. See Notes.

Notes. Tolerance to the anticonvulsant effect of clonazepam may occur in up to one-third of patients within 6 months of starting the drug; dosage increase may result in return to initial therapeutic effect.[122] Clonazepam is indicated for treatment of typical and atypical absence (petit mal), atonic or myoclonic seizures. Despite prominent CNS adverse effects and the development of tolerance, the drug is considered a primary agent for atonic or myoclonic seizures. However, these limitations make the drug an alternative to ethosuximide and valproic acid for therapy of absence seizures.[123] See Anticonvulsants Comparison Chart.

28:12.12 HYDANTOINS
Phenytoin
Dilantin®, Various

Pharmacology. A hydantoin that suppresses the spread of seizure activity mainly by inhibiting synaptic post-tetanic potentiation and blocking the propagation of electrical discharge. Phenytoin may decrease sodium influx and inhibit calcium uptake at the cellular level to produce these actions.

Administration and Adult Dose. **PO maintenance dose** 100 mg tid initially. Using plasma levels as a guide, increase in 50–100 mg/day increments q 5–7 days to effective dose. Due to dose-dependent metabolism, small increases in dosage may produce disproportionate increases in plasma levels. Usual maintenance dose is 300–500 mg/day or 4–7 mg/kg/day in 2 doses.[124] Once daily administration may be considered after a divided dose regimen is established. Presently, only extended phenytoin sodium capsules are recommended for once daily administration. **PO loading dose** 1 g divided into 3 doses (400 mg, 300 mg and 300 mg) administered over a 4 hr period. An individualized regimen of 19 mg/kg in divided doses over 6–12 hr has also been recommended.[125] Using plasma levels as a guide, a maintenance dose can be initiated within 24 hr of starting the loading dose. **IV loading dose** 15–18 mg/kg can be given by direct IV injection, at a rate not greater than 50 mg/min. This dosage range results in therapeutic plasma levels for up to 18–24 hr in most patients.[115,124,126] Alternatively, the loading dose, diluted with 0.45% or 0.9% sodium chloride to a final phenytoin concentration of 20–30 mg/ml, can be infused through an IV volume control set containing an inline filter at a rate not greater than 50 mg/min.[124] See Adverse Reactions and Notes. **IM** administration is painful and results in slow, but complete, absorption over a 5-day period due to deposition of phenytoin crystals in muscle.[127] The IV route is preferred to rapidly attain therapeutic plasma levels or in patients unable to take phenytoin by mouth. If IV route not available, increase the PO phenytoin daily dose by 50% and administer it IM; when returning to PO, give 50% of original PO phenytoin daily dose for the same period of time the patient received IM doses.[240] Routine plasma level monitoring is recommended during conversion.

Dosage Individualization. During pregnancy, phenytoin clearance may increase. During this time and after giving birth, dosage adjustment may be necessary and should be guided by plasma levels and patient status.[114] Renal disease alters phenytoin protein binding due to decreased affinity of plasma proteins and reduced albumin concentration. Increases in fraction unbound are most pronounced in patients with Cl_{cr} below 25 ml/min. Thus, measured total phenytoin levels of 5–10 mcg/ml in patients with Cl_{cr} less than 10 ml/min, and 6–12 mcg/ml in patients with Cl_{cr} 10–24 ml/min, are considered equivalent to the usual therapeutic phenytoin levels of 10–20 mcg/ml.[128] Ideally, dosage adjustment should be guided by patient status and actual measurement of unbound and total phenytoin levels.

Pediatric Dose. **PO maintenance dose** 5 mg/kg/day initially in 2–3 divided doses. Increase by no more than 15–30% of initial dose q 5–7 days to effective dose.[124] Due to dose-dependent metabolism, small increases in dosage may produce disproportionate increases in plasma levels. Usual maintenance dose is 5–8 mg/kg/day in 2–3 divided doses.[123] **IV loading dose** same as adult dose.

Dosage Forms. (Phenytoin) **Chew Tab** 50 mg; **Susp** 6, 25 mg/ml; (phenytoin sodium) **Cap** 30, 100 mg; **Inj** 50 mg/ml. Phenytoin sodium is 92% phenytoin.

Patient Instructions. Good dental hygiene and regular dental visits may prevent gum tenderness, bleeding or enlargement (especially in children). Shake oral suspension well prior to each dose. See also Class Instructions.

Pharmacokinetics. *Onset and Duration.* Steady-state plasma levels are attained within 5–10 days.[110] See Notes.

Plasma Levels. 10–20 mcg/ml. Nystagmus, slurred speech, ataxia, blurred vision and dizziness appear between 20–40 mcg/ml,[110] confusional states and mood changes above 40 mcg/ml.[108] See also Dosage Individualization.

Fate. Peak plasma levels occur in 4–12 hr with extended release capsules;[108,110] rapid release capsules are absorbed more quickly. Patient and plasma level monitoring are suggested when changing phenytoin dosage form or brand. Time to peak level is also prolonged with large oral doses.[129] Oral phenytoin absorption is slow and incomplete in infants up to 3 months.[108] Absorption of suspension is impaired in patients receiving concurrent enteral tube feedings.[130] Stopping the feeding before and after the dose, diluting the suspension, and irrigating the tube are recommended to improve absorption.[130,131] IM injection is slowly absorbed over 5 days.[127] V_d is 0.52–0.78 L/kg; V_{max} is 6–8 mg/kg/day; K_m is 5.4–6.8 mg/L;[109] 88–93% plasma protein bound. Hypoalbuminemia, chronic liver or renal disease or nephrotic syndrome alter binding and increase fraction of unbound phenytoin.[109] 5-(p-hydroxyphenyl)-5-phenylhydantoin is the major metabolite and is inactive. 5% of drug excreted in urine unchanged.[109]

$t_{1/2}$. 7–42 hr (average 22),[108] dependent on dose. Liver's ability to metabolize drug is limited and saturation occurs when capacity is exceeded.

Adverse Reactions. See Plasma Levels. Burning, aching or pain at IV site, ataxia, confusion, dizziness and drowsiness occur frequently with IV phenytoin. Bradycardia or hypotension due to IV phenytoin are reported occasionally; slowing the rate of administration may minimize these complications.[132] Morbilliform rash occurs frequently and with a marked seasonal variation.[133] Other hypersensitivity reactions are rare, usually occur within 2 months and include fever, abnormal liver function tests, lymphoid hyperplasia, eosinophilia, erythema multiforme, exfoliative dermatitis, Stevens-Johnson syndrome, leukopenia, anemia, thrombocytopenia or serum sickness.[134] Occasionally, with chronic administration, hypertrichosis, gingival hypertrophy (especially in children and adolescents), coarsening of facial features or folate deficiency occur.[110,123] Hepatocellular necrosis has been reported.[243] See Drugs in Pregnancy chapter.

Precautions. Pregnancy. Use with caution in patients with severe liver disease. Abrupt withdrawal of the drug in patients with epilepsy may precipitate status epilepticus. See Drug Interactions chapter.

Parameters to Monitor. Plasma level monitoring, after attaining steady-state (5–10 days), is useful in evaluating therapeutic efficacy or potential for adverse effects.[109] Nystagmus or ataxia may represent mild, tolerable toxicity. CBC and liver function tests should be monitored periodically with chronic therapy.

Notes. Although crystal formation occurs when phenytoin sodium injection is mixed with 0.45 or 0.9% sodium chloride, phenytoin concentrations between 4.6–18.4 mg/ml in an admixture appear to be stable for at least 24 hr.[135] In tonic-clonic status epilepticus, phenytoin's anticonvulsant effect appears 20–30 min after start of infusion. Thus, concurrent use of phenytoin with a rapid acting benzodiazepine (diazepam or lorazepam) is recommended in this situation.[112] Phenytoin is recommended, as is carbamazepine, as a drug of first choice for single-drug therapy of partial (focal or psychomotor) or generalized tonic-clonic (grand mal) seizures.[119] See Anticonvulsants Comparison Chart.

28:12.20 SUCCINIMIDES

Ethosuximide
Zarontin®

Pharmacology. A succinimide anticonvulsant that protects against pentylenetetrazol seizures in animals and suppresses three cycle per second spike and wave activity in humans.

Administration and Adult Dose. PO for epilepsy 250 mg bid initially; increase in 250 mg/day increments q 4 days to effective dose, to maximum of 1.5 g/day. Usual maintenance dose is 20-40 mg/kg/day in 2 doses.[110]

Pediatric Dose. PO for epilepsy (3-6 yr) 250 mg/day initially; increase in 250 mg/day increments q 4 days to effective dose, to maximum of 1.5 g/day. Usual maintenance dose is 20-40 mg/kg/day in 2 doses;[110] (over 6 yr) same as adult dose.

Dosage Forms. Cap 250 mg; Syrup 50 mg/ml.

Patient Instructions. This drug may be taken with food or milk to minimize stomach upset. See also Class Instructions.

Pharmacokinetics. *Onset and Duration.* Steady-state plasma levels are attained in 5-8 days.[110]

   Plasma Levels. 40-100 mcg/ml.[110]

   Fate. Well absorbed orally with peak plasma level in 1-4 hr. V_d is 0.6-0.7 L/kg; Cl is 0.01 L/hr/kg; plasma protein binding is less than 10%. Metabolized to three inactive metabolites. 10-20% of drug is excreted unchanged in the urine.[109,110]

   $t_{1/2}$. (Adults) 60 hr; (children) 30 hr.[110]

Adverse Reactions. Nausea, vomiting, drowsiness and dizziness occur frequently during initiation of therapy and usually diminish with time. Occasionally, behavior changes or rashes occur. Rarely, systemic lupus erythematosus, leukopenia, aplastic anemia or Stevens-Johnson syndrome are reported.

Precautions. Pregnancy. Frequency of generalized tonic-clonic (grand mal) seizures may increase in patients with mixed seizure types who are treated with ethosuximide alone. Abrupt withdrawal of the drug may precipitate absence (petit mal) status.

Parameters to Monitor. Periodic plasma level monitoring, after attaining steady-state (5-8 days), is useful in evaluating therapeutic efficacy or potential for adverse effects.[109] CBC should be monitored periodically during chronic therapy.

Notes. Ethosuximide is only indicated for treatment of absence (petit mal) seizures. Because of the drug's low potential for developing serious or chronic toxicity and its proven efficacy, ethosuximide is considered the drug of choice for absence seizures.[123] See Anticonvulsants Comparison Chart.

28:12.92 MISCELLANEOUS ANTICONVULSANTS

Carbamazepine
Tegretol®, Various

Pharmacology. An iminostilbene compound related structurally to the tricyclic antidepressants. In animals, carbamazepine produces anticonvulsant effects by depressing neuronal synaptic transmission and penicillin-induced cortical discharges. The former mechanism may also be responsible for its analgesic effect.

Administration and Adult Dose. PO for epilepsy 200 mg bid initially; increase in increments of up to 200 mg/day at daily intervals to effective dose, to maximum of 1.2 g/day. Usual maintenance dose is 10-20 mg/kg/day[108] or 800-1200 mg/day in 3-4 divided doses. **PO for trigeminal neuralgia** 100 mg bid initially; increase by 200 mg/day in 100 mg increments q 12 hr until relief of pain, to maximum of 1.2 g/day. Usual maintenance dose is 400-800 mg/day in 2-3 divided doses.

Dosage Individualization.   During pregnancy, increases in carbamazepine clearance may occur. During this time and after giving birth, dosage adjustments may be necessary and should be guided by plasma levels and patient status.[114]

Pediatric Dose. PO for epilepsy (6-12 yr) 100 mg bid initially; increase gradually in 100 mg/day increments to effective dose, to maximum of 1 g/day. Usual maintenance dose is 15-25 mg/kg/day or 400-800 mg/day in 3-4 divided doses.[123] Safety and efficacy under 6 yr not established.

Dosage Forms. Chew Tab 100 mg; Susp 20 mg/ml; Tab 200 mg.

Patient Instructions. Sore throat, fever or oral lesions may be an early sign of a severe, but rare, blood disorder and should be reported immediately. See Class Instructions.

Pharmacokinetics. *Onset and Duration.* Steady-state plasma levels are attained within 2-4 days.[110]

   Plasma Levels. (Anticonvulsant) 6-12 mcg/ml. Variability exists in relationship between plasma levels and CNS side effects. Plasma levels of 10, 11-epoxide metabolite range from 20-40% of carbamazepine level.[108] See Notes.

   Fate. Oral bioavailability is 75-85%; peak plasma levels occur 6-12 hr after dose. V_d is 0.82-1.43 L/kg; Cl is 0.016-0.132 L/hr/kg; 72-76% plasma protein bound. Metabolized to pharmacologically active carbamazepine-10, 11-epoxide. See Notes. Up to 2% of drug is excreted unchanged in the urine.[108-110]

   $t_{1/2}$. 18-54 hr after a single dose; 10-25 hr after multiple doses, related to auto-induction of metabolism.[108]

Adverse Reactions. Dizziness, drowsiness, unsteadiness, nausea and vomiting occur frequently with initiation of therapy and are minimized by slow titration of dose. Occasionally, headache, confusion, visual disturbances, stomatitis or rash occur. Hyponatremia and water intoxication have been reported and may be related to elevated plasma levels.[136] Leukopenia has been observed in 10% of patients and may be transient.[137] Rare effects include aplastic anemia, hepatic damage, lenticular opacities, thrombocytopenia and arrhythmias.

Contraindications.   History of previous bone marrow depression; hypersensitivity to tricyclic antidepressants.

Precautions. Pregnancy. Because of structural similarities to tricyclic compounds, MAO inhibitors should be discontinued for a minimum of 14 days before carbamazepine is begun. Abrupt withdrawal of the drug in patients with epilepsy may precipitate status epilepticus. Exacerbation of atypical absence seizures may occur in children receiving carbamazepine for mixed seizure disorders.[138]

Parameters to Monitor. Baseline CBC and platelets, repeated q 2 weeks during the first 2 months and then q 3 months.[137] Liver function tests should be monitored periodically during chronic therapy. Plasma levels should be monitored at least twice during the first month of therapy, because metabolism is auto-induced.[108] Periodic plasma level monitoring is useful in evaluating therapeutic efficacy or potential adverse effects.[109]

Notes. The carbamazepine-10, 11-epoxide metabolite may contribute to the therapeutic and adverse effects associated with carbamazepine.[108] Carbamazepine is recommended, as is phenytoin, as a drug of first choice for single drug therapy of partial (focal or psychomotor) or generalized tonic-clonic (grand mal) seizures.[119] See Anticonvulsants Comparison Chart.

Valproic Acid   Depakene®
Divalproex Sodium   Depakote®

Pharmacology. A carboxylic acid compound whose anticonvulsant activity may be mediated by an inhibitory neurotransmitter, γ-aminobutyric acid (GABA). Valproic acid may increase GABA levels by inhibiting GABA metabolism or enhancing postsynaptic GABA activity.

Administration and Adult Dose. PO for epilepsy 15 mg/kg/day initially in 3 divided doses, increase in 5–10 mg/kg/day increments q 7 days to effective dose, to maximum of 60 mg/kg/day. Usual maintenance dose is 20–40 mg/kg/day in 3 divided doses.[139] In patients previously receiving valproic acid, divalproex can be initiated at the same daily dose and, in selected patients, can be given bid.

Pediatric Dose. Same as adult dose.

Dosage Forms. (Valproic acid) **Cap** 250 mg; **Syrup** 50 mg/ml; (divalproex) **EC Tab** 125, 250, 500 mg.

Patient Instructions. This drug may be taken with food or milk to minimize stomach upset. Do not chew, break or crush the tablet or capsule, because this may irritate your mouth or throat. Weakness, tiredness, repeated vomiting or loss of seizure control may be an early sign of a severe, but rare, liver disorder and should be reported immediately.

Pharmacokinetics. *Onset and Duration.* Steady-state plasma levels are attained in 2–4 days.[110]
   Plasma Levels. 50–100 mcg/ml. Minimum therapeutic level of 70 mcg/ml may be necessary for certain seizure types.[140] Tremor, irritability, confusion, restlessness or alopecia are observed above 100 mcg/ml.[140] See Notes.
   Fate. Oral bioavailability is 78%.[139] Valproic acid peak levels occur 1–2 hr after dose; divalproex in 4 hr;[141] both are delayed by food.[139] With rectal administration peaks occur in 2–4 hr.[142] See Notes. V_d is 0.14–0.16 L/kg,[109] up to 0.3 L/kg in children;[143] Cl is 0.008–0.023 L/hr/kg;[109,143] plasma protein binding is 84–96%. Increasing plasma concentrations, hypoalbuminemia, severe liver or renal disease and pregnancy reportedly increase the unbound fraction.[139] Metabolized to at least 10 metabolites with valproic acid glucuronide accounting for 40%.[108] 1.8–3.2% of drug is excreted unchanged in urine.[108]
   $t_{1/2}$. 8–17 hr;[139,143] 17–19 hr in hepatitis or cirrhosis.[139]

Adverse Effects. See Plasma Levels. Nausea, vomiting, diarrhea and abdominal cramps occur frequently during initiation of therapy and are minimized by slow titration. Drowsiness, ataxia, tremor, behavioral disturbances, transient hair loss, minor elevations in liver function tests, asymptomatic hyperammonemia or weight gain occur occasionally. Drowsiness and ataxia are more prominent in patients taking valproic acid together with other anticonvulsants.[139] Rarely, thrombocytopenia, acute pancreatitis, abnormal coagulation parameters or hyperglycinemia occur. Liver failure has occurred during the first 6 months of therapy; children with severe neurologic disease or receiving multiple anticonvulsants appear to be at greatest risk.[139]

Contraindications. Hepatic dysfunction.

Precautions. Pregnancy. The drug may alter results of urine ketone tests. Absence status reported in patients also receiving clonazepam.

Parameters to Monitor.   Baseline liver function tests and platelets; repeat periodically, especially during the first 6 months. Monitor coagulation tests prior to surgery. Periodic plasma level monitoring, after attaining steady-state (2–4 days), is most useful in evaluating potential for adverse effects.[139,140]

Notes. Large intra-individual diurnal fluctuations in valproic acid plasma levels are reported and predose sampling at standard times is recommended.[139] Administration of valproic acid syrup, diluted 1:1 with water, as a retention enema in a single dose of 17–20 mg/kg produces plasma levels of 45–50 mcg/ml.[142] Due to the potential for serious toxicity, valproic acid is considered a secondary, yet effective, choice for absence (petit mal) seizures.[123] Clinical experience with valproic acid in atonic, myoclonic and generalized tonic-clonic (grand mal) seizures has been reported. Some clinicians recommend the drug as a primary agent for atonic or myoclonic seizures and as an alternative to primary agents in generalized tonic-clonic seizures.[109,123,144] See Anticonvulsants Comparison Chart.

Anticonvulsants Comparison Chart

| | CHOICE OF ANTICONVULSANT FOR CLINICAL SEIZURE TYPE[a] | | | | | | ANTICONVULSANT DOSAGE RANGE AND PLASMA LEVELS | | |
| | GENERALIZED SEIZURES[b] | | | | PARTIAL SEIZURES[c] | | USUAL DAILY DOSAGE RANGE (MG/KG) | | THERAPEUTIC PLASMA LEVELS (MCG/ML) |
DRUG	TONIC-CLONIC	ABSENCE	MYOCLONIC	ATONIC	SIMPLE	COMPLEX	ADULT	CHILD	
Carbamazepine	1	W	–	–	1	1	10–20	15–25	6–12
Clonazepam	W	3	1	1	–	–	0.05–0.2	0.05–0.2	0.025–0.075
Ethosuximide	W	1	–	–	–	–	20–40	20–40	40–100
Phenobarbital	2	W	–	–	2	2	2–3	3–5	15–40
Phenytoin	1	–	–	–	1	1	4–7	5–8	10–20
Primidone	2	–	–	–	2	2	10–25	10–25	6–12
Valproic Acid	3	2	1	1	–	–	15–60	15–60	50–100

a. Choice of anticonvulsant based on available information regarding relative and comparative efficacy and potential for serious or chronic toxicity. Final choice of agent should consider individual patient factors. See references 109, 119, 122, 123, 139, 144.

b. Common names: tonic-clonic (grand mal), absence (petit mal), atonic ("drop attacks").

c. Common names: simple (focal, Jacksonian), complex (psychomotor, temporal lobe).

KEY:

1 = Drug of first choice; initial agent; given as monotherapy.

2 = Drug of second choice; alternative to first choice; given as monotherapy or in combination with first choice.

3 = Drug of third choice; alternative to first or second choice; given as monotherapy or in combination with first or second choice.

W = May worsen clinical seizure type.

28:16 PSYCHOTHERAPEUTIC AGENTS

General References: 145-147

Class Instructions. This drug may cause drowsiness. Until the extent of this effect is known, caution should be used when driving, operating machinery or performing other tasks requiring mental alertness. Avoid excessive concurrent use of alcohol and other drugs which cause drowsiness. This drug may also cause dry mouth, blurring of vision or constipation.

28:16.04 ANTIDEPRESSANTS

Heterocyclic Antidepressants

Pharmacology. Heterocyclic antidepressants are not general CNS stimulants, but rather have a very specific effect on neurotransmitters and receptor sensitivity. Antidepressants differ greatly in their effect on neurotransmitters—see Heterocyclic and Related Antidepressants Comparison Chart.

Administration and Adult Dose. See Heterocyclic and Related Antidepressants Comparison Chart for dosage ranges. Initiate dosing at lower limit of range. Use divided dosing schedule to assess tolerance to side effects, then once daily dosing at bedtime can be used. "Long-acting" forms (eg, imipramine pamoate) offer no advantages. **IM** rarely used (eg, surgical patient NPO for 1-2 days).

Dosage Individualization. Initial dose and rate of titration should be reduced in patients with cardiovascular or hepatic disease and in adolescent or geriatric patients.

Pediatric Dose. Not recommended in children under 12 yr. Imipramine, however, is indicated for childhood enuresis. **PO for enuresis** (under 12 yr) 25-50 mg/day; (12 yr and over) up to 75 mg/day.[148]

Dosage Forms. See Heterocyclic and Related Antidepressants Comparison Chart.

Patient Instructions. See Class Instructions. These drugs usually take 2 weeks for a noticeable response and up to 4 weeks for full therapeutic benefit. If you have small children, be sure to keep this medication in a secure place.

Pharmacokinetics. *Onset and Duration.* Peak plasma levels do not correlate with onset of therapeutic effect. Physiologic symptoms of depression (eg, insomnia, anorexia, decreased energy) should show some response after 1 week, while mood (eg, pessimism, hopelessness, anhedonia) often requires 2-4 weeks for response.

Plasma Levels. Nortriptyline has a well established therapeutic range and shows a curvilinear relationship of plasma levels and response ("therapeutic window"). Other antidepressants show a linear relationship, but their therapeutic ranges are not well established.[149] See Heterocyclic and Related Antidepressants Comparison Chart.

Fate. Bioavailability is variable due to first-pass metabolism (protriptyline 15%, imipramine 53% and doxepin 73%).[150,151] Major metabolites are desmethyl (for tertiary amines) and hydroxy compounds; rate may be genetically determined.[152]

Adverse Reactions. Sedation, postural hypotension and anticholinergic effects (dry mouth, blurred vision, constipation, urinary retention, aggravation of narrow angle glaucoma and prostatic hypertrophy) are frequent. Nortriptyline is the least likely to cause postural hypotension. See Heterocyclic and Related Antidepressants Comparison Chart for relative differences in frequency of common adverse reactions. Occasionally fine hand tremor, hypomanic or manic episodes in bipolar patients and cardiac effects (EKG changes, first degree heart block, arrhythmias) occur. Cholestatic jaundice and blood dyscrasias are rare.

Contraindications. Pregnancy; congestive heart failure; angina pectoris; cardiovascular disease; cardiac arrhythmias.

Precautions. Use with caution in the elderly, or in patients with epilepsy, glaucoma, prostatic hypertrophy, renal or liver disease. Many drug interactions occur. 10-25% of manic-depressive patients may be "switched" into a manic or hypomanic state by antidepressants; concurrent lithium therapy may prevent this switch.[153]

Notes. Ingestion of 1-2 g of an antidepressant constitutes a life-threatening medical emergency.[154] Quantities dispensed to depressed patients with suicidal ideation should be limited. Newer antidepressants offer few advantages over standard tricyclic antidepressants. Amoxapine has a metabolite with dopamine blocking activity, resulting in extrapyramidal effects and occasional tardive dyskinesia. Maprotiline has a higher frequency of seizures, which caused its maximum daily dosage to be reduced from 300 mg to 225 mg. Neither drug offers greater safety in overdose than standard tricyclic antidepressants.

Bupropion Hydrochloride   Wellbutrin®
(Investigational - Burroughs Wellcome)

Bupropion is a unique monocyclic antidepressant. Its effect on neurotransmitters is also unique compared to available antidepressants since it is a dopamine uptake inhibitor with no direct effect on norepinephrine or serotonin reuptake. Potential advantages of this drug include virtual lack of autonomic and cardiovascular effects, lack of sedation, no interaction with alcohol and lack of weight gain seen with other antidepressants. Disadvantages include the tid dosage schedule, seizure potential at higher therapeutic doses, CNS activation, stimulation and insomnia in some patients. The effective dosage range is 300-750 mg/day, but an increased frequency of seizures at higher doses will likely result in a maximum dosage of 450 mg/day. Most studies have utilized a divided, tid schedule, and no data are available concerning once or twice daily dosing.[155,156] See Heterocyclic and Related Antidepressants Comparison Chart.

Fluoxetine Hydrochloride   Prozac®

Fluoxetine is a chemically unique antidepressant with selective inhibition of serotonin uptake, and no significant effect on muscarinic, serotonergic or noradrenergic receptors. Fluoxetine is most similar to trazodone as a drug with selective serotonergic activity, but trazodone's predominant effect on the serotonergic system is as a receptor antagonist. Nausea, nervousness and insomnia are the most common adverse effects, occurring more frequently than with the standard tricyclic antidepressants. Anticholinergic effects are rare, there is no effect on cardiac conduction, it appears to have no epileptogenic potential, and it consistently causes weight loss. Thus far, most published studies with fluoxetine have been done in outpatient settings. The recommended starting dose is 20 mg/day in one morning dose. Dosage may be increased at intervals of several weeks to a maximum of 80 mg/day. Doses over 20 mg/day should be divided into morning and noon doses. Fluoxetine has also been used in the treatment of obesity.[157-160] Related serotonin uptake inhibitors include **sertraline** (Pfizer) and **rianserin** (Janssen). See Heterocyclic and Related Antidepressants Comparison Chart. Available as 20 mg capsules.

Trazodone Hydrochloride   Desyrel®, Various

Pharmacology. Trazodone has effects similar to other antidepressants in causing β-receptor subsensitivity, and causes selective inhibition of serotonin reuptake without significant effect on norepinephrine reuptake—see Heterocyclic and Related Antidepressants Comparison Chart.

Administration and Adult Dose. See Heterocyclic and Related Antidepressants Comparison Chart. Trazodone is less potent than most other antidepressants, and a trial of trazodone should not be abandoned without reaching a dose of 400–600 mg/day. Dosing after meals minimizes sedation and postural hypotension.[161]

Dosage Individualization. Initial dose and rate of titration should be reduced in geriatric patients. Dosage adjustments in patients with hepatic or renal impairment may be prudent although limited experience thus far does not suggest major dosage adjustments are necessary.[162,163]

Pediatric Dose. Safety and efficacy under 18 yr not established.

Dosage Forms. See Heterocyclic and Related Antidepressants Comparison Chart.

Patient Instructions. See Class Instructions. Trazodone should be taken after a meal.

Pharmacokinetics. *Onset and Duration.* Trazodone has a delayed onset of effect similar to other antidepressant drugs.
Plasma Levels. Not established; clinical efficacy does not correlate with peak plasma levels, but adverse effects do.
Fate. Peak plasma levels are reduced by about one-third and are delayed with food, while bioavailability is slightly higher when the drug is taken with food. Extensively metabolized.

Adverse Reactions. Sedation and postural hypotension are most frequent, but anticholinergic effects are infrequent and mild — see Heterocyclic and Related Antidepressants Comparison Chart. Cardiac effects that occur with tricyclic antidepressants (eg, tachycardia, slowed AV conduction, EKG changes) rarely occur with trazodone. However, trazodone may aggravate pre-existing arrhythmias. Very rarely, trazodone causes priapism, with one-third of cases requiring pharmacological or surgical intervention.

Contraindications. Pregnancy; cardiac arrhythmia; initial recovery phase of myocardial infarction.

Notes. Trazodone is much safer in overdosage than other antidepressant drugs. Trazodone also is a useful drug for patients who cannot tolerate anticholinergic effects or who have CHF, angina pectoris or bundle branch block in which other antidepressants are contraindicated.

Heterocyclic and Related Antidepressants Comparison Chart[a]

DRUG CLASS DRUG	DOSAGE FORMS	USUAL DAILY ADULT DOSAGE RANGE (MG) (A) ACUTE (M) MAINTENANCE	THERAPEUTIC PLASMA LEVELS (NG/ML)	BIOCHEMICAL EFFECTS[b,c] (N) NOREPINEPHRINE (S) SEROTONIN	SEDATION	ANTI-CHOLINERGIC
TRICYCLICS **Amitriptyline** Elavil® Endep® Amitril® Various	Tab 10, 25, 50, 75, 100, 150 mg Inj 10 mg/ml.	(A) 150–300 (M) 75–150	125–250[c]	(N) + (S) +	High	High
Desipramine Norpramin® Various	Cap 25, 50 mg Tab 10, 25, 50, 75, 100, 150 mg.	(A) 150–300 (M) 75–150	>175	(N) + (S) 0	Low	Low
Doxepin Sinequan® Various	Cap 10, 25, 50, 75, 100, 150 mg Soln 50 mg/5 ml.	(A) 150–300 (M) 75–150	110–250[c]	(N) + (S) +	High	Moderate
Imipramine Tofranil® SK-Pramine® Janimine® Various	Tab 10, 25, 50 mg Inj 12.5 mg/ml. Cap (as pamoate) 75, 100, 125, 150 mg.	(A) 150–300 (M) 75–150	>200[c]	(N) + (S) +	Moderate	Moderate
Nortriptyline Aventyl® Pamelor®	Cap 10, 25, 75 mg Soln 10 mg/5 ml.	(A) 100–200 (M) 75–150	50–150	(N) + (S) +	Moderate	Moderate

Continued

Heterocyclic and Related Antidepressants Comparison Chart[a]

DRUG CLASS DRUG	DOSAGE FORMS	USUAL DAILY ADULT DOSAGE RANGE (MG) (A) ACUTE (M) MAINTENANCE	THERAPEUTIC PLASMA LEVELS (NG/ML)	BIOCHEMICAL EFFECTS[b,c] (N) NOREPINEPHRINE (S) SEROTONIN	RELATIVE FREQUENCY OF SIDE EFFECTS SEDATION	ANTI-CHOLINERGIC
Protriptyline Vivactil®	Tab 5, 10 mg.	(A) 30–60 (M) 20–40	70–260	(N)[d] (S)[d]	Very Low	Low
Trimipramine Surmontil® Various	Cap 25, 50, 100 mg.	(A) 150–300 (M) 75–150	d	(N) 0 (S) +	Moderate	Moderate
TETRACYCLICS **Maprotiline** Ludiomil®	Tab 25, 50, 75 mg.	(A) 150–225 (M) 75–150	200–300	(N) + (S) 0	Moderate	Moderate
DIBENZOXAZEPINES **Amoxapine** Asendin®	Tab 25, 50, 100, 150 mg.	(A) 300–600 (M) 150–300	d	(N) + (S) +	Low	Low
TRIAZOLOPYRIDINES **Trazodone** Desyrel® Various	Tab 50, 100, 150 mg.	(A) 200–600 (M) 100–400	d	(N) 0 (S) +	High	Lowest
TRIAZOLOBENZODIAZEPINES **Alprazolam** Xanax®	Tab 0.25, 0.5, 1 mg.	(A) 4–10 (M) —	d	(N) 0 (S) 0	High	None

Continued

Heterocyclic and Related Antidepressants Comparison Chart[a]

DRUG CLASS DRUG	DOSAGE FORMS	USUAL DAILY ADULT DOSAGE RANGE (MG) (A) ACUTE (M) MAINTENANCE	THERAPEUTIC PLASMA LEVELS (NG/ML)	BIOCHEMICAL EFFECTS[b,c] (N) NOREPINEPHRINE (S) SEROTONIN	RELATIVE FREQUENCY OF SIDE EFFECTS SEDATION	RELATIVE FREQUENCY OF SIDE EFFECTS ANTI-CHOLINERGIC
BICYCLICS **Fluoxetine** Prozac®	Cap 20 mg.	(A) 20–80 (M) 20–40	d	(N) 0 (S) +	None	Very Low
CHLOROPROPIOPHENONES **Bupropion** Wellbutrin® (Investigational - Burroughs Wellcome)	—	(A) 300–450 (M) —	d	(N) 0 (S) 0	None	None

a. From references 149, 164–170.
b. Blocks reuptake of (N) Norepinephrine, (S) Serotonin.
c. Includes active metabolites.
d. Not well established.

Monoamine Oxidase Inhibitors

Pharmacology. The antidepressant action of monoamine oxidase inhibitors (MAOIs) is thought to be due to alterations in adrenergic and serotonergic receptor sensitivity. The most consistent findings during long-term MAOI therapy include up-regulation of α_1-adrenergic function and down-regulation of β-adrenergic and adenyl cyclase activity.

Administration and Adult Dose. See MAOIs Comparison Chart for oral dosage range. Phenelzine dose is 1 mg/kg/day.[171] Doses should be initiated at the lower limit and titrated upward depending on tolerance to side effects. Dosage schedule should remain divided, usually bid or tid.

Dosage Individualization. Initial dosage and rate of upward dosage titration should be reduced if the patient has taken a heterocyclic antidepressant within 7–10 days.

Pediatric Dose. Not recommended in children under 16 yr.

Dosage Forms. See MAOIs Comparison Chart.

Patient Instructions. This drug usually takes 2 weeks for significant response and up to 4 weeks for full therapeutic benefit to occur. This drug may cause faintness or dizziness, especially after rising suddenly, standing for prolonged periods or after exertion or alcohol intake. Nausea and vomiting, sweating, severe occipital headache and stiff neck may be a sign of a serious adverse effect and should be reported immediately. Avoid concurrent use of diet pills, cough and cold remedies and restrict consumption of aged foods high in tyramine (see Tyramine Content of Foods and Beverages in the Dietary Considerations chapter). See also Class Instructions.

Pharmacokinetics. *Onset and Duration.* Onset 2 weeks, while maximum improvement occurs after 4 weeks.[171,172]
   Plasma Levels. Not used clinically.
   Fate. Termination of drug action is dependent upon MAO regeneration, because the drugs or their active metabolites chemically combine with the MAO enzyme.

Adverse Reactions. Autonomic effects are frequent and are not necessarily dose-dependent; these include postural hypotension, dry mouth and constipation. Drowsiness is more frequent with phenelzine, while overstimulation and agitation is more likely with tranylcypromine. Occasionally delayed ejaculation, edema, skin rash, urinary retention and blurred vision occur.[148,150] Although overstated as a problem, hypertensive crisis may result from concurrent use of sympathomimetic amines or ingestion of high tyramine-content food and drinks.[173]

Contraindications. Patients over 60 yr; patients with confirmed or suspected cerebrovascular defect; cardiovascular disease; hypertension; pheochromocytoma; history of liver disease or abnormal liver function tests.

Precautions. Combinations with sympathomimetic drugs, meperidine, heterocyclic antidepressants and other MAOIs should be avoided; postural hypotension may be increased when phenothiazine, heterocyclic antidepressant or antihypertensive drugs are co-administered. Avoid diets high in tyramine content—see Tyramine Content of Foods and Beverages in the Dietary Considerations chapter. Like other antidepressant drugs, MAOIs may switch bipolar patients to a hypomanic or manic state. The possibility of suicide should always be considered in depressed patients and adequate precautions taken.

Notes. MAOIs are effective in major depressive disorder and in panic disorder, and are drugs of choice for atypical depression.[171,174] Phenelzine is the preferred MAOI, because it has been more recently and thoroughly studied in terms of indications, efficacy, dosage and safety.[171]

Monoamine Oxidase Inhibitors Comparison Chart[a]

DRUG	DOSAGE FORMS	USUAL EFFECTIVE DAILY ADULT DOSAGE RANGE (MG)	COMMENTS
Isocarboxazid Marplan®	Tab 10 mg.	10–30	Mild stimulating effect; hydrazine.
Phenelzine Nardil®	Tab 15 mg.	60–90	Most sedating MAOI; hydrazine.
Tranylcypromine Parnate®	Tab 10 mg.	20–40	Most stimulating MAOI; nonhydrazine.

a. From references 171, 175.

28:16.08 TRANQUILIZERS

Neuroleptic Drugs

Pharmacology. The antipsychotic efficacy is most likely related to blockade of postsynaptic dopaminergic receptors in the mesolimbic area of the brain, although other neurotransmitter systems may also be involved.[156]

Administration and Adult Dose. See Neuroleptic Drugs Comparison Chart for oral dosage ranges. Initiate therapy with divided doses until therapeutic dosage is found, then, for most patients, once daily dosing at bedtime is preferred. For maintenance therapy, decrease acute dosage by 25% q 3 months, with a target maintenance dose being 50–67% of the acute treatment dose.[176,177] Recent concern has focused on the need to establish a minimum effective dose for neuroleptic drugs, and low-dose treatment regimens are likely to become prevalent.[185] **Rapid IM** neuroleptization is indicated for rapid control of aggressive, combative, psychotic patients; one to four IM injections of 2.5–10 mg of haloperidol, fluphenazine or thiothixene is usually sufficient.[178] **IM depot** fluphenazine decanoate and haloperidol decanoate indicated only for drug-responsive patients with an established history of noncompliance.

Dosage Individualization. Doses in the lower range are sufficient for most elderly patients and the rate of dosage titration should be slower.[177]

Pediatric Dose. As with adults, dosage is primarily determined by titration and adjustment to the individual. No precise dosage ranges exist, but in general, initial dosage is lower and should be increased more gradually in children.

Dosage Forms. See Neuroleptic Drugs Comparison Chart.

Patient Instructions. See Class Instructions. These drugs usually take several weeks for clinical response and up to 6 weeks for full therapeutic response.

Pharmacokinetics. *Onset and Duration.* Onset of antipsychotic activity is variable, with significant response requiring days to weeks.[177]

Plasma Levels. Not used clinically.[177-179]

Fate. During chronic oral chlorpromazine therapy, peak plasma levels occur within 3 hr. Oral SR products have poor bioavailability. Peak plasma levels can be delayed up to 6 hr after IM administration. IM injection of chlorpromazine gives plasma levels several times higher than an equivalent PO dose, while haloperidol can be used in a PO:IM ratio of 1–1.5:1.[180,181] Prior to extensive hepatic metabolism, a significant portion of chlorpromazine is metabolized crossing the intestinal wall to the portal circulation. Phenothiazines have many active metabolites, while haloperidol has inactive metabolites.[182] Chlorpromazine is 95–98% protein bound.[180]

$t_{1/2}$. Plasma half-lives have no clinical correlation to biologic half-lives for neuroleptic drugs. Chlorpromazine plasma half-life has been reported as 2–31 hr, thioridazine 4–10 hr, thiothixene 34 hr and haloperidol 13–35 hr. Of more clinical importance than half-life is the attainment of steady-state CNS levels and tissue saturation which allows once daily dosing.

Adverse Reactions. See Neuroleptic Drugs Comparison Chart for relative frequency of the common adverse reactions. Frequently sedation, extrapyramidal effects (eg, parkinsonism, dystonic reactions, akathisia), anticholinergic effects (eg, dry mouth, blurred vision, constipation, urinary retention) and postural hypotension occur. Occasionally weight gain, amenorrhea, galactorrhea, ejaculatory disturbance, photosensitivity and skin rash. Rarely cholestatic jaundice, seizures, thermoregulatory impairment, agranulocytosis, quinidine-like effect and skin or eye pigmentation occur. Tardive dyskinesia is a long-term adverse effect, sometimes irreversible and untreatable.[183,184]

Contraindications. Coma; circulatory collapse or severe hypotension; bone marrow depression; history of blood dyscrasias.

Precautions. Use cautiously in patients with myasthenia gravis, Parkinson's disease, seizure disorders or hepatic disease.

Notes. No neuroleptic drug has been shown to possess greater safety or efficacy for any subgroup of schizophrenic patients or any target symptom.[177] See also Prochlorperazine (56:22) for anti-emetic uses.

Haloperidol Decanoate   Haldol Decanoate®

Haloperidol decanoate (HD) represents an alternative to fluphenazine decanoate as a long-acting depot neuroleptic drug. Although fluphenazine and haloperidol are very similar in efficacy, potency and adverse effect profile, there are several major differences in these two drugs as depot formulations. Fluphenazine decanoate is typically given once every 2 weeks, while HD is recommended to be given once every 4 weeks. Because HD has only recently been introduced into clinical practice, little is known about its dose-response relationship and frequency of adverse effects compared to oral neuroleptic drugs. All patients should be stabilized on an oral neuroleptic drug before HD is considered. Most studies suggest monthly administration in doses of 10–15 times the daily oral haloperidol dose or its equivalent. Initial HD dosage should not exceed 100 mg, and experience with monthly doses greater than 300 mg is limited. Steady-state haloperidol plasma concentrations are achieved by the third or fourth dose of monthly HD. When oral neuroleptic supplements are necessary for control of psychotic symptoms between injections, the HD dose should be increased at the next scheduled injection interval. Despite the convenience of monthly injections, dosage and dosing interval must be individualized as with oral neuroleptic drug therapy.[186,187] Available as a 50 mg/ml injection.

Neuroleptic Drugs Comparison Chart[a]

DRUG CLASS DRUG	DOSAGE FORMS	ORAL DOSAGE RANGE (MG/DAY)	ORAL EQUIVALENT ANTI-PSYCHOTIC DOSE	RELATIVE FREQUENCY OF SIDE EFFECTS			
				SEDATION	ANTI-CHOLINERGIC	EXTRA-PYRAMIDAL	POSTURAL HYPOTENSION
PHENOTHIAZINES							
Chlorpromazine Thorazine® Various	Soln 30, 100 mg/ml Syrup 10 mg/5 ml Tab 10, 25, 50, 100, 200 mg Inj 25 mg/ml Supp 25, 100 mg SR cap not recommended.	50–1200	100	High	Moderate	Moderate	High
Fluphenazine Permitil® Prolixin® Various	Elxr 0.5 mg/ml Soln 5 mg/ml Tab 1, 2.5, 5, 10 mg Inj 2.5 mg/ml.	2–40 +	2	Low	Low	Very High	Low
Fluphenazine Decanoate Prolixin® Various	Inj 25 mg/ml.	12.5–75 (IM) q 2 weeks	—	Low	Low	Very High	Low

Continued

Neuroleptic Drugs Comparison Chart[a]

| DRUG CLASS DRUG | DOSAGE FORMS | ORAL DOSAGE RANGE (MG/DAY) | ORAL EQUIVALENT ANTI-PSYCHOTIC DOSE | RELATIVE FREQUENCY OF SIDE EFFECTS | | | |
				SEDATION	ANTI-CHOLINERGIC	EXTRA-PYRAMIDAL	POSTURAL HYPOTENSION
Perphenazine Trilafon® Various	Soln 16 mg/5 ml Tab 2, 4, 8, 16 mg Inj 5 mg/ml SR not recommended.	12–64	8	Low	Low	High	Low
Thioridazine Mellaril®	Soln 30, 100 mg/ml Susp 25, 100 mg/5 ml Tab 10, 15, 25, 50, 100, 150, 200 mg.	50–800	100	High	High	Low	High
Trifluoperazine Stelazine®	Soln 10 mg/ml Tab 1, 2, 5, 10 mg Inj 2 mg/ml	5–40 +	5	Low	Low	High	Low
THIOXANTHENES **Thiothixene** Navane® Various	Cap 1, 2, 5, 10, 20 mg Soln 5 mg/ml Inj 2, 5 mg/ml.	5–60	4	Low	Low	High	Low

Continued

Neuroleptic Drugs Comparison Chart[a]

DRUG CLASS DRUG	DOSAGE FORMS	ORAL DOSAGE RANGE (MG/DAY)	ORAL EQUIVALENT ANTI-PSYCHOTIC DOSE	RELATIVE FREQUENCY OF SIDE EFFECTS			
				SEDATION	ANTI-CHOLINERGIC	EXTRA-PYRAMIDAL	POSTURAL HYPOTENSION
BUTYROPHENONES							
Haloperidol Haldol® Various	Soln 2 mg/ml Tab 0.5, 1, 2, 5, 10, 20 mg Inj 5 mg/ml.	2–100	2	Low	Very Low	Very High	Low
Haloperidol Decanoate Haldol Decanoate®	Inj 50 mg/ml.	50–300 (IM) monthly	—	Low	Very Low	Very High	Low
DIBENZOXAZEPINES							
Loxapine Daxolin® Loxitane®	Cap 5, 10, 25, 50 mg Soln 25 mg/ml Inj 50 mg/ml.	20–250	15	Low	Low	High	Low
DIHYDROINDOLONES							
Molindone Moban®	Tab 5, 10, 25, 50, 100 mg Soln 20 mg/ml.	50–225	10	Low	Low	High	Low

a. From references 164, 176, 177, 184.

Pimozide   Orap®

Pimozide is an "orphan drug" indicated for the treatment of Tourette's disorder. Although structurally different from other neuroleptic drugs, pimozide shares the ability to block dopaminergic receptors. Its lack of effect on norepinephrine receptors led to the hope that pimozide would have a much more favorable adverse effect profile compared to other neuroleptic drugs. Haloperidol is considered the drug treatment of choice for Tourette's disorder. Thus far, their relative frequency of adverse effects is very similar and pimozide remains an alternative to haloperidol rather than a first-line drug. Initial oral dosage is 1–2 mg/day in divided doses, with dosage increased every other day up to a maximum of 20 mg/day. Most patients who respond require 10 mg/day or less.[188] Available as 2 mg tablets.

28:24 ANXIOLYTICS, SEDATIVES, AND HYPNOTICS

General References: 189–193

Class Instructions. This drug causes drowsiness and may produce sleep. Do not exceed prescribed dosage and use caution when driving, operating machinery or performing other tasks requiring mental alertness. Avoid concurrent use of alcohol and other drugs which cause drowsiness or sleep.

28:24.04 BARBITURATES

Phenobarbital   Various

Pharmacology. A "long-acting" barbiturate which depresses a wide range of cellular functions in many organ systems, although its central depressant action is desired for sedative-hypnotic effect. See also Phenobarbital, 28:12.04.

Administration and Adult Dose. See Sedatives and Hypnotics Comparison Chart. **PO hypnotic dose,** although rarely indicated, is 100–200 mg. See Phenobarbital, 28:12.04 for anticonvulsant dosage.

Dosage Individualization. Dosage reduction may be necessary in severe chronic liver disease or in renal impairment.[118,194]

Pediatric Dose. **PO for sedation** 2 mg/kg/day in 4 divided doses.

Dosage Forms. See Sedatives and Hypnotics Comparison Chart.

Patient Instructions. See Class Instructions.

Pharmacokinetics. *Onset and Duration.* PO onset of sedation 20–60 min; duration 6–8 hr.[195]
   Plasma Levels. (Anticonvulsant) 15–40 mcg/ml.[108,110]
   Fate. About 80% oral absorption, although variable, with 49–58% plasma protein bound. V_d is 0.6–1 L/kg; Cl is 0.0038–0.0053 L/hr/kg. Peak plasma levels after oral dosage occur in 6–18 hr.[197,198] There is much individual variation in metabolism and elimination; about 65% is converted to the inactive metabolite para-hydroxyphenobarbital. 35% is excreted unchanged in the urine; acidic urine may increase, and alkaline urine decrease half-life.[108-110,118,119,200]
   $t_{1/2}$. (Adults) 2–5 days; (children) 1.6–2.9 days.[199] In one study, half-life increased to 5.4 days in chronic liver disease, while remaining unchanged in acute liver disease.[200]

Adverse Reactions. Most frequent dose-related side effect is sedation, to which tolerance usually develops. Children and the elderly may become paradoxically excited and hyperactive. Occasionally skin rashes, disturbances in motor function and megaloblastic anemia may occur. Rarely, Stevens-Johnson syndrome, exfoliative dermatitis, photosensitivity, hepatitis and jaundice have been reported. SC or intra-arterial administration may result in necrosis or sloughing; IV administration may cause injury to adjacent nerves and extravasation can produce tissue necrosis.[195]

Contraindications. Respiratory disease where dyspnea or obstruction is present; porphyria.

Precautions. Pregnancy. Use with caution in severe cardiac disease and IV in patients with pulmonary or cardiovascular disease. Severe liver disease might be expected to decrease metabolism to the drug's inactive metabolite, although information is limited. In patients with renal disease, increased toxicity has been observed.[199] See Barbiturates in Drug Interactions Chapter.

Notes. Do not mix with other injectables. In overdosage, excretion may be enhanced by alkalinizing the urine. See also Phenobarbital 28:12.04.

Secobarbital Sodium   Seconal®, Various

Pharmacology. A "short-acting" barbiturate, capable of producing all levels of CNS depression.

Administration and Adult Dose. PO for sleep 100-200 mg; PO for preoperative sedation 200-300 mg 1-2 hr before surgery. IM for sedation 1-2 mg/kg. IV for preanesthesia basal sleep up to 250 mg, at a rate not to exceed 50 mg/15 sec.

Pediatric Dose. PO for sedation 2 mg/kg/day in 4 divided doses; PO for preoperative sedation 50-100 mg.

Dosage Forms. See Sedatives and Hypnotics Comparison Chart.

Patient Instructions. See Class Instructions.

Pharmacokinetics. *Onset and Duration.* Oral or rectal onset 10-30 min; duration 6-8 hr.[195]
   Fate. Well absorbed following oral, rectal or parenteral administration; 52-57% plasma protein bound.[201] Metabolized to active and inactive compounds; less than 0.1% excreted in urine unchanged.[198]
   $t_{1/2}$. See Sedatives and Hypnotics Comparison Chart.

Adverse Reactions. CNS depression, sedation and morning hangover are dose-related. Rarely, hypersensitivity reactions (eg, skin rashes, Stevens-Johnson syndrome, photosensitivity, blood dyscrasias) occur.

Contraindications. See Phenobarbital. Also, parenteral secobarbital is contraindicated in obstetric deliveries.

Precautions. See Phenobarbital. Although secobarbital is not harmful in renal disease, the parenteral polyethylene glycol vehicle may irritate the kidneys.

Notes. Refrigerate injection; do not mix with other injectables. Hypnotic efficacy is significantly reduced after 1-2 weeks of continuous use.[202,203]

28:24.08 BENZODIAZEPINES

Benzodiazepines

Pharmacology. Benzodiazepines have a more specific anxiolytic effect than other sedatives such as barbiturates. Benzodiazepines facilitate gamma aminobutyric acid (GABA)-mediated transmission and mimic the actions of glycine at its receptor sites. Barbiturates share the GABA effect, but have negligible effects on the glycine receptor.[204]

Administration and Adult Dose. See Benzodiazepines and Related Drugs Comparison Chart. Optimal oral dosing requires individual titration to clinical response. The long-acting drugs can be dosed once daily at bedtime, while the short-acting drugs require multiple daily dosing—see Benzodiazepines and Related Drugs Comparison Chart. Dosing schedule should be determined by the individual patient's degree of dysfunction from daytime anxiety versus insomnia. **PO for alcohol withdrawal** chlordiazepoxide 25–100 mg or diazepam 5–20 mg q 6 hr (not prn) for agitation, tremor and anxiety. Many patients need oral chlordiazepoxide 100–200 mg the first day; occasionally 300 mg or more is necessary; unusual cases may require up to 1600 mg the first day. **IV for extreme agitation of withdrawal** chlordiazepoxide 12.5 mg/min or diazepam 2.5 mg/min slow push until patient is calm. After the first day, dose can be decreased by 25% daily and discontinued on the 5th day. Published withdrawal protocols are only guidelines; dosage may need to be adjusted upward for withdrawal breakthrough or decreased due to toxicity. Higher doses may be necessary in heavy smokers; lower doses may be needed in patients with severe liver disease and decreased serum albumin; **IM chlordiazepoxide is not recommended** because of slow, erratic absorption, pain and muscle damage.[205] See Fate and Notes.

Dosage Individualization. Patients with liver disease or elderly patients may have reduced clearance and/or enhanced CNS sensitivity which requires dosage reduction. Alcoholic patients with reduced plasma proteins may require a lower dosage due to decreased protein binding.

Pediatric Dose. PO (diazepam) 1–2.5 mg tid-qid. Most benzodiazepines are not recommended in children due to insufficient clinical experience.

Dosage Forms. See Benzodiazepines and Related Drugs Comparison Chart.

Patient Instructions. See Class Instructions, 28:24.

Pharmacokinetics. *Fate.* Oral diazepam and chlordiazepoxide administration gives faster and more complete drug absorption than IM injection.[206] Lorazepam has rapid and reliable IM absorption.[207] Midazolam and flunitrazepam also offer good IM absorption.[208] See also Benzodiazepines and Related Drugs Comparison Chart.

Adverse Reactions. Frequent effects include drowsiness, dizziness, ataxia and disorientation; these effects rarely require drug discontinuation and are easily managed by dosage reduction. Occasionally, agitation and excitement may occur; this "paradoxical rage reaction" is usually attributed to the long-acting drugs and a short-acting drug is preferred for patients with a history of aggressive, hostile behavior.[209] Hypotension and respiratory depression are occasionally observed with parenteral therapy. Rarely, hepatic disease and blood dyscrasias occur.

Contraindications. Acute narrow angle glaucoma.

Precautions. Pregnancy; impaired hepatic function. Abrupt drug withdrawal may result in rebound insomnia, an abstinence syndrome similar to barbiturate withdrawal, seizures or, rarely, psychosis.[210]

Notes. Benzodiazepines are preferred over barbiturates, phenothiazines or paraldehyde for alcohol withdrawal because they are equally efficacious, provide superior anticonvulsant activity and are less toxic. No evidence suggests superiority of any benzodiazepine over others in withdrawal efficacy, although chlordiazepoxide has been most well studied and is most often used. Pharmacokinetic differences may be important in some patients (eg, oxazepam may be preferred in severe liver disease).[205]

Alprazolam   Xanax®

Alprazolam is a triazolobenzodiazepine used as an anxiolytic and antidepressant. Compared to diazepam, it has as rapid an onset, an earlier peak plasma level and a much shorter duration of action. Studies in mixed anxious-depressed outpatients have shown alprazolam to be more effective than diazepam. There is also evidence that alprazolam is effective in the treatment of panic disorders. Adverse effects are similar to other benzodiazepines, but may be less severe (eg, sedation and ataxia, which are dose-related). Alprazolam is 3–5 times more potent than diazepam; initial oral dose is 0.25–0.5 mg tid, which can be increased up to 4 mg/day. The lower dosage range is recommended for anxiety, while the higher doses are recommended for neurotic depression and mild anxious depression.[211,212] It is available as 0.25, 0.5 and 1 mg tablets.

Flurazepam Hydrochloride   Dalmane®, Various

Pharmacology. Flurazepam's hypnotic effect is probably related to its facilitation of gamma aminobutyric acid-mediated neurotransmission, but the exact mechanism is unknown.

Administration and Adult Dose. See Benzodiazepines and Related Drugs Comparison Chart. An oral 30 mg initial dose is preferred for young healthy patients, because 15 mg may be less effective.[213] Elderly patients, particularly over 70 yr, should be given an initial dose of 15 mg PO at bedtime.[214,215]

Pediatric Dose. Not recommended in children under 15 yr.

Dosage Forms. See Benzodiazepines and Related Drugs Comparison Chart.

Patient Instructions. See Class Instructions, 28:24. The full benefit of hypnotic effect may not be seen until after several nights' use.

Pharmacokinetics. *Onset and Duration.* Clinical effect increases on the second and third night of continuous use and persists for several nights after drug discontinuation.

**   *Fate.*** Rapidly absorbed after oral administration and rapidly metabolized to N_1-hydroxyethylflurazepam and N-desalkylflurazepam. Flurazepam levels are too low to detect within a few hours after ingestion.[213] The hydroxyethyl metabolite is measurable only in the early hours after ingestion; the major active metabolite is N-desalkylflurazepam.[216]

    $t_{1/2}$. (N-desalkylflurazepam) 47–100 hr, reaching steady-state in 7–10 days.[216]

Adverse Reactions. Unwanted morning drowsiness or hangover are frequent; prevalence of hangover is about 5% with the 30 mg dose in young patients, rising to 39% with the 30 mg dose in patients over 70 yr.[214,215] Occasional effects include impairment of motor function and intellectual performance, dry mouth, nightmares, delirium and confusion.[213]

Precautions. Pregnancy; impaired hepatic function.

Notes. Flurazepam is preferred to nonbenzodiazepine hypnotics, because it is much safer in overdosage, interferes less with sleep physiology and remains effective beyond one week of continuous use.[213,217] There are no differences which favor flurazepam over other benzodiazepines for insomnia, but others have not been as well studied for this indication.

Midazolam Hydrochloride   Versed®

Midazolam is a short-acting triazolobenzodiazepine for use in insomnia and in anesthesia. It is unique in its physicochemical properties; at a pH of < 4.0 the drug exists as a highly water soluble, stable compound, but at a physiologic pH it becomes lipophilic. This allows for IV administration of a water soluble, rapid acting drug with a very low frequency of venous irritation. Midazolam is currently indicated for IM preoperative sedation and IV for induction of anesthesia or for conscious sedation for endoscopy and other procedures. Usual adult IM dose is 0.07–0.08 mg/kg one hour before surgery. Induction of anesthesia typically requires 0.15–0.35 mg/kg IV depending upon age and presence of premedication. For endoscopy and other conscious sedation procedures, dosage must be individualized and not administered by rapid bolus. Titrate *slowly* to desired effect; some patients may respond to as little as 1 mg. No more than 2.5 mg should be given over at least 2 minutes as the 1 mg/ml (or more dilute) solution; in elderly, debilitated or chronically ill patients, the initial dose should be limited to 1.5 mg. Further small doses may be given after waiting at least 2 min. The drug should never be given IV without oxygen and resuscitation equipment immediately available. Midazolam, in an oral dose of 15 mg, is an effective hypnotic for patients experiencing difficulty falling asleep. Its very short duration of effect would not make midazolam a drug of choice for patients with early morning awakening. In geriatric patients, the minimum effective hypnotic dose is 7.5 mg PO, and doses of up to 30 mg at bedtime are well tolerated. A comparison of midazolam 30 mg and triazolam 1 mg demonstrated equal hypnotic efficacy and less residual effect the next morning from midazolam. The extent and degree of rebound adverse effects from midazolam upon treatment withdrawal is not known.[218-220] Available as 1 and 5 mg/ml injection.

Triazolam   Halcion®

Triazolam is a triazolobenzodiazepine compound with hypnotic efficacy equal to flurazepam. It differs from flurazepam, because it has a rapid onset of effect and very short half-life. Its short-term efficacy is established, but efficacy beyond 2–4 weeks has not been established. Of some concern are reports of rebound insomnia when triazolam is discontinued after only several days' use. Common adverse effects include drowsiness, dry mouth and ataxia which are dose-related; less common is anterograde amnesia. Triazolam is 30–60 times more potent than flurazepam; initial oral hypnotic dose is 0.25 mg; in geriatric or debilitated patients the initial dose is 0.125 mg.[193,221] Available as 0.125 and 0.25 mg tablets.

Benzodiazepines and Related Drugs Comparison Chart[a]

DRUG	DOSAGE FORMS	ORAL DOSAGE RANGE	PEAK ORAL PLASMA LEVELS (HOURS)	HALF-LIFE (HOURS)	MAJOR ACTIVE METABOLITES (HALF-LIFE IN HOURS)
ANXIOLYTICS					
LONG-ACTING					
Chlordiazepoxide Librium® Libritabs® Various	Cap 5, 10, 25 mg Tab 5, 10, 25 mg Inj 100 mg.	15–100 mg/day	2–4	5–30	Desmethylchlordiazepoxide; demoxepam; desmethyl-diazepam (30–60).
Clorazepate Tranxene® Various	Cap 3.75, 7.5, 15 mg Tab 3.75, 7.5, 11.25, 15, 22.5 mg.	15–60 mg/day	b	30–60[a]	Desmethyldiazepam (30–60).
Diazepam Valium® Various	SR Cap 15 mg Tab 2, 5, 10 mg Soln 1, 5 mg/ml Inj 5 mg/ml.	6–40 mg/day	1–2	20–50	Desmethyldiazepam (30–60).
Halazepam Paxipam®	Tab 20, 40 mg.	60–160 mg/day	1–3	7	n-3-Hydroxyhalazepam; desmethyldiazepam.
Prazepam Centrax® Various	Cap 5, 10, 20 mg Tab 10 mg.	20–60 mg/day	6	78	3-Hydroxyprazepam; desmethyldiazepam.

Continued

Benzodiazepines and Related Drugs Comparison Chart[a]

DRUG	DOSAGE FORMS	ORAL DOSAGE RANGE	PEAK ORAL PLASMA LEVELS (HOURS)	HALF-LIFE (HOURS)	MAJOR ACTIVE METABOLITES (HALF-LIFE IN HOURS)
SHORT-ACTING					
Alprazolam[e] Xanax®	Tab 0.25, 0.5, 1 mg.	0.75–4 mg/day	0.7–1.6	12–19	α-Hydroxyalprazolam.
Lorazepam[c] Ativan® Various	Tab 0.5, 1, 2 mg Inj 2, 4 mg/ml.	2–6 mg/day	2	10–20	None.
Oxazepam Serax® Various	Cap 10, 15, 30 mg Tab 15 mg.	30–120 mg/day	1–2	5–10	None.
HYPNOTICS **LONG-ACTING**					
Flurazepam Dalmane® Various	Cap 15, 30 mg.	15–60 mg	d	d	Desalkylflurazepam (50–100).
Quazepam Dormalin®	Tab 7.5 mg.	7.5–30 mg	—	40	2-Oxo-quazepam (40); desalkylflurazepam (50–100).

Continued

Benzodiazepines and Related Drugs Comparison Chart[a]

DRUG	DOSAGE FORMS	ORAL DOSAGE RANGE	PEAK ORAL PLASMA LEVELS (HOURS)	HALF-LIFE (HOURS)	MAJOR ACTIVE METABOLITES (HALF-LIFE IN HOURS)
Flunitrazepam[c] Rohypnol® (Investigational - Roche)	—	1–2 mg	<1	24	7-Aminoflunitrazepam (23); N-desmethylflunitrazepam (31).
SHORT-ACTING **Midazolam**[c,e] Versed®	Inj 1, 5 mg/ml.	7.5–30 mg (Investigational)	0.4–0.7	1.8	None.
Temazepam Restoril® Various	Cap 15, 30 mg.	15–30 mg	2–3	9–12	None.
Triazolam[e] Halcion®	Tab 0.125, 0.25 mg.	0.125–0.5 mg	0.5–1.5	2.3	α-Hydroxytriazolam.

a. From references 192, 208, 211, 221–224.
b. Hydrolyzed to desmethyldiazepam before absorption.
c. Also used as an IV anesthetic; well absorbed IM.
d. Rapidly and completely metabolized to desalkylflurazepam.
e. Not a true benzodiazepine, but a closely related triazolobenzodiazepine.

28:24.92 MISCELLANEOUS ANXIOLYTICS, SEDATIVES, AND HYPNOTICS

Buspirone   BuSpar®

Buspirone is a nonbenzodiazepine anxiolytic drug. Its mechanism of action is unknown, and it does not directly affect the GABA-benzodiazepine receptor complex. Buspirone antagonizes striatal dopamine autoreceptors, thus acting as a mild dopamine agonist. It lacks anticonvulsant activity, does not interact or have cross-tolerance with alcohol or other CNS depressants, produces no muscle relaxation or euphoriant effect, and has little potential for dependence and addiction. Buspirone is rapidly absorbed, has high first-pass metabolism and is extensively metabolized, with an elimination half-life of 2–3 hr. In anxiolytic efficacy, buspirone is equipotent to diazepam. Its onset of anxiolytic effect requires several days with maximum efficacy seen after several weeks, making buspirone an ineffective prn anxiolytic or hypnotic. Headache, GI distress, dizziness and nervousness are the most frequent side effects. Sedation is possible, but rarely occurs with doses less than 30 mg/day. Patients being switched from a benzodiazepine to buspirone should be tapered off the benzodiazepine slowly since buspirone may enhance withdrawal effects. Buspirone should be used with caution in patients receiving monoamine oxidase inhibitors. The initial dose is 5 mg tid, increasing in 5 mg/day increments at 2–3 day intervals, to a maximum of 60 mg. Most patients are maintained on doses of 15–30 mg/day.[225-228] Available as 5 and 10 mg tablets.

Chloral Hydrate   Noctec®, Somnos®, Various

Pharmacology.   A chlorinated aliphatic alcohol, rapidly reduced to trichloroethanol which is responsible for CNS depression.

Administration and Adult Dose. **PO or PR for sleep** 500 mg–1 g hs, to maximum of 2 g. **PO or PR for sedation** 250 mg tid after meals, to maximum of 2 g/day. **PO for alcohol withdrawal** 500 mg–1 g q 6 hr (often given with paraldehyde).

Pediatric Dose. **PO or PR for sleep** 50 mg/kg to maximum of 1 g/dose. Sedative dose is one-half the hypnotic dose, given in divided doses.

Dosage Forms. See Sedatives and Hypnotics Comparison Chart.

Patient Instructions. Capsules should be taken with a full glass of liquid; syrup should be mixed in a half glass of water, juice or ginger ale. See also Class Instructions.

Pharmacokinetics. *Onset and Duration.* Onset 30–60 min.
    Fate. Rapidly and well absorbed from GI tract; rapidly reduced to active metabolite trichloroethanol, with a smaller fraction oxidized to the inactive trichloroacetic acid. Metabolites and their glucuronides excreted in urine.[196]
    $t_{1/2}$. (Trichloroethanol) 8 hr.[199]

Adverse Reactions. Occasionally, gastric irritation and nausea occur; rarely, excitement, delirium, disorientation, erythematous and urticarial allergic reactions are reported.

Contraindications. Marked hepatic or renal impairment.

Precautions. Pregnancy; gastritis or ulcers; severe cardiac disease.

Notes. Chloral hydrate is a useful agent for prn use, but loses its hypnotic efficacy by the second week of use.[202] Unlike barbiturates, chloral hydrate causes no significant enzyme induction and there is no significant effect on REM sleep or difficulty with REM rebound for most patients.[202]

Sedatives and Hypnotics Comparison Chart[a]

DRUG CLASS DRUG	DOSAGE FORMS	ORAL DOSE	HALF-LIFE (HOURS)
SEDATIVES			
BARBITURATES			
Amobarbital Amytal® Various	Cap 65, 200 mg Tab 15, 30, 50, 100 mg Pwdr for Inj 250, 500 mg.	30–50 mg bid-tid.	14–42
Phenobarbital Various	Cap 16 mg Elxr 15, 20 mg/5 ml Tab 16, 32, 65, 100 mg Inj 30, 65, 130 mg/ml Pwdr for Inj 120 mg.	15–30 mg bid-qid.	48–120
PROPANEDIOLS			
Meprobamate Equanil® Miltown® Various	Tab 200, 400, 600 mg SR Cap 200, 400 mg.	400 mg tid-qid.	6–16
HYPNOTICS			
BARBITURATES			
Pentobarbital Nembutal® Various	Cap 50, 100 mg Elxr 20 mg/5 ml Supp 30, 60, 120, 200 mg Inj 50 mg/ml.	100–200 mg.	21–42
Secobarbital	Cap 50, 100 mg	100–200 mg.	19–34

Continued

Sedatives and Hypnotics Comparison Chart[a]

DRUG CLASS DRUG	DOSAGE FORMS	ORAL DOSE	HALF-LIFE (HOURS)
Seconal® Various	Tab 100 mg Inj 50 mg/ml.		
CHLORAL DERIVATIVES			
Chloral Hydrate Noctec® Various	Cap 250, 500 mg Supp 324, 500, 648 mg Syrup 250, 500 mg/5 ml.	500 mg–1 g.	8 (Trichloroethanol)
PIPERIDINEDIONES			
Glutethimide Doriden® Various	Cap 500 mg Tab 250, 500 mg.	500 mg–1 g.	5–22
Methyprylon Noludar®	Cap 300 mg Tab 50, 200 mg.	200–400 mg.	4
ACETYLINIC ALCOHOLS			
Ethchlorvynol Placidyl®	Cap 200, 500, 750 mg.	500 mg–1 g.	6
OTHER			
L-Tryptophan Various	Cap 500 mg Tab 500 mg, 1 g.	0.5–4 g.	—
Zolpidem (Investigational)	—	10–30 mg.	3.5–5

a. From references 199, 229, 230.

28:28 ANTIMANIC AGENTS

Lithium Carbonate	Various
Lithium Citrate	Cibalith-S®, Lithonate-S®

Pharmacology. The mechanism of antimanic effect is unknown; lithium may substitute for Na^+, K^+, Mg^{++} and Ca^{++} at various cellular sites and alter the synthesis and function of various neurotransmitters.

Administration and Adult Dose. Individualize dosing according to plasma levels and clinical response. Acute manic episodes typically require 1.2-2.4 g/day, while maintenance therapy requires 900 mg-1.5 g/day.[231] A loading dose of 30 mg/kg, in 3 divided doses, can be given to achieve the desired plasma level within 12 hr.[232]

Dosage Individualization. Dosage must be more carefully adjusted in patients with decreased renal function (eg, renal disease and the elderly) and in patients receiving thiazide diuretics.

Pediatric Dose. Not recommended in children under 12 yr.

Dosage Forms. **Cap** 300 mg (8 mEq); **Tab** 300 mg; **SR Tab** 300, 450 mg (12 mEq); **Syrup** 8 mEq/5ml (as citrate).

Patient Instructions. This drug may be taken with food, milk or antacid to minimize stomach upset. Report immediately if signs of toxicity occur, such as persistent diarrhea, vomiting, hand tremor, drowsiness or slurred speech, or prior to beginning any diet. In hot weather, ensure adequate water and salt intake.

Pharmacokinetics. *Onset and Duration.* Onset 7-10 days.[233]

  Plasma Levels. For acute mania or hypomania 0.8-1.5 mEq/L. For prophylaxis 0.6-1.2 mEq/L.[231,234] Levels above 1.5 mEq/L are regularly associated with some signs of toxicity and levels above 2.0 mEq/L result in serious toxicity. See Adverse Reactions.

  Fate. Virtually total absorption within 8 hr after oral administration, with peak levels occurring in 2-4 hr. Distribution is throughout total body water, but tissue uptake is not uniform. Not protein bound or metabolized, but freely filtered through the glomerulus with about 80% being reabsorbed.[235]

  $t_{1/2}$. 18-20 hr; up to 36 hr in the elderly.[236]

Adverse Reactions. Dose-related: (therapeutic plasma levels) nausea, vomiting, diarrhea, polyuria, polydipsia, fine hand tremor, muscle weakness; (1.5-2.0 mEq/L) coarse hand tremor, persistent GI effects, muscle hyperirritability, slurred speech, confusion; (over 2.0 mEq/L) stupor, seizures, increased deep tendon reflexes, irregular pulse, hypotension, coma.

  Non dose-related: Nontoxic goiter, nephrogenic diabetes insipidus-like syndrome, folliculitis, acneiform eruptions, cogwheel rigidity, leukocytosis. Possible long-term adverse effect is histochemical evidence of renal damage.[231,237]

Contraindications. Fluctuating renal function; significant renal impairment.

Precautions. Use with caution in patients with significant cardiac disease, dehydration, sodium depletion, organic brain disease or the elderly.[238]

Parameters to Monitor. Pre-lithium workup should include thyroid function tests, Cr_s and BUN, CBC (for baseline white count), urinalysis (for baseline specific gravity), electrolytes and EKG (if over 40 yr).[231,239] During therapy, obtain plasma lithium levels (drawn 8-12 hr after last dose) q week during initiation and monthly during maintenance.

References, 28:00 Central Nervous System Agents

1. Fuster V, Chesebro JH. Antithrombotic therapy: role of platelet-inhibitor drugs (3 parts). Mayo Clin Proc 1981;56:102-12;185-95;265-73.

2. Yu TF, Gutman AB. Study of the paradoxical effects of salicylate in low, intermediate and high dosage on the renal mechanisms for excretion of urate in man. J Clin Invest 1959;38:1298-1315.

3. Borga O, Odar-Cederlof I, Ringberger V-A et al. Protein binding of salicylate in uremic and normal plasma. Clin Pharmacol Ther 1976;20:464-75.

4. Netter P, Faure G, Regent MC et al. Salicylate kinetics in old age. Clin Pharmacol Ther 1985;38:6-11.

5. Davison C. Salicylate metabolism in man. Ann NY Acad Sci 1971;179:249-68.

6. Mongan E, Kelly P, Nies K et al. Tinnitus as an indication of therapeutic serum salicylate levels. JAMA 1973;226:142-5.

7. Done AK. Aspirin-overdosage: incidence, diagnosis, and management. Pediatrics 1978;62(Suppl):890-7.

8. Levy G, Tsuchiya T, Amsel LP. Limited capacity for salicyl phenolic glucuronide formation and its effect on the kinetics of salicylate elimination in man. Clin Pharmacol Ther 1972;13:258-68.

9. Rowland M, Riegelman S, Harris PA et al. Absorption kinetics of aspirin in man following oral administration of an aqueous solution. J Pharm Sci 1972;61:379-85.

10. Levy G. Pharmacokinetics of salicylate elimination in man. J Pharm Sci 1965;54:959-67.

11. Levy G, Yaffe SJ. Clinical implications of salicylate-induced liver damage. Am J Dis Child 1975;129:1385-6.

12. Jusko WJ, Gretch M. Plasma and tissue protein binding of drugs in pharmacokinetics. Drug Metab Rev 1976;5:43-140.

13. Stevenson DD, Mathison DA. Aspirin sensitivity in asthmatics. When may this drug be safe? Postgrad Med 1985;78:111-9.

14. Mielke CH, Heiden D, Britten AF et al. Hemostasis, antipyretics, and mild analgesics: acetaminophen vs aspirin. JAMA 1976;235:613-6.

15. Anon. Surgeon General's advisory on the use of salicylates and Reye syndrome. Morbid Mortal Wkly Rep 1982;31:289-90.

16. Rahwan GL, Rahwan RG. Aspirin and Reye's syndrome: the change in prescribing habits of health professionals. Drug Intell Clin Pharm 1986;20:143-5.

17. Housholder GT. Intolerance to aspirin and the nonsteroidal anti-inflammatory drugs. J Oral Maxillofac Surg 1985;43:333-7.

18. Anon. Is all aspirin alike? Med Lett Drugs Ther 1974;16:57-9.

19. Lanza FL, Royer GL, Nelson RS. Endoscopic evaluation of the effects of aspirin, buffered aspirin, and enteric-coated aspirin on gastric and duodenal mucosa. N Engl J Med 1980;303:136-8.

20. Mills RFN, Adams SS, Cliffe EE et al. The metabolism of ibuprofen. Xenobiotica 1973;3:589-98.

21. Kaiser DG, Vangiessen GJ. GLC determination of ibuprofen in plasma. J Pharm Sci 1974;63:219-21.

22. Gryfe CI, Rubenzahl S. Agranulocytosis and aplastic anemia possibly due to ibuprofen. Can Med Assoc J 1976;114:877.

23. Stempel DA, Miller JJ. Lymphopenia and hepatotoxicity with ibuprofen. J Pediatr 1977;90:657-8.

24. Bernstein RF. Ibuprofen-related meningitis in mixed connective tissue disease. Ann Intern Med 1980;92:206-7.

25. Alvan G, Orme M, Bertilsson L et al. Pharmacokinetics of indomethacin. Clin Pharmacol Ther 1975;18:364-73.

26. Duggan DE, Hogans AF, Kwan KC. The metabolism of indomethacin in man. J Pharmacol Exp Ther 1972;181:563-75.

27. O'Brien WM. Indomethacin: a survey of clinical trials. Clin Pharmacol Ther 1968;9:94-107.

28. Ansell BM, Hanna DB, Stoppard M. Naproxen absorption in children. Curr Med Res Opin 1975;3:46-50.

29. Simon LS, Mills JA, Nonsteroidal antiinflammatory drugs (2 parts). N Engl J Med 1980;302:1179-85;1237-43.

30. Day RO et al. Relationship of serum naproxen concentration to efficacy in rheumatoid arthritis. Clin Pharmacol Ther 1982;31:733-40.

31. Runkel R, Chaplin M, Boost G et al. Absorption, distribution, metabolism, and excretion of naproxen in various laboratory animals and human subjects. J Pharm Sci 1972;61:703-8.

32. Segre EJ. Naproxen metabolism in man. J Clin Pharmacol 1975;15:316-23.

33. Runkel R, Forchielli E, Boost G et al. Naproxen-metabolism, excretion and comparative pharmacokinetics. Scand J Rheumatology (Suppl)1973;2:29-36.

34. Runkel R, Forchielli E, Sevelius H et al. Nonlinear plasma level response to high doses of naproxen. Clin Pharmacol Ther 1974;15:261-6.

35. Williams RL, Upton RA, Cello JP et al. Naproxen disposition in patients with alcoholic cirrhosis. Eur J Clin Pharmacol 1984;27:291-6.

36. Brogden RN, Pinder RM, Sawyer PR et al. Naproxen: a review of its pharmacological properties and therapeutic efficacy and use. Drugs 1975;9:326-63.

37. Brezin JH, Katz SM, Schwartz AB et al. Reversible renal failure and nephrotic syndrome associated with nonsteroidal anti-inflammatory drugs. N Engl J Med 1979;301:1271-3.

38. Cartwright KC, Trotter TL, Cohen ML. Naproxen nephrotoxicity. Ariz Med 1979;36:124-6.

39. Special symposium on piroxicam. Eur J Rheumatol Inflammation 1981;4:275-377.

40. Ishizaki T et al. Pharmacokinetics of piroxicam, a new nonsteroidal anti-inflammatory agent, under fasting and postprandial states in man. J Pharmacokinet Biopharm 1979;7:369-81.

41. Bigby M, Stern R. Cutaneous reactions to nonsteroidal anti-inflammatory drugs: a review. J Am Acad Dermatol 1985;12:866-76.

42. Brogden RN et al. Diflunisal: a review of its pharmacological properties and therapeutic use in pain and musculoskeletal strains and sprains and pain in osteoarthritis. Drugs 1980;19:84-106.

43. Goulton J, Baker PG. Ketoprofen (Orudis) in the treatment of inflammatory arthritic conditions: a multicenter

study in general practice. Curr Med Res Opin 1980;6:423-30.

44. Ishizaki T, Sasake T, Suganuma T et al. Pharmacokinetics of ketoprofen following single oral, intramuscular and rectal doses and after repeated oral administration. Eur J Clin Pharmacol 1980;18:407-14.

45. Hart FD, Huskisson EC. Non-steroidal anti-inflammatory drugs. Current status and rational therapeutic use. Drugs 1984;27:232-55.

46. Marsh CC, Schuna AA, Sundstrom WR. A review of selected investigational nonsteroidal antiinflammatory drugs of the 1980s. Pharmacotherapy 1986;6:10-25.

47. Lewis AJ. The pharmacologic profile of oxaprozin. Semin Arthritis Rheum 1986;15(Suppl 2):11-7.

48. McEvoy G, ed. American Hospital Formulary Service. Bethesda, MD: American Society of Hospital Pharmacists, 1959-87.

49. Schmerzler E, Yu W, Hewitt MI et al. Gas chromatographic determination of codeine in serum and urine. J Pharm Sci 1966;55:155-7.

50. Way EL, Adler TK. The pharmacologic implications of the fate of morphine and its surrogates. Pharmacol Rev 1968;12:383-446.

51. Gilman AG, Goodman LS, Rall TW et al, eds. Goodman and Gilman's the pharmacological basis of therapeutics. 7th ed. New York: Macmillan, 1985.

52. Mather LE, Tucker GT. Systemic availability of orally administered meperidine. Clin Pharmacol Ther 1976;20:535-40.

53. Edwards DJ, Svensson CK, Visco JP et al. Clinical pharmacokinetics of pethidine: 1982. Clin Pharmacokinet 1982;7:421-33.

54. Gourlay GK, Cousins MJ. Strong analgesics in severe pain. Drugs 1984;28:79-91.

55. Fochtman FW, Winek CL. Therapeutic serum concentrations of meperidine (Demerol®). J Forensic Sci 1969;14:213-8.

56. Klotz U, McHorse TS, Wilkinson GR et al. The effect of cirrhosis on the disposition and elimination of meperidine in man. Clin Pharmacol Ther 1974;16:667-75.

57. McHorse TS, Wilkinson GR, Johnson RF et al. Effect of acute viral hepatitis in man on the disposition and elimination of meperidine. Gastroenterology 1975;68:775-80.

58. Tang R, Shimomura SK, Rotblatt M. Meperidine-induced seizures in sickle cell patients. Hosp Formul 1980;15:764-72.

59. Inturrisi CE. Role of opioid analgesics. Am J Med 1984;77:27-35.

60. Fultz JM, Senay EC. Guidelines for the management of hospitalized narcotic addicts. Ann Intern Med 1975;82:815-8.

61. Dalton WS. Rational use of narcotic analgesics. Hosp Ther 1985;(Sept):45-60.

62. Holmstrand J, Anggard E, Gunne L-M. Methadone maintenance: plasma levels and therapeutic outcome. Clin Pharmacol Ther 1978;23:175-80.

63. Berkowitz BA. The relationship of pharmacokinetics to pharmacological activity: morphine, methadone and naloxone. Clin Pharmacokinet 1976;1:219-30.

64. Gourlay GK, Cousins MJ. Strong analgesics in severe pain. Drugs 1984;28:79-91.

65. Verebely K, Volavka J, Mule S et al. Methadone in man: pharmacokinetic and excretion studies in acute and chronic treatment. Clin Pharmacol Ther 1976;18:180-90.

66. Olsen GD, Wendel HA, Livermore JD et al. Clinical effects and pharmacokinetics of racemic methadone and its optical isomers. Clin Pharmacol Ther 1977;21:147-57.

67. Beauclair TR, Stoner CP. Adherence to guidelines for continuous morphine sulfate infusions. Am J Hosp Pharm 1986;43:671-6.

68. Holmes AH. Morphine IV infusion for chronic pain. Drug Intell Clin Pharm 1978;12:556-7.

69. Bollish SJ, Collins CL, Kirking DM et al. Efficacy of patient-controlled versus conventional analgesia for postoperative pain. Clin Pharm 1985;4:48-52.

70. Baumann TJ, Batenhorst RL, Graves DA et al. Patient-controlled analgesia in the terminally ill cancer patient. Drug Intell Clin Pharm 1986;20:297-301.

71. Berkowitz BA, Ngai SH, Yang JC et al. The disposition of morphine in surgical patients. Clin Pharmacol Ther 1975;17:629-35.

72. Stanski DR, Greenblatt DJ, Lowenstein E. Kinetics of intravenous and intramuscular morphine. Clin Pharmacol Ther 1978;24:52-9.

73. Brunk SF, Delle M. Morphine metabolism in man. Clin Pharmacol Ther 1974;16:51-7.

74. Melzack R, Mount BM, Gordon JM. The Brompton mixture versus morphine solution given orally: effects on pain. Can Med Assoc J 1979;120:435-8.

75. Twycross RG. Value of cocaine in opiate-containing elixirs. Br Med J 1977;4:1348.

76. Miller RR. Evaluation of nalbuphine hydrochloride. Am J Hosp Pharm 1980;37:942-9.

77. Anon. Reevaluation of parenteral pentazocine. Med Lett Drugs Ther 1976;18:46-7.

78. Berkowitz B. Influence of plasma levels and metabolism on pharmacological acitivty: pentazocine. Ann NY Acad Sci 1971;179:269-81.

79. Ehrnebo M, Boreus LO, Lonroth U. Bioavailability and first-pass metabolism of oral pentazocine in man. Clin Pharmacol Ther 1977;22:888-92.

80. Burt RAP, Beckett AH. The absorption and excretion of pentazocine after administration by different routes. Br J Anesth 1971;43:427-35.

81. Keeri-Szanto M, Pomeroy JR. Atmospheric pollution and pentazocine metabolism. Lancet 1971;1:947-9.

82. Oh SJ, Rollins JL, Lewis I. Pentazocine-induced fibrous myopathy. JAMA 1975;231:271-3.

83. Brogden RN, Speight TM, Avery GS. Pentazocine: a review of its pharmacologic properties, therapeutics, efficacy and dependence liability. Drugs 1973;5:6-91.

84. Beaver WT. A clinical comparison of the effects of oral and intramuscular administration of analgesics: Pentazocine and phenazocine. Clin Pharmacol Ther 1968;9:582-97.

85. Reed DA, Schnoll SH. Abuse of pentazocine-naloxone combination. JAMA 1986;256:2562-4.

86. Miller RR. Dosage and choice of parenteral strong analgesics. Am J Hosp Pharm 1974;31:780-2.

87. Beaver WT. The pharmacologic basis for the choice of an analgesic. I. potent analgesics. Pharmacol for Physi-

cians 1970;4(10):1-7.

88. Ameer B, Salter FJ. Drug therapy reviews: evaluation of butorphanol tartrate. Am J Hosp Pharm 1979;36:1683-91.

89. Rubin TN. Tomosada WP. The pain cocktail as an adjunctive agent in the treatment of spine pain patients. Drug Intell Clin Pharm 1981;15:958-63.

90. Koch-Weser J. Acetaminophen. N Engl J Med 1976;295:1297-1300.

91. Cote J, Moriarty RW, Rumack BH. Facing toxic overdose of acetaminophen. Patient Care 1979;13:16-33.

92. Slattery JT, Levy G. Acetaminophen kinetics in acutely poisoned patients. Clin Pharmacol Ther 1979;25:184-94.

93. Mitchell JR, Thorgeirsson SS, Potter WZ et al. Acetaminophen-induced hepatic injury: protective role of glutathione in man and rationale for therapy. Clin Pharmacol Ther 1974;16:676-84.

94. Albert KS. Pharmacokinetics of orally administered acetaminophen in man. J Pharmacokinet Biopharm 1974;2:381-93.

95. Finlayson NDC, Prescott LF, Adjepon-Yamoah KK et al. Antipyrine, lidocaine, and paracetamol metabolism in chronic liver disease. Gastroenterology 1974;67:790. Abstract.

96. Prescott LF, Roscoe P, Wright N et al. Plasma-paracetamol half-life and hepatic necrosis in patients with paracetamol overdosage. Lancet 1971;1:519-22.

97. Barker JD, de Carle DJ, Anuras S. Chronic excessive acetaminophen use and liver damage. Ann Intern Med 1977;87:299-301.

98. Longnecker DE, Grazis PA, Eggers GWN. Naloxone for antagonism of morphine-induced respiratory depression. Anesth Analg 1973;52:447-53.

99. Evans JM, Hogg MIJ, Lunn JN et al. Degree and duration of reversal by naloxone of effects of morphine in conscious subjects. Br Med J 1974;2:589-91.

100. Fishman J, Roffwarg H, Hellman L. Disposition of naloxone-7,8-^{3}H in normal and narcotic-dependent men. J Pharmacol Exp Ther 1973;187:575-80.

101. Ngai SH, Berkowitz BA, Yang JC et al. Pharmacokinetics of naloxone in rats and in man: basis for its potency and short duration of action. Anesthesiology 1976;44:398-401.

102. Moreland TA, Brice JEH, Walker CHM et al. Naloxone pharmacokinetics in the newborn. Br J Clin Pharmacol 1980;9:609-12.

103. Bonnet F, Bilaine J, Lhoste F et al. Naloxone therapy of human septic shock. Crit Care Med 1985;13:972-5.

104. Hughes GS, Porter RS, Marx R et al. Naloxone and septic shock. Ann Intern Med 1983;98:559. Letter.

105. Verebey K, Volavka J, Mule SJ et al. Naltrexone: disposition, metabolism, and effects after acute and chronic dosing. Clin Pharmacol Ther 1976;20:315-28.

106. Crabtree BL. Review of naltrexone, a long-acting opiate antagonist. Clin Pharm 1984;3:273-80.

107. Meyer MC, Straughn AB, Lo M-W et al. Bioequivalence, dose-proportionality, and pharmacokinetics of naltrexone after oral administration. J Clin Psychiatry 1984;45(9, Sec. 2):15-9.

108. Woodbury DM, Penry JK, Pippenger CE, eds. Antiepileptic drugs. 2nd ed. New York: Raven Press, 1982.

109. Eadie MJ. Anticonvulsant drugs — an update. Drugs 1984;27:328-63.

110. Penry JK, Newmark ME. The use of antiepileptic drugs. Ann Intern Med 1979;90:207-18.

111. Goldberg MA, McIntyre HB. Barbiturates in the treatment of status epilepticus. In: Delgado-Escueta AV, Wasterlain CG, Treiman DM et al, eds. Advances in neurology, Vol 34: Status epilepticus. New York: Raven Press, 1983;499-503.

112. Delgado-Escueta AV, Wasterlain C, Treiman DM et al. Management of status epilepticus. N Engl J Med 1982;306:1337-40.

113. Alvin J, McHorse T, Hoyumpa A et al. The effect of liver disease in man on the disposition of phenobarbital. J Pharmacol Exp Ther 1975;192:224-35.

114. Levy RH, Yerby MS. Effects of pregnancy on antiepileptic drug utilization. Epilepsia 1985;26(Suppl 1):S52-7.

115. Rothner AD, Erenberg G. Status epilepticus. Pediatr Clin North Am 1980;27:593-602.

116. Nelson E, Powell JR, Conrad K et al. Phenobarbital pharmacokinetics and bioavailability in adults. J Clin Pharmacol 1982;22:141-8.

117. Reynolds EH, Trimble MR. Adverse neuropsychiatric effects of anticonvulsant drugs. Drugs 1985;29:570-81.

118. Theodore WH, Porter RJ. Removal of sedative-hypnotic antiepileptic drugs from the regimens of patients with intractable epilepsy. Ann Neurol 1983;13:320-4.

119. Mattson RH, Cramer JA, Collins JF et al. Comparison of carbamazepine, phenobarbital, phenytoin, and primidone in partial and secondarily generalized tonic-clonic seizures. N Engl J Med 1985;313:145-51.

120. Cloyd JC, Miller KW, Leppik IE. Primidone kinetics: effects of concurrent drugs and duration of therapy. Clin Pharmacol Ther 1981;29:402-7.

121. Pisani F, Richens A. Pharmacokinetics of phenylethylmalonamide (PEMA) after oral and intravenous administration. Clin Pharmacokinet 1983;8:272-6.

122. Browne TR. Clonazepam. N Engl J Med 1978;299:812-6.

123. Dreifuss FE. Treatment of the nonconvulsive epilepsies. Epilepsia 1983;24(Suppl 1):S45-S54.

124. Cloyd JC, Gumnit RJ, McLain LW. Status epilepticus — the role of intravenous phenytoin. JAMA 1980;244:1479-81.

125. Record KE, Rapp RP, Young AB et al. Oral phenytoin loading in adults: rapid achievement of therapeutic plasma levels. Ann Neurol 1979;5:268-70.

126. Salem RB, Wilder BJ, Yost RL et al. Rapid infusion of phenytoin sodium loading doses. Am J Hosp Pharm 1981;38:354-7.

127. Kostenbauder HB, Rapp RP, McGovren JP et al. Bioavailability and single-dose pharmacokinetics of intramuscular phenytoin. Clin Pharmacol Ther 1975;18:449-56.

128. Liponi DF, Winter ME, Tozer TN. Renal function and therapeutic concentrations of phenytoin. Neurology 1984;34:395-7.

129. Jung D, Powell JR, Walson P et al. Effect of dose on phenytoin absorption. Clin Pharmacol Ther

1980;28:479-85.

130. Bauer LA. Interference of oral phenytoin absorption by continuous nasogastric feedings. Neurology 1982;32:570-2.

131. Cacek AT, DeVito JM, Koonce JR. In vitro evaluation of nasogastric administration methods for phenytoin. Am J Hosp Pharm 1986;43:689-92.

132. Earnest MP, Marx JA, Drury LR. Complications of intravenous phenytoin for acute treatment of seizures: recommendations for usage. JAMA 1983;249:762-5.

133. Leppik IE, Lapora J, Loewenson R. Seasonal incidence of phenytoin allergy unrelated to plasma levels. Arch Neurol 1985;42:120-2.

134. Haruda F. Phenytoin hypersensitivity: 38 cases. Neurology 1979;29:1480-5.

135. Cloyd JC, Bosch DE, Sawchuk RJ. Concentration-time profile of phenytoin after admixture with small volumes of intravenous fluids. Am J Hosp Pharm 1978;35:45-8.

136. Lahr MB. Hyponatremia during carbamazepine therapy. Clin Pharmacol Ther 1985;37:693-6.

137. Hart RG, Easton JD. Carbamazepine and hematological monitoring. Ann Neurol 1982;11:309-12.

138. Snead OC, Hosey LC. Exacerbation of seizures in children by carbamazepine. N Engl J Med 1985;313:916-21.

139. Rimmer EM, Richens A. An update on sodium valproate. Pharmacotherapy 1985;5:171-84.

140. Turnbull DM, Rawlins MD, Weightman D et al. Plasma concentrations of sodium valproate: their clinical value. Ann Neurol 1983;14:38-42.

141. Wilder BJ, Karas BJ, Hammond EJ et al. Twice-daily dosing of valproate with divalproex. Clin Pharmacol Ther 1983;34:501-4.

142. Snead OC, Miles MV. Treatment of status epilepticus in children with rectal sodium valproate. J Pediatr 1985;106:323-5.

143. Chiba K, Suganuma T, Ishizaki T et al. Comparison of steady-state pharmacokinetics of valproic acid in children between monotherapy and multiple antiepileptic drug treatment. J Pediatr 1985;106:653-8.

144. Delgado-Escueta AV, Treiman DM, Walsh GO. The treatable epilepsies. (Second of two parts). N Engl J Med 1983;308:1576-84.

145. Klein DF, Gittleman R, Quitkin F et al, eds. Diagnosis and drug treatment of psychiatric disorders: adults and children. 2nd ed. Baltimore: Williams and Wilkins, 1980.

146. Jarvick ME. Psychopharmacology in the practice of medicine. New York: Appleton-Century-Crofts, 1977.

147. Eisdorfer C. Fann WE. Psychopharmacology of aging. New York: Spectrum Publications, 1980.

148. Rapoport JL, Mikkelsen EJ, Zavadil A et al. Childhood enuresis II. Psychopathology, tricyclic concentration in plasma, and antienuretic effect. Arch Gen Psychiatry 1980;37:1146-52.

149. Van Brunt N. The clinical utility of tricyclic antidepressant blood levels: a review of the literature. Ther Drug Monit 1983;5:1-10.

150. Ziegler VE, Biggs JT, Wylie LT et al. Protriptyline kinetics. Clin Pharmacol Ther 1978;23:580-4.

151. Gram LF, Christiansen J. First-pass metabolism of imipramine in man. Clin Pharmacol Ther 1975;17:555-63.

152. Taska RJ. Clinical laboratory aids in the treatment of depression. Curr Concepts Psychiatry 1977;3:12-20.

153. Bunney WE. Psychopharmacology of the switch process in affective illness. In: DiMascio A, Kollam KF, eds. Psychopharmacology: a generation of progress. New York: Raven Press, 1978;1249-59.

154. Bailey DN, van Dyke C, Langou RA et al. Tricyclic antidepressants: plasma levels and clinical findings in overdose. Am J Psychiatry 1978;135:1325-8.

155. Preskorn SH, Othmer SC. Evaluation of bupropion hydrochloride: the first of a new class of atypical antidepressants. Pharmacotherapy 1984;4:20-34.

156. Richelson E. Pharmacology of neuroleptics in use in the United States. J Clin Psychiatry 1985;46(8, Sec. 2):8-14.

157. Stark P, Fuller RW, Wong DT. The pharmacologic profile of fluoxetine. J Clin Psychiatry 1985;46(3, Sec. 2):7-13.

158. Stark P, Hardison CD. A review of multicenter controlled studies of fluoxetine vs. imipramine and placebo in outpatients with major depressive disorder. J Clin Psychiatry 1985;46(3, Sec. 2):53-8.

159. Wernicke JF. The side effect profile and safety of fluoxetine. J Clin Psychiatry 1985;46(3, Sec. 2):59-67.

160. Nelson EB, Pool JL. Fluoxetine in the treatment of obesity. Clin Pharmacol Ther 1987;41:198. Abstract.

161. Bryant SG, Ereshefsky L. Antidepressant properties of trazodone. Clin Pharm 1982;1:406-17.

162. Brogden RN, Heel RC, Speight TM et al. Trazodone: a review of its pharmacological properties and therapeutic use in depression and anxiety. Drugs 1981;21:401-76.

163. Georgotas A, Forsell TL, Mann JJ et al. Trazodone hydrochloride: a wide spectrum antidepressant with a unique pharmacological profile. Pharmacotherapy 1982;2:255-65.

164. Klein DF, Gittleman R, Quitkin F et al, eds. Diagnosis and drug treatment of psychiatric disorders: adults and children. 2nd ed. Baltimore: Williams and Wilkins, 1980.

165. Gelenberg AJ. Prescribing antidepressants. Drug Ther 1979;9:95-112.

166. Stimmel GL. Maprotiline (Ludiomil®). Drug Intell Clin Pharm 1980;14:585-90.

167. Coccaro EF, Siever LJ. Second generation antidepressants: a comparative review. J Clin Pharmacol 1985;25:241-60.

168. Pi EH, Simpson GM. New antidepressants: a review. Hosp Formul 1985;20:580-8.

169. Richelson E. Pharmacology of antidepressants in use in the United States. J Clin Psychiatry 1982;43:(11, Sec. 2):4-11.

170. Salzman C. Clinical guidelines for the use of antidepressant drugs in geriatric patients. J Clin Psychiatry 1985;46:(10, Sec. 2):38-44.

171. Robinson DS, Nies A, Ravaris L et al. Clinical pharmacology of phenelzine. Arch Gen Psychiatry 1978;35:629-35.

172. Goodman WK, Charney DS. Therapeutic applications and mechanisms of action of monoamine oxidase inhibitor and heterocyclic antidepressant drugs. J Clin Psychiatry 1985;46(10, Sec.2):6-22.

173. Walker JI, Davidson J, Zung WWK. Patient compliance with MAO inhibitor therapy. J Clin Psychiatry 1984;45(7, Sec. 2):78-80.

174. Nies A. Differential response patterns to MAO inhibitors and tricyclics. J Clin Psychiatry 1984;45(7, Sec. 2):70-7.

175. Davidson J, Turnbull C. The importance of dose in isocarboxazid therapy. J Clin Psychiatry 1984;45(7, Sec 2):49-52.

176. Coyle JT. The clinical use of antipsychotic medications. Med Clin North Am 1982;66:993-1009.

177. Kessler KA, Waletzky JP. Clinical use of the antipsychotics. Am J Psychiatry 1981;138:202-9.

178. Donlon PT, Hopkins J, Tupin JP. Overview: efficacy and safety of the rapid neuroleptization method with injectable haloperidol. Am J Psychiatry 1979;136:273-8.

179. Simpson GM, Yadalam K. Blood levels of neuroleptics: state of the art. J Clin Psychiatry 1985;46(5, Sec. 2):22-8.

180. Curry SH, Davis JM, Janowski DS, et al. Factors affecting chlorpromazine plasma levels in psychiatric patients. Arch Gen Psychiatry 1970;22:209-16.

181. Mason AS, Granacher RP. Basic principles of rapid neuroleptization. Dis Nerv Syst 1976;37:547-51.

182. DiMascio A, Shader RI. Butyrophenones in psychiatry. New York: Raven Press, 1972;11-23.

183. Anon. Tardive dyskinesia: summary of a Task Force Report of the American Psychiatric Association. Am J Psychiatry 1980;137:1163-72.

184. Simpson GM, Pi EH, Sramek JJ. Adverse effects of antipsychotic agents. Drugs 1981;21:138-51.

185. Johnson EAW. Antipsychotic medication: clinical guidelines for maintenance therapy. J Clin Psychiatr 1985;46(5, Sec 2):6-15.

186. Kane JM. Dosage strategies with long-acting injectable neuroleptics, including haloperidol decanoate. J Clin Psychopharmacol 1986;6:20S-3S.

187. Nair NPV, Suranyi-Cadotte B, Schwartz G et al. A clinical trial comparing intramuscular haloperidol decanoate and oral haloperidol in chronic schizophrenic patients: efficacy, safety, and dosage equivalence. J Clin Psychopharmacol 1986;6:30S-7S.

188. Colvin CL, Tankanow RM. Pimozide: use in Tourette's syndrome. Drug Intell Clin Pharm 1985;19:421-4.

189. Consensus Conference. Drugs and insomnia: the use of medications to promote sleep. JAMA 1984;251:2410-4.

190. Schuckit MA. Current therapeutic options in the management of typical anxiety. Clin Psychiatry 1981;42(11, Sec. 2):15-26.

191. Meyer BR. Benzodiazepines in the elderly. Med Clin North Am 1982;66:1017-35.

192. Sussman N. The benzodiazepines: selection and use in treating anxiety, insomnia, and other disorders. Hosp Formul 1985;20:298-305.

193. Wincor MZ. Insomnia and the new benzodiazepines. Clin Pharm 1982;1:425-32.

194. Hvidberg EF, Dam M. Clinical pharmacokinetics of anticonvulsants. Clin Pharmacokinet 1976;1:161-88.

195. Anon. Current drug therapy-barbiturates. Am J Hosp Pharm 1976;33:333-9.

196. Marshall EK Jr, Owens AH Jr. Absorption, excretion, and metabolic fate of chloral hydrate and trichloroethanol. Bull Johns Hopkins Hosp 1954;95:1-18.

197. Lous P. Plasma levels and urinary excretion of three barbituric acids after oral administration to man. Acta Pharmacol Toxicol 1954;10:147-65.

198. Parker KD, Elliott HW, Wright JA et al. Blood and urine concentrations of subjects receiving barbiturates, meprobamate, glutethimide, or diphenylhydantoin. Clin Toxicol 1970;3:131-45.

199. Breimer DD. Clinical pharmacokinetics of hypnotics. Clin Pharmacokinet 1977;2:93-109.

200. Hvidberg EF, Dam M. Clinical pharmacokinetics of anticonvulsants. Clin Pharmacokinet 1976;1:161-88.

201. Jusko WJ, Gretch M. Plasma and tissue protein binding of drugs in pharmacokinetics. Drug Metab Rev 1976;5:43-140.

202. Kales A, Bixler EO, Kales JD et al. Comparative effectiveness of nine hypnotic drugs: sleep laboratory studies. J Clin Pharmacol 1977;17:207-13.

203. Kales A, Hauri P, Bixler EO et al. Effectiveness of intermediate—term use of secobarbital. Clin Pharmacol Ther 1976;20:541-5.

204. Snyder SH, Enna SJ, Young AB. Brain mechanisms associated with therapeutic actions of benzodiazepines: focus on neurotransmitters. Am J Psychiatry 1977;134:662-5.

205. Sellers EM, Kalant H. Alcohol intoxication and withdrawal. N Engl J Med 1976;294:757-62.

206. Hillestad L, Hansen T, Melsom H et al. Diazepam metabolism in normal man: I. Serum concentrations and clinical effects after IV, IM, and oral administration. Clin Pharmacol Ther 1974;16:479-84.

207. Greenblatt DJ, Joyce TH, Comer WH et al. Clinical Pharmacokinetics of lorazepam. II. Intramuscular injection. Clin Pharmacol Ther 1977;21:222-30.

208. Dundee JW. New IV anaesthetics. Br J Anaesth 1979;5:641-8.

209. Brown CR. The use of benzodiazepines in prison populations. J Clin Psychiatry 1978;39:219-22.

210. Dominguez RA, Goldstein BJ. 25 years of benzodiazepine experience: clinical commentary on use, abuse, and withdrawal. Hosp Formul 1985;20:1000-14.

211. Evans RL. Alprazolam. Drug Intell Clin Pharm 1981;15:633-8.

212. Fawcett JA, Kravitz HM. Alprazolam: pharmacokinetics, clinical efficacy, and mechanism of action. Pharmacotherapy 1982;2:243-54.

213. Greenblatt DJ, Shader RI, Koch-Weser J. Flurazepam hydrochloride, a benzodiazepine hypnotic. Ann Intern Med 1975;83:237-41.

214. Marttila JK, Hammel RJ, Alexander B et al. Potential untoward effects of longterm use of flurazepam in geriatric patients. J Am Pharm Assoc 1977;NS17:692-5.

215. Greenblatt DJ, Allen MD, Shader RI. Toxicity of high-dose flurazepam in the elderly. Clin Pharmacol Ther 1977;21:355-61.

216. Kaplan SA, deSilva JAF, Jack ML et al. Blood level profile in man following chronic oral administration of flurazepam hydrochloride. J Pharm Sci 1973;62:1932-5.

217. Kales A, Bixler EO, Kales JD et al. Comparative effectiveness of nine hypnotic drugs: sleep laboratory studies. J Clin Pharmacol 1977;17:207-13.

218. Dundee JW, Halliday NJ, Harper KW et al. Midazolam: a review of its pharmacological properties and

therapeutic use. Drugs 1984;28:519-43.

219. Reves JG, Fragen RJ, Vinik HR et al. Midazolam: pharmacology and uses. Anesthesiology 1985;62:310-24.

220. Kanto JH. Midazolam: the first water-soluble benzodiazepine — pharmacology, pharmacokinetics and efficacy in insomnia and anesthesia. Pharmacotherapy 1985;5:138-55.

221. Roth T, Roehrs TA, Zorick FJ. Pharmacology and hypnotic efficacy of triazolam. Pharmacotherapy 1983;3:137-48.

222. Mattila MAK, Larni HM. Flunitrazepam: a review of its pharmacological properties and therapeutic use. Drugs 1980;20:353-74.

223. Mitler MM. Evaluation of temazepam as a hypnotic. Pharmacotherapy 1981;1:3-13.

224. Greenblatt DJ, Shader RI, Divoll M et al. Benzodiazepines: a summary of pharmacokinetic properties. Br J Clin Pharmacol 1981;11:11S-6S.

225. Goa KL, Ward A. Buspirone: a preliminary review of its pharmacological properties and therapeutic efficacy as an anxiolytic. Drugs 1986;32:114-29.

226. Kastenholz KV, Crismon LM. Buspirone, a novel nonbenzodiazepine anxiolytic. Clin Pharm 1984;3:600-7.

227. Goldberg HL. Buspirone hydrochloride: a unique new anxiolytic agent. Pharmacokinetics, clinical pharmacology, abuse potential and clinical efficacy. Pharmacotherapy 1984;4:315-24.

228. Eison AS, Temple DL. Buspirone: review of its pharmacology and current perspectives on its mechanism of action. Am J Med 1986;80(Suppl 3B):1-9.

229. Kadak D, Inaba T, Endrenyl L et al. Comparative drug elimination capacity in man-glutethimide, amobarbital, antipyrine, and sulfinpyrazone. Clin Pharmacol Ther 1973;14:552-60.

230. Hartmann E. L-tryptophan: a rational hypnotic with clinical potential. Am J Psychiatry 1977;134:366-70.

231. Stimmel GL. Affective disorders. J Contin Educ Hosp Clin Pharm 1979;1:27-39.

232. Kook KA, Stimmel GL, Wilkins JN et al. Accuracy and safety of a prior lithium loading. J Clin Psychiatry 1985;46:49-51.

233. Goodwin FK, Zis AP. Lithium in the treatment of mania. Arch Gen Psychiatry 1979;36:840-4.

234. Grof P. Some practical aspects of lithium treatment. Arch Gen Psychiatry 1979;36:891-3.

235. Schou M. Biology and pharmacology of the lithium ion. Pharmacol Rev 1957;9:17-58.

236. Amidsen A. Serum level monitoring and clinical pharmacokinetics of lithium. Clin Pharmacokinet 1977;2:73-92.

237. Ramsey TA, Cox M. Lithium and the kidney: a review. Am J Psychiatr 1982;139:443-9.

238. Donaldson IMG, Cuningham J. Persisting neurologic sequelae of lithium carbonate therapy. Arch Neurol 1983;40:747-51.

239. Salem RB. Recommendations for monitoring lithium therapy. Drug Intell Clin Pharm 1983;17:346-50.

240. Wilder BJ, Ramsay RE. Oral and intramuscular phenytoin. Clin Pharmacol Ther 1976;19:360-4.

241. Hall AH, Smolinske SC, Conrad FL et al. Ibuprofen overdose: 126 cases. Ann Emerg Med 1986;15:1308-13.

242. Adams SS, Cliffe EE, Lessel B et al. Some biological properties of 2-(4-isobutylphenyl)-propionic acid. J Pharm Sci 1967;56:1686.

243. Prosser TR, Lander RD. Phenytoin-induced hypersensitivity reactions. Clin Pharm 1987;6:728-34.

40:00 ELECTROLYTIC, CALORIC AND WATER BALANCE

40:12 REPLACEMENT SOLUTIONS

General References: 1-4

Class Instructions.   Oral products should be taken with (tablets) or diluted in (liquids and powders) 3/4 to 1 glass of water or juice to avoid GI injury or laxative effect; may be taken with food or after meals if upset stomach occurs.

Calcium Salts   Various

Pharmacology. Calcium is a structural element of bone, essential for normal nerve and muscle function, excitation-contraction coupling process, maintenance of membrane integrity and coagulation.[5]

Administration and Adult Dose. **PO as dietary supplement** 500–2000 mg elemental calcium bid-qid.[6-8] **IV for emergency elevation of serum calcium** 7–14 mEq, may repeat q 1–3 days depending upon response. **IV for hypocalcemic tetany** 4.5–16 mEq, may repeat until tetany is controlled; infuse slowly at a rate of 0.5–2 ml/min.

Dosage Individualization. Maintenance doses should be based on serum calcium and diet; adolescence, renal impairment and the postmenopausal state may increase requirements.[9,10]

Pediatric Dose. **PO as dietary supplement** (children) 45–64 mg/kg elemental calcium daily. **PO for neonatal hypocalcemia** 50–150 mg/kg elemental calcium daily, to maximum of 1 g/day. RDA (0–0.5 yr) 360 mg/day; (0.5–1 yr) 540 mg/day; (1–10 yr) 800 mg/day; (11–18 yr) 1200 mg/day.[8] **IV for emergency elevation of serum calcium** (infants) less than 1 mEq repeated q 1–3 days, depending on response; (children) 1–7 mEq repeated q 1–3 days, depending on response. **IV for hypocalcemic tetany** (infants) 2.4 mEq/day in divided doses; (children) 0.5–0.7 mEq/kg tid-qid or more until tetany controlled.

Dosage Forms. See Oral Calcium Products Comparison Chart. **Inj** (chloride) 1 g/10 ml (contains 272 mg or 13.6 mEq Ca); (gluconate) 1 g/10 ml (contains 90 mg or 4.5 mEq Ca); (gluceptate) 1.1 g/5 ml (contains 90 mg or 4.5 mEq Ca).

Patient Instructions. See Class Instructions. Do not take within 2 hours of oral tetracycline products.

Pharmacokinetics. *Plasma Levels.* 8.5–10.5 mg/dl (2.1–2.6 mM). Calcium is 45% plasma protein bound and 10% diffusable, but complexed to citrate, phosphate and other anions; the remaining 45% is diffusable and physiologically active. For each 1 g/dl alteration of albumin from normal (4.0–4.4 g/dl), total calcium changes by 0.8 mg/dl.[5]
   Fate. The amount of calcium absorbed is dependent on intake, vitamin D and parathyroid hormone, but in general, approximately one-third of ingested calcium is absorbed.[11] See Notes. Normal intake varies from 200–2500 mg/day.[5] Calcium is primarily eliminated in the stool with a small, nearly constant amount excreted in the urine.[6]

Adverse Reactions. GI symptoms are rare, but constipation or flatulence may occasionally occur with the carbonate form, especially with high doses. The gluconate salt is a less constipating alternative, but is more expensive.[12] Calcium overload due to oral calcium supplementation is rare.[8,12] The following conditions may contribute to hypercalcemia, hypercalciuria or renal lithiasis during concomitant oral supplementation: immobilization, doses in excess of 2 g/day, vitamin D therapy and renal impairment.[12] Symptoms of hypercalcemia include nausea, vomiting, constipation, abdominal pain, dry mouth and polyuria.

Contraindications. Hypercalcemia; sarcoidosis; severe cardiac disease; digitalis glycoside therapy; renal lithiasis.

Precautions. Concomitant thiazide diuretic therapy and states of sodium depletion or metabolic acidosis may increase tubular reabsorption of calcium.[12] Avoid extravasation of parenteral calcium products.

Parameters to Monitor. Serum calcium regularly, with frequency determined by condition of patient; BUN and/or Cr_s, serum phosphate and magnesium periodically.

Notes. Calcium supplementation can also be achieved by dietary measures (eg, skim milk provides approximately 1200 mg calcium/quart, cheeses 200 mg calcium/oz, yogurt 350 mg calcium/cup).[12] The bioavailability of calcium from various salt forms does not appear to differ significantly;[7] however, those salts with a higher calcium content require fewer dosage units and may increase compliance.

Oral Calcium Products Comparison Chart

PRODUCT	PERCENT CALCIUM	BRAND NAMES	CALCIUM CONTENT
Calcium Glubionate	6.5	Neo-Calglucon®	5 ml Syrup = 115 mg Ca.
Calcium Gluconate	9	Various	500 mg Tab = 45 mg Ca. 650 mg Tab = 58.5 mg Ca. 1000 mg Tab = 90 mg Ca.
Calcium Lactate	13	Various	325 mg Tab = 42.25 mg Ca. 650 mg Tab = 84.5 mg Ca.
Dibasic Calcium Phosphate	23	Dibasic Calcium Phosphate	486 mg Tab = 112 mg Ca.
	31	Various	500 mg Tab = 155 mg Ca.

Calcium Carbonate	40	Titralac®
		Tums®
		BioCal® (Chewable)
		Various
		Calciday®-667
		Cal-Sup®, Tums EX®
		BioCal®, Os-Cal® 500,
		  Oystercal® 500
		Caltrate® 600, Gencalc® 600,
		  Suplical® (Chewable)
			5 ml Susp = 400 mg Ca.
			500 mg Tab = 200 mg Ca.
			625 mg Tab = 250 mg Ca.
			650 mg Tab = 260 mg Ca.
			667 mg Tab = 266.8 mg Ca.
			750 mg Tab = 300 mg Ca.
			1250 mg Tab = 500 mg Ca.
			1500 mg Tab = 600 mg Ca.

Magnesium Salts

Various

Pharmacology. Magnesium is the second most abundant intracellular cation, essential for transfer, storage and utilization of intracellular energy and an integral component of bone matrix.[13] Extracellular magnesium is important in neuromuscular transmission.

Administration and Adult Dose. **PO as dietary supplement** 20–130 mg elemental magnesium daily-bid; **PO for chronic deficiency** 240–600 mg/day elemental magnesium in divided doses. **IM for mild deficiency** 1 g $MgSO_4$ q 6 hr for 4 doses; **IM for severe hypomagnesemia** up to 250 mg/kg $MgSO_4$ within a period of 4 hr if necessary; a 25–50% solution is generally used IM. **IV for severe hypomagnesemia** 8–12 g $MgSO_4$ in divided doses followed by 4–5 g/day for 3–4 days;[14] alternatively, **IV** 6 g over 3 hr, followed by 10 g during the first 24 hr and 6 g q 24 hr for 3 days.[15] Dilute IV infusion solutions to a concentration of 20% or less in D5W or NS and do not exceed an infusion rate of 150 mg/min; **IV for acute emergencies such as ventricular tachy-dysrhythmias** 1–2 g $MgSO_4$ (as a 20–25% solution) over 1 min, followed if necessary by a continuous infusion of 1 mg/min $MgSO_4$.[16,17] Larger doses are used in pre-eclampsia. See Notes.

Dosage Individualization. Maintenance doses should be based on serum magnesium and diet. Renal impairment decreases requirements. In renal failure, reduce dose to one-fourth recommended amount and monitor serum magnesium daily.[16]

Pediatric Dose. **IV push for hypomagnesemia** 25 mg/kg $MgSO_4$ as a 25% solution over 3–5 min q 6 hr for 3–4 doses. **IM for seizures** 20–40 mg/kg $MgSO_4$ as a 20% solution as needed. **IV for severe seizures** 100–200 mg/kg $MgSO_4$ as a 1–3% solution infused slowly with close monitoring of blood pressure. Administer one-half the dose during the initial 15–20 min and the total dose within 1 hr.

Dosage Forms. See Magnesium Products Comparison Chart.

Patient Instructions. See Class Instructions.

Pharmacokinetics. *Onset and Duration.* Therapeutic levels are achieved immediately with IV, 1 hr with IM. Duration (anticonvulsant) 30 min with IV, 3–4 hr post-onset with IM.

Plasma Levels. (Normal) 1.5–2.2 mEq/L; (anticonvulsant) 4.0–7.0 mEq/L. Intracellular and extracellular concentrations can vary independently, hence, serum magnesium levels may not be indicative of total body stores.

Fate. Absorption varies inversely with intake; on average, one-third of dietary magnesium is absorbed, principally in the upper small intestine. Normal dietary intake is borderline deficient (170–308 mg/day).[18] Total body store is about 25 mg/kg, of which 1% is extracellular, 31% is intracellular and 68% is in bone.[2] 20–30% plasma protein bound. Eliminated primarily by the kidneys with minimal amount (1–2%) by the fecal route. A renal threshold for magnesium excretion exists; therefore, replacement therapy must be continued slowly over several days; raising the serum value above normal exceeds the maximum tubular reabsorption capacity with subsequent excretion of excess.[14]

Adverse Reactions. Serum level-related (4–10 mEq/L) muscle weakness, loss of deep tendon reflexes and hypotension; (12–15 mEq/L) respiratory paralysis; (over 15 mEq/L) altered cardiac conduction (lengthening of QRS interval, dysrhythmias) and complete heart block.[5] Pain on IM injection.

Contraindications. Hypermagnesemia; heart block; myocardial damage.

Precautions. Use with caution in patients with renal impairment (especially Cl_{cr} less than 30 ml/min)[19] and those on concomitant digitalis glycosides. With bolus $MgSO_4$ administration, 10 ml of 10% calcium gluconate IV should be available if apnea or heart block occurs.[18]

Parameters to Monitor. Serum magnesium regularly, frequency determined by condition of patient; BUN and/or Cr_s and serum calcium periodically. Deep tendon reflexes, respiratory rate, EKG periodically.

Notes. For mild deficiencies, dietary supplementation may be sufficient to normalize magnesium stores. Green vegetables and cereals are rich in magnesium as are meat and fish; however, the large content of protein, calcium and phosphate in the latter foods interfere with magnesium absorption.[20] Patients on chronic diuretic therapy who are prone to hypomagnesemia may benefit from using the minimally effective dose of diuretic and 20–30 mEq/day of magnesium orally or changing to a magnesium-sparing agent (eg, amiloride, triamterene or spironolactone).[13,15] Drugs known to produce hypomagnesemia include aminoglycosides, amphotericin B, diuretics, alcohol, carbenicillin and cisplatin.[21] Addition of 3 g $MgSO_4$ IV to high-dose cisplatin chemotherapy has been recommended.[13] The correction of refractory hypocalcemia and hypokalemia with concurrent hypomagnesemia requires magnesium replacement to restore mineral balance.[22] To avoid the precipitation reaction when $MgSO_4$ and calcium chloride are added to TPN mixtures, use of calcium gluceptate has been recommended because it reacts more slowly than calcium chloride and a precipitate does not form.[22]

Magnesium Products Comparison Chart

PRODUCT	DOSAGE FORMS[a]	MAGNESIUM CONTENT[b] (MEQ/G)	COMMENTS
Magnesium Carbonate	Tab 500 mg.	23.7	Poorly soluble; low absorption.
Magnesium Chloride	Soln 200 mg/ml.	9.8	Used IV or orally as a 5% solution. Alternative to parenteral MgSO$_4$.
Magnesium Citrate	Soln 297 mg/5 ml.	4.4	Oral use only.
Magnesium Gluconate	Tab 300, 500 mg.	4.8	Very soluble; well absorbed; produces no diarrhea.
Magnesium Hydroxide	Susp 200–400 mg/5 ml Tab 300, 600 mg.	34.0	Readily available in combination antacid formulations. Start with 5 ml susp or 1 tab, increase as tolerated to qid.[16] Requires gastric acid to be absorbed. Inexpensive.
Magnesium Oxide	Cap 140 mg Tab 250, 400, 420, 500 mg.	49.6	Poorly soluble; net absorption low especially in malabsorptive states.
Magnesium Sulfate	Soln 10, 12.5, 50%.	8.1	Use IV, IM or PO.

a. Magnesium products exhibit variable absorption; dose patient incrementally until no further rise in serum magnesium occurs or until diarrhea ensues. Oral magnesium alleviates diarrhea in some patients with malabsorption.[16]

b. 1 mEq = 12 mg = 0.5 mmol Mg.

Phosphate Salts

Various

Pharmacology. Phosphate is a structural element of bone and is involved in carbohydrate metabolism, energy transfer, muscle contraction and as a buffer in the renal excretion of hydrogen ion.

Administration and Adult Dose. PO 250–500 mg (8–16 mmol) of phosphorus qid initially, adjusted according to serum phosphate and calcium. IV replacement (recent and uncomplicated hypophosphatemia) 0.08 mmol/kg, to maximum of 0.2 mmol/kg; (prolonged and multiple causes) 0.16 mmol/kg, to maximum of 0.24 mmol/kg. Doses should be infused over 6 hr and additional doses guided by serum levels. Alternatively, IV 0.5 mmol/kg (serum phosphorus below 0.5 mg/dl) or 0.25 mmol/kg (serum phosphorus 0.5–1 mg/dl) infused over 4 hr and repeated based on serum levels has been recommended.[23] When serum level reaches 2 mg/dl, change to oral dosing.

Dosage Individualization. Renal impairment decreases requirements. The salt form should be carefully chosen based on patient's sodium and potassium requirements. Needs are increased during alcohol withdrawal, diabetic ketoacidosis, respiratory alkalosis, aluminum antacid therapy, burns and anabolism.[3]

Pediatric Dose. PO (under 4 yr) 250 mg (8 mmol) of phosphorus qid initially; (4 yr and over) same as adult dose. IV same as adult dose.

Dosage Forms. See Phosphate Products Comparison Chart.

Patient Instructions. Do not take capsules whole, but dissolve contents in 3/4 glass of water before taking. Powder must be dissolved in one gallon of water before using. Chilling solution may improve palatability. See Class Instructions.

Pharmacokinetics. *Plasma Levels.* (As phosphorus) adults 3.0–4.5 mg/dl (0.1–0.15 mmol/dl); children 4.0–7.0 mg/dl (0.13–0.23 mmol/dl). Normal serum phosphorus levels may vary by as much as 2 mg/dl throughout the day, secondary to changes in transcellular distribution.[3] Levels below 1 mg/dl are dangerous and require replacement.

Fate. About 80% is absorbed from the GI tract. Normal daily adult intake is 800–1200 mg phosphorus with about 90% excreted in urine and 10% in feces.[3]

Adverse Reactions. Frequently diarrhea and stomach upset occur with oral dosage forms.[3,24] Dose-related hyperphosphatemia,[25] metastatic calcium deposition, dehydration, hypotension, hypomagnesemia and hyperkalemia or hypernatremia (depending on salt used) can occur.

Contraindications. Hyperphosphatemia; hypocalcemia; hyperkalemia (potassium salt); hypernatremia (sodium salt).

Precautions. Use cautiously in patients with renal impairment and in those with hypercalcemia. Dilute IV forms before use and administer slowly. Administer the potassium salt no faster than 10 mEq/hr to avoid vein irritation.[24]

Parameters to Monitor. Serum phosphorus regularly, frequency determined by condition of patient; BUN and/or Cr_s and serum calcium and magnesium periodically.[5,23,26] Monitor serum sodium and/or potassium periodically, depending on salt form used.

Notes. Phosphate salts may precipitate in the presence of calcium salts in IV solutions; add no more than 40 mmol phosphate and 5 mEq calcium per liter. Calcium supplementation may be necessary to prevent hypocalcemic tetany during phosphate repletion. IV calcium gluconate or calcium chloride may be given until tetany subsides.[3]

Phosphate Products Comparison Chart[a]

| PRODUCT | PHOSPHORUS | | SODIUM | | POTASSIUM |
	MG	MMOL	MG	MEQ	MEQ
ORAL					
Fleet's Phospho-Soda® (per ml)	128	4.1	111	4.8	0
K-Phos® Modified Formula (per tablet)	125	4	67	2.9	1.4
K-Phos® Neutral (per tablet)	250	8.1	301	13.1	1.1
Neutra-Phos® Plain (per cap or 75 ml)	250	8.1	164	7.1	7.1
Neutra-Phos® K (per cap or 75 ml)	250	8.1	0	0	14.3
Skim Milk (per quart)	1000	32	552	24	40
INTRAVENOUS					
Potassium Phosphate Abbott (per ml) Various	94	3	0	0	4.4
Sodium Phosphate Abbott (per ml)	94	3	93	4	0

a. From reference 27 and product information.

Potassium Salts   Various

Pharmacology. Potassium is the major intracellular cation essential for nerve impulse transmission, muscle contraction, acid-base balance and glucose utilization.[28] The chloride salt is preferred for most uses, because concomitant chloride loss and metabolic alkalosis frequently accompany hypokalemia. Nonchloride salts are preferred in acidosis (eg, secondary to amphotericin B or carbonic anhydrase inhibitor therapy and in chronic diarrhea with bicarbonate loss.[29]

Administration and Adult Dose. Variable, must be adjusted to needs of patient. **PO** 40-100 mEq/day prevents hypokalemia in most patients on long-term diuretic therapy. For nonedematous, ambulatory patients with uncomplicated hypertension, generally no supplementation is needed; however, if serum potassium falls below 3 mEq/L, 50-60 mEq/day is recommended. For edematous patients (eg, CHF, cirrhosis with ascites) 40-80 mEq/day (mild deficit) or 100-120 mEq/day (severe deficit), with careful monitoring of serum potassium.[29] **IV** (serum potassium greater than 2.5 mEq/L) up to 10 mEq/hr may be infused; a maximum concentration of 40 mEq/L and maximum dose of 200 mEq/day should not be exceeded; (serum potassium less than 2 mEq/L) up to 40 mEq/hr may be given; a maximum concentration of 80 mEq/L and a maximum dose of 400 mEq/day should not be exceeded. Infusion into a central vein requires use of a volume control device — potassium concentration should not exceed 40 mEq/L unless the infusion site is via a large vein distal to the heart (eg, femoral vein).

Dosage Individualization. Maintenance doses should be based on serum potassium; renal impairment decreases requirements.

Pediatric Dose. **PO** 1-2 mEq/kg/day during diuretic therapy.

Dosage Forms. **PO**—see Oral Potassium Products Comparison Chart; **Inj** (potassium chloride) 2 mEq/ml; (potassium acetate) 2, 2.5 mEq/ml; (potassium phosphate)—see Phosphate Products Comparison Chart.

Patient Instructions. See Class Instructions. Do not chew or crush tablets. The expanded wax matrix of sustained-release forms may be found in the stool.

Pharmacokinetics. *Onset and Duration.* Peak elevation of serum potassium levels following SR preparations is slightly delayed (2 hr) compared to liquid form (1 hr). Effect on serum potassium is generally confined to the first 3 hr after dosing.[30]
   Plasma Levels. (May vary depending on laboratory) 3.5-5 mEq/L (adult and child); 5-7.5 mEq/L (newborn); total body stores are approximately 50 mEq/kg or 3500 mEq.[31] As a general rule, a decrease of 1 mEq/L in serum potassium reflects a 10-20% total body deficit; however, there is considerable variation;[29] signs of hypokalemia appear below 2.5 mEq/L; levels above 7 mEq/L are dangerous. Clinical signs of hyperkalemia are not reliable indicators of serum levels. Alkalosis decreases levels and acidosis increases levels.
   Fate. When initially administered, the rates of absorption and excretion are more rapid with the liquid than the SR forms; however, bioavailability is the same when administered long-term (78-90%).[30,32,33] Approximately 10 mEq/day are eliminated in feces; 7.5 mEq/L in sweat and 60-90 mEq/day in urine.[31]

Adverse Reactions. Bad taste, nausea, vomiting, diarrhea and abdominal discomfort may occur frequently with oral liquids. Small bowel and occasional gastric ulceration may occur with enteric-coated tablets and they should not be used.[29] Hyperkalemia may occur. Local tissue necrosis may occur if IV solution extravasates.

Contraindications. Severe renal impairment with oliguria or azotemia; untreated Addison's disease; adynamia episodica hereditaria; acute dehydration; heat cramps; hyperkalemia. Additionally, all solid dosage forms (including SR products) are contraindicated in patients in whom delay or arrest of the tablet through the GI tract may occur.

Precautions. Use with caution (if at all) in patients receiving potassium-sparing diuretics, in patients with digitalis-induced atrioventricular conduction disturbances and in renal failure.

Parameters to Monitor. Serum potassium regularly, with frequency determined by condition of patient; BUN and/or Cr_s periodically. For supplementation in patients on long-term diuretic therapy, obtain a pretreatment serum potassium, reassess after 2–3 weeks and then monthly to determine pattern of potassium loss. Once steady-state or normokalemia is achieved, assess quarterly or as condition requires.[29]

Notes. A potassium-sparing diuretic may be preferable to potassium supplementation when large supplements are needed, when aldosterone levels are elevated or when enhanced therapeutic response is desired.[29] See also Potassium Content of Selected Foods, Beverages and Salt Substitutes in the Dietary Considerations chapter.

Oral Potassium Products Comparison Chart[a]

DOSAGE FORMS	POTASSIUM SALT	BRAND NAMES	POTASSIUM CONTENT	COMMENTS
Liquid	Potassium Chloride	Various	Soln 10, 20, 30, 40 mEq/15 ml.	Rapid absorption; low frequency of GI ulceration; unpleasant taste.
	Potassium Acetate/Bicarbonate/Citrate	Trikates®, Tri-K®	Soln 45 mEq/15 ml.	Preferred forms in patients with delayed GI transit time; avoid nonchloride salts in metabolic alkalosis.
	Potassium Gluconate	Kaon®	Soln 20 mEq/15 ml.	
Powder	Potassium Chloride	Various	Packet 15, 20, 25 mEq.	
	Potassium Bicarbonate/Citrate	K-Lyte® K-Lyte® DS	Packet 25 mEq. Packet 50 mEq.	Must be dissolved in water before use; avoid nonchloride salts in metabolic alkalosis.
Effervescent Tablets	Potassium Chloride	Kaochlor-Eff®, Klorvess® K-Lyte/Cl® K-Lyte/Cl® 50	Tab 20 mEq. Tab 25 mEq. Tab 50 mEq.	
Sustained-Release Capsules, Tablets	Potassium Chloride	Kaon-Cl® Micro-K®, Slow-K® Kaon® Cl 10, K-Tab®, Klotrix® K-Dur®	Tab 6.7 mEq. Cap 8 mEq. Tab 10 mEq. Tab 20 mEq.	Wax matrix or polymer-coated crystals in gelatin capsule; bioequivalent to liquid forms; avoid in patients with delayed GI transit time.
Salt Substitutes[b]	Potassium Chloride	Adolph's®, Morton's®, NuSalt®, No Salt®, Various	Pwdr 50–70 mEq/tsp.	Inexpensive dietary source;[34] prescribe specific amount to avoid hyperkalemia; contraindicated in oliguria, severe renal disease.

a. Adapted in part from reference 29.
b. See also Potassium Content of Salt Substitutes, page 55.

Oral Rehydration Solutions   Various

Pharmacology. Oral rehydration solutions supply sodium, chloride, potassium and water to prevent or replace mild to moderate fluid loss in diarrhea,[4,35] postoperative states, or when food and liquid intake are temporarily discontinued. Glucose is present to aid in sodium transport and subsequent water absorption.[36]

Administration and Adult Dose. PO 1900–2850 ml (2–3 quarts)/day. Give only enough solution to supply the calculated water requirement.

Dosage Individualization. Adjust intake based on fluid status and serum electrolytes. When electrolyte-containing foods are restarted, adjust solution intake accordingly.

Pediatric Dose. PO (infants) 150 ml/kg/day (one-half in the first 8 hr if possible, the remainder over the ensuing 16 hr) offered in frequent, small amounts (not to exceed 100 ml in a 20 min period).[37] Once the solution is well tolerated, it may be given less frequently (q 3–4 hr). To avoid hypernatremia, infants who finish the prescribed amount of solution in less than 24 hr should be offered plain tap water;[38] PO (5–10 yr) 950–1900 ml (1–2 quarts)/day; (11 yr and over) same as adult dose.

Dosage Forms. See Oral Rehydration Solutions Comparison Chart.

Patient Instructions. These products are not for fluid replacement in prolonged or severe diarrhea. Reconstitute powdered products in tap water; do not mix with milk or fruit juices. If additional fluids are desired, drink water or other nonelectrolyte-containing fluids to quench thirst.

Adverse Reactions. Hypernatremia, hyperkalemia and acid-base disturbances may occur, especially in renal insufficiency or if errors in reconstituting bulk powders are made.

Contraindications. Intractable vomiting; adynamic ileus; intestinal obstruction; perforated bowel; renal dysfunction (anuria, oliguria).

Precautions. Use parenteral replacement to correct electrolyte imbalances due to severe fluid loss (10–15% of body weight), inability to take oral fluids, severe gastric distention or severe vomiting. A 5–8% acute weight loss has successfully responded to oral replacement.[39] Errors in reconstituting or diluting commercial powders may lead to severe consequences.

Parameters to Monitor. Serum sodium, potassium, chloride and bicarbonate regularly, with frequency determined by condition of patient; BUN and/or serum creatinine periodically; weight daily.

Notes. To prevent dehydration early in the course of diarrhea or to maintain hydration following parenteral replacement in adults and children, 90 mEq/L of sodium is acceptable.[40] For infants, however, who have a higher insensible water loss, dilute solutions containing 50–60 mEq/L of sodium have been suggested.[38] Alternatively, solutions of higher sodium concentration may be used in a ratio of 2:1 with additional free water.[41]

Oral Rehydration Solutions Comparison Chart[a]

| SOLUTION | ELECTROLYTES (MEQ/L)[b] | | | | | CARBOHYDRATE | DOSAGE FORMS |
	Na$^+$	K$^+$	Cl$^-$	BASE	OTHER		
Gastrolyte®	90	20	80	30 Citrate	—	Glucose 2%	Powder
Hydralyte®	84	10	59	10 Bicarbonate 20 Citrate	—	Glucose + Sucrose: 2%	Powder
Infalyte®	50	20	40	30 Bicarbonate	—	Glucose 2%	Powder
Lytren®	30	25	25	36 Citrate	4 Ca^{++} 4 Mg^{++} 4 SO$_4^=$ 5 HPO$_4^=$	Dextran, Corn syrup solids	Soln 946 ml
Oral Electrolyte Solution	30	20	30	23 Citrate	4 Ca^{++} 4 Mg^{++} 5 HPO$_4^=$	Glucose 7.5%	Soln
Pedialyte®	45	20	35	30 Citrate	—	Dextrose 2.5%	Soln 237, 946 ml
Rehydralyte®	75	20	65	30 Citrate	—	Dextrose 2.5%	Soln 237 ml
WHO Oral Rehydration Salts[c]	90	20	80	30 Bicarbonate	—	Glucose 2%	Powder

a. Adapted in part from reference 38.
b. Optimal solution (mEq): Na$^+$ 75–100, K$^+$ 20–30, Cl$^-$ 65–100, base 20–30, carbohydrate 1.5–2%.[36]
c. WHO = World Health Organization Oral Rehydration Salts; available from Jianas Brothers Packaging, Kansas City, MO.

40:18 POTASSIUM-REMOVING RESINS

General References: 42,43

Sodium Polystyrene Sulfonate   Kayexalate®, Various

Pharmacology. A cation exchange resin that exchanges potassium for sodium with about 33% exchange efficiency. Each gram of resin binds 0.5–1 mEq of potassium and liberates 2–3 mEq of sodium.[44] Sorbitol is present in some formulations to induce diarrhea and to reduce the potential for fecal impaction. See Notes.

Administration and Adult Dose. PO 15 g 1–4 times daily, although doses up to 40 g have been recommended;[42,45] total dose and duration of therapy depend on patient response. Powder should be given with, or suspended in, a sorbitol solution (eg, 15 ml of 70% sorbitol).[42] PR as enema 30–50 g qid as an emulsion in 100 ml aqueous solution retained for 4–10 hr, if possible; alternatively, enema may be retained for 30–60 min and repeated at 6 hr intervals until serum potassium is in a safe range.[5,46]

Dosage Individualization. In severe situations, such as ongoing tissue damage or rapidly rising serum potassium in renal failure, an increase in dose to 80–100 g for every mEq/L of potassium above 5.0 mEq/L has been recommended.[45]

Pediatric Dose. For small children and infants, calculate dose on the basis of one gram of resin binding 1 mEq of potassium.

Dosage Forms. Pwdr 454 g; Susp (in 70% sorbitol) 15 g/60 ml.

Pharmacokinetics. *Onset.* PO 2–12 hr, PR somewhat longer.

  Fate. Not absorbed from GI tract; binds potassium and liberates sodium as it passes through intestine.

Adverse Reactions. Anorexia, nausea and vomiting occur frequently with large doses; gastric irritation, constipation and fecal impaction (especially in the elderly) occur occasionally. These effects may be avoided by using the enema. However, intestinal necrosis due to the enema has been reported. See Notes.

Precautions. Use with caution in patients who cannot tolerate any additional sodium load (eg, severe CHF, severe hypertension, marked edema). In addition to potassium, other cations (such as magnesium and calcium) may bind to the resin, causing electrolyte imbalances. If rapid potassium lowering is required, other measures should be employed.

Parameters to Monitor. Serum potassium at least daily and more frequently if indicated; serum magnesium and calcium periodically; electrocardiogram and patient signs may be useful in evaluating status.

Notes. On average, 50 g resin will lower serum potassium by 0.5–1 mEq/L.[44] Rectal administration is less effective than oral use. Heating may alter the exchange properties of the resin. Sodium polystyrene sulfonate-induced constipation may be treated with 70% sorbitol in doses sufficient to produce 1–2 watery stools/day (ie, 10–20 ml/2 hr). Use of sorbitol in the enema may predispose uremic patients to potentially fatal intestinal necrosis.[135]

40:28 DIURETICS

General References: 47–52

Class Instructions. If divided doses are taken, the last dose should usually be taken in the afternoon or early evening to avoid having to void urine during the night. If no potassium supplement or no potassium-sparing diuretic has been prescribed, some foods high in potassium should be taken each day (see Potassium Content of Selected Foods in Chapter 3). Highly salted foods should be avoided, but rigid salt restriction is not necessary. Excessive water intake should be avoided. Dizziness or lightheadedness (especially upon arising from sitting or lying), muscle cramps, weakness, lethargy, dry mouth, thirst or low urine output should be reported.

Amiloride Hydrochloride

Midamor®

Amiloride is a potassium-sparing diuretic with a mechanism and site of action resembling triamterene. It has antihypertensive activity equivalent to the thiazides and a longer duration of action than triamterene. Adverse reactions are generally similar to triamterene. Dosage is 10 mg/day in 1 or 2 doses, to a maximum of 20 mg daily. It is available as 5 mg tablets and also in Moduretic® 5–50 and generic products which contain hydrochlorothiazide 50 mg and amiloride 5 mg.[53]

Bumetanide

Bumex®

Bumetanide is a loop diuretic similar to furosemide. Over the usual dosage range, it is 40 times more potent than furosemide. This potency ratio may not apply with the higher doses used in renal failure. Indications are similar to furosemide. It has a rapid onset of 30 min and peak effect in 1 hr with a duration of 3–6 hr orally. Greater than 90% plasma protein bound; elimination half-life is 1–3.5 hr. Overall, the frequency of adverse effects is similar to furosemide: hypochloremia and hypokalemia are more frequent with bumetanide; whereas, hyperglycemia and ototoxicity are less frequent. Myalgias have been reported with the higher doses used in renal failure. Bumetanide may be preferred over furosemide for diabetics and for patients at risk for ototoxicity (those receiving concomitant ototoxic drugs and renal failure patients). Dosage is 0.5–2 mg/day PO, IM or IV. If response is inadequate, additional doses may be given at 4–5 hr intervals, to a maximum of 10 mg/day. Up to 15 mg/day may be needed in renal failure. Alternate day dosing or dosing for 3–4 days followed by a 1–2 day rest period may be used for control of edema.[54-56] Available as 0.5 and 1 mg tablets and 0.25 mg/ml injection.

Furosemide

Lasix®, Various

Pharmacology. Inhibits active chloride transport in the ascending limb of the loop of Henle, causing markedly enhanced excretion of chloride and its attendant sodium and water. Medullary hypertonicity is decreased, thus interfering with the countercurrent multiplier system and resulting in large volumes of dilute urine. Potassium, magnesium, calcium and phosphate excretion are also increased. IV doses increase venous capacitance independent of diuretic effect, producing rapid improvement in pulmonary edema.[60]

Administration and Adult Dose. PO for edema 20-80 mg as a single morning dose initially, increasing successive doses by 20-40 mg in 6-8 hr until response is obtained or to maximum of 600 mg/day (although doses this large probably indicate need for sodium restriction and/or addition of other diuretics to regimen). After response, effective dosage is given in 1-2 doses daily; usual maintenance dose is 40-120 mg/day. **PO for chronic renal failure** 240 mg bid, increasing to maximum of 500 mg bid.[61] **PO for hypertension** 40 mg bid. **IV** should be used only when oral administration is not feasible. Doses can be given over 1-2 min, except rate should not exceed 4 mg/min when large doses are given to patients in renal failure. **IM or IV for edema** 20-40 mg as a single dose; additional doses of 20 mg greater than previous dose may be given q 2 hr until desired response is obtained. This dose is then given in 1-2 doses daily for maintenance; change to PO as soon as feasible. **IV for acute pulmonary edema** 40 mg initially, may repeat in 1 hr with 80 mg if necessary.

Pediatric Dose. PO for edema 2 mg/kg in 1 dose initially, increasing by 1-2 mg/kg in 6-8 hr if necessary, to maximum of 6 mg/kg/day. **IM or IV** 1 mg/kg in 1 dose initially, increasing by 1 mg/kg q 2 or more hr until desired response is obtained or to maximum of 6 mg/kg/day. See Notes.

Dosage Individualization. See Hydrochlorothiazide.

Dosage Forms. Soln 8, 10 mg/ml; Tab 20, 40, 80 mg; Inj 10 mg/ml.

Patient Instructions. See Class Instructions.

Pharmacokinetics. *Onset and Duration.* (Venous capacitance) IV onset 5 min, duration over 1 hr. (Diuresis) PO onset 30-60 min, peak 1-2 hr, duration 6 hr; IV onset 15 min, peak 30-60 min, duration 1-2 hr; duration may be prolonged in severe renal impairment. (Hypertension) maximum effect may not occur for several days.[60,62]

Plasma Levels. No relationship between plasma levels and therapeutic effect.[63]

Fate. Much discrepancy among studies because of the lack of reliable assay techniques; 60-69% bioavailable in normals with much variability; 43-46% in uremia; absorption may be markedly impaired in patients with edematous bowel caused by CHF or nephrotic syndrome. 91-98% plasma protein bound; reduced in hypoalbuminemia and azotemia. Furosemide appears to be conjugated with glucuronic acid and excreted primarily in the urine by filtration and secretion as unchanged drug and glucuronide. Some studies indicate an increase in hepatic clearance in renal impairment, while others show a decrease.[64-66]

$t_{1/2}$. About 50 min in normals, increasing to about 120 min in CHF and up to several hr in renal impairment.[64]

Adverse Reactions. Dehydration, hypotension, hypochloremic alkalosis and hypokalemia are frequent, although hyperkalemia may occur when potassium supplements or potassium-sparing diuretics are also given. Hyperglycemia, glucose intolerance and hyperuricemia occur as with thiazides—see Hydrochlorothiazide.[57,58,67] Hearing loss, occasionally permanent, has been reported, usually associated with too rapid IV injection of large doses in patients with renal impairment. Rarely thrombocytopenia, neutropenia, jaundice, pancreatitis and a variety of skin reactions have been reported.

Contraindications. Anuria (except for single dose in acute anuria); pregnancy.

Precautions. Furosemide is extremely potent and profound dose-related diuresis and fluid and electrolyte disturbances can occur if the drug is used indiscriminately. Use caution in patients with severe or progressive renal disease; discontinue if renal function worsens. Use with caution in liver disease, cirrhosis and ascites (may precipitate hepatic encephalopathy),[68] or history of diabetes or gout. Dosage of potent hypotensive agents may have to be reduced if furosemide is added to regimen. Caution should be used in patients allergic to other sulfonamides.

Parameters to Monitor. Monitor serum potassium closely, other electrolytes periodically and serum glucose, uric acid, BUN and Cr_s occasionally. Observe for clinical signs of fluid or electrolyte disturbance—see Hydrochlorothiazide.

Notes. Total body potassium is not depleted during long-term use in essential hypertension with or without renal disease; potassium supplementation is not needed unless other factors warrant it.[58,69] Slightly less effective antihypertensive agent than the thiazides.[70] Furosemide has been used IV in hypercalcemia[71] and IV and PO in the treatment of SIADH;[72,73] these techniques require careful monitoring and replacement of fluid and electrolytes—consult literature for details. Furosemide is light-sensitive; oral solution must be refrigerated and protected from light; discard an open bottle after 60 days. Do not use injection if solution is yellow; slight discoloration of tablets does not affect potency.

Hydrochlorothiazide

Esidrix®, HydroDiuril®, Oretic®, Various

Pharmacology. Thiazides increase sodium and chloride excretion by interfering with their reabsorption in the cortical diluting segment of the nephron; a mild diuresis of slightly concentrated urine results. Potassium, bicarbonate, magnesium, phosphate and iodide excretion are also increased, while calcium is decreased. Antihypertensive efficacy is primarily due to a decrease in extracellular fluid volume, although direct vasodilation may also occur. Urine output is decreased in diabetes insipidus.[5,74,75]

Administration and Adult Dose. PO for edema 25–200 mg/day in 1–3 doses initially; 25–100 mg/day or intermittently for maintenance, to a maximum of 200 mg/day. **PO for hypertension** 12.5–50 mg bid initially; 12.5–100 mg/day in one dose for maintenance, to a maximum of 200 mg/day. Use the minimum dose required for effectiveness; larger doses increase side effects with little additional benefit.

Dosage Individualization. Thiazides and related diuretics (except metolazone and xipamide) are not effective as diuretics with a Cl_{cr} less than 20–30 ml/min.[5,69,74]

Pediatric Dose. PO (under 6 months) may require up to 3.3 mg/kg/day in 2 doses; (over 6 months) 2.2 mg/kg/day in 2 doses.

Dosage Forms. Tab 25, 50, 100 mg.

Patient Instructions. See Class Instructions. If stomach upset occurs, take drug with meals. Report persistent anorexia, nausea or vomiting.

Pharmacokinetics. *Onset and Duration.* Onset of diuresis within 2 hr; peak in 3–6 hr; duration 6–12 hr. Onset of hypotensive effect in 3–4 days; duration one week or less after discontinuing therapy.[74]
   Plasma Levels. No relationship between levels and therapeutic effect.[63]
   Fate. 71 ± 15% oral absorption in normals;[76] increased slightly when given with food and considerably when given with an anticholinergic; decreased by one-half after intestinal shunt surgery.[77] No differences in absorption among formulations. 40–64% plasma protein bound.[63,76] More

than 95% excreted unchanged by filtration and secretion.[63]

$t_{1/2}$. α phase 5.2 hr, β phase 5.6–14.8 hr; prolonged in uncompensated CHF or renal impairment.[63,76]

Adverse Reactions. Volume depletion, hypotension and weakness may occur with high doses and salt restriction. Dilutional hyponatremia may occur in patients with excessive fluid intake; hypochloremic alkalosis may occur.[58] Hypokalemia is frequent; however, its treatment in otherwise healthy hypertensive patients is usually unnecessary.[58,78] Potassium chloride supplementation or potassium-sparing diuretic therapy is needed in older patients, those with cirrhosis, those on digitalis glycosides, those taking other potassium-wasting drugs or if serum potassium falls below 3.0 mEq/L.[58,74] Hyperuricemia frequently occurs, but is reversible and treatment is unnecessary unless prior personal or family history of gout exists.[58] Hyperglycemia and alterations in glucose tolerance (usually reversible), loss of diabetic control and precipitation of diabetes occur occasionally.[58] Decreased glucose tolerance may increase in prevalence after several years of therapy.[58,79] Thrombocytopenia and pancreatitis occur rarely. Elevation of serum cholesterol and triglycerides occurs, but significance is unknown.[80]

Contraindications. Anuria; pregnancy, unless accompanied by severe edema; allergy to sulfonamide derivatives.

Precautions. Use with caution in patients with renal function impairment, liver disease (may precipitate hepatic encephalopathy),[68] history of diabetes or gout. Dosage of potent hypotensive agents may have to be reduced if a thiazide is added to the regimen.

Parameters to Monitor. Serum potassium weekly to monthly initially; every 3–6 months when stable.[78,81] Other serum electrolytes periodically. Monitor all electrolytes more closely when other losses occur (eg, vomiting, diarrhea). Clinical signs of fluid or electrolyte depletion such as dry mouth, thirst, weakness, lethargy, muscle pains or cramps, hypotension, oliguria, tachycardia and GI upset.

Thiazides and Related Diuretics Comparison Chart[a]

DRUG	DOSAGE FORMS	DAILY DOSAGE RANGE FOR EDEMA	DAILY DOSAGE RANGE FOR HYPERTENSION	MAXIMUM DAILY DOSAGE	DURATION OF DIURESIS (HOURS)
Bendroflumethiazide Naturetin®	Tab 5, 10 mg.	2.5–5 mg.	2.5–15 mg.	20 mg.	18–24
Benzthiazide Various	Tab 25, 50 mg.	50–150 mg.	50–100 mg.	200 mg.	12–18
Chlorothiazide Diuril®	Susp 50 mg/ml Tab 250, 500 mg Inj 500 mg.[b]	1–2 g.	1–2 g.	2 g.	6–12 (PO) 2 (IV)
Chlorthalidone[c] Hygroton® Various	Tab 15 mg (Thalitone®),[d] 25, 50, 100 mg (Hygroton®, Various).	50–200 mg daily or on alternate days.	25–100 mg.	200 mg.	48–72
Cyclothiazide Anhydron®	Tab 2 mg.	1–2 mg on alternate days.	2 mg.	6 mg.	24–36
Hydrochlorothiazide Various	Tab 25, 50, 100 mg.	25–100 mg.	12.5–100 mg.	200 mg.	6–12
Hydroflumethiazide Diucardin® Saluron®	Tab 50 mg.	25–100 mg.	50–100 mg.	200 mg.	10–12
Indapamide[c] Lozol®	Tab 2.5 mg.	2.5–5 mg.	2.5–5 mg.	5 mg.	36

Continued

Thiazides and Related Diuretics Comparison Chart[a]

DRUG	DOSAGE FORMS	DAILY DOSAGE RANGE FOR EDEMA	DAILY DOSAGE RANGE FOR HYPERTENSION	MAXIMUM DAILY DOSAGE	DURATION OF DIURESIS (HOURS)
Methyclothiazide Aquatensen® Enduron®	Tab 2.5, 5 mg.	2.5–5 mg.	2.5–5 mg.	10 mg.	24
Metolazone[c] Diulo® Microx® Zaroxolyn®	Tab 0.5 mg (Microx®),[d] 2.5, 5, 10 mg (Diulo®, Zaroxolyn®).	5–10 mg.[e]	2.5–5 mg.	20 mg.	12–24
Polythiazide Renese®	Tab 1, 2, 4 mg.	1–4 mg.	2–4 mg.	4 mg.	24–36
Quinethazone[c] Hydromox®	Tab 50 mg.	50–100 mg.	50–100 mg.	200 mg.	18–24
Trichlormethiazide Various	Tab 2, 4 mg.	1–4 mg.	2–4 mg.	4 mg.	24
Xipamide[c] Diurexan® (Investigational - Mead Johnson)	—	10–80 mg.[e]	5–40 mg.	80 mg.	12–24

a. From references 74, 82, 83; patients unresponsive to maximal dose of one agent are unlikely to respond to another agent,[74] except as in e. below.
b. There is no therapeutic advantage in giving the drug parenterally.
c. Not a thiazide, but similar in structure and mechanism of action.
d. Thalitone® and Microx® are more bioavailable than previous formulations.
e. In high doses (up to 20 mg/day), metolazone is more effective than other thiazide-like diuretics in patients with chronic renal failure and Cl$_{cr}$ less than 20 ml/minute.[74,84] Xipamide 20–40 mg/day has been effective in patients with marked renal insufficiency.[85]

Mannitol

Osmitrol®, Various

Pharmacology. An osmotic diuretic that inhibits sodium and chloride reabsorption in the proximal tubule and ascending loop of Henle. Sodium, potassium, calcium and phosphate excretion are increased and GFR decreases slightly. Mannitol increases serum osmolality, expanding intravascular volume and decreasing intra-ocular and intracranial pressures. It also appears to disrupt the blood-brain barrier, enhancing penetration of other drugs into the CNS.[86]

Administration and Adult Dose. Never administer IM or SC, or add to whole blood for transfusion. **IV as diagnostic evaluation of acute oliguria** (*after* blood pressure and CVP are normal and cardiac output is maximized) give test dose of 12.5-25 g of 20-25% solution over 3-5 min (often along with furosemide 80-120 mg IV), repeat in 1 hr if urine output is less than 50 ml/hr. If no response after 2 doses, give no more mannitol and treat for acute tubular necrosis. If response occurs, look for underlying cause of oliguria (eg, hypovolemia). **IV for prevention of acute renal failure** give test dose as above to a total dose of 50 g or more in 1 hr as a loading dose, then maintain urine output at 50 ml/hr with continuous infusion of 5% solution, 20 mEq/L sodium chloride and 1 g/L calcium gluconate. **IV for promotion of excretion of toxins** give test and loading doses as above, then maintain urine output at 150-500 ml/hr with continuous infusion of 5% solution, 45 mEq/L sodium chloride, 24 mEq/L sodium acetate, 1 g/L calcium gluconate, 1 g/L magnesium sulfate and 20 mEq/L potassium acetate. To alkalinize urine to enhance excretion of acidic toxins (eg, phenobarbital, myoglobin), use less chloride and more acetate as sodium salt or use sodium bicarbonate.[87] **IV for reduction of intracranial or intraocular pressure** 1.5-2 g/kg over 30-60 min as a 15-25% solution. **IV to decrease nephrotoxicity of cisplatin** 12.5 g push just prior to cisplatin, then 10 g/hr for 6 hr with 20% solution. Replace fluids with 0.45% sodium chloride with 20-30 mEq/L potassium chloride at 250 ml/hr for 6 hr. Maintain urine output greater than 100 ml/hr with mannitol infusion.[88] See Notes.

Pediatric Dose. **IV for oliguria or anuria** give test dose of 200 mg/kg as above; therapeutic dose 2 g/kg over 2-6 hr as a 15-20% solution. **IV for reduction of intracranial or intraocular pressure** 2 g/kg over 30-60 min as a 15-25% solution. **IV for intoxications** 2 g/kg as 5-10% solution as needed to maintain a high urinary output. See Notes.

Dosage Forms. **Inj** 5, 10, 15, 20, 25%; **Inj** as 5, 10, 15% solution with 0.45% NaCl; **Inj** as 5, 15% solution with 5% dextrose and 0.12% or 0.45% NaCl.

Pharmacokinetics. *Onset and Duration.* (Diuresis) onset 1-3 hr. (Decrease in intraocular pressure) onset in 30-60 min; duration 4-6 hr. (Decrease in intracranial pressure) onset within 15 min; peak 60-90 min; duration 3-8 hr after stopping infusion.[62,87]

Fate. 17% absorbed orally.[62] A 200 g/70 kg IV dose increases serum osmolality to 380 mOsm/kg, expands extracellular volume by 2+ liters and decreases serum sodium to 115 mEq/L.[89] Given IV, drug is distributed in extracellular space primarily, but it can slowly penetrate intracellularly. Excreted unchanged in urine, primarily by filtration; 7-10% metabolized by liver.[87]

$t_{1/2}$. 15 min.[87]

Adverse Reactions. Most serious are fluid and electrolyte imbalance, particularly symptoms of fluid overload such as pulmonary edema, hypertension, water intoxication and CHF. Necrosis of skin can occur if solution extravasates. Anaphylaxis has been reported rarely.[59]

Contraindications. Patients with well established anuria due to severe renal disease or impaired renal function who do not respond to test dose; severe pulmonary congestion, frank pulmonary edema or severe congestive heart failure; severe dehydration; edema not due to renal, cardiac or hepatic disease which is associated with abnormal capillary fragility or membrane permeability; active intracranial bleeding, except during craniotomy.

Precautions. Pregnancy. Observe solution for crystals before administering; see Notes. Water intoxication may occur if fluid input exceeds urine output; masking of inadequate hydration or hypovolemia may occur by drug-induced sustaining of diuresis.

Parameters to Monitor. Monitor urine output closely and discontinue drug if it is low. Monitor serum electrolytes closely, taking care not to misinterpret low serum sodium as a sign of hypotonicity; see Fate. If serum sodium is low, measure serum osmolality.[89]

Notes. Mannitol may crystallize out of solution at concentrations above 15%—crystals may be redissolved by warming in hot water and shaking or by autoclaving; cool to body temperature before administration. Solutions of 20% or greater should be administered through an inline filter. Addition of electrolytes to solutions of 20% or greater may cause precipitation.

Piretanide (Investigational - Hoechst)   Arelix®

Piretanide is a loop diuretic similar to furosemide and bumetanide. Its saluretic potency is 2-4 times that of furosemide and one-tenth that of bumetanide. Onset of diuresis is 1-2 hr orally and 0.25-1 hr IV; duration is 4-6 hr orally and 2-3 hr IV. V_d is 0.3 L/kg and is increased in renal failure to 0.4-0.5 L/kg. Piretanide is over 90% plasma protein bound. Elimination half-life is 1-1.7 hr in normals and 1.7-9 hr in renal failure. Ototoxicity has been reported in animals, but further testing in humans is needed. An increased frequency of side effects such as pronounced diuresis, nausea or thirst has been reported with the conventional tablet form of piretanide compared with furosemide or bumetanide; the frequency is lower with a sustained-release formulation. A potential for hypokalemia exists, but preliminary evidence suggests that kaliuresis is less with piretanide compared to furosemide or chlorothiazide in CHF or to hydrochlorothiazide in hypertension. Dosage used in investigational studies have ranged from 6-12 mg/day. Up to 192 mg has been used in moderate to severe renal failure.[90-96] See Furosemide Precautions and Parameters to Monitor.

Spironolactone   Aldactone®, Various

Pharmacology. A competitive aldosterone antagonist that blocks sodium-potassium exchange at the distal tubule, producing a very mild diuresis. Diuretic effect is maximal in states of hyperaldosteronism. Sodium, chloride and calcium excretion are increased, while potassium and magnesium excretion are decreased. Antihypertensive activity is equal to thiazides and it also has a direct positive inotropic action on the heart.[5,58,97]

Administration and Adult Dose. PO for edema 25-200 mg/day (usually 100 mg) initially, adjusting dose after 5 days. If response is inadequate, a thiazide, furosemide, or ethacrynic acid should be added to the regimen. PO for essential hypertension 50-100 mg/day initially, adjusting dose after 2 weeks; up to 100 mg/day combined with a thiazide.[98] Dose of 100 mg bid has been used in low renin hypertension[99] and doses up to 400 mg/day have been used in primary aldosteronism.[100] PO for ascites 100 mg/day initially, increasing to 200-400 mg/day. Restrict sodium to 2 g/day or less and, if necessary, fluid to 1 L/day. Doses of up to 1 g/day have been used, but such high doses are expensive and are an indication for adding a thiazide or loop diuretic.[101] See Parameters to Monitor. Daily or bid dosing is as effective as multiple doses.[97,100,102] To eliminate delay in onset, a loading dose of 2 to 3 times the daily dose may be given on the first day of therapy.[97]

Pediatric Dose. PO 3.3 mg/kg/day, readjust dose after 5 days; dose may be increased up to triple this value. Restrict duration of therapy to 1 month.

Dosage Forms. **Tab** 25, 50, 100 mg; **Tab** 25 mg with hydrochlorothiazide 25 mg (Aldactazide®, Various); **Tab** 50 mg with hydrochlorothiazide 50 mg (Aldactazide® 50/50).

Patient Instructions. Avoid excessive amounts of high potassium foods or salt substitutes. See also Class Instructions.

Pharmacokinetics. *Onset and Duration.* Onset gradual, peak 2-3 days with continued dosing;[81] onset can be hastened by giving loading dose;[97] duration 2-3 days after cessation of therapy.[81]

Fate. Low bioavailability of unchanged drug due to extensive first-pass metabolism to active metabolite, canrenone, which accounts for 30-70% of antimineralocorticoid activity of spironolactone.[63,97,103-106] Canrenone levels are greater when spironolactone is taken with food, possibly indicating increased bioavailability.[63] Canrenone is 98% plasma protein bound and is in equilibrium with canrenoate; a total of less than 10% of these metabolites are excreted unchanged in urine.[97,103] Sulfur-containing metabolites probably contribute to activity.[104]

$t_{1/2}$. (Canrenone) 13-26 hr (average 19) when given in 1 or 2 doses daily; 9-16 hr (average 12.5) when given in 4 divided doses daily.[97,102]

Adverse Reactions. Hyperkalemia may occur, most frequently in patients with renal function impairment and those receiving potassium supplements.[107,108] Dehydration and hyponatremia occur occasionally, especially when drug is combined with other diuretics. Hyperchloremic acidosis has been reported in cirrhosis.[109] Occasionally, estrogen-like side effects occur including gynecomastia (dose and duration related and usually reversible), decreased libido and relative impotence in males; menstrual irregularities and breast tenderness in females.[107,110]

Contraindications. Anuria; acute renal insufficiency; rapidly deteriorating renal function; Cr_s greater than 2.5 mg/dl; serum potassium greater than 5.5 mEq/L.

Precautions. Pregnancy. Caution in patients with renal function impairment (Cr_s over 1.5 mg/dl) or hepatic disease.[58,107] Dosage of potent hypotensives may have to be decreased if spironolactone is added to the regimen. Potassium supplements should be given only to those with demonstrated hypokalemia who are taking a proximally acting diuretic and a corticosteroid concurrently with spironolactone or only for very short periods in treating cirrhosis and ascites. Do not give with triamterene or amiloride. Spironolactone is tumorigenic in animals and its use should be restricted to patients in whom other therapy is inadequate or inappropriate.

Parameters to Monitor. Serum electrolytes, particularly potassium, should be measured periodically, especially early in the course of therapy.[81] BUN and/or Cr_s should be measured periodically. In ascites, obtain daily weight and urinary electrolytes in addition to above, maintaining weight loss at no greater than 0.5-1 kg/day and urinary Na^+/K^+ ratio at greater than 1.[101]

Notes. Useful in patients with diabetes or gout because it causes no impairment of glucose tolerance and minimal hyperuricemia. Used in the diagnosis of primary aldosteronism and may be used in the management of the condition in patients unable to undergo surgery.[100] More expensive, yet more effective than potassium supplements.[98] Suspension of drug in cherry syrup is stable for 1 month if refrigerated.

Triamterene   Dyrenium®

Pharmacology. Triamterene acts directly on distal tubular transport of sodium exchange for potassium and hydrogen, producing a mild diuresis that is independent of aldosterone levels. Sodium, chloride, calcium and possibly bicarbonate excretion are increased, while potassium and possibly magnesium excretion is decreased. Antihypertensive activity is inconsistent and less pronounced than with thiazides or spironolactone.[5,58]

Administration and Adult Dose. PO initially 100 mg bid after meals if used alone; lower dose if used with another diuretic. Maintenance dosage should be adjusted to needs of the patient and may range from 100 mg/day to 100 mg every other day; maximum dosage is 300 mg/day.

Pediatric Dose. PO 4 mg/kg/day initially, may increase to 6 mg/kg/day in 1 or 2 doses after meals; maximum dose is 300 mg daily. Decrease dose if used with another diuretic.

Dosage Forms. **Cap** 50, 100 mg; **Cap** 50 mg with hydrochlorothiazide 25 mg (Dyazide®, Various); **Tab** 75 mg with hydrochlorothiazide 50 mg (Maxzide®, Various); 37.5 mg with hydrochlorothiazide 25 mg (Maxzide®-25).

Patient Instructions. This drug may be taken with food or milk to minimize stomach upset. Report persistent loss of appetite, nausea or vomiting. Avoid eating excessive amounts of high potassium foods or salt substitutes. See also Class Instructions.

Pharmacokinetics. *Onset and Duration.* Onset 2–4 hr; full therapeutic effect may not occur for several days; duration 7–9 hr.
   Fate. 30–70% absorbed orally.[111] 43–53% plasma protein bound; V_d is 2.5 L/kg.[63] Metabolized to para-hydroxy metabolite, which is partly further metabolized to sulfate conjugate; these two compounds, triamterene glucuronide and a small amount of free triamterene are excreted in the urine and bile.[111-113]
   $t_{1/2}$. 1.9–3.7 hr (average 2.8); increased in uremia.[63]

Adverse Reactions. Nausea, vomiting, diarrhea and dizziness occur frequently. Dehydration and hyponatremia with an increase in BUN occur occasionally, especially when drug is combined with other diuretics. Hyperkalemia occurs occasionally, especially in diabetics and in patients with renal function impairment; metabolic acidosis has been reported. Megaloblastic anemia can occur in alcoholic cirrhosis. Triamterene renal stones reported rarely.[58,82,108]

Contraindications. Severe or progressive renal disease or dysfunction (except possibly nephrosis); Cr_s greater than 2.5 mg/dl; severe hepatic disease; serum potassium greater than 5.5 mEq/L or development of hyperkalemia while taking the drug; concomitant potassium supplementation.

Precautions. Pregnancy. May cause elevation in serum uric acid in patients predisposed to gout. Should not be used with spironolactone or amiloride. Use with extreme caution with Cr_s greater than 1.5 mg/dl.

Parameters to Monitor. Serum electrolytes, particularly potassium, should be measured periodically, especially early in the course of therapy;[81] BUN and/or Cr_s should be measured periodically.

Notes. Appears to be less effective than spironolactone in sparing potassium,[108] but is less expensive.

Diuretics of Choice Comparison Chart[a]

CONDITION	ETHACRYNIC ACID	FUROSEMIDE	OSMOTIC	SPIRONOLACTONE	THIAZIDES	TRIAMTERENE/ AMILORIDE	COMMENTS AND OTHER TREATMENTS	REFERENCES
Hypertension	C	B	—	D,E	A	E	Loop diuretic may be added to thiazide for a few days to overcome refractoriness.	82,83
Right Heart Failure	B	B	—	E	A	E	Treat underlying pathology; digitalis.	82,83
Left Heart Failure	B	B	—	—	A	—	Digitalis.	82
Pulmonary Edema	A(IV)	A(IV)	—	—	—	—	Digitalis, O_2, aminophylline, morphine; consult literature.	82,83
Cirrhotic Edema and Ascites	C	C	—	A,E	B	C,E	Sodium and water restriction; albumin, mannitol if severe; slow diuresis preferable.	68,82,83
Acute Renal Failure	C	C	C	—	—	—	Hydration; dialysis.	81–83
Chronic Renal Failure	C	A	—	—	—	—	Diet; dialysis.	58,82,83
Nephrotic Syndrome	A	A	—	—	D	—	Corticosteroids, increase protein intake, plasma expanders, mannitol.	82
Diabetes Insipidus	—	—	—	E	A	E	Thiazides most useful in nephrogenic form; long-acting agent preferred.	75

Continued

Diuretics of Choice Comparison Chart[a]

CONDITION	ETHACRY-NIC ACID	FURO-SEMIDE	OSMOTIC	SPIRONO-LACTONE	THIAZIDES	TRIAM-TERENE/AMILORIDE	COMMENTS AND OTHER TREATMENTS	REFERENCES
Drug Poisoning	C	C	C	—	—	—	Fluids; urinary acidification or alkalinization; dialysis.	75,82
Hypercalcemia	—	A	—	—	—	—	Replace fluid loss; many other drugs useful.	71,75
Hypercalciuria	—	—	—	—	A	—		75,82
Relative Maximal Potency[b]	>15%	>15%	10–15%	<5%	5–10%	<5%	Total diuresis is also determined by the duration of action and fluid and electrolyte balance of patient.	83,89

a. This table is a guide to the selection of the most appropriate diuretic for the condition listed, but is not an all-inclusive guide to therapy. Consult references 81–83 for further information.

b. Numbers refer to maximum fraction of filtered sodium that is excreted following maximally effective dose of drug.

KEY:

A = Diuretic of choice.
B = Diuretic of second choice if patient unresponsive to first choice.
C = Useful in some circumstances.
D = May be useful alone, but low potency limits usefulness.
E = Useful as an adjunct to a more potent diuretic to reduce potassium loss and possibly enhance therapeutic effect.

40:40 URICOSURIC AGENTS

(SEE ALSO ANTI-GOUT AGENTS 92:00)

General References: 114-118

Probenecid
Benemid®, Various

Pharmacology. An organic acid that inhibits renal tubular reabsorption of urate, thereby increasing the urinary excretion of uric acid and lowering serum urate. Probenecid also interferes with renal tubular secretion of many drugs causing an increase or prolongation in their plasma levels. See Notes.

Administration and Adult Dose. PO for chronic gout 250 mg bid for 1 week, then 500 mg bid. Prophylactic colchicine, in doses of 0.5–1.5 mg/day for the first 6–12 months after initiation of treatment effectively diminishes the exacerbation of uricosuric-induced gouty attacks in patients with chronic tophaceous gout.[114,118] A liberal fluid intake and alkalinization of the urine (to prevent hematuria, renal colic, costovertebral pain and urate stone formation) is recommended, at least until serum uric acid levels normalize and tophaceous deposits disappear. If an acute gouty attack is precipitated during therapy, add colchicine to control the attack. **PO to prolong penicillin or cephalosporin action** 2 g/day in 4 divided doses.

Dosage Individualization. For chronic gout in renal impairment (although probably ineffective when Cl_{cr} is 30 ml/min or less), increase initial dose of 500 mg bid in 500 mg/day increments monthly to the dosage that maintains normal serum uric acid levels, to maximum of 2 g/day in divided doses.

Pediatric Dose. Contraindicated in children under 2 yr. **PO to prolong penicillin or cephalosproin action** (under 50 kg) 25 mg/kg initially, then maintain at 40 mg/kg/day in 4 divided doses; (over 50 kg) same as adult dose.

Dosage Forms. Tab 500 mg.

Patient Instructions. This drug may be taken with food, milk or an antacid to minimize stomach upset. Drink a large amount (10–12 full glasses) of fluids each day and avoid the use of aspirin-containing products unless directed otherwise.

Pharmacokinetics. *Fate.* Rapidly and well-absorbed from GI tract; 93–99% plasma protein bound, mostly to albumin.[119,120] Extensively metabolized or conjugated, such that about 40% is excreted in the urine as monoacyl glucuronide, less than 5% as unchanged drug and the remainder as hydroxylated metabolites which may have uricosuric activity.[121,122]

$t_{1/2}$. Dose-dependent (increases with increasing dose), with a range of 4–17 hr (usually 6–12 hr).[123]

Adverse Reactions. Headache, GI upset and skin rash occasionally. Exacerbation of gout and uric acid stones have been reported.[118] Nephrotic syndrome and hepatic necrosis may be part of a hypersensitivity reaction; aplastic anemia and hemolytic anemia (possibly related to G-6-PD deficiency) occur rarely.

Contraindications. Children under 2 yr; known blood dyscrasias or uric acid kidney stones; initiation of therapy during an acute gouty attack.

Precautions. Hypersensitivity reactions require drug discontinuation. Use with caution in patients with a history of peptic ulcer. Salicylates antagonize the uricosuric action of probenecid. Probenecid may increase the plasma concentration of indomethacin, naproxen, methotrexate, sulfonamides, sulfonylureas and rifampin. See Notes.

Parameters to Monitor. Serum uric acid; pretreatment 24-hour urinary uric acid excretion.[117] When alkali is administered, periodically determine acid-base balance.[117] Occasionally determine plasma levels of sulfa drugs when co-administered with probenecid for prolonged periods.

Notes. Ineffective in prolonging the half-life of β-lactams that are not preferentially excreted by tubular secretion (eg, cephalexin, ceftazidime and moxalactam).[124] Decreases clearance of some NSAIAs by competitively inhibiting either formation or renal excretion of acylglucuronide metabolites.[125]

Sulfinpyrazone   Anturane®

Sulfinpyrazone, an analogue of phenylbutazone, is a uricosuric agent with a mechanism and site of action resembling that of probenecid. It also has antiplatelet activity. Rapid and complete oral absorption, with peak 1–2 hr; V_d is 0.25–0.35 L/kg. Hepatic metabolism yields four metabolites. The parent compound is mainly responsible for uricosuric activity while the sulfide metabolite produces the antiplatelet effect. Half-life is 4–6 hr (sulfinpyrazone), 11–14 hr (sulfide metabolite). Adverse effects are similar to probenecid with the addition of rarely reported blood dyscrasias and occasional acute renal insufficiency, possibly due to precipitation of uric acid in renal tubules or decrease in prostaglandin synthesis. May not be effective and should be avoided when Cl_{cr} is less than 50 ml/min. Dosage as a uricosuric agent is 200–400 mg/day orally in 2 divided doses, to a maximum of 800 mg/day. A guided incremental dosing schedule has been proposed to increase renal tolerance in elderly, azotemic cardiovascular patients: therapy is initiated at 200 mg/day and increased in 200 mg/day increments q 4 days or kept constant for another 4 days depending upon Cr_s and uric acid, to a maximum maintenance dose of 800 mg/day.[118,126-131] See also Antiplatelet Drug Therapy Summary 20:12.04. Available as 100 mg tablets and 200 mg capsules.

Uricosuric Agents Comparison Chart[a]

DRUG	DOSAGE FORMS	DOSAGE	COMMENTS	REFERENCES
Apazone (Investigational - A. H. Robins)	—	600–1200 mg bid.[b]	Provides analgesic and anti-inflammatory activity. 1800–2400 mg/day is comparable to 1 g probenecid as a uricosuric.	132,133
Diflunisal Dolobid®	Tab 250, 500 mg.	500 mg bid.	A salicylate derivative; antihyperuricemic activity may be secondary to xanthine-oxidase inhibition in overexcretors, and uricosuria in normo-excretors.	134
Probenecid Benemid® Various	Tab 500 mg.	250 mg bid for 1 week, then 500 mg bid.	May decrease clearance of NSAIAs when used concurrently.	See Monograph.
Sulfinpyrazone Anturane® Various	Cap 200 mg Tab 100 mg.	100–200 mg bid.	Most potent uricosuric.	See Monograph.

a. Avoid uricosuric therapy in patients with inadequate urine volume (under 1400 ml/day); past history of renal calculi or renal insufficiency (Cl_{cr} less than 60 ml/min). Increase in urinary excretion of urate is generally greatest during the first few weeks after institution of therapy. An alkaline diuresis is desirable to avoid urate crystalluria.

b. Dosage used in investigational studies.

References, 40:00 Electrolytic, Caloric and Water Balance

1. Brass EP, Thompson WL. Drug-induced electrolyte abnormalities. Drugs 1982;24:207-28.

2. Knochel JP. Hypokalemia. Adv Intern Med 1984;30:317-35.

3. Stoff GS. Phosphate homeostasis and hypophosphatemia. Am J Med 1982;72:489-95.

4. Sack DA. Treatment of acute diarrhoea with oral rehydration solution. Drugs 1982;23:150-7.

5. Gilman AG, Goodman LS, Rall TW et al, eds. Goodman and Gilman's the pharmacological basis of therapeutics. 7th ed. New York: Macmillan, 1985.

6. Keyler D, Peterson CD. Oral calcium supplements: how much of what, for whom, and why? Postgrad Med 1985;78:123-5.

7. Spencer H, Kramer L, Lesniak M et al. Calcium requirements in humans: report of original data and a review. Clin Orthop 1984;184:270-80.

8. National Research Council. Recommended dietary allowances. 9th rev. ed. Washington, DC: National Academy of Sciences, 1980.

9. Heaney RP, Gallagher JC, Johnston CC et al. Calcium nutrition and bone health in the elderly. Am J Clin Nutr 1982;36:986-1013.

10. Nordin BEC. Calcium requirement and the menopause. Med J Aust 1984;141:144-5.

11. Allen LH. Calcium bioavailability and absorption: a review. Am J Clin Nutr 1982;35:783-808.

12. Anon. Calcium for postmenopausal osteoporosis. Med Lett Drugs Ther 1982;24:105-6.

13. Berkelhammer C, Bear RA. A clinical approach to common electrolyte problems: 4. hypomagnesemia. Can Med Assoc J 1985;132:360-8.

14. Cronin RE, Knochel JP. Magnesium deficiency. Adv Intern Med 1983;28:509-33.

15. Juan D. Clinical review: the clinical importance of hypomagnesemia. Surgery 1982;91:510-7.

16. Flink EB. Magnesium deficiency: etiology and clinical spectrum. Acta Med Scand 1981;Suppl 647:125-37.

17. Tzivoni D, Keren A, Cohen AM et al. Magnesium therapy for torsades de pointes. Am J Cardiol 1984;53:528-30.

18. Morgan KJ, Stampley GL, Zabik ME et al. Magnesium and calcium dietary intakes of the U.S. population. J Am Coll Nutr 1985;4:195-206.

19. Leary WP, Reyes AJ. Prophylaxis and treatment of magnesium depletion. S Afr Med J 1983;64:281-2.

20. Wester PO, Dyckner T. The importance of the magnesium ion. Magnesium deficiency-symptomatology and occurrence. Acta Med Scand 1982;Suppl 661:3-4.

21. Nanji AA, Denegri JF. Hypomagnesemia associated with gentamicin therapy. Drug Intell Clin Pharm 1984;18:596-8.

22. Chernow B, Smith J, Rainey TG et al. Hypomagnesemia: implications for the critical care specialist. Crit Care Med 1982;10:193-6.

23. Kingston M, Al-Siba'i MB. Treatment of severe hypophosphatemia. Crit Care Med 1985;13:16-8.

24. Baker WL. Hypophosphatemia. Am J Nurs 1985;85:999-1003.

25. Chernow B, Rainey TG, Georges LP et al. Iatrogenic hyperphosphatemia: a metabolic consideration in critical care medicine. Crit Care Med 1981;9:772-4.

26. Vannatta J, Whang R, Papper S. Efficacy of intravenous phosphorus therapy in the severely hypophosphatemic patient. Arch Intern Med 1981;141:885-7.

27. Benderev K. Hypophosphatemia and phosphorus supplementation. Hosp Pharm 1980;15:611-3.

28. Martin ML, Hamilton R, West MF. Potassium. Emerg Med Clin North Am 1986;4:131-44.

29. Stanaszek WF, Romankiewicz JA. Current approaches to management of potassium deficiency. Drug Intell Clin Pharm 1985;19:176-84.

30. Toner JM, Ramsay LE. Pharmacokinetics of potassium chloride in wax-based and syrup formulations. Br J Clin Pharmacol 1985;19:489-94.

31. Poole-Wilson PA. Hypokalaemia induced by thiazide diuretics in the treatment of hypertension: a cause for concern, not nihilism. Postgrad Med J 1983;59(Suppl 3):137-9.

32. Skoutakis VA, Acchiardo SR, Wojciechowski NJ et al. The comparative bioavailability of liquid, wax-matrix, and microencapsulated preparations of potassium chloride. J Clin Pharmacol 1985;25:619-21.

33. Skoutakis VA, Acchiardo SR, Wojciechowski NJ et al. Liquid and solid potassium chloride: bioavailability and safety. Pharmacotherapy 1984;4:392-7.

34. Riccardella D, Dwyer J. Salt substitutes and medicinal potassium sources: risks and benefits. J Am Diet Assoc 1985;85:471-4.

35. Sack RB, Pierce NF, Hirschhorn N. The current status of oral therapy in the treatment of acute diarrheal illness. Am J Clin Nutr 1978;31:2251-7.

36. Hirschhorn N. The treatment of acute diarrhea in children: an historical and physiological perspective. Am J Clin Nutr 1980;33:637-63.

37. Swedberg J, Steiner JF. Oral rehydration therapy in diarrhea. Postgrad Med 1983;74:335-41.

38. Anon. Oral rehydration solutions. Med Lett Drugs Ther 1983;25:19-20.

39. Pizarro D, Posada G, Mata L. Treatment of 242 neonates with dehydrating diarrhea with an oral glucose-electrolyte solution. J Pediatr 1983;102:153-6.

40. Santosham M, Daum RS, Dillman L et al. Oral rehydration therapy of infantile diarrhea. N Engl J Med 1982;306:1070-6.

41. Dibley M, Phillips F, Mahoney TJ et al. Oral rehydration fluids used in the treatment of diarrhoea. Med J Aust 1984;140:341-7.

42. Rovner DR. Use of pharmacologic agents in the treatment of hypokalemia and hyperkalemia. Ration Drug Ther 1972;6(2):1-6.

43. Williams ME, Rosa RM, Epstein FH. Hyperkalemia. Adv Intern Med 1986;31:265-91.

44. Alvo M, Warnock DG. Hyperkalemia. West J Med 1984;141:666-71.

45. Elms JJ. Potassium imbalance: causes and prevention. Postgrad Med 1982;72:165-71.

46. Lavelle KJ, Luft FC, Aronoff GR. Disorders of potassium balance. J Indiana State Med Assoc 1983;76:684-7.

47. Lant A. Diuretics: clinical pharmacology and therapeutic use (2 parts). Drugs 1985;29:57-87, 162-88.

48. Kokko JP. Site and mechanism of action of diuretics. Am J Med 1984;77(5A):11-7.

49. Narins RG, Chusid P. Diuretic use in critical care. Am J Cardiol 1986;57:26A-32A.

50. Gifford RW. The role of diuretics in the treatment of hypertension. Am J Med 1984;77(4A):102-6.

51. Witte MK, Stork JE, Blumer JL. Diuretic therapeutics in the pediatric patient. Am J Cardiol 1986;57:44A-53A.

52. Leary WP, Reyes AJ. Drug interactions with diuretics. S Afr Med J 1984;65:455-61.

53. Macfie HL, Colvin CL, Anderson PO. Amiloride. Drug Intell Clin Pharm 1981;15:94-8.

54. Halstenson CE, Matzke GR. Bumetanide: a new loop diuretic. Drug Intell Clin Pharm 1983;17:786-97.

55. Ward A, Heel RC. Bumetanide: a review of its pharmacodynamic and pharmacokinetic properties and therapeutic use. Drugs 1984;28:426-64.

56. Pentikäinen PJ, Pasternack A, Lampainen E et al. Bumetanide kinetics in renal failure. Clin Pharmacol Ther 1985;37:582-8.

57. Cooperman LB, Rubin IL. Toxicity of ethacrynic acid and furosemide. Am Heart J 1973;85:831-4.

58. Offerhaus L. Diuretic drugs. In: Dukes MNG, ed. Meyler's side effects of drugs, 10th ed. Amsterdam: Elsevir 1984;369-85.

59. McNeill IY. Hypersensitivity reaction to mannitol. Drug Intell Clin Pharm 1985;19:552-3.

60. Dikshit K, Vyden JK, Forrester JS et al. Renal and extrarenal hemodynamic effects of furosemide in congestive heart failure after acute myocardial infarction. N Engl J Med 1973;288:1087-90.

61. Anderton JL, Kincaid-Smith P. Diuretics II. clinical considerations. Drugs 1971;1:141-65.

62. McEvoy GK, ed. AHFS American hospital formulary service. Drug Information 87. Bethesda, MD: American Society of Hospital Pharmacists, 1959-87.

63. Beerman B, Groschinsky-Grind M. Clinical pharmacokinetics of diuretics. Clin Pharmacokinet 1980;5:221-45.

64. Benet LZ. Pharmacokinetics/pharmacodynamics of furosemide in man: a review. J Pharmacokinet Biopharm 1979;7:1-27.

65. Cutler RE, Blair AD. Clinical pharmacokinetics of furosemide. Clin Pharmacokinet 1979;4:279-96.

66. Odlind BG, Beerman B. Diuretic resistance: reduced bioavailability and effect of oral furosemide. Br Med J 1980;2:1577.

67. Spino M, Sellers EM, Kaplan HL et al. Adverse biochemical and clinical consequences of furosemide administration. Can Med Assoc J 1978;118:1513-8.

68. Sherlock S, Senewiratne B, Scott A et al. Complications of diuretic therapy in hepatic cirrhosis. Lancet 1966;1:7446-53.

69. Anderson RJ, Schrier RW, eds. Clinical use of drugs in patients with kidney and liver disease. Philadelphia. WB Saunders, 1981.

70. Anderson J, Godfrey BE, Hill DM et al. A comparison of the effects of hydrochlorothiazide and of furosemide in the treatment of hypertensive patients. Q J Med 1971;NS40:541-60.

71. Suki WN, Yium JJ, Von Minden M et al. Acute treatment of hypercalcemia with furosemide. N Engl J Med 1970;283:836-40.

72. Hantman D, Rossier B, Zohlman R et al. Rapid correction of hyponatremia in the syndrome of inappropriate secretion of antidiuretic hormone. Ann Intern Med 1973;78:870-5.

73. Decaux G, Waterlot Y, Genette F et al. Treatment of the syndrome of inappropriate secretion of antidiuretic hormone with furosemide. N Engl J Med 1981;304:329-30.

74. Anderson PO et al. Current drug therapy—thiazide diuretics. Am J Hosp Pharm 1975;32:473-80.

75. Martinez-Maldonado M, Eknoyan G, Suki WN. Diuretics in nonedematous states — physiological basis for the clinical use. Arch Intern Med 1973;131:797-808.

76. Benet LZ, Sheiner LB. Design and optimization of dosage regimens; pharmacokinetic data. In Gilman AG, Goodman LS, Rall TW et al, eds. Goodman and Gilman's the pharmacological basis of therapeutics. 7th ed. New York: Macmillan, 1985;1663-733.

77. Backman L, Beerman B, Groschinsky-Grind M et al. Malabsorption of hydrochlorothiazide following intestinal shunt surgery. Clin Pharmacol 1979;4:63-8.

78. Wilkinson PR, Hesp R, Issler H et al. Total body and serum potassium during prolonged thiazide therapy for essential hypertension. Lancet 1975;1:759-62.

79. Amery A, Bulpitt C, de Schaepdryver A et al. Glucose intolerance during diuretic therapy. Lancet 1978;1:681-3.

80. Grimm RH, Leon AS, Hunninghake DB et al. Effects of thiazide diuretics on plasma lipids and lipoproteins in mildly hypertensive patients. Ann Intern Med 1981;94:7-11.

81. Frazier HS, Yager H. The clinical use of diuretics (2 parts). N Engl J Med 1973;288:246-9,455-9.

82. Anderton JL, Kincaid-Smith P. Diuretics II. clinical considerations. Drugs 1971;1:141-65.

83. Davies DL, Wilson GM. Diuretics: mechanism of action and clinical application. Drugs 1975;9:178-226.

84. Stern A. Metolazone, a diuretic agent. Am Heart J 1976;91:262-3.

85. Prichard BNC, Brogden RN. Xipamide: a review of its pharmacodynamic and pharmacokinetic properties and therapeutic efficacy. Drugs 1985;30:313-32.

86. Gunby P. Mannitol opens pathway for brain tumor chemotherapy. JAMA 1981;245:1802. News.

87. Nissenson AR, Weston RE, Kleeman CR. Mannitol. West J Med 1979;131:277-84.

88. Hoffman DM, Grossano D. Use of mannitol diuresis to reduce cis-platinum nephrotoxicity. Drug Intell Clin Pharm 1978;12:489-90.

89. Gennari FJ, Kassirer JP. Osmotic diuresis. N Engl J Med 1974;291:714-20.

90. McNabb WR, Noormohamed FH, Brooks BA et al. Renal actions of piretanide and three other ''loop'' diuretics. Clin Pharmacol Ther 1984;35:328-37.

91. Lawrence JR, Ansari AF, Elliott HL et al. Kinetic and dynamic comparison of piretanide and furosemide. Clin Pharmacol Ther 1978;23:558-65.

92. Brater DC, Anderson S, Baird B et al. Effects of piretanide in normal subjects. Clin Pharmacol Ther 1983;34:324-30.

93. Clissold SP, Brogden RN. Piretanide: a preliminary review of its pharmacodynamic and pharmacokinetic properties, and therapeutic efficacy. Drugs 1985;29:489-530.

94. Walter U, Rockel A, Lahn W et al. Pharmacokinetics of the loop diuretic piretanide in renal failure. Eur J Clin Pharmacol 1985;29:337-43.

95. Marone C, Reubi FC, Perisic M et al. Pharmacokinetics of high doses of piretanide in moderate to severe renal failure. Eur J Clin Pharmacol 1984;27:589-93.

96. Berg KJ, Walstad RA, Bergh K. The pharmacokinetics and diuretic effects of piretanide in chronic renal insufficiency. Eur J Clin Pharmacol 1983;15:347-53.

97. Sadee W, Schroder R, Leitner E et al. Multiple dose kinetics of spironolactone and canrenoate-potassium in cardiac and hepatic failure. Eur J Clin Pharmacol 1974;7:195-200.

98. Ramsay LE, Hettiarachchi J, Fraser R et al. Amiloride, spironolactone, and potassium chloride in thiazide-treated hypertensive patients. Clin Pharmacol Ther 1980;27:533-43.

99. Karlberg BE, Kagedal B, Teyler L et al. Controlled treatment of primary hypertension with propranolol and spironolactone. Am J Cardiol 1976;37:642-9.

100. Brown JJ, Davies DL, Ferriss JB et al. Comparison of surgery and prolonged spironolactone therapy in patients with hypertension, aldosterone excess, and low plasma renin. Br Med J 1972;2:729-34.

101. Eggert RC. Spironolactone diuresis in patients with cirrhosis and ascites. Br Med J 1970;4:401-3.

102. Karim A, Zagarella J, Hutsell TC et al. Spironolactone. III. Canrenone—maximum and minimum steady-state plasma levels. Clin Pharmacol Ther 1976;19:177-82.

103. Karim A, Zagarella J, Hribar J et al. Spironolactone. I. Disposition and metabolism. Clin Pharmacol Ther 1976;19:158-69.

104. Ramsay L, Shelton J, Harrison I et al. Spironolactone and potassium canrenoate in normal man. Clin Pharmacol Ther 1976;20:167-77.

105. Huston GJ, Turner P. Antagonism of fludrocortisone by spironolactone and canrenone. Br J Clin Pharmacol 1976;3:201-4.

106. Ramsay L, Asbury M, Shelton J et al. Spironolactone and canrenoate-K: relative potency at steady state. Clin Pharmacol Ther 1977;21:602-9.

107. Greenblatt DJ, Koch-Weser J. Adverse reactions to spironolactone: a report from the Boston Collaborative Drug Surveillance Program. JAMA 1973;225:40-3.

108. Anon. Potassium-sparing diuretics: spironolactone v. triamterene and amiloride. Drug Ther Bull 1972;10:30-2.

109. Gabow PA, Moore S, Schrier RW. Spironolactone-induced hyperchloremic acidosis in cirrhosis. Ann Intern Med 1979;90:338-40.

110. Loriaux DL, Menard R, Taylor A et al. Spironolactone and endocrine dysfunction. Ann Intern Med 1976;85:630-6.

111. Pruitt AW, Winkel JS, Dayton PG. Variations in the fate of triamterene. Clin Pharmacol Ther 1977;21:610-9.

112. Pruitt AW, Dayton PG, Steinhorst J. Fate of triamterene in man. Clin Res 1974;22:77a.

113. Lehmann K. Separation, isolation and identification of metabolic products of triamterene. Arzneim Forsch 1965;15:812-6.

114. German DC, Holmes EW. Hyperuricemia and gout. Med Clin North Am 1986;70:419-36.

115. Emmerson BT. Therapeutics of hyperuricaemia and gout. Med J Aust 1984;141:31-6.

116. Littman BH. Asymptomatic hyperuricemia: the case for benign neglect. Postgrad Med 1985;77:221-4.

117. Boss GR, Seegmiller JE. Hyperuricemia and gout: classification, complications and management. N Engl J Med 1979;300:1459-68.

118. Mangini RJ. Drug therapy reviews: pathogenesis and clinical management of hyperuricemia and gout. Am J Hosp Pharm 1979;36:497-504.

119. Jusko WJ, Gretch M. Plasma and tissue protein binding of drugs in pharmacokinetics. Drug Metab Rev 1976;5:43-140.

120. Koch-Weser J, Sellers EM. Binding of drugs to serum albumin (2 parts). N Engl J Med 1976;294:311-6,526-31.

121. Israili ZH, Perel JM, Cunningham RF et al. Metabolites of probenecid. Chemical, physical, and pharmacological studies. J Med Chem 1972;15:709-13.

122. Perel JM, Cunningham RF, Fales HM et al. Identification and renal excretion of probenecid metabolites in man. Life Sci 1970;9:1337-43.

123. Dayton PG, Yu TF, Chen W et al. The physiological disposition of probenecid, including renal clearance, in man, studied by an improved method for its estimation in biological material. J Pharmacol Exp Ther 1963;140:278-86.

124. Anon. Plugging the penicillin leak with probenecid. Lancet 1984;2:499. Editorial.

125. Smith PC, Langendijk PNJ, Bosso JA et al. Effect of probenecid on the formation and elimination of acyl glucuronides: studies with zomepirac. Clin Pharmacol Ther 1985;38:121-7.

126. Hood WB. More on sulfinpyrazone after myocardial infarction. N Engl J Med 1982;306:988-9.

127. Palummeri E, Borghi C, DiRuvo R et al. Sulphinpyrazone in cardiovascular elderly azotemic patients: a proposal of a guided incremental dose schedule. J Int Med Res 1984;12:271-6.

128. Mahoney C, Wolfram KM, Nash PV et al. Kinetics and metabolism of sulfinpyrazone. Clin Pharmacol Ther 1983;33:491-7.

129. Schlicht T, Staiger C, deVries J et al. Pharmacokinetics of sulfinpyrazone and its major metabolites after a single dose and during chronic treatment. Eur J Clin Pharmacol 1985;28:97-103.

130. Orlandini G, Brognoli M. Acute renal failure and treatment with sulfinpyrazone. Clin Nephrol 1983;20:161-2.

131. Rosenkranz B, Fejes-Toth G, Diener U et al. Effects of sulfinpyrazone on renal function and prostaglandin formation in man. Nephron 1985;39:237-43.

132. Higgins CS, Scott JT. The uricosuric action of azapropazone: dose-response and comparison with probenecid. Br J Clin Pharmacol 1984;18:439-43.

133. Templeton JS. Azapropazone or allopurinol in the treatment of chronic gout and/or hyperuricaemia: a preliminary report. Br J Clin Pract 1982;36:353-8.

134. Ferraccioli G, Spisni A, Ambanelli U. Hypouricemic action of diflunisal in gouty patients: in vitro and in vivo

studies. J Rheumatol 1984;11:330-2.
    135. Lillemoe KD, Romolo JL, Hamilton SR et al. Intestinal necrosis due to sodium polystyrene (Kayexalate) in sorbitol enemas: clinical and experimental suppoort for the hypothesis. Surgery 1987;101:267-72.

48:00 ANTITUSSIVES, EXPECTORANTS, AND MUCOLYTIC AGENTS

48:08 ANTITUSSIVES

General References: 1–3

Class Instructions. **Antitussives.** This drug should not be used to suppress productive cough; see your physician or pharmacist if cough persists. **Expectorants.** This drug should be taken with a large quantity of fluid to ensure proper drug action; see your physician or pharmacist if cough persists.

Codeine Salts   Various

See Section 28:08.08.

Dextromethorphan Hydrobromide   Various

Pharmacology. The nonanalgesic, nonaddictive d-isomer of the codeine analogue of levorphanol. With usual antitussive doses, the cough threshold is elevated centrally with little effect on the respiratory, cardiovascular or GI systems.

Administration and Adult Dose. **PO as cough suppressant** 10–30 mg q 4–8 hr, to maximum of 120 mg/day; **SR** 60 mg bid.

Pediatric Dose. **PO as cough suppressant** (2–6 yr) 2.5–5 mg q 4 hr or 7.5 mg q 6–8 hr, to maximum of 30 mg/day; (6–12 yr) 5–10 mg q 4 hr or 15 mg q 6–8 hr, to maximum of 45–60 mg/day; (over 12 yr) same as adult dose. **SR** (2–5 yr) 15 mg bid; (6–12 yr) 30 mg bid.

Dosage Forms. **Lozenges** 5, 15 mg; **SR Susp** 6 mg/ml; **Syrup** 1, 1.5, 2, 3 mg/ml; (available in many combination products in variable concentrations).

Patient Instructions. See Class Instructions for antitussive use.

Pharmacokinetics. *Onset and Duration.* PO onset 1–2 hr; duration up to 6 hr or more.[4]

Adverse Reactions. Mild and infrequent drowsiness and GI upset.[3] Intoxication, bizarre behavior, CNS depression and respiratory depression can occur with extremely high doses. Naloxone may be effective in reversing these effects.[5-7]

Contraindications. MAO inhibitor therapy.

Precautions. Generally, do not use in patients with chronic cough or cough associated with excessive secretions.

Notes. Approximately equipotent with codeine in antitussive effectiveness.[1,4]

48:16 EXPECTORANTS

Guaifenesin

2/G®, Robitussin®,
Various

Pharmacology.   The proposed expectorant action of guaifenesin is through an increased output of respiratory tract fluid, enhancing the flow of less viscid secretions, promoting ciliary action and facilitating the removal of inspissated mucus. Evidence of the effectiveness of guaifenesin is largely subjective and not established clinically.[8-11]

Administration and Adult Dose. **PO as expectorant** 200–400 mg q 4 hr, to a maximum of 2.4 g/day has been proposed.[1]

Pediatric Dose. **PO as expectorant** (2–6 yr) 50 mg q 4 hr, to maximum of 300 mg/day; (6–12 yr) 50–100 mg q 4–6 hr, to maximum of 600 mg/day.

Dosage Forms. **Cap** 200 mg; **Syrup** 13.4, 20 mg/ml; **Tab** 100, 200 mg.

Patient Instructions. See Class Instructions for expectorant use.

Adverse Reactions.   Occasional drowsiness, nausea and possibly vomiting.

Notes.   May produce a color interference with certain laboratory determinations of 5-hydroxyindoleacetic acid (5-HIAA) and vanilmandelic acid (VMA).[12] May lower serum uric acid;[13] may have a mild, transitory antiplatelet action (without affecting bleeding time) which is of little clinical importance.[14]

References, 48:00 Antitussives, Expectorants and Mucolytic Agents

1. Anon. Establishment of a monograph for OTC cold, cough, allergy, bronchodilator and antiasthmatic products. Fed Regist 1976;41:38312-424.
2. Anon. Over-the-counter cough remedies. Med Lett Drugs Ther 1979;21:103-4.
3. Bryant BG, Cormier JF. Cold and allergy products. In: Feldmann EG, ed. Handbook of nonprescription drugs. 8th ed. Washington, DC: American Pharmaceutical Association, 1986;127-74.
4. Matthys H, Bleicher B, Bleicher U. Dextromethorphan and codeine: objective assessment of antitussive activity in patients with chronic cough. J Int Med Res 1983;11:92-100.
5. Committee on Drugs. Use of codeine- and dextromethorphan-containing cough syrups in pediatrics. Pediatrics 1978;62:118-22.
6. Shaul WL, Wandell M, Robertson WO. Dextromethorphan toxicity: reversal by naloxone. Pediatrics 1977;59:117-9.
7. Katona B, Wason S. Dextromethorphan danger. N Engl J Med 1986;314:993. Letter.
8. Boyd EM, Sheppard EP, Boyd CE. The pharmacological basis of the expectorant action of glyceryl guaiacolate. Appl Ther 1967;9:55-9.
9. Hirsch SR, Viernes PF, Kory RC. The expectorant effect of glyceryl guaiacolate in patients with chronic bronchitis. Chest 1973;63:9-14.
10. Heilborn H, Pegelow K-O, Odeblad E. Effect of bromhexine and guaiphenesine on clinical state, ventilatory capacity and sputum viscosity in chronic asthma. Scand J Resp Dis 1976;57:88-96.
11. Anon. Guaiphenesin and iodide. Drug Ther Bull 1985;23:62-4.
12. Hansten PD. Drug interactions. 4th ed. Philadelphia: Lea & Febiger, 1979.
13. Ramsdell CM, Kelley WN. The clinical significance of hypouricemia. Ann Intern Med 1973;78:239-42.
14. Buchanan GR, Martin V, Levine PH et al. The effects of ''anti-platelet'' drugs on bleeding time and platelet aggregation in normal human subjects. Am J Clin Pathol 1977;68:355-9.

56:00 GASTROINTESTINAL DRUGS

General References: 1–3

56:04 ANTACIDS AND ADSORBENTS

General References: 1–4

Activated Charcoal   Various

Pharmacology. A nonspecific GI adsorbent with a surface area of 1000–3000 M^2/g used primarily in the management of acute poisonings.[5]

Administration and Adult Dose. **PO or via gastric tube** dispersed in liquid 30–120 g as soon as possible after ingestion of poison (the FDA suggests 240 ml diluent/30 g activated charcoal). If syrup of ipecac-induced emesis is contemplated, delay administration of activated charcoal until after emesis; repeat administration of activated charcoal after gastric lavage.

Pediatric Dose. **PO or via gastric tube** dispersed in liquid (up to 12 yr) 15–30 g or 1–2 g/kg; (over 12 yr) same as adult dose.[6]

Dosage Forms. **Pwdr** (plain, or dispersed in water or sorbitol-water mixture).

Patient Instructions. This drug causes the stools to turn black.

Pharmacokinetics. *Onset and Duration.* Onset immediate; duration continual while it remains in the GI tract.
   Fate. Eliminated unchanged in the feces.

Adverse Reactions. Stools will turn black; gritty consistency may cause emesis in some patients.

Parameters to Monitor. Passage of activated charcoal in the stools. If sorbitol or other cathartics are administered, their doses should be limited to prevent excessive fluid and electrolyte losses.

Notes. A suspension of activated charcoal in 70% sorbitol may increase palatability of the drug.[7] Substances *not* adsorbed by activated charcoal include mineral acids, alkalis, boric acid, DDT, ferrous sulfate, cyanide, lithium and other small ions, and alcohols.[5,8] Repeated oral doses of activated charcoal (eg, q 4 hr) have been used to enhance the elimination of some drugs which undergo enterohepatic circulation, most notably phenobarbital and theophylline.

Antacids

Pharmacology. Antacids are weakly basic inorganic salts whose primary action is to neutralize gastric acid. Antacid-induced pH above 4 inhibits the proteolytic activity of pepsin. Gastric juice and acid secretion may be increased by gastrin release due to elevated pH. Antacids may increase urine pH. Aluminum salts bind phosphate in the GI tract, decreasing the serum phosphate level.

Administration and Adult Dose. **PO for symptomatic relief of gastroesophageal reflux disease** 10–30 ml prn or 1 and 3 hr after meals and hs.[1,2] **PO for peptic ulcer disease** 100–160 mEq of acid-neutralizing capacity per dose given 1 and 3 hr after meals and hs for 4–8 weeks until healing is complete. Additional doses may be taken if pain persists.[1,4,9] There is some evidence that lower doses may heal peptic ulcers.[10] **PO or NG for prevention of stress-related mucosal bleeding** titrate hourly to maintain intragastric pH above 4 at the end of each hour.[11] **PO for phosphate binding in renal failure** (aluminum hydroxide or carbonate) titrate dose based on serum phosphate.

Pediatric Dose. **PO for peptic ulcer disease** (up to 12 yr) maximum dose of 5–15 ml as often as q 1 hr.

Dosage Forms. See Antacid Products Comparison Chart.

Patient Instructions. Ulcer pain may be relieved initially; however, it is necessary to take this medication for a full 4–8 weeks to ensure ulcer healing. Diarrhea may occur with magnesium-containing antacids; this may be minimized by alternating doses with aluminum-containing antacids. Antacids may interfere with other medications; take any other medications 1–2 hours before or after antacids unless otherwise directed. If tablets are used, chew thoroughly before swallowing.

Pharmacokinetics. *Onset and Duration.* Onset of acid neutralizing is immediate; duration is 20–40 min taken on an empty stomach and 2–3 hr if ingested after meals.[1,2,9]

Fate. Antacids are absorbed to varying degrees. Calcium is significantly absorbed and can result in hypercalcemia and/or systemic alkalosis; magnesium is 15–30% absorbed; aluminum is slightly absorbed. Calcium, magnesium and aluminum are excreted renally with normal renal function.[1,2] The unabsorbed portion is excreted in the feces.

Adverse Reactions. Calcium-containing antacids can cause rebound acid secretion, metabolic alkalosis and hypercalcemia ("milk-alkali syndrome") which can lead to nephrolithiasis. Magnesium-containing antacids frequently cause a dose-related laxative effect;[12] hypermagnesemia can occur in patients with renal impairment. Aluminum- and calcium-containing antacids occasionally cause constipation. Prolonged administration and/or large doses of aluminum hydroxide or carbonate can result in hypophosphatemia; encephalopathy has been reported in dialysis patients receiving aluminum antacids.[13]

Precautions. Use with caution in patients with renal impairment, edema, hypertension or CHF. See Drug Interactions chapter.

Parameters to Monitor. Observe for diarrhea or constipation and relief of epigastric pain. Obtain periodic serum magnesium levels in patients with renal impairment and serum phosphate during chronic use.

Notes. Tablet formulations are generally not as effective as liquids; however, thoroughly chewed magnesium-containing antacid tablets might be effective.[1]

Continued

Antacid Products Comparison Chart[a]

ANTACID	ACID NEUTRALIZING CAPACITY		SODIUM CONTENT			
	MEQ/5 ML	MEQ/TABLET	MEQ/5 ML	MG/5 ML	MEQ/TABLET	MG/TABLET
Aluminum Carbonate Gel, Basic						
Basaljel®	11.5	12.5 (Tab)	0.13	3.0	0.12	2.8
		12.0 (Cap)		—	0.12	2.8
Basaljel® Extra Strength	22.0	—	1.0	23.0	—	—
Aluminum Hydroxide Gel						
ALternaGel®	16.0	—	0.11	2.5	—	—
Amphojel®	10.0	8.0 (300 mg Tab)	0.10	2.3	0.08	1.8
		16.0 (600 mg Tab)		—	0.13	3.0
Aluminum Hydroxide with Magnesium Hydroxide						
Aludrox®	12.0	9.5	0.10	2.3	0.06	1.4
Maalox®	13.3	9.7 (#1 Tab)	0.06	1.4	0.03	0.7
		11.7 (#2 Tab)		—	0.06	1.4
Maalox®Therapeutic Concentrate	27.2	28.0	0.03	0.8	0.02	0.5
WinGel®	11.6	12.3	b	b	b	b
Aluminum Hydroxide with Magnesium Hydroxide and Calcium Carbonate						
Camalox®	18.5	18.4	0.05	1.2	0.04	1.0

Antacid Products Comparison Chart[a]

ANTACID	ACID NEUTRALIZING CAPACITY		SODIUM CONTENT			
	MEQ/5 ML	MEQ/TABLET	MEQ/5 ML	MG/5 ML	MEQ/TABLET	MG/TABLET
Aluminum Hydroxide with Magnesium Hydroxide and Simethicone						
Di-Gel®[c]	9.0	9.0	0.37	8.5	<0.22	<5.0
Gelusil®	12.0	11.0	0.03	0.7	0.03	0.8
Gelusil-M®	15.0	12.5	0.05	1.2	0.06	1.3
Gelusil II®	24.0	21.0	0.06	1.3	0.09	2.1
Maalox Plus®	13.4	11.4	0.05	1.2	0.03	0.8
Mylanta®	12.7	11.5	0.03	0.68	0.03	0.77
Mylanta II®	25.4	23.0	0.05	1.14	0.06	1.3
Calcium Carbonate with Glycine						
Titralac®	—	7.5	—	—	0.01	<0.3
Titralac Plus® (with Simethicone)	11.0	7.5	0.00002	<0.0005	0.001	<0.03
Magaldrate						
Riopan® and Riopan Plus® (with Simethicone)	15.0	13.5	0.004	0.1	0.004	0.1
Extra Strength Riopan Plus® (with Simethicone)	30.0	—	0.013	0.3	—	—

a. Product formulations, and hence neutralizing capacity and sodium content, are subject to change by manufacturer.
b. Information not available.
c. Contains aluminum hydroxide-magnesium carbonate gel, magnesium hydroxide and simethicone.

56:08 ANTIDIARRHEA AGENTS

General References: 14, 15

Diphenoxylate Hydrochloride and Atropine Sulfate

Lomotil®,
Various

Pharmacology. Diphenoxylate is a narcotic-like agent that slows GI motility; atropine is added in subtherapeutic amounts to decrease abuse potential.

Administration and Adult Dose. PO 1–2 tablets or 5–10 ml 3–6 times daily for 24–48 hr initially to control diarrhea, then 1 tablet or 5 ml daily-tid prn.

Pediatric Dose. Use liquid only. Not recommended under 2 yr. PO (2–5 yr) 4 ml tid; (5–8 yr) 4 ml qid; (8–12 yr) 4 ml 5 times daily. Reduce dosage once diarrhea is controlled.

Dosage Forms. Syrup 2.5 mg diphenoxylate and 25 mcg atropine/5 ml; **Tab** 2.5 mg diphenoxylate and 25 mcg atropine.

Patient Instructions. This drug may cause blurred vision, drowsiness or dizziness. Until the severity of these reactions is known, caution should be used when performing tasks that require mental alertness.

Pharmacokinetics. *Onset and Duration.* Onset 45–60 min; duration 3–4 hr.

** *Fate.*** Diphenoxylate is well absorbed from the GI tract and metabolized to an active metabolite, diphenoxylic acid. Both drug and metabolite attain peak plasma levels in 2 hr; their conjugates are excreted primarily in the urine.[16]

  $t_{1/2}$. (Diphenoxylate) 2.5 hr; (diphenoxylic acid) 12–24 hr.[16]

Adverse Reactions. Drowsiness, dizziness and headache occur occasionally. Anticholinergic symptoms such as dry mouth, blurred vision, fever or tachycardia may occur with high doses (over 12–15 tablets) in adults, or occasionally with usual doses in children.

Contraindications. Children under 2 yr; advanced liver disease.

Precautions. Use with caution in children due to variable response and potential for toxicity, and in patients with acute ulcerative colitis or cirrhosis.

Parameters to Monitor. Frequency and volume of bowel movements; observe for signs of atropine toxicity.[14]

Notes. Diphenoxylate 2.5 mg has equivalent efficacy to 5 ml of paregoric.

Loperamide

Imodium®

Pharmacology. A synthetic antidiarrheal, structurally similar to haloperidol that causes a dose-related inhibition of colonic motility without significant opiate activity.

Administration and Adult Dose. PO for acute diarrhea 4 mg initially, then 2 mg after each unformed stool, to a maximum of 16 mg/day.[15] PO for chronic diarrhea initiate therapy as above, then individualize dosage; usual maintenance dosage is 4–8 mg/day in single or divided doses.

Pediatric Dose. Not recommended under 2 yr. PO for acute diarrhea (2–5 yr) 1 mg tid as liquid; (5–8 yr) 2 mg bid; (8–12 yr) 2 mg tid. After first day of therapy, give 1 mg/10 kg after each loose stool to a maximum of above initial dose.

Dosage Forms. **Cap** 2 mg; **Liquid** 1 mg/5 ml.

Patient Instructions. This drug may cause drowsiness or dizziness. Until the severity of these reactions is known, caution should be used when performing tasks that require mental alertness.

Pharmacokinetics. *Onset and Duration.* Onset 45-60 min; duration 4-6 hr.

    Fate. Absorption from GI tract is insignificant; less than 2% of a dose is recovered in the urine.[15]

    $t_{1/2}$. 7-15 hr (average 11).[15]

Adverse Reactions. Abdominal cramping occurs occasionally; nausea, rash, dizziness and dry mouth are rare.

Precautions. Use with caution in patients with ulcerative colitis.

Parameters to Monitor. Frequency and volume of bowel movements.

Notes. Adverse reactions may be less frequent than with diphenoxylate with atropine.

56:12 CATHARTICS AND LAXATIVES

General References: 17-21

Bisacodyl   Dulcolax®, Various

Pharmacology. A stimulant cathartic structurally similar to phenolphthalein that produces its effect by direct contact with colonic mucosa. Net water and electrolyte absorption may also be inhibited.

Administration and Adult Dose. **PO as a laxative/cathartic** 5-20 mg; **PR** 10-20 mg. Dosage is variable, and should be adjusted based on response.

Pediatric Dose. **PO** (over 6 yr) 5-10 mg; **PR** (under 2 yr) 5 mg; (over 2 yr) 10 mg.

Dosage Forms. **EC Tab** 5 mg; **Supp** 10 mg.

Patient Instructions. Tablets should be swallowed whole (not chewed or crushed) and should not be taken within 1 hour of antacids or dairy products.

Pharmacokinetics. *Onset and Duration.* Onset PO 6-8 hr; PR 15 min-1 hr.[17]

    Fate. Absorption is less than 5% by oral or rectal route. Rapidly converted by intestinal and bacterial enzymes to its active desacetyl metabolite.[19]

Adverse Reactions. Abdominal cramps occur occasionally; excessive use of suppositories can cause rectal irritation.

Contraindications. Acute surgical abdomen; fecal impaction; intestinal or biliary tract obstruction; abdominal pain of unknown origin; acute hepatitis; intestinal perforation.[17]

Notes. Useful for preoperative or radiographic bowel preparation. Cathartic effect can be overcome by the application of a local anesthetic.[17]

Docusate Salts   Various

Pharmacology. An anionic surfactant that lowers the surface tension of the oil-water interface of the stool, allowing fecal material to be penetrated by water and fat, thereby softening the stool. The emulsifying action also enhances the absorption of many fat-soluble drugs.[17,18,22]

Administration and Adult Dose. **PO as a stool softener** 50–500 mg/day in single or divided doses.[17] **PR as enema** 50–100 mg in water.

Pediatric Dose. **PO** (under 3 yr) 10–40 mg/day; (3–6 yr) 20–60 mg/day; (6–12 yr) 40–120 mg/day.

Dosage Forms. (Sodium salt-Colace®, Various) **Cap** 50, 60, 100, 240, 250, 300 mg; **Soln** 10, 50 mg/ml; **Syrup** 3.3, 4 mg/ml; **Tab** 50, 100 mg. (Calcium salt-Surfak®, Various) **Cap** 50, 240 mg. (Potassium salt-Dialose®, Various) **Cap** 100, 240 mg.

Patient Instructions. This drug should be taken with a full glass of fluid; liquid or solution should be taken in milk, fruit juice or infant formula to mask bitter taste.

Pharmacokinetics. *Onset and Duration.* Onset of effect on stools 1–3 days after first dose with continuous use.[19]
   Fate. May be partially absorbed in the duodenum and jejunum and secreted in the bile.[17]

Adverse Reactions. Occasional abdominal cramps.

Contraindications. Undiagnosed abdominal pain; intestinal obstruction. Theoretically, absorption of mineral oil is enhanced by these drugs and therefore long-term concurrent use with mineral oil should be avoided.[17,18]

Precautions. Concurrent use with oxyphenisatin or danthron (both removed from US market) may cause chronic active hepatitis by enhancing their absorption.[23-25] Concurrent use with aspirin results in greater mucosal damage than when either agent is given separately.[17]

Parameters to Monitor. Frequency and consistency of stools; ease of defecation.

Notes. Surfactant cathartic useful for hard dry stools and in lessening the strain of defecation. Use of 200 mg or less daily in the hospital setting may be ineffective in altering the prevalence of constipation.[17,22,25] These agents may change intestinal morphology, cellular function and cause fluid and electrolyte accumulation in the colon.[17,22]

Hydrocolloid Mucilloid   Effersyllium®, Metamucil®,
                                                      Various

Pharmacology. Bulk-forming cathartic which absorbs water and provides an emollient mass.

Administration and Adult Dose. **PO for constipation** 2.5–7.5 g bid-qid, stirred in a full glass of water, followed by an additional glass of liquid. **PO for diarrhea**—see Notes.

Pediatric Dose. **PO for constipation** (6–12 yr) 2.5–3.75 g 1–4 times/day with fluid as above.

Dosage Forms. **Pwdr** 210, 250, 420, 630 g; **Pwdr** (effervescent) 3.7, 6.4, 7 g packets.

Patient Instructions. Mix with a full glass of water before taking and follow with another glass of liquid.

Pharmacokinetics. *Onset and Duration.* Onset 12-24 hr, but 2-3 days may be required for full effect.[18,26]

Adverse Reactions. Flatulence occurs frequently. Serious side effects are rare, but intestinal obstruction has been reported.[17]

Contraindications. Acute surgical abdomen; fecal impaction; intestinal obstruction; abdominal pain of unknown origin; intestinal perforation.[17]

Precautions. Use with caution in patients who require fluid restriction, because constipation may occur unless fluid intake is adequate. Use effervescent Metamucil® formulation (packet) with caution in patients who require potassium restriction. The noneffervescent formulation of Metamucil® should be used cautiously in diabetics, because it contains 50% dextrose (14 kcal/7 g). Sugar-free preparations include Metamucil® Sugar Free and Effersyllium®.

Notes. Useful in lessening the strain of defecation and for inpatients who are on low residue diets and/or constipating medications. May relieve symptoms in patients with diverticular disease.[18,19] Large doses may be used to "firm up" effluent from an ileostomy or ascending colostomy or diarrhea caused by tube feedings.[19]

Lactulose   Cephulac®, Chronulac®

Pharmacology. A synthetic derivative of lactose which is metabolized by colonic bacteria to lactic and small amounts of acetic and formic acids, resulting in acidification of colonic contents, decreased ammonia absorption and an osmotic catharsis.[21,27]

Administration and Adult Dose. **PO as a cathartic** 15-30 ml (10-20 g), to maximum of 60 ml; **PO for hepatic encephalopathy** 30-45 ml (20-30 g) q 1 hr until laxation, then 30-45 ml tid-qid, titrated to produce about 3 + stools per day. **PR for hepatic encephalopathy as an enema** 300 ml with 700 ml water or NS retained for 30-60 min, may repeat q 4-6 hr.

Dosage Individualization. Elderly patients may require reduced doses.[19]

Pediatric Dose. **PO for hepatic encephalopathy** (infants) 2.5-10 ml/day in divided doses; (older children and adolescents) 40-90 ml/day in divided doses.

Dosage Forms. **Syrup** 10 g/15 ml.

Patient Instructions. In the treatment of hepatic encephalopathy, 3-4 loose stools per day are common, but a worsening of diarrhea should be reported.

Pharmacokinetics. *Onset and Duration.* (Catharsis) onset 12-24 hr; duration 24-36 hr. (Hepatic encephalopathy) onset and duration variable.

Fate. After oral administration, less than 3% is absorbed and most reaches the colon unabsorbed and unchanged. The small amount absorbed is excreted in the urine unchanged.[19]

Adverse Reactions. Flatulence, belching and abdominal discomfort are frequent initially. Excessive diarrhea and fecal water loss may result in hypernatremia.[28]

Contraindications. Patients requiring a low galactose diet.

Precautions. Use with caution in diabetics due to small amounts of free lactose and galactose in the drug.

Parameters to Monitor. Observe for changes in hepatic encephalopathy, number of stools per day and stool pH (maintain at about pH 5).[19] Periodically obtain serum sodium, potassium and bicarbonate levels during prolonged use.

Notes. Neomycin has been used concurrently in hepatic encephalopathy.[27] Lactulose is effective in hepatic encephalopathy, but as a laxative it offers no advantage over less expensive agents.[20,29]

Magnesium Salts   Various

Pharmacology. A saline cathartic that inhibits fluid and electrolyte absorption by increasing osmotic forces in the gut lumen; it has also been suggested that part of its action may be due to cholecystokinin release which stimulates small bowel motility and inhibits fluid and electrolyte absorption from the jejunum and ileum.[17]

Administration and Adult Dose. **PO as a laxative/cathartic** (citrate) 200–300 ml; (sulfate) 20–30 ml of 50% solution (10–15 g) in a full glass of water; (milk of magnesia) 15–60 ml.

Pediatric Dose. PO citrate (2–5 yr) 2.5–5 g; sulfate (2–5 yr) 2.5–5 g, (6–12 yr) 5–10 g in one-half glass or more of water; milk of magnesia (2–5 yr) 0.4–1.2 g, (6–12 yr) 1.2–2.4 g.[18]

Dosage Forms. **Soln** (citrate) 77 mEq/dl magnesium; (sulfate) 50%; **Susp** (milk of magnesia) 7–8.5%, see Notes (also available as a concentrate with 10 ml = 30 ml of susp); **Pwdr** (citrate and sulfate) 454 g.

Patient Instructions. Milk of magnesia and magnesium sulfate should be taken with at least one full glass of liquid; magnesium sulfate may be taken with fruit juice to partially mask its bitter taste.

Pharmacokinetics. *Onset and Duration.* Onset dose-dependent: cathartic dose 0.5–3 hr; laxative dose 6–8 hr.[18,19]

Fate. Slow absorption of 15–30% of a dose from the GI tract. Absorbed magnesium is rapidly excreted in the urine in normal renal function.[17]

Adverse Reactions. Chronic use in patients with renal impairment may lead to hypermagnesemia, CNS depression and hypotension. Excessive use can lead to electrolyte abnormalities; dehydration may occur if taken with insufficient fluids.[17]

Contraindications. Acute surgical abdomen; fecal impaction; intestinal obstruction; abdominal pain of unknown origin; intestinal perforation; nausea; vomiting.[17]

Precautions. Use with caution in patients with impaired renal function.

Parameters to Monitor. Periodic serum magnesium levels in patients with impaired renal function.

Notes. Magnesium salts are useful for preparing the bowel for radiologic examination and surgical procedures. The following amounts of various magnesium salts are approximately equivalent to 80 mEq of magnesium: 100 ml citrate; 2.4 g (30 ml) milk of magnesia; and 10 g sulfate. The sulfate salt is the most potent cathartic, but is the least palatable.

PEG Electrolyte Lavage Solution   Golytely®, Various

Polyethylene glycol (PEG) electrolyte lavage solution is an isosmotic solution containing 5.69 g/L sodium sulfate, 1.69 g/L sodium bicarbonate, 1.47 g/L sodium chloride, 743 mg/L potassium chloride and 59-60 g/L PEG 3350 used for total bowel cleansing prior to GI examination. PEG acts as an osmotic cathartic and the electrolyte concentrations are such that there is little net fluid or electrolyte movement into or out of the bowel. This method of bowel cleansing is well suited for colonoscopy, but, because of some residual lavage fluid retained in the colon, other cleansing methods may be preferred prior to barium enema. The solution should be used at least 4 hr before the examination, allowing the patient 3 hr for drinking and a 1 hr waiting period to complete bowel evacuation. Solid food should be withheld 2 hr before the solution is administered. The first bowel movement usually occurs after 1 hr, with total bowel cleansing 3-5 hr after starting. Side effects include nausea, abdominal fullness, bloating and occasional cramps and vomiting. PEG electrolyte lavage solution should not be used in patients with GI obstruction, gastric retention or bowel perforation; however, the solution appears safe for patients with liver, kidney or heart disease. The usual dosage for adults is 200-300 ml orally or by NG tube q 10 min, until about 4 liters is consumed or the rectal effluent is clear. A one liter trial before the full dosage should be used in patients suspected of having bowel obstruction. Chilling the solution may improve its palatability.[30-32] Available as powder for reconstitution.

56:14 CHOLELITHOLYTIC AGENTS

Chenodiol   Chenix®

Chenodiol (chenodeoxycholic acid) is a bile acid used to dissolve radiolucent cholesterol gallstones. Its exact mechanism of action is unknown, but it increases chenodiol in bile from 33% to 60-90% and reduces both absolute and relative biliary cholesterol secretion. This results in a lowering of cholesterol saturation, allowing solubilization of cholesterol and eventual gallstone dissolution. Radiopaque gallstones consisting primarily of calcium do not respond to treatment. The drug appears to be most effective in patients who have small stones, a serum cholesterol above 227 mg/dl and in women. Complete dissolution rates of 50-80% have been reported when optimal doses are used. The safety of chenodiol has not been established beyond 24 months. Dose-related diarrhea occurs in up to 50% of patients receiving 15 mg/kg/day. The severity of the diarrhea is minimized if the initial dose is increased gradually. Total serum cholesterol and low-density lipoprotein may increase about 10% over baseline during therapy. Dose-related increases in AST (SGOT) and ALT (SGPT) occur in 30% of patients within the first 3 months of therapy and may require drug discontinuation. Hepatotoxicity occurs in 3% of patients receiving 750 mg/day. A dose of 13-17 mg/kg/day is usually recommended, beginning initially with 250 mg bid for the first few weeks, increasing the daily dosage by 250 mg at weekly intervals until the recommended dose is reached or intolerance develops. Obese patients may require higher doses of 18-20 mg/kg/day. Doses of less than 10 mg/kg/day are generally ineffective. Gallstone dissolution usually requires 6-24 months of treatment. Therapy should be continued for 3 months after apparent dissolution. Gallstones recur in up to 50% of patients within 5 yr following drug discontinuation. Low-dose prophylactic therapy following dissolution is ineffective and not recommended.[52,53] Available as 250 mg tablets.

Ursodiol   Actigall®

Ursodiol (ursodeoxycholic acid) is a bile salt chemically similar to chenodiol. It appears to act by a slightly different mechanism from chenodiol, dispersing cholesterol throughout the bile and decreasing biliary cholesterol secretion. Its advantages over chenodiol include lack of diarrhea and hepatotoxicity. Combined therapy with ursodiol and chenodiol may be more effective than either drug alone. The usual dose of ursodiol is 10 mg/kg/day in 2-3 divided doses; its efficacy may be increased by administration of the entire dose at bedtime.[52,53] Available as 300 mg capsules.

56:20 EMETICS

Apomorphine Hydrochloride   Various

Pharmacology. A morphine derivative which induces vomiting by stimulation of the chemoreceptor trigger zone in the CNS.

Administration and Adult Dose. SC for emesis 0.1 mg/kg to maximum of 10 mg. Repeat dosing is *not* recommended. Precede use with 240 ml water orally. Hypodermic tablet requires dissolution in sterile water immediately prior to use. Reconstituted solution is unstable and should not be used if a green or brown color or a precipitate develops.

Pediatric Dose. SC for emesis 0.1 mg/kg or 3 mg/M^2.

Dosage Forms. Hyp Tab 6 mg.

Pharmacokinetics. *Onset and Duration.* Onset 2-15 min; duration up to 40 min.[33,34]

Adverse Reactions. Prolonged or violent emesis; CNS depression and respiratory depression possibly requiring reversal with naloxone may occur. Excessive doses may cause cardiac depression and death.

Contraindications. Hypersensitivity to morphine or other opiates.

Precautions. Use with caution in: children, debilitated persons, or patients with cardiac disease; overdosage with alcohol, sedative-hypnotics or other drugs with CNS depression as a major symptom; impending shock or unconsciousness; convulsions or impending convulsions; ingestion of corrosive or caustic substances. Use in petroleum distillate ingestion is controversial.

Parameters to Monitor. Onset and frequency of emesis; signs of CNS or respiratory depression; presence of poison in the vomitus.

Notes. Apomorphine depressant and emetic effects may be terminated by the narcotic antagonist naloxone which should be immediately available whenever apomorphine is used; patients who fail to vomit with apomorphine should be considered for gastric lavage. Apomorphine is difficult to prepare, potentially more toxic, and only marginally more rapid in onset than syrup of ipecac; therefore, it is not the emetic of choice in most patients. It has the advantage of being useful in uncooperative patients and not being inhibited by co-administration of activated charcoal. An experimental stable solution of apomorphine has been described.[35]

Ipecac Syrup   Various

Pharmacology. A mixture of plant alkaloids, including emetine and cephaeline, which induces emesis through stimulation of the stomach and the chemoreceptor trigger zone in the CNS.

Administration and Adult Dose. PO for emesis 30 ml, followed by 240 ml or more of water; may repeat once in 20–30 min if no effect.

Pediatric Dose. PO for emesis (6 mo–1 yr) 10 ml; (1–5 yr) 15 ml given as above; (over 5 yr) same as adult dose. Give with at least 120 ml of water.

Dosage Forms. Syrup 70 mg/ml.

Patient Instructions. This drug should be taken with at least one or more glasses of water. Save vomitus in a bowl for later inspection. Do not take without first consulting poison information center or physician.

Pharmacokinetics. *Onset and Duration.* Onset about 15–20 min; duration usually about 25 min, but may last several hr.[33,34]

Adverse Reactions. Mild drowsiness and diarrhea may occur after emesis.[33] Protracted vomiting with GI damage. Cardiotoxicity, manifested by tachycardia and EKG abnormalities has occurred after toxic doses of fluidextract[44] and myopathy has occurred with chronic use in binge-purge eating disorders.[45] Cardiotoxicity is unlikely with normal doses of the syrup.

Contraindications. Present or anticipated CNS depression; convulsions or anticipated convulsions; ingestion of corrosives or caustics.

Precautions. Do not administer activated charcoal until emesis has occurred. If emesis does not occur, gastric lavage should be considered as an alternative. Use in petroleum distillate ingestion is controversial.

Parameters to Monitor. Onset and frequency of emesis; presence of poison in the vomitus.

Notes. Syrup of ipecac is the emetic of choice in most toxic ingestions and is useful for inducing emesis at home. It appears effective in antiemetic drug ingestions,[46,47] although the prescribing information for some phenothiazine drugs specifically recommends against its use in phenothiazine poisoning.

56:22 ANTIEMETICS

Dronabinol   Various

Pharmacology. Also known as delta-9-tetrahydrocannabinol (THC), the most active antinauseant component of cannabis products. Its mechanism of action is complex and poorly understood, but probably includes inhibition of the chemoreceptor trigger zone in the medulla.

Administration and Adult Dose. PO as antiemetic during cancer chemotherapy 5 mg/M^2 1–3 hr before chemotherapy, then q 2–4 hr after chemotherapy for a total of 4–6 doses/day. Dose may be increased in 2.5 mg/M^2 increments to a maximum of 15 mg/M^2/dose.

Pediatric Dose. PO as antiemetic during cancer chemotherapy same as adult dose in mg/M^2.

Dosage Forms. Cap 2.5, 5, 10 mg.

Patient Instructions. This drug may cause drowsiness. Until the extent of this effect is known, caution should be used when driving, operating machinery or performing other tasks requiring mental alertness. Avoid excessive concurrent use of alcohol or other drugs which cause drowsiness.

Pharmacokinetics. ***Onset and Duration.*** Onset 30-60 min after ingestion; peak 2-4 hr; duration 4-6 hr.[36,37]

Fate. Only 10-20% oral bioavailability. Primarily metabolized by hydroxylation to active and inactive metabolites. Ultimately, 35% of metabolites are found in feces and 15% in urine.[38,39]

$t_{1/2}$. 20-30 hr; may be longer in inexperienced users.[38-40]

Adverse Reactions. Drowsiness is the most frequent adverse reaction. It may be accompanied by dizziness, ataxia, loss of balance and disorientation to the point of being disabling. Other side effects include dry mouth, orthostatic hypotension, tachycardia and conjunctival injection. The cannabis "high" experienced by some is not always well tolerated, especially in older patients.[41]

Contraindications. Nausea and vomiting from causes other than cancer chemotherapy.

Precautions. Lactation; patients with hypertension or heart disease.

Parameters to Monitor. Frequency of emesis.

Notes. Dronabinol is at least as effective as phenothiazines for chemotherapy-induced nausea and vomiting,[42] but may not be as effective as IV metoclopramide.[43] It is not particularly effective for cisplatin-induced nausea and vomiting.[43]

Nabilone   Cesamet®

Nabilone is an orally active cannabinoid antiemetic used in the management of nausea and vomiting associated with cancer chemotherapy in patients who have failed to respond adequately to conventional antiemetic treatment. The drug is rapidly and almost completely (96%) absorbed after oral administration and is metabolized to possibly active metabolites. The parent compound has a half-life of about 2 hr, but the metabolites are longer lived. Side effects are similar to those of other cannabinoids and include drowsiness, dizziness or vertigo, dry mouth, and a cannabis "high". Nabilone appears to be superior to prochlorperazine for the control of chemotherapy-induced gastrointestinal side effects. The usual adult starting dose is 1-2 mg PO bid, with the first dose being given 1-3 hr before chemotherapy. The dose may be increased in 1-2 mg increments as needed, to a maximum dosage of 2 mg tid. Dosing may be continued for up to 48 hr after chemotherapy.[103,104] Available as 1 mg capsules.

Prochlorperazine Salts   Compazine®, Various

Pharmacology. A phenothiazine tranquilizer which is used mainly for its antiemetic properties. It suppresses the chemoreceptor trigger zone in the CNS; not effective for the treatment of motion sickness or vertigo. See Antiemetic Agents Comparison Chart.

Administration and Adult Dose. **PO as an antiemetic** 5-10 mg tid-qid; **PR as an antiemetic** 25 mg bid; **IM as an antiemetic** (deep in upper outer quadrant of buttock) 5-10 mg q 4-6 hr, to maximum of 40 mg/day. **IM presurgically** (given as above) 5-10 mg 1-2 hr before induction, may repeat once before or after surgery; **IV presurgically** 5-10 mg 15-30 min before induction or as infusion (20 mg/L) started 15-30 min before induction. **SC not recommended.**

Dosage Individualization. Use the lower end of the recommended dosage range in elderly patients.

Pediatric Dose. Not to be used in surgery or in patients under 9 kg or 2 yr. **PO or PR as an antiemetic** (9–13 kg) 2.5 mg daily-bid; (14–18 kg) 2.5 mg bid-tid; (19–39 kg) 2.5 mg tid–5 mg bid. **IM as an antiemetic** (deep in upper outer quadrant of buttock) 0.13 mg/kg. **SC not recommended.**

Dosage Forms. **Inj** 5 mg/ml; **Supp** 2.5, 5, 25 mg; **Syrup** 1 mg/ml; **Tab** 5, 10 mg. Larger dose tablets are available for psychiatric use. **SR Cap** not recommended.

Patient Instructions. This drug may cause drowsiness. Until the extent of this effect is known, caution should be used when driving, operating machinery or performing other tasks requiring mental alertness. Avoid excessive concurrent use of alcohol or other drugs which cause drowsiness.

Pharmacokinetics. *Onset and Duration.* PO onset 30–40 min; PR onset 60 min; IM onset 10–20 min. Duration for all routes 3–4 hr.[48]
  Fate. Primarily eliminated by liver metabolism.[49]

Adverse Reactions. Extrapyramidal reactions, especially dystonias and dyskinesias occur occasionally (other extrapyramidal reactions are less likely because of the short duration of therapy when used as an antiemetic). Anticholinergic effects such as dry mouth, mydriasis, cycloplegia, urinary retention, decreased GI motility and tachycardia have been reported.[50,51] SC use can cause local reactions at injection site.

Contraindications. Pediatric surgery; children under 9 kg or 2 yr; comatose or greatly depressed states due to CNS depressants.

Precautions. Antiemetic action may mask signs and symptoms of overdose with other drugs and may mask the diagnosis and treatment of other conditions such as intestinal obstruction, brain tumor or Reye's syndrome. Use with caution in conditions in which the drug's anticholinergic effects might be detrimental, in children with acute illnesses or dehydration or in patients with a history of allergy to phenothiazine derivatives (eg, blood dyscrasias, jaundice). Avoid getting the concentrate or injection solutions on hands or clothing, due to possibility of contact dermatitis.

Notes. The solution should be protected from light; slight yellowish discoloration will not alter potency, but markedly discolored solution should be discarded. Protect suppositories from heat.

Antiemetic Agents Comparison Chart

| DRG | DOSAGE FORMS | INITIAL DOSE[a] | | INDICATIONS | | |
		ADULT	PEDIATRIC	NAUSEA AND VOMITING	MOTION SICKNESS	VERTIGO
ANTIHISTAMINES						
Buclizine Bucladin®	Tab 50 mg.	PO 50 mg.	—		X	
Cyclizine Marezine®	Tab 50 mg Inj 50 mg/ml.	PO, IM 50 mg.	PO (6–12 yr) 25 mg.		X	
Dimenhydrinate Dramamine® Various	Tab 50 mg Liquid 12.5 mg/4 ml Inj 50 mg/ml.	PO, IM, IV 50–100 mg.	PO, IM (over 2 yr) 1.25 mg/kg.	X	X	X
Diphenhydramine Benadryl® Various	Cap 25, 50 mg Elxr 12.5 mg/5 ml Syrup 12.5, 13.3 mg/5 ml Tab 25, 50 mg Inj 10, 50 mg/ml.	PO 50 mg; IM, IV 10–50 mg.	PO (over 9 kg) 12.5–25 mg; IM, IV (over 9 kg) 1.25 mg/kg.		X	
Meclizine Antivert® Bonine® Various	Tab 12.5, 25, 50 mg Chew Tab 25 mg.	PO 25–50 mg.	—		X	b

Continued

Antiemetic Agents Comparison Chart

DRUG	DOSAGE FORMS	INITIAL DOSE[a] ADULT	INITIAL DOSE[a] PEDIATRIC	INDICATIONS NAUSEA AND VOMITING	INDICATIONS MOTION SICKNESS	INDICATIONS VERTIGO
CANNABINOIDS						
Dronabinol® Marinol®	Cap 2.5, 5, 10 mg.	PO 5 mg/M².	PO 5 mg/M².	X		
Nabilone Cesamet®	Cap 1 mg.	PO 1–2 mg.	—	X		
PHENOTHIAZINES						
Chlorpromazine Thorazine® Various	Liquid 30, 100 mg/ml Syrup 2 mg/ml Tab 10, 25, 50 mg Inj 25 mg/ml.	PO 10–25 mg; PR 100 mg; IM 25 mg.	PO, IM (over 6 months) 0.55 mg/kg; PR (over 6 months) 1.1 mg/kg.	X		
Perphenazine Trilafon®	Liquid 16 mg/5 ml Tab 2, 4 mg Inj 5 mg/ml.	PO 2–4 mg; IM 5 mg.	—	X		
Prochlorperazine Compazine® Various	Syrup 1 mg/ml Tab 5, 10, 25 mg Supp 2.5, 5, 25 mg Inj 5 mg/ml.	PO, IM 5–10 mg; PR 25 mg.	PO, PR (over 9 kg or 2 yr) 2.5 mg; IM (over 9 kg or 2 yr) 0.13 mg/kg.	X		

Continued

Antiemetic Agents Comparison Chart

| DRUG | DOSAGE FORMS | INITIAL DOSE[a] | | INDICATIONS | | |
		ADULT	PEDIATRIC	NAUSEA AND VOMITING	MOTION SICKNESS	VERTIGO
Promethazine Phenergan® Various	Syrup 6.25, 25 mg/5 ml Tab 12.5, 25, 50 mg Supp 12.5, 25, 50 mg Inj 25, 50 mg/ml.	PO, PR 25 mg; IM 12.5–25 mg.	PO, PR, IM 0.25–0.5 mg/kg.	X	X	X
Thiethylperazine Torecan®	Tab 10 mg Supp 10 mg Inj 5 mg/ml.	PO, IM 10 mg.	—	X		
Triflupromazine Vesprin®	Inj 10, 20 mg/ml.	IM 5–15 mg; IV 1 mg.	IM (over 2½ yr) 0.07 mg/kg.	X		
MISCELLANEOUS						
Benzquinamide Emete-Con®	Inj 50 mg/ml.	IM 50 mg; IV 25 mg.	—	X		
Diphenidol Vontrol®	Tab 25 mg.	PO 25–50 mg.	PO (over 6 months or 12 kg) 0.9 mg/kg.	X		X
Droperidol Inapsine®	Inj 2.5 mg/ml.	IM, IV 2.5 mg.	—	d		

Continued

Antiemetic Agents Comparison Chart

DRUG	DOSAGE FORMS	INITIAL DOSE[a] ADULT	INITIAL DOSE[a] PEDIATRIC	INDICATIONS NAUSEA AND VOMITING	INDICATIONS MOTION SICKNESS	INDICATIONS VERTIGO
Metoclopramide Reglan®	Syrup 1 mg/ml Tab 5, 10 mg Inj 5 mg/ml.	PO, IM 2 mg/kg; IV 1–2 mg/kg.	—	X		
Scopolamine Transderm-Scop® Various	Cap 0.25 mg SR Patch 0.5 mg/day.	PO 0.6–1.2 mg; SR Patch 1.5 mg.[c]	—		X	
Trimetho-benzamide Tigan® Various	Cap 100, 250 mg Supp 100, 200 mg Inj 100 mg/ml.	PO 250 mg; PR 200 mg; IM 200 mg.	PO (14–40 kg) 100–200 mg; PR (under 14 kg) 100 mg; (14–40 kg) 100–200 mg.	X		

a. Initial dose only, check prescribing information for subsequent dosing.
b. Possibly effective.
c. Provides continuous drug release for 3 days; a total of 0.5 mg is released.
d. Effective, but not FDA approved for this use.

56:40 MISCELLANEOUS GI DRUGS

Cimetidine

Tagamet®

Pharmacology. Cimetidine competitively inhibits the action of histamine at the H_2-receptors of the parietal cell and reduces basal, nocturnal, pentagastrin- and food-stimulated gastric acid secretion.

Administration and Adult Dose. **PO for short-term treatment of duodenal ulcer** 300 mg qid or 400 mg bid or 800 mg hs for 4–8 weeks. Certain patients (eg, heavy cigarette smokers with ulcers larger than 1 cm in diameter) may require a dose of 1600 mg hs. **PO for prophylaxis of recurrent duodenal ulcer** 400 mg hs. **PO for short-term treatment of gastric ulcer** 300 mg qid. **PO for gastroesophageal reflux disease** 300 mg qid.[54] **PO for hypersecretory conditions** 300 mg qid initially, administered more frequently prn to maximum of 2.4 g/day. Adjust dosage to individual patient requirement and continue as long as needed. **IM** 300 mg q 6–8 hr. **IV for hospitalized patients with hypersecretory states, intractable ulcers or patients unable to take oral medication** 300 mg q 6–8 hr initially, frequency of administration may be increased to a maximum dosage of 2.4 g/day. Dilute doses to 20 ml and inject over a period of not less than 2 min; alternatively, dilute to at least 50 ml and infuse over 15–20 min. See Notes. **IV for prevention of bleeding from stress-related mucosal lesions in acutely ill patients** adjust the dose or frequency of intermittent therapy or the rate of continuous infusion to maintain the intragastric pH above 4.[55,56]

Dosage Individualization. Adjust dosage in renal impairment as follows: with Cl_{cr} 20–40 ml/min, give 300 mg q 8 hr; with Cl_{cr} below 20 ml/min, give 300 mg q 12 hr. Give doses at the end of scheduled hemodialysis; an extra dose is apparently not necessary in CAPD. Further dosage reduction may be necessary with concomitant liver impairment. Use the lowest dosing frequency that permits an adequate response.[57,58]

Pediatric Dose. Not well established. **PO, IM or IV** (newborn) 10–20 mg/kg/day; (older children) 20–40 mg/kg/day. Divide into 4 doses daily.[59]

Dosage Forms. **Tab** 200, 300, 400, 800 mg; **Liq** 300 mg/5 ml; **Inj** 150 mg/ml.

Patient Instructions. The effectiveness of cimetidine in inhibiting nighttime gastric acid secretion may be decreased by cigarette smoking. Discontinue smoking altogether or avoid smoking after the last dose of the day. Antacids may be used as needed for relief of ulcer pain. Even though ulcer symptoms may improve, treatment should be continued for 4 to 8 weeks unless instructed otherwise.

Pharmacokinetics. *Onset and Duration.* (Antisecretory effect) onset PO within 1 hr, IM or IV within 15 min; peak PO occurs within 1–3 hr, IM or IV within 30 min; duration PO with 300 and 400 mg dose is 5–6 hr, IM or IV with 300 mg dose is 4–6 hr.[58]

Plasma Levels. 0.5–1 mcg/ml inhibits 50% of pentagastrin-stimulated acid secretion in healthy subjects.[58] Plasma concentrations remain above this level for about 4–6 hr after a 300 mg oral or IM/IV dose. CNS changes have been associated with concentrations of 1.25 mcg/ml in critically ill patients and 0.25–0.5 mcg/ml in hepatic failure.[58]

Fate. Oral bioavailability is 60–70%; IM bioavailability is 90–100%. Peak plasma concentrations of 1.2 and 1.8 mcg/ml occur 1–3 hr after 300 and 400 mg oral doses, respectively; a peak of 5.25 mcg/ml occurs after 300 mg IV. The drug is 15–20% plasma protein bound; V_{dss} is 0.8–1.2 L/kg; distribution into the CNS increases in hepatic failure. Cimetidine is hepatically metabolized 15% to the sulfoxide, 1% to the 5-hydroxymethyl derivative and to guanylurea derivatives. About 2–10% is eliminated in the feces.

Renal clearance is 24–36 L/hr, indicating renal tubular secretion; 75% of a parenteral dose is excreted unchanged in urine in 24 hr.[58]

$t_{1/2}$. 2 hr in healthy subjects; 4–5 hr in renal failure; 2.9 hr in hepatic failure; 6.7 hr in renal and hepatic failure.[58]

Adverse Reactions. Adverse reactions are generally mild and occur infrequently. GI effects occur most frequently;[60] dizziness, somnolence, headache and rash have also been reported. Reversible confusional states occur predominantly in patients with renal and/or liver disease. Cardiac arrhythmias and hypotension may occur following rapid IV bolus administration; bradycardia has been reported with both IV and oral administration. Impotence occurs occasionally. Leukopenia, thrombocytopenia, agranulocytosis and aplastic anemia occur rarely as do interstitial nephritis, hepatitis and pancreatitis. Mild increases in serum transaminases may occur, but resolve upon drug discontinuation. Small increases in Cr_s may occur, but are thought to result from competitive inhibition of renal creatinine secretion by cimetidine. Gynecomastia develops in less than 1% of all patients and in 4% of patients treated for pathological hypersecretory states.

Precautions. Pregnancy; lactation. Dosage adjustment may be required in severe renal and/or hepatic dysfunction. Cimetidine inhibits the cytochrome P 450 mixed function oxidase system and may produce clinically significant drug interactions with warfarin, phenytoin, theophylline, lidocaine, nifedipine and other drugs metabolized by this system.[61] Cimetidine inhibits the renal elimination of procainamide and NAPA.[61] Symptomatic response to therapy does not preclude the possibility of gastric malignancy.

Parameters to Monitor. Improvement in epigastric pain; however, pain relief does not correlate directly with endoscopic evidence of ulcer healing. Monitor Cr_s, CBC, AST (SGOT), ALT (SGPT), CNS status and potential drug interactions. When used to prevent stress-related GI bleeding in the acutely ill patient, the intragastric pH should be measured periodically.

Notes. Clinical trials have shown cimetidine to be as effective as intensive antacid regimens and standard doses of sucralfate, ranitidine or famotidine for healing duodenal ulcers and as ranitidine for the prophylaxis of recurrent duodenal ulcers or in healing gastric ulcers.[54, 62-67] Cimetidine appears to prevent stress-related GI bleeding and may have a gastroprotective effect independent of its antisecretory action.[55, 56] Cimetidine is stable in D5W, D10W, NS, TPN, Lactated Ringers, or 5% sodium bicarbonate for 48 hr at room temperature.

Cisapride (Investigational - Janssen)   Propulsion®

Cisapride is a cholinergic prokinetic drug which acts primarily by facilitating the release of acetylcholine via postganglionic nerve endings in the myenteric plexus (indirect cholinergic action). It has no dopamine antagonist activity. The drug is a potent stimulant of esophageal, gastric, small intestinal and colonic motility. Its motor-stimulating action is at least 100 times more potent than metoclopramide. Gastric secretion and prolactin release are not affected. Clinical trials suggest that the drug is effective in treating reflux esophagitis, postprandial dyspepsia, gastroparesis, postoperative ileus and severe chronic constipation. The drug has no direct antiemetic effects because it lacks anti-dopaminergic activity. In most clinical situations, cisapride compares favorably with metoclopramide and domperidone, differing in its effect on the large bowel and its lack of antidopaminergic and nonspecific cholinergic side effects. When treating constipation, optimal effects may require 2–3 months of therapy. Once constipation is resolved and laxatives are not needed, cisapride may be stopped without relapse occurring. If maintenance treatment is necessary, a single daily dose is often sufficient. The absolute oral bioavailability of cisapride is 40–50%. Metabolites are excreted in the urine and feces, each route eliminating 50% of the dose. Mean pharmacokinetic parameters after IV administration include a terminal half-life of 14.9 hr, V_{dss} of 1.95 L/kg and a Cl of 7.86 L/hr. The drug is 98% plasma protein bound. Cisapride does not appear to affect antipyrine clearance. Acceleration of gastric emptying may affect the rate of absorption of other orally administered drugs. The main adverse effect is diarrhea and abdominal cramps occurring occasionally. Cisapride should be administered 15 min before meals in an oral dose of 5–10 mg tid-qid, depending on the severity of the condition. Single doses of up to 20 mg PO or 10 mg IV have been given.[68,69]

Domperidone (Investigational - Janssen)   Motilium®

Domperidone is a peripheral-acting dopamine antagonist which possesses antiemetic and GI prokinetic properties similar to those of metoclopramide. Unlike metoclopramide, domperidone does not readily enter the CNS and reports of extrapyramidal side effects are infrequent. Preliminary studies suggest that the drug may be effective in the treatment of diabetic gastroparesis, reflux esophagitis and as an adjunct in preventing the nausea and vomiting induced by the antiparkinsonian drugs bromocriptine and levodopa.

Domperidone appears to be as effective as metoclopramide for the symptoms of postprandial dyspepsia and in preventing nausea and vomiting induced by moderately emetic cytotoxic drugs. Because it is well tolerated and has a lower potential for extrapyramidal effects, domperidone may become the drug of choice in conditions for which it is as effective as metoclopramide. Cardiac arrhythmias and arrest have occurred after IV administration of domperidone when used to control chemotherapy-induced vomiting. Oral bioavailability of domperidone is only 13–17% because of extensive gut wall and hepatic metabolism.

Prior administration of cimetidine 300 mg or sodium bicarbonate have been reported to decrease the absorption of oral domperidone. The drug has a V_d of 5.7 L/kg after IV administration and is 92% plasma protein bound. The usual dose in adults with postprandial dyspepsia is 10 mg tid, 15–30 min before meals and, if necessary, at bedtime. In severe dyspepsia the dose may be increased to 20 mg qid. When used as an antiemetic, the adult oral dose is 20–40 mg tid-qid and the rectal dose is 60 mg bid-qid. Dosage reduction in severe renal dysfunction does not appear to be necessary.[70-73]

Famotidine   Pepcid®

Pharmacology. See Cimetidine.

Administration and Adult Dose. **PO for short-term treatment of duodenal ulcer** 40 mg hs or 20 mg bid for 4–8 weeks. **PO for prophylaxis of recurrent duodenal ulcer** 20 mg hs. **PO for short-term treatment of gastric ulcer** 40 mg hs.[67,74] **PO for hypersecretory conditions** 20 mg q 6 hr initially, up to 200 mg q 6 hr in patients with severe Zollinger-Ellison syndrome.[74] Adjust dosage to individual requirement and continue as long as needed. **IV for hospitalized patients with hypersecretory states, intractable ulcers or patients unable to take oral medication** 20 mg q 12 hr initially. Dilute to 5–10 ml and inject over a period of not less than 2 min; alternatively, dilute to 100 ml and infuse over 15-30 min. See Notes.

Dosage Individualization. To avoid excess accumulation of the drug with a Cl_{cr} less than 10 ml/min, the manufacturer recommends that the daily dosage be reduced to 20 mg hs or the dosing interval prolonged to 36-48 hr. One independent investigator recommends the following: Cl_{cr} 30-60 ml/min, give one-half the usual dose; Cl_{cr} less than 30 ml/min, give one-quarter the usual dose. Severe hepatic impairment may decrease hepatic clearance.[67,75]

Pediatric Dose. Safety and efficacy not established.

Dosage Forms. Tab 20, 40 mg; Inj 10 mg/ml; Susp 8 mg/ml.

Patient Instructions. See Cimetidine.

Pharmacokinetics. Onset and Duration. (Antisecretory effect) onset PO within 1 hr, IV within 15 min; peak PO occurs within 1-3 hr, IV within 30 min; duration PO with doses of 20-40 mg is 10-18 hr, IV with doses of 10-20 mg is 10-12 hr. The 20 mg IV dose is associated with the longer duration of action.[67]

Plasma Levels. 13 ng/ml inhibits 50% of tetragastrin-stimulated acid secretion in healthy subjects.[67] Plasma concentrations remain above this level for about 18 hr after a 40 mg oral dose, and for 7-9 hr following a 20 mg oral dose.[67]

Fate. Oral bioavailability is 37-45%. Peak plasma levels of 50-60 and 78 ng/ml occur 1-3 hr after 20 and 40 mg oral doses, respectively. The drug is 15-20% plasma protein bound; V_{dss} is 1.14-1.42 L/kg. Famotidine is hepatically metabolized to the S-oxide. Renal clearance is 15-27 L/hr, indicating tubular secretion; 65-70% of an IV dose is excreted unchanged in urine in 24 hr.[67,75]

$t_{1/2}$. 2.5-3.5 hr in normals; may exceed 20 hr in severe renal impairment.[67,75]

Adverse Reactions. Adverse reactions occur in 3-7% of patients receiving 20-60 mg/day.[67] Frequent effects include headache, diarrhea, dizziness and constipation. To date, famotidine has not been shown to exert CNS, cardiovascular, respiratory or endocrine effects. No anti-androgenic activity has been detected.

Precautions. Pregnancy; lactation. Famotidine does not appear to interfere with drugs metabolized via the cytochrome P 450 mixed function oxidase system.[76] Symptomatic response to therapy does not preclude the possibility of gastric malignancy.

Parameters to Monitor. Improvement in epigastric pain. However, pain relief does not correlate directly with endoscopic evidence of ulcer healing. Monitor Cr_s, AST (SGOT), ALT (SGPT) periodically.

Notes. Clinical trials have shown famotidine to be as effective as standard doses of ranitidine for healing duodenal and gastric ulcers.[67,74] Store famotidine injection at 2-8° C. Famotidine is stable in D5W, D10W, NS, Lactated Ringer's, or 5% sodium bicarbonate for 48 hr at room temperature.

Metoclopramide Hydrochloride   Reglan®, Various

Pharmacology. Metoclopramide antagonizes central and peripheral dopamine effects, sensitizes receptors in the GI tract to acetylcholine and/or exerts a direct effect on smooth muscle.

Administration and Adult Dose. PO for short-term treatment of symptomatic gastroesophageal reflux disease in patients who fail to respond to conventional therapy up to 10-15 mg qid 30 min before each meal and hs for 4-12 weeks or intermittent single doses up to 20 mg; **PO, IM or IV for diabetic gastroparesis** 10 mg qid 30 min before each meal and hs for 2-8 weeks; **IV to facilitate small bowel intubation or to aid in radiological examinations** 10 mg over 1-2 min; **IV for prevention of cancer chemotherapy-induced emesis** 2 mg/kg 30 min before cisplatin and q 2 hr for 2 doses, then q 3 hr for 3 doses. If emesis is suppressed after the initial 2 doses, reduction of subsequent doses to 1 mg/kg may be tried. Dilute IV doses in excess of 10 mg to 50 ml and infuse over at least 15 min. See Notes.

Dosage Individualization. With a Cl_{cr} under 40 ml/min, begin therapy at one-half the initial dose and increase or decrease based on efficacy and side effects. Give scheduled doses at the end of hemodialysis; an extra dose is apparently not needed in CAPD.[77-79]

Pediatric Dose. **IV to facilitate small bowel intubation or to aid radiologic examination** (under 6 yr) 0.1 mg/kg; (6-14 yr) 2.5-5 mg.

Dosage Forms. **Tab** 5, 10 mg; **Syrup** 1 mg/ml; **Inj** 5 mg/ml.

Patient Instructions. Take doses 30 minutes before meals and at bedtime. This drug may cause drowsiness. Until the degree of drowsiness is known, caution should be used when driving, operating machinery or performing other tasks requiring mental alertness. Avoid excessive concurrent use of alcohol or other drugs which cause drowsiness. Involuntary movements (eg, muscle spasms and jerky movements of the head and face) may occur, especially in children and the elderly.

Pharmacokinetics. *Onset and Duration.* (GI effects) onset PO 30-60 min, IM 10-15 min, IV 1-3 min; peak PO 2 hr, but may be delayed with impaired gastric emptying; duration 3 hr.

Plasma Levels. Levels over 850 ng/ml appear necessary for optimal antiemetic effect in patients receiving cisplatin.[80]

Fate. Oral bioavailability is 30-100% due to first-pass metabolism, and 74-96% following IM administration.[77] Peak plasma concentrations are 32-44 ng/ml and 72-87 ng/ml, following 10 and 20 mg oral doses, respectively, and 221 ng/ml following a 20 mg IV dose.[77,81] The drug is 25-30% plasma protein bound; V_{dss} is 2.2-3.5 L/kg. About 85% of an oral dose of metoclopramide is recovered in the urine after 72 hr as unchanged drug, sulfate and glucuronide conjugates. About 5% is eliminated in the feces.

$t_{1/2}$. α phase 5 min; β phase 5-6 hr, increasing to about 14 hr in severe renal impairment.[77,78]

Adverse Reactions. Drowsiness, restlessness, fatigue and lassitude occur in 10% of patients receiving doses of 10 mg qid. The frequency of drowsiness is about 70% with doses of 1-2 mg/kg. Extrapyramidal symptoms, primarily acute dystonic reactions, occur in 0.2% of patients receiving 30-40 mg/day, in 2% of patients over 35 yr and in 25% of children receiving antiemetic doses. Parkinsonian-like symptoms, tardive dyskinesia and akathisia occur less frequently. Transient flushing of the face and/or diarrhea frequently occur following large IV doses. Endocrine disturbances secondary to hyperprolactinemia and fluid retention related to elevations of aldosterone have been reported.[81]

Contraindications. GI hemorrhage, mechanical obstruction or perforation; pheochromocytoma; epilepsy; concurrent use of drugs likely to cause extrapyramidal effects.

Precautions. Pregnancy. Use with caution in patients with hypertension or those receiving MAO inhibitors, sympathomimetics or heterocyclic antidepressants. Absorption of drugs from the stomach or small bowel may be altered by metoclopramide. Anticholinergics and narcotics may antagonize

GI effects of metoclopramide. Additive sedation can occur with alcohol or other CNS depressants.

Parameters to Monitor. Symptomatic relief of gastroesophageal reflux or diabetic gastroparesis. Efficacy in controlling chemotherapy-induced emesis. Monitor Cr_s periodically.

Notes. If extrapyramidal symptoms occur, administer diphenhydramine 50 mg IM or benztropine 1-2 mg IM. Metoclopramide is stable in D5W, NS, D5NS, Ringer's and Lactated Ringer's solution for 24 hr at room temperature and up to 48 hr if protected from light. High-dose metoclopramide appears to have greater antiemetic activity than prochlorperazine in patients receiving cisplatin.[81]

Omeprazole   Losec®
(Investigational - Merck Sharp & Dohme)

Omeprazole is a substituted benzimidazole derivative which inhibits basal and stimulated acid secretion by binding to parietal cell hydrogen/potassium adenosine triphosphatase. The drug's unique mechanism of action produces a profound and prolonged antisecretory effect by irreversibly blocking the proton pump of the parietal cell at the terminal stage of acid secretion. An oral dose of 20-40 mg once daily heals 60-100% of duodenal ulcers within 2 weeks and between 90-100% within 4 weeks, even in patients resistant to H_2-receptor antagonist therapy. Compared with cimetidine 1 g/day or ranitidine 150 mg bid, omeprazole produces significantly more rapid duodenal ulcer healing. Preliminary studies suggest that once daily doses are also effective in treating gastric ulcers, reflux esophagitis and Zollinger-Ellison syndrome. The potency of omeprazole following oral administration appears to be less than when given IV, possibly due to its instability at low pH. Various oral formulations are under investigation in an attempt to improve its systemic bioavailability. Omeprazole is almost completely metabolized by the liver with little or no unchanged drug recovered in the urine. Studies suggest that omeprazole inhibits hepatic microsomal mixed function oxidase enzymes and, therefore, may inhibit the metabolism of drugs metabolized by this pathway. Long-term toxicological studies in animals receiving high doses of omeprazole have been reported to cause morphological changes in the gastric mucosa which may lead to gastric cancer. The significance of these findings in humans is unknown. When the drug has been used in studies of short duration (2-8 weeks) for the treatment of peptic ulcer, no significant side effects or changes in laboratory parameters have been noted. The usual adult dose of omeprazole is 20 mg once daily until confirmed ulcer healing or for 2-4 weeks in duodenal ulcers or 4-8 weeks in gastric ulcers. In Zollinger-Ellison syndrome, the dose should be individualized so that the smallest dose is administered which will reduce gastric acid secretion to less than 10 mEq/hr for the last hour before the next dose. Total daily doses of up to 180 mg have been used in these patients. Because of its potent antisecretory effect, omeprazole may be the drug of choice in the treatment of Zollinger-Ellison syndrome.[82,83]

Prostaglandin Analogues

The prostaglandin analogues of the PGE_1 and PGE_2 series are potent inhibitors of basal and stimulated acid secretion and withstand degradation when administered by the oral route. These agents are thought to accelerate gastroduodenal ulcer healing by their gastric acid antisecretory action and/or mucosal protective effects. Their antisecretory action probably results from a reduction in the formation of parietal cell cyclic AMP, thus removing the major pathway for stimulation of the parietal cells by histamine, acetylcholine or gastrin. Although the precise mechanism by which nonacid-reducing doses afford mucosal protection is unclear, proposed actions include increased mucosal blood flow, increased gastric and duodenal mucus secretion, increased mucosal bicarbonate secretion and enhanced mucosal cell repair. Prostaglandin PGE analogues undergoing clinical trials in the US include **misoprostol** (Cytotec® - Searle), **arbaprostil** (Arbacet® - Upjohn), and **enprostil** (Gardrin® - Syntex). Initial studies indicate that these agents significantly improve gastric and duodenal ulcer healing when given in multiple daily antisecretory doses, and that the healing rates appear to be similar to those seen with cimetidine and ranitidine. Of concern is the increased frequency of diarrhea reported with some of the higher antisecretory doses and the potential abortifacient effects of these agents. Lower, nonantisecretory doses, although not as effective in healing peptic ulcers, are reported to protect the gastric mucosa from aspirin and nonsteroidal anti-inflammatory agent injury. It is possible that prostaglandins may not become first-line agents for treating peptic ulcer disease. However, they may be useful for treating patients in whom mucosal defense mechanisms appear to play a predominant role (ie, cigarette smokers, aspirin-induced ulcers and the prevention of stress-related GI bleeding).[84,85]

Ranitidine   Zantac®

Pharmacology. See Cimetidine.

Administration and Adult Dose. **PO for short-term treatment of duodenal ulcer** 150 mg bid or 300 mg hs for 4–8 weeks. **PO for prophylaxis of recurrent duodenal ulcer** 150 mg hs. **PO for short-term treatment of gastric ulcer** 150 mg bid. **PO for gastroesophageal reflux disease** 150 mg bid. **PO for hypersecretory conditions** 150 mg bid initially, administered more frequently if necessary; up to 6 g/day has been administered to patients with severe Zollinger-Ellison syndrome. Adjust dosage to individual patient requirement and continue as long as needed. **IM** 50 mg q 6–8 hr. **IV for hospitalized patients with hypersecretory states, intractable ulcers or patients unable to take oral medication** 50 mg q 6–8 hr initially, frequency of administration may be increased to a maximum dosage of 400 mg/day. Dilute doses to 20 ml and inject over a period of not less than 5 min; alternatively, dilute to 100 ml and infuse over 15–20 min. See Notes. **IV for prevention of bleeding from stress-related mucosal lesions in acutely ill patients** adjust the dose or frequency of intermittent therapy or the rate of continuous infusion to maintain the intragastric pH above 4.[86,87]

Dosage Individualization. Adjust dosage in renal impairment as follows: with Cl_{cr} below 50 ml/min, give 150 mg q 24 hr PO or 50 mg q 18–24 hr IM or IV. The dosing interval may be decreased to 12 hr cautiously if necessary. Give doses at the end of scheduled hemodialysis; an extra dose is apparently not necessary in CAPD.[88-90]

Pediatric Dose. Safety and efficacy not established.

Dosage Forms. **Tab** 150, 300 mg; **Inj** 25 mg/ml.

Patient Instructions. See Cimetidine.

Pharmacokinetics. *Onset and Duration.* (Antisecretory effect) onset PO within 1 hr, IM/IV within 15 min; peak PO occurs within 1–3 hr, IM/IV within 30 min; duration PO with 150 mg dose is up to 12 hr, IM/IV with 50 mg dose is 6-8 hr.[88]

Plasma Levels. 36-94 ng/ml inhibit 50% of pentagastrin-stimulated acid secretion in healthy subjects. Plasma concentrations are maintained above this level for about 12 hr after a 150 mg oral dose, and for 6-8 hr following an IM or IV dose.

Fate. Oral bioavailability is 50-60%, possibly increased by cirrhosis; IM bioavailability is 90-100%. Peak plasma concentrations of 440-545 ng/ml occur 1-3 hr after a 150 mg oral dose; a peak of 576 ng/ml occurs after 50 mg IM. The drug is 15% plasma protein bound; V_{dss} is 1.2-1.9 L/kg; distribution into the CNS is minimal. Ranitidine is hepatically metabolized 4% to the N-oxide, 1% to the S-oxide and 1% to desmethylranitidine. Renal clearance is 24.6-31.8 L/hr, indicating renal tubular secretion; 70% of an IV dose is excreted unchanged in urine in 24 hr. The remainder is eliminated in the feces.[88]

$t_{1/2}$. 2.5-3 hr in normals; 4-10 hr in renal failure; 2.8 hr in liver disease.[88]

Adverse Reactions. Adverse reactions are usually minor and occur infrequently. Headache occurs in about 3% of patients; rash, abdominal pain, dizziness, nausea and constipation or diarrhea occur occasionally. Rare cases of reversible CNS effects have been reported, predominantly in severely ill elderly patients. Increases in ALT (SGPT) to at least twice pretreatment values have been reported in 6 of 12 healthy volunteers receiving 100 mg qid IV for 7 days and in 4 of 24 subjects receiving 50 mg qid IV for 5 days. There have been occasional reports of reversible hepatitis and hepatotoxicity (with or without jaundice) with oral ranitidine. Small increases in Cr_s may occur, but are thought to be a result of competitive inhibition of creatinine secretion by ranitidine.

Precautions. Pregnancy; lactation. Ranitidine does not appear to interfere significantly with drugs metabolized via the cytochrome P 450 mixed function oxidase system.[91] Symptomatic response to therapy does not preclude the possibility of gastric malignancy.

Parameters to Monitor. Improvement in epigastric pain. However, pain relief does not correlate directly with endoscopic evidence of ulcer healing. Monitor Cr_s, AST (SGOT), ALT (SGPT). In patients receiving IV doses of 400 mg/day or more for 5 days or longer, it is advisable to monitor the ALT daily from the fifth day to the remainder of IV therapy. When used to prevent stress-related GI bleeding in the acutely ill patient, measure the intragastric pH periodically.

Notes. Clinical trials have shown ranitidine to be as effective as standard doses of cimetidine and famotidine for healing duodenal ulcers. It is possibly more effective than cimetidine 400 mg hs for the prophylaxis of recurrent duodenal ulcers, and as effective as cimetidine 300 mg qid or famotidine 40 mg hs for healing gastric ulcers.[62,65-67] Ranitidine appears to prevent stress-related GI bleeding when the intragastric pH is maintained above pH 4.0.[86,87] Ranitidine is stable in D5W, D10W, NS, Lactated Ringer's or 5% sodium bicarbonate for 48 hr at room temperature, and in TPN for 24 hr at room temperature.

Sucralfate   Carafate®

Pharmacology. Sucralfate is an aluminum salt of a sulfated disaccharide which is only minimally absorbed from the GI tract. Its exact mechanism of action is not known; however, it is thought to form an ulcer-adherent complex with proteinaceous exudates at the ulcer site, thereby protecting against further attack by acid, pepsin and bile salts. Sucralfate inhibits pepsin activity, adsorbs bile salts and has negligible acid-neutralizing capacity.

The drug also appears to enhance mucosal defense.[92]

Administration and Adult Dose. **PO for short-term treatment of duodenal ulcer** 1 g qid on an empty stomach, 1 hr before meals and hs, or 2 g bid for 4–8 weeks.[64] **PO for prophylaxis of recurrent duodenal ulcer** 1 g bid or 2 g hs.[62,64] **PO for short-term treatment of gastric ulcer** 1 g qid.[63]

Pediatric Dose. Safety and efficacy not established.

Dosage Forms. Tab 1 g.

Patient Instructions. This drug should be taken with water on an empty stomach, 1 hour before each meal and at bedtime. Antacids may be used as needed for relief of ulcer pain but should not be taken within one-half hour before or after sucralfate. Even though ulcer symptoms may decrease, treatment should be continued for 4 to 8 weeks unless directed otherwise.

Pharmacokinetics. *Onset and Duration.* Onset (attachment of sucralfate to ulcer site) within 1 hr; duration usually 6–8 hr.
   Fate. Sucralfate is a nonsystemic drug with more than 90% of an administered dose recovered unchanged in the feces. 3–5% of an oral dose is absorbed and excreted primarily unchanged in urine.[93] Aluminum absorption is increased in uremia.[94]

Adverse Reactions. Adverse reactions to sucralfate are minor and infrequent. Constipation occurs occasionally; diarrhea, nausea, gastric discomfort, indigestion, dry mouth, rash, pruritus, backache, dizziness, drowsiness and vertigo occur rarely.

Precautions. Pregnancy. Since duodenal ulcer is a chronic, recurrent disease, successful short-term therapy should not be expected to alter the post-healing frequency of recurrence or the severity of the duodenal ulcerations.

Parameters to Monitor. Improvement in epigastric pain. However, pain relief does not correlate directly with endoscopic evidence of ulcer healing. Observe for constipation.

Notes. Sucralfate is as effective as cimetidine in the short-term treatment of duodenal ulcer.[63,64] Combination therapy with sucralfate and an H_2-receptor antagonist offers no significant advantage over single-drug therapy when used to treat uncomplicated duodenal ulcer.[95] Sucralfate appears to prevent gastric mucosal aspirin-induced erosions.[96,97] Evidence suggests that sucralfate may be effective in preventing stress-related GI bleeding and when compared to antacids or H_2-receptor antagonists appears to be associated with a lower frequency of pneumonia in patients on mechanical ventilation.[98,99] Sucralfate has been used to bind phosphate in uremic patients.[94] A sucralfate suspension may be used for administration via NG tube or topically for treatment of stomatitis due to cancer chemotherapy.[100-102]

Histamine H₂-Receptor Antagonists Comparison Chart[a]

DRUG	DOSAGE FORMS	ADULT DOSE	ORAL BIOAVAIL-ABILITY (PERCENT)	ELIMINATION HALF-LIFE (HOURS)		PERCENT EXCRETED UNCHANGED IN URINE	RING STRUCTURE[b]
				NORMAL	ANURIC		
Cimetidine Tagamet®	Tab 200, 300, 400, 800 mg Liquid 60 mg/ml Inj 150 mg/ml.	PO 300 mg qid, 400 mg bid, or 800 mg hs; IV 300 mg q 6–8 hr initially.	60–70	2	4–5	75	Imidazole.
Famotidine Pepcid®	Tab 20, 40 mg Susp 8 mg/ml Inj 10 mg/ml.	PO 20 mg bid, or 40 mg hs; IV 20 mg q 12 hr initially.	40–45	2.5–3.5	20 +	65–70	Thiazole.
Nizatidine Axid®	Cap 150, 300 mg.	PO 150 mg bid or 300 mg hs.	90–100 (75% in renal failure)	1.6	6–8.5	65–75	Thiazole.
Ranitidine Zantac®	Tab 150, 300 mg Inj 25 mg/ml.	PO 150 mg bid or 300 mg hs; IV 50 mg q 6–8 hr initially.	50–60	2.5–3	4–10	70	Furan.

a. From references 58, 67, 75, 88, 105–107.
b. The imidazole ring structure is associated with inhibition of the cytochrome P450 hepatic enzyme system, resulting in a reduction in clearance of drugs metabolized by this system.

References, 56:00 Gastrointestinal Drugs

1. Feldmann EG, ed. Handbook of nonprescription drugs. 8th ed. Washington, DC: American Pharmaceutical Association, 1986.

2. Sleisenger MH, Fordtran JS, eds. Gastrointestinal disease: pathophysiology, diagnosis, management. 3rd ed. Philadelphia: WB Saunders, 1983.

3. Siepler JK, Mahakian K, Trudeau WT. Current concepts in clinical therapeutics: peptic ulcer disease. Clin Pharm 1986;5:128-42.

4. Ritschel WA. Antacids. In: Ritschel WA. Antacids and other drugs in gastrointestinal diseases. Hamilton, IL: Drug Intelligence Publications, 1984:42-124.

5. Neuvonen PJ. Clinical pharmacokinetics of oral activated charcoal in acute intoxications. Clin Pharmacokinet 1982;7:465-89.

6. Rodgers GC, Matyunas NJ. Gastrointestinal decontamination for acute poisoning. Pediatr Clin North Am 1986;33:261-85.

7. Scholtz EC, Jaffe JM, Colaizzi JL. Evaluation of five activated charcoal formulations for inhibition of aspirin absorption and palatability in man. Am J Hosp Pharm 1978;35:1355-9.

8. Greensher J, Mofenson HC, Picchioni AL et al. Activated charcoal updated. JACEP 1979;8:261-3.

9. Berstad A, Weberg R. Antacids in the treatment of gastroduodenal ulcer. Scand J Gastroenterol 1986;21:385-91.

10. Bianchi Porro G, Parente F, Lazzaroni M et al. Medium-dose antacids versus cimetidine in the short-term treatment of duodenal ulcer. J Clin Gastroenterol 1986;8:141-5.

11. Shuman RB, Schuster DP, Zuckerman GR. Prophylactic therapy for stress ulcer bleeding: a reappraisal. Ann Intern Med 1987;106:562-7.

12. Strom M. Antacid side-effects on bowel habits. Scand J Gastroenterol 1982;17(Suppl 75):54-5.

13. Herzog P, Holtermuller K-H. Antacid therapy—changes in mineral metabolism. Scand J Gastroenterol 1982;17(Suppl 75):56-62.

14. Barowsky H, Schwartz SA. Method for evaluating diphenoxylate hydrochloride. JAMA 1962;180:1058-61.

15. Heel RC, Brogden RN, Speight TM et al. Loperamide: a review of its pharmacological properties and therapeutic efficacy in diarrhea. Drugs 1978;15:33-52.

16. Karin A, Raney RE, Evensen KL. Pharmacokinetics and metabolism of diphenoxylate in man. Clin Pharmacol Ther 1972;13:407-19.

17. Pietrusko RG. Use and abuse of laxatives. Am J Hosp Pharm 1977;34:291-300.

18. Curry CE. Laxative products. In: Feldmann EG, ed. Handbook of nonprescription drugs. 8th ed. Washington, DC: American Pharmaceutical Association, 1986;75-97.

19. Brunton LL. Laxatives. In: Gilman AG, Goodman LS, Rall TW et al, eds. Goodman and Gilman's the pharmacological basis of therapeutics. 7th ed. New York: Macmillan, 1985;994-1003.

20. Tedesco FJ et al. Laxative use in constipation. Am J Gastroenterol 1985;80:303-9.

21. Fraser CL, Arieff AI. Hepatic encephalopathy. N Engl J Med 1985;313:865-73.

22. Anon. Laxative stool softeners. Med Lett Drugs Ther 1977;19:45-6.

23. Godfrey H. Dangers of dioctyl sodium sulfosuccinate in mixtures. JAMA 1971;215:643.

24. Goldstein GB, Lam KC, Mistilis SP. Drug-induced active chronic hepatitis. Am J Dig Dis 1973;18:177-84.

25. Tolman KG, Hammar S, Sannella JJ. Possible hepatotoxicity of Doxidan®. Ann Intern Med 1976;84:290-2.

26. Anon. Laxatives and dietary fiber. Med Lett Drugs Ther 1973;15:98-100.

27. Crossley IR, Williams R. Progress in the treatment of chronic portasystemic encephalopathy. Gut 1984;25:85-98.

28. Nelson DC, McGrew WRG, Hoyumpa AM. Hypernatremia and lactulose therapy. JAMA 1983;249:1295-8.

29. Anon. Lactulose (Chronulac) for constipation. Med Lett Drugs Ther 1980;22:2-4.

30. Michael KA, DiPiro JT, Bowden TA et al. Whole-bowel irrigation for mechanical colon cleansing. Clin Pharm 1985;4:414-24.

31. Davis GR, Santa Ana CA, Morawski SG et al. Development of a lavage solution associated with minimal water and electrolyte absorption or secretion. Gastroenterology 1980;78:991-5.

32. Anon. Oral electrolyte solutions for colonic lavage before colonoscopy or barium enema. Med Lett Drugs Ther 1985;27:39-40.

33. MacLean WC. A comparison of ipecac syrup and apomorphine in the immediate treatment of ingestion of poisons. J Pediatr 1973;82:121-4.

34. Corby DG, Decker WJ, Moran MJ et al. Clinical comparison of pharmacologic emetics in children. Pediatrics 1968;42:361-4.

35. deCastro FJ, Jaeger RW, Peters A et al. Apomorphine: clinical trial of stable solution. Clin Toxicol 1978;12:65-8.

36. Lemberger L, Weiss JL, Watanabe AM et al. Delta-9-tetrahydrocannabinol. Temporal correlation of the psychologic effects and blood levels after various routes of administration. N Engl J Med 1972;286:685-8.

37. Hollister LE, Gillespie HK, Ohlsson A et al. Do plasma concentrations of Δ^9-tetrahydrocannabinol reflect the degree of intoxication? J Clin Pharmacol 1981;21:171S-7S.

38. Wall ME, Sadler BM, Brine D et al. Metabolism, disposition, and kinetics of delta-9-tetrahydrocannabinol in men and women. Clin Pharmacol Ther 1983;34:352-63.

39. Agurell S, Halldin M, Lindgren J-E et al. Pharmacokinetics and metabolism of Δ^1-tetrahydrocannabinol and other cannabinoids with emphasis on man. Pharmacol Rev 1986;38:21-43.

40. Lemberger L, Silberstein SD, Axelrod J et al. Marihuana: studies on the disposition and metabolism of delta-9-tetrahydrocannabinol in man. Science 1970;170:1320-2.

41. Anon. Synthetic marijuana for nausea and vomiting due to cancer chemotherapy. Med Lett Drugs Ther 1985;27:97-8.

42. Bakowski MT. Advances in anti-emetic therapy. Cancer Treat Rev 1984;11:237-56.

43. Gralla RJ, Tyson LB, Bordin LA et al. Antiemetic therapy: a review of recent studies and a report of a random assignment trial comparing metoclopramide with delta-9-tetrahydrocannabinol. Cancer Treat Rep 1984;68:163-72.

44. Miser JS, Robertson WO. Ipecac poisoning. West J Med 1978;128:440-3.

45. Palmer EP, Guay AT. Reversible myopathy secondary to abuse of ipecac in patients with major eating disorders. N Engl J Med 1985;313:1457-9.

46. Manoguerra AS, Krenzelok EP. Rapid emesis from high-dose ipecac syrup in adults and children intoxicated with antiemetics or other drugs. Am J Hosp Pharm 1978;35:1360-2.

47. Thoman ME, Verhulst HL. Ipecac syrup in antiemetic ingestion. JAMA 1966;196:433-4.

48. McEvoy GK, ed. AHFS American hospital formulary service drug information 87. Bethesda MD: American Society of Hospital Pharmacists, 1987:1543-4.

49. Anderson RJ, Schrier RW, eds. Clinical use of drugs in patients with kidney and liver disease. Philadelphia: WB Saunders, 1981.

50. Drugs for psychiatric disorders. Med Lett Drugs Ther 1980;22:77-84.

51. Side effects of antipsychotic drugs and their treatment. In: Klein DF, Gittelman R, Quitkin F et al. Diagnosis and drug treatment of psychiatric disorders. 2nd ed. Baltimore: Williams and Wilkins, 1980:177-90.

52. Abate MA. Medical management of cholesterol gallstones. Drug Intell Clin Pharm 1986;20:106-15.

53. Tangedahl T. The present status of agents for dissolving gallstones. Am J Gastroenterol 1985;80:64-6.

54. Freston JW. Cimetidine I. Developments, pharmacology, and efficacy. Ann Intern Med 1982;97:573-80.

55. Ostro MJ, Russell JA, Soldin SJ et al. Control of gastric pH with cimetidine: boluses versus primed infusions. Gastroenterology 1985;89:532-6.

56. Peura DA, Johnson LF. Cimetidine for prevention and treatment of gastroduodenal mucosal lesions in patients in an intensive care unit. Ann Intern Med 1985;103:173-7.

57. Luk GD, Luk WJ, Hendrix TR. Cimetidine and impaired renal function. Ann Intern Med 1979;90:991-2.

58. Somogyi A, Gugler R. Clinical pharmacokinetics of cimetidine. Clin Pharmacokinet 1983;8:463-95.

59. Chhattriwalla Y, Colon AR, Scanlon JW. The use of cimetidine in the newborn. Pediatrics 1980;65:301-2.

60. Freston JW. Cimetidine II. Adverse reactions and patterns of use. Ann Intern Med 1982;97:728-34.

61. Nazario M. The hepatic and renal mechanisms of drug interactions with cimetidine. Drug Intell Clin Pharm 1986;20:342-8.

62. Berardi RR, Savitsky ME, Nostrant TT. Maintenance therapy for prevention of recurrent peptic ulcers. Drug Intell Clin Pharm 1987;21:493-501.

63. Brogden RN, Heel RC, Speight TM et al. Sucralfate. A review of its pharmacodynamic properties and therapeutic use in peptic ulcer disease. Drugs 1984;27:194-209.

64. Marks IN. Sucralfate: worldwide experience in recurrence therapy. J Clin Gastroenterol 1987;9(Suppl 1):18-22.

65. Zeldis JB, Friedman LS, Isselbacher KJ. Ranitidine: a new H_2-receptor antagonist. N Engl J Med 1983;309:1368-73.

66. Silvis SE et al. Final report on the United States multicenter trial comparing ranitidine to cimetidine as maintenance therapy following healing of duodenal ulcer. J Clin Gastroenterol 1985;7:482-7.

67. Berardi RR, Tankanow RM, Nostrant TT. Comparison of famotidine with cimetidine and ranitidine. Clin Pharm 1988;7:271-84.

68. First International Cisapride Investigators' Meeting. Abstracts. Digestion 1986;34:137-60.

69. Reyntjens A, Verlinden M, Schuurkes J et al. New approach to gastrointestinal motor dysfunction: non-antidopaminergic, non-cholinergic stimulation with cisapride: an introductory survey. Curr Ther Res 1984;36:1029-37.

70. Brogden RN, Carmine AA, Heel RC et al. Domperidone. A review of its pharmacological activity, pharmacokinetics and therpaeutic efficacy in the symptomatic treatment of chronic dyspepsia and as an antiemetic. Drugs 1982;24:360-400.

71. Emanuel MB. The pharmacology and clinical uses of domperidone. Clin Res Rev 1983;3:15-33.

72. Horowitz M, Harding PE, Chatterton BE et al. Acute and chronic effects of domperidone on gastric emptying in diabetic autonomic neuropathy. Dig Dis Sci 1985;30:1-9.

73. Osborne RJ, Slevin ML, Hunter RW et al. Cardiotoxicity of intravenous domperidone. Lancet 1985;2:385.

74. Texter EC, ed. Famotidine: clinical applications of a new H_2-receptor antagonist. Am J Med 1986;81(Suppl 4B):1-64.

75. Takabatake T, Ohta H, Maekawa M et al. Pharmacokinetics of famotidine, a new H_2-receptor antagonist, in relation to renal function. Eur J Clin Pharmacol 1985;28:327-31.

76. Somerville KW, Kitchingman GA, Langman MJS. Effect of famotidine on oxidative drug metabolism. Eur J Clin Pharmacol 1986;30:279-81.

77. Bateman DN. Clinical pharmacokinetics of metoclopramide. Clin Pharmacokinet 1983;8:523-9.

78. Lehmann CR, Heironimus JD, Collins CB et al. Metoclopramide kinetics in patients with impaired renal function and clearance by hemodialysis. Clin Pharmacol Ther 1985;37:284-9.

79. Berardi RR, Cornish LA, Hyneck ML. Metoclopramide removal during continuous ambulatory peritoneal dialysis. Drug Intell Clin Pharm 1986;20:154-5. Letter.

80. Meyer BR, Lewin M, Drayer DE et al. Optimizing metoclopramide control of cisplatin-induced emesis. Ann Intern Med 1984;100:393-5.

81. Albibi R, McCallum RW. Metoclopramide: pharmacology and clinical application. Ann Intern Med 1983;98:86-95.

82. Clissold SP, Campoli-Richards DM. Omeprazole: a preliminary review of its pharmacodynamic and pharmacokinetic properties, and therapeutic potential in peptic ulcer disease and Zollinger-Ellison syndrome. Drugs 1986;32:15-47.

83. Delchier J-C, Soule J-C, Mignon M et al. Effectiveness of omeprazole in seven patients with Zollinger-Ellison syndrome resistant to histamine H_2-receptor antagonists. Dig Dis Sci 1986;31:693-9.

84. Sontag SJ. Prostaglandins in peptic ulcer disease: an overview of current status and future directions. Drugs 1986;32:445-57.

85. Konturek SJ, Pawlik W. Physiology and pharmacology of prostaglandins. Dig Dis Sci 1986;31(Suppl):6S-19S.

86. Albin M, Friedlos J, Hillman K. Continuous intragastric pH measurement in the critically ill and treatment with parenteral ranitidine. Intensive Care Med 1985;11:295-9.

87. Morris DL, Markham S, Beachey A et al. Bolus or infusion ranitidine for the control of intragastric pH in critically ill patients. Am J Gastroenterol 1985;80:865. Abstract.

88. Roberts CJC. Clinical pharmacokinetics of ranitidine. Clin Pharmacokinet 1984;9:211-21.

89. Sica D, Harford A, Comstock T et al. Ranitidine pharmacokinetics in chronic hemodialysis. Clin Pharmacol Ther 1985;37:229. Abstract.

90. Sica DA, Harford A, Comstock T et al. Ranitidine pharmacokinetics in continuous ambulatory peritoneal dialysis (CAPD). Clin Pharmacol Ther 1985;37:229. Abstract.

91. Kirch W, Hoensch H, Janisch HD. Interactions and non-interactions with ranitidine. Clin Pharmacokinet 1984;9:493-510.

92. Ligumsky M, Karmeli F, Rachmilewitz D. Sucralfate stimulation of gastric PGE$_2$ synthesis—possible mechanism to explain its effective cytoprotective properties. Gastroenterology 1984;86:1164. Abstract.

93. Giesing D, Lanman R, Runser D. Absorption of sucralfate in man. Gastroenterology 1982;82:1066. Abstract.

94. Leung ACT, Henderson IS, Halls DJ et al. Aluminum hydroxide versus sucralfate as a phosphate binder in uraemia. Br Med J 1983;286:1379-81.

95. Van Deventer GM, Schneidman D, Walsh JH. Sucralfate and cimetidine as single agents and in combination for treatment of active duodenal ulcers; a double-blind, placebo-controlled trial. Am J Med 1985;79(Suppl 2C):39-44.

96. Sabesin SM, Lak SK, eds. International sucralfate research conference. Am J Med 1987;83(Suppl 3B):1-128.

97. Shea-Donahue T, Steel L, Montcalm E et al. Gastric protection by sucralfate: role of mucus and prostaglandins. Gastroenterology 1986;91:660-6.

98. Borrero E, Bank S, Margolis I et al. Comparison of antacid and sucralfate in the prevention of gastrointestinal bleeding in patients who are critically ill. Am J Med 1985;79(Suppl 2C):62-4.

99. Driks MR, Craven DE, Celli BR et al. Nosocomial pneumonia in intubated patients given sucralfate as compared with antacids or histamine type 2 blockers: the role of gastric colonization. N Engl J Med 1987;317:1376-82.

100. Schneider JS, Ouellette SM. Sucralfate administration via nasogastric tube. N Engl J Med 1984;310:990. Letter.

101. Ferraro JM, Mattern JQA. Sucralfate suspension for stomatitis. Drug Intell Clin Pharm 1984;18:153. Letter.

102. Adams S, Toth B, Dudley BS. Evaluation of sucralfate as a compounded oral suspension for the treatment of stomatitis. Clin Pharmacol Ther 1985;37:178. Abstract.

103. Ward A, Holmes B. Nabilone. A preliminary review of its pharmacological properties and therapeutic use. Drugs 1985;30:127-44.

104. Ahmedzai S, Carlyle DL, Calder IT et al. Anti-emetic efficacy and toxicity of nabilone, a synthetic cannabinoid, in lung cancer chemotherapy. Br J Cancer 1983;48:657-63.

105. Knadler MP, Bergstrom RF, Callaghan JT et al. Nizatidine, an H$_2$-blocker. Its metabolism and disposition in man. Drug Metab Dispos 1986;14:175-82.

106. Aronoff GR, Sloan RS, Bopp RJ et al. Nizatidine kinetics in patients with renal insufficiency. Clin Pharmacol Ther 1986;39:178. Abstract.

107. Callaghan JT, Bergstrom RF, Rubin A et al. A pharmacokinetic profile of nizatidine in man. Scand J Gastroenterol 1987;22(Suppl 136):9-17.

68:00 HORMONES AND SYNTHETIC SUBSTITUTES

68:04 ADRENALS

General References: 1-4, 28-31

Class Instructions. These drugs may be taken with food, milk or antacid to minimize stomach upset. Single daily doses or alternate-day doses should be taken in the morning prior to 9 AM. Multiple doses should be taken at evenly spaced intervals during the day. Report unusual weight gain, lower extremity swelling, muscle weakness, facial swelling, menstrual irregularities, prolonged sore throat, fever, cold, infection or serious injury. Patients on chronic steroid therapy should carry appropriate identification. Do not discontinue this medication without medical approval; tell any new physician that you are taking a corticosteroid.

Beclomethasone Dipropionate Beconase®, Beclovent®, Vancenase®, Vanceril®

Pharmacology. Potent topical glucocorticoid—see Prednisone.

Administration and Adult Dose. **Inhal for asthma** 42–84 mcg (1–2 inhalations) tid-qid, to maximum of 840 mcg/day (20 inhalations). In severe cases, start with 504–672 mcg/day (12–16 inhalations); after patient is symptom-free for 30 days and pulmonary function tests are normalized, decrease daily dose by 84 mcg (2 inhalations) at weekly intervals until minimum dose necessary to control patient has been defined.[4-7] See Notes. **Intranasal for nasal congestion** not responsive to maximally tolerated doses of antihistamine-decongestant combination 42–84 mcg/nostril bid-qid (168–336 mcg/day total dose) for several days, then decrease dose (if symptoms do not recur) to minimum amount necessary to control stuffiness.[8]

Pediatric Dose. **Inhal for asthma** (6–12 yr) 42–84 mcg (1–2 inhalations) tid-qid to maximum of 420 mcg/day; (over 12 yr) same as adult dose.[8] **Intranasal for nasal congestion** not responsive to maximally tolerated doses of antihistamine-decongestant combination (under 6 yr) not recommended; (6–12 yr) 42 mcg/nostril bid-tid.[9]

Dosage Forms. **Inhal** (Beclovent®, Vanceril®) 42 mcg/inhalation (200 doses/inhaler); **Nasal Inhal** (Beconase®, Vancenase®) 42 mcg/spray (200 doses/inhaler); (Beconase® AQ Aq Susp 42 mcg/spray (200 doses/bottle).

Patient Instructions. (Metered dose inhaler). Shake thoroughly, place mouthpiece into mouth with teeth and tongue out of the way. Tilt head back and actuate inhaler during *slow* deep breath and hold breath for 5–10 seconds. Allow at least 1 minute between inhalations. Use inhaled sympathomimetics (if prescribed) a few minutes prior to beclomethasone to prevent bronchospasm and to enhance penetration of the steroid into the bronchial tree. The use of "spacers" with steroid inhalers decreases the frequency of local side effects, hoarseness and oropharyngeal candidiasis.[7,8] Rinsing mouth and gargling with water or mouthwash following administration may also be beneficial. This medication is for preventive therapy and should not be used to treat acute asthma attacks.

Pharmacokinetics. *Onset and Duration.* Clinical effect is usually evident within a few days, but it may take 2–4 weeks for maximum improvement.[5-7]

Fate. Only 10% or less of an inhaled dose is deposited in the lung, while most (90%) is deposited in the mouth and swallowed. Oral absorption is slow and incomplete (61–90%) and undergoes significant first-pass metabolism resulting in oral bioavailability of less than 5%.[4,10] Well absorbed from the lung. Extensively metabolized with 65% excreted in the bile and less than 10% of drug and metabolites excreted in urine.[4,10]

$t_{1/2}$. See Inhaled Aerosol Corticosteroids Comparison Chart.

Adverse Reactions. Deaths due to adrenal insufficiency during and after transfer from systemic corticosteroids to aerosol may occur. After oral use, localized growth of *Candida* in the mouth occurs frequently, but clinically apparent infections are less common. Hoarseness and dry mouth occur occasionally; minimal to no suppression of the pituitary-adrenal axis occurs at the usual recommended doses; however, significant dose-dependent suppression occurs at higher dosages.[7,8] After intranasal use, irritation and burning of the nasal mucosa and sneezing occur occasionally; intranasal and pharyngeal *Candida* infections, nasal ulceration and epistaxis occur rarely.

Contraindications. Status asthmaticus or other acute episodes of asthma in which intensive measures are required; beclomethasone-exacerbated symptoms.

Precautions. During stress or severe asthmatic attacks, patients withdrawn from systemic corticosteroids should resume them (in large doses) immediately and contact their physician.

Parameters to Monitor. For treatment of asthma, frequency of asthmatic symptoms during day; nocturnal use of prn sympathomimetic inhaler. For nasal congestion, relief of symptoms.

Notes. Oral inhalation is indicated only for patients (including those already receiving oral corticosteroids) who require chronic treatment with corticosteroids in conjunction with other anti-asthmatic therapy. Patients needing chronic steroids should be continued on therapeutic doses of a bronchodilator. Prior to use, a patient should be as free of symptoms as possible, which can be achieved with a one-week course of oral prednisone. Start at maximum dose and titrate down after the patient is stabilized. After stabilization, many patients can be controlled on a bid dosing schedule.[5-7] The nasal inhalation provides effective, prompt relief of nasal congestion when maximally tolerated doses of oral sympathomimetics are inadequate. See also Inhaled Aerosol Corticosteroids Comparison Chart.

Dexamethasone   Decadron®, Hexadrol®, Various

Pharmacology. A potent, long-acting glucocorticoid lacking sodium-retaining activity with low to moderate doses—see Oral Corticosteroids Comparison Chart.

Administration and Adult Dose. Total daily dose is variable depending on the clinical disorder. **PO for acute, self-limited allergic disorders or exacerbation of chronic allergic disorders** 0.75–10 mg/day in 2–4 divided doses initially, tapered over 7 days and discontinued. **IV for cerebral edema** 10 mg (as the sodium phosphate) initially, followed by 4 mg IM or IV q 6 hr for 2–4 days, then taper dose over 5–7 days and discontinue. **IV for septic shock** not recommended because of lack of efficacy and possible increased mortality.[12-14] **PO as the dexamethasone suppression test to screen for Cushing's disease** 1 mg at 11 PM; measure serum cortisol at 8 AM the next day. A cortisol concentration above 5 mcg/dl is abnormal. Alternatively, PO 0.5 mg q 6 hr for 48 hr, with 24-hr urine collected for 17-hydroxy-corticosteroids (17-OHCS) during the second 24-hr period. A normal response for the second 24-hr period is less than 3 mg 17-OHCS.[15] See Notes. **PO or IV as an antiemetic with cancer chemotherapy** (usually in combination with other antiemetics) 10–30 mg before therapy; optionally, up to 40 mg may be given after chemotherapy.[16,17] See also Inhaled Aerosol Corticosteroids Comparison Chart.

Pediatric Dose. PO, IM or IV 0.024–0.34 mg/kg/day in 4 divided doses.

Patient Instructions. See Class Instructions.

Dosage Forms. **Elxr** 0.1 mg/ml; **Soln** 0.1, 1 mg/ml; **Tab** 0.25, 0.5, 0.75, 1, 1.5, 2, 4, 6 mg; **Inj** 4, 10, 20, 24 mg/ml.

Pharmacokinetics. *Onset and Duration.* See Oral Corticosteroids Comparison Chart.
   Plasma Levels. Therapeutic effects are not directly correlated with plasma concentration.
   Fate. Readily absorbed after oral administration; V_d is 0.7–0.8 L/kg; eliminated primarily by hepatic metabolism with about 2–3% excreted unchanged in urine.[18]
   $t_{1/2}$. (Males) 3.4 hr; (females) 2.4 hr.[18]

Adverse Reactions. See Prednisone. Perineal itching or burning may occur after IV administration.[19a]

Contraindications. Systemic fungal infections; administration of live virus vaccines to patients receiving immunosuppressive doses of dexamethasone.

Precautions. See Prednisone.

Parameters to Monitor. See Prednisone.

Notes. The dexamethasone suppression test for diagnosis of depression is of unproven value.[19] Decadron® injection contains 8 mg/ml of creatinine which can complicate the evaluation of creatinine clearance; Hexadrol® injection and some generic products contain no creatinine.

Methylprednisolone Sodium Succinate Solu-Medrol®, Various

Methylprednisolone sodium succinate is an injectable glucocorticoid that is about 1.25 times as potent as prednisone and prednisolone—see Oral Corticosteroids Comparison Chart. It is commonly used when oral therapy is not possible and in situations in which large parenteral doses are necessary. Side effects are similar to prednisone in equivalent doses. Evidence of efficacy in improving the outcome of septic shock is lacking and, because of increased mortality in some patient groups, the use of methylprednisolone in septic shock is not recommended. Large doses should be infused cautiously, because arrhythmias and sudden death have occurred with rapid infusions.[12-14,20] The drug is available in 40, 125, 500 mg, 1, 2 g vials.

Prednisone   Deltasone®, Orasone®, Various

Pharmacology. A synthetic glucocorticoid with minimal sodium-retaining activity. At the cellular level, glucocorticoids appear to act by controlling the rate of protein synthesis. Clinically, these drugs are used primarily for their anti-inflammatory and immunosuppressant effects.

Administration and Adult Dose. Total daily dose is variable, depending on the clinical disorder and patient response.[1,21] Daily divided high-dose therapy for initial control of more severe disease states may be necessary until satisfactory control is obtained, usually 4–10 days for many allergic and collagen diseases. Administration of a short-acting preparation given as a single dose in the morning (eg, 6–8 AM) is likely to produce fewer side effects and less pituitary-adrenal suppression than either a divided daily dose regimen with the same agent or an equivalent dose of a long-acting agent.[2,22] Alternate-day therapy (ie, total 48-hr dose administered every other morning) further reduces the prevalence and degree of steroid side effects. However, it may not be uniformly effective in treating all disease states,[2,22-25] unless large doses are used (eg, 40–60 mg every other day for adults requiring chronic steroid therapy for asthma). Complete adrenal suppression may not occur with single daily doses given either in the morning or evening if the dose is not more than 15 mg of prednisone,[26] but Cushing's syndrome may still occur,[3] and patients should receive supplemental steroids during periods of unusual stress. Protocols for withdrawal from glucocorticoid therapy have been published.[1,27]

 Common initial doses are: PO for arthritis 10 mg/day; **PO for collagen diseases** 1 mg/kg/day; **PO for rheumatic carditis** 40 mg/day; **PO for nephrotic syndrome** 60 mg/day; **PO for skin disorders** 40 mg/day, up to 240 mg/day in pemphigus;[25] **PO for ulcerative colitis** 60–120 mg/day; **PO for thrombocytopenia** 0.5 mg/kg/day; **PO for organ transplantation** 50–100 mg/day;[21,24] **PO for acute asthma exacerbations** in adults and adolescents 40 mg 2–6 times/day for 3–5 days;[28] hospitalized patients may need a parenteral preparation.[28-31] In all cases, reduce dose to minimum effective maintenance dose as soon as possible.

Pediatric Dose. Dose depends on disease state and patient response. **Common initial doses are: PO** 2 mg/kg/day; **PO for nephrosis** (1.5-4 yr) 30-40 mg/day; (4-10 yr) 60 mg/day; (over 10 yr) 80 mg/day. **PO for asthma exacerbations** (under 1 yr) 10 mg 2-6 times/day depending on severity (status asthmaticus, q 4 hr); (1-3 yr) 20 mg 2-6 times/day for 3-5 days; (3 yr-adolescent) 30 mg 2-6 times/day for 3-5 days; (adolescent and older) 40 mg 2-6 times/day for 3-5 days.[28,29]

Dosage Forms. Soln 1, 5 mg/ml; **Syrup** 1 mg/ml; **Tab** 1, 2.5, 5, 10, 20, 25, 50 mg.

Patient Instructions. See Class Instructions. If a dose is missed and the proper schedule is *every other day*, take it as soon as possible and resume the schedule unless it is past noon. In that case, wait until the next morning and resume every other day dosing. If the proper schedule is *once a day*, take the dose as soon as possible. If not remembered until the next day, do not double that day's dose; skip the missed dose. If the proper schedule is *several times a day*, take the dose as soon as possible and resume the normal schedule. If not remembered until the next dose is due, then take that regular dose and skip the missed dose; resume the normal dosing schedule.[32]

Pharmacokinetics. *Onset and Duration.* See Oral Corticosteroids Comparison Chart.
  Plasma Levels. Therapeutic effects are not directly correlated with plasma concentration; however, the half-life of the effect on serum corticosterone is 1.5-2 times the plasma half-life.[33,34]
  Fate. Bioavailability differences between products have been reported.[35] 70-95% plasma protein bound, depending on plasma concentration; V_d of prednisolone is 1.5 L/kg.[21] Prednisone and cortisone must be metabolized in the liver to their active forms, prednisolone and hydrocortisone, respectively;[36] liver disease does not impair conversion to active metabolites. In fact, patients with liver disease and hypoalbuminemia are more likely to suffer major side effects of prednisone as a result of decreased protein binding and delayed clearance of prednisolone.[37-39] Prednisolone is eliminated primarily by hepatic metabolism, with greater than 90% of metabolites found in the urine. About 7-15% of a dose of prednisone or prednisolone is excreted as unchanged prednisolone in urine.[37]
  $t_{1/2}$. (Prednisone) 3.3-3.8 hr; (prednisolone) 2.5-3.5 hr; may exhibit dose-dependent kinetics—with increasing doses, half-life may increase.[21,37]

Adverse Reactions. Prolonged therapy may lead to suppression of pituitary-adrenal function. Too rapid a withdrawal of long-term therapy can cause acute adrenal insufficiency (eg, fever, myalgia, arthralgia and malaise); suppressed patients are unable to respond to stress. Therapy with prednisone (other adrenocorticoids vary in propensity for certain adverse effects), depending on dose and duration, can result in fluid and electrolyte disturbances (with possible edema and hypertension), hyperglycemia and glycosuria, spread of herpes conjunctivitis, activation of tuberculosis, peptic ulcers,[40] osteoporosis, myopathy, menstrual irregularities, behavioral disturbances,[41] poor wound healing, ocular cataracts, glaucoma, arrest of growth, pseudotumor cerebri (primarily in children)[1] and Cushing's syndrome (moon face, buffalo hump, central obesity, easy bruising, acne, hirsutism and striae).[21] Acute onset reactions in one study occurred in 11.4% of patients and included psychiatric reactions, GI reactions, hyperglycemia, infections and leukocytosis.[41]

Contraindications. Systemic fungal infections (except as maintenance therapy in adrenal insufficiency); administration of live virus vaccines in patients receiving immunosuppressive doses of corticosteroids.

Precautions. Pregnancy; diabetes mellitus; osteoporosis; peptic ulcer; esophagitis; tuberculosis and other acute and chronic bacterial, viral and fungal infections; hypertension or other cardiovascular diseases; immunizations; hypoalbuminemia; psychosis; suppression of TB skin test reactions. See Drug Interactions chapter.

Parameters to Monitor. Observe for psychotic personality changes and signs or symptoms of Cushing's syndrome. With short-term, high-dose therapy, frequently monitor serum potassium and glucose, blood pressure and stool guaiac. With long-term therapy, monitor these parameters occasionally and perform periodic eye examinations. The 24-hr urinary free cortisol is the most sensitive measurement of HPA axis suppression.

Notes. Other more expensive glucocorticoids offer minimal advantages over prednisone in most clinical situations.[22,42] Patients who have received daily steroid therapy for asthma for less than 2 weeks *do not* require dose tapering.[29] In times of stress (eg, surgery, severe trauma, serious illness), patients on chronic adrenal-suppressing doses of corticosteroids (greater than 5 mg/day prednisone or equivalent) should receive supplemental hydrocortisone.[21,27,31]

Oral Corticosteroids Comparison Chart[a]

DURATION AND DRUG	DOSAGE FORMS	EQUIVALENT ANTI-INFLAMMATORY DOSE (MG)	RELATIVE ANTI-INFLAMMATORY POTENCY	RELATIVE MINERALO-CORTICOID ACTIVITY	PLASMA HALF-LIFE (HOURS)	COMMENTS
SHORT-ACTING (biologic activity 8–12 hr)						
Cortisone Various	Tab 5, 10, 25 mg.	25	0.8	0.8	0.5	Must be hydroxylated to active species (hydrocortisone).
Hydrocortisone Various	Tab 5, 10, 20 mg Susp 2 mg/ml.	20	1	1	1.5	Daily secretion in man is 20 mg.
INTERMEDIATE-ACTING (biologic activity 12–36 hr)						
Methylpred-nisolone Medrol® Various	Tab 2, 4, 8, 16, 24, 32 mg.	4	5	0.5	3.3	Minimal sodium-retaining activity.
Prednisolone Various	Tab 5 mg Soln 1 mg/ml Syrup 3 mg/ml.	5	4	0.8	3	Minimal sodium-retaining activity.
Prednisone Various	Tab 1, 2.5, 5, 10, 20, 25, 50 mg Soln 1, 5 mg/ml Syrup 1 mg/ml.	5	4	0.8	3.6	Must be hydroxylated to active species (prednisolone).

Continued

Oral Corticosteroids Comparison Chart[a]

DURATION AND DRUG	DOSAGE FORMS	EQUIVALENT ANTI-INFLAMMATORY DOSE (MG)	RELATIVE ANTI-INFLAMMATORY POTENCY	RELATIVE MINERALO-CORTICOID ACTIVITY	PLASMA HALF-LIFE (HOURS)	COMMENTS
Triamcinolone Aristocort® Kenacort® Various	Tab 1, 2, 4, 8, 16 mg Syrup 400, 800 mcg/ml.	4	5	0	3.3 +	May cause a higher frequency of muscle wasting.
LONG-ACTING (biologic activity 36–54 hr)						
Betamethasone Celestone®	Tab 600 mcg Syrup 120 mcg/ml.	0.6	25	0	5 +	Minimal sodium-retaining activity, but with high doses retention may occur.
Dexamethasone Decadron® Hexadrol® Various	Tab 250, 500, 750 mcg, 1, 1.5, 2, 4, 6 mg Elxr 100 mcg/ml Soln 100 mcg/ml, 1 mg/ml.	0.75	30	0	Males 3.4 Females 2.4	
MINERALOCORTICOID (biologic activity 18–36 hr)						
Fludrocortisone Florinef®	Tab 100 mcg.	—	10	125	—	Mineralocorticoid useful in Addison's disease.

a. From references 1, 3, 21, 37, 43–45.

Inhaled Aerosol Corticosteroids Comparison Chart[a,b]

| DRUG | DOSAGE FORMS | INITIAL DOSAGE[c] | | RELATIVE TOPICAL POTENCY[e] | SYSTEMIC BIOAVAILABILITY[f] (PERCENT) | PLASMA HALF-LIFE (HOURS) |
		ADULT	PEDIATRIC[d]			
Beclomethasone-17, 21-dipropionate Beclovent® Beconase® Vancenase® Vanceril®	Inhal (metered dose) 42 mcg/inhal; Nasal Inhal (metered dose) 42 mcg/spray; (aqueous susp) 42 mcg/spray.	Inhal 1-2 inhal tid-qid; Nasal Inhal 1-2 sprays in each nostril bid-qid.	Inhal 1-2 inhal tid-qid; Nasal Inhal 1 spray in each nostril bid-tid.	500	< 5	15
Dexamethasone Sodium Phosphate Decadron®	Inhal (metered dose) 100 mcg/inhal; Nasal Inhal (metered dose) 100 mcg/spray.	Inhal 3 inhal tid-qid— **not recommended;** Nasal Inhal 2 sprays in each nostril bid-tid— **not recommended.**	Inhal 2 inhal tid-qid— **not recommended;** Nasal Inhal 1-2 sprays in each nostril bid— **not recommended.**	0.8	80	5
Flunisolide Aerobid® Nasalide®	Inhal (metered dose) 250 mcg/inhal; Nasal Inhal (soln) 25 mcg/spray.	Inhal 2 inhal bid up to 8 inhal/day; Nasal Inhal 2 sprays in each nostril bid up to 8 sprays/day in each nostril.	Inhal 1-2 inhal bid up to 4 inhal/day; Nasal Inhal 1 spray in each nostril tid-qid.	>100	20	1.6

Continued

Inhaled Aerosol Corticosteroids Comparison Chart[a,b]

| DRUG | DOSAGE FORMS | INITIAL DOSAGE[c] | | RELATIVE TOPICAL POTENCY[e] | SYSTEMIC BIOAVAILABILITY[f] (PERCENT) | PLASMA HALF-LIFE (HOURS) |
		ADULT	PEDIATRIC[d]			
Triamcinolone-16, 17-acetonide Azmacort®	Inhal (metered dose) 100 mcg/inhal.	Inhal 2 inhal tid-qid up to 16 inhal/day.	Inhal 1–2 inhal tid-qid up to 12 inhal/day.	100	Unknown	0.5–1
Budesonide (Investigational - MSD)	Inhal (metered dose) 50 mcg/inhal; Nasal Inhal (metered dose) 50 mcg/spray.	Inhal 400–1600 mcg/day in 2–4 doses; Nasal Inhal 2 sprays in each nostril bid.	Inhal 200–400 mcg/day in 2–4 doses; Nasal Inhal not established.	1000	10	2–2.8

a. From references 4, 5, 7–11.

b. Although there are differences, comparative trials have not established any product to be clearly superior; however, dexamethasone should *not* be used due to its extensive systemic effects.

c. Recommended starting dosages; higher doses may be used, but they produce dose-dependent systemic effects.

d. Pediatric dosing is for patients 6 to 12 yr; dosages for patients under 6 yr have not been established.

e. Topical potency based on skin vasoconstrictive effect.

f. Reflects oral bioavailability, because 90% of an inhaled dose is deposited in the mouth and swallowed. Most drugs are rapidly and completely absorbed from the respiratory tract.

68:12 CONTRACEPTIVES

(SEE ALSO ESTROGENS 68:16 AND PROGESTINS 68:32)

General References: 46-49

Class Instructions. Estrogens, Progestins and Combinations. Report immediately if any of the following occur: new severe or persistent headache; blurred vision; calf, chest or abdominal pain; or any abnormal vaginal bleeding. This (oral) drug may be taken with food, milk or an antacid to minimize stomach upset.

Oral Contraceptives
(Estrogen-Progestin Combinations)

Pharmacology. These drugs cause inhibition of ovulation, endometrial changes which are hostile to egg implantation and cervical mucus changes which are hostile to sperm migration.

Administration and Adult Dose. PO for contraception 1 tablet daily beginning on the first day of menses[50] and continued for 20–21 days, depending on the product; stop for 7 days and restart the next cycle of 20–21 tablets. Combination 28-day products (7 inert tablets) are taken 1 tablet daily continuously. **PO for contraception postpartum** start 2–4 weeks postpartum; lactation may increase period of infertility. **PO for contraception postabortion** start immediately if gestation is terminated at 12 weeks or less; start in 1 week if gestation terminated at 13–28 weeks. **PO for dysfunctional uterine bleeding (anovulatory cycles)** (any combination agent) 1 tablet qid for 5–7 days for acute bleeding, then 1 tablet daily cyclically as for contraception for 3 months to prevent further bleeding. **PO for dysmenorrhea or endometriosis** 1 tablet cyclically as for contraception for 3–9 months to induce a pseudopregnant state—use minimal estrogen, maximal progestin combination (eg, Ovral®, Demulen®, Norlestrin® 2.5 mg). **PO for emergency postcoital contraception** 2 tablets of Ovral® taken as soon as possible after coitus, and 2 more tablets taken 12 hr later, but within 72 hr after coitus.[51] See Notes.

Dosage Forms. See Oral Contraceptive Agents Comparison Chart.

Patient Instructions. See Class Instructions. (Contraception) If spotting occurs and no doses have been missed, continue to take pills even if spotting continues. If one dose is missed, take it as soon as it is remembered or take 2 tablets the next day; if 2 doses are missed, take 2 tablets daily for the next 2 days. If more than 2 doses are missed and bleeding occurs, consider as a normal period and restart cycle; also use an alternative form of contraception for the remainder of the cycle. Report if no menses occur for 2 months. (Acute anovulatory bleeding) Expect heavy and severely cramping flow 2–4 days after stopping pills with normal periods thereafter.

Pharmacokinetics. *Onset and Duration.* Onset of contraception after one week of regimen. Dysfunctional uterine bleeding should decrease within 12–24 hr of starting regimen.

Fate. Rapidly and well absorbed. Bioavailability of levonorgestrel is complete;[52] norethindrone 65%[52,53] and ethinyl estradiol 40%,[52,54] due to first-pass effect. About 54% of mestranol is converted to ethinyl estradiol in vivo. Mestranol is detectable in plasma 24 hr after a dose, although plasma level of ethinyl estradiol is higher. Norethynodrel and ethynodiol diacetate are rapidly converted to norethindrone in vivo. All are strongly plasma protein bound, concentrated in body fat and endometrium, and penetrate poorly into breast milk. Ethinyl estradiol undergoes enterohepatic recirculation. All are inactivated by the liver, conjugated with glucuronic acid and sulfate and excreted in the urine and feces.[52] See ethinyl estradiol and norethindrone.

$t_{1/2}$. Ethinyl estradiol 6–20 hr;[52,54] norethindrone 5–14 hr;[52,53] levonorgestrel 10–24 hr;[52,55] norethynodrel 45 hr;[52,56] mestranol metabolites 40–60 hr;[57] norethindrone metabolites 42–84 hr.[57]

Adverse Reactions. See Adverse Reactions of Oral Contraceptives and Hormone Excess and Deficiency Symptomatology Comparison Charts.

Contraindications. Presence or history of thrombophlebitis or thromboembolic disorders; known or suspected pregnancy; presence or history of carcinoma of breast, genitals or other estrogen-dependent tumors; cerebral vascular or coronary artery disease; markedly impaired liver function; undiagnosed abnormal genital bleeding; heavy smoking (over 15 cigarettes/day) in women 35 yr or older.[48,49,58-60] See Notes.

Precautions. Use with caution in patients with hyperlipidemia, diabetes, conditions which may be aggravated by fluid retention (eg, hypertension, convulsions, migraine and cardiac or renal dysfunction), severe varicosities, in adolescents in whom regular menses are not established and during lactation. Oral contraceptives may be less effective, resulting in increased breakthrough bleeding and/or pregnancy, when given with rifampin, phenobarbital, ampicillin, penicillin V, phenytoin, chloramphenicol, tetracycline, primidone, nitrofurantoin or neomycin.[61] Caffeine elimination may be impaired by oral contraceptives.[62] Antipyrine clearance (dependent on cytochrome P 450) is impaired by oral contraceptives.[63]

Parameters to Monitor. Complete pretreatment physical examination with special reference to blood pressure, breasts, abdomen, pelvis and Pap smear. Repeat examination every year.

Notes. Contraceptive efficacy is less than 1 pregnancy/100 woman-years with products containing 35 mcg or greater of estrogen and 1–2 pregnancies/100 woman-years for those containing less than 35 mcg estrogen. Initial selection of an oral contraceptive should approximate, as closely as possible, the patient's natural hormone balance. Ortho-Novum® 1/35, Norinyl® 1/35, and Nordette® are balanced agents that are often selected as the initial contraceptive. Prescribing of oral contraceptives in women over 35 who smoke or for all women over 40 requires adequate informed consent because of a doubled risk of cardiovascular disease in these groups. However, the health risks of pregnancy in healthy, nonsmoking women in their forties is greater than those of sub-50 mcg estrogen or progestin-only contraceptives.[60] Noncontraceptive benefits of oral contraceptives include a 33–50% risk reduction of pelvic inflammatory disease after 1 yr of use; reductions in ectopic pregnancy, endometrial cancer, benign breast disease; and symptomatic improvement of dysmenorrhea, premenstrual syndrome, iron deficiency anemia and rheumatoid arthritis.[48] Certain combination contraceptives (ie, Ovral®) are effective as postcoital contraceptives. Compared to estrogens, Ovral® is less expensive, causes less nausea and vomiting, and takes 12 hours rather than 5 days for a course of therapy.[51]

Oral Contraceptive Agents Comparison Chart[a]

PRODUCT	DOSAGE[b] CYCLE	ESTROGEN[c]	PROGESTIN[d]	POTENCY[e] ESTROGENIC[f]	PROGESTATIONAL[g]	ANDROGENIC	BREAKTHROUGH BLEEDING[h] AND SPOTTING(%)
MONOPHASIC COMBINATION AGENTS CONTAINING LESS THAN 50 MCG OF ESTROGEN							
Loestrin®1/20	21,28	Ethinyl Estradiol 20 mcg.	Norethindrone Acetate 1 mg.	+	+ +	+ +	25.2
Loestrin® 1.5/30	21,28	Ethinyl Estradiol 30 mcg.	Norethindrone Acetate 1.5 mg.	+	+ + +	+ + +	30.9
Levlen® Nordette®	21,28	Ethinyl Estradiol 30 mcg.	Levonorgestrel 0.15 mg.	+ +	+	+ +	14
Lo-Ovral®	21,28	Ethinyl Estradiol 30 mcg.	Norgestrel 0.3 mg.	+	+	+ +	9.8
Brevicon® ModiCon® Various	21,28	Ethinyl Estradiol 35 mcg.	Norethindrone 0.5 mg.	+ +	+	+	14.6
Ovcon®-35	21,28	Ethinyl Estradiol 35 mcg.	Norethindrone 0.4 mg.	+ +	+	+	19
Demulen® 1/35	21,28	Ethinyl Estradiol 35 mcg.	Ethynodiol Diacetate 1 mg.	+	+ +	+	37.5

Continued

Oral Contraceptive Agents Comparison Chart[a]

PRODUCT	DOSAGE[b] CYCLE	ESTROGEN[c]	PROGESTIN[d]	POTENCY[e] ESTROGENIC[f]	PROGESTATIONAL[g]	ANDROGENIC	BREAKTHROUGH BLEEDING[h] AND SPOTTING(%)
Norinyl® 1 + 35 **Ortho-Novum® 1/35** Various	21,28	Ethinyl Estradiol 35 mcg.	Norethindrone 1 mg.	++	++	+	14.7

BIPHASIC[i] COMBINATION PRODUCTS CONTAINING LESS THAN 50 MCG OF ESTROGEN

PRODUCT	DOSAGE CYCLE	ESTROGEN	PROGESTIN	ESTROGENIC	PROGESTATIONAL	ANDROGENIC	BREAKTHROUGH
Ortho-Novum® 10/11	21,28	Ethinyl Estradiol 35 mcg (days 1–25).	Norethindrone 5 mg (days 1–10) 1 mg (days 11–21).	++	+	low	19.6

TRIPHASIC[i] COMBINATION PRODUCTS CONTAINING LESS THAN 50 MCG OF ESTROGEN

PRODUCT	DOSAGE CYCLE	ESTROGEN	PROGESTIN	ESTROGENIC	PROGESTATIONAL	ANDROGENIC	BREAKTHROUGH
Ortho-Novum® 7/7/7	21,28	Ethinyl Estradiol 35 mcg (days 1–21).	Norethindrone 0.5 mg (days 1–7); 0.75 mg (days 8–14); 1 mg (days 15–21).	++	+	low	12.2
Tri-Norinyl®	21,28	Ethinyl Estradiol 35 mcg (days 1–21).	Norethindrone 0.5 mg (days 1–7); 1 mg (days 8–16); 0.5 mg (days 17–21).	++	+	low	14.7

Continued

Oral Contraceptive Agents Comparison Chart[a]

PRODUCT	DOSAGE[b] CYCLE	ESTROGEN[c]	PROGESTIN[d]	POTENCY[e] ESTROGENIC[f]	PROGESTATIONAL[g]	ANDROGENIC	BREAKTHROUGH BLEEDING[h] AND SPOTTING(%)
Tri-Levlen® Triphasil®	21,28	Ethinyl Estradiol 30 mcg (days 1–6); 40 mcg (days 7–11); 30 mcg (days 12–21).	Levonorgestrel 0.05 mg (days 1–6); 0.075 mg (days 7–11); 0.125 mg (days 12–21).	+ +	+	low	15.1
MONOPHASIC COMBINATION AGENTS CONTAINING 50 MCG OF ESTROGEN							
Noriny l® 1 + 50 Ortho-Novum® 1/50	21,28	Mestranol 50 mcg.	Norethindrone 1 mg.	+ +	+ +	+	10.6
Demulen®	21,28	Ethinyl Estradiol 50 mcg.	Ethynodiol Diacetate 1 mg.	+	+ +	+	13.4
Norlestrin ®1/50	21,28	Ethinyl Estradiol 50 mcg.	Norethindrone Acetate 1 mg.	+ +	+ +	+ +	13.6
Norlestrin® 2.5/50	21,28	Ethinyl Estradiol 50 mcg.	Norethindrone Acetate 2.5 mg.	+	+ + +	+ + + +	5.1
Ovcon®-50	21,28	Ethinyl Estradiol 50 mcg.	Norethindrone 1 mg.	+ +	+ +	+ +	11.9
Ovral®	21,28	Ethinyl Estradiol 50 mcg.	Norgestrel 0.5 mg.	+ +	+ + +	+ + +	4.5

Continued

Oral Contraceptive Agents Comparison Chart[a]

PRODUCT	DOSAGE[b] CYCLE	ESTROGEN[c]	PROGESTIN[d]	POTENCY[e] ESTROGENIC[f]	PROGESTATIONAL[g]	ANDROGENIC	BREAKTHROUGH BLEEDING[h] AND SPOTTING(%)
MONOPHASIC COMBINATION AGENTS CONTAINING GREATER THAN 50 MCG OF ESTROGEN							
Ortho-Novum® 10	21	Mestranol 60 mcg.	Norethindrone 10 mg.	N/A	++++	++++	3.8
Enovid®-5 mg	20	Mestranol 75 mcg.	Norethynodrel 5 mg.	++++	++	0	7.4
Norinyl® 1 + 80[j] Ortho-Novum® 1/80[j]	21,28	Mestranol 80 mcg.	Norethindrone 1 mg.	++	+	++	4.8
Ovulen®[j]	21,28	Mestranol 100 mcg.	Ethynodiol Diacetate 1 mg.	+++	++	+	6.1
Norinyl® 2 mg[j] Ortho-Novum® 2 mg[j]	20 21	Mestranol 100 mcg.	Norethindrone 2 mg.	++	++	+++	6.1
Enovid-E®[j]	21	Mestranol 100 mcg.	Norethynodrel 2.5 mg.	+++	+	0	10.9
PROGESTIN ONLY							
Micronor® Nor-Q.D.®	Con- tinuous	None	Norethindrone 0.35 mg.	+	+++	+	42.3

Continued

Oral Contraceptive Agents Comparison Chart[a]

PRODUCT	DOSAGE[b] CYCLE	ESTROGEN[c]	PROGESTIN[d]	POTENCY[e] ESTROGENIC[f]	POTENCY[e] PROGESTATIONAL[g]	POTENCY[e] ANDROGENIC	BREAKTHROUGH BLEEDING[h] AND SPOTTING(%)
Ovrette®	Continuous	None	Norgestrel 0.075 mg.	0	+	+	34.9

a. Adapted from reference 46.

b. 28-day cycles contain 7 placebo tablets to complete the 28-day cycle.

c. Estrogen equivalent potency: ethinyl estradiol is 1.5–1.75 times as potent as mestranol, because mestranol must be demethylated to its active form, ethinyl estradiol. Inhibition of ovulation requires 50 mcg of ethinyl estradiol versus 80 mcg mestranol.

d. Norethynodrel has estrogenic properties; norgestrel has estrogen antagonist properties; norethindrone, norethindrone acetate and ethynodiol diacetate have weak estrogenic properties, but also have estrogen antagonist properties. Relative progestogenic potency: norgestrel > ethynodiol diacetate > norethindrone acetate > norethindrone > norethynodrel.

e. Potency designations are based on laboratory tests of individual components. Applicability of these methods for combination products used clinically has been questioned.

f. Overall estrogenic effect as modified by anti-estrogenic/estrogenic effect of progestational component.

g. Progestational potency as measured by delay of menses test.

h. Prevalence of bleeding decreases from the first cycle to third cycle by 50–66% per cycle; these figures represent data submitted to FDA on prevalence of bleeding on third cycle of use.

i. Bi- and triphasic compounds are overall estrogen dominant.

j. No longer available. On recommendation of the FDA, high-dose (over 50 mcg of estrogen) products for contraceptive use were phased out in 1988.

Adverse Reactions of Oral Contraceptives Comparison Chart[a]

REACTION	CLINICAL INFORMATION	CAUSAL FACTORS
Myocardial Infarction	Increased risk 2.8 times that of nonuser; risk is concentrated in women over 35 yr, smokers and presence of other predisposing factors (eg, ↑ lipids, ↑ BP); risk may persist after discontinuation in long-term users.	May be related to progestin/ estrogen ratio: progestins decrease HDL, estrogens increase HDL.
Thromboembolism and Thrombophlebitis	Increased risk 4–11 times that of nonuser; risk is concentrated in smokers, older females and duration of use over 5 yr. Risk may be decreased with estrogen under 50 mcg.	Related to estrogen dose: estrogens decrease antithrombin III and increase coagulation factors and platelet aggregation.
Hepatic Tumors	Both benign and malignant tumors reported. Risk is greater with duration of use over 5 yr. Shock can result from rupture of mass. Surgical intervention may be needed, because tumors are not always reversible with discontinuation of pill.	Unknown, although mestranol and higher dosage formulations are implicated.
Breast Disease	No increase in breast cancer shown; improvement in fibrocystic disease and fibroadenoma with over 2 yr use.	Protection secondary to progestin component. Does not prevent breast cancer.
Endometrial Cancer; Cervical Cancer	Sequentials are implicated in endometrial cancer; no increased prevalence with combinations, but increased cervical erosions and eversions; cervical cancer risk is 1.8–2.1 times that of nonusers; increased with duration of use over 5–10 yr; risk factors include multiple sexual partners and early sexual activity.	Progestin component protective against endometrial adenomatous hyperplasia (which may be precursor to adeno cancer).
Thrombotic Stroke	Risk is 1.5–2.1 times higher in current users, especially with pills containing over 2 mg norethindrone acetate or equivalent.	Related to the progestin component. Continued

Adverse Reactions of Oral Contraceptives Comparison Chart[a]

REACTION	CLINICAL INFORMATION	CAUSAL FACTORS
Subarachnoid Hemorrhage	Risk is increased in both current and previous users, and is increased with age over 35 yr, smoking and hypertension.	Related to estrogen/progestin ratio.
Hypertension	Increased risk 2–3 times that of nonusers; blacks are at less risk.	Related to the progestin component.
Postpill Amenorrhea	Prevalence is 0.2–2.6% after pill use; check for pituitary tumor in presence of galactorrhea.	Presence of irregular menses prior to starting pill. Unrelated to duration or dose.
Metabolic Glucose	Abnormal glucose tolerance found in predisposed individuals (eg, sub-clinical or gestational diabetes) and rare cases of diabetic ketoacidosis. These effects are minimal with combinations containing 35 mcg or less of ethinyl estradiol or equivalent.	Hyperinsulinemia with relative insulin resistance caused by progestins with synergistic effect of estrogen.
Lipids	Elevated triglycerides; may precipitate pancreatitis in patients with underlying hyperlipidemia; LDL is highest with progestin-dominant pills, especially norgestrel and ethynodiol diacetate.	Estrogens increase triglycerides.
Gallbladder Disease	Two-fold increase in gallstones in users compared to nonusers only during the first 4 yr of use, then risk returns to baseline.	Estrogens increase cholesterol saturation.
Infertility	Little risk of permanent sterility. Conception rate after discontinuation may temporarily lag behind that of nonusers for a few months.	Risk concentrated in older women with a long history of contraceptive use.

a. From references 48, 49, 58-60, 190.

Hormone Excess and Deficiency Symptomatology Comparison Chart[a]

CONDITION	SYMPTOMATOLOGY
Estrogen Excess	Estrogen excess may also be a result of progestin deficiency. Symptoms include nausea, vomiting, vertigo, leukorrhea, increase in leiomyoma size, uterine cramps, breast tenderness with fluid retention, cystic breast changes, cholasma, edema and fluid retention resulting in abdominal or leg pain with cyclic weight gain, headaches on pill days, ill-fitting contact lenses and hypertension.
Estrogen Deficiency	Estrogen deficiency may also be a result of progestin excess. Symptoms include irritability, nervousness, decreased libido, hot flashes, early and midcycle breakthrough bleeding and spotting (days 1–7), atrophic vaginitis, dyspareunia, no withdrawal bleeding with continued contraceptive use and decreased amount of withdrawal bleeding.
Progestin Excess	Progestin excess may also be a result of estrogen deficiency. Symptoms include increased appetite and weight gain on non-pill days, tiredness, fatigue, weakness, depression, decreased libido, decreased length of menstrual flow, *Candida* vaginitis, headaches on non-pill days and breast tenderness on non-pill days.
Progestin Deficiency	Progestin deficiency may also be a result of estrogen excess. Symptoms include late breakthrough bleeding (days 8–21), heavy menstrual flow and clots, dysmenorrhea and delayed onset of menses following last pill.
Androgen Excess	Symptoms include increased appetite and weight gain, oily scalp, acne and hirsutism.

a. Adapted from references 46, 47.

68:16 ESTROGENS

General References: 64-67

Diethylstilbestrol　　　　　　　　　　　　Various
Diethylstilbestrol Diphosphate　　　　Stilphostrol®

Pharmacology.　Diethylstilbestrol (DES) is a nonsteroidal stilbene derivative with estrogenic activity and shares actions and uses of other estrogens. See Conjugated Estrogens.

Administration and Adult Dose.　(DES) **PO for postmenopausal symptoms and prevention of osteoporosis** use smallest effective dose in the range of 0.25–1 mg/day, in cycles of 21–25 days/month;[64] administer as with conjugated estrogens. **PO for dysfunctional uterine bleeding** 2 mg q 2 hr until bleeding stops. **PO for suppression of postpartum lactation** most effective when given before lactation begins: 5 mg/day for 5 days. **PO for prostatic cancer** 1–3 mg/day.[68] **PO for breast cancer** 10–20 mg/day.[69] **PO for emergency postcoital contraception** within 72 hr of unprotected intercourse 25 mg bid for 5 days.[70] **Vag Supp for atrophic vaginitis** 0.1–1 mg/day. **IV for prostatic cancer** (DES diphosphate) 250–500 mg 1–2 times/week. **PO for prostatic cancer** (DES diphosphate) 50 mg tid initially, increasing to 200 mg or more tid depending on patient tolerance.

Dosage Forms. **Tab** (DES) 0.1, 0.25, 0.5, 1, 5 mg; (DES diphosphate) 50 mg; **Inj** (DES diphosphate) 50 mg/ml; **Vag Supp** (DES) 0.1, 0.5 mg.

Patient Instructions. See Class Instructions, 68:12.

Pharmacokinetics. *Fate.* See Estrogens, Conjugated. DES and its metabolites undergo enterohepatic circulation. Oxidation of DES results in formation of an active metabolite, dienestrol. About 40% is recovered in the urine in the first 24 hours, 90% as glucuronides (70% of glucuronide is conjugated DES, 10% dienestrol and 20% hydroxydienestrol).[71]

Adverse Reactions. See Estrogens, Conjugated. Increased risk of myocardial infarction in men taking greater than 3 mg/day of DES.[68]

Contraindications. See Estrogens, Conjugated.

Precautions. See Estrogens, Conjugated.

Parameters to Monitor. See Estrogens, Conjugated.

Notes. High-dose postcoital DES is associated with a high frequency of nausea and vomiting, so pretreatment with an antiemetic is desirable. DES diphosphate 1.6 mg contains 1 mg DES.

Estradiol and its Esters

Estinyl®, Estrace®, Estraderm®, Various

Pharmacology. 17β estradiol (E$_2$) is the most potent of the naturally occurring estrogens and is the major estrogen secreted during the reproductive years. Estradiol and its derivatives share the actions of other estrogens. See Estrogens, Conjugated.

Administration and Adult Dose. **PO for postmenopausal symptoms and atrophic vaginitis** use smallest effective dose in the range of (ethinyl estradiol) 0.02–0.05 mg/day or (micronized estradiol) 1–2 mg/day up to a maximum of 4 mg/day in cycles of 21–25 days/month; administer as with conjugated estrogens.[64,72] **Top for postmenopausal symptoms** initiate with 50 mcg/day patch; patch is changed twice weekly and administered cyclically (eg, for 3 weeks followed by 1 week without patch). Dose may be increased to 100 mcg/day patch if symptoms are not controlled. See Notes. **Vag for postmenopausal vasomotor symptoms and atrophic vaginitis** 2–4 g/day of cream for 1–2 weeks, then reduce to 1–2 g/day for 1–2 weeks, then to maintenance of 1 g 1–3 times/week. **PO for prevention of osteoporosis** use minimum effective dose of 25 mcg/day of ethinyl estradiol or equivalent.[73] See Estrogens, Conjugated. **PO for dysfunctional uterine bleeding** 0.05–0.1 mg/day for 3 weeks with addition of progestin the third week. **PO for suppression of postpartum lactation** (ethinyl estradiol) most effective when given before lactation begins 0.1–0.15 mg/day for 5–7 days. **PO for palliation of prostatic cancer** (ethinyl estradiol) 0.05–2 mg/day. **PO for palliation of breast cancer** (ethinyl estradiol) 1 mg tid. **PO for emergency postcoital contraception** within 72 hr of unprotected intercourse (ethinyl estradiol) 2.5 mg bid for 5 days.[70] **IM for postmenopausal symptoms and prevention of osteoporosis** when oral or vaginal therapy does not provide expected response, is poorly tolerated or when noncompliance occurs (estradiol cypionate) 1–5 mg q 3–4 weeks; (estradiol valerate) 10–20 mg q 4 weeks.[64] **IM for dysfunctional uterine bleeding** (estradiol valerate) 20 mg initially, then 5 mg q 2 weeks with addition of progestin. **IM for suppression of postpartum lactation** (estradiol valerate) 10–30 mg immediately after delivery. **IM for palliation of prostatic cancer** (polyestradiol phosphate) 40 mg q 2–3 weeks.

Dosage Forms. **Tab** (ethinyl estradiol) 0.02, 0.05, 0.5 mg; (micronized 17β estradiol) 1, 2 mg; **Inj** (estradiol cypionate in oil) 1, 5 mg/ml; (estradiol valerate in oil) 10, 20, 40 mg/ml; (polyestradiol phosphate) 20 mg/ml. **Vag Crm** (micronized 17β estradiol) 0.1 mg/g; **SR Patch** (17β estradiol) 50, 100 mcg/day.

Pharmacokinetics. **Onset and Duration.** Onset of therapeutic E_2 levels after oral or vaginal administration is 0.5–1 hr with peak levels at 5 hr and progressive decline toward baseline by 12–24 hr. Estrone (E_1) levels are higher and vary widely, but are not related to efficacy.[74-77] Reduction of FSH and LH levels occur within 6 hr and 3 hr, respectively, with a duration of 24 hr.[74,77] Onset of depot products variable following IM injection; duration (cypionate) 14–28 days, (valerate) 14–21 days, (polyestradiol phosphate) 14–28 days.[66]

Plasma Levels. PO administration results in unphysiologic ratio of E_1 to E_2 over 1.[74-76] Therapeutic E_2 levels for relief of vasomotor symptoms are 40–70 pg/ml.[75]

Fate. Estradiol is not orally active because of extensive and rapid first-pass metabolism with the exception of the micronized product in which decreased particle size augments absorption. Addition of ethinyl radical results in an orally active compound that is 15–20 times more active than estradiol. PO administration of 1 mg 17β estradiol yields 25 pg/ml; 2 mg yields 40 pg/ml; 4 mg yields 50 pg/ml.[75] By avoiding the first-pass effect, vaginal administration results in physiologic ratio of E_2 to E_1 over 1; 0.2 mg 17β estradiol yields E_2 levels of 60 ± 18 pg/ml.[77] See Notes. Estradiol is converted in the liver and intestine to estrone and its conjugates (primarily glucuronides and sulfates) and excreted in urine and feces. Less than 1% excreted unchanged in urine and 50–80% as conjugates (estrone 20%, estriol 20%, estradiol 7% as glucuronide).[71,75] Estradiol V_d is 10.9 ± 1.1 L; Cl is 27–37.5 L/hr/M^2.[78]

$t_{1/2}$. (Estradiol) 1 hr;[76] (ethinyl estradiol) 6–20 hr. See Oral Contraceptives.

Adverse Reactions. Pain at injection site occurs frequently. See Estrogens, Conjugated.

Contraindications. See Estrogens, Conjugated.

Precautions. See Estrogens, Conjugated.

Parameters to Monitor. See Estrogens, Conjugated.

Notes. Estradiol has been advocated as the estrogen replacement of choice because it is the principal estrogen of the reproductive years; however, advantages over other estrogens for this use have not been established. Vaginal administration, which results in a physiologic plasma level ratio of E_2 to E_1 may be the preferred route of estrogen replacement in select patients over oral administration of E_2 which results in an unphysiologic ratio of E_2 to E_1. Physiologic E_2 and E_1 levels are also achieved through use of smaller doses delivered continuously by injection, implant or the transdermal route.[78] Because transdermal administration of estradiol avoids the first-pass effect that affects oral estrogens, much lower total doses can be used. These lower doses appear to have the advantage of not causing certain physiologic alterations associated with oral estrogen therapy such as increases in renin substrate, sex hormone-binding globulin, thyroxine-binding globulin and cortisol-binding globulin. Conversely, the lower doses of transdermal estradiol do not have the favorable effects on low- and high-density lipoproteins of the oral estrogens. There are no studies that evaluate the long-term effects of estradiol patch use on bone loss or cardiovascular disease.[79-81] See Estrogens, Conjugated.

Estrogens, Conjugated

Premarin®, Various

Estrogens, Esterified

Estratab®, Menest®, Various

Pharmacology. Hormones capable of producing characteristic effects on specific tissues (such as breast) and causing proliferation of vaginal and uterine mucosa. Estrogens increase calcium deposition in bone and accelerate epiphyseal closing following initial growth stimulation.

Administration and Adult Dose. PO for postmenopausal symptoms and atrophic vaginitis use smallest effective dose in the range of 0.3–1.25 mg/day, in cycles of 21–25 days/month; **PO for prevention of postmenopausal osteoporosis** use minimum effective dose of 0.625 mg/day cyclically (possibly 0.3 mg/day if 1.5 g/day of elemental calcium is also used);[191] higher doses of 1.25 mg/day may be necessary following resultant fractures;[65,82] for patients with intact uterus, monthly administration of progestin is recommended to induce endometrial sloughing and decrease the risk of endometrial cancer.[65-67] For women experiencing migraine or other symptoms during the withdrawal period, a 5 day/week regimen or a shorter withdrawal period may be employed. **PO for dysfunctional uterine bleeding** 2.5–5 mg/day for 7–10 days, then decrease to 1.25 mg/day for 2 weeks with addition of progestin the third week. **PO to prevent postpartum lactation** (most effective given immediately postpartum before lactation begins) 3.75 mg q 4 hr for 5 doses or 1.25 mg q 4 hr for 5 days. **PO for palliation of prostatic cancer** 1.25–2.5 mg tid. **PO for palliation of breast cancer** (patients should be at least 5 yr postmenopause) 10 mg tid. **PO for emergency postcoital contraception** (within 72 hr of unprotected intercourse) 10 mg tid for 5 days.[70] **Vaginally for postmenopausal symptoms and/or atrophic vaginitis** 1.25–2.5 mg/day.[64] **IV for rapid cessation of dysfunctional uterine bleeding** 25 mg of conjugated estrogen q 6–12 hr until bleeding stops.[83]

Dosage Forms. Tab 0.3, 0.625, 0.9, 1.25, 2.5 mg; **Inj** 25 mg; **Vag Crm** 0.625 mg/g.

Patient Instructions. See Class Instructions, 68:12.

Pharmacokinetics. *Onset and Duration.* Onset of therapeutic E_2 levels after vaginal administration is 3 hr, peak of 6 hr with decline over 24 hr to baseline values. PO onset of equilin is 3 hr with a peak of 4 hr; onset of estrone is 3 hr with a peak of 5 hr; duration over 24 hr. Gonadotropin suppression occurs within one month of therapy, although suppression to premenopausal levels may not occur.[84]

Plasma Levels. See Estradiol and its Esters.

Fate. GI absorption of oral estrogens is complete. Both oral and vaginal administration result in an unphysiological E_1 to E_2 ratio over 1, although higher E_2 levels occur orally than vaginally.[85-88] PO (E_2 levels) 0.3 mg yields 20 pg/ml; 0.625 mg yields 50 pg/ml; 1.25 mg yields 35–70 pg/ml; 2.5 mg yields 160 pg/ml.[85,86] Vaginal (E_2 levels) 0.3 mg yields 4 pg/ml; 0.625 mg yields 13–29 pg/ml; 1.25 mg yields 25–27 pg/ml; 2.5 mg yields 32 pg/ml.[87,88] Systemic absorption of 0.3 mg vaginally is low compared to oral.[88] Both conjugated equilin and estrone sulfate are rapidly absorbed and hydrolyzed to unconjugated forms when given orally or vaginally. Wide distribution and concentration in fat.[84] Estrone sulfate is rapidly converted to estrone and estradiol. Inactivation of estrogens occurs mainly in the liver with degradation to less active estrogenic products such as estrone. Metabolites are conjugated with sulfate and glucuronic acid; 70–88% urinary recovery within 5 days after oral administration.[71,78] See Estradiol and its Esters.

Adverse Reactions. Nausea, vomiting, breast tenderness and spotting occur frequently—see Hormone Excess and Deficiency Symptomatology Comparison Chart. Increased risk of endometrial cancer with longer duration of use (over 3 yr), with higher doses and with unopposed estrogen stimulation. Small increase in breast cancer risk with over 15 yr of use.[89] Hypercalcemia occurs occasionally in patients with breast cancer. Thromboembolism, thrombophlebitis, diabetes, hypertension and gall bladder disease may occur—see Adverse Reactions of Oral Contraceptives Comparison Chart.

Contraindications. Pregnancy; history or presence of estrogen-dependent cancer (except in appropriate patients treated for metastatic disease); undiagnosed abnormal genital bleeding; history or presence of thromboembolism or severe thrombophlebitis; active or severe chronic liver disease.

Precautions. Use with caution in patients with disease states which may be exacerbated by increased fluid retention (eg, asthma, epilepsy, migraine and cardiac or renal dysfunction); in women with strong family history of breast cancer or presence of fibrocystic disease, fibroadenoma or abnormal mammogram; in women with fibromyomata, diabetes, hyperlipidemia, severe liver disease or history of jaundice during pregnancy; and in young patients in whom bone growth is not complete. Estrogen can increase thyroid binding globulin and cause false elevations in T_4 and false depression of resin T_3 uptake, while the thyroid index and the patient remain normal.

Parameters to Monitor. Signs and symptoms of side effects, especially abnormal bleeding. Pretreatment physical examination with reference to blood pressure, breasts, pelvic and Pap smear. Baseline laboratory should include glucose, triglycerides and cholesterol, liver function tests and calcium. Repeat examination every year.

Notes. Conjugated estrogens contain a mixture of 50–65% sodium estrone sulfate and 20–35% sodium equilin sulfate obtained from the urine of pregnant mares. Esterified estrogens are a combination of 75–85% sodium estrone sulfate and 6.5–15% sodium equilin sulfate. Postmenopausal women most likely to develop osteoporosis are whites, while blacks seem to be spared.[65-67]

Estrone and its Esters

Ogen®, Theelin®, Various

Pharmacology. Estrone (E_1) is the major estrogen produced in the postmenopausal period. It is one-half as potent as estradiol and shares the actions of other estrogens. See Estrogens, Conjugated.

Administration and Adult Dose. **PO for postmenopausal symptoms and prevention of osteoporosis** (estropipate) use smallest effective dose in the range of 0.625–2.5 mg/day in cycles of 21–25 days/month; administer as with conjugated estrogens.[64] **PO for suppression of postpartum lactation** (estropipate) most effective when given before lactation begins 4.5 mg q 4 hr for 4 doses. **PO for palliation of prostatic cancer** (estropipate) 3–6 mg tid. **PO for emergency postcoital contraception** (estropipate) within 72 hr of unprotected intercourse 5 mg tid for 5 days.[70] **Vaginally for postmenopausal symptoms and/or atrophic vaginitis** (estropipate) 3–8 mg/day. **IM for postmenopausal symptoms and prevention of osteoporosis** (estrone) when oral or vaginal therapy does not provide expected response, is poorly tolerated or when noncompliance occurs 0.1–2 mg weekly.

Dosage Forms. **Tab** (estropipate) 0.625, 1.25, 2.5, 5 mg; **Inj** (estrone) 2, 5 mg/ml; **Vag Crm** (estropipate) 1.5 mg/g.

Patient Instructions. See Class Instructions, 68:12.

Pharmacokinetics. *Fate.* Estrone is not orally active due to enzymatic degradation in the gut and liver. Addition of piperazine moiety increases oral efficacy and stability. Plasma E_2 levels attained after oral administration are similar to those after administration of 17β estradiol (E_2). See Estradiol and its Esters. Estrone is hydroxylated to α-hydroxyestrone, estriol and 2-hydroxyestrone.[71]

Adverse Reactions. See Estrogens, Conjugated.

Contraindications. See Estrogens, Conjugated.

Precautions. See Estrogens, Conjugated.

Parameters to Monitor. See Estrogens, Conjugated.

Notes. See Estrogens, Conjugated.

Estrogens Comparison Chart

DRUG	DOSAGE FORMS	EQUIPOTENT PHYSIOLOGIC DOSE[a,b]	COMMENTS
STEROIDAL AGENTS			
Conjugated Estrogens Premarin® Various	Tab 0.3, 0.625, 0.9, 1.25, 2.5 mg Vag Crm 0.625 mg/g Inj 25 mg.	0.625 mg.	Expensive; nausea is rare; contains mainly estrone.
Esterified Estrogens Estratab® Menest® Various	Tab 0.3, 0.625, 1.25, 2.5 mg.	0.625 mg.	
17β Estradiol, Micronized Estrace®	Tab 1, 2 mg Vag Crm 0.1 mg/g.	1 mg.	Moderate cost; some nausea with oral; pain at site of injection; variable onset with duration of 14–28 days with depot injections; estradiol is the major estrogen secreted during the reproductive years.
17β Estradiol Estraderm®	SR Patch 50, 100 mcg/day.	50 mcg/day.	
Estradiol Cypionate Depo-Estradiol® Various	Inj 1, 5 mg/ml in oil.	—	
Estradiol Valerate Delestrogen® Various	Inj 10, 20, 40 mg/ml in oil.	—	

Continued

Estrogens Comparison Chart

DRUG	DOSAGE FORMS	EQUIPOTENT PHYSIOLOGIC DOSE[a,b]	COMMENTS
Ethinyl Estradiol Estinyl® Feminone®	Tab 0.02, 0.05, 0.5 mg.	0.02 mg.	
Estrone Theelin® Various	Inj 2, 5 mg/ml.	0.9 mg.	No advantage over conjugated/esterified, except tasteless and no urine odor; estrone is the major estrogen of the postmenopausal years.
Estropipate Ogen® Various	Tab 0.625, 1.25, 2.5, 5 mg Vag Crm 1.5 mg/g.	1.5 mg (1.25 mg Ogen®).	Ogen® 0.625 mg = 0.75 mg estropipate. Ogen® 1.25 mg = 1.5 mg estropipate. Ogen® 2.5 mg = 3 mg estropipate. Ogen® 5 mg = 6 mg estropipate.
Polyestradiol Phosphate Estradurin®	Inj 20 mg/ml.	—	Indicated only in treatment of prostatic carcinoma.
Quinestrol Estrovis®	Tab 100 mcg.	—	Promoted for once-a-week estrogen therapy because it is stored in fat and gradually released.

Continued

Estrogens Comparison Chart

DRUG	DOSAGE FORMS	EQUIPOTENT PHYSIOLOGIC DOSE[a,b]	COMMENTS
NONSTEROIDAL AGENTS			
Chlorotrianisene Tace®	Cap 12, 25, 72 mg.	12 mg.	Expensive; weak estrogenic activity, metabolized by liver to a more active compound. Long duration of action because of storage in adipose tissue. Infrequently used because of long duration of activity.
Dienestrol Various	Vag Crm 0.01% Vag Supp 0.7 mg.	—	
Diethylstilbestrol Various	Tab 0.1, 0.25, 0.5, 1, 5 mg Vag Supp 0.1, 0.5 mg.	0.25 mg.	Inexpensive; frequent nausea, drug of choice for prostatic cancer, postcoital contraception, and breast cancer; may be less desirable for estrogen replacement because of its relationship to carcinogenicity.
Diethylstilbestrol Diphosphate Stilphostrol®	Tab 50 mg Inj 50 mg/ml.	0.4 mg.	

a. Potency of estrogens: estradiol > esterone > estriol.
b. See monographs or product information for exact dosing regimens for various uses.

68:20 ANTIDIABETIC AGENTS

68:20.08 INSULINS

General References: 132,133

Insulins

Pharmacology. Insulin promotes cellular uptake of glucose, fatty acids and amino acids and their conversion to storage forms in most tissues.

Administration and Adult Dose. Dosing must be adjusted in response to improvement of clinical symptoms and blood and urine glucose levels. For insulin-dependent diabetes mellitus, requirements may occasionally be as high as 200 units/day due to growth spurts. **Insulin resistance** is usually due to obesity, and weight reduction will improve insulin response.[111,112] Occasionally, resistance is due to insulin destruction at the injection site, and these patients can use only IV insulin; other patients require large doses (up to 200 units/day) due to a decrease in insulin action at the receptor.[112,113] When switching from conventional or "single-peak" insulins to the "highly purified" or human insulins, dosage may need to be reduced; however, in many patients no change is necessary.[114] **IV for diabetic ketoacidosis** 0.1 unit/kg bolus, followed by a continuous IV infusion of 2–3 units/hr. If the serum glucose does not decrease by 75 mg/dl in 1–2 hr, the infusion rate should be doubled. The dose is titrated in this manner to reverse the ketoacidosis. The usual infusion rate is 0.7 units/kg/hr or 5–10 units/hr.[115] This method is effective regardless of the route of administration (SC, IM or IV), but IV is preferred in patients in shock.[116]

Dosage Individualization. Insulin requirements may be decreased in patients with renal or hepatic impairment, or hypothyroidism. Requirements may be increased during pregnancy, especially in the second and third trimesters, in those with high fever, hyperthyroidism, severe infections, and following trauma or surgery.

Dosage Forms. See Insulins Comparison Chart.

Patient Instructions. Patients should be instructed in the following areas: use of insulin syringes and needles, storage and handling of insulin, urine ketone testing, blood glucose testing, adherence to proper diet and regular meals, personal hygiene (especially the feet), and recognition and treatment of hypoglycemia and hyperglycemia—see Sulfonylurea Agents.

Pharmacokinetics. *Onset and Duration.* See Insulins Comparison Chart.

Plasma Levels. Diabetics vary widely in their response to insulin; plasma levels are affected by obesity, diet, degree of activity, pancreatic beta cell activity, growth hormone and circulating antibodies.[117]

Fate. Insulin is primarily metabolized in the liver, although the kidneys appear to have a role in removal of about 18% of the daily insulin output.[118,119]

$t_{1/2}$. (Regular insulin) 4–5 min after IV administration.[120]

Adverse Reactions. Hypoglycemia is dose-related. Local allergic reactions, with an onset of 15 min–4 hr, are usually due to insulin impurities, and 70% of these patients have a history of interrupted treatment. Immune or non-immune insulin resistance occurs occasionally. Lipohypertrophy at the injection site may occur, especially with repeated use of the same site. Lipoatrophy may also occur at the injection site and may be less frequent with the highly purified insulins. Allergy, resistance and lipoatrophy may be overcome by switching to insulin from another animal source or to a more highly purified product (eg, human insulin). In general, pork insulin is less antigenic than beef-pork or pure beef insulin, because it is more structurally similar to human insulin.[113,114,121,122] Human insulin is the least immunogenic and is the insulin of choice for patients with insulin resistance, allergy, new insulin-dependent patients or any patient taking insulin intermittently.

Contraindications.   Hypersensitivity, although desensitization procedures may be warranted in some patients.[123,124]

Precautions. Use with caution in patients with renal or hepatic disease, or hypothyroidism. Insulin requirements may change when switching animal sources or to more purified products.

Parameters to Monitor. Blood glucose should be monitored frequently as a routine—see Blood Glucose Testing Systems Comparison Chart. Long-term diabetic control may best be monitored using hemoglobin A$_{1C}$.[101,102] Subjective symptoms of hypoglycemia and hyperglycemia should be continually monitored by the patient. Observe for signs of lipoatrophy and allergic reactions.

Notes. Insulin is stable for 6 months at constant room temperature and up to 24 months under refrigeration.[125] Insulin adsorbs to glass and plastic IV infusion equipment, with little difference between glass and plastic; maximal adsorption occurs within 15 seconds.[126,127] Adsorption may be minimized by the addition of small amounts (1–2%) of albumin to the infusion container,[126] however, this may be costly and unnecessary because patient response is generally adequate without addition of albumin. Variation can be minimized by flushing all new IV administration equipment with 50 ml of the insulin-containing solution (thereby saturating "binding sites") before it is used.[128]

Pump devices are available to deliver insulin dependently or independently of a measured serum glucose level. "Open-loop" devices can deliver insulin at a constant rate and can be manually controlled. "Closed-loop" devices (the "artificial pancreas") can deliver insulin at variable rates in response to serum glucose. Although the open-loop devices have been used successfully in selected patients, few physicians are placing patients on the pumps due to concern with infection at the injection site, hypoglycemia and relatively high cost.[129-131]

Biosynthetic "human" insulin has been produced by Eli Lilly using recombinant DNA technology. In one double-blind, crossover comparison, requirements of biosynthetic insulin were found to be approximately equal to bovine insulin. Slightly greater doses of biosynthetic insulin were required in patients who were previously stabilized on purified pork insulin. This difference is thought to be due to slightly faster absorption of the biosynthetic insulin from subcutaneous injection sites, resulting in a slightly more rapid onset and shorter duration than with purified pork. No differences in side effects or long-term control of diabetics have been identified between biosynthetic human insulin and highly purified animal insulins.[132] Now available as Humulin®R, Humulin®N, Humulin®L and Humulin®U from Eli Lilly.

Human insulin that is produced by converting pork insulin to human insulin is available from Squibb-Novo as Novolin®R, Novolin®N, and Novolin®L, and from Nordisk as Velosulin® Human and Insulatard® Human. These insulins are referred to as semi-synthetic human insulins.

Insulins Comparison Chart[a]

PRODUCT AND MANUFACTURER	ANIMAL SOURCE AND STRENGTHS (UNITS/ML)	PURITY PRO-INSULIN[b] (PPM)	ONSET[c] (HOURS)	PEAK[c] (HOURS)	DURATION[c] (HOURS)	MIXING COMPATIBILITIES[d]
RAPID-ACTING						
Insulin Injection (Regular)			0.5-1	1-5	5-8	
Humulin® BR (Lilly)	Biosynthetic Human-100	—	e	e	e	For pump use only; do not mix with other insulins.
Humulin® R (Lilly)	Biosynthetic Human-100	—	e	e	e	Mixtures with NPH may result in less regular action; lente mixtures result in regular result in shorter action of lente.
Iletin® I Regular (Lilly)	Beef/Pork-40, 100	10				See Humulin® R above.
Iletin® II Regular (Lilly)	Beef-100	1				See Humulin® R above.
Iletin® II Regular (Lilly)	Pork-100, 500	1				See Humulin® R above.
Novolin® R (Squibb-Novo)	Semisynthetic Human-100	1	e	e	e	See Humulin® R above.
Purified Regular (Squibb-Novo)	Pork-100	1				See Humulin® R above.
Regular Insulin (Squibb-Novo)	Pork-100	10				See Humulin® R above.
Velosulin® (Nordisk)	Pork-100	1				Phosphate buffers used in Velosulin® are incompatible with lente insulins. Stable when mixed with Nordisk's NPH.
Velosulin® Human (Nordisk)	Semisynthetic Human-100	1	e	e	e	See Velosulin® above.

Continued

Insulins Comparison Chart[a]

PRODUCT AND MANUFACTURER	ANIMAL SOURCE AND STRENGTHS (UNITS/ML)	PURITY PRO-INSULIN[b] (PPM)	ONSET[c] (HOURS)	PEAK[c] (HOURS)	DURATION[c] (HOURS)	MIXING COMPATIBILITIES[d]
Prompt Insulin Zinc Suspension (Semilente)			0.5–3	2–10	12–16	
Iletin® I (Lilly)	Beef/Pork-40, 100	10				Regular, lentes; premixture with other lentes stable indefinitely.
Purified Semilente (Squibb-Novo)	Pork-100	1				See Iletin® I above.
Semilente (Squibb-Novo)	Beef-100	10				See Iletin® I above.
INTERMEDIATE-ACTING						
Isophane Insulin Suspension (NPH)			1–4	4–12	24–28	
Humulin® N (Lilly)	Biosynthetic Human-100	—	e	e	e	Regular and NPH interact after 5 min to form a mixture that is less rapid acting than antici-
Iletin® I (Lilly)	Beef/Pork-40, 100	10				pated; after 30 min the mixture is stable.
Iletin® II (Lilly)	Beef or Pork-100	1				
Insulatard® (Nordisk)	Semisynthetic Human or Pork-100	1	e	e	e	Velosulin® with Insulatard® forms a stable mixture; less
Novolin® N (Squibb-Novo)	Semisynthetic Human-100	1	e	e	e	excess protamine or zinc than other brands.
NPH (Squibb-Novo)	Beef-100	10				
Purified NPH (Squibb-Novo)	Pork-100	1				

Continued

Insulins Comparison Chart[a]

PRODUCT AND MANUFACTURER	ANIMAL SOURCE AND STRENGTHS (UNITS/ML)	PURITY PRO-INSULIN[b] (PPM)	ONSET[c] (HOURS)	PEAK[c] (HOURS)	DURATION[c] (HOURS)	MIXING COMPATIBILITIES[d]
Mixtard® (Nordisk)	Pork-100	1				A mixture of 30% Velosulin® and 70% Insulatard®.
Novolin® 70/30 (Squibb-Novo)	Semisynthetic Human-100	1	e	e	e	A mixture of 30% Novolin® R and 70% Novolin® N.
Insulin Zinc Suspension (Lente; 70% Ultralente + 30% Semilente)			1-3	6-15	22-28	
Humulin® L (Lilly)	Biosynthetic Human-100	—	e	e	e	Can mix with any of the other lente type insulins; do not mix with Velosulin®; lente plus regular immediately combine to form a mixture that has a shorter duration than expected; mixture is stable for 2-3 months.
Iletin® I (Lilly)	Beef/Pork-40, 100	10				
Iletin® II (Lilly)	Beef or Pork-100	1				
Novolin® L (Squibb-Novo)	Semisynthetic Human-100	1	e	e	e	
Purified (Squibb-Novo)	Pork-100	1				
Standard Lente (Squibb-Novo)	Beef-100	10				
LONG-ACTING						
Protamine Zinc Insulin Suspension (PZI)			1-6	14-24	36 +	
Iletin® I (Lilly)	Beef/Pork-40, 100	10				May mix with regular, but such mixtures are unpredictable, depending on ratios, and offer no advantages.
Iletin® II (Lilly)	Beef or Pork-100	1				

Continued

Insulins Comparison Chart[a]

PRODUCT AND MANUFACTURER	ANIMAL SOURCE AND STRENGTHS (UNITS/ML)	PURITY PRO-INSULIN[b] (PPM)	ONSET[c] (HOURS)	PEAK[c] (HOURS)	DURATION[c] (HOURS)	MIXING COMPATIBILITIES[d]
Extended Insulin Zinc Suspension (Ultralente)						
Iletin® I (Lilly)	Beef/Pork-40, 100	10	2–8	10–30	36 +	Can be mixed with semilente, lente or regular. Stable indefinitely after mixing.
Purified (Squibb-Novo)	Beef-100	1				
Ultralente (Squibb-Novo)	Beef-100	10				
Humulin® U	Biosynthetic Human-100	—	2–6	7–10	24–26	

a. From references 107, 133 and product information.

b. Other contaminants, such as glucagon-like substances, pancreatic polypeptide, somatostatin and vasoactive intestinal polypeptides, may also be present; levels of these are low in highly purified insulin products.

c. There may be variations within this range among manufacturers; onset and duration may be prolonged in long-standing diabetes and large doses may have prolonged duration of action. Site of injection, depth of injection and whether site is exercised, massaged or has heat applied to it also affects rate of insulin absorption.

d. It is recommended that insulins from different manufacturers not be mixed, due to differences in preservatives, buffers and excess amounts of zinc and protamine.

e. Human insulins have a slightly more rapid onset and a shorter duration of action than animal-derived insulins.

68:20.20 SULFONYLUREAS

Sulfonylurea Agents

Pharmacology. These agents acutely enhance insulin secretion from the pancreatic beta cells and potentiate insulin action on several extrahepatic tissues. Chronically, sulfonylureas increase peripheral utilization of glucose, suppress hepatic gluconeogenesis and possibly increase the sensitivity and/or number of peripheral insulin receptors. In addition, acetohexamide has significant uricosuric activity.[90,96]

Administration and Adult Dose. See Sulfonylurea Agents Comparison Chart.

Dosage Individualization. Dosing alterations of all sulfonylureas may be necessary in patients with severe hepatic dysfunction. With renal disease, especially in geriatric patients, there is an increased duration of action with chlorpropamide and acetohexamide.

Dosage Forms. See Sulfonylurea Agents Comparison Chart.

Patient Instructions. Approved diets should be consistent on a day-to-day basis. Medication should be taken at the same time each morning. Factors which might alter blood glucose levels (eg, infection, fasting states) as well as any side effects should be reported.

Pharmacokinetics. See Sulfonylurea Agents Comparison Chart.
   Plasma Levels. Vary due to rates and completeness of absorption, differing rates of metabolism, renal clearance and degree of protein binding.[90]
   $t_{1/2}$. See Sulfonylurea Agents Comparison Chart—acetohexamide and chlorpropamide half-lives may be prolonged in patients with renal failure.[90,97,98]

Adverse Reactions. Anorexia, nausea, vomiting, diarrhea, allergic skin reactions and hypoglycemic reactions (especially with chlorpropamide) occur occasionally. Hematologic disorders, mild disulfiram-like reaction to alcohol, hyponatremia (most common with chlorpropamide, may occur with tolbutamide), hepatic damage, cholestatic jaundice and bone marrow suppression occur rarely.

Contraindications. Pregnancy; insulin-dependent diabetes; juvenile, unstable or brittle diabetes; diabetes complicated by acidosis, ketosis, diabetic coma, major surgery, severe infection or severe trauma.

Precautions. Although controversial, the data of University Group Diabetes Program (UGDP) suggest that obese patients with mild adult-onset diabetes who are not insulin-dependent are more likely to die from cardiovascular complications when taking fixed doses of tolbutamide than if they relied on diet alone or on insulin.[99] Criticism of the UGDP study has been made.[100] Displacement from protein occurs with high-dose salicylates, phenylbutazone and sulfonamides. Drugs which impair glucose tolerance include oral contraceptives, corticosteroids, thiazides, furosemide, thyroid hormones (large doses) and niacin.[100] Acute ingestion of alcohol produces hypoglycemia, but chronically, it increases metabolism of sulfonylureas.[90] See also Drug Interactions chapter.

Parameters to Monitor. Clinical symptoms of hyperglycemia (mainly polyphagia, polyuria, polydipsia, numbing and/or tingling of feet) and/or hypoglycemia (hunger, nervousness, warmth, sweating, palpitations, headaches, confusion, drowsiness, anxiety, blurred vision and/or paresthesias of lips). Fasting serum glucose levels should be monitored frequently at the initiation of therapy to gauge the adequacy of the dose. Self-monitoring of fasting and selected postprandial blood glucose levels by the patient is also helpful—see Blood Glucose Testing Systems Comparison Chart. Long-term diabetic control may best be monitored using hemoglobin A$_{1c}$.[101,102]

Glyburide

DiaBeta®,
Micronase®

Glyburide is a "second-generation" sulfonylurea with a mechanism of action similar to the older sulfonylureas; in addition, it probably produces a release of an insulinotropic hormone from the gut which stimulates pancreatic beta cells. Second-generation agents have a greater milligram potency than earlier agents, but their maximal effect is essentially the same. The frequency of side effects in general is lower with the newer agents. Most notably absent are the flushing reaction with alcohol, hyponatremia, and a lack of drug-drug interactions with phenylbutazone, salicylates and warfarin. Because of their potency, it is important that these agents be used with caution in elderly or debilitated patients. Other "second-generation" agents include **glipizide, gliclazide, glisoxepide, glibornuride, gliquidone** and the nonsulfonylureas, **glymidine** and **glycodiazine.** Glyburide is relatively short-acting with low doses, but intermediate acting at higher doses. It is primarily metabolized to inactive metabolites, but a clinically insignificant amount of a compound with 1/6th the potency of the parent drug is also formed. Essentially no drug is excreted unchanged in the urine, and dosage modification is unnecessary in renal impairment. For the purpose of conversion among sulfonylureas, equivalent doses are approximately as follows: tolbutamide 500 mg, chlorpropamide 125 mg, glyburide 2.5 mg and glipizide 5 mg. The dose of glyburide is 1.25-20 mg/day in one or two doses. It is available as 1.25, 2.5 and 5 mg tablets.[90,92-95]

Sulfonylurea Agents Comparison Chart[a]

DRUG	DOSAGE FORMS	DAILY DOSAGE[b]	FATE	HALF-LIFE (HOURS)	DURATION (HOURS)
Acetohexamide Dymelor® Various	Tab 250, 500 mg.	250 mg–1.5 g in 2 divided doses.	60% converted to active metabolites; excreted by kidney.	Parent 1.6 Metabolite 5.3	8–12 +
Chlorpropamide Diabinese® Various	Tab 100, 250 mg.	100–500 mg in 1 dose.	Metabolized, as well as 20% excreted unchanged.	25–42 (average 33; urine pH-dependent)	24–72
Glipizide[c] Glucotrol®	Tab 5, 10 mg.	2.5–40 mg in 1–2 divided doses.	Converted to inactive metabolites.	3.3	6–12
Glyburide DiaBeta® Micronase®	Tab 1.25, 2.5, 5 mg.	1.25–20 mg in 1–2 divided doses.	Converted mostly to inactive metabolites.	10	24
Tolazamide Tolinase® Various	Tab 100, 250, 500 mg.	100 mg–1 g in 1–2 divided doses.	Slow absorption and onset; metabolized to partially active metabolites.	7	10–15
Tolbutamide Orinase® Various	Tab 250, 500 mg.	500 mg–2 g in 2–3 divided doses.	Converted to inactive metabolites.	5.6	6–12

a. From references 90, 91, 93, 95, 96, 98, 103-105.

b. Except for chlorpropamide, divided doses should be used when higher doses are required; highest dose listed represents the maximum recommended daily dosage.

c. The only sulfonylurea that must be taken on an empty stomach.

68:20.92 MISCELLANEOUS ANTIDIABETIC AGENTS

Aldose Reductase Inhibitors

With prolonged hyperglycemia causing excess flux of glucose into tissues, glucose is shunted to the polyol pathway, resulting in excess sorbitol production. The excess sorbitol is thought to be a cause of neuropathy, collagen disorders, cataracts and possibly retinopathy in diabetics. Since aldose reductase is the enzyme responsible for this conversion of glucose to sorbitol, aldose reductase inhibitors are being studied in diabetics as a possible means of decreasing the various sorbitol-linked sequelae of diabetes. While this is a promising class of drugs, the side effects, dosing regimens and long-term benefits are yet to be determined. **Tolrestat** (Alredase® - Investigational - Ayerst) has a serum half-life of 10–13 hours and has been used investigationally in doses of 100 mg bid. **Sorbinil** (Investigational - Pfizer) is chemically similar to phenytoin and has similar adverse reactions. About 10% of patients have had allergic reactions, including fevers and myalgias. It has a half-life of 35–52 hours and has been used investigationally in doses of 200–250 mg/day.[134-137]

Blood Glucose Testing Systems Comparison Chart[a]

NAME AND MANUFACTURER	METHOD OF READING	NO. OF TEST PADS ON A STRIP	PROCEDURE[b]	RANGE (MG/DL)	COMPATIBLE METERS
Betascan (OMI)® (Orange Medical Instruments)	Visually or with meter (can use 'dry wipe' process with Glucometer).	1	Blood on strip for 60 sec, blot off with blotter paper or rinse with water.	0–300	Glucometer, Betascan.
Chemstrip® bG (Biodynamics)	Visually or in meter.	2[c]	Blood on strip for 60 sec, wipe with cotton ball, wait 60 sec. For visual: if 240, wait 60 sec more, then compare color again. Color or shades: light tan to dark blue.	20–800	Accu-chek bG, Glucochek,[d] Glucokey,[d] Betascan.[d]
Dextrostix® (Ames)	Primarily for meter readings.	1	Blood on strip 60 sec, then rinse with water, blot.	—	Glucometer, Dextrometer, Eyetone, Glucochek,[d] Betascan,[d] Glucokey.[d]
Glucoscan® Test Strips (LifeScan)	Meter only.	1	Blood on strip 60 sec, blot with blotter paper (strip read by meter after 60 sec). Strips individually foil wrapped.	—	Glucoscan Plus, Glucoscan 2000, Glucoscan 3000.

Continued

Blood Glucose Testing Systems Comparison Chart[a]

NAME AND MANUFACTURER	METHOD OF READING	NO. OF TEST PADS ON A STRIP	PROCEDURE[b]	RANGE (MG/DL)	COMPATIBLE METERS
Glucoscan/GM® Test Strips (LifeScan)	Meter only.	1	Can use 'dry wipe' process; blood on strip 60 sec, blot with blotter paper, read in meter after 60 sec. Comes with calibration strips.	—	Glucometer.
Glucostix® (Ames)	Visually or in meter.	2[e]	Visual: blood on strip 30 sec, blot with tissue or cotton ball, wait 90 sec. Color shades: green (top pad); peach-brick (bottom-pad). Meter: blood on strip 30 sec, blot with tissue or cotton ball, read in meter after 50 sec.	—	Glucometer II, Glucometer II with Memory.
Kyodex® (Kyoto Diagnostics)	Visually or with meter.	2	Blood on strip 60 sec, blot with blotter paper or rinse with water.	0–300	Betascan, Glucometer.
Trendstrips® (Orange Medical Instruments)	Visually or with meter.	2[c]	Blood on strip 60 sec, wipe with cotton ball or tissue. Visual: compare	—	TrendsMeter.

Continued

Blood Glucose Testing Systems Comparison Chart[a]

NAME AND MANUFACTURER	METHOD OF READING	NO. OF TEST PADS ON A STRIP	PROCEDURE[b]	RANGE (MG/DL)	COMPATIBLE METERS
			with chart after 120 sec. Color shades: blue and green. Meter: press button after 120 sec.		
Visidex II[®] (Ames)	Visual only.	2[e]	Blood on strip 30 sec, blot with tissue or cotton ball, wait 90 sec. Color shades: green (top pad); peach-brick (bottom pad).	—	—

a. From references 106–110 and product information.
b. Time given before insertion into meter refers here to total time elapsed.
c. Two pads read simultaneously.
d. Pads read one at a time—the first, for values of 20–140 mg/dl; the second, 140–800 mg/dl.
e. One pad is used for values 20–110 mg/dl; the other for values 140–800 mg/dl.

NOTE: When testing capillary whole blood using the glucose oxidase products described here, a nondiabetic blood glucose level would be 70–140 mg/dl before meals and at bedtime; 2 hour post-prandial levels would be <140–160 mg/dl. There have been no reports of drug interactions altering the accuracy of home blood glucose monitoring, as have been reported with home urine glucose monitoring. Products for blood glucose testing are being developed and/or changed frequently; thus, this list does not represent an exhaustive description of these items. In addition, the manufacturer's directions for use should be reviewed before advising patients on the use of a product.

68:32 PROGESTINS

General References: 138

Medroxyprogesterone Acetate

Depo-Provera®,
Provera®, Various

Pharmacology. A 17-α-acetoxy progesterone derivative. Progesterone transforms an estrogen-primed proliferative endometrium into a secretory endometrium. Progestin-only contraceptives alter the cervical mucus, exert a progestational effect on the endometrium which interferes with implantation, and in some patients, suppresses ovulation.

Administration and Adult Dose. **PO for secondary amenorrhea, dysfunctional uterine bleeding and to induce withdrawal bleeding following postmenopausal estrogen replacement therapy** 5–10 mg/day, depending on degree of endometrial stimulation desired, administered for 5–10 days beginning on the presumed 16th–21st day of cycle (during 3rd week of estrogen administration). In cases of secondary amenorrhea, therapy can be started at any time. **PO for relief of vasomotor symptoms** 20 mg/day; **IM for relief of vasomotor symptoms** 150 mg/day.[139-141] **PO for endometriosis** 10 mg tid for 6–9 months; **IM for endometriosis** 100 mg q 2 weeks for 4 doses, then 100 mg/month for 4 months. **IM for contraception** 150 mg q 3 months;[142,143] **IM for palliation of metastatic endometrial cancer** 400 mg–1 g/week initially, then maintenance dose of 400 mg q month.

Dosage Forms. **Tab** 2.5, 5, 10 mg; **Inj** 100, 400 mg/ml.

Patient Instructions. See Class Instructions, 68:12.

Pharmacokinetics. *Onset and Duration.* Withdrawal bleeding (in estrogen-primed endometrium) occurs 2–7 days after last dose.[138,143] Onset of symptomatic relief of hot flashes within 4–7 days; maximum relief after 1 month; duration 8–20 weeks after discontinuation.[140,141] Duration 3 months or longer when given IM for contraception.[138,142,143]

Fate. Peak levels of medroxyprogesterone occur within a few days of 150 mg IM injection and range between 2 and 12 ng/ml (average 7).[142] E_2 and E_1 levels less than 10 pg/ml. Metabolized by hydroxylation; 20–42% of dose is excreted as glucuronide and sulfate conjugates in urine; 5–13% of dose is excreted in feces.

$t_{1/2}$. α phase 52 min; β phase 3.8 hr; biological half-life 14.5 hr.[143]

Adverse Reactions. See Hormone Excess and Deficiency Symptomatology Comparison Chart. Menstrual irregularities and breakthrough bleeding are very frequent in the first 3 months after IM injection; amenorrhea and infertility (up to 18 months), weight gain, malignant breast nodules in beagle dogs, masculinization of female fetus and congenital anomalies when taken during pregnancy occur.[143]

Contraindications. Pregnancy; presence or history of thrombophlebitis, thromboembolism or stroke; liver dysfunction; known or suspected malignancy of breast or genital organs; undiagnosed vaginal bleeding; missed abortion; as a diagnostic test for pregnancy.

Precautions. Use with caution in patients with a history of depression, diabetes or conditions worsened by fluid retention (eg, epilepsy, migraine, asthma and cardiac or renal dysfunction).

Parameters to Monitor. Pretreatment physical examination with special reference to breast and pelvic organs and Pap smear.

Notes. Concurrent administration of estrogen with progestin may be associated with less breakthrough bleeding than with progestin alone for amenorrhea. IM administration for contraception is not approved in US, but may be a useful alternative for women who cannot use other methods.[138] There is inadequate evidence that progestins are effective in preventing habitual abortion or treating threatened abortion; furthermore, progestins may be harmful to the fetus during the first 4 months of pregnancy.

Norethindrone   Nor-Q.D.®, Micronor®, Norlutin®
Norethindrone Acetate   Aygestin®, Norlutate®

Pharmacology.   Norethindrone and norethindrone acetate are 19-nortestosterone derivatives which share the actions of progestins. Norethindrone acetate differs from norethindrone only in potency; the acetate is twice as potent. See Medroxyprogesterone Acetate.

Administration and Adult Dose. **PO for contraception** (norethindrone) 0.35 mg/day continuously, starting on the first day of menses or immediately postpartum. **PO for dysfunctional uterine bleeding** (norethindrone) 5 mg (norethindrone acetate) 2.5 mg qid for 5 days to stop bleeding; on 5th day decrease dose to 5–20 mg/day of norethindrone or 2.5–10 mg/day of norethindrone acetate and maintain for 21 days to prevent recurrence. **PO for secondary amenorrhea or withdrawal bleeding following postmenopausal estrogen therapy** (norethindrone) 5–20 mg/day (norethindrone acetate) 2.5–10 mg/day starting on the 15th–20th day of the cycle and continued for 10 or 5 days, respectively. In cases of secondary amenorrhea, therapy can be started at any time. **PO for endometriosis** (norethindrone) 10 mg/day (norethindrone acetate) 5 mg/day for 2 weeks, increased in 10 mg/day increments (norethindrone acetate—5 mg/day) q 2 weeks, until maintenance dose of 30 mg/day of norethindrone or 15 mg/day of norethindrone acetate is reached.

Dosage Forms. (Norethindrone) **Tab** 0.35 mg (Micronor®, Nor-Q.D.®); 5 mg (Norlutin®). (Norethindrone acetate) **Tab** 5 mg (Aygestin®, Norlutate®).

Patient Instructions. See Class Instructions, 68:12.

Pharmacokinetics. *Onset and Duration.* Acute bleeding should decrease in 1–2 days and stop in 3–4 days. Withdrawal bleeding occurs in 2–7 days after last dose; onset of contraception after 1 week of therapy.
  Fate. Norethindrone acetate is rapidly converted to norethindrone in vivo. Rapidly and completely absorbed, but only 47–73% (average 65) bioavailability due to first-pass effect.[52,53] Peak plasma levels occur in 0.5–4 hr, are dose-dependent and exhibit considerable interindividual variation. Distributed into fat with minimal amounts detected in breast milk. 50–70% recovered in the urine over 5–7 days as the conjugated glucuronide (25%) and sulfate (40%); less than 5% is excreted as unchanged norethindrone; V_d is 3.6–4.3 L/kg. Cl is 23 L/hr.[52,53]
  $t_{1/2}$. (Norethindrone) 5–14 hr;[52,53] (metabolites) 42–84 hr.[57]

Adverse Reactions. See Medroxyprogesterone Acetate.

Contraindications. See Medroxyprogesterone Acetate.

Precautions. See Medroxyprogesterone Acetate.

Parameters to Monitor. See Medroxyprogesterone Acetate.

Notes.   Contraceptive efficacy is 2.54 pregnancies/100 woman years. Progestin-only contraceptives are the drugs of choice for contraception during breast feeding or in patients with contraindications to estrogen therapy; see Oral Contraceptive Agents Comparison Chart.

Progesterone
Hydroxyprogesterone Caproate

Various
Various

Pharmacology. Progesterone is the natural hormone which induces secretory changes in the endometrium, relaxes uterine smooth muscle and maintains pregnancy. Esterification produces a more potent compound, hydroxyprogesterone caproate.

Administration and Adult Dose. IM for secondary amenorrhea and dysfunctional uterine bleeding (progesterone) 5–10 mg/day for 6–8 days; (hydroxyprogesterone caproate) 375 mg, may repeat in 4 weeks prn. **IM for palliation of metastatic endometrial cancer** (hydroxyprogesterone caproate) 500 mg–1 g 2–3 times/week.

Dosage Forms. Inj (progesterone) 25, 50, mg/ml; (progesterone in oil) 25, 50, 100 mg/ml; (hydroxyprogesterone caproate in oil) 125, 250 mg/ml.

Patient Instructions. Bleeding should stop in a few days after injection; expect a normal period after a few days. The first 48 hr of menses may be excessive, but of normal duration. See also Class Instructions, 68:12.

Pharmacokinetics. *Onset and Duration.* Onset of withdrawal bleeding 2–6 days after IM progesterone and 2 weeks after IM hydroxyprogesterone caproate; duration 12–24 hr with progesterone, 9–17 days with hydroxyprogesterone caproate.

Fate. Rapidly metabolized, reduced and hydroxylated in the gut and liver after oral administration with formation of active metabolites 20-α-hydroxy-4-pregene-3-one, 17-α-hydroxyprogesterone and deoxycorticosterone (a potent mineralocorticoid).[144] Plasma levels of progesterone after oral administration increase rapidly to reach luteal phase values within 1–4 hr and remain elevated after 12 hr.[144] Higher levels of active metabolites occur after IM administration, because gut and liver first-pass effects are avoided. Urinary excretion is 50–60% as pregnanediol and isomers conjugated with glucuronic acid or sulfate; 5–10% excreted in feces.

Adverse Reactions. Local reaction and swelling at the site of progesterone injection. See Medroxyprogesterone Acetate.

Contraindications. See Medroxyprogesterone Acetate.

Precautions. See Medroxyprogesterone Acetate.

Parameters to Monitor. See Medroxyprogesterone Acetate.

Notes. Aqueous injections of progesterone are very irritating and should not be used.

68:36 THYROID AND ANTITHYROID AGENTS

68:36.04 THYROID AGENTS

General References: 145,167

Class Instructions. This medication must be taken regularly to maintain proper hormone levels in the body. Report immediately if chest pain (especially in elderly patients), palpitations, sweating, nervousness or other signs of overactivity occur. Take any missed dose as soon as it is remembered, but if more than one dose is missed, do not double up doses.

Levothyroxine Sodium

Levothroid®, Synthroid®,
Various

Pharmacology. A synthetically prepared hormone identical to the thyroid hormone, T_4. Thyroid hormones are responsible for normal growth, development and energy metabolism.

Administration and Adult Dose. PO for replacement in relatively acute hypothyroidism 50–100 mcg/day initially, increasing if needed and tolerated in 25–50 mcg/day increments at 4 week intervals to a maintenance dose of 75–150 mcg/day to normalize TSH. The usual dosage requirement is 1.2–2.1 (average 1.7) mcg/kg/day.[146,189] Poorly compliant young patients have been maintained on a once-a-week dosing regimen; however, this regimen may be dangerous in cardiac patients.[147] IV for myxedema coma 200–500 mcg or 300 mcg/M^2 initially, then 100–300 mcg in 24 hr; use smaller doses in cardiovascular disease.[149] IM indicated only for replacement therapy if patient cannot take oral medication; parenteral dose is about 80% of oral dose due to bioavailability differences.[189]

Dosage Individualization. In the elderly, patients with cardiovascular disease and those with severe, long-standing myxedema, PO 12.5–25 mcg/day initially, then increase if tolerated in 4–6 weeks by 12.5–25 mcg/day to a maintenance dose necessary to normalize TSH. In the elderly, a lower maintenance dose of 75–100 mcg/day (1.6 mcg/kg/day) is sufficient.[150-152] In patients with cardiovascular disease, particularly angina, increments should be titrated against exacerbation of angina and maintenance of euthyroidism. In some patients with severe coronary disease, incomplete control of hypothyroidism may be necessary to prevent further exacerbation of angina.[153] In pregnancy, usually no dosage adjustment in replacement therapy is necessary.

Pediatric Dose. PO for hypothyroidism (preterm infants and infants at risk for cardiac disease) 25 mcg/day initially, increasing to 50 mcg/day in 4–6 weeks; (full-term neonate to 1 yr) 25–50 mcg/day (average 37.5) initially;[154] (over 1 yr) 3–5 mcg/kg/day (average 3.5).[155] Adjust maintenance dose on the basis of growth, development, T_4 and TSH values.

Dosage Forms. Tab 25, 50, 75, 100, 125, 150, 175, 200, 300 mcg; Inj 200, 500 mcg.

Patient Instructions. See Class Instructions.

Pharmacokinetics. *Onset and Duration.* PO onset 3–5 days; duration after cessation of therapy 7–10 days. IV onset in myxedema coma 6–8 hr, maximum effect in 1 day.[145]

  Plasma Levels. 6–17 mcg/dl (T_4 range in treated patients may be higher than normal, but the serum T_3 is normal).[145,156,157] Many drugs, pathological and physiological states affect binding and, hence, may affect results of some plasma level determinations.[158]

  Fate. Oral bioavailability averages 80% and is affected by many factors (eg, malabsorption, diet, cholesterol-binding resins).[159,160,189] Only 0.03% is unbound in plasma. About 80% is deiodinated in the body; 35% is peripherally converted to the more active T_3 and 45% to inactive reverse T_3.[181] Another 15–20% is conjugated in the liver to form glucuronides and sulfates which undergo an enterohepatic recirculation with reabsorption or excretion in the feces.[158,160] V_d is 10–12 L;[160] fractional turnover rate is 10%/24 hr.[158,160]

  $t_{1/2}$. Euthyroid 6.5–7 days,[162] may increase to 9–10 days in hypothyroidism, decrease to 3–4 days in hyperthyroidism. Protein binding affects half-life (increased binding retards elimination and decreased binding increases elimination).[158]

Adverse Reactions. All are dose-related and can be avoided by increasing the initial dose slowly to the minimum effective maintenance dose. Signs of overdosage include headache, palpitations, chest pain, heat intolerance, sweating, leg cramps, weight loss, diarrhea, vomiting and nervousness.

Contraindications. Thyrotoxicosis; acute myocardial infarction; uncorrected adrenal insufficiency.

Precautions. Initiate and increase dosage with caution in patients with cardiovascular disease, the elderly and in long-standing hypothyroidism. In myxedema coma, corticosteroids should be given concurrently.[149] The status of other metabolic diseases, including diabetes, adrenal insufficiency, hyperadrenalism and panhypopituitarism may be affected by changes in thyroid status. Drugs such as phenytoin and cholestyramine may increase thyroxine requirements while others (eg, digoxin, warfarin, insulin) may be altered by changing thyroid status.[145,158]

Parameters to Monitor. Free T_4, T_3, TSH and clinical status of the patient q 4-6 weeks initially. After stabilized, monitor free T_4, TSH and clinical status at 6-12 month intervals; in children, q 4 weeks initially and q 3-4 months after stabilization. In congenital hypothyroidism free T_4 should be monitored, because TSH may remain elevated despite adequate replacement doses.[163] In patients over 40 yr, the replacement dosage of thyroxine should be evaluated every year and adjusted downward, as necessary, because dosage requirements decrease with age.[150-152]

Notes. Drug of choice for thyroid replacement because of purity, standardization, long half-life, large body pool and close simulation to normal physiologic hormone levels. Protect from light. Significant bioinequivalence between generic products has been reported, although the reformulated Synthroid® and Levothroid® are similar, but not bioequivalent.[164,189] It should be noted that Synthroid® was reformulated in 1982 so that a 20-30% reduction in previously recommended dosage requirements is necessary.[146,157,189] Physiologic doses of thyroid hormones in euthyroid patients are ineffective for weight reduction; larger doses may result in toxicity. See Thyroid Replacement Products Comparison Chart.

Liothyronine Sodium   Cytomel®, Various

Pharmacology. A synthetically prepared hormone identical to the thyroid hormone T_3, which is 4 times as potent as T_4. See Levothyroxine.

Administration and Adult Dose. **PO for mild hypothyroidism** 25 mcg/day initially, increasing, if tolerated, in 12.5-25 mcg/day increments at 1-2 week intervals to a maintenance dose of 25-75 mcg/day to normalize TSH. **PO for severe hypothyroidism** 5 mcg/day initially, increasing in 5-10 mcg/day increments at 1-2 week intervals until 25 mcg/day is reached, then increase in 12.5-25 mcg/day increments at 1-2 week intervals until euthyroid. Dividing daily dosage into 2-3 doses may prevent wide plasma level fluctuations.[146,165] **IV for myxedema coma** 200 mcg initially, then 25 mcg q 6-12 hr. A way to prepare IV liothyronine from tablets has been published.[180] **PO for T_3 suppression test** 75-100 mcg/day for 7 days, then repeat ^{131}I thyroid uptake test.

Dosage Individualization. In the elderly and those with cardiovascular disease, start at PO 5 mcg/day and increase in 5 mcg/day increments at 2 week intervals, if tolerated, until desired response is obtained. Liothyronine is not recommended in patients with cardiac disease or in the elderly, due to potential for greater cardiotoxicity. See Levothyroxine.

Pediatric Dose. **PO for hypothyroidism** 5 mcg/day initially, increasing in 5 mcg/day increments at weekly intervals until desired effect is obtained. Usual maintenance dose is (under 1 yr) 20 mcg/day; (1-3 yr) 50 mcg/day; (over 3 yr) 25-75 mcg/day. Levothyroxine is the drug of choice in congenital hypothyroidism, however.[154,155,163]

Dosage Forms. **Tab** 5, 25, 50 mcg; **Inj** (available by special request from manufacturer only).

Patient Instructions. See Class Instructions.

Pharmacokinetics. *Onset and Duration.* PO onset 1-3 days; duration after cessation of therapy 3-5 days.
   Plasma Levels. During T_3 replacement, T_4 is 1 mcg/dl or less, T_3 has a peak of 450-700 ng/dl 1-2 hr after dose, returning to 100-180 ng/dl prior to the next dose 24 hr later.[165] Plasma T_3 levels are age-related and can be decreased by a wide variety of pharmacological agents (eg, amiodarone, iodinated contrast dyes, corticosteroids, propylthiouracil) or clinical circumstances (eg, malnutrition, chronic renal, hepatic, pulmonary or cardiac disease or acute sepsis) which impair either peripheral or pituitary T_4 to T_3 conversion.[158]
   Fate. Usually complete oral absorption, but may be decreased in CHF.[161] Excreted in the urine as deiodinated metabolites and their conjugates.[166] V_d is 35-45 L; metabolic Cl is 24 L/day. Fractional turnover is 60%/24 hr.[160]
   $t_{1/2}$. Euthyroid 1 day; may increase to 1.4 days in hypothyroidism, or decrease to 0.6 day in hyperthyroidism.[162]

Adverse Reactions. Dose-related (see Levothyroxine Sodium), but may appear more rapidly than with levothyroxine.

Contraindications. See Levothyroxine Sodium.

Precautions. See Levothyroxine Sodium.

Parameters to Monitor. See Levothyroxine Sodium, keeping T_3 plasma level data in mind.

Notes. Liothyronine is not considered the drug of choice for replacement therapy in hypothyroidism, due to its greater expense, shorter half-life (necessitating more frequent dosing) its greater potential for cardiotoxicity and greater difficulty of monitoring. Claimed by some to be useful in patients with cardiac disease, because adverse effects will dissipate faster; however, adverse effects are more likely, because regulation of dosage is more difficult than with longer acting preparations.[167,168] Liothyronine and its mixtures (eg, thyroid, liotrix) cause "unphysiologic" peaks in plasma T_3 levels not found during levothyroxine replacement therapy.[165,169] Liothyronine is the preparation of choice when impairment of T_4 to T_3 conversion is suspected or when thyroid supplements must be stopped prior to isotope scanning. After scanning, maintenance therapy with levothyroxine is recommended. See Thyroid Replacement Products Comparison Chart.

Thyroid Replacement Products Comparison Chart

DRUG	DOSAGE FORMS	EQUIVALENT DOSE	CONTENTS	RELATIVE ONSET AND DURATION[a]	COMMENTS
Levothyroxine Levothroid® Synthroid® Various	Tab 25, 50, 75, 100, 125, 150, 175, 200, 300 mcg. Inj 200, 500 mcg.	60 mcg	T_4	Long	Preparation of choice; bioinequivalence between brands reported.[164]
Liothyronine Cytomel® Various	Tab 5, 25, 50 mcg Inj 114 mcg/ml (available by special request from manufacturer).	37.5 mcg	T_3	Short	Expensive; difficult to monitor; preparation of choice if thyroid supplements are to be stopped for isotope scanning.
Liotrix Euthroid® Thyrolar®	Tab ¼, ½, 1, 2, 3.[b]	#1 Tab[c]	T_4 & T_3 in 4:1 ratio	Intermediate	No advantages; more costly than others and confusing variation in tablet strengths exists.
Thyroglobulin Proloid® Various	Tab 16, 32, 65, 100, 130, 200 mg.	65 mg	T_4 & T_3 in 2.5:1 ratio	Intermediate	Similar to thyroid, but more purified, standardized and costly.

Continued

Thyroid Replacement Products Comparison Chart

DRUG	DOSAGE FORMS	EQUIVALENT DOSE	CONTENTS	RELATIVE ONSET AND DURATION[a]	COMMENTS
Thyroid Various	Tab 15, 30, 60, 90, 120, 180, 240, 300 mg.	60 mg	T_4 & T_3 in variable ratio	Intermediate	Cheapest product; rarely, allergy to animal protein occurs; supraphysiologic elevations in T_3 levels and T_3-toxicosis may occur.[165,169]

a. With equivalent doses.
b. Numbers represent equivalent dose of thyroid in grains.
c. 20% difference in hormone content between manufacturers; Euthroid®-1 contains T_4 60 mcg and T_3 15 mcg; Thyrolar®-1 contains T_4 50 mcg and T_3 12.5 mcg, other strengths are in same proportion.

68:36.08 ANTITHYROID AGENTS

General Reference: 176

Iodides

Various

Pharmacology. Iodide inhibits the synthesis and release of thyroid hormone and preoperatively decreases the size and vascularity of the hyperplastic thyroid gland. Large doses block the uptake of radioactive iodine by the thyroid gland.

Administration and Adult Dose. PO for hyperthyroidism, as adjunct to antithyroid agents or for preoperative thyroidectomy preparation 50–100 mg q 8 hr diluted in a glass of water, milk or juice; doses as high as 500 mg/day have been used. Use for 7–10 days prior to surgery. **PO for thyroid storm** 200 mg q 6 hr. **IV for thyroid storm** 1–2 g/24 hr—see Notes. **PO for prophylaxis in a radiation emergency** 130 mg (100 mg iodine) immediately before or within 1–2 hr after exposure and daily for 3–7 days, to a maximum of 10 days after exposure. However, administration of smaller doses of 30–50 mg iodine and continued suppression with doses of 15–50 mg/day may also be effective.[170]

Pediatric Dose. PO for thyrotoxicosis 300 mg (6 drops SSKI) q 8 hr diluted as above. **PO for prophylaxis in a radiation emergency** (under 1 yr) 65 mg (50 mg iodine) immediately before or after exposure and daily for 3–7 days, to a maximum of 10 days after exposure; (over 1 yr) same as adult dose.

Dosage Forms. Soln (SSKI) 50 mg/drop; **Soln** Lugol's or Strong Iodine (5% iodine/10% potassium iodide) 8 mg/drop; **Soln** (potassium iodide) 21 mg/drop; **Tab** 130 mg; **EC Tab** 300 mg; **Inj** (sodium iodide) 1 g/10 ml.

Patient Instructions. Dilute solution in a glass of liquid before taking; may be taken with food, milk or an antacid to minimize stomach upset. Do not use if breast feeding; advise physician if pregnant. Do not use if solution turns brownish-yellow. If crystals form in the solution, they may be dissolved by warming the closed container in warm water. Dissolve tablets in 1/2 glass of water or milk before taking. Discontinue use and report any symptoms of fever, skin rash, epigastric pain or joint swelling.

Pharmacokinetics. *Onset and Duration.* Onset 24–48 hr in hyperthyroidism with maximum effect in 10–15 days—see Notes.

Plasma Levels. Iodide levels greater than 50 ng/ml inhibit iodide binding by thyroid in hyperthyroidism; greater than 200 ng/ml inhibit iodide uptake by normal thyroid.[168]

Fate. Iodides are absorbed readily throughout GI tract and concentrated in the thyroid, stomach and salivary glands. Renal clearance is 2.22 L/hr in males and 1.5 L/hr in females.[171]

Adverse Reactions. Any adverse reactions warrant drug discontinuation. Hypersensitivity occurs occasionally and is manifested by angioedema, cutaneous hemorrhages and symptoms resembling serum sickness. Iodism is indicated by metallic taste, GI upset, soreness of teeth and gums, coryza, frontal headache, painful swelling of salivary glands, diarrhea, acneiform skin eruptions and erythema of face and chest. Rarely, prolonged use can lead to goiter with hypothyroidism or hyperthyroidism with underlying thyroid disease.[171] See Precautions.

Contraindications. Pulmonary tuberculosis; pulmonary edema.

Precautions. Pregnancy, because fetal goiter, asphyxiation and death may occur;[173] lactation—see Drugs and Breast Feeding chapter. Small bowel lesions are associated with enteric-coated potassium-containing tablets, which can cause obstruction, hemorrhage, perforation and possible death—this dosage form is not recommended. Iodides are not recommended for use as expectorants due to their potential to induce acneiform eruptions, exacerbate existing lesions and adversely affect the thyroid. Use with caution in patients with untreated Hashimoto's thyroiditis, in patients on lithium or amiodarone, in iodide-deficient patients, in children with cystic fibrosis and in euthyroid patients with Graves' disease after treatment with radioactive iodine or surgery, because they may be particularly sensitive to iodide-induced hypothyroidism.[171] Patients with nontoxic multinodular goiters may be prone to development of hyperthyroidism.[172] Iodides should be avoided entirely in patients with toxic nodular goiter or toxic nodules, because thyrotoxicosis may be further aggravated.[171]

Parameters to Monitor.   Signs of iodism, hypothyroidism, hyperthyroidism and parotitis should be monitored occasionally during chronic use. Monitor thyroid function tests at least q 6–12 months if used chronically in patients with a family history of thyroid disease or goiter. Monitor serum potassium frequently in patients who are taking other drugs which may also affect serum potassium (eg, diuretics).

Notes.   Iodides either orally or IV have the most rapid onset of any treatment for hyperthyroidism. In thyroid storm, iodides should theoretically be given 1 hr after the thionamide dose, but should not be withheld if oral thionamides cannot be given. The therapeutic effects of iodide are transient, with "escape" occurring after 10–14 days; iodides should not be used alone in the therapy of hyperthyroidism. Iodide prevents uptake of ^{131}I for several weeks and delays onset of thionamide action if given alone prior to a thionamide. Pharmacological amounts of iodides can be present in serum from vaginal douches such as povidone-iodine.[174]

Methimazole   Tapazole®

Pharmacology.   An antithyroid drug which interferes with the synthesis of thyroid hormones by inhibiting iodide organification. Unlike propylthiouracil (PTU), methimazole does not block peripheral conversion of T_4 to T_3. Titers of thyroid stimulating immunoglobulin fall during therapy. Methimazole is 10 times more potent than PTU on a weight basis.

Administration and Adult Dose.   PO 10–20 mg (depending on the severity of the hyperthyroidism) q 8 hr initially until euthyroid (usually 6–8 weeks), then decrease by 33–50% over several weeks to a maintenance dose of 5–15 mg/day in a single dose. Mild disease may respond initially to a single daily dose regimen. **PO for thyroid storm** 25 mg q 6 hr until euthyroid; maintenance dose must be individualized. See Propylthiouracil for treatment duration.

Dosage Individualization.   In pregnancy, doses should be as small as possible to maintain a mildly hyperthyroid state: initially 30 mg/day orally in 3 divided doses for 4–6 weeks, then decrease to 5–15 mg/day in a single dose.[175]

Pediatric Dose.   PO 0.4 mg/kg/day given in three doses with a maintenance dose of one-half the initial dose.

Dosage Forms.   Tab 5, 10 mg. Can be formulated for rectal administration.[176,177]

Patient Instructions.   See Propylthiouracil.

Pharmacokinetics. *Onset and Duration.*   PO onset about 2–3 weeks which is consistent with the elimination of existing T_4 stores. Duration of 40 hr intrathyroidally.[176,178]

Plasma Levels.   Less than 0.2 mcg/ml inhibit iodide organification.[178]

Fate. Well absorbed orally; plasma level after a 30 mg oral dose is 0.5 mcg/ml, with peak at 1–2 hr.[178] Actively concentrated in thyroid gland, with peak intrathyroidal levels of 1–10 μM within 1 hr.[176,178] V_d is 40 L with minimal plasma protein binding. There are no active metabolites; 7–12% is excreted unchanged in urine, 6% excreted as inorganic sulfate, 1.5% as sulfur metabolites and 50% as unknown metabolites.[178,179]

$t_{1/2}$. 4–6 hr in normal and hyperthyroid patients, increased to 21 hr in cirrhosis.[178] Intrathyroidal half-life is 20 hr.

Adverse Reactions. See Propylthiouracil. Agranulocytosis is more frequent with doses greater than 30 mg/day.[180] Cholestatic jaundice, nephrotic syndrome, loss of taste or spontaneous appearance of circulating antibodies to insulin or glucagon occur rarely.[181]

Precautions. Pregnancy, since methimazole crosses the placenta 4 times better than propylthiouracil and has been associated with scalp defects (aplasia cutis).[176] Lactation—see Drugs and Breast Feeding chapter. Use with caution in patients allergic to other thionamides. See Propylthiouracil.

Parameters to Monitor. See Propylthiouracil.

Notes. Methimazole is often not the drug of choice, because PTU may act more rapidly in thyrotoxicosis and thyroid storm. Methimazole can be considered an alternative to PTU in patients who develop only a rash while on PTU. Methimazole may be preferable in the noncompliant patient, because its long half-life allows single daily dosing.

Propylthiouracil   Various

Pharmacology. Propylthiouracil (PTU) is an antithyroid drug which interferes with the synthesis of thyroid hormones and decreases peripheral conversion of T_4 to T_3.

Administration and Adult Dose. **PO for hyperthyroidism** 100–200 mg (depending on the severity of hyperthyroidism) q 6 hr initially until euthyroid (usually 6–8 weeks), then decrease by 33–50% over several weeks to a maintenance dose of 100–150 mg/day in a single dose. Rarely, initial doses of 1–1.2 g/day (maximum dose) in 3–4 doses may be necessary.[178] **PO for thyroid storm** 250 mg q 6 hr until euthyroid; maintenance dose is determined by patient response.[149] Treatment duration is 1–2 yr traditionally, although shorter courses of 6 months may also be effective in mild disease.[176,182,183] Treatment may be continued indefinitely if necessary to control the disease and no toxicity occurs.[176,184]

Dosage Individualization. In pregnancy, doses should be as small as possible to maintain a mildly hyperthyroid maternal state; initially 300 mg/day orally in 3 divided doses for 4–6 weeks, then decrease to 50–150 mg/day in a single dose.[175,176]

Pediatric Dose. PO 120–175 mg/M^2/day. Alternatively, **PO (6–10 yr)** 50–150 mg/day initially; **(10 yr and over)** 150–300 mg/day initially. Maintenance dose is determined by patient response.

Dosage Forms. **Tab** 50 mg.

Patient Instructions. Sore throat, fever or oral lesions may be an early sign of a severe, but rare blood disorder and should be reported immediately. Also report any skin eruptions, itching, yellowing of eyes and skin. Be sure to take at prescribed dosage intervals. If a dose is missed, take it as soon as possible. If it is time for the next dose, take both doses. Tell any new physician that you are taking this medicine.

Pharmacokinetics. *Onset and Duration.* PO onset of therapeutic effect 2-3 weeks, consistent with the elimination of existing thyroxine stores.[179,185]

Plasma Levels. 3 mcg/ml reduces thyroid function by 50%.[179,185]

Fate. Oral bioavailability is 80-95%. Plasma level after a 300 mg oral dose is 6 mcg/ml, with peak at 1-2 hr.[176,179,185] Actively concentrated in thyroid gland, with peak intrathyroidal levels of 1-10 μM within 1 hr.[176,179] V_d is 0.3-0.4 L/kg; 80% plasma protein bound. Less than 10% excreted unchanged in urine. 85% is excreted in 24 hr, 61% as glucuronides, 8-9% as inorganic sulfates and 8-10% as unknown sulfur metabolites.[179]

$t_{1/2}$. 1-1.6 hr in normal patients and hyperthyroidism.[176,179,185]

Adverse Reactions. Skin rashes, fever, urticaria and arthralgias occasionally occur; prevalence is dose-dependent.[176,180,186] Agranulocytosis occurs in 0.5% of patients, usually in the first 3 months of therapy. Risk of agranulocytosis may be greater in patients over 40 yr.[180] Transient leukopenia is frequent, but does not predispose to agranulocytosis and is not an indication to discontinue the drug.[176,180,186] Mild leukopenia occurs frequently in untreated Graves' disease.[187] Rarely, hepatocellular toxicity, vasculitis, lupus-like syndrome, hypoprothrombinemia, aplastic anemia or thrombocytopenia occur and are indications for cessation of therapy.

Contraindications. Manufacturer states contraindicated in nursing mothers, but if necessary it can be used due to low breast milk drug levels.[188] See Drugs and Breast Feeding chapter.

Precautions. Although it crosses the placenta poorly (1/4 that of methimazole), it can cause fetal hypothyroidism and goiter. Therefore, minimal doses (less than 300 mg/day) should be used during pregnancy.[175,176] Thyroid dysfunction may diminish as pregnancy progresses, allowing a reduction in dosage and, in some cases, a withdrawal of therapy 2-3 weeks before delivery. Adjunctive therapy with thyroid hormone prevents maternal hypothyroidism, but because of minimal placental transfer, has little effect on the fetus.[175] Obtain WBC and differential counts if patient reports signs of agranulocytosis such as fever, sore throat or malaise. Use with caution prior to surgery or during treatment with anticoagulants because of hypoprothrombinemic effect. Obtain an AST (SGOT), ALT (SGPT), total bilirubin and alkaline phosphatase if patient reports signs of hepatitis. A low prevalence of cross-sensitivity occurs between thionamide compounds for skin rashes; so if these occur, another thionamide can be substituted. However, a 50% chance of cross-sensitivity exists for severe reactions (ie, agranulocytosis, hepatitis) so do not substitute another thionamide.[176,186] Iodine, if used before propylthiouracil, may result in a delayed response to PTU.[21]

Parameters to Monitor. Clinical status of patient; plasma free T_4, T_3 and TSH q month initially, then q 2-3 months. Prothrombin time monitoring is advisable, particularly prior to surgery. Occasional liver function tests and CBC with differential (but these are not recommended routinely, because they are not predictive of toxicity).

Notes. Because propylthiouracil decreases peripheral conversion of T_4 to T_3, it is considered the thionamide of choice in treating thyrotoxic crisis. It is also the drug of choice in pregnancy, in breast feeding,[188] and in young adults. Remission rates of 20-40% are common after cessation of therapy. Favorable remission rates correlate with longer duration of therapy, higher doses, mild disease, shrinkage of goiter size with therapy, disappearance of thyroid stimulating immunoglobulin titers after discontinuation of therapy and initial presentation with T_3 toxicosis.[176,184] Most patients eventually require surgery or treatment with radioactive iodine; however, a trial of PTU may be worthwhile in patients with minimal thyroid enlargement or very mild hyperthyroidism.[21] PTU may decrease mortality due to alcoholic liver disease.[193]

References, 68:00 Hormones and Synthetic Substitutes

1. Azarnoff DL, ed. Steroid therapy. Philadelphia: WB Saunders, 1975.

2. Fauci AS, Dale DC, Balow JE. Glucocorticosteroid therapy: mechanisms of action and clinical considerations. Ann Intern Med 1976;84:304-15.

3. Axelrod L. Glucocorticoid therapy. Medicine 1976;55:39-65.

4. Harding SM. Corticosteroids. In: Buckle DR, Smith H, eds. Development of anti-asthma drugs. London: Butterworths, 1984:297-313.

5. Morris HG. Mechanisms of action and therapeutic role of corticosteroids in asthma. J Allergy Clin Immunol 1985;75:1-13.

6. Spector SL. The use of corticosteroids in the treatment of asthma. Chest 1985;8/(Suppl):73S-8S.

7. Toogood JH, Jennings B, Baskerville JC. Aerosol corticosteroids. In: Weiss EB, Segal MS, Stein M, eds. Bronchial asthma: mechanisms and therapeutics. 2nd ed. Boston: Little, Brown, 1985:698-713.

8. Brogden RN, Heel RC, Speight TM et al. Beclomethasone dipropionate: a reappraisal of its pharmacodynamic properties and therapeutic efficacy after a decade of use in asthma and rhinitis. Drugs 1984;28:99-126.

9. Meltzer EO, Zeiger RS, Schatz M et al. Chronic rhinitis in infants and children: etiologic, diagnostic, and therapeutic considerations. Pediatr Clin North Am 1983;30:847-71.

10. Brogden RN. Inhaled steroids: pharmacology and toxicology. In: Clark TJH, ed. Steroids in asthma: a reappraisal in the light of inhalation therapy. Auckland: ADIS Press, 1983:121-34.

11. Clissold SP, Heel RC. Budesonide: a preliminary review of its pharmacodynamic properties and therapeutic efficacy in asthma and rhinitis. Drugs 1984;28:485-518.

12. Bone RC, Fisher CJ, Clemmer TP et al. A controlled clinical trial of high-dose methylprednisolone in the treatment of severe sepsis and shock. N Engl J Med 1987;317:653-8.

13. Hinshaw L, Peduzzi P, Young E et al. Effect of high-dose glucocorticoid therapy on mortality in patients with clinical signs of systemic sepsis. N Engl J Med 1987;317:659-65.

14. Kass EH. High-dose corticosteroids for septic shock. N Engl J Med 1984;311:1178-9.

15. Gold EM. The Cushing syndromes: changing views of diagnosis and treatment. Ann Intern Med 1979;90:829-44.

16. Markman M, Sheidler V, Ettinger DS et al. Antiemetic efficacy of dexamethasone: randomized, double-blind, crossover study with prochlorperazine in patients receiving cancer chemotherapy. N Engl J Med 1984;311:549-52.

17. Cersosimo RJ, Karp DD. Adrenal corticosteroids as antiemetics during cancer chemotherapy. Pharmacotherapy 1986;6:118-27.

18. Tsuei SE, Moore RG, Ashley JJ et al. Disposition of synthetic glucocorticoids. I. Pharmacokinetics of dexamethasone in healthy adults. J Pharmacokinet Biopharm 1979;7:249-64.

19. Health and Public Policy Committee, American College of Physicians. The dexamethasone suppression test for the detection, diagnosis, and management of depression. Ann Intern Med 1984;100:307-8.

20. Barry M. The use of high-dose pulse methylprednisolone in rheumatoid arthritis: unproved therapy. Arch Intern Med 1985;145:1483-4.

21. Gilman AG, Goodman LS, Rall TW et al, eds. Goodman and Gilman's the pharmacological basis of therapeutics. 7th ed. New York: Macmillan, 1985.

22. Thorn GW. Clinical considerations in the use of corticosteroids. N Engl J Med 1966;274:775-81.

23. Harter JG, Reddy WJ, Thorn GW. Studies on an intermittent corticosteroid dosage regimen. N Engl J Med 1963;269:591-6.

24. Breitenfield RV, Hebert LA, Lemann J et al. Stability of renal transplant function with alternate-day corticosteroid therapy. JAMA 1980;244:151-6.

25. Bystryn J-C. Adjuvant therapy of pemphigus. Arch Dermatol 1984;120:941-51.

26. Klinefelter HF, Winkenwerder WL, Bledsoe T. Single daily dose prednisone therapy. JAMA 1979;241:2721-3.

27. Byyny RL. Withdrawal from glucocorticoid therapy. N Engl J Med 1976;295:30-2.

28. Ahrens RC, Hendeles L, Weinberger M. The clinical pharmacology of drugs used in the treatment of asthma. In: Yaffe SJ, ed. Pediatric pharmacology: therapeutic principles in practice. New York: Grune & Stratton, 1980:233-80.

29. Iafrate RP, Massey KL, Hendeles L. Current concepts in clinical therapeutics: asthma. Clin Pharm 1986;5:206-27.

30. Haskell RJ, Wong BM, Hansen JE. A double-blind, randomized clinical trial of methylprednisolone in status asthmaticus. Arch Intern Med 1983;143:1324-7.

31. Siegel SC. Corticosteroid agents: overview of corticosteroid therapy. J Allergy Clin Immunol 1985;76:312-20.

32. United States Pharmacopeial Convention Inc. United States Pharmacopia Dispensing Information 1987. Easton: Mack Publishing Co., 1987.

33. Liddle GW. Clinical pharmacology of the anti-inflammatory steroids. Clin Pharmacol Ther 1961;2:615-35.

34. Meikle AW, Tyler FH. Potency and duration of action of glucocorticoids. Am J Med 1977;63:200-7.

35. Sugita ET, Niebergal PJ. Bioavailability monograph: prednisone. J Am Pharm Assoc 1975;NS15:529-32.

36. Jenkins JS, Sampson PA. Conversion of cortisone to cortisol and prednisone to prednisolone. Br Med J 1967;2:205-7.

37. Gambertoglio JG, Amend WJC, Benet LZ. Pharmacokinetics and bioavailability of prednisone and prednisolone in healthy volunteers and patients: a review. J Pharmacokinet Biopharm 1980;8:1-52.

38. Uribe M, Go VLW. Corticosteroid pharmacokinetics in liver disease. Clin Pharmacokinet 1979;4:233-40.

39. Lewis GP, Jusko WJ, Burke CW et al. Prednisone side-effects and serum-protein levels. Lancet 1971;2:778-81.

40. Messer J, Reitman D, Sacks HS et al. Association of adrenocorticosteroid therapy and peptic-ulcer disease. N Engl J Med 1983;309:21-4.

41. The Boston Collaborative Drug Surveillance Program. Acute adverse reactions to prednisone in relation to dosage. Clin Pharmacol Ther 1972;13:694-8.

42. Anon. Oral corticosteroids. Med Lett Drugs Ther 1975;17:99-100.

43. Pagliaro LA, Benet LZ. Critical compilation of terminal half-lives, percent excreted unchanged, and changes of half-life in renal and hepatic dysfunction for studies in humans with references. J Pharmacokinet Biopharm 1975;3:333-83.

44. Melby JC. Clinical pharmacology of systemic corticosteroids. Ann Rev Pharmacol Toxicol 1977;17:511-27.

45. Tsuei SE, Moore RG, Ashley JJ et al. Disposition of synthetic glucocorticoids. I. Pharmacokinetics of dexamethasone in healthy adults. J Pharmacokinet Biopharm 1979;7:249-64.

46. Dickey RP. Managing contraceptive pill patients. 5th ed. Durant, OK: Creative Infomatics, 1987.

47. Williams NB, ed. Contraceptive technology 1986-1987. 13th revised ed. New York: Irvington Publishers, 1986.

48. Smith MA, Youngkin EQ. Current perspectives on combination oral contraceptives. Clin Pharm 1984;3:485-96.

49. Population Information Program. Oral contraceptives in the 1980's, Baltimore. The Johns Hopkins University series A, number 6, 1982.

50. Loudon NB, Potts M, Hatcher R. Instructions for starting the use of oral contraceptives. N Engl J Med 1984;311:1634-5.

51. Yuzpe AA, Smith RP, Rademaker AW. A multicenter clinical investigation employing ethinyl estradiol combined with dl-norgestrel as a postcoital contraceptive agent. Fertil Steril 1982;37:508-13.

52. Orme ML′E, Back DJ, Breckenridge AM. Clinical pharmacokinetics of oral contraceptive steroids. Clin Pharmacokinet 1983;8:95-136.

53. Back DJ, Breckenridge AM, Crawford FE et al. Kinetics of norethindrone in women. Clin Pharmacol Ther 1978;24:448-53.

54. Back DJ, Breckenridge AM, Crawford FE et al. An investigation of the pharmacokinetics of ethynylestradiol in women using radioimmunoassay. Contraception 1979;20:263-73.

55. Sisenwine SF, Kimmel HB, Liu AL et al. The presence of DL-, D-, and L-norgestrel and their metabolites in the plasma of women. Contraception 1975;12:339-51.

56. Laumas KR, Murugesan K, Hingorani V. Disappearance in plasma and tissue uptake of radioactivity after an intravenous injection of [(6,7-³H)] norethynodrel in women. Acta Endocrinol 1971;66:385-400.

57. Mills TM, Lin TJ, Braselton WE et al. Metabolism of oral contraceptive drugs. Am J Obstet Gynecol 1976;126:987-92.

58. Stadel BV. Oral contraceptives and cardiovascular disease (first of two parts). N Engl J Med 1981;305:612-8.

59. Stadel BV, idem (second of two parts), ibid:672-7.

60. Kay CR. The Royal College of General Practitioners' oral contraception study: some recent observations. Clin Obstet Gynaecol 1984;11:759-86.

61. D'Arcy PF. Drug interactions with oral contraceptives. Drug Intell Clin Pharm 1986;20:353-62.

62. Patwardhan RV, Desmond PV, Johnson RF et al. Impaired elimination of caffeine by oral contraceptives. J Lab Clin Med 1980;95:603-8.

63. Abernethy DR, Greenblatt DJ. Impairment of antipyrine metabolism by low-dose oral contraceptive steroids. Clin Pharmacol Ther 1981;29:106-10.

64. Greenblatt RB, Nezhat C, Karpas A. The menopausal syndrome hormone replacement therapy. In: Eskin BA, ed. The menopause. Comprehensive management. New York: Masson Publishing, 1980:151-72.

65. Haber RJ. Should postmenopausal women be given estrogen? West J Med 1985;142:672-7.

66. Hammond CB, Maxson WS. Estrogen replacement therapy. Clin Obstet Gynecol 1986;29:407-30.

67. Gambrell RD. The menopause: benefits and risks of estrogen-progestogen replacement therapy. Fertil Steril 1982;37:457-74.

68. Catalona WJ, Scott WW. Carcinoma of the prostate: a review. J Urol 1978;119:1-8.

69. Ingle JN, Ahmann DL, Green SJ et al. Randomized clinical trial of diethylstilbestrol versus tamoxifen in postmenopausal women with advanced breast cancer. N Engl J Med 1981;304:16-21.

70. Yuzpe AA. Postcoital contraception. Clinics Obstet Gynaecol 1984;11:787-97.

71. Bolt HM. Metabolism of estrogens—natural and synthetic. Pharmacol Ther 1979;4:155-81.

72. Callantine MR, Martin PL, Bolding OT et al. Micronized 17β-estradiol for oral estrogen therapy in menopausal women. Obstet Gynecol 1975;46:37-41.

73. Horsman A, Jones M, Francis R et al. The effect of estrogen dose on postmenopausal bone loss. N Engl J Med 1983;309:1405-7.

74. Yen SSC, Martin PL, Burnier AM et al. Circulating estradiol, estrone and gonadotropin levels following the administration of orally active 17β-estradiol in postmenopausal women. J Clin Endocrinol Metab 1975;40:518-21.

75. Dada DA, Laumas V, Landgren B-M et al. Effect of graded oral doses of oestradiol on circulating hormonal levels. Acta Endocrinol 1978;88:754-67.

76. Nichols KC, Schenkel L, Benson H. 17β-estradiol for postmenopausal estrogen replacement therapy. Obstet Gynecol Survey 1984;39:230-45.

77. Martin PL, Greaney MD, Burnier AM et al. Estradiol, estrone, and gonadotropin levels after use of vaginal estradiol. Obstet Gynecol 1984;63:441-4.

78. Longcope C, Williams KIH. The metabolism of estrogens in normal women after pulse injections of ³H-estradiol and ³H-estrone. Clin Endocrinol Metab 1974;38:602-7.

79. Chetkowski RJ, Meldrum DR, Steingold KA et al. Biological effects of transdermal estrogen. N Engl J Med 1986;314:1615-20.

80. Steingold KA, Laufer L, Chetowski RJ et al. Treatment of hot flashes with transdermal estradiol administration. J Clin Endocrinol Metab 1985;61:627-32.

81. Place VA, Powers M, Darley PE et al. A double-blind comparative study of Estraderm and Premarin in the amelioration of postmenopausal symptoms. Am J Obstet Gynecol 1985;152:1092-8.

82. Lindsay R, Hart DM, Clark DM. The minimum effective dose of estrogen for the prevention of postmenopausal bone loss. Obstet Gynecol 1984;63:759-63.

83. Keye WR, Jaffe RB. Hirsutism and dysfunctional uterine bleeding. In: Glass RH, ed. Office gynecology. Baltimore: Williams and Wilkins, 1976:208-26.

84. Bhavnani BR, Sarda IR, Woolever CA. Radioimmunoassay of plasma equilin and estrone in postmenopausal

women after the administration of Premarin. J Clin Endocrinol Metab 1981;52:741-7.

85. Utian WH, Katz M, Davey DA et al. Effect of premenopausal castration and incremental dosages of conjugated equine estrogens on plasma follicle-stimulating hormone, luteinizing hormone, and estradiol. Am J Obstet Gynecol 1978;132:297-302.

86. Whittaker PG, Morgan MRA, Dean PDG et al. Serum equilin, oestrone, and oestradiol levels in postmenopausal women receiving conjugated equine oestrogens ('Premarin'). Lancet 1980;1:14-6.

87. Mandel FP, Geola FL, Meldrum DR et al. Biological effects of various doses of vaginally administered conjugated equine estrogens in postmenopausal women. J Clin Endocrinol Metab 1983;57:133-9.

88. Deutsch S, Ossowski R, Benjamin I. Comparison between degree of systemic absorption of vaginally and orally administered estrogens at different dose levels in postmenopausal women. Am J Obstet Gynecol 1981;139:967-8.

89. Hoover R, Gray LA, Cole P et al. Menopausal estrogens and breast cancer. N Engl J Med 1976;295:401-5.

90. Feldman JM. Glyburide: a second generation sulfonylurea hypoglycemic agent. Pharmacotherapy 1985;5:43-62.

91. Baker DE, Campbell RK. The second generation sulfonylureas: glipizide and glyburide. Diab Educ 1985;11:29-36.

92. Raptis S, Pfeiffer EF. Progress in oral therapy of diabetes mellitus with sulphonylurea of the second generation. Acta Diabetol Lat 1972;2:865-78.

93. Brogden RN, Heel RC, Pakes GE et al. Glipizide: a review of its pharmacological properties and therapeutic use. Drugs 1979;18:32-53.

94. Blohme G, Waldenstrom J. Glibenclamide and glipizide in maturity onset diabetes. Acta Med Scand 1979;206:263-7.

95. Anon. Which sulfonylurea in diabetes mellitus? Drug Ther Bull 1981;19:49-51.

96. Yu T-F, Berger L, Gutman AB. Hypoglycemia and uricosuric properties of acetohexamide and hydroxyhexamide. Metabolism 1968;17:309-15.

97. Cohen BD, Galloway JA, McMahon RE et al. Carbohydrate metabolism in uremia: blood glucose response to sulfonylurea. Am J Med Sci 1976;254:608-18.

98. Petitpierre B, Perrin L, Rudhardt M et al. Behavior of chlorpropamide in renal insufficiency and under the effect of associated drug therapy. Int J Clin Pharmacol Ther Toxicol 1972;6:120-4.

99. University Group Diabetes Program. A study of the effects of hypoglycemic agents on vascular complications in patients with adult-onset diabetes: II. Mortality results. Diabetes 1970;19(Suppl. 2):789-830.

100. Kilo C. The use of oral hypoglycemic agents. Hosp Prac 1979;14:103-10.

101. Bunn HF, Gabbay KH, Gallop PM. The glycosylation of hemoglobin: relevance to diabetes mellitus. Science 1978;200:21-7.

102. Boden G, Master RW, Gordon SS et al. Monitoring metabolic control in diabetic outpatients with glycosylated hemoglobin. Ann Intern Med 1980;92:357-60.

103. Breidahl HD, Ennis GC, Martin FIR et al. Insulin and oral hypoglycaemic agents II: clinical and therapeutic aspects. Drugs 1972;3:204-26.

104. Taylor JA. Pharmacokinetics and biotransformation of chlorpropamide in man. Clin Pharmacol Ther 1972;13:710-8.

105. Nelson E. Rate of metabolism of tolbutamide in test subjects with liver disease or with impaired renal function. Am J Med Sci 1964;248:657-9.

106. Yarborough MC, Campbell RK. CE Module 2: Developing a diabetes program for your pharmacy. Am Pharm 1986;NS26:1-11.

107. Koda-Kimble MA. Diabetes mellitus. In: Katcher BS, Young LY, Koda-Kimble MA eds. Applied therapeutics for clinical pharmacists. 3rd ed. San Francisco: Applied Therapeutics, 1983.

108. Christiansen C, Sachse M. Home blood glucose monitoring. Diab Educ 1980;6:13-21.

109. Shapiro B, Savage PJ, Lomatch D et al. A comparison of accuracy and estimated cost of methods for home blood glucose monitoring. Diabetes Care 1981;4:396-403.

110. Clements RS, Keane NA, Kirk KA et al. Comparison of various methods for rapid glucose estimation. Diabetes Care 1981;4:392-5.

111. Rearen GM, Olefsky JM. Role of insulin resistance in the pathogenesis of hyperglycemia. Adv Med Nutr 1978;2:229-66.

112. Savage PJ, Bennion LJ, Flock EV et al. Diet-induced improvement of abnormalities in insulin and glucagon secretion and in insulin receptor binding in diabetes mellitus. J Clin Endocrinol Metab 1979;48:999-1007.

113. Galloway JA. When the patient is resistant or allergic to insulin. Med Times 1980;108:91-101.

114. Yue DK, Turtle JR. New forms of insulin and their use in the treatment of diabetes. Diabetes 1977;26:341-5.

115. Skordis N, Winter WE, Maclaren NK. Acute onset diabetes: reversing diabetic ketoacidosis. Drug Ther (Dec) 1986:26-41.

116. Fisher JN, Shahshahani MN, Kitabchi AE. Diabetic ketoacidosis: low-dose insulin therapy by various routes. N Engl J Med 1977;297:238-41.

117. Ginsberg S, Block MB, Mako ME et al. Serum insulin levels following administration of exogenous insulin. J Clin Endocrinol Metab 1973;36:1175-9.

118. Rubenstein AH, Spitz I. Role of the kidney in insulin metabolism and excretion. Diabetes 1968;17:161-9.

119. Rabkin R, Simon NM, Steiner S et al. Effect of renal disease on renal uptake and excretion of insulin in man. N Engl J Med 1970;282:181-7.

120. Alberti KGMM, Nattrass M. Severe diabetic ketoacidosis. Med Clin North Am 1978;62:799-814.

121. Andreani D, Iavicoli M, Tamburrano G et al. Comparative trials with monocomponent (MC) and monospecies (MS) pork insulins in the treatment of diabetes mellitus. Influence on antibody levels, on insulin requirement and on some complications. Horm Metab Res 1974;6:447-54.

122. Teuscher A. Treatment of insulin lipoatrophy with monocomponent insulin. Diabetologia 1974;10:211-4.

123. Mattson JR, Patterson R, Roberts M. Insulin therapy in patients with systemic insulin allergy. Arch Intern Med 1975;135:818-21.

124. Marble A. Allergy and diabetes in the treatment of diabetes mellitus. In: Joslin EP, Root HF, White P et al, eds. Diabetic Manual. 10th ed. Philadelphia: Lea and Febiger, 1959:395-406.

125. Storvick WO, Henry HJ. Effect of storage temperature on stability of commercial insulin preparations. Diabetes 1968;17:499-502.

126. Petty C, Cunningham NL. Insulin adsorption by glass infusion bottles, polyvinylchloride infusion containers, and intravenous tubing. Anesthesiology 1979;36:330-7.

127. Whalen FJ, LeCain WK, Latiolais CJ. Availability of insulin from continuous low-dose insulin infusions. Am J Hosp Pharm 1979;36:330-7.

128. Peterson L, Caldwell J, Hoffman J. Insulin adsorbance to polyvinylchloride surfaces with implications for constant-infusion therapy. Diabetes 1976;25:72-4.

129. Albisser AM, Leibel BS, Ewart TG et al. Clinical control of diabetes by the artificial pancreas. Diabetes 1974;23:397-404.

130. Santiago JV, Clemens AH, Clarke WL et al. Closed-loop and open-loop devices for blood glucose control in normal and diabetic subjects. Diabetes 1979;28:71-81.

131. Rizza RA, Gerich JE, Haymond MW et al. Control of blood sugar in insulin-dependent diabetes: comparison of an artificial endocrine pancreas, continuous subcutaneous insulin infusion, and intensified conventional insulin therapy. N Engl J Med 1980;303:1313-8.

132. Clark AJL, Adeniyi-Jones RO, Knight G et al. Biosynthetic human insulin in the treatment of diabetes. Lancet 1982;2:354-7.

133. Kimble MA. CE Module 3: Current concepts in diabetes therapy. Am Pharm 1986;NS26:1-12.

134. Fagius J, Brattberg A, Jameson S et al. Limited benefit of treatment of diabetic neuropathy with an aldose reductase inhibitor: a 24-week controlled trial. Diabetologia 1985;28:323-9.

135. Cogan DG, moderator. Aldose reductase and complications of diabetes. Ann Intern Med 1984;101:82-91.

136. Raskin P, Rosenstock J, Challis P et al. Effect of tolrestat on red blood cell sorbitol levels in patients with diabetes. Clin Pharmacol Ther 1985;38:625-30.

137. Weintraub M, Standish R. Tolrestat: an aldose reductase inhibitor for diabetic peripheral neuropathy. Hosp Formul 1986;21:912-6.

138. Nash HA. Depo-Provera. A review. Contraception 1975;12:377-93.

139. Lobo RA, McCormick W, Singer F et al. Depo-medroxyprogesterone acetate compared with conjugated estrogens for the treatment of postmenopausal women. Obstet Gynecol 1984;63:1-5.

140. Albrecht BH, Schiff I, Tulchinsky D et al. Objective evidence that placebo and oral medroxyprogesterone acetate therapy diminish menopausal vasomotor flushes. Am J Obstet Gynecol 1981;139:631-5.

141. Morrison JC, Martin DC, Blair RA et al. The use of medroxyprogesterone acetate for relief of climacteric symptoms. Am J Obstet Gynecol 1980;138:99-104.

142. Elder MG. Injectable contraception. Clin Obstet Gynaecol 1984;11:723-41.

143. Vecchio TJ. Long acting injectable contraceptives. In: Briggs MH, Christie GA, eds. Advances in steroid biochemistry and pharmacology, 1976;5:1-64.

144. Ottoson UB, Carlstrom K, Damber J-E et al. Serum levels of progesterone and some of its metabolites including deoxycorticosterone after oral and parenteral administration. Br J Obstet Gynaecol 1984;91:1111-9.

145. Sawin CT. Hypothyroidism. Med Clin North Am 1985;69:989-1003.

146. Hennessey JV, Evaul JE, Tseng Y-C et al. L-thyroxine dosage: a reevaluation of therapy with contemporary preparations. Ann Intern Med 1986;105:11-5.

147. Sekadde CB, Slaunwhite WR, Aceto T et al. Administration of thyroxine once a week. J Clin Endocrinol Metab 1974;39:759-64.

148. Greenspan FS. Thyroid nodules and thyroid cancer. West J Med 1974;121:359-65.

149. Nicoloff JT. Thyroid storm and myxedema coma. Med Clin North Am 1985;69:1005-17.

150. Davis FB, LaMantia RS, Spaulding SW et al. Estimation of a physiologic replacement dose of levothyroxine in elderly patients with hypothyroidism. Arch Intern Med 1984;144:1752-4.

151. Rosenbaum RL, Barzel US. Levothyroxine replacement dose for primary hypothyroidism decreases with age. Ann Intern Med 1982;96:53-5.

152. Sawin CT, Herman T, Molitch ME et al. Aging and the thyroid: decreased requirement for thyroid hormone in older hypothyroid patients. Am J Med 1983;75:206-9.

153. Levine HD. Compromise therapy in the patient with angina pectoris and hypothyroidism: a clinical assessment. Am J Med 1980;69:411-8.

154. Committee on Drugs. Treatment of congenital hypothyroidism. Pediatrics 1978;62:413-7.

155. Rezvani I, DiGeorge AM. Reassessment of the daily dose of oral thyroxine for replacement therapy in hypothyroid children. J Pediatr 1977;90:291-7.

156. Rendell M, Salmon D. 'Chemical hyperthyroidism': the significance of elevated serum thyroxine levels in L-thyroxine treated individuals. Clin Endocrinol 1985;22:693-700.

157. Sawin CT, Surks MI, London M et al. Oral thyroxine: variation in biologic action and tablet content. Ann Intern Med 1984;100:641-5.

158. Cavalieri RR, Pitt-Rivers R. The effects of drugs on the distribution and metabolism of thyroid hormones. Pharmacol Rev 1981;33:55-80.

159. Maxon HR, Ritschel WA, Volle CP et al. Pilot study on the absolute and relative bioavailability of Synthroid and Levothroid, two brands of sodium levothyroxine. Int J Clin Pharmacol Ther Toxicol 1983;21:379-82.

160. Brennan MD. Clinical pharmacology. Series on pharmacology in practice. 5. Thyroid hormones. Mayo Clin Proc 1980;55:33-44.

161. Surks MI, Schadlow AR, Stock JM et al. Determination of iodothyronine absorption and conversion of L-thyroxine (T_4) to L-triiodothyronine (T_3) using turnover rate techniques. J Clin Invest 1973;52:805-11.

162. Nicoloff JT, Low JC, Dussault JH et al. Simultaneous measurement of thyroxine and triiodothyronine peripheral turnover kinetics in man. J Clin Invest 1972;51:473-83.

163. Schultz RM, Glassman MS, MacGillivray MH. Elevated threshold for thyrotropin suppression in congenital hypothyroidism. Am J Dis Child 1980;134:19-20.

164. Hennessey JV, Burman KD, Wartofsky L. The equivalency of two L-thyroxine preparations. Ann Intern Med 1985;102:770-3.

165. Surks MI, Schadlow AR, Oppenheimer JH. A new radioimmunoassay for plasma L-triiodothyronine:

measurements in thyroid disease and in patients maintained on hormonal replacement. J Clin Invest 1972;51:3104-13.

166. Pittman CS, Buck MW, Chambers JB. Urinary metabolites of ^{14}C-labeled thyroxine in man. J Clin Invest 1972;51:1759-66.

167. Refetoff S. Thyroid hormone therapy. Med Clin North Am 1975;59:1147-62.

168. DeGroot LJ, Stanbury JB. The thyroid and its diseases. 4th ed. New York: J Wiley and Sons, 1975.

169. Penny R, Frasier SD. Elevated serum concentrations of triiodothyronine in hypothyroid patients. Values for patients receiving USP thyroid. Am J Dis Child 1980;134:16-8.

170. Sternthal E, Lipworth L, Stanley B et al. Suppression of thyroid radioiodine uptake by various doses of stable iodide. N Engl J Med 1980;303:1083-8.

171. Silva JE. Effects of iodine and iodine-containing compounds on thyroid function. Med Clin North Am 1985;69:881-97.

172. Fradkin JE, Wolff J. Iodide-induced thyrotoxicosis. Medicine 1983;62:1-20.

173. Galina MP, Avnet ML, Einhorn A. Iodides during pregnancy: an apparent cause of neonatal death. N Engl J Med 1962;267:1124-7.

174. Safran M, Braverman LE. Effect of chronic douching with polyvinylpyrrolidone-iodine on iodine absorption and thyroid function. Obstet Gynecol 1982;60:35-40.

175. Burrow GN. The management of thyrotoxicosis in pregnancy. N Engl J Med 1985;313:562-5.

176. Cooper DS. Antithyroid drugs. N Engl J Med 1984;311:1353-62.

177. Nabil N, Miner DJ, Amatruda JM. Methimazole: an alternative route of administration. J Clin Endocrinol Metab 1982;54:180-1.

178. Cooper DS, Bode HH, Nath B et al. Methimazole pharmacology in man: studies using a newly developed radioimmunoassay for methimazole. J Clin Endocrinol Metab 1984;58:473-9.

179. Kampmann JP, Hansen JM. Clinical pharmacokinetics of antithyroid drugs. Clin Pharmacokinet 1981;6:401-28.

180. Cooper DS, Goldminz D, Levin AA et al. Agranulocytosis associated with antithyroid drugs: effects of patient age and drug dose. Ann Intern Med 1983;98:26-9.

181. Hirata Y. Methimazole and insulin autoimmune syndrome with hypoglycaemia. Lancet 1983;2:1037-8.

182. Greer MA, Kammer H, Bouma DJ. Short-term antithyroid drug therapy for the thyrotoxicosis of Graves' disease. N Engl J Med 1977;297:173-6.

183. Bing RF, Rosenthal FD. Early remission in thyrotoxicosis produced by short courses of treatment. Acta Endocrinol (Copenh) 1982;100:221-3.

184. Tamai H, Nakagawa T, Fukino O et al. Thionamide therapy in Graves' disease: relation of relapse rate to duration of therapy. Ann Intern Med 1980;92:488-90.

185. Cooper DS, Saxe VC, Meskell M et al. Acute effects of propylthiouracil (PTU) on thyroidal iodide organification and peripheral iodothyronine deiodination: correlation with serum PTU levels measured by radioimmunoassay. J Clin Endocrinol Metab 1982;54:101-7.

186. Rosove MH. Agranulocytosis and antithyroid drugs. West J Med 1977;126:339-43.

187. Irvine WJ, Wu FCW, Urbaniak SJ et al. Peripheral blood leucocytes in thyrotoxicosis (Graves' disease) as studied by conventional light microscopy. Clin Exp Immunol 1977;27:216-21.

188. Kampmann JP, Johansen K, Hansen JM et al. Propylthiouracil in human milk: revision of a dogma. Lancet 1980;1:736-8.

189. Fish LH, Schwartz HL, Cavanaugh J et al. Replacement dose, metabolism, and bioavailability of levothyroxine in the treatment of hypothyroidism. N Engl J Med 1987;316:764-70.

190. Helmrich SP, Rosenberg L, Kaufman DW et al. Venous thromboembolism in relation to oral contraceptive use. Obstet Gynecol 1987;69:91-5.

191. Ettinger B, Genant HK, Cann CE. Postmenopausal bone loss is prevented by treatment with low-dosage estrogen with calcium. Ann Intern Med 1987;106:40-5.

192. Baharav E, Harpaz D, Mittelman M et al. Dexamethasone-induced perineal irritation. N Engl J Med 1986;314:515-6. Letter.

193. Orrego H, Blake JE, Blendis LM et al. Long-term treatment of alcoholic liver disease with propylthiouracil. N Engl J Med 1987;317:1421-7.

86:00 SMOOTH MUSCLE RELAXANTS

86:16 RESPIRATORY SMOOTH MUSCLE RELAXANTS

General References: 1-5

Theophylline   Theo-dur®, Slo-bid®, Various

Pharmacology. Directly relaxes smooth muscle of bronchial airways and pulmonary blood vessels to act as a bronchodilator and pulmonary vasodilator; also is a diuretic, coronary vasodilator, cardiac stimulant, cerebral stimulant, and it improves diaphragmatic contractility and lessens diaphragmatic fatigue.[1-3] The exact cellular mechanism is unknown.[2,6]

Administration and Adult Dose. PO (theophylline), IV (aminophylline) **loading dose for acute asthma symptoms** 5 mg/kg (6 mg/kg aminophylline), if patient has taken no theophylline in previous 24 hr. In emergencies, 2.5 mg/kg (3 mg/kg aminophylline) may be given if an immediate plasma level cannot be obtained. Each 1 mg/kg (1.25 mg/kg aminophylline) results in about a 2 mcg/ml increase in plasma theophylline. Infuse IV aminophylline no faster than 25 mg/min. **Maintenance Dose**—see Maintenance Dose for Acute Symptoms Comparison Chart below. **PO for chronic asthma** (theophylline) initial dose 400 mg/day in divided doses, then increase if tolerated in approximately 25% increments at 3-day intervals to 13 mg/kg/day or 900 mg/day, whichever is less. Use plasma concentrations for subsequent dosage adjustment. For patients with CHF, liver dysfunction or cor pulmonale, initial dose must not exceed 400 mg/day unless plasma levels are measured.[2,3] **IM, PR suppositories not recommended.**

Maintenance Dose for Acute Symptoms[a]

POPULATION GROUP	ORAL THEOPHYLLINE[b] (MG/KG/DAY)	IV AMINOPHYLLINE[c] (MG/KG/HR)
Newborn up to 24 days (for apnea/bradycardia)	2	0.1
Newborn 24 days and older (for apnea/bradycardia)	3	0.15
Infants 6 weeks–1 yr	0.2 × (age in weeks) + 5	0.05 × calculated daily theophylline
Children 1–9 yr	20	1
Children 9–12 yr, and adolescent daily smokers of cigarettes or marijuana, and otherwise healthy adult smokers under 50 yr	16	0.83
Adolescents 12–16 yr (nonsmokers)	13	0.68
Otherwise healthy nonsmoking adults (including elderly patients)	10	0.52
Cardiac decompensation, cor pulmonale and/or liver dysfunction[d]	5	0.26

a. To maintain a plasma concentration of 10 mcg/ml, except 5 mcg/ml for newborn apnea/bradycardia.
b. In patients with less severe symptoms, a rapidly absorbed oral formulation may be used. The total daily dose is divided equally and administered q 4 hr in children, q 6 hr in infants and adults and q 12 hr in newborns.
c. Adjust infusion rate to maintain plasma concentration in the range of 10–20 mcg/ml.
d. Accumulation may occur over 5–7 days; do not exceed 400 mg/day unless plasma levels are measured.

Dosage Individualization. All dosage recommendations are based on the average theophylline clearance for a given population group. There is a wide interpatient variability (often greater than twofold) within all patient groups.[7] Therefore, it is essential that plasma concentrations be monitored in all patients. If no doses have been missed or extra doses taken during previous 48 hr and if peak plasma concentrations have been obtained (1–2 hr after liquid or plain uncoated tablet and 4–6 hr after most SR products), adjust dose using Theophylline Dosage Adjustment Guide which follows.

Theophylline Dosage Adjustment Guide[a]

PLASMA CONCENTRATION[b] (MCG/ML)	ACTION
Therapeutic	
10–20	Maintain dosage if tolerated; recheck plasma level at 6–12 month intervals.
Too High	
20–25	Decrease dosage by 10%.
25–30	Skip next dose and decrease subsequent doses by 25%; recheck level.
Over 30	Skip next 2 doses and decrease subsequent doses by 50%; recheck level.
Too Low	
7.5–10	Increase dosage by 25%.
5–7.5	Increase dosage by 25%; recheck level.

a. Adapted from reference 8.
b. Appropriately measured peak—see Dosage Individualization.

Pediatric Dose. **PO or IV (infused over 20–30 min) for acute symptoms** same as adult dose. **PO for chronic asthma** (theophylline) initial dose (6–24 weeks) 8 mg/kg/day; (over 24 weeks) 16 mg/kg/day or 400 mg/day (whichever is less) in divided doses, then increase, if tolerated, in approximately 25% increments at 3-day intervals to: (6 weeks–1 yr) (0.3) × (age in weeks) + 8 mg/kg/day; (1–9 yr) 24 mg/kg/day; (9–12 yr) 20 mg/kg/day; (12–16 yr) 18 mg/kg/day.[1,8] **IM, PR suppositories not recommended.**

Dosage Forms. See Theophylline Products Comparison Chart.

Patient Instructions. Do not chew or crush SR tablets or capsules. Take at equally spaced intervals around the clock. Report any nausea, vomiting, GI pain, headache or restlessness. Contents of SR bead-filled capsules may be mixed with a vehicle (applesauce or jam) and swallowed without chewing for patients who have difficulty swallowing capsules.

Pharmacokinetics. *Onset and Duration.* IV onset within 15 min with loading dose.[1,2]

Plasma Levels. Well correlated with clinical effects: therapeutic 10–20 mcg/ml;[2,8] toxicity increases over 20 mcg/ml—see Adverse Reactions. Saliva concentration is an unreliable predictor of plasma concentration.[8]

Fate. Plain uncoated tablets and solution well absorbed orally; enteric coated tablets and some SR dosage forms may be unreliably absorbed.

Food may affect rate, but not extent of absorption. Rectal suppository absorption is slow and erratic and not recommended under any circumstances.[8] Rectal solutions may result in plasma concentrations comparable to oral solution. About 60% plasma protein bound (less in neonates); V_d 0.5 L/kg (greater in neonates). Extensively metabolized in the liver to several inactive metabolites; 10% excreted unchanged in the urine.[3] Clearance decreased in elderly, patients with CHF, significant hepatic dysfunction, pulmonary edema and prolonged high fever. There may be significant intrapatient variability in clearance over time.[7] Numerous drugs alter theophylline's metabolic clearance.[5] Smoking increases theophylline metabolism; this effect may last for 3 months to 2 yr after cessation of smoking.[5] Dose-dependent kinetics in therapeutic range occur in children and rarely in adults.[8] Rate of metabolism progressively increases in infants during the first year of life.

$t_{1/2}$. 3–16 hr (average 8) in adult nonsmokers, 4.4 hr in adult smokers (1–2 packs per day) and 3–5 hr in children over 1 yr. Newborn infants, older patients with chronic obstructive pulmonary disease or cor pulmonale and patients with CHF or liver disease may have a half-life greater than 24 hr.

Adverse Reactions. Local GI irritation may occur. Reactions occur more frequently at plasma concentrations over 20 mcg/ml and include anorexia, nausea, vomiting, epigastric pain, diarrhea, restlessness, irritability, insomnia and headache. Serious arrhythmias and convulsions (frequently leading to death or permanent brain damage) may occur at levels over 35 mcg/ml and may *not* be preceded by less serious toxicity; cardiovascular reactions include sinus tachycardia and life-threatening ventricular arrhythmias with PVCs. Rapid IV administration may be associated with hypotension, syncope, cardiac arrest (particularly if administered directly into CVP line) and death.[9] IM is painful and offers no advantage.

Contraindications. Hypersensitivity to ethylenediamine (aminophylline).

Precautions. Use ideal body weight for dosage calculations in obese patients.[3,8] Use caution in severe cardiac disease, hypoxemia, hepatic disease, acute myocardial injury, cor pulmonale, CHF, peptic ulcer, underlying seizure disorder, migraine and neonates. The alcohol in oral liquid preparations may cause side effects in infants. Do not give with other xanthine preparations.

Parameters to Monitor. Plasma theophylline concentrations before starting therapy (if patient previously taking theophylline) and 1, 4, 12 and 24 hr after start of infusion and daily during continuous infusion.[2,8]

Notes. The oral theophylline preparations of choice for chronic use, to achieve both sustained therapeutic concentrations and improved compliance, are completely and slowly absorbed SR formulations that are minimally affected by food and pH[4]—See Theophylline Products Comparison Chart. Combination products containing ephedrine increase CNS toxicity and have no therapeutic advantage over adequate plasma concentrations of theophylline alone.[1] Combination products with iodides are not recommended.[1] **Dyphylline** is chemically related to, but not a salt of, theophylline; the amount of dyphylline equivalent to theophylline is unknown. It is significantly less potent than theophylline, requiring larger doses; half-life of 2 hr requires more frequent dosing.[1,8]

Theophylline Products Comparison Chart[a]

PRODUCT	ANHYDROUS THEOPHYLLINE CONTENT	MEASURABLE DOSE INCREMENT[b] (MG)	COMMENTS
RAPIDLY ABSORBED (for acute therapy)			
Plain Uncoated Tablets			
Slo-Phyllin®	Tab 100 mg scored	50	Plasma level fluctuations are 459%/117%.[c]
Various	Tab 200 mg scored.	100	
Oral Liquids (Alcohol Free)			
Somophyllin®	18 mg/ml.	9	Contains aminophylline.[d]
Slo-Phyllin® 80 Syrup	5.3 mg/ml.	5	Sugar-free.
Theolair® Liquid	5.3 mg/ml.	2.5	
Rectal Solution			
Somophyllin®[d]	51 mg/ml.	16	Only acceptable rectal dosage form; measure dose carefully.
Intravenous Solution			
Aminophylline[d]	20 mg/ml.	5	Use rubber stoppered vials to avoid glass particles from the breaking of ampules.
Theophylline	800 mg/L.	—	Available in large volume solutions only.
SLOW-RELEASE PRODUCTS[e] (for chronic asthma)			
Slo-Phyllin®	Cap 60 mg	30	Plasma level fluctuations are 225%/69%;[c] beads can be sprinkled on food for administration to infants.
Gyrocaps®	Cap 125 mg		
	Cap 250 mg.		

Continued

Theophylline Products Comparison Chart[a]

PRODUCT	ANHYDROUS THEOPHYLLINE CONTENT	MEASURABLE DOSE INCREMENT[b] (MG)	COMMENTS
Slo-bid® Gyrocaps®	Cap 50 mg Cap 100 mg Cap 200 mg Cap 300 mg.	25	Excellent bioavailability in young infants; beads can be sprinkled on small amount of food; plasma level fluctuations are 43%/18%.[c]
Quibron-T/SR®	Tab 300 mg multi-scored (100, 150, 200, 300 mg).	100	Plasma level fluctuations are 128%/46%,[c] may require q 8 hr dosing in children.
Theo-dur®	Tab 100 mg scored Tab 200 mg scored Tab 300 mg scored Tab 450 mg scored.	25 100 150 225	Some rapid metabolizers may require 8-hr dosing intervals to avoid break-through of symptoms; plasma level fluctuations are 38%/16% for 200, 300 and 450 mg and 87%/34% for 100 mg tablets.[c]

a. Only products with documented bioavailability that are minimally affected by food and with dosage forms that permit incremental changes in dose are listed.
b. Accuracy of measurement decreases below 0.5 ml with suspensions and syrups, because of viscosity; smaller amounts cannot be accurately measured. All liquid dosage forms should be measured with a syringe.
c. Predicted fluctuation between peak and trough (%) for 12-hr dosing interval; average child $t_{1/2}$ = 3.7 hr, average adult $t_{1/2}$ = 8.2 hr.[4]
d. The ethylenediamine portion of aminophylline causes urticaria or exfoliative dermatitis rarely.
e. Only Slo-bid® Gyrocaps® and Theo-dur® tablets have sufficiently slow and complete absorption to allow 12-hr dosing with minimal plasma concentration fluctuations in most patients.[4] Many products advertised for bid dosage (eg, LaBID®, Phyllocontin®) do not maintain plasma concentrations within the therapeutic range in many patients, especially children.[4] Once daily dosage products (eg, Theo-24®, Uniphyl®) are affected by food and may be unreliable.[10,11]

References, 86:16 Respiratory Smooth Muscle Relaxants

1. Hendeles L, Weinberger M. Theophylline: a "state of the art" review. Pharmacotherapy 1983;3:2-44.
2. Jenne JW. Theophylline use in asthma: some current issues. Clin Chest Med 1984;5:645-58.
3. Bukowskyj M, Nakatsu K, Munt PW. Theophylline reassessed. Ann Intern Med 1984;101:63-73.
4. Hendeles L, Iafrate RP, Weinberger M. A clinical and pharmacokinetic basis for the selection and use of slow release theophylline products. Clin Pharmacokinet 1984;9:95-135.
5. Jonkman JHG, Upton RA. Pharmacokinetic drug interactions with theophylline. Clin Pharmacokinet 1984;9:309-34.
6. Kelly HW. Controversies in asthma therapy with theophylline and the β_2-adrenergic agonists. Clin Pharm 1984;3.386-95.
7. Slaughter RL. Theophylline commentary. In: Evans WE, Schentag JJ, Jusko WJ, eds. Applied pharmacokinetics: principles of therapeutic drug monitoring. 2nd ed. Spokane: Applied Therapeutics, 1986:1189-1209.
8. Hendeles L, Massanari M, Weinberger M. Theophylline. Ibid:1105-88.
9. Gaudreault P, Guay J. Theophylline poisoning: pharmacological considerations and clinical management. Med Toxicol 1986;1:169-91.
10. Hendeles L, Weinberger M, Milavetz G et al. Food-induced "dose-dumping" from a once-a-day theophylline product as a cause of theophylline toxicity. Chest 1985;87:758-65.
11. Karim A, Burns T, Wearley L et al. Food-induced changes in theophylline absorption from controlled-release formulations. II. Importance of meal composition and dosing time relative to meal intake in assessing changes in absorption. Clin Pharmacol Ther 1985;38:642-7.

88:00 VITAMINS

88:24 VITAMIN K ACTIVITY

Phytonadione

AquaMephyton®, Konakion®, Mephyton®

Pharmacology. A required cofactor for the hepatic microsomal enzyme system that carboxylates glutamyl residues in precursor proteins to γ-carboxyglutamyl residues. These proteins are present in vitamin K-dependent clotting factors (II, VII, IX and X), as well as noncollagen bone protein, some plasma proteins and the protein of several organs.[1]

Administration and Adult Dose. PO, SC or IM (Konakion® may only be given IM) 2.5–10 mg up to 25 mg initially. A single dose of 1–5 mg is usually sufficient to normalize PT during anticoagulant therapy, but in the presence of severe bleeding, 20–40 mg may be needed.[2-4] The initial dose may be repeated, based on PT and clinical response, after 12–48 hr if given PO and 6–8 hr if given parenterally. The smallest dose possible should be used to reverse anticoagulant effect, to obviate possible refractoriness to further anticoagulant therapy.[4,5] The normal daily nutritional requirement is about 0.03–1.5 mcg/kg.[6,9] AquaMephyton® should be used IV only if absolutely essential.

Pediatric Dose. IM for prophylaxis of hemorrhagic disease of the newborn 0.5–1 mg. SC or IM for treatment of hemorrhagic disease of the newborn 1 mg; more if mother has been receiving an oral anticoagulant.

Dosage Forms. Tab (Mephyton®) 5 mg; Inj (AquaMephyton®, Konakion®) 2, 10 mg/ml.

Pharmacokinetics. *Onset and Duration.* Reversal of anticoagulant effect is variable among individuals; parenteral onset often within 6 hr; peak and duration variable among individuals and with dose. A 5 mg dose IV usually returns PT to normal in 24–48 hr.[3] Large doses may cause prolonged refractoriness to oral anticoagulants.[4,5]

Fate. Absorbed from the GI tract via intestinal lymphatics only in the presence of bile; well absorbed after parenteral administration. Metabolized in the liver to hydroquinone form and epoxide form which are interconvertible with the quinone.[1] Little storage in the body occurs. In the absence of bile, hypoprothrombinemia develops over a period of several weeks.[4,5,7]

Adverse Reactions. The drug itself appears to be nontoxic; however, severe reactions (flushing, dyspnea, chest pain) and occasionally deaths have occurred after IV administration of AquaMephyton®, possibly due to emulsifying agents.[4,8,9] This product should rarely be used IV, and only when other routes of administration are not feasible. A transient flushing sensation, peculiar taste and pain and swelling at the injection site have been reported. Large parenteral doses in neonates have caused hyperbilirubinemia.

Contraindications. Konakion® is contraindicated for other than IM use.

Precautions. Temporary refractoriness to oral anticoagulants may occur, especially with large doses of vitamin K. Reversal of anticoagulant activity may restore previous thromboembolic conditions. Either no effect or worsening of hypoprothrombinemia may occur in severe liver disease and repeated doses are not warranted if response to the initial dose is unsatisfactory.[4,8]

Parameters to Monitor. PT before, and at intervals after, administration of the drug. The testing interval depends on the route of administration, the condition being treated and the patient's status. See Administration and Adult Dose.

Notes. Protect drug from the light at all times. Drug of choice for reversal of oral anticoagulant therapy, but has no antagonist activity against heparin. Parenteral phytonadione and oral menadione and its derivatives are equally effective in treating hypoprothrombinemia caused by malabsorption.[2,8] See Vitamin K Activity Comparison Chart.

Vitamin K Activity Comparison Chart

DRUG	SYNONYMS	ORAL ABSORPTION	USES	SOURCES
Phytonadione AquaMephyton® Konakion® Mephyton®	Vitamin K₁; phylloquinone	Via lymph; bile salts needed.	Hypoprothrombinemia due to oral anticoagulants, antibacterials and salicylates; hemorrhagic disease of the newborn; malabsorption (parenteral or oral with bile salts).	Dietary & synthetic.
Not commercially available.	Vitamin K₂; mena-quinone(s)	No good evidence for absorption in humans.[10]	—	Formed by bacteria in GI tract.
Menadione Not commercially available.	Vitamin K₃	Direct; bile salts not needed.	—	Synthetic.
Menadiol Sodium Diphosphate Kappadione® Synkayvite®	—	Direct; bile salts not needed; converted to menadione in body; about one-half as potent as menadione.	Hypoprothrombinemia due to antibacterials and salicylates; malabsorption due to lack of bile salts.	Synthetic.

References, 88:24 Vitamin K Activity

1. Suttie JW. The metabolic role of vitamin K. Fed Proc 1980;39:2730-5.
2. Gamble JR, Dennis EW, Coon WW et al. Clinical comparison of vitamin K₁ and water-soluble vitamin K. Arch Intern Med 1955;95:52-8.
3. Zieve PD, Solomon HM. Variation in the response of human beings to vitamin K₁. J Lab Clin Med 1969;73:103-10.
4. Mandel HG, Cohn VH. Fat-soluble vitamins; vitamins A, K, and E. In: Gilman AG, Goodman LS, Gilman A, eds. Goodman and Gilman's the pharmacological basis of therapeutics. 6th ed. New York: Macmillan, 1980:1583-601.
5. Koch-Weser J, Sellers EM. Drug interactions with coumarin anticoagulants (2 parts). N Engl J Med 1971;285:487-9, 547-58.
6. Frick PG, Riedler G, Brogli H. Dose response and minimal daily requirement for vitamin K in man. J Appl Physiol 1967;23:387-9.
7. Woolf IL, Babior BM. Vitamin K and warfarin. Am J Med 1972;53:261-7.
8. Finkel MJ. Vitamin K₁ and the vitamin K analogues. Clin Pharmacol Ther 1961;2:794-814.
9. Mattea EJ, Quinn K. Adverse reactions after intravenous phytonadione administration. Hosp Pharm 1981;16:224-35.
10. Rodriguez-Erdmann F, Hoff JV. Interaction of antibiotics with vitamin K. JAMA 1981;246:937. Letter.

92:00 UNCLASSIFIED THERAPEUTIC AGENTS

ANTIGOUT AGENTS

(SEE ALSO URICOSURIC AGENTS 40:40)

General References: 1-6

Allopurinol

Lopurin®, Zyloprim®, Various

Pharmacology. A structural analogue of the purine base hypoxanthine which competitively inhibits xanthine oxidase. This reduces both serum and urinary uric acid levels by blocking the conversion of hypoxanthine and xanthine to uric acid and by decreasing purine synthesis.[2]

Administration and Adult Dose. PO for gout 100 mg/day initially, then increase in 100 mg/day increments at weekly intervals until a serum uric acid level of 6 mg/dl or less is attained; dose within the following guidelines: **PO for maintenance of mild gout** 200–300 mg/day in single or divided doses; **PO for moderately severe tophaceous gout** 400–600 mg/day, to maximum of 800 mg–1 g/day for resistant cases.[3,4] Give dosages which exceed 300 mg/day in divided doses. Prophylactic maintenance doses of colchicine (0.5 mg bid) and/or a nonsteroidal anti-inflammatory agent should be given with allopurinol for several months after initiation of therapy due to an initial increased risk of gouty attacks.[6] A fluid intake sufficient to yield a daily urinary output of at least 2 L and the maintenance of a neutral or slightly alkaline urine are desirable. In transferring from a uricosuric agent to allopurinol, reduce the uricosuric dosage over a period of several weeks, while gradually increasing the dose of allopurinol. **PO for secondary hyperuricemia associated with vigorous treatment of malignancies** 600–800 mg/day for 2–3 days is advisable with a high fluid intake; maintenance dose is 100–200 mg/day, to maximum of 800 mg/day. **PO for recurrent calcium oxalate stones in hyperuricosuria** 200–300 mg/day adjusted up or down based on control of hyperuricosuria.[7]

Dosage Individualization. Reduce dosage in renal impairment as follows: 250 mg/day with a Cl_{cr} of 80 ml/min; 200 mg/day with a Cl_{cr} of 60 ml/min; 150 mg/day with a Cl_{cr} of 40 ml/min; 100 mg/day with a Cl_{cr} of 20 ml/min; 100 mg q 2 days with a Cl_{cr} of 10 ml/min; 100 mg q 3 days with a Cl_{cr} below 10 ml/min.[8]

Pediatric Dose. PO for secondary hyperuricemia associated with malignancies (under 6 yr) 150 mg/day; (6–10 yr) 300 mg/day; evaluate response after 48 hr and adjust dosage as needed.

Dosage Forms. Tab 100, 300 mg. See Notes.

Patient Instructions. This drug may be taken with food, milk or an antacid to minimize stomach upset. Adults should drink at least 10–12 full glasses (240 ml each) of fluid each day. Report any skin rash, itching, chills, fever, nausea or vomiting while taking this drug.

Pharmacokinetics. *Onset and Duration.* A measurable decrease in uric acid occurs in 2–4 days; normal serum uric acid is achieved in 1–3 weeks.

Fate. Well absorbed from the GI tract and rapidly oxidized to oxipurinol, an active, but less potent, inhibitor of xanthine oxidase. 6–10% of a single dose is excreted in the urine as unchanged allopurinol and 45–65% as oxipurinol.[9,10]

$t_{1/2}$. (Allopurinol) 0.5–2 hr. (Oxipurinol) 14–26 hr (average 20) with normal renal function; 5–10 days in renal failure.[8-12]

Adverse Reactions. Most frequent is a maculopapular skin rash, but exfoliative, urticarial, purpuric and erythema multiforme lesions are also reported. Such reactions necessitate drug discontinuation because more severe hypersensitivity reactions such as vasculitis, toxic epidermal necrolysis, renal impairment and hepatic damage can occur. Hypersensitivity reactions, frequently marked by fever and eosinophilia, usually begin 2–4 weeks after start of therapy and appear related to pre-existing renal dysfunction, elevated oxipurinol plasma levels and/or concurrent thiazide therapy.[8] Occasionally, nausea, vomiting and abdominal pain occur. Rarely, alopecia, cataract formation, bone marrow depression, leukopenia, leukocytosis or renal xanthine stones occur.

Contraindications. Children (except for hyperuricemia secondary to malignancy). Patients who have developed a severe reaction should not be restarted on the drug.

Precautions. Pregnancy; lactation. Should not be given to immediate relatives of patients with idiopathic hemochromatosis. Use with caution in renal impairment in reduced doses. Thiazide diuretics may contribute to allopurinol toxicity, although a cause-and-effect relationship has not been established. Adjust dosage conservatively in patients with impaired renal function who are on a thiazide concomitantly.[8]

Parameters to Monitor. Serum uric acid levels; pretreatment 24-hour urinary uric acid excretion.[2] Periodic determination of liver function (particularly in patients with pre-existing liver disease). Renal function studies and CBC should be performed, especially during the first few months of therapy. Monitor renal function in patients on concurrent thiazide therapy.[8]

Notes. Drug of choice for patients with impaired renal function who respond poorly to uricosuric agents; however, these patients should be monitored closely because of an increased frequency of adverse reactions.[5,8] Current data do not support the routine treatment of asymptomatic hyperuricemia in patients other than those receiving vigorous treatment of malignancies.[6,8] Uricosuric drugs enhance the renal clearance of oxipurinol and diminish the degree of xanthine oxidase suppression; however, in appropriate cases the net effect of combined treatment facilitates mobilization of uric acid deposits.[5,9] Concurrent use of salicylates, for their antirheumatic effect, does not compromise the action of allopurinol. Because of limited studies showing very poor or no absorption of extemporaneously compounded allopurinol suppositories, this dosage form is not recommended.[12] IV drug is available from manufacturer for investigational use.

Colchicine

Various

Pharmacology. An anti-inflammatory agent relatively specific for gout, with activity probably due to the impairment of leukocyte chemotaxis and synovial cell phagocytosis of urate crystals present in the synovial fluid.

Administration and Adult Dose. **PO for acute gout** 0.5–1.2 mg initially, then 0.5–1.2 mg q 1–2 hr until pain is relieved or GI toxicity occurs (ie, nausea, vomiting or diarrhea), to maximum total dose of 8 mg. An interval of 3 days is advised if a second course is required. **PO for prophylaxis in chronic gout** 0.5–1.8 mg/day or every other day, depending on severity of the case. **Slow IV for acute gout** 1–2 mg initially, diluted (if desired) in non-bacteriostatic NS, then 0.5 mg q 6–24 hr prn, to maximum of 4 mg in 24 hr. Some clinicians recommend a single IV dose of 3 mg over 5 min. If pain recurs, 1–2 mg IV daily for several days. IV colchicine is very irritating and extravasation must be avoided to prevent tissue and nerve damage. Transfer to PO therapy at a similar dose as soon as possible. **Do not administer by SC or IM routes.** See Notes.

Dosage Individualization. During prolonged use, reduce both oral and IV doses in the presence of renal impairment.

Dosage Forms. **Granules** 500 mcg; **Tab** 500, 600 mcg; **Inj** 500 mcg/ml.

Patient Instructions. A supply of this drug should always be at hand and it should be taken promptly at the earliest symptoms of a gouty attack. Relief of gout pain or occurrence of nausea, vomiting or diarrhea indicate that full therapeutic dose has been attained and no more drug should be taken. Black tarry stools or bright red blood in the stools may indicate gastrointestinal bleeding and should be reported immediately. Sore throat, fever or oral lesions may be an early sign of a severe, but rare, blood disorder and should be reported immediately.

Pharmacokinetics. *Fate.* Well absorbed after oral administration, with partial hepatic deacetylation; V_d is 1–2 L/kg; 31% plasma protein bound.[13-16] Extensive leukocyte uptake with significant levels found up to 10 days. Both urinary (10–36%, in part unchanged) and fecal elimination occur.[14-16]

$t_{1/2}$. 35–90 min (average 58) following a single 2 mg IV dose in normals; slightly shorter in patients with severe liver disease and longer in patients with gout or severe renal impairment.[14,15]

Adverse Reactions. Overdosage can cause hemorrhagic gastroenteritis, vascular damage leading to shock, nephrotoxicity and paralysis. As little as 7 mg has proved fatal, but much larger doses have been survived.[16,17] Nausea, vomiting and diarrhea are frequent and may occur several hours after oral or IV drug administration; discontinue drug at first signs. Prolonged administration may cause bone marrow depression with agranulocytosis, aplastic anemia or thrombocytopenia; peripheral neuritis, purpura, myopathy, alopecia and reversible azoospermia also reported.

Precautions. Use with great caution in elderly or debilitated patients, especially those with hepatic, renal, GI or heart disease. Reduce dosage if weakness, anorexia, nausea, vomiting or diarrhea occurs.

Notes. Colchicine may be an effective anti-inflammatory agent in the therapy of the arthritis of pseudogout.[18] For acute gout, a nonsteroidal anti-inflammatory agent may be preferred, but daily colchicine is still frequently given for prophylaxis against recurrent gouty attacks during the first 6–12 months of allopurinol or uricosuric treatment.[2,3,6] Continuous prophylactic colchicine therapy can be effective in suppressing the acute attacks and renal dysfunction of familial Mediterranean fever.[19] Colchicine therapy may also be effective for refractory idiopathic thrombocytopenic purpura and certain inflammatory dermatoses.[20,21]

ANTIPARKINSONIAN AGENTS

(SEE ALSO BENZTROPINE AND TRIHEXYPHENIDYL 12:08.04 AND BROMOCRIPTINE 92:00)

General References: 22-24

Amantadine Hydrochloride   Symmetrel®, Various

Pharmacology. Amantadine is an antiviral compound which appears to prevent the release of viral nucleic acid into the host cell. In Parkinson's disease, the drug may augment dopamine activity by increasing presynaptic dopamine release.

Administration and Adult Dose. PO for Parkinson's disease usual maintenance dose 100 mg bid. In patients with serious medical illnesses or who are receiving other antiparkinson drugs 100 mg/day initially, increasing in 100 mg/day increments q 7–14 days to effective dose, to maximum of 400 mg/day in 2 divided doses. **PO for drug-induced extrapyramidal reactions** 100 mg bid, to maximum of 300 mg/day in 3 divided doses. **PO for prophylaxis or treatment of influenza A illness** 200 mg/day in 1 or 2 divided doses. For prophylaxis, continue for at least 10 days following exposure or for 2-3 weeks after giving influenza A vaccine. For treatment, continue for 24–48 hr after symptoms disappear.

Dosage Individualization. Reduce dosage in renal impairment as follows: give loading dose of 200 mg, then 150 mg/day with Cl_{cr} of 60 ml/min; 100 mg/day with Cl_{cr} of 40–50 ml/min; 200 mg twice/week with Cl_{cr} of 30 ml/min; 100 mg three times/week with Cl_{cr} of 20 ml/min; and 150 mg/week with Cl_{cr} of 10 ml/min or less. No additional doses needed after hemodialysis.[25] Renal clearance is diminished in elderly (over 60 yr) men; therefore, lower the initial dose for influenza prophylaxis.[26]

Pediatric Dose. PO for prophylaxis or treatment of influenza A illness (under 1 yr) safety and efficacy not established; (1-9 yr) 4.4–8.8 mg/kg/day in 2 divided doses, to maximum of 150 mg/day; (9–12 yr) 100 mg bid.

Dosage Forms. Cap 100 mg; **Syrup** 10 mg/ml.

Patient Instructions. Stopping this medication suddenly may cause your Parkinson's disease to worsen quickly. This medication may cause dizziness, confusion or difficulty in concentrating. Until the extent of these effects are known, caution should be used when driving, operating machinery or performing other tasks requiring mental alertness. Avoid excessive concurrent use of alcohol.

Pharmacokinetics. *Onset and Duration.* Peak antiparkinson effect occurs within 14 days.[27] Tolerance to the therapeutic effects of amantadine occurs in most patients after 3 months.[22]

Plasma Levels. (Therapeutic, antiviral) 300–500 ng/ml.[28] Neurotoxicity above 1.5 mcg/ml.[25]

Fate. Peak plasma levels occur in 4–8 hr. Steady-state plasma levels occur in healthy adults within 3 days.[28] V_d is 6–10 L/kg; Cl is 2.37–10.53 L/hr. 90% excreted unchanged in urine.[25,26]

$t_{1/2}$. 9.7–14.5 hr; (over 60 yr) 23–45 hr; (during chronic hemodialysis) 8.3 days.[25,26]

Adverse Reactions. Occasionally, dose-related dizziness, confusion, hallucinations, anxiety, restlessness, irritability, nausea, peripheral edema or livedo reticularis occur. Rarely, depression, psychosis, CHF, orthostatic hypotension, seizures or leukopenia are reported.

Precautions. Pregnancy; lactation. Use with caution in patients with CHF, seizures, renal disease, peripheral edema, orthostatic hypotension, affective disorders, a history of eczematoid rash or those receiving CNS stimulants. Abrupt withdrawal of the drug in patients with Parkinson's disease may result in rapid return of symptoms.

Parameters to Monitor. Monitor renal function and clinical signs of neurotoxicity periodically.

Notes. In Parkinson's disease, amantadine produces clinical improvements in akinesia and rigidity to a lesser degree than levodopa,[27] but greater than anticholinergics.[22] However, anticholinergics appear to reduce tremor to a greater degree than amantadine.[29]

Carbidopa and Levodopa   Sinemet®

Pharmacology. See Levodopa. Carbidopa inhibits extracerebral DOPA decarboxylase. This action prevents the peripheral decarboxylation of levodopa, thereby increasing the amount available to the brain.

Administration and Adult Dose. PO for Parkinson's disease in patients not receiving levodopa 25 mg carbidopa/100 mg levodopa tid initially, increasing in 1 tablet/day increments q 1-2 days to effective dose, to maximum of 6 tablets/day. Alternatively, 10 mg carbidopa/100 mg levodopa tid initially, to maximum of 8 tablets/day. Initial dosing with 10 mg carbidopa/100 mg levodopa may result in more nausea and vomiting, because the 70-100 mg/day of carbidopa needed to saturate DOPA decarboxylase is not provided. If initial dosage maximum is reached and further titration is necessary, substitute 25 mg carbidopa/250 mg levodopa tid or qid, increase in 0.5-1 tablet/day increments q 1-2 days to effective dose, to maximum of 8 tablets/day. **PO for Parkinson's disease in patients receiving levodopa** discontinue levodopa at least 8 hr before starting carbidopa/levodopa. Daily dose of carbidopa/levodopa should provide approximately 25% of the previous levodopa daily dose and 70-100 mg/day of carbidopa.

Pediatric Dose. Safety not established under 18 yr.

Dosage Forms. Tab 10 mg carbidopa/100 mg levodopa, 25 mg carbidopa/100 mg levodopa, 25 mg carbidopa/250 mg levodopa.

Patient Instructions. Stopping this medication suddenly may cause your Parkinson's disease to worsen quickly. Report bothersome or unusual side effects. Unless prescribed, do not take levodopa in addition to this drug.

Pharmacokinetics. _Onset and Duration._ Peak therapeutic effect 7-10 days.[30] 50-80% of patients lose initial therapeutic effect after 5 yr.[24] See Notes.

Fate. About 40-70% of carbidopa is absorbed. 30% of carbidopa is excreted unchanged in urine.[31] Carbidopa inhibits peripheral decarboxylation of levodopa which increases levodopa plasma levels; thus, more drug passes into the brain. Carbidopa allows 75% reduction in the amount of levodopa needed for therapy.[30] See Levodopa.

$t_{1/2}$. (Carbidopa) 2-3 hr.[30]

Adverse Reactions. See Levodopa. Compared to levodopa alone, carbidopa/levodopa markedly reduces GI effects and causes less orthostatic hypotension and sinus tachycardia. However, mental disturbances are not eliminated and abnormal involuntary muscle movements (dyskinesias) may appear earlier in therapy.[30] See Notes.

Contraindications. See Levodopa.

Precautions. See Levodopa. In addition, levodopa must be discontinued at least 8 hr before carbidopa/levodopa is started.

Parameters to Monitor. See Levodopa.

Notes. Pyridoxine (vitamin B_6) can be given safely to patients receiving carbidopa/levodopa. Compared to levodopa, carbidopa/levodopa allows a more rapid titration and smoother response in many patients. Loss of therapeutic effect is manifested by fluctuations in clinical response ("on-off" phenomenon). The occurrence of certain fluctuations, "end-of-dose" akinesia, "wearing-off" response or peak dose dyskinesia are related to time of drug administration. Others, such as rapid unpredictable fluctuations between dyskinesia and akinesia ("on-off" or "yo-yo" effect), may respond to smaller and more frequent carbidopa/levodopa doses or the introduction of bromocriptine.[24] A drug-free interval ("drug holiday") of 7-10 days may transiently relieve disease fluctuations or psychiatric disturbances in some patients receiving chronic therapy. Complete withdrawal of carbidopa/levodopa must be undertaken in the hospital and may lead to development of infectious or thrombotic complications.[22]

Levodopa   Larodopa®, Dopar®, Various

Pharmacology. Levodopa is a precursor of the neurotransmitter dopamine. Levodopa is decarboxylated in the brain to dopamine which is deficient in the basal ganglia of patients with Parkinson's disease.

Administration and Adult Dose. **PO for Parkinson's disease** 250 mg bid-qid initially. Depending upon patient tolerance, increase in 125-750 mg/day increments q 3-7 days to effective dose, to maximum of 8 g/day. Usual maintenance dose is 2-6 g/day in 4 divided doses.[32]

Pediatric Dose. Safety not established under 12 yr.

Dosage Forms. **Cap** 100, 250, 500 mg; **Tab** 100, 250, 500 mg.

Patient Instructions. Stopping this medication suddenly may cause your Parkinson's disease to worsen quickly. This medication should be taken with food or milk to minimize stomach upset. Avoid foods or vitamins containing pyridoxine (vitamin B_6). Report bothersome or unusual side effects.

Pharmacokinetics. *Onset and Duration.* Onset of therapeutic effect determined by patient tolerance. Usually, initial onset is after 10 days; peak is 4-8 weeks as dose reaches 2-4 g/day.[32] 50-80% of patients lose initial therapeutic effect after 5 yr.[24] See Notes.

Fate. Peak plasma levels occur in 1 hr. Peak level is reduced an average of 29% and delayed 34 min by meals.[33] DOPA decarboxylase metabolizes 99% of levodopa to dopamine outside the CNS. Pyridoxine enhances decarboxylation of levodopa.[22] 1% of levodopa is transported into CNS and converted to dopamine. High protein meals (65-104 g protein) may reverse clinical response to levodopa by inhibiting its transport into the CNS.[33] Drug is excreted in urine, 85% as metabolites and 1% as unchanged drug.[32]

$t_{1/2}$. 1-1.75 hr.[22]

Adverse Reactions. Anorexia, nausea, vomiting, abdominal distress, postural hypotension, dystonic or choreiform muscle movements (dyskinesias), confusion, memory changes, depression and hallucinations occur frequently, and are generally reversible with dosage reduction.[23] Occasionally, anxiety, insomnia or sinus tachycardia occur. Rarely, psychosis, hemolytic anemia, leukopenia or agranulocytosis are reported. See Notes.

Contraindications.   MAO inhibitors concurrently or 2 weeks prior to levodopa; narrow angle glaucoma; lactation; history of melanoma.

Precautions.   Pregnancy. Use with caution in patients with history of myocardial infarction complicated by arrhythmias, active peptic ulcer disease, severe cardiovascular, pulmonary, renal, hepatic or endocrine disease, open angle glaucoma, bronchial asthma or psychosis. Also, caution in patients receiving antihypertensives. Symptoms resembling neuroleptic malignant syndrome have been reported when levodopa or carbidopa/levodopa in combination with other antiparkinson agents have been withdrawn abruptly.[34]

Parameters to Monitor.   CBC, renal and liver function tests should be monitored periodically during chronic therapy. In patients with glaucoma, monitor intraocular pressure.

Notes.   Levodopa reduces all symptoms of Parkinson's disease: tremor, rigidity and bradykinesia.[24] Levodopa is best administered combined with carbidopa, a DOPA decarboxylase inhibitor. Compared to use of levodopa as a single agent, the combination significantly reduces GI and cardiac adverse effects and attains higher levels of dopamine in the CNS.[31] Loss of therapeutic effect is manifested by fluctuations in clinical response ("on-off" phenomenon). See Carbidopa and Levodopa.

BROMOCRIPTINE

Bromocriptine Mesylate   Parlodel®

Pharmacology.   An ergot alkaloid which directly stimulates dopamine receptors. This results in reduction of prolactin and growth hormone release from the pituitary gland and improves motor function in Parkinson's disease.

Administration and Adult Dose.   **PO for Parkinson's disease** 1.25 mg bid initially with food, increase in 2.5 mg/day increments q 14–28 days to effective dose. When given to patients concurrently receiving carbidopa/levodopa, usual maintenance dose is 10–20 mg/day in 2–3 divided doses.[35,36] See Notes. **PO for prevention of lactation** 2.5 mg bid with food starting no sooner than 4 hr postpartum. Usual dose is 2.5 mg bid-tid for 14–21 days. **PO for amenorrhea with or without galactorrhea or infertility** 1.25 mg/day or bid initially with food, increase in 2.5 mg/day increments q 3–7 days to effective dose, to maximum of 15 mg/day. Usual maintenance dose is 2.5 mg bid-tid. **PO for acromegaly** 1.25 mg/day or bid initially with food, increase in 1.25–2.5 mg/day increments q 3–7 days to effective dose, to maximum of 100 mg/day. Usual maintenance dose is 20–30 mg/day in 2–3 divided doses.

Pediatric Dose.   Safety and efficacy not established under 15 yr.

Dosage Forms.   **Cap** 5 mg; **Tab** 2.5 mg.

Patient Instructions.   This drug may cause dizziness or drowsiness. Until the extent of these effects is known, caution should be used when driving, operating machinery or performing tasks requiring mental alertness. This drug should be taken with food to minimize stomach upset. A barrier contraceptive should be used in female patients taking this drug to induce ovulation.

Pharmacokinetics. *Onset and Duration.* (Parkinsonism) peak improvement in symptoms occurs in 15 weeks;[35] (amenorrhea) normal menstrual function may return within 1 month; (lactation suppression) lactation may be blocked within 48 hr.[37]

Fate. About 28% absorbed and plasma levels peak in 1–3 hr.[37] 90–96% bound to albumin. The majority of drug is metabolized and excreted via bile; about 7% is excreted as metabolites in urine.[38]

$t_{1/2}$. About 2 days.[38]

Adverse Reactions. Nausea, vomiting, symptomatic hypotension, dizziness and headache occur frequently. Hypotension is most frequent in postpartum patients. Occasionally, abdominal cramps, diarrhea, fatigue, drowsiness or syncope may occur. Rarely, hypertension, stroke, seizures, pulmonary infiltrates or pleural effusions reported. Hallucinations, insomnia, erythromelalgia or dyskinesias are rare, but may be more prominent in parkinsonism.[35,36]

Contraindications. Pregnancy; hypersensitivity to ergot alkaloids; severe ischemic heart disease; peripheral vascular disease.

Precautions. In patients with amenorrhea, galactorrhea or infertility, a barrier contraceptive should be used. Discontinue drug as soon as pregnancy is detected. Use with caution in patients with history of pulmonary disease, myocardial infarction, severe angina or psychiatric disease. Concurrent use with dopamine antagonist drugs (eg, phenothiazines) may cause decreased efficacy of bromocriptine.

Notes. As an adjunct to levodopa in Parkinson's disease, bromocriptine, in doses up to 20 mg/day, may provide improvement in clinical symptoms. Greatest improvement occurs in patients with mild to moderate disease. Bromocriptine may improve some of the fluctuations in disease ("on-off" phenomenon) seen with long-term levodopa therapy.[36]

CROMOLYN

Cromolyn Sodium   Intal®, Nasalcrom®, Opticrom®

Pharmacology. Cromolyn stabilizes the mast cell membrane, inhibiting release and production of soluble mediators (eg, histamine, leukotrienes) that produce inflammation and bronchospasm. The mechanism appears to be the inhibition of calcium ion influx through the cell membrane. Cromolyn inhibits both the early and late responses to specific allergen and exercise challenges. It also prevents the increase in nonspecific bronchial hyperreactivity that occurs during a specific allergen season in atopic asthmatics.[39,40]

Administration and Adult Dose. **Inhal for asthma** 20 mg qid at regular intervals via Spinhaler® or powered nebulizer (1 ampule inhalant solution) or 1–2 mg qid via a pressurized metered-dose inhaler. See Notes. **Inhal for prevention of exercise-induced bronchospasm** single dose (as above) just prior to exercise. **Intranasal for prophylaxis of allergic rhinitis** 5.2 mg/nostril 3–6 times/day at regular intervals. **Ophth for allergic ocular disorders** 1–2 drops (1.6–3.2 mg) in each eye 4–6 times/day at regular intervals.[41] For chronic conditions the drug must be used continuously to be effective.

Dosage Individualization. It may require 4–6 weeks to achieve maximal response, although most asthmatics have a clinically significant response within 2 weeks.[42,43] Initial therapy should be started in conjunction with an aerosolized β_2-agonist. The therapeutic effect is dose-dependent and patients with more severe disease may require more frequent administration initially.[43] After a patient becomes symptom-free, the frequency of administration may be reduced to bid-tid.

Pediatric Dose. **Inhal** (under 2 yr) dosage not established; (2 yr and over) same as adult dose. **Intranasal or Ophth** same as adult dose.

Dosage Forms. **Inhal Cap** (not for oral use) 20 mg; **Inhal Soln** 10 mg/ml; **Inhal** 800 mcg/metered dose (112 or 200 doses/inhaler); **Nasal Inhal** 40 mg/ml (100 doses/inhaler); **Ophth Drops** 40 mg/ml (250 drops/container).

Patient Instructions. Do not stop therapy abruptly, except on medical advice. Do not swallow capsule; capsules must be inhaled using the special inhaler. This medication must be used regularly and continuously to be effective. Carefully follow directions for inhaler use included with the device. A rapid deep inhalation with the head tilted back is the best method for the Spinhaler®.[40] Actuate (metered-dose device) during a *slow* deep inhalation, then hold breath for 5–10 seconds.[41] Discontinue using the Spinhaler® during acute asthmatic attacks. Do not discontinue the use of the nebulizer solution during acute asthmatic attacks. You may mix the nebulizer solution with any bronchodilator inhalant solution.

Pharmacokinetics. *Onset and Duration.* Onset within 1 min for prevention of allergen-induced mast cell degranulation; duration dose-dependent, 2–5 hr.[40]

   Fate. Oral bioavailability is 0.5–1%. Amount absorbed after inhalation is dependent on the delivery system—approximately 10% of the dose from a Spinhaler® and less than 2% with the nebulizer solution.[40] Peak plasma levels occur 15–20 min after inhalation. V_d is 0.2 L/kg; Cl is 0.35 L/hr/kg. Rapidly excreted unchanged in equal portions in the bile and urine.[39,40]

   $t_{1/2}$. 11–20 min.[39,40]

Adverse Reactions. Bronchospasm and pharyngeal irritation occur occasionally with inhalation capsules, but not following nebulizer solution or metered-dose aerosol. Rarely, allergic reactions reported.[42] Mild burning or stinging may occur with ophthalmic solution.[41]

Precautions. Do not discontinue cromolyn during acute asthmatic exacerbations; if the capsules for inhalation cause irritation and worsening, switch the patient temporarily to the nebulizer solution. Caution in patients with lactose sensitivity (capsules only). Watch for worsening of asthma in patients discontinuing the drug. Children under 5 yr should receive cromolyn as the nebulizer solution. The ophthalmic solution contains 0.01% benzalkonium chloride; therefore, soft contact lenses should not be worn during therapy.[41]

Parameters to Monitor. Relief of asthmatic symptoms and the proper dose and inhalation technique should be monitored. Patient noncompliance and/or inappropriate inhalation technique often contribute to treatment failures. The measurement of peak expiratory flow rate with a Wright peak flow meter is useful in severe chronic asthma. Periodic standard pulmonary function tests are indicated q 1–6 months in less severe asthma.

Notes. Comparative studies have shown cromolyn and theophylline to be equally effective for the prophylaxis of chronic asthma, although cromolyn produces fewer side effects.[39,40,42,43] Before beginning cromolyn, it is important that the patient is not symptomatic. The inhalant solution is stable with all β_2-agonist and anticholinergic solutions for nebulization and can be used as the diluent for these in place of NS.[40] The nasal spray is most effective if started 1 week prior to the allergen season; however, patients receive benefit even if begun after symptoms occur.[42]

CYCLOSPORINE

Cyclosporine
Sandimmune®

Pharmacology. Cyclosporine is a cyclic polypeptide immunosuppressant agent whose exact mechanism of action is unknown. It appears to inhibit cells from making or releasing interleukin-2, to block interleukin-2-mediated activation of resting T-lymphocytes and to selectively inhibit activated T-lymphocytes. It has little effect on B-cells.[44]

Administration and Adult Dose. **PO for prophylaxis of organ rejection** 15 mg/kg/day initially, given 4–12 hr before transplantation and continued for 1–2 weeks. Taper the dose by about 5% weekly to a maintenance dose of 5–10 mg/kg/day. Mix the solution with milk, chocolate milk or orange juice and administer immediately after mixing. **IV for patients unable to take oral solution** 5–6 mg/kg/day initially, given as a dilute solution of 50 mg/20–100 ml and infused over 2–6 hours. This dose should be continued daily until patient can tolerate oral dosing as above.

Dosage Individualization. Adjust dosage in patients with renal impairment. Frequent blood/plasma level monitoring is required in hepatic transplant patients.

Pediatric Dose. Safety and efficacy not established, although children as young as 6 months have received the drug with no unusual effects. Infants and children may require larger weight-adjusted doses than adults.[45]

Dosage Forms. **Soln** 100 mg/ml; **Inj** 50 mg/ml.

Patient Instructions. Take this medication daily and do not discontinue its use unless directed. Mixing oral solution with milk, chocolate milk or orange juice improves its palatability. Take it immediately after mixing. Report fever, sore throat, tiredness or unusual bleeding or bruising.

Pharmacokinetics. *Plasma Levels.* Not well established; dependent on assay, biologic fluid and time post-transplant.[46] Therapeutic trough levels (HPLC, whole blood) 150 ng/ml for first 2 months post-renal transplant, then 50–100 ng/ml; levels over 300 ng/ml with slowly rising Cr_s suggest nephrotoxicity.[46] Other methods are as follows: (RIA, whole blood) 250–800 ng/ml; (RIA, plasma) 100–250 ng/ml.[44,46] Lower levels may be associated with increased risk of rejection and higher levels with overimmunosuppression and an increased frequency of nephrotoxicity.[44,46] See Notes.

Fate. Poor and erratic oral bioavailability ranging from 4–60%. Peak plasma concentration occurs 1–8 hr after the dose. Food decreases peak level and delays the time to peak. Diarrhea may also decrease absorption. Cyclosporine is widely distributed in tissues with a V_{dss} averaging 3.5–4.5 L/kg.[47] In blood, the drug is distributed 55% in red blood cells, 10% in white cells and 30% in plasma where it is highly protein bound. Red cell binding is time-, temperature- and hematocrit-dependent, with about 2 hr required for equilibration at room temperature. The drug is extensively metabolized by the liver to inactive metabolites, with a negligible amount excreted unchanged in the urine. Cl (HPLC, whole blood) averages about 0.36 L/hr/kg.[44,45,48]

$t_{1/2}$. 4–60 hr.[44]

Adverse Reactions. Dose-dependent nephrotoxicity is relatively frequent and is indicated by a greater than 25% increase in Cr_s over a few days with no fever and maintenance of urine output. It is usually responsive to dosage reduction, but persistent elevations in BUN and Cr_s are an indication to discontinue the drug. Hypertension occurs frequently; it is sometimes associated with convulsions, and is occasionally difficult to control. Hepatotoxicity, indicated by increased liver enzymes and serum bilirubin, occurs occasionally and is responsive to dosage reduction. Hypotension, hirsutism, tremors and paresthesias have also been reported. Rarely, hyperkalemia, hyperuricemia, sensitivity to temperature extremes and allergy to the drug or to the emulsifying agent in the IV product have been reported. Too rapid IV infusion may cause warmth, flushing, headache and abdominal discomfort. As with other immunosuppressive agents, there is an increased risk of lymphoproliferative malignancies.

Contraindications. Allergy to drug or polyethoxylated castor oil.

Precautions. Pregnancy. Use with caution in patients with renal function impairment.

Parameters to Monitor. Renal and hepatic function tests should be monitored repeatedly during therapy. Blood/plasma drug trough level monitoring has been suggested as follows: twice weekly immediately post-transplant, weekly for 3 months, then monthly.[46]

Notes. A new RIA assay is being developed which is more specific for cyclosporine than earlier assays. Serum level ranges with the new assay should be similar to those of the HPLC assay.

References, 92:00 Unclassified Therapeutic Agents

1. Rodnan GP, Robin JA, Tolchin SF et al. Allopurinol and gouty hyperuricemia: efficacy of a single daily dose. JAMA 1975;231:1143-7.

2. Boss GR, Seegmiller JE. Hyperuricemia and gout: classification, complications and management. N Engl J Med 1979;300:1459-68.

3. Simkin PA. Management of gout. Ann Intern Med 1979;90:812-6.

4. Mangini RJ. Drug therapy reviews: pathogenesis and clinical management of hyperuricemia and gout. Am J Hosp Pharm 1979;36:497-504.

5. Yu TF. Milestones in the treatment of gout. Am J Med 1974;56:676-85.

6. German DC, Holmes EW. Hyperuricemia and gout. Med Clin North Am 1986;70:419-36.

7. Ettinger B, Tang A, Citron JT et al. Randomized trial of allopurinol in the prevention of calcium oxalate calculi. N Engl J Med 1986;315:1386-9.

8. Hande KR, Noone RM, Stone WJ. Severe allopurinol toxicity: description and guidelines for prevention in patients with renal insufficiency. Am J Med 1984;76:47-56.

9. Elion GB, Yu TF, Gutman AB et al. Renal clearance of oxipurinol, the chief metabolite of allopurinol. Am J Med 1968;45:69-77.

10. Elion GB, Kovensky A, Hitchings GH. Metabolic studies of allopurinol, an inhibitor of xanthine oxidase. Biochem Pharmacol 1966;15:863-80.

11. Hande K, Reed E, Chabner B. Allopurinol kinetics. Clin Pharmacol Ther 1978;23:598-605.

12. Appelbaum SJ, Mayersohn M, Dorr RT et al. Allopurinol kinetics and bioavailability: intravenous, oral and rectal administration. Cancer Chemother Pharmacol 1982;8:93-8.

13. Jusko WJ, Gretch M. Plasma and tissue protein binding of drugs in pharmacokinetics. Drug Metab Rev 1976;5:43-140.

14. Ertel NH, Mittler JC, Akgun S et al. Radioimmunoassay for colchicine in plasma and urine. Science 1976;193:233-5.

15. Wallace SL, Omokoku B, Ertel NH. Colchicine plasma levels: implications as to pharmacology and mechanism of action. Am J Med 1970;48:443-8.

16. Wallace SL. Colchicine. Semin Arthritis Rheum 1974;3:369-81.

17. Freeman DL. Frequent doses of intravenous colchicine can be lethal. N Engl J Med 1983;309:310. Letter.

18. Tabatabai MR, Cummings NA. Intravenous colchicine in the treatment of acute pseudogout. Arthritis Rheum 1980;23:370-4.

19. Zemer D, Pras M, Sohar E et al. Colchicine in the prevention and treatment of the amyloidosis of familial Mediterranean fever. N Engl J Med 1986;314:1001-5.

20. Strother SV, Zuckerman KS, LoBuglio AF. Colchicine therapy for refractory idiopathic thrombocytopenic purpura. Arch Intern Med 1984;144:2198-200.

21. Aram H. Colchicine in dermatologic therapy. Int J Dermatol 1983;22:566-9.

22. Quinn NP. Anti-parkinsonian drugs today. Drugs 1984;28:236-62.

23. Parkes JD. Adverse effects of antiparkinsonian drugs. Drugs 1981;21:341-53.

24. Burton K, Calne DB. Pharmacology of Parkinson's disease. Neurol Clin 1984;2:461-72.

25. Horadam VW, Sharp JG, Smilack JD et al. Pharmacokinetics of amantadine hydrochloride in subjects with normal and impaired renal function. Ann Intern Med 1981;94(part 1):454-8.

26. Aoki FY, Sitar DS. Amantadine kinetics in healthy elderly men: implications for influenza prevention. Clin Pharmacol Ther 1985;37:137-44.

27. Mawdsley C, Williams IR, Pullar IA et al. Treatment of parkinsonism by amantadine and levodopa. Clin Pharmacol Ther 1972;13:575-83.

28. Aoki FY, Stiver HG, Sitar DS et al. Prophylactic amantadine dose and plasma concentration—effect relationships in healthy adults. Clin Pharmacol Ther 1985;37:128-36.

29. Koller WC. Pharmacologic treatment of parkinsonian tremor. Arch Neurol 1986;43:126-7.

30. Boshes B. Sinemet and the treatment of parkinsonism. Ann Intern Med 1981;94:364-70.

31. Pinder RM, Brogden RN, Sawyer PR et al. Levodopa and decarboxylase inhibitors: a review of their clinical pharmacology and use in the treatment of parkinsonism. Drugs 1976;11:329-77.

32. Brogden RN, Speight TM, Avery GS. Levodopa: a review of its pharmacological properties and therapeutic uses with particular reference to parkinsonism. Drugs 1971;2:262-400.

33. Nutt JG, Woodward WR, Hammerstad JP et al. The ''on-off'' phenomenon in Parkinson's disease—relation to levodopa absorption and transport. N Engl J Med 1984;310:483-8.

34. Friedman JH, Feinberg SS, Feldman RG. A neuroleptic malignantlike syndrome due to levodopa therapy withdrawal. JAMA 1985;254.2792-5.

35. Teychenne PF, Bergsrud D, Racy A et al. Bromocriptine: low-dose therapy in Parkinson disease. Neurology 1982;32:577-83.

36. Maier Hoehn M, Elton RL. Low dosages of bromocriptine added to levodopa in Parkinson's disease. Neurology 1985;35:199-206.

37. Vance ML, Evans WS, Thorner MO. Bromocriptine. Ann Intern Med 1984;100:78-91.

38. Friis ML, Gron U, Larsen N-E et al. Pharmacokinetics of bromocriptine during continuous oral treatment of Parkinson's disease. Eur J Clin Pharmacol 1979;15:275-80.

39. Shapiro GG, Konig P. Cromolyn sodium: a review. Pharmacotherapy 1985;5:156-70.

40. Murphy S, Kelly HW. Cromolyn sodium: a review of mechanisms and clinical use in asthma. Drug Intell Clin Pharm 1987;21:22-35.

41. Sorkin EM, Ward A. Ocular sodium cromoglycate: an overview of its therapeutic efficacy in allergic eye disease. Drugs 1986;31:131-48.

42. Berman BA. Cromolyn: past, present, and future. Pediatr Clin North Am 1983;30:915-30.

43. Bernstein IL. Cromolyn sodium in the treatment of asthma: changing concepts. J Allergy Clin Immunol 1981;68:247-53.

44. Ptachcinski RJ, Burckart GJ, Venkataramanan R. Cyclosporine. Drug Intell Clin Pharm 1985;19:90-100.

45. Yee GC, Lennon TP, Gmur DJ et al. Age-dependent cyclosporine: pharmacokinetics in marrow transplant recipients. Clin Pharmacol Ther 1986;40:438-43.

46. Burckart GJ, Canafax DM, Yee GC. Cyclosporine monitoring. Drug Intell Clin Pharm 1986;20:649-52.

47. Ptachcinski RJ, Burckart GJ, Venkataramanan R. Cyclosporine concentration determinations for monitoring and pharmacokinetic studies. J Clin Pharmacol 1986;26:358-66.

48. Burkle WS. Cyclosporine pharmacokinetics and blood level monitoring. Drug Intell Clin Pharm 1985;19:101-5.

INDEX

DRUGS IN THE INDEX are listed by nonproprietary name; drug classes are also used as index terms and some information may be indexed under the drug class entry only. Therefore, to gain access to the maximum amount of information on a drug in the *Handbook*, the entries for both the specific agent and its drug class should be consulted. British Approved Names, where different from United States Adopted Names (USAN), are listed with the designation (**BAN**) following the nonproprietary name. Canadian brand names, where different from US brand names, are listed with the designation (**Can**) following the name.

A

P